FITNESS FOR WORK
The Medical Aspects

THIRD EDITION

Edited by
R. A. F. Cox
Consultant Occupational Physician
Previously Chief Medical Officer, CEGB and National Power

WITH

F. C. Edwards
Previously Senior Medical Adviser, Health and Safety Executive

K. Palmer
Honorary Consultant Occupational Physician
Southampton Universities NHS Trust

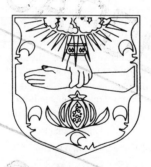

A publication of the
Faculty of Occupational
Medicine of the Royal College
of Physicians of London

OXFORD
UNIVERSITY PRESS

OXFORD
UNIVERSITY PRESS

Great Clarendon Street, Oxford OX2 6DP

Oxford University Press is a department of the University of Oxford.
It furthers the University's objective of excellence in research, scholarship,
and education by publishing worldwide in

Oxford New York

Athens Auckland Bangkok Bogotá Buenos Aires Calcutta
Cape Town Chennai Dar es Salaam Delhi Florence Hong Kong Istanbul
Karachi Kuala Lumpur Madrid Melbourne Mexico City Mumbai
Nairobi Paris São Paulo Singapore Taipei Tokyo Toronto Warsaw
with associated companies in Berlin Ibadan

Oxford is a registered trade mark of Oxford University Press
in the UK and in certain other countries

Published in the United States
by Oxford University Press Inc., New York

First edition published 1987
Second edition published 1995
Reprinted 1996
Third edition published 2000

British Library Cataloguing in Publication Data

Data available

Library of Congress Cataloging in Publication Data

Fitness for work: the medical aspects / edited by R.A.F Cox, F.C. Edwards,
K. Palmer.—3rd ed.
p. cm.—(Oxford medical publications)
'A publication of the Faculty of Occupational Medicine of the Royal College of Physicians of London.'
Includes bibliographical references and index.
1. Disability evaluation. 2. Chronically ill—Employment.
3. Handicapped—Employment. 4. Industrial medicine. I. Cox, R.A.F. (Robin Anthony
Frederick), 1935– II. Edwards, Felicity. III. Palmer, K. (Keith). IV. Royal College of
Physicians of London. Faculty of Occupational Medicine. V. Series.
[DNLM: 1. Occupational Medicine. 2. Disability Evaluation. WA 400 F546 2000]
RC963.4 F57 2000 616.9'803—dc21 99–059593

ISBN 0–19–263043–1 (pbk.)

Typeset by
J&L Composition Ltd, Filey, North Yorkshire
Printed in Great Britain
on acid-free paper by
Biddles Ltd, Guildford and King's Lynn

Foreword

During the 20th century, working life has undergone great changes. Today there is a growing understanding that a good working environment should not only be healthy and safe; it should also encourage personal and professional development and well-being at the job, which all contribute to improved work quality and higher productivity.

However, chemical and physical threats to health still need to be well identified and controlled. We need to investigate the effects of new chemicals and new technologies, and should be alert to adverse interactions between exposures, chemical as well as physical. To promote health and well-being we also need to consider the total life situation and to see the work environment as part of our total environment. In the future we can expect further changes in working life: fewer people will work in production and more people will be engaged in providing services. Furthermore, working conditions have changed with increasing computerisation and new work tasks. The age distribution in populations is changing; there will be more elderly in the future work force. Gender differences at work have been recognised, for example, differences between men and women in their work tasks and reaction to occupational stresses. It is also likely that employees will more often change their occupation and place of work. While such mobility may have advantages, there is a need for new methods to establish which factors in the workers' total environment may cause signs of discomfort or ill-health.

Another question will concern the employment of the work force: in hard times with high unemployment rates a well-educated, often permanently employed élite will profit. Another 'just-in-time' group steps in whenever, and wherever there is need for it, but always under uncertain and often very stressful conditions. A third group is the real loser: the unemployed for whom it is a trauma. However, those still at work also feel the consequences of high unemployment. Enterprises downsize and work pace and work stress increase. Nobody complains because of the risk of losing their job. They worry for their own position in the company. As a paradox sick leave diminishes because of fear of losing their job if they stay home sick.

Thus, occupational health today is a growing field. It covers a wide panorama of different topics, where research, practice, and prevention go hand in hand. In an overall perspective musculo–skeletal diseases, asthma and other allergies, and mental stresss are the most prevalent work-related diseases. However, it should be mentioned that there are one million different chemical compounds in our immediate environment; that several hundred new chemicals are introduced each year into the environment; and that the long-term toxicity of extremely low environmental concentrations of these chemicals are unknown. New work technologies means exposures to 'new' physical factors, for example electromagnetic fields, the effects of which we do not fully understand.

In this time of rapid working life developments basic knowledge of the medical disciplines concerned is of the utmost importance. All disciplines within medicine have their own developments; new knowledge means better diagnosis and therapy, and a better foundation for the proper prevention of all diseases including occupational diseases. Already when first published *Fitness for work* marked a breakthrough in this respect— seen from the viewpoint of occupational health professionals. The third edition takes some important new steps with additional contributions on ethics, no-fault compensation, rehabilitation, the ageing work force, and the UK Disability Discrimination Act.

I welcome this new edition of *Fitness for work*, because I am convinced that it will be an invaluable help to occupational health professionals in their work. *Fitness for work* will undoubtedly contribute to the better health and well-being of workers in a changing world of work. I congratulate the editors and the authors for their contribution to improving the working ability of both those who are fit and those who are temporarily or pemanently medically handicapped.

Bengt Knave
President Elect of ICOH
National Institute for Working Life, Stockhom, Sweden

Acknowledgements

Altogether so many people have helped with the production of this book that there is a danger, in compiling a list of acknowledgements, that someone will be omitted. If there is anyone who feels affronted, however slightly, because their name is not mentioned please accept our apologies and assurance that no offence was intended.

First, we would particularly like to thank the authors of the second edition, some of whom have not contributed to the third edition, because their original work provided the foundations for the new chapters. A particular example is Chapter 10, which is mostly the work of Dr A. Sinclair and Dr R.R.A. Coles, the original authors who have now retired.

Secondly, whether chapters have been simply brought up to date, whether they have been completely re-written, or whether they are totally new chapters, all the authors have responded willingly and helpfully to our cajoling and criticisms which has made our job so much easier. For that we are extremely grateful. Several authors have 'contributed twice' by reviewing other chapters where there have been parts relevant to their specialties and to them we owe special thanks. We are also particularly conscious that both the occupational physicians and the clinical specialists, who have worked together on most of the chapters, have contributed their expertise in spite of the almost impossible work commitments which now afflict all members of our profession. This generous contribution of their time and expertise is even more magnanimous when neither the authors nor the editors of this or previous editions receive any remuneration for their efforts as all royalties from this book accrue to the Faculty of Occupational Medicine. We would also like to thank the officers and staff of the Faculty who have given their support whenever we have needed it.

The Department of Social Security has very generously assisted with the funding of the production costs of this enterprise. We are also indebted to the Department of Health and Safety Executive, who have agreed to provide sponsorship towards the conference at which the book will be launched on September 18, 2000. The Faculty is also particularly grateful to Esso Petroleum for their continuing donations in support of the publication of standards in occupational medicine of which this book is a prime example.

Some individuals have given us assistance with specific topics and their help is especially appreciated. In Chapter 8 Mr C.G.D. Bradley LLb, solicitor, Dr R.J.M. Irvine of the Medical Advisory Branch of the DVLA and Wing Commander J. Aitken, Surgeon General's Department of the Ministry of Defense have given particular help. Others are Emeritus Professor Michael Warren for his help and advice in the preparation of statistics on disability in Chapter 1; Dr Gill Lea of the travel Section of the PHLS Communicable Disease Surveillance Centre, Colindale, London NW9 and Trailfinders Travel Clinic, Kensington High Street, London W8, for help with the preparation of Appendix 5; Emeritus Professor Ian McCallum, a previous editor of this book, for additional editorial assistance; Dr Nerys Williams, Senior Employment Medical Adviser with the HSE, for updating the section on EMAS in Chapter 4; the staff of the Department for Education and Employment for help with the section on the Careers Service in Chapter 4; Dr Philip Sawney for updating the references to the DSS in Chapter 4; and Anna McNeil for the preparation of Appendix 7.

In addition to her work on Appendix 7, Anna has been our executive secretary again and without her the book would never have been completed. We wish to thank her for her indefatigability, dedication, and great efficiency. We know that every contributor would also wish us to thank Anna for her courtesy and unfailing good humour on the frequent occasions when she has had cause to communicate with them. It has been a pleasure for us all to work with her and she will be greatly missed now the project is complete.

R.A.F.C.
F.C.E.
K.P.

June 2000

Preface to the third edition

Fitness for work is now an established textbook for those doctors in training or practising as occupational physicians and an essential source of reference for non-medical professionals such as lawyers, personnel officers, and general managers who need information on the medical aspects of fitness for work. It is also mandatory reading for all occupational health nurses who may often work in isolation.

The words of the preface to the first edition of this book remain relevant:

Most firms, particularly small ones, still have no occupational health service or medical advice of their own. Medical guidance on fitness for work usually comes from the patient's family or hospital doctor. Unfortunately, inappropriate advice may be given, either because not enough is known by doctors about the jobs their patients do, or because employers are unaware of the way in which advances in medical treatment have improved prognosis.

The up-to-date specialist opinion and background information given here on a number of medical conditions should improve both the relevance and consistency of advice. It should also reduce discrimination, often on irrelevant health grounds, against those who are at work or seeking work. As with any clinical judgement, the medical advice that is given on a patient remains the responsibility of the doctor concerned, and the general guidance contained in this book must always be interpreted in the light, not only of the effect of the illness or disability on the individual patient, but also of the special requirements of the job.

Although access to occupational health services is still not as complete as it should be, the benefits of occupational health services are more generally recognized today by employers, employees, unions, and government. Indeed, through recent initiatives of the Health and Safety Executive (see *Developing an occupational health strategy for Great Britain*, Health and Safety Executive discussion document, 1998), the government has accorded very high priority to occupational health. As the demand for these services expands, more doctors and nurses trained in the specialty are required and there is a need to keep standard texts, such as *Fitness for work*, up-dated; it is equally important to take account of recent advances in medical practice. Of the 27 chapters on clinical topics, 26 have been written jointly by an occupational physician and by a clinician practising in the appropriate specialty. This new, revised edition includes a number of contributions from new authors.

The second main motivating force for revision has been the Disability Discrimination Act 1995, which came in to force in the UK in December 1996 and upon which sufficient experience and case law have now accrued to enable specific advice to be proffered. Each chapter refers to the Act where relevant, and a whole chapter is devoted entirely to this topic. It is hoped that the advice contained in the book will assist tribunals when considering cases brought before them under the Act.

The editors feel that the subject of ethics in occupational medicine is not only of great importance but is also often misunderstood by employers and even by occupational physicians. The previous edition of *Fitness for work* included the Faculty's *Ethics for occupational physicians* but, in this edition, a whole chapter has been devoted to ethical issues in occupational medicine written by the current Chairman of the Ethics Committee of the Faculty of Occupational Medicine. This is one of five new chapters. Another is a chapter on work and the older employee written in response to the increasing trend towards working in a self-employed capacity after the normal age of retirement. Older workers have special problems, particularly in adapting to change, which are addressed in this chapter. The other new chapters have been created by re-arranging the chapters on musculoskeletal disorders, the biggest single group of medical conditions affecting the working population, into separate chapters on spinal and general orthopaedic disorders, trauma, and rheumatology. Although this creates some overlap, the new format has allowed us to deal with the wide range of individual conditions in greater detail.

We have also included in the Introduction a contribution about no-fault compensation and the New Zealand experience of this practice in the hope that this wider publicity will give impetus to its implementation elsewhere, and so reduce the demands for prolonged and expensive litigation. Compensation and rehabilitation can both be expedited by the use of vocational assessment and so a new section on that subject is included in Chapter 4.

The Appendix on European Directives which appeared in the second edition has been excluded from the third edition because all the directives, where relevant, are referred to in the general text.

Although the contents of this book will be of particular use to doctors, managers, nurses, and personnel staff in the United Kingdom, we feel that most of the topics are covered in such a general way that they will help others elsewhere in the world who need to make informed decisions about the medical aspects of fitness for work; both of the previous editions have been shown to be of value in Europe and many other countries. It is particularly with this wider readership in mind that we are delighted that Professor Bengt Knave, Professor of Occupational Medicine at the National Institute of Working Life in Stockholm and the President Elect of the International Commission on Occupational Health (ICOH) has written the Foreword to this edition.

R. A. F. Cox
F. C. Edwards
K. Palmer

June 2000

Preface to the second edition

The first edition of this book was published as a Report of the Royal College of Physicians in 1988. It clearly fulfilled a very real need and we have been greatly encouraged by the favourable comments and reviews which it received. With changes both in clinical medicine and in employment practice the contents of the Report required updating. In so doing, the book has become a reference textbook and is no longer a report of a large steering group. The general format has been retained with each chapter written by an occupational physician and a practising clinician in the respective specialty, but some of the chapters in the first edition have been divided for functional convenience. For example, a separate chapter on trauma has replaced part of the previous chapter on orthopaedics, while disorders of the spine now have a chapter to themselves. In addition, there are new appendices on fitness for work overseas, European Community legislation, ill-health retirement and ethics. All the addresses referred to in each chapter will be found in the appendix of useful addresses (Appendix 9).

The editors feel that the subject of ethics in occupational medicine is not only of great importance but is also often misunderstood by employers and even by occupational physicians. The Faculty of Occupational Medicine's *Ethics for occupational physicians*, has recently been published and we believed that this should be included in its entirety apart from some minor editing to save space (see Appendix 6). Copies of the booklet are available from the Faculty of Occupational Medicine.

A further concession to the need to keep the size of the book within the publisher's limits was to prune the number of references. The references which the editors have included, therefore, are selected for their interest and relevance and we have abandoned any attempt to make the list at the end of each chapter comprehensive. We apologize to any authors who may be offended by this decision and to any readers who may feel that the style of the book has been diminished but the limitation of references has enabled us to expand the breadth of the book.

Although it will be of particular value to doctors, nurses, managers, and personnel staff in the United Kingdom, we feel that most of the topics are covered in such a general way that it will also be a great help wherever in the world there is a need to make informed dicisions about the medical aspects of fitness for work. It is particularly with this wider readership in mind that we are delighted that Professor Jean-François Caillard, Professor of Occupational Medicine, Director of Occupational Medicine in the University of Rouen, Chairman of the French Federation of Occupational Medicine, and the current President of the International Commission on Occupational Health (ICOH), has written the Foreword to this edition. We also feel that the book will have an even greater relevance and application in the United Kingdom in the light of the new DSS proposals on the medical assessment for Incapacity Benefit.

In fact, this book will be invaluable to anyone practising occupational medicine.

Although occupational medicine is one of the most rapidly expanding medical disciplines, and more doctors enter training for the specialty every year, the advice of occupational physicians is still not available widely enough, in the United Kingdom, to workers in industry and commerce, and to the self-employed. We hope that this book will, therefore, be of particular value to those people, whether general practitioners, nurses, personnel managers, trade unionists, or others such as the staff of the employment and careers services who need guidance on the medical aspects of employment and may not be able to obtain it from a specialist occupational physician.

R.A.F. Cox
F.C. Edwards
R.I. McCallum

February 1995

Preface to the first edition

The stimulus for this report came originally from the Health and Safety Executive's Medical Division, who approached the Royal College of Physicians of London and its Faculty of Occupational Medicine. A steering group, under the Chairmanship of the late Dr Peter Taylor, was set up by the College and the Faculty to plan and produce the report, with the requirements of hospital specialists, general practitioners, and occupational physicians particularly in mind.

Apart from specific activities for which detailed guidelines exist, such as heay goods vehicle drivers, airline pilots, and professional divers, the vast majority of jobs have no clear criteria of fitness and precise guidelines cannot be laid down. Thus the need for informed advice on medical aspects of fitness for work covering a wide range of medical conditions is evident. Some chronic diseases, while not excluding work altogether, can clearly limit the scope of employment, but the restrictions that may be imposed on such patients are often unnecessary and without any rational basis. While it must be accepted that there may be diverse views on employability in many medical conditions, such problems should always be the subject of informed discussion between the employer, occupational medical adviser, the patient's own doctor, and the patient. This report provides a basis for such discussions.

Occupational medicine is often thought of as being concerned only with the effects of work on health, i.e. the prevention of occupational disease and of the effects of exposure to various environmental hazards, but equally it is about the effects of health on work, the fitness for work, and the rehabilitation of the individual. Occupational medicine is essentially a clinical speciality and throughout this book authors emphasize the need for close collaboration between occupational physicians and their clinical colleagues. Each chapter has been written jointly by a clinician practising in the specialty and an occupational physician, and it is hoped that one outcome will be that clinicians and occupational physicians will be brought closer together, enabling them to see each other's point of view.

Most firms, particularly small ones, still have no occupational health service or medical advice of their own. Medical guidance on fitness for work usually comes from the patient's family or hospital doctor. Unfortunately, inappropriate advice may be given, either because not enough is known by doctors about the jobs their patients do, or because employers are unaware of the way in which advances in medical treatment have improved prognosis.

The up-to-date specialist opinion and background information given here on a number of medical conditions should improve both the relevance and consistency of advice. It should also reduce discrimination, often on irrelevant health grounds, against those who are at work or seeking work. As with any clinical judgement, the medical advice that is given on a patient remains the responsibility of the doctor concerned, and the general guidance contained in this book must always be interpreted in the light, not only of the effect of the illness or disability on the individual patient, but also of the special requirements of the job.

We hope that the report will be of use not only to doctors in occupational medicine, but also to those in general practice or hospital medicine, and of interest to occupational health nurses, managers, and personnel staff. It will provide an essential core of information and advice on the effects of health on work for doctors in training for the examination for Associateship of the Faculty of Occupational Medicine (AFOM).

It was decided to retain some overlapping sections in different chapters, for example those on haemophilia, cervical spondylosis, and ankylosing spondylitis, because these reflected the different approaches and expertise of the authors. In spite of the speed with which the picture of Acquired Immune Deficiency Syndrome (AIDS) is changing as further knowledge of the disease develops, the steering group felt strongly that it should be included in the book because of its importance in relation to public concern about employability and safety at work.

F.C.E.

April 1988   R.I.McC.

Contents

Contributors

C. Astbury
Occupational Physician, Essex County Council

P. J. Baxter
University of Cambridge, Addenbrooke's NHS Trust Hospital, Cambridge

H. A. Bird
Professor of Pharmacological Rheumatology, Chapel Allerton Hospital, Leeds

D. Black
Specialist Occupational Physician, Enviromedix, Auckland.
Senior Lecturer in Occupational Medicine, Department of Medicine,
University of Auckland

D. Bracher
Formerly Manager Medical Services BP Exploration Europe

I. Brown
Consultant Occupational Health Physician and Toxicologist,
Honorary Senior Lecturer, Institute of Occupational Health,
University of Birmingham

A. Cockroft
Director, Occupational Health and Safety Unit, Royal Free Hospital, London

C. C. H. Cook
Professor of the Psychiatry of Alcohol Misuse,
Kent Institute of Medicine and Health Science, University of Kent at Canterbury

R. A. F. Cox
Consultant Occupational Physician, formerly Chief Medical Officer,
CEGB and National Power

N. F. Davies
Chief Medical Officer, Magnox Electric plc, Gloucester

P. A. M. Diamond
Formerly Chief Medical Adviser, Department of Transport

K. Edgington
Chief Medical Officer, Civil Aviation Authority

F. C. Edwards
Formerly Senior Employment Medical Adviser, Medical Division,
Health and Safety Division

P. M. Emerson
Formerly Consultant Haematologist, John Radcliffe Hospital, Oxford

C. J. English
Consultant in Occupational Health, North Tees and Hartlepool NHS Trust

A. L. Fingret
Formerly Consultant Physician, Occupational Medicine,
Royal Marsden Hospital, London

M. Floyd
Director, Rehabilitation Resource Centre, City University, London

F. B. Gibberd
Consultant Neurologist, Chelsea and Westminster Hospital, London

G. Gill
Senior Lecturer and Consultant Physician,
University Clinical Department of Medicine, Fazakerley Hospital, Liverpool

W. J. A. Goedhard
Professor, Department of Occupational Health and Ageing,
Free University, Amsterdam

R. Gokal
Consultant Nephrologist, Honorary Lecturer, University of Manchester

P. Griffiths
Professor of Virology, Royal Free and University College Medical School, London

I. Haslock
Professor of Rheumatology, South Cleveland Hospital, Middlesbrough

J. Hobson
Occupational Physician, Michelin Tyre plc

G. S. Howard
Honorary Fellow of the Faculty of Occupational Medicine. Employment Lawyer

K. B. Hughes
Consultant Otolaryngologist, The Doncaster Royal and Montagu Hospital
NHS Trust

C. M. Jones
Senior Medical Officer, British Steel Engineering Steels, part of the Corus Group

L. H. Kapadia
Occupational Health Physician, Marks & Spencer plc

J. L. Kearns
Consultant Occupational Physician.
Late Medical Director, BUPA Occupational Health Limited, formerly Head of Health
and Safety, J. Lyons Group of Companies

D. Landymore
Vocational Rehabilitation Adviser

M. S. Lipsedge
Consultant Psychiatrist, Keat's House, Guy's Hospital. Head of Section of Occupational Psychiatry, Department of Psychiatry and Psychology, Guy's, King's and St Thomas's Hospitals Medical and Dental School, London

E. B. Macdonald
Senior Lecturer in Occupational Health, University of Glasgow

Professor The Lord McColl
Professor of Surgery, Guy's Hospital, London

G. T. McInnes
Senior Lecturer in Medicine and Therapeutics, University of Glasgow

N. K. I. McIver
Director, North Sea Medical Centre, Gorleston, Great Yarmouth, Norfolk

G. Munton
Consultant Ophthalmic Surgeon, formerly (1989–94) Visual Standards Sub-Committee, Royal College of Ophthalmologists, London

I. Nugent
Consultant Orthopaedic Surgeon, Royal Berkshire Hospital, Reading

P. Owen
Consultant Obstetrician and Gynaecologist,
Glasgow Royal Maternity Hospital and Stobhill Hospital, Glasgow

K. Palmer
Clinical Scientist, MRC Environmental Epidemiology Unit,
University of Southampton, Honorary Consultant Occupational Physician, Southampton Universities Hospitals Trust, Southampton

S. Pearson
Consultant Physician and Senior Clinical Lecturer,
Department of Respiratory Medicine, Leeds General Infirmary, Leeds

M. C. Petch
Consultant Cardiologist, Papworth Hospital, Cambridge

K. J. Pilling
Consultant in Occupational Medicine, Managing Director, Occhea Ltd

B. Povlsen
Consultant Orthopaedic Surgeon, Guy's and St Thomas' Hospital, London.
Associated Professor in Hand Surgery at University of Linkoping, Sweden

I. G. Rennie
Chief Medical Officer, Kodak Ltd

A. Ross
Consultant Occupational Health Physician, West Berkshire Occupational Health, Reading

R. J. G. Rycroft
Consultant Dermatologist, St John's Institute of Dermatology,
St Thomas' Hospital, London

M. Samuel
Group Occupational Physican, London Electricity plc

S. D. Shorvon
Professor of Clinical Neurology and Chairman of the Department of Neurology,
Institute of Neurology, University College London. Consultant Neurologist,
National Hospital for Neurology and Neurosurgery, Queen Square, London

G. Smith
Consultant Occupational Physician, formerly Chief Medical Officer,
British Railways Board

D. Snashall
Clinical Director, Occupational Health Services, Guy's and St Thomas' Trust, London

E. Waclawski
Consultant Occupational Physician, Renfrewshire Healthcare NHS Trust,
Honorary Senior Lecturer, University of Glasgow

R. Willcox
Consultant in Occupational Medicine, Occupational Health Solutions.
Formerly Group Medical Officer, Cable and Wireless

D. S. Wright
Chairman, Ethics Committee of the Faculty of Occupational Medicine,
Royal College of Physicians, London

R. J. Wyke
Consultant Physician and Gastroenterologist, The Ipswich Hospital NHS Trust,
Ipswich, Suffolk

P. A. Wynn
Clinical Lecturer in Occupational Medicine, Institute of Occupational Health,
University of Birmingham

1

Introduction

R. A. F. Cox and F. C. Edwards

This book on medical aspects of fitness for work gathers together specialist advice on the medical aspects of employment and the majority of medical conditions likely to be encountered in the working population. Though personnel managers and others will find it of great help it is primarily written for doctors so that family practitioners, hospital consultants, and occupational physicians, as well as other doctors and occupational health nurses can best advise managers and others who may need to know how a patient's illness might affect their work. Although decisions on return to work or on placement must depend on many factors, it is hoped that this book, which combines best current clinical and occupational health practice, will be used by doctors and others as a source of reference and will remind them about the occupational implications of illness.

It must be emphasized that, apart from relieving suffering and prolonging life, the objective of much medical treatment, whether it be a course of antibiotics or a renal transplant, is to return the patient to work. Much of the benefit of modern medical technology and the skills of physicians and surgeons will have been wasted if patients who have been successfully treated are denied work by employers, or doctors acting on their behalf, through ignorance or prejudice. A main aim of this book is to remove the excuse for denying work to those who have overcome injury and disease and deserve to work.

The book is arranged in chapters according to specialty or topic, each chapter having been written jointly by a clinician and an occupational physician. For each specialty the chapter outlines the conditions covered; notes relevant statistics; discusses clinical aspects, including treatment that may affect work capacity; notes rehabilitation requirements or special needs at the workplace; discusses problems that may arise at work and any necessary work restrictions; notes any current advisory or statutory medical standards; and makes recommendations on the employment aspects of the conditions covered. A chapter on the possible effects of medication on work performance and additional chapters on ethics and the ageing worker (see below) are also included. Appendices on medical standards for driving, civil aviation, merchant shipping, offshore work and diving, fitness for work overseas, ill health retirement, and useful addresses conclude the book.

The first four chapters are applicable to any condition. This introductory chapter deals mainly with the principles underlying medical assessments of fitness for work, contacts between medical practitioners and the workplace, and confidentiality of medical information. Chapter 2 covers legal aspects, Chapter 3 focuses on the Disability Discrimination Act 1995 (DDA), Chapter 4 outlines the vocational rehabilitation services and benefits currently available to assist with employment, and the ethical aspects are discussed in Chapter 5.

The Disability Discrimination Act 1995

Since the second edition of this book was published in 1995, the UK Disability Discrimination Act (DDA) has come into effect (December 1996); this Third Edition takes account of the Act and its implications.

In the Act, disability is not defined in terms of working ability or capacity but in terms of 'an adverse effect on the ability to carry out normal day to day activities'. Work itself does not, therefore, have to be considered in deciding whether an individual is disabled or not but it does have to be considered when a disabled person is in a work situation. It is in this circumstance that the opinion of the occupational physician will be required. The physician may be asked

* whether an individual's disability falls within the definition of the Act
* if it does, what adjustments may be needed to accommodate the disabled individual in the workplace.

Adjustments may be to the physical and psychological nature of the work or to the methods by which the work is accomplished. It is for management, not the occupational physician, to decide in each individual case whether such adjustments are reasonable. Before offering such opinions the occupational physician must make an accurate determination of the individual's disability, not in medical but in functional terms; this requires a precise knowledge and detailed understanding of the work and the workplace in question.

In addition to a whole chapter (Chapter 3) devoted to the DDA and its application, references to the effects of the Act in clinical situations are made throughout the rest of the book. This edition of *Fitness for work* provides expert guidance to occupational physicians and other people who have to consider the consequences of disability on employment and employability.

The ageing worker

Despite the radical changes which have affected industry and commerce in recent years and the consequent reduction in the number of employed people ('downsizing', 'right-sizing', 'empowerment', 're-structuring', and other euphemisms for reducing the payroll) the number of older people who continue to work is increasing. This may be because many people, having taken early retirement from full-time employment, continue to offer their skills and experience in their particular fields as self-employed 'consultants'. In this role, unlike that of a full-time employee, there is no upper retirement age and people can continue to work, choosing their own pace, as long as they are fit and able to do so. For this and for other demographic reasons, more people are working to greater ages with consequences both for themselves and for their work. The declining ability of the ageing worker to adapt to change or to learn new technologies are just two of these consequences. The problems of the ageing worker will continue to grow, and are now of such importance that a whole chapter (Chapter 27) has been devoted to the subject in this edition.

No-fault compensation

The question of compensation for people who suffer injuries or ill health as a consequence of their work is one which frequently comes up for debate and is a cause of argument and expense in the courts. The long delay in making settlements, however they are reached, is also a cause of much distress and hardship to the victim. A system of no-fault compensation, which may not be perfect, but does have the benefit of quick settlement of claims without recourse to the courts, has been in operation in New Zealand for 25 years. An account of the experience gained from this policy appears as an appendix to this chapter in the hope that some of the benefits gained and lessons learned may be applied elsewhere.

Contacts between the patient's medical advisers and the workplace

The importance of contact between the patient's own medical advisers and the workplace cannot be overemphasized. We suggest that consultants, as well as family practitioners, should ask the patient if there is an occupational health service at the workplace and, if so, obtain written consent to contact the occupational physician, or the occupational health nurse in the absence of a physician.

Where there is no occupational health service, early contact between the patient's doctor and management (usually the personnel manager) may also be valuable. It helps the employer to know when the patient is likely to return to work, and whether some work adjustment will be needed, while family practitioners and consultants will be helped by having a better understanding of their patient's job.

Occupational health services (OHS)

All employees should have access to occupational health advice, whether this is provided from within a company or by external consultants. Such advice may be provided by occupational health trained nurses or by specialist occupational physicians but, for some problems advice from one of the latter practitioners will be essential—e.g. in providing evidence for industrial tribunals or in other medico-legal cases. The exact nature and size of the occupational health service to which any company needs access depends on the size of the company and the hazards of the activities in which it is engaged. Some companies find it advantageous to share occupational health services.

The local Employment Medical Advisory Service (EMAS) of the Health and Safety Executive (HSE) is able to advise on the availability and sources of local occupational health services and occupational health practitioners. EMAS may give advice to individual employees, although the main role their medical inspectors (doctors) and occupational health inspectors (nurses) now fulfil is to support the general inspectors of the HSE.

Control of sickness absence

Some employers consider that the main function of an occupational health service is to control sickness absence. Although occupational health professionals, whether nurses or physicians, can help both management and individuals to reduce sickness absence, its control is the responsibility of management; occupational health practitioners have no role to play in the policing of employees who are absent for reasons attributed to sickness (see also Chapter 5, Ethics).

Confidentiality

Usually, any recommendations and advice on placement or return to work are based on the functional effects of the medical condition, the diagnosis itself normally being unnecessary. A simple statement that the patient is medically 'fit' or 'unfit' for a particular job often suffices, but occasionally further information may need to be disclosed, particularly if limitations on work are being imposed. The certificated reason for any sickness absence is usually known by personnel departments, who maintain their own confidential records.

The patient's consent must be obtained, preferably in writing, before disclosure of confidential health information to third parties, including other doctors, occupational health nurses, employers, or other people such as staff of the careers or employment services. The purpose of this should be made clear to the patient; it may be to help with suitable work, and/or to maintain health and safety (their own and that of others). A patient who is found to be medically unfit for certain employment should be given a full explanation of why the disclosure of unfitness is necessary. Further advice may be found in the Faculty of Occupational Medicine's Guidance on Ethics for Occupational Physicians 1999[1] (see also Chapter 5).

Medical reports

When a medical report is requested on an individual, the person should be informed of the purpose for which the report is being sought. The person requesting the report should put the request in writing and should also give a copy to the subject. Likewise the doctor, on completing the report, should also give a copy to the subject. If a medical report is being sought from an employee's general practitioner or specialist, then the employer is required, under the Access to Medical Reports Act 1988, to inform the employee of their rights under that Act (which include the right to see the report before it is sent to the employer and the right to refuse to allow the report to be sent to the employer). If the report is sought from an occupational physician it will also come under the Access to Medical Reports Act if the occupational physician has ever had clinical care of the patient. Even if the occupational physician has not cared for the patient clinically, it is good ethical practice to follow the legal requirements of the Access to Medical Reports Act. Employees are also now entitled to see their medical records, including their occupational health records, which would include any medical reports.

Any doctor being asked for a medical report should insist that the originator of the request writes a referral letter containing full details of the individual, a description of their job, an outline of the problem, and the matters on which the doctor's opinion is sought.

At the outset the doctor should obtain the patient's consent, preferably in writing, to examine him and furnish the report. Even if the patient has given consent the report should not contain clinical information, unless it is absolutely essential, and the contents should be confined to addressing the questions posed in the letter of referral and advising on interpreting the person's medical condition in terms of functional capability and their ability to meet the requirements of their employment. Gratuitous comment should be avoided, but the employer is entitled to be sufficiently informed to make a clear decision about the individual's work ability, both currently and in the future, and any adjustments, modifications, restrictions, or prohibitions which may be required. The doctor should express an opinion clearly and unequivocally and should give a copy of the report to the employee. The employee can then request the doctor to correct any factual errors which they consider may have been included, but they are not entitled to require the doctor to modify the opinion expressed, even if they strongly disagree with it.

When writing any medical report the occupational physician should always remember that the document will be discoverable if litigation subsequently ensues. It should be clear from the report, either from its content, the letter heading, or the affiliation under the signature, why the doctor is qualified to address the subject in question. For example, a doctor who does not possess recognized qualifications in occupational medicine should not purport to be an occupational physician.

Impairment, disability, and handicap*

Workers with disabilities are commonly found to be highly motivated, often with excellent work and attendance records. When medical fitness for work is assessed, what matters is often not the medical condition itself, but the associated loss of function, and any resulting disability or handicap. It should be borne in mind that a disability seen in the consulting room may be irrelevant to the performance of a particular job. **The patient's condition should be interpreted in functional terms and in the context of the job requirements**. Handicap may result directly from an impairment (for instance, severe facial disfigurement), or more usually, from the resulting disability.

To be consistent in the use of these terms, the simplified scheme of the *International classification of impairments, disabilities, and handicaps*[2,3] should be used as follows.

- A disease, disorder or injury produces an **impairment** (change in normal structure or function).
- A **disability** is a resulting reduction or loss of an ability to perform an activity—for example climbing stairs, or manipulating a keyboard.
- A **handicap** is a social disadvantage resulting from an impairment or disability, which limits or prevents the fulfilment of a normal role.

As examples:

- A relatively minor impairment, the loss of a finger, would be both a major disability and an occupational handicap to a pianist, although not to a labourer.
- A relatively common impairment, defective colour vision, limits the ability to discriminate between certain hues. This may occasionally be a handicap at work,

---

* See also p. 66.

although there are in fact very few occupations for which defective colour vision is a significant handicap.

Prevalence of disability in populations of working age

Figures on the prevalence of disability and/or handicap in different populations vary according to the definitions and methods used and the groups sampled. Much of the uncertainty about the numbers of disabled people in the workforce, or seeking work, arises from variations in definition and ascertainment and the reluctance of people to admit their disability. Differences between surveys may also be due to the inclusion of non-physical handicaps, and to different methods of reporting and sampling. Common to all is the rise in prevalence of disability with increasing age and, to a lesser extent, with manual as opposed to non-manual workers, social class, and/or occupational groups.

A major national population survey was undertaken in Great Britain in 1985–87 by the Social Survey Division of the Office of Population Censuses and Surveys (OPCS). Six reports were published. The first described the prevalence of disability among adults[4], the fourth dealt with services for transport and the employment of disabled adults,[5] and the fifth described their financial circumstances. The other report was concerned with disabled children and their families.

From the survey's findings it was estimated that there were about 6.5 million people of all ages in Great Britain with physical, sensory and/or mental disabilities, of whom 6.2 million (11.3% of the whole population) were aged 16 years or more, and almost 2 million (3.5% of the whole population) were aged between 16 and 59 years. The survey classified the severity of disability into 10 categories, category 1 being the least severe and category 10 the most. The survey found that 20% of disabled adults aged between 16 and 59 years were classified in the five highest categories—that is, they were considered to be severely or very severely disabled. Put another way, the findings suggest that there were about 17 severely or very severely disabled people per 1000 people aged 16–59 years and another 45 with minor or less severe disabilities. (For a description of the scales of severity and of the methods used in the OPCS Surveys see the first report,[4] and for a summary of the prevalence figures see Warren.[6])

The OPCS report on employment[5] indicated that, of disabled adults under pension age living at home, about one-third were working, one-third were permanently unable to work; and 1 in 10 was looking for work, but the remainder were not. Severity of disability was strongly related to employment status.

Specific work forces have also been studied in Britain[7–9] and in Scandinavia.[10,11] Taylor and Fairrie[8] found that the prevalence of disability was about 10% of men working in the refinery they studied. A markedly increased prevalence of disability/handicap was found with age, particularly over 50 years. Substantial proportions of the workforce were found to be sufficiently incapacitated to need 'rehabilitation measures' such as work accommodation, and/or would have been restricted in their ability to perform if their jobs had been more demanding. The commonest causes of disablement in all four studies were circulatory, respiratory, and musculoskeletal disorders. These were the main causes of ill health retirement over a 2 year period in British Steel.[12] The main causes of ill health retirement in coal-miners (between 1981 and 1983) were musculoskeletal, psychological, cardiovascular, and respiratory conditions, in that order (Dr Roy Archibald, personal communication). The two earlier British studies[7,8] highlighted the inadequacies of the Register of Disabled Persons and the Quota Scheme, both of which have now become obsolete with the implementation of the DDA.

Fitness for work

The primary purpose of a medical assessment of fitness for work is to make sure that an individual is fit to perform the task involved effectively and without risk to their own or others' health and safety.

Why an assessment may be needed

1 The patient's condition may limit, reduce, or prevent them from performing the job effectively (e.g. musculoskeletal conditions that limit mobility, or manipulative ability).

2 The patient's condition may be made worse by the job (e.g. excessive physical exertion in some cardiorespiratory conditions; exposure to certain allergens in asthma).

3 The patient's condition is likely to make it unsafe for them to do certain jobs (e.g. liability to sudden unconsciousness in a hazardous situation; risk of damage to the remaining eye or ear in a patient with monocular vision, or monaural hearing in some work environments).

4 The patient's condition is likely to make it unsafe both for themselves and others, whether fellow workers and/or the community, in some occupational roles (e.g. road or railway driving in someone who is liable to sudden unconsciousness or to behave abnormally).

5 The patient's condition may pose a risk to the community (e.g. for consumers of the product, if a food handler transmits infection).

There is usually a clear distinction between the first-party risks of 2 and 3 and the third-party risks of 5. In 4, first- and third-party risks may both be present.

Thus, when assessing a patient's fitness for work, the doctor must consider the following factors:

• The level of skill, physical and mental capacity, sensory acuity, etc. needed for effective performance of the work.

• Any possible adverse effects of the work itself or of the work environment on the patient's health.

• The possible 'health and safety' implications of the patient's medical condition when undertaking the work in question, for themselves, fellow workers, and/or the community.

For some jobs it should also be remembered that there may be an 'emergency' component in addition to the 'routine' job structure, and higher standards of fitness may thus be needed, on occasion, for the former.

Medical standards

Medical standards may be advisory or statutory. Standards are often laid down where work entails entering a new environment that may present some hazard to the individual, such as the increased or decreased atmospheric pressures encountered in compressed-air work, diving and flying, or work in the high temperatures of nuclear reactors. Standards are also laid down for work where there is a potential risk of a medical condition causing an accident, as in transport; or transmitting infection, as in food handling. For onerous or arduous work such as in mines rescue or in firefighting, very high standards of physical fitness are needed. Specific medical standards will need to be met in such types of work: where relevant, such advisory and/or statutory standards are noted in each specialty chapter.

Pension schemes

Many doctors and personnel managers in industry still believe that their company pension fund requires high standards of medical fitness for new entrants. Direct enquiry to the pension fund administrators themselves usually demonstrates that this is not the case. Fortunately, most pension funds follow the general principle recommended by the Occupational Pensions Board: 'Fit for employment—fit for the pension fund'.[13] It was the Board's view that 'The concern of an employer, when assessing a prospective employee, should be with ability to perform the job efficiently. There is no reason why pension scheme considerations should influence the employer's decision whether to employ him.' In general, a disease or disability should not be a reason *per se* for exclusion from pension schemes, nor should it be used as an excuse to deny employment, unless it adversely affects job performance or health and safety. For an approach to the calculation of disability pensions and current thinking on life underwriting the reader is referred to Brackenridge and Elder.[14] Where company schemes still operate against people with disabilities, attempts should be made to amend them. However, with recent changes in legislation pensions can now be personal, flexible, and mobile; anyone with a medical disability may be well advised to negotiate a personal policy which they can retain permanently irrespective of their employer.

When an assessment of medical fitness is needed

An assessment of medical fitness may be needed for those who are:

1   unemployed, or employed, but being considered for a particular job (i.e. at recruitment or transfer or pre-placement assessment)

2   already in employment

3   unemployed and seeking work or training, but without a specific job in mind.

For 1 and 2, the assessment will be related to a particular job, or to a defined range of alternative work in a given workplace. The assessment is needed to help both employer and employee, and should be clearly related to the job in question. However, after a pre-placement or pre-employment medical examination, employers are entitled to know if there may be consequences from a medical condition which may curtail or restrict a potential employee's working life in the future. But, for 3, where there may be no specific job in view, the assessment must inevitably be more open-ended: health assessments may be required, for instance, by the employment or careers services in their attempt to find suitable work for unemployed disabled people. It is thus all the more important to avoid unnecessary medical restrictions or labels (such as 'epileptic'), as these tend to follow individuals in their search for work and may limit their future choice unduly.

Recruitment and disclosure

Employers often use health questionnaires as part of their recruitment process. Such questionnaires should be marked 'medically confidential' and should be read and interpreted only by an occupational physician or nurse. A questionnaire which has to be returned to a non-medical person —because an employer does not have an occupational health service, for example—is not protected by medical confidentiality and should not be so described. Some individuals may be reluctant to disclose a medical condition to a future employer (sometimes with their own doctor's support) for fear that this may lose them the job. Although understandable, it must be pointed out that, should work capability be impaired or an accident arise due to the concealed condition, dismissal on medical grounds may follow. An industrial tribunal would be likely to support the dismissal if the employee had failed to disclose the relevant condition (see p. 32). It is not in the patient's interest to conceal any medical condition which could adversely affect their work, but it would be entirely reasonable for the applicant to request that the details will be disclosed only to an occupational physician or nurse.

It is noted above that for some jobs (e.g. driving) there are statutory medical standards, and that for others employing organizations lay down their own advisory medical standards (e.g. food handling or work in the offshore oil and gas industry). For the majority of jobs, however, no agreed advisory medical standards exist, and for many jobs there need be no special health requirements. Job application forms should be accompanied by a clear indication of any health standards or physical qualifications that are required and of any medical conditions that would be a bar to certain types of job, but no questions about health or disabilities should be included on job application forms themselves. If health information is necessary, applicants should be asked to complete a separate health declaration form or questionnaire, which should be inspected and interpreted only by health professionals, and only after the candidate has been selected, subject to satisfactory health.

Employees

The stages at which a health appraisal may become necessary for someone in employment are as follows:

- **Job change**, although still working for the same employer, possibly for transfer or promotion. The employee should be told of any special health requirements or qualifications for the new post and the health appraisal should relate to these. Job change may include more seniority or responsibility, for instance, or include overseas posting with a considerable increase in travel. All of these factors may have to be taken into account.

- **Periodic review** of individual health may be undertaken in some circumstances and will relate to specific requirements (for instance, regular assessment of visual acuity in some jobs).
- **Return to work after illness or injury** usually merits a health assessment and is discussed further below.
- Employees returning to work after **prolonged absence** often have special needs that should be taken into account where possible.
- The question of **retirement on grounds of ill health** may need to be considered. (See also Appendix 6).

In any of the above situations there is a legal requirement to consider 'reasonable adjustment' if the individual has a disability within the definition of the DDA, and it is good occupational health practice to do so in any case.

Young people

Medical advice on occupation or training given to a young person who has not yet started a career often has a different slant from that given to an adult developing the same medical condition late in an established career. The later stages of a particular vocation may involve jobs incompatible with the young person's medical condition, or its foreseeable development. Conversely, a mature adult's work experience may enable them to overcome obstacles posed by a disease or disability in ways that a young worker could not. It is particularly important that young people entering employment are given appropriate and consistent medical advice when it is needed. For instance, although a school-leaver with epilepsy might be eligible for an ordinary driving licence at the time of recruitment, it would be most inadvisable for them to take up a position where vocational driving was likely to become an essential requirement for career progression.

Severely disabled people

Where a medical condition has so reduced an individual's employment abilities or potential that they are incapable either of continuing in their existing work or of working in any open competitive employment, even with all appropriate adjustments, then sheltered work of some kind may be the only alternative to premature medical retirement, on the one hand, or to continued unemployment on the other. Further details of sheltered employment are given in Chapter 4 (see p. 74).

The assessment of medical fitness for work

General framework for the assessment

The clinician's assessment should always be reported in terms of functional capacity; the actual diagnosis need not be given. Even so, an opinion on the medical fitness of an individual is being conveyed to others and the patient's written consent is needed for the information to be passed on, in confidence.

To estimate the individual's level of function, general assessments of all systems should be made, with special attention both to those that are disordered and to those that may be relevant to the work. As well as physical systems, sensory and perceptual abilities should be noted, as well as psychological reactions, such as responsiveness, alertness, and other features of the general mental state. The effects of different treatment regimes on work suitability should also be considered; the possible effects of some medication on alertness, or the optimal position of an arthrodesis, are only two of many examples. Each of the specialty chapters which follow outlines the main points to be considered in the respective conditions, but a summary of the main features relevant to an assessment of fitness for work for use as a general framework, is listed here.

Framework for assessing fitness for work

An evaluation of general physical and mental health forms the background to more specific assessments. Guiding principles throughout will be the **patient's residual abilities in terms of likely requirements at the workplace**. Many of these aspects are listed below. Not all will be relevant to any one individual, while some are relevant to more than one type of condition, or to more than one system or specialty.

Assessment should always include the results of relevant tests.

- **General**: stamina; ability to cope with full working day, or shiftwork; liability to fatigue, etc.
- **Mobility**: ability to get to work, and exit safely; to walk, climb, bend, stoop, crouch, etc.
- **Locomotor**: general/specific joint function and range; reach of arms; gait; back/spinal function, etc.
- **Posture**: ability to stand or sit for certain times; any postural constraints; work in confined spaces, etc.
- **Muscular**: specific palsies or weakness; tremor; ability to lift, push or pull, with weight/time abilities if known; strength tests, etc.
- **Manual skill**: any defects in dexterity, ability to grip, or grasp, etc.
- **Co-ordination**: including hand–eye co-ordination if relevant.
- **Balance**: ability to work at heights; vertigo.
- **Cardiorespiratory limitations**, including exercise tolerance, and how this was tested; respiratory function and reserve; sub-maximal exercise tests, aerobic work capacity, if relevant.
- **Liability to unconsciousness**, including nature of episodes, timing, any precipitating factors, etc.
- **Sensory aspects**: may be relevant for the actual work, or in order to get about a hazardous environment safely.
    Vision: ability for fine/close work, distant vision, visual standards corrected or uncorrected, any aids in use or needed. Visual fields. Colour vision defects may occasionally be relevant. Is the eyesight good enough to cope with a difficult working environment with possible hazards?
    Hearing: level in each ear; can warning signals or instructions be heard?

- For both **vision** and **hearing** it is very important that if only one eye or one ear is functioning, this should be noted, so that the remaining organ can be adequately protected against possible damage.
- **Communication/speech**: two-way communication; hearing or speech defects; reason for limitation.
- **Cerebral function** will be very relevant after head injury, cerebrovascular accident, some neurological conditions, and in those with some intellectual deficit: the presence of any confusion; disorientation; impairment of memory, intellect, verbal, or numerical aptitudes, etc.
- **Mental state**: psychiatric assessments may mention anxiety, relevant phobias, mood, withdrawal, relationships with other people, etc.
- **Motivation**: may well be the most important determinant of work capacity. With it, impairments may be surmounted; without it, difficulties may not be overcome. It can be particularly difficult to assess by a doctor who has not previously known the patient.
- **Treatment of the condition**: special effects of treatment may be relevant, e.g. drowsiness, inattention, as side-effects of some medication; implications of different types of treatment in one condition (e.g. insulin as opposed to oral treatment for diabetes).
- **Further treatment**: if further treatment is planned, e.g. further orthopaedic or surgical procedures, these may need to be mentioned.
- **Prognosis**: if the clinical prognosis is likely to affect work placement, e.g. likely improvements in muscle strength, or decline in exercise tolerance, these should be indicated.
- **Special needs**: these may be dietary; need for a clean area for self-treatment, e.g. injection; or relate to time, e.g. frequent rest pauses, no paced or shiftwork, etc.
- **Aids or appliances** in use or needed. Implanted artificial aids may be relevant in the working environment (pacemakers and artificial joints). Aids to mobility may have implications for work (e.g. wheelchair). Prostheses/orthoses should be mentioned. Artificial aids or appliances that could help at the workplace should be indicated.
- **Specific third-party risks** that could be conferred on other workers or members of the community, e.g. via the product such as infection in food handlers, etc.

Requirements of the task

The requirements of the task may relate not only to the individual's present job but also to their future career. Always considering the possibility of 'reasonable adjustment', some of the following aspects may be relevant:

- **Work demands**: physical (e.g. mobility needs; strength for certain activities; lifting/carrying; climbing/balancing; stooping/bending; postural constraints; reach requirements; dexterity/manipulative ability, etc.—see next section for further detail); intellectual/perceptual demands; types of skill involved in tasks.
- **Work environment**: physical aspects, risk factors (e.g. fumes/dust; chemical or biological hazards; working at heights).

- **Organizational/social aspects**, e.g. working in small groups or alone; intermittent or regular pressure of work; need for tact in public relations, etc.
- **Temporal aspects**, e.g. need for early start; type of shiftwork; day or night work; arrangements for rest pauses or breaks, etc.
- **Ergonomic aspects**: workplace (e.g. need to climb stairs; distance from toilet facilities; access for wheelchairs, etc.); workstation (e.g. height of workbench; adequate lighting; type of equipment or controls used, etc.). Adaptations of equipment that could help at the workplace should be indicated.
- **Travel**, e.g. need to work in areas remote from healthcare or where there are risks not found in the UK (see Appendix 5).

Factors influencing work performance

The ability to perform physical work, and even intellectual occupations involve some physical work, depends ultimately on the ability of muscle cells to transform chemically bound energy from food into mechanical energy. This in turn depends on the intake, storage, and mobilization of nutrient (fuel), and the uptake of oxygen and its delivery by the cardiovascular system to the muscles where it is oxidized to release energy. This chain of activities and processes is influenced at every juncture by other factors, both endogenous and external or environmental.

Factors which may influence work performance, directly or indirectly, include:

- training and adaptation
- the general state of health of the individual
- sex (e.g. the maximal strength of women's leg muscles is only 65–75% of that of men)
- body size
- age (the maximal muscle strength of a 65 year old man is, on average, only 75–80% of that when he was 20 and at his peak)
- nutritional state—particularly important when working in cold environments
- individual differences
- attitude
- motivation
- sleep deprivation (this causes a marked deterioration in mental performance and releases emotional effects)
- stress
- type of work (physical or mental)
- the work itself
- workload
- fatigue
- work schedules
- the environment (heat, cold, humidity, air velocity, altitude, hyperbaric pressure, noise, vibration, air pollution)

These factors are summarized in Fig. 1.1 which is taken from *The physiology of work* by Rodahl.[15]

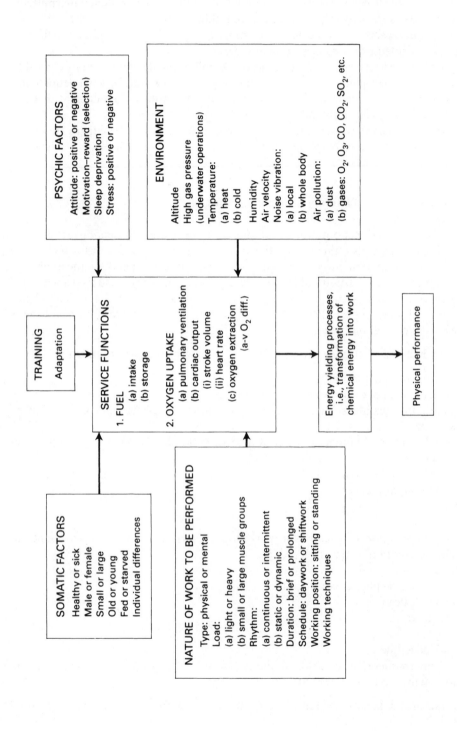

Fig. 1.1 Requirements for the job (from Rodahl 1989).

Too often, medical statements simply state 'fit for light work only'. The dogmatic separation of work into 'light', 'medium', and 'heavy' has often resulted in individuals being unduly limited in their choice of work. A refinement of this broad grading is adopted by the US Department of Labor in its *Dictionary of occupational titles.*[16] Jobs are graded according to physical demands, environmental conditions, certain levels of skill and knowledge, and specific vocational preparation (training time) required, but current occupational health practice requires more specific adjustment of the job to the individual.

If the energy or metabolic requirements of a particular task are known, the individual's work capacity may be estimated and, if expressed in the same units, a comparison between the energy demands of the work and the physiological work capacity of the individual may be made. This has been used in assessing work capacity of patients with heart disease.[17] (See also Chapter 18, p. 358). Energy requirements of various tasks have been estimated and are often expressed in metabolic equivalents, or Mets. (The Met is an arbitrary unit recommended by the American Heart Association: 1 Met is the approximate energy expended while sitting at rest, and is defined as the rate of energy expenditure requiring an oxygen consumption of 3.5 ml per kilogram of body weight per minute.) The metabolic demands of many working activities have been published and the equivalents for the five grades of physical demands in terms of muscular strength adopted by the US Department of Labor are listed below. Work physiology assessments in occupational medicine provide a quantitative way of matching patients to their work[18] and are commonly used in Scandinavia and the US.

Physical demands

The physical demands listed below (taken from the selected characteristics of occupations defined in the *Dictionary of Occupational Titles*[16]) serve as a means of expressing both the physical requirements of the job and the physical capacities (specific physical traits) that a worker must have to meet those required by many jobs, e.g. perceiving by the sense of vision. The worker must possess a physical capacity that at least matches the physical demands made by the job.

1. Strength

This factor is expressed in terms of sedentary, light, medium, heavy, and very heavy. It is measured by involvement of the worker with one or more of the following activities:

(a) Worker position(s):

  (i) standing: remaining on one's feet in an upright position at a workstation without moving about

  (ii) walking: moving about on foot

  (iii) sitting: remaining in the normal seated position.

(b) Worker movement of objects (including extremities used):

  • (i) lifting: raising or lowering an object from one level to another (includes upward pulling)

- (ii) carrying: transporting an object, usually holding it in the hands or arms or on the shoulder

- (iii) pushing: exerting force upon an object so that the object moves away from the force (includes slapping, striking, kicking, and treadle actions)

- (iv) pulling: exerting force upon an object so that the object moves toward the force (includes jerking).

The five degrees of Physical Demands Factor No. 1 (strength) (estimated equivalents in Mets) are as follows:

S **Sedentary work (under 2 Mets)**: lifting 10 lbs (4.5 kg) maximum and occasionally lifting and/or carrying such articles as dockets, ledgers, and small tools. Although a sedentary job is defined as one which involves sitting, a certain amount of walking and standing is often necessary in carrying out job duties. Jobs are sedentary if walking and standing are required only occasionally and other sedentary criteria are met.

L **Light work (2–3 Mets)**: lifting 20 lbs (9 kg) maximum with frequent lifting and/or carrying of objects weighing up to 10 lbs (4.5 kg). Even though the weight lifted may be only a negligible amount, a job is in this category when it requires walking or standing to a significant degree, or when it involves sitting most of the time with a degree of pushing and pulling of arm and/or leg controls.

M **Medium work (4–5 Mets)**: lifting 50 lbs (23 kg) maximum with frequent lifting and/or carrying of objects weighing up to 25 lbs (11.5 kg).

H **Heavy work (6–8 Mets)**: lifting 100 lbs (45 kg) maximum with frequent lifting and/or carrying of objects weighing up to 50 lbs (23 kg).

V **Very heavy work (8 Mets)** lifting objects in excess of 100 lbs (45 kg) with frequent lifting and/or carrying of objects weighing 50 lbs (23 kg) or more.

2. Climbing and/or balancing

(a) **Climbing**: ascending or descending ladders, stairs, scaffolding, ramps, poles, ropes, and the like, using the feet and legs and/or hands and arms.

(b) **Balancing**: maintaining body equilibrium to prevent falling when walking, standing, crouching, or running on narrow, slippery, or erratically moving surfaces; or maintaining body equilibrium when performing gymnastic feats.

3. Stooping, kneeling, crouching, and/or crawling

(a) **Stooping**: bending the body downward and forward by bending the spine at the waist.

(b) **Kneeling**: bending the legs at the knees to come to rest on the knee or knees.

(c) **Crouching**: bending the body downward and forward by bending the legs and the spine.

(d) **Crawling**: moving about on the hands and knees or hands and feet.

4. Reaching, handling, fingering, and/or feeling

(a) **Reaching**: extending the hands and arms in any direction.

(b) **Handling**: seizing, holding, grasping, turning, or otherwise working with the hand or hands (fingering not involved).

(c) **Fingering**: picking, pinching, or otherwise working with the fingers primarily (rather than with the whole hand or arm as in handling).

(d) **Feeling**: perceiving such attributes of objects and materials as size, shape, temperature, or texture, by means of receptors in the skin, particularly those of the fingertips.

5. Talking and/or hearing

(a) **Talking**: expressing or exchanging ideas by means of the spoken word.

(b) **Hearing**: perceiving the nature of sounds by the ear.

6. Seeing

Obtaining impressions through the eyes of the shape, size, distance, motion, color or other characteristics of objects. The major visual functions are defined as follows:

(a) **acuity**

- far—clarity of vision at 20 feet (6 m) or more
- near—clarity of vision at 20 inches (50 cm) or less

(b) **depth perception**: three-dimensional vision; the ability to judge distance and space relationships so as to see objects where and as they actually are

(c) **field of vision**: the area that can be seen up and down or to the right or left while the eyes are fixed on a given point

(d) **accommodation**: adjustment of the lens of the eye to bring an object into sharp focus; especially important for doing near-point work at varying distances from the eye

(e) **color vision**: the ability to identify and distinguish colors.

Objective tests

The result of any objective tests of function relevant to the working situation should be noted. For instance, the physical work capacity of an individual may be estimated ergometrically using standard exercise tests, step tests, or different task simulations. Cardiorespiratory function may be relevant. Muscular strength and lifting ability can be assessed objectively by using either dynamic or static strength tests.

Presentation of the assessment

If a written report is needed it should be legible, clearly laid out, signed, and dated. The report should mention any functional limitations and outline activities that may, or may not, be undertaken. Any health or safety implications should be noted and the assessment should aim at a positive statement about the patient's abilities. Any adaptations, ergonomic alterations or 'reasonable adjustments' to the work that would be helpful or required by the DDA should be indicated (work accommodation is discussed on p.51). Recommendations on restriction or limitation of employment, particularly for health and/or safety reasons, should be unambiguous and precise, and should be made only if definitely indicated.

Many standard functional profiles of individual abilities have been used in North America, Scandinavia, and the UK (mainly in the armed services). These profiles, which resemble each other, are known by acronyms of the initial letters of the parts of the body assessed, e.g. PULHEEMS, GULHEMP, PULSES. In the case of the GULHEMP profile each division is graded from 1 to 7. Other profiles have combined the evaluation of physical abilities with indications of the frequency with which certain activities may be undertaken. Although such profiles are relatively objective and systematic, and allow for consistent recordings on the same individual over a period of time, they take time to complete and much of the information may not be needed. Many doctors in industry who have tried to introduce a PULHEEMS type of system have found that it does not always help when dealing with the practical, and often complex, problems affecting individual employees.

Other simpler classifications are often used in clinical settings, e.g. the New York Heart Association's Impairment of Cardiac Functions. Graded in terms of symptoms, such classifications are of less use in assessing occupational fitness than in recording clinical progress or deterioration. Other scales (e.g. the Barthel Index) used to grade degree of damage or recovery after stroke, for instance, are used to assess outcome after different rehabilitation procedures, and often form part of occupational therapy assessments.

Matching the individual with the job

A functional assessment of the individual's capacities will be of most use when as much is known about the job as about the individual assessed. Sophisticated equipment is now available to make a functional capacity assessment (FCA) that will match an individual to a task (further discussed in Chapter 4). Less formally, the requirements of the task can be categorized, so that a match can be made with the individual's capacity. There are wide variations in the practice of occupational medicine in different countries. In both France and Germany job matching is used formally in some work settings, but systematic job analysis and matching is currently rarely done at the workplace in the UK. However, an activity matching ability system (AMAS), which was developed in the UK, has been used by Remploy in a sheltered work setting. A comparable instrument is the work ability index (WAI), developed in Finland (see Chapter 27, p. 524 *et seq*). In British industry, however, a pragmatic solution emerges when personnel staff and managers, company doctors, and supervisors discuss the placement needs of their disabled employees and, as both worker abilities and task requirements are well known to them, a theoretical match is often superfluous. Outside the workplace itself, more formal assessments may be made in medical rehabilitation or occupational therapy departments (see Chapter 4).

A comprehensive review of current approaches to the analysis of both the physical demands of jobs and the physical abilities of individuals, job matching and functional capacity assessment was published by Fraser in 1992.[19] Accommodation at the workplace is also discussed, and appendices include details of physiological and biomechanical techniques for work capacity measurement, as well as some schemata and scales in current use.

It is essential that the occupational physician or nurse who is assessing medical suitability for employment has an intimate understanding of the job in question.

Recommendations following assessment

- **If the patient is employed,** it should be possible to make a medical judgement on whether they are:

1 capable of performing the work without any ill effects

2 capable of performing the work but with reduced efficiency or effectiveness

3 capable of performing the work although this may adversely affect their medical condition

4 capable of performing the work but not without unacceptable risks to the health and safety of themselves, other workers, or the community

5 physically or mentally incapable of performing the work in question.

For the employed patient, where the judgement is 2–5, the options of 'reasonable adjustment' may include work accommodation; alternative work on a temporary or permanent basis; sheltered work; or, in the last resort, retirement on medical grounds.

- **If the patient is unemployed but is being given a pre-employment assessment** for recruitment to a particular job, options 1–5 will still be appropriate.
- However, **if the unemployed patient is not being considered for a specific job**, then the recommendation following the assessment cannot relate to specific job requirements and it is particularly important that **no unnecessary medical restrictions are imposed.**

The return to work

Even if the patient is assessed as medically fit for a return to their previous job without modification, medical advice may still be needed on the timing of return to work. A clear indication by the consultant or family practitioner to the patient, or to the employer or occupational physician, on when work may be resumed should be given wherever possible. Work should be resumed as soon as the individual is physically and mentally fit enough, having regard to their own and others' health and safety. Return to work at the right time can assist recovery, whereas undue delay can aggravate the sense of uselessness and isolation that so often accompanies incapacity due to major illness or injury.

The contact between the patient's doctor and their employer or occupational physician, stressed earlier in this chapter, will ensure that preparations for the patient's return to work can be put in hand. Recommendations on when work may be resumed and on the patient's functional and work capacities should be clear and specific.

Patients who have been treated for cancer may have particular difficulties in integrating on their return to work, but, with modern treatment, many cancer patients return to full and productive employment. The advice of an occupational physician will be especially valuable in helping workers with cancer to return to their jobs as well as helping their employers and work colleagues to make any necessary adjustments. Close friends and relatives may also need advice when working at the same time as caring for a cancer patient. Many, but not all, patients who have been treated for cancer will be disabled, by definition, under the DDA. Doctors, employers, patients and their carers can obtain information and advice on all aspects of cancer and including working with cancer, from CancerBACUP, whose address and telephone numbers are included in Appendix 7. They have recently introduced a support service for occupational health departments supporting workers with cancer.

Work accommodation

The patient's condition which may or may not come within the DDA, may be such that their previous work needs to be modified. In either case, both the physical and organizational aspects of the job must be considered. Simple features such as bench height, type of chair or stool, or lighting may need adjustment, or more sophisticated aids or adaptations may be required. The workplace environment may need to be adapted, for example by building a ramp or widening a doorway to improve access for wheelchairs. Financial assistance may be available from the Employment Service. Further details are included in Chapter 4 (see p.74).

Information on equipment may be available from several voluntary organizations such as the Royal Association for Disability and Rehabilitation (RADAR), the Disabled Living Foundation (DLF) and the Disability Information Trust (DIT) (see list of addresses in Appendix 7). The DIT has published a comprehensive volume, *Employment and the Workplace*.[20]

Certain organizational features of the work may need adjustment—for instance adjustment of objectives, more flexible working hours, more frequent rest pauses, job sharing, alterations to shiftwork or arrangements to avoid rush-hour travel. A short period of unpaced work may be necessary before resuming paced work. Sometimes the way in which the patient relates to fellow workers may need attention.

Alternative work

In many occupations, work accommodation or job restructuring is not possible and some type of suitable alternative work, possibly only temporary, may have to be recommended. This is usually judged on an individual basis by the occupational physician who can keep the employee under regular review. Where there are no occupational health services, the Employment Service's Disability Employment Advisers (DEAs) can visit the workplace to advise on work accommodation or alternative work (see Chapter 4); EMAS may be able to provide some advice to individual employees.

Premature medical retirement

Medical retirement is a last resort, if further treatment is impossible or ineffective, if suitable alternative or sheltered work cannot be provided, or if the employee will not accept such initiatives. If the 'threshold of employability for a particular job' (K. H. Nikol, personal communication) cannot be reached, either through recovery of fitness, or adjustment of work, retirement on medical grounds may have to be considered. **A management decision on premature retirement on grounds of ill health should never be made without a supporting medical opinion that has taken the requirements of the job fully into account.** Medical retirement is discussed more fully in Appendix 6. Other aspects of premature medical retirement in relation to the law are discussed in Chapter 2.

The future

In 1998 the Government published a Green Paper, *New ambitions for our country: a new contract for welfare* which is driven by the motive of encouraging work for those who can and providing security for those who cannot. In October 1998 the Government had set out details of its reform proposals in *A new contract for welfare: support for disabled people*. Among these reforms were measures to help disabled people back to work where possible. In order to obtain this objective:

- The medical assessment for claimants of state incapacity benefits (the All Work Test) is to be reformed so that it provides information about their capacities as well as their incapacities. The information will be used to support a possible return to work. In addition, and where appropriate, the assessment will provide advice on positive measures to help the individual overcome those barriers to work that are created by their disease or disability. There will be no change in the way the test acts as a gateway to benefit. Entitlement to state benefit will be determined by the same functional criteria of incapacity as now.
- There will also be a new requirement on people with long-term illness or disability claiming incapacity benefit to have an interview with a personal job adviser. The adviser will help the disabled person plan how they can achieve independence, supported by the information gathered at the reformed medical assessment (Dr R. Thomas, Medical Policy Adviser, personal communication).

The maintenance of fitness

From the viewpoint of the occupational physician, fitness for work does not end with medical assessment; an employee must remain fit, which means attention to those factors that will prevent the deterioration of health. These may include policies or advice on smoking, exercise, diet, and alcohol consumption.

The subjects of health promotion, health screening, and general prevention of ill health are not discussed in this book, although these matters are important aspects of the activities of doctors in the workplace. The prevention of vascular disease—cardiac, cerebral, and peripheral—is particularly important because these diseases take a very high toll of the working population and because simple initiatives can be very effective.

The 1998 Department of Health document *Our healthier nation*[21] mentions some of the factors which can be addressed by occupational physicians, although the booklet unfortunately contains insufficient emphasis on the importance of the work environment in the prevention of ill health.

Doctors have a duty to discourage smoking at work and smoking should be banned absolutely, on health grounds, in places where non-smoking employees would be subject to the tobacco fumes of others. Smoking causes more than a quarter of all deaths in men and women of working age and it is the cause of more than half the total deaths of those who indulge in the habit. Most of the deaths are from vascular diseases.

Diet is also important in the prevention of vascular disease Cholesterol and high intakes of animal fat are notable risk factors. The occupational physician should, therefore, be concerned not only with the education of employees on these matters, but also with ensuring that healthy food is available in eating places at work and—perhaps especially—in executives' dining rooms.

Employers should also be encouraged to provide facilities for employees to take regular exercise. This does not necessarily mean the provision of exercise gymnasia but it does mean ensuring that changing and showering facilities are available for those employees who wish to pursue their own exercise programmes, whether these are cycling to and from work or running in the lunch break.

The long-term prevention of ill health, by whatever means, is as important to the prudent employer as ensuring that a new employee is fit for work.

Conclusion

Medical fitness is relevant when illness or injury reduce performance, or affect health and safety in the workplace; it may also be specifically relevant to certain onerous or hazardous tasks for which medical standards exist. Medical fitness should always be judged in relation to the work, and not simply the pension scheme. It has little relevance in a wide range of employment: very many medical conditions, and virtually all minor health problems, have minimal implications for work and should not debar from employment. Medical fitness for employment is not an end in itself. It must be maintained.

Annexe: Accident compensation

D. Black

Outstanding or delayed compensation following an industrial injury or illness is often thought to delay recovery and rehabilitation. In an endeavour to overcome this problem New Zealand introduced a 'no fault' compensation scheme in 1974. Since then the scheme known as Accident Compensation (now ACC) has been generally successful and has evolved to cover all accidents of any cause. Variations on this approach have been used elsewhere, particularly for medical misadventure insurance.

The merit of the idea depends on the many disadvantages associated with the inevitable administrative overhead of a system requiring common law demonstration of fault in causation of an accident. At the time of the accident, access to funding for treatment and particularly rehabilitation may be delayed by legal proceedings to establish blame, and this at a time when support is most needed. When the matter is eventually decided, the overall cost may be greatly inflated by these proceedings even in apparently straightforward cases. In a no fault system, it is only necessary to demonstrate that an accident within the definition of the scheme has actually occurred. Any issue of fault is irrelevant to the prescribed entitlements.

Before 1974, New Zealand had operated an insurance-based workers compensation system, with employers required to hold cover for workers underwritten by private insurers. The original ACC scheme was designed by the initiative of a National (conservative) government and was eventually introduced by a Labour administration. Funding was achieved by redirecting the existing resource of premiums away from the private sector companies, effectively nationalizing workers compensation to support a government owned corporation, the Accident Compensation Corporation (ACC).

Early experience with the scheme was generally positive, and soon it was extended to cover personal injury occurring outside work, funded by top-up from central government.

The scheme also had to cover occupational diseases which were defined as diseases arising out of the nature of employment, although there was no specific schedule of such diseases, except noise-induced hearing loss which was covered by a specific part of the Act. Various difficulties arose during practical implementation, for example the problem of defining cover for diseases with long latency, or gradual onset. This was resolved by defining the date of diagnosis as the date of commencement of the disease for the purpose of ascribing causation. As the scheme extended into injuries outside work, additional issues such as medical misadventure and sexual abuse came under the umbrella of ACC. By the 1980s the ACC scheme was coming under scrutiny from employer groups who considered that their funds were being applied to matters not related to employment, and who advocated reform. These concerns were hard to substantiate objectively, as the average cost of insurance to employers still remained low compared to other jurisdictions with common law systems. Nevertheless, by 1992, there was sufficient pressure to change the scheme and to bring back some requirement to assess causation, so that the ACC now operates separate accounts for different groups: employer, personal, motor vehicle, etc.

In addition, the original actuarial basis for funding the scheme had been changed in the early 1980s to a pay-as-you-go system which allowed normal reserves expected of an insurance company to flow out on the basis that there was government backing for the scheme anyway. This meant that for periods during the 1980s some premiums had been artificially low, and, in addition, the scheme was no longer that of a stand-alone insurance company which effectively limited any potential for competition.

Since 1992, the scheme has continued under the new legislation, which defines occupational disease as 'disease by gradual process' and assesses every claim as to whether the precipitating event was work-related or not. The scheme still comes in for some criticism by employers who believe the result could be achieved for less cost, and some substantial organizations have been permitted to underwrite the first year of claims themselves for reduced premiums. This experiment has had limited success, if only in some cases to demonstrate the existing integrity of the scheme.

Overall, the New Zealand experience with ACC would have to be seen as a success, particularly in terms of the underlying ideology and concept. Some of the most difficult hurdles have been caused by political interference with the scheme (for example changing the basis of funding and reintroducing the need for assigning an accident to the party at fault) but despite this it has survived robustly and has substantial support both from the public and across the political spectrum in New Zealand.

The major advantages of the scheme are, as predicted, immediate access to financial support after an accident and also effectively unlimited support—for example in the case of lifetime disability. Support is limited to earnings-related compensation; regular payments which are based on 80% of earnings before the accident up to a prescribed maximum. The scheme will also pay for reasonable medical costs, and now makes significant contributions to private treatment particularly where this can enable earlier return to work. Though compensation is the primary responsibility of the ACC it has statutory responsibilities in accident prevention and rehabilitation, and is active in both of these areas.

There is no provision now for any lump sum benefit to be paid, although until 1992 limited payouts were possible. This change had both desirable and undesirable effects. On the positive side, the lack of lump sums means that there is little incentive to make a claim which cannot be substantiated by a continuing disability. On the other hand, there is no opportunity to use a single payout to send a message to an injured person that compensation is now complete, which was often a valuable tool in motivating rehabilitation. Various attempts have been tried, for instance to limit continued compensation when a prescribed level (80%) of ability to work was reached. This was largely motivated by a belief that some people remain on ACC when they are really unemployed and therefore are receiving the wrong benefit. Again this approach has met with legal challenge, limited success, and considerable patient hostility. Nonetheless, the problem is real.

The main concern which has persisted amongst the business community is that, as an effective government monopoly, the ACC scheme does not find a market level of cost by ordinary competitive forces. In December 1998 an amendment to the legislation was passed by parliament which allows the entry of commercial insurers to compete with ACC for cover from 1 July 1999. This now means that some employers will be able to operate in a no fault environment by a combination of self cover (for the first year) and private cover thereafter.

There is little doubt that the no fault compensation system for accidents and occupational illness will continue in New Zealand, whatever future political direction. There is frequent interest from other jurisdictions in the New Zealand approach and there is no reason why this experience cannot be applied to jurisdictions elsewhere.

Selected references

1 *Guidance on ethics for occupational physicians*, 5th edn. London: Faculty of Occupational Medicine, Royal College of Physicians, 1999.
2 *International classification of impairments, disabilities and handicaps*. Geneva: World Health Organization, 1980.
3 Wood PHN. The language of disablement: a glossary relating to disease and its consequences. *Int Rehabil Med* 1980;**2**: 86–92.
4 Martin J, Meltzer H, Elliot D. *The prevalence of disability among adults*. OPCS surveys of disability in Great Britain. Report 1. London: HMSO, 1988.
5 Martin J, White A, Meltzer H. *Disabled adults: services, transport and employment*. OPCS surveys of disability in Great Britain. Report 4. London: HMSO, 1989.
6 Warren MD. The prevalence of disability. *J Roy Coll Phys London* 1989;**23**: 171–5.
7 Taylor PJ, Fairrie AJ. Chronic disabilities and capacity for work (A study of 3299 men aged 16–24 in a general practice and an oil refinery.) *Br J Prev Soc Med* 1968;**22**: 86–93.
8 Taylor PJ, Fairrie AJ. Chronic disability in men of middle age. A study of 165 men in a general practice and a refinery. *Br J Prev Soc Med* 1968;**22**: 183–92.
9 Taylor PJ with Barrett JD, Fletcher GC *et al*. A combined survey of chronic disability in industrial employees. *Trans Soc Occup Med* 1970;**20**: 98–102
10 Heijbel CA. Occurrence of personal handicaps in an industrial population, survey and appraisal: Physical demands and the disabled. *Scand J Rehab Med* 1978;suppl 6: 182–92.
11 Jarvikoski A, Tuunainen K. The need for early rehabilitation among Finnish municipal employees. *Scand J Rehab Med* 1978;**10**: 115–20.
12 Fanning D. Ill health retirement as an indicator of morbidity. *J Soc Occup Med* 1981;**31**: 103–11.
13 *Occupational pension scheme cover for disabled people*. Cmnd 6849. London: HMSO, 1977.
14 Brackenridge RDC, Elder WJ. *Medical selection of life risks*, 4th edn. London: Macmillan, 1998.
15 Rodahl K. *The physiology of work*. London: Taylor & Francis, 1989.
16 US Department of Labor. *Selected characteristics of occupations defined in the Dictionary of Occupational Titles*. Washington: US Government Printing Office, 1981.
17 Long C (ed.). *Prevention and rehabilitation in ischemic heart disease*. Baltimore: Williams and Wilkins, 1980.
18 Erb BD. Applying work physiology to occupational medicine. *Occup Health Saf* 1981;**50**: 20–4.
19 Fraser TM. *Fitness for work: the role of physical demands analysis and physical capacity assessment*. London: Taylor & Francis, 1992.
20 *Employment and the Workplace*. Oxford: Disability Information Trust, 1994.
21 *Our healthier nation: a contract for health*. London: Stationery Office, 1998.

2

Legal aspects of fitness for work

G. Howard

This chapter outlines some of the ways in which the law may affect the employment of people with health problems. There are three major legal sources—the common law, statute law, and European Directives.

Common law

The English legal system is based on the common law.[*] This system developed from the decisions of judges whose rulings over the centuries have created precedents for other courts to follow and these decisions were based on the 'custom and practice of the Realm'. The common law can be contrasted with statute law (passed by Parliament) and equity (the body of rules administered by the Court of Chancery).

The system of binding precedent means that any decision of the House of Lords (the highest court in the United Kingdom) will bind all the lower courts, unless the lower courts are able to distinguish the facts of the current case and argue that the old decision cannot apply because of differences in the facts of the two cases.

However, since the UK joined the European Union (EU), the decisions of the European Court of Justice (ECJ) now supersede any decisions of the domestic courts and require the national courts to follows its decisions.[1] A human rights bill was introduced in 1997 in order to incorporate the provisions of the European Convention on Human Rights into UK law.

The common law covers both the criminal and civil law. The law of negligence has grown out of the common law and forms part of the civil law of torts (civil wrongs). For centuries, the common law courts have held employers liable for negligence if the employer had not taken reasonable care for the health and safety of their workers.

Common law duties of employers

At common law, employers have an obligation to take **reasonable care** of all their employees and to guard against reasonably foreseeable risks of injury. These duties are judged in the light of the 'state of the art' of knowledge of the employer—what they either knew or ought to have known.

---

[*] See footnote on p. 39.

Standard of care of occupational physicians

The **standard of care** expected of a professional, e.g. an occupational health specialist, is set out in a case which established the so-called 'Bolam' test[2]. McNair J held that the test of the ordinary person's standard of care is judged by the action of the 'man in the street'. However, in the case of a medical specialist, such as an occupational physician, the standard of care is higher because the occupational physician is considered to be an expert in that particular field of medicine.

Duty to inform and warn of risks to health and safety

Employers are obliged to inform their workers, including prospective employees, of inherent risks of the job so that they can accept or decline employment having made an informed choice. Any warning does not of course relieve the employer of the duty to take all reasonable care to guard against reasonably foreseeable risks of injury. What it does is to provide employees with information they would otherwise have lacked. Sometimes, and possibly most effectively, this information is imparted through the company's medical advisers.

The principle of *volenti non fit injuria*, i.e. that the individual knew about the risk, understood the exact nature of that risk, and accepted that risk may conceivably be used by an employer in defence of a negligence claim. However, it has rarely proved to be a successful defence because the risk has to be accepted freely and without duress. If the only choice was between dismissal or accepting a particular risk at the workplace, the courts would not be slow to disallow the defence of *volenti*.

In one of the several cases brought against Bernard Matthews for work-related upper limb disorders (WRULDs), it was successfully argued by Mrs Mountenay and others[3] that she had not been given sufficient warning of the inherent risk of WRULDs associated with eviscerating chickens on a paced production line.

In another leading case, *Stokes* v. *Guest Keen and Nettlefold*,[4] the company was found liable for the scrotal cancers which eventually killed several of its workers. The company had employed a doctor who lectured in industrial medicine. This doctor had failed to warn the men of the dangers of cancer associated with the oils which contaminated their overalls, as he had not wanted 'to alarm the men'. He could, and should, have circulated a leaflet to the men warning of the dangers of scrotal warts, and should have instituted periodic medical examinations. The employer was held to be vicariously liable for this act of negligence on the doctor's part.

In summary, the employer's duties include obligations to:
- take positive and practical steps to ensure the safety of their employees in the light of the knowledge which they have, or ought to have
- follow current recognized practice, unless in the light of common sense or new knowledge this is clearly unsound
- keep reasonably abreast of developing knowledge and not be too slow in applying it
- take greater than average precautions where the employer has greater than average knowledge of the risk
- weigh up the risk (in terms of the likelihood of the injury and the possible consequences) against the effectiveness and the cost and inconvenience of the precautions to be taken to meet the risk.

Balancing the risk

In deciding what is 'reasonably practicable' to do in terms of eliminating risk and in determining what is reasonably foreseeable in terms of injury, the courts have determined a test which balances the quantum of risk against the time, trouble, and expense that the employer must go to to avert that risk. The greater the risk to health or safety, the greater the time, trouble, and expense the law expects the employer to devote to mitigating that risk. In a leading case involving the National Coal Board,[5] the Court of Appeal held that the employer' obligation to discharge their duty of care would only be satisfied when the time, trouble, and expense required to avert the risk was grossly disproportionate to the risk involved.

Ignorance is no defence in law. Furthermore if one member of the employer's staff knows about a risk or a health or safety problem, then (whether this is shared with the employer or not) the employer is deemed to know about it. This is called **constructive knowledge**.

The state of the art

The courts will look at the state of knowledge at the time of the alleged act of negligence in judging whether the employer ought to have acted or not.

Employers are not expected to be prophets, nor are they expected to remain ignorant of the growing knowledge of health and safety matters. Nor are they permitted to ignore advice and information given to them by their occupational health experts merely because other employers do not know about or concern themselves with these issues.

In cases concerning noise-induced hearing loss, the courts have investigated the state of knowledge among employers in the 1950s, even though the Ministry of Labour pamphlet *Noise and the worker* was not published until 1963. In *Baxter* v. *Harland and Wolff plc*,[6] **the employer was held liable for noise-induced deafness as far back as 1953 because the employer failed to 'seek out knowledge of facts which are not in themselves obvious'.**

Harland and Wolff had not sought or heeded medical, scientific and legal advice between 1953 and 1963, despite there being evidence of several incidents of noise-induced deafness problems in the naval shipyards in Devon before the Second World War and medical reports and papers on this in the early 1950s. Evidence was produced that an advertisement in the *Lancet* on 28 April 1951 had featured a protective earplug.

The employer was held to be negligent because of its 'lack of interest and apathy . . . The defendants, knowing that noise was causing deafness among their workmen, should have applied their minds to removing or reducing the risk . (and) . . sought advice . . .'

Greater duty of care: 'eggshell skull' principle

The employer owes a higher duty of care to any particularly vulnerable employee with a known, pre-existing medical condition. Those with an 'eggshell skull physique' are more vulnerable to serious injury than others of robust physical health. Those with a fragile personality may suffer far greater psychological damage than those with a robust personality. This is defined as the 'eggshell skull' principle[7] and a classic example of this can be seen in the case of *Paris* v. *Stepney Borough Council*. Here the Council employed a labourer with only one eye. They failed to ensure that he was wearing eye goggles and as a result he suffered an injury to his other eye at work and was blinded. The courts held that his employers owed him a much higher duty of care as he was an individual with extra risk of serious injury.

It is therefore important for employers to take informed advice from qualified occupational health professionals on fitness and placement decisions and the need for special arrangements or precautions. Failure to consider whether pre-employment medical checks are required and, if they are indicated, to arrange for them to be done by properly qualified and trained occupational health staff, may lead to a successful claim for negligence against the employer.

Duty owed in mental illness

In several recent cases the courts have extended the principle of the employer's common law duty to psychiatric injury. In a case which went to the House of Lords[8] the negligent party was held liable for the onset of chronic fatigue syndrome precipitated by a car accident.

Although not the first case to establish an employer's duty of care to look after the mental well-being of employees, *Walker* v. *Northumberland County Council* (1995) IRLR 35 was the first successful claim for damages. In this case John Walker, a senior social worker in charge of child abuse cases, was eventually forced to leave his job, after suffering two mental breakdowns. The Council was held liable for the second of his nervous breakdowns and ordered to pay damages of over £250,000 for his lost career and permanent psychological impairment. The High Court held that it was reasonably foreseeable that in returning to his former post without adequate help and resources, Mr Walker would again become mentally ill—especially in the light of the medical experts' opinions that the nature and the volume of his work was the major contributory factor for his first nervous breakdown.

Employees' duties

In common law employees have implied duties, including the duty to work with reasonable care and competence and to serve their employer loyally and faithfully. They are also under a duty to be reasonably competent, to co-operate with their employer, and to obey reasonable lawful instructions.

Statute law

Health and Safety at Work Act 1974

The Health and Safety at Work Act 1974 (HSAWA) is superimposed on earlier Acts and the duties imposed by some of these (e.g. the Mines and Quarries Act 1954, the Factories Act 1961, and the Offices, Shops and Railway Premises Act 1963) must still be met, although most of their enforcement provisions have been replaced in the new legislation.

The Health and Safety Commission (HSC) was set up by the Act and is responsible for policy; the Health and Safety Executive (HSE), together with local authority environmental health officers, are responsible for enforcing the Act's requirements.

HSAWA imposes criminal liability, and the company, individual managers, and employees can be prosecuted for breaches of their statutory duties. Lesser criminal cases brought under the HSAWA can be heard in the Magistrates Courts which have the power to impose fines or commit a person to prison for up to 6 months. With the passage of the Offshore Safety Act 1992 the fines were increased to a maximum of £5000 for breaches of sections 2–6 of the HSAWA and £20 000 for breaches of improvement or prohibition notices. If the HSE consider the breaches to be sufficiently serious, then the matter can be tried in the Crown Court which has the power to impose an unlimited fine or a term of imprisonment.

There is provision in Section 47 of HSAWA to extend the jurisdiction of the Act to permit employees injured at work to sue for their injuries in the civil courts under the Act, but this Section has not been implemented to date. Employees who are injured at work as a result of a breach of any other statutory duties can sue in the civil courts, as the other statutory enactments impose both civil and criminal liability.

The Act covers everyone at work, including independent contractors and their employees, the self-employed, and visitors, but excludes domestic servants in private households.

Employers' statutory duties

HSAWA imposes general duties on employers under Section 2 to ensure, so far as is reasonably practicable, the health, safety and welfare at work of their employees. This specifically includes ensuring that:

- there is a safe system of work
- there is a safe place of work
- staff are given information, instruction, and training on matters of health and safety, and are adequately supervised
- there is a safe system for the handling, storage, and transport of substances and materials
- there is a safe working environment.

Although there is no specific mention of a duty to conduct pre-employment medical examinations, part of a safe system of work could be interpreted as ensuring that the staff who have been recruited are fit to perform their duties where there is any question of medical fitness impinging on the work requirements. Adequate medical data on new members of staff is essential. However, due care must be taken to observe the employer's duties under the Disability Discrimination Act 1995 (DDA) (see Chapter 3).

Employees' statutory duties

Employees have duties under Sections 7 and 8 of the Act to 'take reasonable care' of their own health and safety, and the safety of others; to co-operate on any matter of health and safety; and to do nothing which could endanger their health and safety or that of others.

This duty could be taken to include the disclosure of a relevant medical condition when questioned. For example, an employee who failed to disclose that they had epilepsy, when working in a job where this could pose a hazard, might be in breach of their duty under Section 7 of the Act. Failing to disclose material health information on request may also constitute grounds for lawful dismissal (see 'Unfair Dismissal', below).

The institutions

The HSC was set up under the HSAWA as a tripartite body—Government, Confederation of British Industry (CBI) and Trades Union Congress (TUC)—and is responsible for national health and safety policy. The HSE is responsible for enforcing health and safety legislation, including the HSAWA. There are several divisions, the largest of which is the Factory Inspectorate (HMFI). The Employment Medical Advisory Service (EMAS) is the field force of the medical division of HSE, and will be described in Chapter 4.

Enforcement of the Act in offices, shops, railway premises and warehouses is carried out by environmental health officers, who are employed by the local authorities. Their powers are the same as those of factory inspectors.

Employment protection legislation

Employees have been given statutory protection from being unfairly dismissed; the relevant provisions can be found in the Employment Rights Act 1996.[9] Several aspects of these measures are important for those who develop illnesses or injuries while at work.

Employees have been given protection from unfair dismissal provided that they satisfy certain qualifying conditions, such as 2 years' continuous service, being under the normal retirement age, ordinarily employed in Great Britain, etc.

Claims for unfair dismissal are heard by industrial tribunals. The tribunals are chaired by a legally qualified solicitor or barrister of at least 15 years' standing and a panel of two lay members (one appointed by employers' organizations such as the CBI and one appointed by the TUC or other trades union bodies).

The lay members advise the chairman as to good industrial practice. The chairman directs the lay members as to points of law. Appeals on points of law or a perverse decision lie with the Employment Appeal Tribunal (EAT), then with the Court of Appeal and the House of Lords on points of law only and where leave has been given.

In cases involving questions of European Community law, cases may be referred directly from industrial tribunals to the ECJ. Whether transsexuals and gay men or women fall within the meaning of the word 'sex' under the Sex Discrimination Act 1975 and the Equal Treatment Directive and Article 119 of the Treaty of Rome are questions that have recently been determined by the ECJ. The decision has been that they are not covered by any antidiscrimination legislation in the Equal Treatment Directive.[10]

Grounds for dismissal

Section 98 of the Employment Rights Act 1996 sets out five potentially fair grounds for dismissal. They are conduct, capability, redundancy, illegality, and 'some other substantial reason'.

Capability cases

Dismissal on grounds of 'capability' covers both ill health and poor performance. As far as ill health is concerned, the Act defines this matter as being 'assessed in relation to health or any other physical or mental quality'. Employers must advance factual evidence of the ill health preventing the individual from performing the jobs which they were employed to do, in order to justify the dismissal. Tribunals also have to be satisfied that the employer acted reasonably in treating that reason as sufficient for dismissal. The tribunals have given guidance as to what constitutes reasonable conduct on the part of the employer in this regard (see below).

The mere fact that the individual is not prevented from performing all the duties does not affect a decision to dismiss for ill health as long as the individual is unfit to perform some of the duties. This was stated in the case of *Shook* v. *London Borough of Ealing* (1986), IRLR 46. Miss Shook was employed as a trainee residential care assistant who strained her back and was off work for some 9 months. She was declared unfit to carry out her duties as a residential social worker because of the bending and lifting which was involved in her job and this was confirmed by both her general practitioner and the Council's medical officer. She was eventually dismissed after having been offered alternative posts which she had rejected.

She argued that her employers did not have any fair reason to dismiss her because she was not disabled from all her contractual duties since her contract actually contained a very wide flexibility and mobility clause and she worked in numerous posts within the Social Services Department of the Council.

The Court of Appeal ruled that the dismissal was fair and rejected this argument:

. . . The Tribunal were entitled to reject the submission that an employee is not incapacitated from performing . . . the work that they are employed to do unless he is incapacitated from performing every task which the employers are entitled by law to call on him to discharge. . . .

. . . However widely that contract was construed, her disabilities related to her performance of her duties thereunder, even though her performance of all of them may not have been affected.

Lying about previous health conditions

Lying, as opposed to failing to volunteer information about material health problems, has been accepted as being a potentially fair reason for dismissal in claims for unfair dismissal under the Employment Protection (Consolidation) Act.[11]

The tribunals have distinguished between lying on a pre-employment medical questionnaire and failing to volunteer the information. There is a subtle but important distinction. In some cases it has been held that there is no duty on employees to offer voluntarily medical information about themselves.[12] It follows that prospective employees need to be asked direct questions in any pre-employment questionnaire, which should be designed on the advice of an occupational physician.

Medical evidence and medical reports

In assessing fitness for work most employers rely initially on medical statements (MED 3) from the employee's general practitioner. The tribunals, however, require full medical evidence including reports from either the general practitioner, the consultant (where applicable), and the occupational physician.

However, the tribunals have made it clear that employers should not rely on medical certificates alone. A full medical report should be sought by the employer from the occupational health physician or nurse (if there is one). The employer is required to inform the doctor and the employee of the purpose of the medical report sought.[13] In most cases the employer will state that the report is required in order to plan for the work in the department and administer the sick pay scheme(s).

Doctors should always ensure that every employee who presents for an assessment clearly understands its purpose and the intended use of the report. In case of doubt, the occupational physician should explain the situation to the patient prior to any examination. If necessary, the doctor should write to the originator of the request seeking clarification.

When employers without any occupational health staff seek advice from an independent occupational physician they should advise the doctor as to the purpose of their enquiry, the basic job functions of the individual, and the length of the absence to date. The employer should obtain prior, written informed consent to do this from the employee. If a medical report is being sought from the employee's general practitioner or own specialist, then the employer is required under the Access to Medical Reports Act 1988 to inform the employee of their rights under that Act (which include the right to see the report before it is sent to the employer and the right to refuse to allow the report to be sent to the employer).

By virtue of the Access to Health Records Act 1990 (effective from 1 November 1991) employees are now entitled to see their medical records, which include occupational health records as well as general practitioner and hospital records.

Employers may ask the specialist or general practitioner a range of questions. Answers should be limited to the list taken from the British Medical Association's model letter (Box 2.1).[14]

Box 2.1 British Medical Association's model letter
1. When is the likely date of return to work?
2. Will there be any residual disability on return to work?
3. If so, will it be permanent or temporary?
4. Will the employee be able to render regular and efficient service?
5. If the answer is 'Yes' to question 2, what duties would you recommend that your patient does not do and for how long?
6. Will your patient require continued treatment or medication on return to work?

Under the Access to Medical Reports Act 1988, employees are entitled to see any medical report which relates to them, if it has been prepared by a medical practitioner who is or has been responsible for their clinical care. It is clear that once an occupational physician (or a member of their staff) has treated an employee the Act will apply to all subsequent medical reports,[15] but it is less clear whether this may apply to other clinical reports such as fitness and placement assessments.

The Court may order an individual's clinical notes to be disclosed, including any correspondence between the occupational physician, the consultant, and the management of the company.[16]

Conflicting medical advice

In some cases employers receive conflicting medical opinions—the employee's own specialist or general practitioner stating that the individual is unfit to return to work and the occupational health practitioner confirming that the individual is fit to return to work. In such a dilemma, the tribunals have made it clear that employers are entitled to rely on the view of their occupational physician **unless**:

- the occupational physician has not personally examined the individual but has merely written a report on the basis of the medical notes
- the occupational physician's report is 'woolly' and indeterminate
- the continued employment of the individual would pose a serious threat to the health or safety of the individual or to others
- the individual has been treated or is being treated by a specialist and the occupational physician has not received a report from that specialist.

The tribunals have accepted that an unreasonable refusal by an individual to return to work following the advice of the occupational physician constitutes misconduct on the part of the employee. Here the reason for dismissal is refusing to obey a lawful and reasonable instruction.

Consultation with the employee

The tribunals have ruled that in ill health dismissal, the employer should normally contact the employee, either by telephone or personally, ideally by visiting them at home by appointment. The purpose of this contact is to consult the employee about the incapacity, to discuss any possible return date, the continuation or otherwise of company benefits and State benefits, the employment of a temporary or permanent replacement, and the future employment or termination of employment. Consultation in this case takes the place of warnings which employees are entitled to receive in poor performance or misconduct cases. This was stated in a number of leading cases.[17]

There may, however, be exceptional cases where the tribunal views the lack of consultation as still rendering a subsequent dismissal fair. In one such case, *Eclipse Blinds Ltd* v. *Wright*,[18] the managing director received a very pessimistic medical opinion concerning the state of health of, and improbability of a return to work of the company's receptionist, Mrs Wright, who had been off sick for some time with a bad back. The managing director felt it was not in her best interests to speak to her personally since Mrs Wright had no appreciation of the seriousness of her illness. The managing director decided instead to write to Mrs Wright to inform her that a permanent replacement had been employed and that her services were to be terminated.

Seeking suitable alternative employment

The tribunals expect an employer to consider all alternatives other than dismissal, and this includes looking for suitable alternative employment within the organization or with any associated employers. The duty also includes considering whether any modification to the original job would be possible.

The leading cases cited above of Daubney and Spencer[17] confirm that failure by the employer to seek alternative employment will normally render any dismissal for ill health unfair. This proposition has received judicial approval in the Court of Appeal in the case of *P* v. *Nottinghamshire County Council*[19] where Balcombe LJ stated:

In an appropriate case and where the size and administrative resources of the undertaking permit, it may be unfair to dismiss an employee without the employer first considering whether the employee can be offered some other job notwithstanding that it may be clear that the employee cannot be allowed to continue in his original job . . .

This duty has now been made more explicit, since Section 6 of the DDA requires employers to make 'reasonable adjustments' to the workplace. In this situation occupational physicians may offer valuable advice to employers (see Chapter 3).

Permanent health insurance benefits

Practitioners who advise employers offering long-term disability (LTD) or permanent health insurance (PHI) schemes as part of their contractual benefits ought to be aware that a failure to consider offering such benefits in an appropriate case could well be challenged in the common law courts as a breach of the contract of employment, i.e. breach of the implied obligations of good faith.

In a recent House of Lords case[20] the House of Lords ruled that there was a positive duty on employers rather than their medical advisers to inform their staff of those benefits for which the employee must make an application. This includes the option of making additional voluntary contributions (AVCs) to the pension, claiming sick pay and PHI or LTD, maternity rights, etc. In the context of PHI and LTD schemes, it is essential for the management of any employer to inform any member of staff that they may be eligible for participation in such schemes. Consideration of eligibility for an LTD scheme or PHI scheme may also be viewed by the industrial tribunals as an important factor in any unfair dismissal case since the tribunals could well decide that there was an alternative to dismissal which was not properly considered by the employer—thus rendering the dismissal unfair. Company medical advisers should make themselves aware whether such benefits are offered so that they can advise effectively and appropriately. If such a scheme exists, the doctor (whether general practitioner or occupational physician) ought to enquire of the employer whether the patient has been considered for such a scheme.

Early retirement on medical grounds

In some cases where the employee is permanently incapacitated from any further full-time, permanent employment with the employer, the individual may be dismissed and given an early retirement pension. The common law courts have also indicated that the employer must act in good faith in deciding such cases.[21]

It is essential for medical practitioners to read the exact wording of any pension scheme in this regard, particularly if a medical examination is to be performed in order to assess eligibility. It would be wise for medical practitioners to require a copy of the sick pay scheme, PHI scheme, and pension fund rules as they apply to early medical pensions.

Management's role in sickness decisions

The tribunals have emphasized that the option to dismiss an employee off sick and unable to work is a management decision and not a medical one. Doctors should therefore not allow themselves to be pressured into making such decisions for management. The doctor's role is to provide and interpret the medical information which managers will need, so that they can make decisions about the employee's position.

Pre-employment medical assessments

Pre-placement medical questionnaires should ask suitable and relevant questions and gather only information which is pertinent (see also Chapter 5).

Duty of care

A recent case in the Court of Appeal has clarified to whom the occupational physician owes a duty of care when writing a report on the fitness for work of the job applicant. A ruling in 1998[22] made it clear that the person commissioning the report (i.e. the potential employer) was the only person to whom the occupational physician owed a duty of care when writing the report on the potential employee's fitness for work.

This was because there is no special relationship between a job applicant and the examining occupational physician. The disappointed job applicant will never see the pre-employment medical report nor would they rely on it for any purpose. Therefore the only person who could properly sue, if the report was negligent, is the employer as it would be he who had commissioned it and he who would rely on it.

This case overturned an earlier decision of the High Court[23] which found that the occupational physician did owe a prospective job candidate a duty of care when performing a pre-employment assessment and writing the report.

Although the Kapfunde ruling has now clarified the occupational physician's duty *vis a vis* their pre-employment medical report, the doctor still owes to the patient the normal standard of care and expertise in clinical matters. This includes ensuring that the actual examination and any tests carried out are conducted to the highest professional standards and that any abnormalities detected are notified to the patient and/or to his general practioner with the subject's informed consent.

Duty to be honest

In a case brought before the ECJ,[24] it was ruled that prospective job candidates have the right to be informed of the exact nature of the tests to be carried out and to refuse to participate if they so wish.

A man had applied for a temporary post of a typist with the European Commission. He had undergone a medical examination but refused to be screened for HIV antibodies. After giving blood, undergoing the medical examination, and disclosing his medical records, the medical officer ordered blood tests to determine the T4 and T8 lymphocyte counts. When these were below the normal ratio, the medical officer concluded that Mr X was suffering from a significant immunodeficiency constituting a case of full-blown AIDS and his application was rejected on health grounds.

Mr X complained to the Court that he had been subjected to an AIDS test without his consent. The ECJ held that the manner in which the appellant had been medically examined and declared physically unfit constituted an infringement of his right to respect for his private life as guaranteed by Article 8 of the European Convention on Human Rights. The right to respect for private life requires that a person's refusal to undergo a test be respected in its entirety, but, equally, the employer cannot be obliged to take the risk of recruitment.

Confidentiality

Ethical questions including the duty of confidentiality are covered in detail in Chapter 5. Suffice it to say here that although there is little legal protection in the UK from the invasion of privacy, medical staff are under very strict ethical codes of conduct and can be struck off the medical register for serious breaches.

Employers are not entitled to require their staff to undergo medical examinations without obtaining, **on each occasion**, the informed written consent of the individual. This means ensuring that the employee understands the nature of the examination and tests and the reasons for them. Medical staff should ensure that written consent forms are completed. Employers must also, **on each occasion**, obtain the employee's written, informed consent to disclosure of the results or outcome to a senior named individual in the company.

In the absence of written consent no medical examination or disclosure should take place.

Pregnancy, discrimination, and the law

Any form of discrimination on the grounds of a woman's pregnancy is unlawful; this has been settled in case law and statute law. All aspects are covered, including her intention to take maternity leave, the taking of maternity leave, and intention to return to work following maternity leave. Under the Sex Discrimination Act 1975 there is no ceiling on compensation for such discriminatory acts.

More recent legislative provisions[25] have covered the health and safety risks to pregnant workers, requiring risk assessments to be carried out and adequate control measures to be taken where possible.

European law

Directives which are adopted by the Council of Ministers are binding on Member States and any emanations of the State including former state bodies, such as nationalized industries, public utilities, and state schools are bound by the Directives.

Their employees may sue for breach of an article of the Directive directly in the UK tribunals. Employers in the private sector are not directly bound by a Directive, but Member States are required to adopt the Directive into their national legislation within a defined time scale.

The Council of Ministers is represented by the appropriate minister from each Member State. Each Member State has a block vote, the number of votes depending on the size of its population. Four member states (UK, Italy, Germany, and France) have 10 votes each. Except on matters of health and safety and product safety, voting must be unanimous for a Directive to be adopted. However, in 1987 under the Single European Act, two articles of the Treaty of Rome were altered, Article 188A (worker health and safety) and Article 110A (product safety). These matters can now be resolved by a process of 'qualified majority voting'. Under this system only 62 of 87 possible votes are required to carry a motion.

The Council of Ministers can also make recommendations. Recommendations are generally adopted by the institutions of the Community when they do not have the power to adopt binding acts or when they think that it is not appropriate to issue more constraining rules under the Treaty. Although not legally binding, EU resolutions and recommendations have legal effect in particular when they clarify the interpretation of national provisions or supplement binding Community measures.

Working time directive

The Working Time Directive, which was adopted under the QMV system, requires member states to legislate for a maximum of 48 working hours in any 7 day period, with rest breaks and restrictions on the number of hours of work that can be performed at night. It was adopted on 23 November 1993, with the UK abstaining. Draft regulations embraced by the Working Time Directive were published in April 1998 and became law in the UK in October 1998.

The Working Time Regulations 1998 (SI 1998/1833) provided workers with an entitlement to:

* a rest break where the working day exceeds 6 hours
* at least one whole hour off in each 24 hours
* at least 24 hours off in every week.

Other provisions include at least 4 weeks paid annual leave (from 23rd November 1999); restrictions on night work, (including an average limit of 8 hours in 24); organization of work patterns to take account of health and safety requirements, and the adaptation of work to the worker; an average working limit of 48 hours over each 7 day period, calculated over a reference period of 17 weeks (Regulation 4(3) of the Working Time Regulations 1998).

A further Statutory Instrument, amending the first Working Time Regulations became law on 17 December 1999 - The Working Time Regulations 1999. These Regulations simplified the meaning of the unmeasured hours and those workers who work unmeasured hours are now exempt from the 48 hour week; it also amended the requirement for employers to keep records of the hours worked by workers who had opted out of the 48 hour maximum working week.

The Directive is littered with 'derogations' which exempt certain types of worker. There are some general exceptions which exclude workers in air, sea, rail and road, inland waterways and lake transport, sea fishing and other work at sea, as well as doctors in training. The major provisions for which there are no derogations are the 4 weeks of paid annual leave and the 48 hour working week.

Other exemptions may arise through national legislation or collective agreements for those whose working time is self-determined or flexible (e.g. senior managers or workers with autonomous decision-taking powers, family workers, and workers officiating at religious ceremonies). In addition, workers may agree voluntarily to work longer hours than those laid down in the Directive. In other cases, the workers must be permitted compensatory rest breaks if they work for more than 48 hours in a week (e.g. those whose job involves a great deal of travelling; security and surveillance workers; those whose jobs involve a foreseeable surge in activity such as tourism and agriculture; and emergency rescue workers).

The former Conservative government mounted a legal challenge to this Directive,[26] but this proved unsuccessful. The present government is committed to implementing it but has yet to produce national legislation.

Other health and safety directives

In January 1992, the UK introduced the 'Six Pack'[27] implementing EU Directives on a range of health and safety matters. These regulations made it mandatory for employers to carry out risk assessments in situations where there were 'significant and substantial' risks to health or safety and to appoint 'competent' people to assist them in this task. Employers are required to maintain and update these risk assessments and to document them.

Notes and references[*]

1 *Marleasing* v. *La Comercial Internacional De Alimentacion*. The ECJ ruled that Spanish Company law had to be interpreted to comply with EC Directives which pre-dated Spain joining the European Community—i.e. existing law may need reinterpretation to meet the provisions of a subsequent Directive.

For example, in the case of *Halford* v. *United Kingdom* [1997] IRLR 471, the European Court of Human Rights held that the interception by an employer of telephone calls made from an office amounted to an unjustifiable interference with an employee's right to respect for her private life and correspondence, in accordance with the European Convention on Human Rights. Furthermore UK domestic law failed to provide the employee with an effective remedy for this breach of her rights. The Court awarded her £10 000 for the intrusion into her private life, £600 towards her personal expenses in bringing the proceedings, and £25 000 towards her legal costs.

[*] In contrast to the English legal system the legal system in Scotland is based on Roman Law. However employment protection legislation applies in Scotland, the same as in the rest of Great Britain.

2   *Bolam* v. *Friern Hospital Management Committee* [1957] 1 WLR 582. The High Court held that 'Where you get the situation which involves the use of some special skill or competence, then the test whether there has been negligence or not is not the test of the man on the top of the Clapham omnibus, because he has not got this special skill. The test is the standard of the ordinary skilled man exercising and professing to have that special skill. . .'

3   *Mountenay (Hazzard) and others* v. *Bernard Matthews Plc* (Unreported) 4.5.93 Norwich County Court (HSIB 215, Nov 1993).

4   *Stokes and others* v. *Guest Keen & Nettlefold* [1968] 1 WLR 1776.

5   *Edwards* v. *National Coal Board* 1 ALL ER 743, Court of Appeal.

6   *Baxter* v. *Harland & Wolff plc* [1990] IRLR 516.

7   *Paris* v. *Stepney Borough Council* [1951] 1 ALL ER 42.

8   *Page* v. *Smith—The Times* 4 May 1994. Here a negligent motorist was held liable for the victim's nervous shock and for his 'chronic fatigue syndrome' which he had previously had in a mild form but which he argued had been exacerbated by the accident. As a result, he recovered damages for mental distress due to an exacerbation of his current condition.

9   Employment Rights Act 1996, formerly contained in Employment Protection (Consolidation) Act 1978 and Trade Union Reform and Employment Rights Act (1992).

10 Grant v. *South-West Trains Ltd* [1998] IRLR 188. The ECJ ruled that it was not contrary to Article 119 of the Treaty of Rome or Equal Treatment Directive to deny a lesbian railway clerk a free travel concession for her cohabiting female partner.

Another case to be heard by the ECJ, *R* v. *Secretary of State for Defence* ex parte *Perkins* (C-168/97) concerns the Ministry of Defence's policy of dismissing homosexual employees from the Armed Forces. The ECJ has been asked to consider whether the policy is in breach of the EU Equal Treatment Directive (No 76/207).

11 *O'Brien* v. *The Prudential Assurance Co Ltd* [1979] IRLR 140. Here the Employment Appeal Tribunal held that it was reasonable to dismiss Mr O'Brien for lying about his medical condition (past mental history): 'He had deliberately misled his employers about it in order to obtain employment. The practice of the employer of not employing as district agents persons with long histories of serious mental illness (he had a long-standing history of psychosis and periods of hospitalisation) was not in itself an unreasonable policy.

Whether an employer acts unreasonably in stipulating for a particular employment the conditions which he seeks to establish must depend upon the facts of the case. The Tribunal was satisfied on the evidence that this was a reasonable condition for the job of district agent which involved going into people's homes not only for the company to impose in their selection procedure but also for it to enforce in the case of someone who had misled them as to facts which they regarded as important. . .'.

12 *Walton* v. *TAC Constructions Materials Ltd* [1981] IRLR 357. The EAT held that: '. . . it could not be said that there is any duty on the employee in the ordinary case, though there may be exceptions, to volunteer information about himself otherwise than in response *to a direct question.* . .'.

13 *Whitbread & Co plc* v. *Mills* [1988] IRLR 501. In this case an EAT criticized the employer for failing to make it clear to the employee that the purpose of requiring her to be examined by their medical adviser and in seeking a medical report related to her sickness absence and not her claim for personal injuries: 'The Company did not explain to the Applicant why they wanted this examination or that it was usual practice for this consultant to carry out full medical examination on any employee referred to him. The Tribunal found that she believed that she was examined because of the claim that she was making against the company for the injury to her back. . .'

This case was further complicated because Ms Mills went on to make serious allegations of impropriety against the consultant who had examined her. These were dismissed as false when the consultant denied absolutely her allegations. The Company then dismissed Ms Mills for making false allegations against the consultant.

The dismissal was held to have been unfair because of the defects in the disciplinary procedure. These were that following her initial appeal against dismissal on grounds of ill health and after she had made the allegations of misconduct against the consultant, she was only then informed that she was being dismissed summarily for making 'scandalous and malicious allegations against a senior medical practitioner'.

14 *Discipline at work.* Advisory Conciliation and Arbitration Service advisory handbook. London: ACAS, 1987.
15 Advice from the British Medical Association, 1988 and 26 June 1989.
16 *Ford Motor Company Ltd* v. *Nawaz* [1987] IRLR 163.
17 *East Lindsey District Council* v. *Daubney* (1977), IRLR 181; *Spencer* v. *Paragon Wallpapers Ltd* (1976), IRLR 373; *Williamson* v. *Alcan Foils* (unreported).
18 *Eclipse Blinds Ltd* v. *Wright* (1992), IRLR 133.
19 *P* v. *Nottinghamshire County Council* (1992), IRLR 362.
20 *Scally* v. *Southern Health and Social Services Board* (1991) IRLR 522.
21 *Mihlenstedt* v. *Barclays Bank International* (1989) IRLR 522.
22 *Kapfunde* v. *Abbey National plc and Daniel* (1998) IRLR 583.
23 *Baker* v. *Kaye* (1997) IRLR 219.
24 *X* v. *European Commission* (1995) IRLR 320.
25 Management of Health and Safety at Work (Amendment) Regulations 1994 (SI 1994 No 2865) and Suspension from Work (on Maternity Grounds) Order 1994 (SI 1994 No 2930).
26 *United Kingdom of Great Britain and Northern Ireland* v. *Council of the European Union*, Case C - 84/94 [1997] IRLR 30.
27 The Management of Health and Safety at Work Regulations 1992; Health and Safety (Display Screen Equipment) Regulations 1992; Personal Protective Equipment at Work Regulations 1992; Provision and Use of Work Equipment regulations 1992; Manual Handling Operations Regulations 1992; Workplace (Health, Safety and Welfare) Regulations 1992.

3

The Disability Discrimination Act 1995

G. S. Howard and R. A. F. Cox

The law

There are some 6.5 million disabled people in the UK and 10–15% of the working population are disabled. The passing of the Disability Discrimination Act 1995 (DDA)[1] was a milestone for disabled people who for many years had lobbied for legislation to root out and destroy stereotyped ideas about disabled people and to stop unlawful discrimination in areas such as employment, the provision of goods and services, and education and transport. Nevertheless those lobbying for the disabled were still not entirely satisfied with the new Act, which removes the quota scheme from employers as well as any requirement to register as a disabled person.

One amendment to the Act has already been implemented (since 1 December 1998). Exclusion from the Act of small employers was changed to those employers with fewer than 15 employees (instead of fewer than 20 employees). A Disability Rights Commission has been set up under the Disability Rights Commission Act. This became law in 1999 and the Commission opened for business in April 2000.

Some misconceptions

There are two common misconceptions about disability.

The 'medical model'

The medical model encapsulates the myths that being disabled means not being able to work, and that disabled people are ill and 'suffer' from a medical condition which may be cured or ameliorated by medication or treatment. Neither is true.

The 'tragedy model'

Some able-bodied individuals believe that being disabled is a tragedy and that the best way of dealing with disabilities is to leave disabled people in the care of others, such as charitable organizations. There is also a belief in some quarters that disabled people can play no role in a society or workplace of able-bodied people and should therefore be kept quite separate. This is extended to the view that the able-bodied can discharge their responsibility to the disabled by making financial contributions to the caring organizations set up to look after the disabled.

The 'social model'

The social model assumes that disabled people only become so because of the barriers erected by society. For example, a lawyer who happens to be a tetraplegic is not disabled from working *per se*. However, if his employer provides no wheelchair access or specially adapted equipment, that individual will effectively be disabled at work but through no fault of his own.

History of the DDA

The first official UK recommendation for legislation to give disabled people rights against discrimination was made by the Committee on Restrictions against Disabled People (CORAD) in 1982. This Committee was chaired by Alf Morris, MP.

Numerous attempts to introduce private members' bills followed. The Government responded to these unsuccessful private members' bills by introducing the Disability Discrimination Bill after the publication in 1995 of a White Paper.[2] Over 1000 representations were made in response to the White Paper, but the Bill rejected some of these ideas.

In 1998 the Council of Europe passed a resolution to promote a Code of Practice for the recruitment of disabled people (OJC 12 13.1.1997).

The Act and its Regulations

The Act is drafted so as to leave many of the provisions to be 'interpreted' by Regulations, Guidance Notes, and Codes of Practice. The employment provisions of the DDA came into force on 2 December 1997 and the Code of Practice[3] and Guidance Notes[4] were published in November 1996. Two sets of Regulations—the Meaning of Disability Regulations 1996 and the Disability Discrimination (Employment) Regulations 1996[5]— also came into force in 1996.

Summary of the Act

In order to qualify for protection under the DDA, a person must have, or have had in the past, a physical or mental impairment causing a substantial and long-term adverse effect on their ability to carry out 'normal day to day activities'. An impairment will only affect normal day to day activities if it affects one or more of the following:

* mobility
* manual dexterity
* physical co-ordination
* continence

- the ability to lift, carry, or otherwise move everyday objects
- hearing, speech, or corrected eyesight
- memory or ability to concentrate, learn or understand
- perception of risk of physical danger.

'Long-term' is defined (Schedule 2 (1) (2)) as:

- lasting, or likely to last, for 12 months or more or
- for the rest of the affected person's lifetime
- or likely to recur if in remission.

The Act makes it unlawful for employers to treat a person less favourably for a reason related to the person's present or past disability than they treat (or would treat) a person to whom that reason does not (or would not) apply. However, an employer may be able to defend a complaint of discrimination, even if the disabled person is treated less favourably for reasons relating to disability, if the employer can show that no reasonable adjustments could be made and that the treatment was justified for a reason which is both material to the circumstances of the case and substantial.

Where any arrangement made by an employer, or any physical feature of an employer's premises put a disabled person at a substantial disadvantage in comparison with an able-bodied person, then the employer is under an obligation to make reasonable adjustments to prevent that disadvantage arising. An unjustified failure to meet this duty amounts to unlawful discrimination.

Provision is also made in the Act to enable employers who lease their property to obtain the landlord's permission to make alterations, in order to comply with their duty to make reasonable adjustments.[6]

Discrimination against a disabled worker by other employees acting in the course of their employment will render employers vicariously liable unless they can show that they took all reasonably practicable steps to prevent the discrimination occurring.[7]

Enforcement of the Act requires an individual to bring a complaint to an industrial tribunal.

Unlike other antidiscriminatory legislation, the DDA was not originally supported by a statutory enforcement agency like the Equal Opportunities Commission (EOC) or the Commission for Racial Equality (CRE). However, a new Disability Rights Commission was set up in April 2000 which will remedy this omission.

Meaning of disability

The Act defines a 'disability' as having a 'substantial and long-term adverse effect on that person's ability to carry out normal day to day activities'. **The definition does not include a person's ability to work unless the disability also affects 'normal day to day activities'.**

In an important case concerning disability discrimination (*Goodwin* v. *The Patent Office*, 1999—IRLR 4), the Employment Appeal Tribunal (EAT) gave guidance on how tribunals should interpret a normal day to day activity and how, in general, tribunals should approach disability discrimination cases and what questions they should address. In this case the EAT ruled that, although Mr. Goodwin was able to cope with ordinary, everyday activities at home, he was still disabled within the meaning of the Act because he was unable to hold a normal conversation and he had hallucinations and paranoid delusions which impaired his ability to concentrate, learn and understand (Sched.1. Para.4(g)) and may have impaired his perception of the risk of physical danger (Sched.1. Para.4(h)). (See also p. 52.)

The EAT held that:

The words of Section 1 required a tribunal to look at the evidence by reference to four different conditions:

(1) impairment,

(2) adverse effect,

(3) substantiality and

(4) long-term effect.

Tribunals might find it helpful to address each, while being aware of the risk of taking their eye off the whole picture.

The EAT made a number of recommendations as to how tribunals should deal with this type of case and referred to the definition of disability issued by the Secretary of State on 25 July 1996 in the Code of Practice[3]. Tribunals are now required to refer explicitly to any relevant provision of the guidance or code taken into account in arriving at a decision.

The loss of a little finger in a professional violinist would seriously impair their work, but it would not be a disability within the meaning of the Act because it would not substantially impair their ability to carry out 'normal day to day activities'. The guidance on matters to be taken into account in determining questions relating to the definition of disability, which accompanies the Act, unhelpfully defines the word 'substantial' in this context as 'more than minor'. Numerous examples of adverse effects on the conduct of normal day to day activities are provided in the Guidance Notes, which are recommended reading.[4]

Terminal illness and recurrent illness

The definition of disability also encompasses those with terminal illnesses who are not expected to recover within the next 12 months and those with serious physical or mental disabilities who may become asymptomatic for part of the time but whose symptoms are likely to recur. Such periods of remission will form part of the requisite 12 month period.

Severe disfigurement

The definition also includes people with 'severe disfigurements' such as facial scars or burns. The Code of Practice suggests that in deciding whether a severe disfigurement ought to be regarded as a disability, account should be taken of its location (e.g. whether it is on the back or on the face).

Exceptions

The Act excludes from the scope of 'severe disfigurements' deliberately acquired disfigurements. The Meaning of Disability Regulations exclude people with tattoos which have not been removed and piercings of the body for decorative or non-medical purposes, including any objects which may be attached through such piercings.

Perceived disability

One Minister's view was that the Act would apply 'only once symptoms have appeared'. This is not, however, made explicit in the Act. There appears to be confusion between the symptoms and clinical signs of a condition which has not yet produced any impairment (and may never do so), and asymptomatic carriers of conditions such as HIV or Huntington's chorea who will inevitably become impaired in due course. However, the Government has stated that people who are perceived to have a disability but who have no symptoms will not be protected by the Act. This means, for example, that a person with mild cerebral palsy or a diagnostically confirmed but latent neurological condition or someone genetically destined to develop Huntington's chorea or a person infected with HIV will not be protected until the condition causes an impairment of normal day to day activities.

If this interpretation of the statute is applied by employment tribunals, the Act will not afford protection, for example, to HIV-infected but asymptomatic workers who may be subject to emotional harassment by colleagues at work.

Unlawful discrimination

It will be unlawful for employers to discriminate at recruitment, during employment or to dismiss a disabled person (Section 5(1) of the Act):

(1) (a) for a reason which relates to the person's disability, if he treats him less favourably than he treats (or would treat) others to whom that reason does not (or would not) apply; and

    (b) he cannot show that the treatment in question is justified.

The first element of the definition clearly requires that the disability should be a factor in the employer's decision. The reason for an alleged discrimination must be related to a person's disability, so if an employer treats disabled and able-bodied alike, there can be no 'reason relating to the person's disability.'

In order to establish a case against an employer, the reason for the less favourable treatment has only to relate to the disability in a wide term, thus avoiding the problem of causation that arises under the sex discrimination and race relations legislation.

Able-bodied comparator not required

Unlike the Sex Discrimination Act 1975 and Race Relations Act 1976, a like for like comparison of the treatment of disabled people and of others in similar circumstances is not required under the DDA.

The test under the DDA is based on the reasons for the treatment of the disabled person and not on the fact of their disability (*Clark* v. *Novacold*, [1999] IRLR 318). Darren Clark's absence from work was due to a disability, i.e. a chronic back complaint following an accident at work. The fact of and the length of his absence was taken into account as part of the criteria for his selection for redundancy. Since he would not be resuming work for some time, his employers selected him for redundancy.

The employment tribunal and EAT concluded that no discrimination had occurred because someone who was not disabled, with the same or a similar record of absence, would also have been dismissed. Mr. Clark argued that this conclusion was wrong. The Court of Appeal overruled both the lower tribunals and ruled that the only comparison required by a disabled person complaining of disability discrimination was with someone to whom the reason for the treatment did not or would not apply.

Mr Clark's treatment was his dismissal. The reason for it was that he was unable to perform the main functions of his job because of his disability. The correct comparator was therefore a person able to perform those functions, and such a person would not have been dismissed.

However the Court of Appeal also ruled that the employer's actions in dismissing Mr Clark did not automatically mean that Mr Clark had been discriminated against. The employer had a right to show that the dismissal was justified. Finally, the Court of Appeal ruled that the lower tribunals had ignored the recommendations of the Code of Practice and the case was remitted to a fresh tribunal for the determination of these questions.

The word 'relates' would also enable a complainant to challenge policies that give rise to indirect discrimination. For example, a rule that an employer will not employ anyone who needs time off for medical treatment or rehabilitation would constitute unlawful discrimination and the employer would be required to justify such a requirement or condition.[8]

Additional duty on employer

The Act (Section 5(2)) states that an employer also discriminates against a disabled person if:

(a) he fails to comply with a Section 6 duty (the duty to make reasonable adjustments) imposed on him in relation to the disabled person; and

(b) he cannot show his failure to comply with that duty is justified.[9]

In two cases (*Morse* v. *Wiltshire County Council* [1998] IRLR 352, *Ridout* v. *TC Group* [1998] IRLR 628) the Appellate Tribunal gave guidance on the duty to make reasonable adjustments. In Morse's case, the EAT ruled that the tribunal should go through a number of sequential steps:

1 The words in section 6(2) (b) 'any ... arrangements on which employment is afforded' were wide enough to cover arrangements in relation to whether employment continued or was terminated.

2 Tribunals are entitled to take a purposive view of section 6 and to bear in mind that the protective value of obliging an employer to investigate reasonable alternatives is particularly intended in cases where the vulnerable disabled are threatened with dismissal through redundancy.

3 Sections 5(2) (employers discriminate if they fail to comply with the section 6 duty to make reasonable adjustments to the workplace) and section 6 required the tribunal to go through a series of sequential steps.

4   The tribunal must first decide whether there is a duty under section 6(1) and that the individual has been placed at a substantial disadvantage in comparison to an able-bodied person; if so it also has to decide if the employer exercised their duty to make reasonable adjustments to the workplace.

5   If such a duty is imposed the tribunal must then decide whether the employer has taken such steps, as were reasonably practicable in all the circumstances of the case for them to take, in order to prevent the arrangements or physical features of the workplace having the effect of placing the disabled person at a substantial disadvantage in comparison with people who were not disabled.

6   That in turn involves the tribunal inquiring whether the employer could have taken any steps that were reasonable and practicable to eliminate the disadvantage faced by the person with the disability.

7   At the same time, the tribunal must have regard to factors such as effectiveness of the adjustments, financial factors, and the practicability of taking such steps.

8   If, but only if, the tribunal finds that the employers have failed to comply with their section 6 duty in respect of the disabled appellant, does the tribunal finally have to decide whether the employer has shown that their failure to comply with their duty to make reasonable adjustments was justified. To be justified the reason for the failure to comply must be material to the circumstances of the particular case and substantial.

9   In taking these steps the tribunal must apply an objective test.

10   In progressing through these steps the tribunal should pay considerable attention to the factors the employer has considered or failed to consider. It must always scrutinize the explanation for selection for redundancy put forward by the employer, but it has to reach its own decision on what, if any, steps were reasonable and what was objectively justified, material and substantial.

Employer's ignorance of the disability—a common sense approach

Section 6(6) makes it clear that an employer has a duty to make reasonable adjustments only when they know, or could reasonably be expected to know, about the disability. This includes both actual and constructive knowledge. In most cases, this will be a matter of fact to be determined by the employment tribunal. Did the employer have enough information about the fact of and the details of the disability, and should they have realized from that knowledge that a duty to make reasonable adjustments existed? Often this will depend on the size of the employing organization and the expertise of the staff that it employs. Small employers are less likely to be expected to have a high standard of constructive knowledge.

The knowledge that occupational health staff may have about the fact of and nature of an employee's disability is often also the key to this question. The Code of Practice provides an example of how a physician should approach the sensitive matter of disclosure to the employer of an employee's disability (Box 3.1).

Box 3.1—Disclosure of a disability to an employer

In a large company, an occupational health officer is engaged by the employer to provide them with information about their employees' health.

- The officer becomes aware of an employee's disability, which the employee's line manager does not know about.
- The employer's working arrangements put the employee at a substantial disadvantage because of the effects of the disability, and the employee claims that a reasonable adjustment should have been made.
- It will not be a defence for an employer to claim that they did not know of the employeee's disability. This is because the information gained by the medical officer on the employer's behalf is imputed to the employer.
- Even if the employee does not want their line manager to know that they have a disability, the occupational health officer's knowledge means that the employer's duty under the Act applies.
- It might even be necessary for the line manager to make the reasonable adjustments without knowing precisely why they have to do so.

(Taken from Para 4.62 of the Code of Practice)[3]

In *Ridout* v. *TC Group* [1998] IRLR 628, the EAT took a pragmatic approach to the question of how much an employer should be expected to find out about a disability and how much it would be realistic to expect a job applicant to disclose before attending an interview. In this case, Ms Ridout had disclosed on her CV that she had 'photosensitive epilepsy controlled with Epilim'. She also reported this in a confidential medical questionnaire. She was interviewed for a post advertised in a national newspaper. The room in which she was interviewed had bright fluorescent lighting without diffusers or baffles. Ms Ridout wore sunglasses round her neck, and as she entered the room made the comment that she might be disadvantaged because of the lighting. It was thought she was referring to her sunglasses which in the event she did not wear. Ms Ridout did not tell the respondent that she felt unwell or was actually disadvantaged. The employer was held not to have discriminated against her when no adjustment was made to the lighting.

The tribunal ruled that

she should have been much more forthcoming with the respondent about what she regarded as being required ... A tribunal is required to measure the extent of the duty, if any, against the actual or assumed knowledge of the employer both as to the disability and its likelihood of causing a substantial disadvantage in comparison with people who are not disabled.

Tribunals should be careful not to impose on disabled people a duty to give a long and detailed explanation as to the effects of their disability merely to cause the employer to make adjustments which it probably should have made in the first place. On the other hand, it is equally undesirable that an employer should be required to ask a number of questions as to whether a person with a disability feels disadvantaged merely to protect themselves from liability.

... The Code will help [tribunals] in resolving questions at issue since the Code sets out the standards to be expected in relatively straightforward language.

Another case (*O'Neill* v. *Symm & Co Ltd* [1998] IRLR 233) illustrated the distinction which tribunals draw between general knowledge of symptoms (which could have many causes) and specific knowledge about a particular disability. In this case, the EAT upheld an earlier finding that there had been no discrimination in the dismissal of an accounts clerk following several episodes of sickness absence for 'viral illness'. She was diagnosed as having 'ME/Chronic Fatigue Syndrome' very shortly before her dismissal. At the tribunal, there was dispute concerning whether the employer had received her Medical Certificate before she was dismissed. The employers denied ever receiving it. The tribunal ruled that the employer knew of her symptoms as a matter of fact even though they did not know what caused them.

"What is material to discrimination on the grounds of disability is the disability and not merely one or other equivocal symptom . . ."

Examples of more subtle discrimination

An example of more subtle, 'institutionalized' discrimination would be a blanket requirement to hold a current, full UK driving licence, whether or not a driving licence was essential for a particular job. This would clearly discriminate against some people with some physical or mental disabilities.

Employers must ensure that only essential requirements are imposed as critical at recruitment. Standard contracts with ill-considered clauses on mobility and requirements for a driving licence render them vulnerable to charges of discrimination.

Practical example

Consider an example of how the Act might apply in practice. A competent secretary who has suffered from rheumatoid arthritis for 15 years applies for a job. She cannot type at a normal speed but she can type with the help of an arm rest and with repeated and constant breaks from the keyboard, although her typing speed is slower than that of an average secretary. Will it be unlawful to refuse to employ this candidate because of her arthritis? It appears so, if she would have been suitable save for her disability.[3] Would it be unlawful to refuse to employ her because she could not type at the normal speed? Again, yes—unless the employer could justify, as an absolute necessity, that this particular job required normal typing speed and that no reasonable modifications could be made to the job, such as sharing some of the duties. This secretary would fall into the definition of someone who was physically disabled, and if she were rejected because she could not type at normal speed, then this would fall within the definition of discrimination under section 5(1) of the Act, namely a reason relating to her disability.

It would not matter for the purposes of the Act if a secretary were recruited who suffered from another disability, say depressive illness, which did not affect her typing speed but did affect her moods and her attendance record. Neither would it matter that all able-bodied recruits who could not type at the normal speed were also rejected for the job. The reason for refusing to employ this particular woman would have related to her disability.

Duty to make reasonable adjustments

One of the central duties on employers under the Act (Section 6(1)) is to make 'reasonable adjustment to the workplace', if the disabled person would be 'at a substantial disadvantage in comparison with persons who are not disabled'[10].

The Act lists examples of the kinds of adjustments that employers might be expected to make, including:

- adjustments to their premises
- allocating some of the duties to able-bodied employees
- transferring the disabled person to another vacancy
- altering the employee's working hours
- assigning the employee to a different workplace
- allowing the employee time off during work for rehabilitation, treatment, or assessment
- giving the employee training, or acquiring or modifying equipment (e.g. a simple device on a telephone for someone who has impaired hearing would suffice if that was all that was needed).

In the example of the typist with rheumatoid arthritis, the applicant could show that she would be at a 'substantial disadvantage' compared with workers who are not disabled. To avoid discrimination it would be necessary to make reasonable adjustments to the workplace[11], such as allocating some of the typing duties to others so that the typing duties were reduced and, perhaps, making this employee responsible for more non-typing duties such as making travel arrangements, keeping the diary, preparing expense claims etc.; or even offering an adapted keyboard if this would overcome the problem. Moving the individual to another vacancy where there is less typing is another adjustment that would avoid potential discrimination.

In other cases more sophisticated adjustments may be necessary, such as providing a voice-operated wordprocessor, modifying manuals and instructions, providing readers or interpreters, providing extra supervision, and so on.

The employer may argue that it is not reasonably practicable to do any of these things. The tribunals will weigh which measures are actually practicable, and whether they would help to overcome the difficulty faced by the disabled person. The cost and disruption to the employer, and the availability of resources and financial assistance, would be taken into account. In one case[12] the EAT confirmed that it was not necessary for an employer to provide a personal carer "to cater for a disabled person's needs in the toilet....."

Employers are not allowed to plead ignorance about external sources of finance and support: they have an obligation to find out about access to agencies and resources for the disabled.

Employer's defence

If no reasonable adjustment can be made, and, as a result, a disabled person receives less favourable treatment, this can be justified but only if the reason for it is both material to the circumstances of the particular case and substantial'. Under equal pay case law, the word 'material' has been held to mean 'significant and relevant'.[13]

Definition of mental impairment

A mental impairment is defined in the Act as a mental illness that is 'clinically well-recognized'.[14] Any mental illness within the Diagnostic and Statistical Manual of Mental Disorders (DSM) and International Classification of Diseases (ICD) would probably be accepted by the industrial tribunals, as these definitions are applied and accepted by courts (e.g. in personal injury cases). When the Bill was in preparation, examples of mental impairment that were given included schizophrenia, manic depression, severe and extended depressive psychoses and 'a range of other conditions well-recognized by clinicians, psychiatrists and psychologists'. The minister indicated that moods or mild eccentricities would not be covered by the Act.[15]

Because of its potential relevance to the DDA, the scope of the definition of 'mental impairment' is especially sensitive. The Meaning of Disability Regulations 1996 (SI 1996/1455) exclude the following conditions even though they are recognized antisocial and psychopathic disorders: a tendency to set fires, a tendency to steal, a tendency to physical or sexual abuse of other people, exhibitionism and voyeurism. Under the Regulations addictions to alcohol, nicotine, drugs or solvents cannot be treated as 'impairments'. However, any addiction which was originally the result of the administration of medically prescribed drugs or other medical treatment will be covered by the Act.

Conditions that may fall within the Act's scope

At any given time there are a number of physical and mental complaints whose clinical basis is not strictly proven or defined. Often such cases arise when emerging conditions engender controversy and a genuine dispute within the medical profession. Sometimes these are regarded as falling within the definition of mental illness. The tribunals have accepted that 'ME' or chronic fatigue syndrome is a mental impairment in the Act, and this condition is now recognized in the ICD and DSM classifications.[14]

Obesity is another example of a condition which may or may not fall within the definition of a physical or mental impairment, though a cautious employer may deem it wise to give a wide meaning to the word 'impairment' and treat conditions such as obesity as falling within the Act.

Other difficult cases

Another example would be the case of someone suffering from schizophrenia, who can do their job perfectly well as long as they take their medication but cause mayhem when they fail to have their monthly injection. Such an employee is definitely disabled within the meaning of the Act, but what adjustments would be reasonable for an employer to make in order to accommodate their occasional lapses in obtaining their regular medication? Perhaps it would be reasonable to make it a term of continued employment that they self-refer every month to the occupational physician or nurse to be given their injection?

The definition of illness encompasses conditions in remission which may recur with lapses of treatment. In Goodwin's case (see above), Mr Goodwin suffered from paranoid schizophrenia. The evidence was that at times he was able to hold down his job as a patent examiner. He lived on his own, did his own shopping and cooking, and saw to his own personal hygiene. However, when he omitted his medication he was unable to hold a normal conversation, imagined that other people could access his thoughts, suffered from auditory hallucinations which caused him to leave the office, and had paranoid thoughts about his work colleagues. The EAT held that this evidence was sufficient to establish that he had a recognized mental illness under the terms of the DDA.

What the Act does not cover

To reiterate a point made earlier, the disability must have an adverse and long-term effect on one of the listed day to day activities (set out in Schedule 1 paragraph 4 of the Act).

The Guidance Notes give advice on how an employer should judge whether an impairment has a 'substantial' effect on the carrying out of 'normal day to day activities' and give several practical examples of substantial effects.[16] Thus, if a person with dyslexia is either unable to write a cheque without assistance or has considerable difficulty in following a short, written sequence such as a simple recipe or a brief list of domestic tasks, then this could constitute a substantial effect. Merely being unable to remember the name of a familiar person once in a while or not being able to concentrate on a task requiring application over several hours, in themselves, would not be seen as having a substantial effect.

However, the Guidance Notes do state that if two or more conditions which, taken individually, would not be regarded as having a substantial effect where present, then their summated consequences might constitute 'a substantial effect'. Further information is provided in the appendix to this chapter.

Effects of medical treatment

Disabled people are still protected against discrimination even if they have successfully controlled or corrected their disability by medication or the use of a prosthesis or other aid. People wearing hearing aids are covered by the Act.[17] (Sched.1. Para.6). Epilepsy corrected by medication or diabetes controlled by insulin are other examples, and the Act would appear to cover people disabled by osteoarthritis of the hip, even when they no longer have any impairment following the successful insertion of a prosthesis.

Exclusion for corrected sight

People whose sight impairments are correctable by spectacles or contact lenses are not protected by the Act. According to the Government 'People who wear spectacles or contact lenses would not generally think of themselves as disabled'. The word 'correctable' implies that those who choose not to wear spectacles or contact lenses and whose sight is consequently impaired will not enjoy the protection of the Act.

What should the employer ask?

Should an employer quiz job candidates or employees returning from sick leave to determine if they have a substantial, long-term disability? If such enquiries are relevant to the job it is entirely appropriate for them to be raised, but the Government's advice is not entirely clear.

The Code of Practice recommends the following:

It will be necessary for employers to consider carefully whether and in what circumstances they may need to ask for information about disabilities and if they do the use they will make of it. Employers should avoid asking about disabilities unless there are sound reasons for needing to know. It should be clearly indicated on application forms that any such information will be treated as confidential. The effects of a disability might be an important factor in deciding how you treat a disabled person and what adjustments ought to be made. However, in asking questions about disability, you should not treat a disabled person less favourably than others without justification.

Dangers of not asking

The employer may subsequently be deemed not to have taken reasonable steps to ascertain whether an employee had a disability within the meaning of the Act.

Dangers of asking

The potential danger of employers asking such questions would be to give to the dissatisfied job applicant or dismissed employee *prima facie* evidence against the employer that the disability, or a reason relating to it, may have been the reason for the non-engagement or the dismissal.

If the job candidate or employee does declare the disability voluntarily, then some employers may seek to marginalize them either into lower graded, less well-paid jobs or may find some other reason not to employ them.

It is also possible that some employers may attempt to look for a 'medical' excuse for refusing to recruit or for dismissing, particularly where there has been a history of 'nervous breakdown' or stress-related illness.

'Warning' on application forms

It might be wise to include a statement on application forms, so that the tribunals may see that the employer has made clear the reason for asking about disabilities. It could read in the following terms:

This organization is committed to its policy of equal opportunities and in particular its duties under the Disability Discrimination Act. This organization seeks to offer employment opportunities irrespective of physical or mental disabilities wherever possible, as long as they do not compromise your health and safety or the health and safety of other workers, contractors or members of the public.

These questions are asked in order to assist any person with a physical or mental disability in order to accommodate their needs.

The answers to any questions on disability will not be used in any way adversely to affect or discriminate against any job candidate in any employment decisions that will be made about you, either now or in the future.

The information contained on this form will be kept strictly confidential within the personnel/occupational health department and will not be used or disclosed to any other people without the written consent of the person to whom the information relates.

Using the appropriate experts

Because the need to establish a medical condition rests with the applicant in disability cases, the evidential burden is very similar to personal injury claims. This means that both parties will wish in many cases to have expert witness evidence.

Unfortunately the tribunals have no power to order an applicant to submit to a medical examination and to stay the proceedings if the applicant refuses. This matter will need to be addressed in the future in order to give those powers to tribunal chairmen.

Taking dyslexia as an example, tribunals would need to address the following matters with the help of expert witnesses:

• Has the Applicant established that they have dyslexia?
• If yes, does the condition have a substantial effect on the carrying out of one or more of the normal day to day activities in Schedule 1, para 4?

The fact that dyslexia is a recognized impairment would be confirmed by reference to the ICD or DSM definitions and its presence in the individual should be tested with the WAIS R test administered by a qualified and expert educational psychologist (a new WAIS III test is due to be published, with new UK norms, in the summer of 2000). Whether the dyslexia has a 'substantial' effect on the ability to learn or concentrate or memorize would depend on the results of the WAIS or any other tests administered. **The tribunals have emphasized the need for employers to take expert occupational health advice in disability cases.**

In *Holmes* v. *Whittington & Porter*, the Tribunal held that:

The General Practitioner should not have signed himself 'Company Medical Adviser' as he was neither a specialist in occupational medicine nor . . . a specialist with regard to epilepsy.

The employer admitted to the tribunal that it did not address its mind as to whether (their medical advice) was the best medical advice, as to whether the doctor had any qualifications in occupational medicine or any speciality with regard to epilepsy and did not address its mind as to whether they should have gone further than their doctor's report and take further advice from a medical professional who was a specialist in occupational medicine and someone who was a specialist in that particular disability, in this case epilepsy, and see whether they had the same view as the company's doctor and particularly, whether it was possible for them to make any suggestions about Mr Holmes, about his treatment and about how he should be treated at work or any adjustments that might be made to his working conditions . . .

The employers had come to the decision that no reasonable adjustments could be made for Mr Holmes

but that decision was made without knowing the full picture because it did not have sufficient information on which to make those sorts of decisions in the absence of specialist and the best medical advice. It is not true to say that it is an enormous imposition on the employer, it just means the requirements of this Act are different from what has been required of employers before and that they just have to take more steps so that employees who are disabled persons are protected.

Disability policies and strategies

A dismissal can be fair in cases of disability, if the reason for dismissal is material and substantial and reasonable accommodation is not possible. Avenues that should have been explored include seeking suitable alternative employment, modifying the duties, hours or place of work, etc. Written advice from the occupational physician will be vital. Such documents may be viewed by the dismissed employee under complaint procedures so it is important to ensure that reports are factual and accurate.

Advice from the occupational physician

At recruitment

Although some disabilities are clearly apparent to anyone, such as the person who is blind, on crutches or in a wheelchair, there are many that may be known only to the disabled people themselves.

The status of some conditions under the DDA will often not be apparent without medical advice. Those with disabilities will need the protection of medical confidentiality when it comes to interpreting the disability in functional terms and in advising on the 'reasonable adjustments' which may be needed to accommodate them.

The overall responsibility for compliance with the employment provisions of the Act rests firmly with the employer, but employers will need professional help in many cases in interpreting the definitions and in determining what adjustments are needed. Employers will normally call on occupational physicians to provide expert advice.

At the recruitment stage, the occupational physician should advise an employer on the pitfalls and how to avoid unlawful discrimination. It would, for example, be discriminatory to examine medically those people who claim to be disabled but not those who did not. If a medical examination, questionnaire, or medical review is a part of the recruitment process then it must be applied to all the candidates, or at least to all the short-listed candidates, and not only to those who seem to have disabilities. The assessment should relate to the job in question: an occupational physician who is not familiar with the job should visit the workplace or obtain a detailed job description in order to make a valid and relevant assessment.

When disabilities are revealed in the recruitment process whether by completion of a medical questionnaire or in an examination, the occupational physician will need to evaluate them and to advise the employer whether the disability will affect the person's work capability or work attendance and, if so, what adjustments are required.

The Act requires an employer to accommodate a higher level of sickness absence in a disabled individual, for example. If a disabled candidate is otherwise suitable in terms of competence, experience and qualifications, and **is no threat to the health and safety of themselves or others** (the Act does not oblige an employer to take on a person whose disability may be a hazard to themselves or others in a particular work situation) then an employer would be in contravention of the Act if they rejected the person solely on the basis of a predicted greater sickness absence.

A possible exception might arise in jobs whose nature required full availability for work at all relevant times (e.g. emergency rescue team members).

In order to give appropriate advice on necessary adjustments, the occupational physician should have an intimate knowledge of the job and its requirements for which the applicant is being recruited and a broad knowledge of the company. The occupational physician is also uniquely placed to determine whether the applicant's disability is compatible with considerations of health and safety.

It is entirely justified to deny employment where a disability may compromise the health and safety of the applicant or third parties where no reasonable adjustments can be made.

In summary, the occupational physician will need to address three questions:

- Does the individual have a disability within the definition of the Act, i.e. a physical or mental impairment which has a substantial and long-term adverse effect on normal day to day activities?
- Is the person fit for the particular employment, i.e. can they fulfil the job requirement without risk to their own health or safety or that of others?
- Are any adjustments needed in the workplace to accommodate the individual's disability?

During employment

There will be occasions when, in order to avoid inadvertent discrimination, management will need to know whether a current employee has a disability within the meaning of the Act. The occupational physician's expertise will be called on in those circumstances and they may need to examine the employee or obtain medical information from other sources such as the employee's general practitioner. **In conveying an opinion to managers, the doctor must observe the normal rules regarding confidentiality and informed consent.**

Confidentiality

At times the occupational physician may be in an ethical dilemma. For example, a disabled person may reasonably refuse to allow the occupational physician to reveal information about their disability to the employer. However, employers are deemed to know what their agents know, and so knowledge of an individual's disability gained by an occupational physician working on behalf of the employer is imputed to the employer. In these circumstances the occupational physician should explain to the disabled person the reasons and benefits of disclosing non-confidential information about the latter's functional ability to the employer. If consent is still refused, careful note of the fact should be recorded in the medical record and a copy given to the individual. If the disability would require adjustments to the workplace, the doctor should inform the employer of that fact alone without revealing the medical diagnosis or the nature of the disability.

A disability need only be disclosed to an employer if it may affect the person's functional performance, or jeopardize health and safety. If, in the occupational physician's opinion, a disability will not affect functional performance and no adjustment is necessary, disclosure to the employer is not needed. Employers may reasonably request to be made aware of any employee who may have a disability within the meaning of the Act so that they can avoid inadvertent discrimination. If that is an employer's policy it should be made plain to all employees or prospective employees so that they can give written, informed consent or withhold permission for disclosure of such information if they wish.

The occupational physician must do everything possible to promote the employment of disabled people and to protect them against discrimination, and should not hesitate to emphasize this. Their role should be that of a scrupulous arbiter, to ensure that the disabled are treated equitably and without discrimination. Their duty is not solely to protect the employer against charges of discrimination, though this will be the natural sequel of an established professional trust between the doctor, employer, and employee.

Justification

It may be entirely justified to treat a disabled person less favourably if the person's disability limits their ability to fulfil the demands of the job effectively, either through physical or mental impairments which affect functional performance or for reasons of health and safety. The occupational physician's assessment will be crucial in these circumstances and they may be required subsequently to justify their opinion in a tribunal. Tribunals that consider cases of alleged discrimination against the disabled are likely to depend heavily on the expert evidence of occupational physicians.

An action may only be brought under the Act if discrimination has occurred. The claimant is most unlikely to bring an action if they have voluntarily chosen to retire on grounds of ill health and such medical retirement has been sanctioned by the doctor advising the pension trustees. If, however, early retirement is proposed on medical grounds by an employer or by a doctor acting on behalf of the employer, then it is essential to ensure that 'reasonable adjustment' has been carefully and rigorously considered and rejected for justified reasons before recommending retirement on grounds of disability. Medical retirement may be discriminatory against a disabled individual unless the reasons for it are substantial and material. The occupational physician will need to establish this before sanctioning retirement to the pension trustees.

In dealing with cases which may be covered under the DDA, occupational physicians must ensure that they have fully investigated and understood the functional implications of an individual's disability. They must also have a full understanding of the job in question so that their advice on adjustment is based on sound information and not speculation. Finally, they must follow the well-defined path of professional ethics at all times while protecting the interest of the disabled individual as their primary responsibility. Occupational physicians should always bear in mind that their actions, advice, and opinions may be the subject of cross-examination in an industrial tribunal at a later date.

Appendix: Definitions

The DDA states that 'an impairment is to be taken to affect the ability of the person concerned to carry out normal day to day activities only if it affects one of the following'.

The Guidance Note expands on the list recorded in the Act by providing definitions as follows.

• **Mobility** covers moving or changing position in a wide sense. Thus account will be taken of the extent to which a person can get around unaided or using an appropriate means of transport, can leave home with or without assistance, walk a short distance, climb stairs, travel in a car or on public transport, sit, stand, bend or reach or get around in an unfamiliar place. An impairment which has a substantial effect on mobility would include an inability to travel a short journey as a passenger in a vehicle; inability to walk other than at a slow pace or with unsteady or jerky movements, and difficulty in going up and down stairs.

- **Manual dexterity** covers ability to use hands and fingers with precision. Account will be taken of ability to pick up and manipulate small objects, write, type, or operate a range of equipment manually. Loss of function in the dominant hand would be expected to have a greater effect than equivalent loss in the non-dominant hand.

  An impairment which has a substantial effect on manual dexterity would be loss of function in one or both hands such that the person cannot use the hand(s); inability to use a knife and fork at the same time; ability to press the buttons on a keyboard or keypad in an ordered way but only much more slowly than is normal for most people.

- **Physical co-ordination** covers balanced and effective interaction of body movement, including hand and eye co-ordination.

  An impairment which has a substantial effect on physical co-ordination would be ability to pour liquid into another vessel only with unusual slowness or concentration; inability to place food into one's own mouth with fork/spoon without unusual concentration or assistance.

  This definition does not cover 'mere clumsiness'.

- **Continence** covers the ability to control urination and/or defecation. Account should be taken of the frequency and extent of loss of control and the age of the person. For example, infrequent loss of control of the bowels or loss of control of the bladder while asleep at least once a month would be regarded as having a substantial effect.

- **Ability to lift, carry, or otherwise move everyday objects**: account should be taken of a person's ability to repeat these functions or, for example, bear weights over a reasonable period of time. Everyday objects might include such items as books, a kettle of water, bags of shopping, briefcase, an overnight bag, a chair, or other piece of light furniture.

  An impairment which has a substantial effect on ability to lift and carry etc. would include ability to pick up an object of moderate weight with one hand but not with the other; inability to carry a loaded tray steadily.

- **Speech, hearing, or eyesight**
  - **Speech**: Account should be taken how far a person is able to speak clearly at normal pace and rhythm and to understand someone speaking normally in their native language. It is necessary to consider any effects on speech patterns or which impede the acquisition or processing of one's native language, for example by someone who has had a stroke.

    An impairment which has a substantial effect on speech if the person is unable to give clear instructions orally to colleagues or providers of a service or is unable to ask specific questions to clarify instructions would be regarded as substantial.
  - **Hearing**: If a person uses a hearing aid or similar device, what needs to be considered is the effect experienced if the person is not using the hearing aid or

device. The level of background noise should be within such a range and of such a type that most people would be able to hear adequately.

An impairment which has a significant effect on hearing where there was an inability to hold a conversation in a noisy place such as on a factory floor or an inability to hear and understand another person speaking clearly over the telephone would be regarded as substantial.

*   **Eyesight**: Schedule 1, paragraph 6 (2) (a) clearly states that where the impairment of a person's sight is 'correctable' by spectacles or contact lenses they will not be deemed to have a physical impairment: **but** a sight impairment which has a substantial effect would be inability to recognize by sight a known person across a moderately-sized room; inability to distinguish colours (i.e. total colour blindness); inability to read ordinary newsprint.
*   **Memory or ability to concentrate, learn or understand:** account should be taken of the person's ability to remember, organize their thoughts, plan a course of action and then execute it, or take in new knowledge. This includes whether the person learns to do things more slowly than others. An impairment which has a substantial effect on memory or ability to concentrate, learn or understand would be persistent inability to remember the names of familiar people such as family or friends; inability to adapt to minor change in work routine.
*   **Perception of the risk of danger:** this includes both the underestimation and overestimation of physical danger, including danger to their well-being. Account should be taken of matters such as whether they are inclined to neglect basic functions such as eating, drinking, sleeping, keeping warm and personal hygiene; reckless behaviour which puts the person at risk; or excessive avoidance behaviour without a good cause.

An impairment which has a substantial effect on perception of the risk of danger would be where there was an inability safely to operate properly maintained machinery or an inability to nourish oneself. Fear of heights, or underestimating dangerous hobbies such as mountaineering would not be regarded as substantial impairment.

The Code of Practice explains that this list is meant to take into account the activities that are normal for most people on a daily or regular basis. It is not intended to include activities which are normal only for a particular person or group of people. The Guidance gives examples which it describes as 'indicators' and not 'tests'. They do not mean that if a person can do an activity listed in the Guidance then they do not experience a substantial effect. The person may be inhibited in other activities and this instead may indicate a substantial effect.

Notes and references

1   *Disability Discrimination Act 1995*. London: The Stationery Office.
2   *Ending discrimination against disabled people*. Command 2729. London: HMSO, 1995.
3   *Disability Discrimination Act 1995*. Code of Practice for the elimination of discrimination in the field of employment against disabled persons or persons who have had a disability. London:The Stationery Office, 1996.
4   *Disability Discrimination Act 1995*. Guidance on matters to be taken into account in determining questions relating to the definition of disability. London: The Stationery Office, 1996.

5 Disability Discrimination (Employment) Regulations 1996. SI No 1456. London: The Stationery Office.

6 The Disability Discrimination (Employment) Regulations 1996 make provision for obtaining the landlord's consent.

7 Disability Discrimination (Meaning of Disability) Regulations: London HMSO 1996.

8 In the case of *Bilka-Kaufhaus* v. *Weber von Hartz* [1986] IRLR 317, the European Court of Justice ruled that if the employer applies a rule, requirement or condition which adversely affects the protected group, the court must find that the means chosen for achieving that objective serve a real need on the part of the undertaking, are appropriate with a view to achieving the objective in question, and are necessary to that end.

9 Mr James Paice, one of the ministers steering the Act through Parliament, stated that the word 'arrangements' in s.4(1) (a) of the Act meant 'the use of standards, criteria, administrative methods, work practices or procedures that adversely affect a disabled person. That applies whether determining who should be employed or dismissed or establishing terms on the basis of which people are employed and their access to opportunities are structured. The broad term 'arrangements' has deliberately been used in both sections 4(1) and 6(1) to cover anything done by or for an employer as part of his recruitment process or in making available opportunities in employment'.

10 Under s.6(3) and 6(4) of the Act examples of reasonable adjustments are given and factors such as how far the step that could be taken would prevent the disadvantage to the disabled person, the internal and external financial resources available and the disruption to others of taking the particular measure, will all be assessed by an industrial tribunal.

11 At p. 9 of the Code of Practice, it states that 'Her typing speed would not in itself be a substantial reason for employing her. Therefore her employer would be unlawfully discriminating against her if on account of her typing speed he did not employ her and provide the adjustment.'

12 *Kenny* v *Hampshire Constabulary* [1999] IRLR 76.

13 Under s.5(3). In *Rainey* v. *Greater Glasgow Health Board* [1987] IRLR 26, the House of Lords held that the word 'material' in an equal pay defence meant 'significant and relevant'.

14 Schedule 1, para 1(1). According to the Minister of State, a mental illness will be regarded as 'clinically well recognised' where a reasonably substantial body of practitioners accepts that a condition exists. 'We do not want to open up the possibility of claims based on obscure conditions unrecognised by reputable clinicians which courts and tribunals would find extremely difficult to assess.'

15 The Joint Report on Chronic Fatigue Syndrome published by the Royal Colleges of Physicians, Psychiatrists and General Practitioners in October 1996 (CR54) makes it clear that its primary cause is not associated with any virus and is not caused by one single agent. It is multifactorial. However, the association between virus infections and psychological disorders is still unknown. Previous personality disorders and psychological distress appear to be more important than common viral infections *per se*, the Report concludes.

16 The term 'substantial' in relation to its adverse effect should take into account the time taken to carry out an activity and the cumulative effects of an impairment—see pp. 4–7 of the Guidance Notes. The words 'adversely affecting ability to carry out normal day-to-day activities' should be interpreted in light of the guidance set out on pp. 10–18 of the Guidance Notes.

17 The Minister announced that: 'At the moment, people wearing hearing aids will be covered by the legislation because hearing aids usually provide only partial correction of a disability. Those people are still usually seen as disabled and should be. But if at some future date, as a result of improved technology, hearing aids become as completely effective as spectacles or contact lenses are today, it might be appropriate to exclude people in that situation from the general definition of disability'.

4

Vocational rehabilitation services

M. Floyd and D. Landymore

This chapter outlines the vocational rehabilitation services currently available in the UK to assist with the rehabilitation, retention, and management of people with disabilities in the workplace. It reviews how vocational rehabilitation services have developed over the 50 years since the Disabled Persons Act 1944, and outlines specific aspects of the current range of services available, including those involved in complying with the Disability Discrimination Act 1995 (DDA).

Historical background

Disabled Persons Act 1944

Vocational rehabilitation services were virtually non-existent in the UK before the Second World War, when the government became increasingly aware of the need for their provision. The Tomlinson Committee was set up in 1941 and its recommendations embodied in the 1944 Disabled Persons Act. This Act has shaped British vocational rehabilitation services during the last 50 years, and no other major legislation was introduced until the Disability Discrimination Act in 1995.

The 1944 Act offered four distinct means for helping disabled people:

- A **quota scheme**, like those adopted in many other European countries, which was very simple in concept; at least 3% of the workforce of employing organizations with more than 20 employees. If organizations failed to comply with the legislation, it was necessary to prosecute and then fine them. Over a period of 50 years only 11 such prosecutions were made and the fines imposed have never been increased from the very low levels set in 1944—just a few hundred pounds.
- **Industrial rehabilitation units** (IRUs) were established in most large cities and by the 1950s there were 27. Each offered a 1 week assessment programme, followed by a rehabilitation programme to be spent in one of a number of workshops. Initially the IRUs were very successful and approximately three-quarters of their clients were successful in finding employment.[1]
- The **resettlement**, or placement services were provided by Disablement Resettlement Officers (DROs), based at the Ministry of Labour's local offices, later known as Job Centres. DROs helped individuals to find job vacancies and to apply for them. They referred clients to the IRUs, determined whether individuals could be registered as disabled, and judged whether they were likely to be capable of working in open employment or needed sheltered work. The government set up an organization,

Remploy, to run a large number of sheltered workshops; like the IRUs, these were found in most cities.

• A few local authorities and large voluntary organizations also set up **sheltered workshops**. Eventually around 15 000 disabled people were employed overall.

Developments in the services, 1950–1980

Initially the quota scheme seems to have been quite successful and the level of compliance by employers was high. Gradually, though, the number of employers achieving the 3% quota declined and, in parallel, the number of disabled people registering as disabled also fell. There was also a steady decline in the proportion of IRU clients securing employment. By the mid 1970s the proportion had dropped below a half. A major evaluation of the IRUs, or Employment Rehabilitation Centres (ERCs), as they were now called, was instituted. The report of this comprehensive evaluation was critical of the ERCs. It pointed out that very few changes had been made in ERC rehabilitation programmes, in spite of major changes both in the range of disabilities their clients had and in the labour market. ERC assessment techniques were also found to be very out of date.

Meanwhile, some more positive developments were put in place to tackle the barriers disabled people faced in the employment situation itself. Over the years a number of special schemes were introduced; help with fares to work; providing advice and financial assistance, with regard to technical aids that enable disabled employees to carry out their job, and with regard to adaptations to premises and equipment; personal reader services for blind and partially sighted employees; a small subsidy to employers for the first few weeks (job introduction scheme, see below).

The Employment Medical Advisory Service (EMAS)

This service was set up under the EMAS Act of 1972. EMAS is part of the regional specialist groups of the Field Operations Directorate of the Health and Safety Executive (HSE) and is based at offices of the HSE throughout the UK. EMAS has about 50 specialist doctors and nurses who advise HSE inspectors, employers, employees, trade unions, and the general public on the occupational health aspects of work and on the development and maintenance of a safe working environment. EMAS has statutory duties under Sections 55 and 56 of the Health and Safety at Work Act and is charged with giving information and advice on health in relation to employment and in regard to training for employment, both to employed persons and to persons seeking or training for employment. Additionally, EMAS provides the medical support to the Employment Services' Disability Services Teams and assists them in the training of their staff and others who are engaged in rehabilitation activities. Finally, EMAS staff investigate cases of ill health and advise employers and employees on maintaining individuals at work and also carry out investigations into accidents, injuries, and occupational diseases.

The HSE produces guidance on all aspects of health and safety at work including advice, in some instances, of health standards for specific jobs. Enquirers can obtain free leaflets from HSE's Infoline or can contact their local office. Telephone numbers are listed in the telephone directory under Health and Safety Executive. It is a legal requirement that the address of the local EMAS office is displayed on Health and Safety at Work posters in all workplaces.

Developments during the 1980s

The serious criticisms of the employment rehabilitation service led to some significant changes in the rehabilitation programmes on offer. The approach to assessment, in particular, was radically altered by the introduction of VALPAR work samples, imported from the US, and of more up-to-date psychometric assessments. Six new centres, known as ASSET centres, were also set up. These centres offered only assessment and were located in areas where access to ERCs was poor. Rehabilitation, which was formerly provided in the artificial environment of a workshop in the ERC, was provided instead by local employers.

These changes represented progress in assessing clients' abilities, although more might have been done in relation to job requirements. In the US a key resource for the vocational guidance and assessment services is an extensive database of occupational information, the *Dictionary of Occupational Titles* (DOT),[2] much of it available in electronic form. This makes it possible to match the functional abilities of the disabled client, as determined using a range of physical and psychological assessments, to the mental and physical requirements of over 20 000 different jobs. In the absence of such information relating to jobs in the UK, the new approach to assessment was inevitably limited in its effectiveness. Furthermore, in the 10 years or so since the changes were brought in, no attempt has been made to address this problem.

Perhaps the most successful of the changes has been the introduction of the **sheltered placement scheme**. The 1944 Act had envisaged the possibility of small groups of more severely disabled people working in an ordinary employing organization, but nonetheless employed by a non-governmental organization (NGO), which received a contribution from the government towards their wages, these being set at a level similar to that of the workshops. This type of provision, sometimes referred to as enclaves or sheltered industrial groups (SIGs), had not proved very successful, and only a few hundred sheltered employment places of this kind existed at the beginning of the 1980s. Eventually a SIG of just one disabled individual was introduced. This came to be known as a sheltered placement. The NGOs employing the disabled people (the sponsoring organization), pay them and receive from the host employing organization (where the individual actually works), an agreed contribution towards wage costs, proportionate to their productivity.

The stronger orientation in the UK towards tackling the barriers disabled people face in the workplace was shown by the Code of Practice for Employers 1993.[3] This publication provided guidance to employers on a wide range of issues relating to disabled people. The Code also provided a valuable reference for the Disability Advisory Service (DAS) teams that were set up at around the same time. These teams took over from the DROs the responsibility for working with employers, advising on technical aids, adaptations, etc. and represented a further strengthening of the emphasis on overcoming barriers in the workplace. Considerable progress was also made towards the range and the amount of training provision that disabled people could access.

More recent developments

In 1990 the Department of Employment published a major review of its services for disabled people.[4] This review was, in part, a response to a fairly critical report produced by the government's National Audit Office.[5]

Soon after the publication of the review, all the ERCs were closed and over 60 Placing, Assessment and Counselling Teams (PACTs) were set up, each serving a population of between half a million and a million people. The PACTs consisted mainly of DROs, now called Disability Employment Advisers (DEAs), but also incorporated some of the staff from the ERCs, together with staff from DAS teams. Each PACT has around 15 staff, most of whom are based at Job Centres (usually more than one) and they are now called Disability Service Teams (DSTs).

Rehabilitation is now done by non-governmental agencies who are contracted by the DSTs to provide a rehabilitation programme similar in length to that offered previously by the ERCs. The rehabilitation providers fall into two fairly distinct categories:

* 'Mainstream' providers provide rehabilitation for disabled people but only as a small part of their activity. Their main function is to provide vocational rehabilitation and /or training for non-disabled people.
* 'Specialist' rehabilitation providers tend to cater solely for disabled people. Information on local rehabilitation providers can be obtained from the local DST.

Working with the Employment Service in each of its seven regions are newly formed Disability Consulting Groups, which arose out of the previous committees for the employment of disabled people (CEDPs). Their remit is to work with DSTs to promote local employment opportunities for disabled people and help create wider awareness among employers of the business benefits of effective disability policies and practices. Membership is made up of local disabled people and employers, between whom the DSTs act as brokers.[6]

The 1990 Department of Employment review also recommended a further shift in sheltered employment provision towards sheltered placements and away from sheltered workshops. At present there are still approximately 14 000 workshop places, but the number of sheltered placements has grown to around 10 000.

The most significant change during the last few years has undoubtedly been the passing of the Disability Discrimination Act 1995 (DDA) (see Chapter 3). The Act is primarily designed to combat discrimination with regard to employment. Unlike the 'Americans with Disabilities Act' (ADA), it does not address to the same extent discrimination experienced by disabled people in accessing education and transport. It does, however:

* give new powers with regard to standards of accessibility to public transport
* amend education legislation with regard to the provision of information.

The major weakness in the DDA, as it stands, was the absence of a body such as the Equal Opportunities or Race Relations Commission to enforce the legislation. The National Disability Council, set up under the Act, had only advisory responsibilities. Under the new Labour government (1997) a Task Force was set up to work out ways in which the Act could be strengthened and made more effective, including a Disability Rights Commission which was established in 1999. The introduction of the DDA highlights the need now for more systematic assessments of fitness for work. One of the roles of the occupational physician is to assist management and human resources staff to establish specific occupational health service policies and procedures to ensure that the Act is complied with.

The Act represents a significant shift in the way in which disability is perceived and addressed by society. Some describe this as a shift from a 'clinical' model to an 'ecological' approach;[7] others as a shift from a 'medical model' of disability to a 'social model' (see p. 43). The different perspectives are best understood in terms of the concepts of impairment, disability, and handicap (see Chapter 1).

Impairment, disability, and handicap*

The terms impairment, disability, and handicap were very clearly defined in a World Health Organization (WHO) report published in 1980. According to the WHO model, the **impairment** experienced by a disabled person refers to the injury or illness that they have. The impairment results in a **disability**, an inability to carry out some function, such as walking, lifting, seeing, etc. This in turn, may result in some kind of **handicap**, that is to say they may be unable to fill some kind of social role. Thus, in the case of someone who loses a limb in an accident, their impairment might be the absence of a leg. This results in an inability to walk—the disability—and this, in turn, may prevent them from doing their previous job, which is an occupational handicap.

The WHO model helps to distinguish two very different, but equally important, kinds of help that can be provided by vocational rehabilitation services. The disabling effect of the impairment can be reduced by various forms of rehabilitation, the provision of an artificial limb for example; or the handicapping effect of the disability can be reduced, or eliminated, by making changes to the working environment, or job, such that not being able to walk is no longer a barrier.

In the past, too much emphasis has been given, by vocational rehabilitation services, to the first kind of help, i.e. reducing the disabling effect of the impairment, and insufficient attention paid to modifying the working environment and overcoming other handicapping barriers that disabled people experience. This has led to the adoption of what is sometimes called the 'social model' of disability by many disabled people and their organizations. In its more extreme form the proponents of the 'social model' argue that the only help disabled people need is the second kind, i.e. the adaptation of the environment and the removal of handicapping barriers that prevent them from doing the things that other people can do. Indeed it is argued that the 'individual' does not have a disability, it is rather that 'society' disables people by not catering for their needs. A balanced view embraces both the 'medical' and the 'social' models, the importance of each obviously varying with the individuals, their impairment and its effects on their work.

In the US there is a much greater awareness of the role of really effective rehabilitation services in implementing their antidiscrimination legislation (ADA). In particular, the importance of ensuring that the staff of rehabilitation centres receive professional training is widely recognized.[8] In the UK both government and the disability organizations have so far failed to address this issue.

Vocational assessment and rehabilitation services

Vocational assessment

Vocational assessment contributes to the whole process of recruitment, prevention of injury in the workplace, and the management of disability. It is the process of determining individual vocational assets, limitations, behaviours, and physical tolerances in a work

---

* See also p. 5.

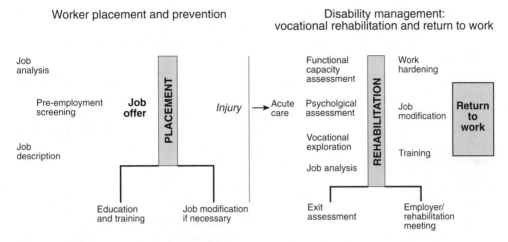

Fig. 4.1 An ideal vocational rehabilitation system.

environment. Career objectives and plans can be formulated as a result of performance in functional capacity assessments, psychometric tests, and vocational exploration. There is no point in assessing an individual's functional ability unless the core requirements and tasks of the job are also analysed and used to match the suitability of the person to the job. Employers have realised that rehabilitating injured workers is more cost-effective than paying long-term disability costs or hiring, training, or transferring other workers to fill the post. The prime objective therefore is to return injured workers to their pre-injury employment status.

Figure 4.1 summarizes an ideal 'seamless' rehabilitation process, where the medical and vocational elements are phased into one another with assessment as a continuous part of these activities. The aims of the rehabilitation process are directed at maximum health gain, the (re)establishment of skills, and job placement or retention in open employment.

In recent years, and particularly in the light of the DDA, there has been a greater focus on the use of standardized practices and procedures for the assessment of employees' abilities to perform in the workplace.

The field of rehabilitation is an area of increasing economic significance in both the private and public sectors. On-site rehabilitation in the management of work-related injury leads to a more intimate awareness of each job, highlighting the risk factors, the worker's capabilities and the psychosocial issues within the workplace. In some cases the client can remain at work during the rehabilitation process and biomechanical and ergonomic advice can be given on site. A planned gradual return of the worker to full duties (graded return to work programme) can be implemented and monitored by the occupational health team.

The benefits of vocational rehabilitation are thus threefold: to enable earlier return to work; to limit disability payments; and to ensure earlier and more fully restored productivity.

According to the former Under Secretary of State for Employment, sections 3(1) and (2) of the DDA are intended to cover:

The use of standards, criteria, administrative methods, work practices or procedures that adversely affect a disabled person. That applies whether determining who should be employed or dismissed or establishing terms on the basis of which people are employed and their access to opportunities are structured. The broad term 'arrangements' had deliberately been used in both section 4(1) and 7(1) to cover anything done by or for an employer as part of his recruitment process or in making available opportunities in employment.'

It is essential for the occupational physician to have objective information on the physical and psychological demands of the jobs within the organization. In a model occupational health service, members of the team should be able to analyse job requirements, identify the risks of work-related injuries, educate on prevention of injury, evaluate employees' capabilities to perform tasks, establish the injured worker's work capabilities, and assist the employee to return to suitable duties.

Job description

The job description is a description of the tasks of the job as outlined by the employer. It should be objective, thorough, and complete and must delineate the requirements of the job. It must be reviewed regularly. It differs from the job analysis[9] (see below) in that it does not include factors that might be measured or assessed, i.e. the physical demand characteristics of the job. The job description must include core medical criteria, any statutory criteria, and essential health and safety requirements (e.g. food industry requirements, or group 2 driving licence).

Job analysis

Under the DDA the employer cannot discriminate against disabled people in recruitment, promotion, training, working conditions, and dismissal. It is essential, therefore, for employers to be fully aware of the requirements and physical demands of each job, before that job is advertised. This can be achieved by ensuring that each individual post has a job analysis, an objective ergonomically based evaluation of the workplace. There are a number of job analysis methods in use which generate this information and assist employers to create functional job descriptions. The job analysis provides a standardized format for identifying and quantifying essential functions of a job and an objective analysis of heavy physical and repetitive tasks such as:[10]

- basic physical demands—strength, endurance, and range of movement (lifting, carrying, pushing, pulling)
- mobility requirements (walking and climbing)
- sensory and perceptual demands (hearing and vision)
- vocational requirements and environmental conditions (exposure to heat, cold, vibrations, etc.)

The job analysis provides a standardized format for identifying and quantifying the core (essential) functions of a job, as well as the non-core (peripheral) functions. It includes the systematic reporting and objective analysis of tasks. Only when one understands the essential or core elements of the job (those tasks that are a fundamental physical demand that the worker must be able to perform unassisted) can one realistically recruit to that post. To do this objectively, overall safe physical capabilities for work-related tasks, such as use of hands, lifting, bending, and special sensory requirements must be determined. This can be achieved by using a standardized and objective assessment tool—a **functional capacity assessment** (see below).

Thereafter, medical examination results may be used to disqualify an applicant only if a medical condition would present an unacceptable risk in respect of the material and substantial duties specified in the job analysis and/or the core medical criteria.

A job analysis helps in the prevention of injury in the workplace by:

- identifying work tasks associated with frequent injuries
- proposing recommendations to modify the job or the way of working i.e. posture, work heights, etc.
- identifying physical demands for pre-employment screening or job rotation.

A job analysis facilitates the return to work of the injured worker by:

- allowing direct comparison of job demands with physical capabilities (ideally as identified in a functional capacity assessment[11])
- identifying critical job demands to establish realistic work conditioning goals
- identifying where the job needs to be modified in order to return to work safely identifying job method/equipment modifications to prevent re-injury

Under the DDA there is a duty on the employer to make reasonable adjustments to working conditions or to the physical working environment if these would help to overcome the practical effects of a disability. A job analysis enables the rehabilitation specialist to suggest changes to work routines or to the workplace to accommodate the person's disability (see p. 71).

In many situations a structured approach to assessment may be required (i.e. in litigation). The development of standardized methods for determining an individual's functional ability has taken place mainly in the US and they are now widely used there, in Australia, Canada, and the Netherlands. The aim of these techniques is to provide objective unbiased and independent evaluation of functional ability.

Functional capacity assessments

A functional capacity assessment (FCA) describes the evaluation of an employee in terms of their capacity to perform the essential duties of the job. Standardized FCAs have been developed which use highly sophisticated apparatus that provides the referrer with high levels of objectivity, validity, reliability, and predictability.[12] The assessments are based on well-researched data and give an unbiased and independent evaluation of an individual's functional ability, not a diagnostic analysis of a specific injury or illness. Task requirements dictate what part of the body is the main focus for the FCA. If a person lifts and carries, then the assessment will concentrate on the whole body; in the case of a receptionist the focus may be more specifically on the upper extremities; and for a heavy machine operator whose job entails moving pedals with the feet and levers with hands while remaining in the sitting position, the focus could be on both the upper and lower extremities.

Assessments which are reliable and valid are essential when measuring functional ability. The tests used should produce measures which exhibit high intra-tester reliability (give similar findings when the same person measures the same thing repeatedly) and a high inter-tester reliability (gives similar findings if different individuals measure the same thing sequentially).[13] An FCA is valid only if its results accurately represent the person's true capabilities to perform job functions.

Dr Leonard Matheson of the Employment and Rehabilitation Institute of California has done considerable work in this area and provides a rationale for the interdisciplinary approach to work functional assessment, defines strength testing protocols and presents a coefficient of variation as part of functional capacity testing.[14,15]

Ideally the FCA is administered by an occupational therapist or other therapist qualified in the method of FCA used. Dynamic assessment of the whole body will measure whether the patient can safely perform various job-related functions. It takes about 4 hours and follows strict protocols to evaluate up to 27 work performance measures including:

- walking/climbing
- standing/sitting
- lifting/carrying
- repetitive hand and foot movements
- squatting/kneeling/crouching
- fine finger movements.

Combined with the analysis of torque patterns, variations in heart rate, pain behaviours and reports, and physiological variables the assessment is able to identify objectively the patient's level of ability and determine whether it is a genuine reflection of their current level.

An increase in the number and severity of complaints such as backache, visual fatigue, stiffness and pain in the hands and arms, headache, depression, and stiffness and pain in the neck and shoulders will result in employees who are off sick regularly and may have to leave the company because of their physical or psychological difficulties.

In these cases the occupational physician will be asked to substantiate a decision in order to protect employees and employers. The FCA is useful in helping the occupational physician to make decisions as to whether the employee can perform the tasks of the job, whether they can return to their own job, or what modifications need to be made to the job or the workplace to enable them to continue working. The FCA defines objectively an individual's 'physical ability' irrespective of subjective issues and helps employers to avoid discrimination in recruitment and employment.

The FCA results can be used for determining:

- if the individual can return to work
- compensation entitlements
- claims/benefits approval
- alternative career options
- modifications to the workplace.

The FCA provides a starting point from which to set achievable goals for rehabilitation, and by using serial FCAs the progress and end point of rehabilitation can be measured.

The FCA can be used to match an individual's physical ability to a job analysis in, for example:

- pre-employment screening
- safe return to work
- alternative job placement.

Occupational physicians should have access to this evidence-based approach to assessment in this country but as yet few UK centres are offering these services, and they are fairly costly per assessment. The greater the demand for these types of services, the more competitive will the rates become. At present a 3–4 hour FCA costs £600–800. The main clients at present are lawyers and insurance companies who are using the assessments for claims management.

Psychological assessment

Assessment by an occupational psychologist can determine the impact of psychological disability on an individual's ability to perform their occupation and can, with an FCA, give a complete picture of an individual's ability to return to work after accident or injury and highlight rehabilitation needs.

A psychological assessment is indicated not only when the individual is away from work for a mental health reason but also where the motivation of the individual to return to work is in question, or where the injury/disability may have a physical and a psychological component i.e. a closed head injury, stroke, chronic fatigue syndrome (CFS), irritable bowel syndrome (IBS), work-related upper limb disorder (WRULD), etc.

Work hardening

Vocational assessments can be augmented by a work hardening programme which simulates dynamic job functions and weights to ensure that the relevant musculoskeletal capabilities are properly developed to meet job demands. This may be done by using work samples or 'on the job'.

In addition there should be an ongoing programme of evaluation and employment counselling for employees who are at risk of developing work-related injuries and for those who are unable to carry out their present job owing to injury or illness.

Reasonable accommodation

The DDA declares that people with disabilities should be treated with equity and that where possible they should be able to remain in, or gain employment. It imposes an obligation on organizations to make reasonable adjustment to facilitate the employment of people with disabilities wherever it is reasonable to do so (DDA Part II Section 6).

One of the objectives of carrying out job analysis and FCA is to determine if an individual is able to carry out the essential elements of their job. Another is to determine what, if any, adjustments need to be made to the job in order that they may carry it out effectively. These may include:

- **Adjustments to premises**: Provision of ergonomically considered work space; ramps; car parking close to the building; dropped kerbs for wheelchairs; steps edged in white or yellow to assist visually impaired people; clearer marking of fragile glass doors; lift control buttons marked and lowered; induction loops; widening of doorways; colour-coded corridors; lowered door handles, light switches, etc.
- **Acquiring or modifying equipment**: Procuring the correct equipment such as voice-controlled computer, chair, armrests, and wheelchair with raiser for each individual (an FCA may highlight areas of difficulty).
- **Provision of support staff, readers and interpreters**
  - few jobs require someone to read/attend meetings all day so part-time readers, sign language support, etc. may be a cost-effective accommodation

- for people with mental health problems consider job coaching, befriending (peer support), flexibility in working practice, providing quiet working space if distractions are a problem, working from home on occasions, flexitime to accommodate medical appointments, phased return to work after time off, keeping job open during sick leave, self-paced workload, etc.
- providing and training a helper.

- **Allocating some of the disabled person's duties to another person**: After a job analysis and an FCA it is possible to identify which aspects of the job the disabled person has difficulty with or cannot do. If these are not essential job functions it may be possible to allocate them to another employee.

- **Altering working hours**: The FCA will indicate how many hours per day the individual can work and when they should take breaks; allowing the employee to come in or leave later so they do not have to travel during the rush hour; working flexitime or split shifts; working from home on occasions; time off for medical treatment appointments which can be made up later.

- **Providing training**
  - the FCA will highlight specific training needs and how to manage the disability effectively
  - providing accessible training sites, advertising training in different ways so that all members of the workforce can see it, i.e. e-mail, notice board, leaflets
  - providing extra assistance to people with learning difficulties
  - work hardening programmes—a graduated programme of work duties to improve concentration, stamina, etc.

- **Modifying procedures for recruitment, testing, or assessment**
  - making application forms user friendly—shorter words, bigger print, etc.
  - demonstrating the job
  - making job descriptions clear and concise
  - adjusting the length of interview to suit the applicant
  - asking the applicant how they would prefer to fill in an application form—verbally, on site, at home, or, if they can't hold a pencil, by other means, (speech, word processor, etc.)
    - if the applicant has hearing problems, conducting the interview in a quiet room (and, if requested, using a professional sign language interpreter).
    - unless you are specifically testing a skill which is job-related try to use a format that does not use the impaired skill; for example, if the applicant is dyslexic conduct an oral rather than a written test.

- **Assigning the applicant to a different workplace**: A vocational exploration programme for those people unable to return to their previous job to help identify alternative occupations for which they are suited. It may include a FCA, psychometric tests to assess the individual's vocational abilities, personal strengths and employment potential, and a supported placement programme.

An example where the employer has adjusted the workplace and the job

An FCA and psychological assessment were conducted on a woman with a work-related upper limb disorder (WRULD). It was found that she could perform most of the duties of the job, but in an 8 hour working day she could not:

- sit for more than 5.5 hours
- reach forward and overhead for more than 3 hours
- handle (i.e. turn pages, photocopy etc.) for more than 5.5 hours
- type for more than 5.5 hours.

The psychological assessment indicated that although she had good problem-solving abilities in relation to work tasks, personality indicators suggested general inflexibility in managing change. She showed high levels of anxiety, associated particularly with anticipated/actual experience of pain. Throughout the period of her incapacity there was a fluctuating and generalized level of depression which had not been in evidence previously and had not been identified in previous examinations.

Recommendations were made regarding job modifications, equipment, workstation alterations, and education to enable her to return to her previous job. It was also recommended that she follow a brief course of cognitive-behavioural therapy and symptom management training.

Her work space was assessed and alterations were made to limit:

- how often she had to reach forward and sideways, by placing the computer monitor on a swivel arm so that she did not have to lean forward to avoid the glare on the screen and did not have to lean sideways to write or use the telephone
- how often she had to reach while bending, by placing objects that were used frequently on a higher level
- how much she used her hands during typing, by installing a voice control system to operate the computer to be used for a part of the day, using a more ergonomically designed keyboard, and using headphones for telephoning
- discomfort when sitting, by using a more ergonomically designed chair and lowering the height of the desk surface.

Her daily duties were modified as follows:

- to limit the amount of sitting she stood every 60 minutes to photocopy, fax, and mail items for herself and her colleagues
- keyboarding in the 'normal' way was restricted to 2.5 hours a day, with a break every 45 minutes; additional keyboard work was carried out using the voice control. Handling was limited to 2.5 hours, with a break every 45 minutes and in the additional time she could work with customers at the reception desk or handle incoming calls, using a head phone only.

Over a period of 3 months she gradually built up her hours to a full 8 hour day under the close supervision of her doctor and her therapist.

- She attended a workshop on management of WRULD to prevent re-injury and optimize her work potential.
- She attended eight sessions of brief integrative psychotherapy.
- She followed a programme of symptom management training including graded return to work, learning coping skills, working with her employer to clarify role responsibilities and to provide realistic goals and to help her manage her time more effectively.
- She attended a pain management course.

She has continued to work full time and has had no return of her symptoms. She has greater awareness of her emotional needs and is learning to manage her time more effectively and productively.

Access to work

The Employment Service's Access to Work programme was introduced in 1994 and brought together, under one programme, a range of pre-existing services. In 1995–96 £19 million was allocated to assist employees (part-time or full-time) and employers with the costs of:

- special equipment or adaptations to existing equipment
- a reader at work for a blind or partially sighted person
- a communicator for deaf people.

Access to Work can also be used to help with the expenditure incurred by an employer in making the work environment more accessible. Included under this heading are:

- alterations to premises
- modifications to the job
- deaf awareness training for co-workers
- a support worker if help is needed either at work or in getting to work
- transport to work if public transport cannot be used because of the individual's disability.

Access to Work will pay for 100% of the costs in the case of a disabled person who was previously unemployed but only 80% in the case of an existing employee. Employers also have to pay the first £300 in such cases, but where costs exceed £10 000, Access to Work may cover 100% of these additional costs.

Access to Work funding is accessed via the DST and can be discussed with the local DEA. The DST team also includes technical consultants who can advise on such matters as special equipment and adaptations to buildings.

Job Introduction Scheme (JIS)

Direct financial assistance to private sector employers is available through the Job Introduction Scheme (JIS). The employer is paid £45 a week for a 'trial period', which is usually of 6 weeks duration. In exceptional circumstances, it may be paid for a longer period, the maximum being 13 weeks. Assistance is available in the case of both part-time and full-time work but the expectation must be that the job is going to last at least 6 months after the trial period ends.

Supported Placement Scheme (SPS)

The Supported Placement Scheme (SPS), previously known as the Sheltered Placement Scheme, has become an increasingly important means for getting more severely disabled people into open employment. There are now approximately 10 000 disabled people employed in such placements. Around 8000 of these are employed by a 'sponsor', usually a local authority or voluntary organization. Budgetary constraints on the size of the

Employment Service grant mean that it seldom covers more than a third of the total wage, even in the case of low-wage occupations. The scheme is therefore of only limited value in the case of very severely disabled people and/or those seeking more skilled and higher wage occupations.

Remploy, which runs most of the sheltered workshops in the UK, also operates a similar scheme called Interwork and employs around 2000 disabled people. To qualify for the SPS scheme, the disabled person must be judged to be between 30% and 70% productive. There are, however, no objective means for assessing 'productivity', so this criterion is fairly meaningless: the main test of eligibility, now that registration has been abolished, is simply whether or not the individual comes within the definition of disability contained in the DDA.

Workplace rehabilitation

A recent comparison of disability support services in a number of European countries observed that

workplace rehabilitation has never been a feature of UK provision. There are no obligations on employers to ensure the retention of employees who become disabled . . . and the notion of disability management at the workplace is only now gaining some limited currency, mainly through the activities of voluntary sector bodies and some large employers.[16]

Good employers will endeavour to re-assign or relocate people who are unable to continue in their own jobs and all employers can obtain detailed help with the provision of all types of assistance from the Employers' Forum on Disability (see Appendix 7 for address).

Vocational training

As in the case of rehabilitation, vocational training provision has tended to be primarily for unemployed, disabled people. Such training is provided under the 'mainstream' Training for Work (TfW) programme which is funded through the Training and Enterprise Councils (TECs).

Just as the Employment Service contracts with rehabilitation providers, so too do the TECs contract with training providers. Again a useful distinction can be drawn between 'mainstream' providers, who cater mainly for non-disabled people, and 'specialist' providers who provide training only for disabled people. TfW training courses usually last for 12 months.

Residential training is also available in residential training colleges. These colleges are able to provide additional support and tend to cater for a particular type of disability. (For example, there are ten colleges which provide training for people with sensory disabilities.)

Voluntary organizations

A great deal of vocational rehabilitation and training services, as well as sheltered employment, is provided by the voluntary sector. The major disability organizations, such as the Royal National Institute for the Blind and SCOPE (previously the Spastics Society), manage several rehabilitation and training centres and offer employment in both workshops and supported placements. There are also a multitude of small, local charitable organizations which are responsible for just one or two centres. Both small and large organizations of this kind are often very innovative in their approach.

The names and locations of such local voluntary providers may be obtained from the local DST, but unfortunately there is no single reference guide to services. A very useful source of information, however, is the Directory for Disabled People.[17]

Disability benefits

State benefit system

Responsibility for administration of claims and payment of state benefits for sick or disabled people rests with the Benefits Agency, an executive agency of the Department of Social Security (DSS). Entitlement to benefit is determined by non-medical staff, who until September 1998 obtained medical advice from DSS doctors in Benefits Agency Medical Services. Since September 1998, the provision of medical advice has been contracted out to a private sector company, SEMA Group. The role of medical services is to give objective advice either on the basis of documentary evidence or, when appropriate, by undertaking medical examination and assessment of claimants on the functional effects of disablement.

The main state benefit for people unable to work as a result of illness or disability is Incapacity Benefit (IB), introduced in 1995 to replace Sickness Benefit and Invalidity Benefit. Short-term IB is payable for the first 28 weeks of incapacity for those people who are unable to claim Statutory Sick Pay (SSP). The basic entitlement condition for short-term IB is incapacity for the person's own occupation. After 28 weeks, the basis for assessing entitlement to IB is the Personal Capability Assessment (PCA), which replaced the All Work Test (AWT) in April 2000. The PCA assesses the extent to which a person, by reason of some specific disability is capable of performing certain everyday tasks as set out in legislation. The threshold for benefit entitlement reflects the point at which the person's ability to perform work-related activities is substantially reduced, rather than the point at which work becomes impossible.

The Welfare Reform and Pensions Act 1999 enables the PCA to provide an additional assessment of a person's residual functional capability, with the intention of providing more help to people with disabilities who are capable of some work. The government's 'New Deal for Disabled People' approach will subsume and widen the scope of the present Employment Service (part of the Department for Education and Employment) in providing personal advice to disabled people to enable them to return to work or to find suitable alternative employment.

Other benefits for people of working age include Industrial Injury Disablement Benefit (IIDB) and Disability Living Allowance (DLA). IIDB is a benefit for people in employment who become disabled as a result of an injury arising out of and during the course of their employment. It can also be claimed by people disabled as a result of contracting certain occupational diseases arising out of work in specified prescribed occupations. In both cases the threshold for benefit is disability amounting to at least 14% (except in the case of certain prescribed respiratory diseases, where benefit may be payable above 1%), assessed with reference to certain scheduled levels of disability which are prescribed in legislation.

DLA is a non-means-tested, non-contributory benefit payable to people of any age up to 65 years, if as a result of illness or disability they require specific levels of help with personal care; or if they have significant restriction of walking ability; or if they require continual supervision to avoid danger to themselves or others.

Many disabled people under 65 years of age are eligible for DLA; for those over 65 years there is a similar benefit known as Attendance Allowance (AA).

If their disability is such that they are deemed to be unable to work they are also entitled to IB or Severe Disablement Allowance (SDA). In order to qualify for the former they must also have paid enough National Insurance contributions whilst previously in work. If they have not they may still be eligible for SDA, but they have to be assessed as at least 80% disabled. The Welfare Reform and Pensions Act 1999 contains proposals to replace SDA with IB for young adults from April 2001.

In order to qualify for either of these the disabled person must also be assessed by the PCA. This was introduced in order to target these benefits more effectively. The PCA is a functional assessment and takes no account of the individual's education, work experience, or the state of the national or local labour market. A score is given, according to their level of disability, for 14 physical and 4 mental activities. If they score at least 15 points on the physical disabilities scale or both physical and mental disabilities scale, or 10 points for mental disabilities only, they are considered to be incapable of any kind of work and therefore entitled to benefit.

In a Green Paper[18] the government acknowledged that the AWT was unsatisfactory and has implemented new legislation (Welfare Reform and Pensions Act 1999) which focuses on what disabled people can do, not on what they cannot'.

Disabled Person's Tax Credit (DPTC)

Most social security benefits for disabled people are targeted on those who are unemployed. In 1992 the Disability Working Allowance (DWA) was introduced which was designed to encourage people who were capable of part-time work, but whose earnings in such work would be less than the benefits they would receive were they to remain unemployed.

The government has recently introduced a new means tested tax credit for people with illness or inability who are in work depending on their circumstances. This is known as the Disabled Person's Tax Credit (DPTC), which has replaced the former Disability Working Allowance (DWA), and is administered by the Inland Revenue. DPTC is for people with an illness or disability who work at least 16 hours a week and have one of a number of qualifying benefits. The government also propose a 'Fast Track' gateway to DPTC to help people who become disabled while working to keep their job.

A 'disability test' is required when someone wishes to renew their entitlement to the benefit. The test assesses 20 areas of 'difficulty'. Difficulty in any of these areas qualifies the individual to continue on the benefit.

Students with disabilities

Skill, the National Bureau for Students with Disabilities is an independent organization which aims to develop opportunities in further, higher, and continuing education for students with disabilities. Its work covers the whole range of disability whether physical, sensory or learning difficulty.

Its activities include a number of specialist careers officers and learning support co-ordinators in colleges who have frequent contact with the Bureau. Membership is open to any institution, TEC/LEC, or individual with an interest in its work. The Bureau is a registered charity.

The Careers Service

The Employment and Training Act 1973[19] places a duty on the Secretary of State to secure the provision of careers guidance and placing services for people attending schools and colleges and for those ceasing to undergo such education. The Act also gives the Secretary of State powers to arrange for the provision of such services for other people. These services are collectively termed 'careers services'.

Funded by Government, there are 66 careers services operating in local areas through-out the country. Most careers services are separate legal entities with boards of directors. Each careers service is accountable to the Secretary of State for Education and Employment, with whom it has a contract, and they work very closely with schools and colleges to provide help to clients in full-time education. Qualified careers advisers together with teachers and careers co-ordinators can ensure that young people have access to information and advice on the full range of opportunities available to them.

Clients of the Careers Service are:

- people undergoing full-time education at any educational institution, other than an educational institution within the higher education sector;
- people undergoing part-time education at any educational institution, other than an education institution within the higher education sector, which is the education people commonly receive to fit them for employment;
- other people aged under 21.

Not included are persons studying higher education courses in colleges of further education, unless their course is funded by the Further Education Funding Council (FEFC). However, the client group does encompass all people falling within its terms of reference, including those in independent schools; those in and leaving care; those who are taught at home; and those in and leaving Young Offenders Institutions (YOIs).

There is no specific age or time restriction in respect of people with disabilities (i.e. those who come within the definition of disability set out in the DDA). They remain part of the client group until settled in their career intention.

Each young person in full-time education or in part-time vocational education may use the free advice and guidance provided by their local careers service. The staff offer impartial advice, based on the needs of each individual, on the requirements of further education courses, training opportunities, and the demands and availability of jobs locally. They will also offer advice on the financial support available while people are in education or training, or if they are unemployed. They have a particular responsibility to provide services to people with disabilities.

Further and higher education

Following the Further and Higher Education Acts of 1992, a number of changes have taken place in post-compulsory education. The main effect for further education is that all further education colleges and sixth-form colleges have become independent, and outside local education authority control since April 1993. In higher education, the distinction between universities and polytechnics has already disappeared, and the Council for National Academic Awards has been disbanded.

Potential students who have a disability should always let their preferred institutions know well in advance of their intended admission so that any special or additional provision needed might be discussed. Skill: The National Bureau for Students with Disabilities (see above) has produced a *Guide to Higher Education* for intending students going to university, and this includes details of facilities available and contact names. The choice of institution should be based on academic criteria, however, not on such matters as physical access most of which can be dealt with on or after acceptance, but before admission.

References

1   Cornes, P. *Employment rehabilitation: the aims and achievements of a service for disabled people.* London: HMSO, 1982.
2   *Dictionary of occupational titles,* Vol 2, 4th edn. Washington, DC: US Department of Labor, Employment and Training Administration, 1991
3   *Code of Practice for Employers.* Sheffield: Manpower Services Commission, 1993.
4   *Employment and training for people with disabilities.* Sheffield: Employment Department, 1990.
5   National Audit Office, Department of Employment, Manpower Services Commission. *Employment assistance to disabled adults..* London: HMSO, 1987.
6   Williams, C. Life after the consultative document. *ReHab NetWork,* Summer, 1993.
7   Stubbins J. The clinical model in rehabilitation and its alternatives. *ReHab NetWork,* Summer, 1986.
8   Menz F, Eggars J, Wehmann P, Brooke V. *Lessons for improving the employment of people with disabilities.* Vocational Rehabilitation Research, Wisconsin: Stout Vocational Rehabilitation Institute, 1997.
9   Lytel B, Botterbusch K. *Physical demands job analysis: another approach.* Menomonie: University of Wisconsin, 1981.
10 US Department of Labor. *Handbook for analysing jobs.* Washington, DC: Manpower Administration, US Dept of Labor, 1972.
11 Livy B. *Job evaluation: a critical view.* London: Allen & Unwin, 1975.
12 Krebs, DE. Measurement in physical theory. *Phys Ther* 1987; **67**(12): 1834–9.
13 Key, G. *Industrial therapy.* St Louis, MO: Mosby, 1995.
14 Matheson LN. How do you know that he tried his best. The reliability crisis in industrial relations. *Industrial Rehabil Qu* 1988;1(1), Spring.
15 Matheson LN. *Work capacity evaluation. a training manual for occupational therapists.* Anaheim, CA: ERIC, 1982.

16 Thornton P, Sainsbury R, Barnes H. *Helping disabled people to work*. London: HMSO, 1997.
17 Darnborough A, Kinrade D. *Directory for disabled people*. London: Prentice Hall, 1995.
18 Department of Social Security. *A new contract for welfare*. London: HMSO, 1998.
19 Employment and Training Act 1973 (Sections 8–10) and Trade Union Reform and Employment Rights Act 1993 (Sections 45 and 46). HMSO.

Further reading

DSS publications

A guide for registered medical practitioners (booklet IB 204), revised April 2000.
Disability living allowance (leaflet DS 704).
Ill or disabled because of work (leaflet SD4).
Incapacity benefit (booklet IB 214), revised April 2000.
Industrial injuries disablement benefit (leaflet NI 6).
Longterm ill or disabled (leaflet SD3).
Sick and unable to work (leaflet SD4).
Sick or disabled (leaflet SD1).
Which benefit—a guide to social security and NHS benefits (booklet FB 2).

Disability Information Trust publications (see Appendix 7 for address)

Employment and the workplace, 1994.
Communication and access to computer technology, 1995.

Other publications

Code of practice for the elimination of discrimination in the field of employment against disabled persons or persons who have had a disability. Department for Education and Employment. London 1996.
Disability Manual. Croner CCH, Telford Rd., Bicester OX6 0XT
Doyle, B. *Disability discrimination—the new law*, 2nd edn. London: Jordans, 1996.
Floyd, M. Pre-employment screening and disabled people. *Occup Health Rev* 1995: May/June.
Society of Occupational Medicine. *Guidelines for occupational physicians on the Disability Discrimination Act 1995*.
The Disability Discrimination Act 1995 with its guidance notes and code of practice. London: HMSO, 1995.
The Employers' Action File on Disability. London: Employers' Forum on Disability.

5

Ethics for occupational physicians

D. S. Wright

Background and scope

Occupational physicians work within a particular environment, which is influenced by legal, temporal, historical, and philosophical factors as well as medical teaching and practice. Ethics is a code of conduct which is only applicable in context. In occupational medicine it will be influenced by the legal code, the regulatory system, and the attitudes and organization of society in the country concerned, as well as by the different professional associations and other controls in place. There are few codes of behaviour that are accepted everywhere, but there is much that is widely accepted throughout the industrialized world. Even within Europe, however, where most health and safety legislation now stems from single Directives from the European Commission, there are fundamental differences in approach to some basic issues in occupational medicine, such as the need and criteria for regular medical examinations. These differences stem from the varied ways in which the specialty has developed in different countries, as well as from its legal framework and regulatory approaches. As a result, attitudes and behaviour may vary, even when working within the same basic set of rules.

Ethical practice does not, therefore, constitute a fixed and universally applicable code of conduct. Even within a single country, regulations and attitudes constantly change, and so the rules of 'acceptable practice' must be re-appraised regularly. Nevertheless, there are some basic principles which underpin the ethical practice of occupational physicians. The International Commission on Occupational Health (ICOH) has published a Code of Ethics that applies to all occupational health professionals,[1] and which forms a valuable basis for a national approach. The International Labour Office (ILO)[2] also gives guidance in which it recommends national associations to prepare and review their own codes of ethics.

The Faculty of Occupational Medicine of the Royal College of Physicians of London has recently reviewed its *Guidance on Ethics for Occupational Physicians*,[3] which was first published in 1980. The review forms the basis for this chapter. Although that means, inevitably, that it focuses on law and practice in the UK, many of the principles espoused will be more widely applicable.

General principles

In the UK, the General Medical Council (GMC) has prime responsibility for the ethical standards of medical practice. It sets out the 'standards that the public have a right to expect of their doctors' in several booklets.[4,5] Occupational physicians also need to be aware of other national publications, such as those from the British Medical Association,[6] and from the medical Royal Colleges.

The need for a special consideration of ethical standards arises because occupational physicians adopt different roles from other specialists or from general practitioners. In addition to their traditional contacts with patients, they give advice on the health aspects of products, processes and practices of companies to managers and employees—including their representatives. In their relationships with people in the workplace, occupational physicians must demonstrate, by their behaviour and their conduct, that they clearly appreciate in which capacity they are acting at the time, and should ensure that others fully understand the position.

Ethics, as a code of conduct, must take account of change including changing attitudes and behaviour in society, changes in the law, and changes as a result of research and technical developments. In recent years in the UK there have also been fundamental changes in the organization and management of occupational health practice. Many more independent practitioners offer services on a contract basis, and fewer physicians are directly employed by companies. Because of these changes, and because of the different roles they are required to play in respect of their patients, their employer, the patient's employer, trade unions and the public, occupational physicians may find that they face conflicts of interest and loyalty. As ethical axioms are not universally agreed, the resolution of such conflicts can be difficult. There may be more than one 'correct' course of action—or there may appear to be none.

Ethical behaviour is largely self-imposed, and each doctor makes decisions and acts according to their own conscience, based on personal experience and training. Guidelines may help in many problem areas, but ethical questions cannot always be codified, and ones with legal implications may have no precedent in a legal system which relies heavily on case law, as opposed to prescriptive regulations. Ethical behaviour thus depends on the exercise of judgement, but the views of experienced colleagues may prove invaluable in such circumstances.

A senior UK judge, Lord Woolf, has stated: [7]

The courts are very conscious that in many fields of litigation they depend on expert medical advice in order to come to a final decision. . . . The general approach of the courts is to apply the standards that the medical profession adopts. Thus we judge whether there has been negligence in the treatment of a patient by asking whether or not the medical treatment which is the subject of the complaint, accords with standards which any recognized section of the medical profession regards as acceptable . . . the courts do not impose their ethical standards on the medical professions. Wisely, they leave the medical profession to determine what is, and what is not, ethical behaviour.

National codes of ethics may, therefore, influence the law, as well as being influenced by it. Experience indicates that such codes not only inform the decisions of occupational physicians, but are used by individual workpeople, managers, lawyers, and other occupational health professionals.

Sometimes doctors find themselves in a position where they give occupational medical advice to companies and, at the same time, provide primary medical care to some or all of the employees of that company, which may give rise to a conflict of interest. In these circumstances they should put the interests of the individual patient first. They should invite the company to seek alternative occupational health advice, rather than jeopardize the primary care doctor–patient relationship.

Occupational physicians may be called on to advise on the nature or extent of work-related health risk to individuals, to the environment, or to the public. It is their responsibility to assist in the risk assessment process, but not to decide on the acceptability of the risk. They are also likely to be part of a team that determines the means whereby such risks may be controlled, but will commonly not lead in such activity. Some doctors may find a subsidiary role less comfortable than the primacy which is normally assumed in general practice. Acting as one of a team is an essential part of the role of any occupational physician.

There is increasing pressure from society for greater openness. Legislation on access to medical records and reports, and on data protection, has followed in recent years, though the lack of case law does not always make the interpretation straightforward. The advice of senior colleagues and the use of national professional guidelines are valuable in such circumstances. As a general principle, physicians should be as open as possible in the disclosure of records and reports to the subjects, always taking account of the effect such openness may have on the patient's health. Employers should be advised that the subjects of reports will normally be told of the contents. Where medical practitioners act as independent advisers (and, therefore, outwith the Access to Medical Reports Act 1988) to third parties such as insurance companies, employers, or lawyers, it is not normally appropriate for the subject of the report to receive a copy of it, unless this is required by a court or has been agreed in advance by the third party.

The occupational physician in an organization must act as an impartial professional adviser, concerned primarily with safeguarding the health of employed people and others who may be affected by work activity. Demonstrable professional competence, independence and integrity, as well as openness in matters of concern, are necessary to command the confidence and respect of management, employees, and their representatives. Without these the doctor cannot be effective.

Guidance on ethics inevitably strays into areas of practice, because advice on behaviour is seldom readily available in technical publications. Occupational health advice is commonly given not only by specialist occupational physicians, but by general practitioners and by doctors in other specialties. All must ensure that they have the necessary competence. Acting outside the limits of professional competence is likely to place the practitioner's career at risk, as well as compromising the health and safety of the individual or organization to whom advice is given.

Occupational physicians commonly have responsibilities for staff working in another country, have themselves to work abroad, or are accountable to business or occupational health management based in another country. Legal and ethical standards vary from country to country. Occupational physicians must ensure that practices and standards imposed from abroad conform, at the minimum, to those in the country in which they are working. When they are working abroad themselves, the standards must be compatible with those of the host country, ensuring that the highest standards prevail.

Medical records and confidentiality

General principles

The occupational physician or nurse is responsible for all clinical information, whether it is held manually or electronically, and must ensure the security of that information at all times. The principles of confidentiality within medical practice, on which guidance is issued by the GMC,[8] apply equally in occupational health.

Medical records

Occupational physicians should take and maintain full, factual, contemporaneous, and dated notes. Not only is this good practice, but these notes may be required for disclosure or litigation.

Although unrestricted access to clinical data should be confined to the doctor and the nurse, other members of an occupational health department will have, and need, some access. All such staff must be made fully aware of their personal responsibility to keep all clinical information confidential, and they should sign an undertaking that they understand this. Temporary staff must be included.

The informed written consent of the subject is required before access to clinical information may be granted to others. 'An informed consent occurs if, and only if, a patient or subject with substantial understanding and in substantial absence of control by others, intentionally authorizes a professional to do something'.[9] Clinical data and other information obtained by occupational physicians may only be disclosed with such consent unless:

- the disclosure is clearly in the patient's interest, but it is not possible or it is undesirable to seek consent
- it is required by law
- it is in the public interest
- in certain circumstances, for the purposes of medical research.

Disclosure, other than with consent or where required by law, needs careful consideration. It may often be relevant to consult with others including, where appropriate, a research ethics committee or medical defence organization. In considering the public interest, the physician needs to assess the risk of serious harm, or death, to the patient or others, national security, and the prevention or detection of serious crime. A decision to disclose clinical information without consent may need to be justified at some time in the future.

It is the responsibility of the physician to ensure that the patient has personally given informed consent. A signature on a paper presented by a third party is no guarantee that it is even genuine or that consent has been obtained by due process and is fully informed.

Access to records

Within the European Union the protection and confidentiality of personal information is the subject of a Data Protection Directive.[10] In the UK this has been implemented by a revised and extended Data Protection Act 1998. This repeals all the provisions of the Access to Health Records Act 1990 as they relate to living people. These Acts are a manifestation of the increasing tendency towards greater openness and more rights for individuals in relation to information held about them. The law has been extended from electronic data to all data held manually in filing systems, and also extends the rights of subjects to access information held about them and control its processing. Processing includes obtaining the data in the first place and covers its handling in many ways, including its transfer to another data controller.

There may be some confusion initially over the applicability of some of this legislation. Not only will there be no case law but, although some of the Data Protection Act 1998 applied from its introduction in October 1998, some parts affecting current records will not be fully effective until October 2007. Occupational physicians should have some understanding of the law relating to records, their confidential maintenance, and the rights of individuals to access and control, and should ensure that their own behaviour conforms to the ethos underpinning this approach. Although professional associations can give more detailed guidance as case law and experience develop, there remains an onus on the individual to develop a broad understanding of the issues and to act appropriately.

Access to reports for employment or insurance purposes provided by medical practitioners who are responsible for the clinical care of a patient is the subject of the Access to Medical Reports Act 1988. When an occupational physician seeks such a report from a general practitioner or hospital specialist, this Act will apply, and the employee's rights under the Act must be explained and respected as a part of the process of obtaining informed consent.

Occupational physicians should develop a clear policy to cover requests for access to reports or records, whether or not these may be covered by the law. They should recognize the possible legal implications, and the tendency towards greater openness. In most circumstances occupational physicians will be regarded as providing clinical care, as defined by the Access to Medical Reports Act 1988, so that it is not only good practice to ensure that the subject of a report is aware of the contents, it also ensures the occupational physician will be covered by the provisions of the Act.

Occupational physicians may act as line managers within their own department. They must claim no special privilege of access to medical information about colleagues and staff over and above that available to other line managers. If a report is required an independent occupational medical assessment of a member of staff may well be appropriate to ensure the protection of the individual's privacy and confidentiality.

Disclosure in legal cases

There are many circumstances where medical records may be required for legal purposes. The procedures to be adopted by occupational physicians will vary from country to country, depending on local regulation, and it is commonly prudent for physicians to seek advice from their medical defence organization or professional association. As a general rule clinical information on individuals should not be released without written informed consent. There may well be pressure from lawyers on either side of a case to allow greater access to an individual's complete medical records, and the physician should ensure that the person concerned understands exactly what is to be released and to whom. In general, however, the consent should relate to records relevant only to the case.

A court of law, an employment tribunal, or similar body may require the disclosure of all or part of a patient's medical records. In that case the physician must comply, but must inform the individual.

Transfer, retention, and archiving of records

Occupational health records should be stored in such a way as to facilitate their transfer to another occupational health provider, their archiving, or their destruction. The detail will vary, but consideration must be given to the possibility of the individual changing employer, dying, or transferring to a different part of the same company, as well as to any changes of occupational health provider. It is necessary also to take account of the circumstances in which a company ceases to exist, or is taken over by another company. Storage and transfer arrangements must ensure security and confidentiality, and must take account of the rights of individuals in respect of data protection and access, and the requirement for consent to any change. The physician must ensure that the new holder of the records is an appropriate person for this role.

Some occupational health records may be required, by law, to be retained for a set period. These may be the records of the results of health assessments such as those for asbestos or lead workers, rather than the actual clinical record. It is the employer's responsibility to retain such records, rather than that of the physician, and they should be kept separate from the clinical records.

Fitness for work

Pre-employment health assessment

Pre-employment health questionnaires are often the only health screening undertaken at the time of employment. Several legal and ethical issues arise over the wording, interpretation, and handling of such questionnaires. If applicants have to post them back, obscurities cannot be clarified by direct questioning, so the design must take this into account. The content and format of the questions must be scrutinized carefully to ensure that they do not encourage any form of discrimination or contravention of the Disability Discrimination Act 1995 (DDA). Applicants should not be expected to reveal clinical details to those who are not bound to observe medical confidentiality. **Only if questionnaires are returned to qualified medical or nursing staff can there be any assurance that clinical details will be handled with appropriate confidentiality.**

Questionnaires should seek only information relevant to the job, and should be sent for completion only when a conditional offer of employment has been made. This may include general information on disabilities, as this may be necessary if the employers are to fulfil their obligations under the DDA. These obligations include consideration of reasonable adjustments to the workplace to enable a disabled person to work. If there are specific medical conditions which would preclude employment, these should be defined.

This may include reference to drugs, whether prescribed or not. It is at the pre-employment stage that the employer should advise potential applicants if health screening will include drug tests, and whether a positive result would be a bar to employment. Potential applicants then have the option to proceed on an informed basis.

Sometimes it may be necessary to apply to an applicant's general practitioner or specialist medical adviser for specific information relevant to employment. This should only happen with the individual's informed consent. It can never be justified to ask for disclosure of the applicant's medical records in general. The request must specify the information, and the purpose for which it is required. The consent applies only at the time it is given.

At a pre-employment health assessment, the primary responsibility of the occupational physician is to the employer. The UK Court of Appeal has ruled that the doctor owes no duty of care to the applicant.[11] Although this ruling clarifies the legal situation, ethically the physician has a professional duty to act with due care and competence in undertaking a pre-employment health assessment. This includes taking appropriate action if an abnormality is discovered, even if this has no relevance to employment.

The physician should ensure that the applicant understands the role of the doctor or nurse in acting for the employer. Medical examination by a physician is justified ethically only where risk assessment, which may include financial risk to the potential employer, shows it to be appropriate, though the laws relating to such examinations vary in different countries, and must be adhered to. If the work requires a specified and justifiable standard of physical or mental health, or the health of the applicant may affect the health or safety of others, a medical examination is likely to be necessary. Rarely, there may be a need for a medical examination by a physician to ascertain fitness for a company pension scheme, or to advise the trustees of any limitations, although normal practice is 'fit for employment, fit for the pension scheme'.

Sickness absence

The control of absence from work, including that attributed to sickness, is a management responsibility. The occupational physician may help to monitor sickness absence and has a role in providing the medical advice necessary to enable managers to discharge their responsibility equitably to the employee and the organization, and in accordance with their statutory obligations. The physician's dual responsibility to the employer and to the employee requires objectivity and impartial, evidence-based medical advice. The physician's assessment will determine to what extent an employee's absence is caused by ill health, the prognosis with regard to return to work, any work adjustments which may be necessary, and any medical steps which could be taken to expedite the return to work. The occupational physician has no role to play in 'policing' sickness absence.

Retirement on health grounds

In order to advise on ill health retirement, the occupational physician must be fully conversant with the rules relating to pay during sickness absence, the rules and definitions of the company pension scheme, and the fitness requirements of the job. The physician's task includes the determination of disability and its likely duration, in relation to the requirements of the individual's work. Wherever possible this should be done by personal examination of the employee, and after having consulted the family doctor or attending specialist. Having confirmed the nature of the condition and the degree of disability, and before making a recommendation, the physician should consult with the management on what reasonable adjustments can be made to the workplace to accommodate the employee, or whether alternative employment is available. This is required under the DDA. The physician should ensure that the advice given is impartial and objective, and related to the medical facts, rather than to any other employment considerations (see also Appendix 6).

It is often helpful for physicians to anticipate likely problems relating to ill health and employment or retirement, and to have discussed these in advance with personnel and pension staff. Difficulties arising over the employment of people with chronic conditions or serious communicable diseases (see below) can often be resolved in advance, ensuring the optimum placement of such staff and satisfactory arrangements for early retirement, should this become necessary.

Health screening and special tests during employment

Health promotion*

Occupational physicians may undertake a variety of health screening tests, often unconnected with the risks of work. Voluntary health promotion programmes must be clearly differentiated from those which are required by law, or as a condition of employment. There should be clear procedures for the handling of results and for the employment consequences of any abnormalities discovered. If the anonymized and grouped results of such programmes are to be passed onto the employer, this should be agreed with the participants in advance *(See also Chapter 1, p. 21).

Biological monitoring

Programmes for biological monitoring and biological effect monitoring must have a clear purpose and be well planned and implemented. The outcome should be improved control of hazards and reduction of risk. Participation should include informed consent, even when monitoring is required by law.

Although the purpose of the programme may be to use the grouped results to assess and improve control measures, individual results falling outside agreed parameters will require specialist interpretation. Arrangements should be in place to refer, if considered necessary.

Planning such programmes must include the communication of results. The release of grouped results to all those with an interest in the control of the risks must be agreed in advance. Occasionally it may be necessary to release an individual's results to a third party to achieve the objective, but this can only be with their informed consent.

Genetic screening

Genetic screening has had little impact in the field of employment so far, but it is a rapidly advancing science. Its only known application in the UK is in the armed forces, where candidates for flying are screened for the sickle cell trait, because of the risk hypoxia may pose.

The Nuffield Council on Bioethics' Working Party on Genetic Screening[12] expressed the view that

... genetic screening of a workforce for increased occupational risks ought to be contemplated in our view only where:

(i)   there is strong evidence of a clear connection between the working environment and the development of the condition for which the screening is conducted;

(ii)   the condition in question is one which seriously endangers the health of the employee, or is one in which an affected employee is likely to present a serious danger to third parties;

(iii) the condition is one for which the dangers cannot be eliminated or significantly reduced by reasonable measures taken by the employer to modify or respond to the environmental risks.

This view has been supported at an international conference of occupational health experts[13] and by the Employment Working Group of the Human Genetics Advisory Commission in the UK.[14]

Serious communicable diseases

The UK GMC[15] has published guidance on the ethical considerations of dealing, particularly, with those with HIV, hepatitis B or C, and tuberculosis. Guidance has also been published by the Department of Health.[16,17] Occupational physicians in the healthcare industry should be conversant with such publications. Wherever occupational physicians work, they are themselves healthcare workers and must therefore follow national guidance. Even when they believe their own work will not jeopardize patients, they must not rely on their own assessment of the risk, but must seek and follow professional advice. Policies and procedures must be in place to ensure that their own staff comply with guidance.

Some countries require proof of freedom from infection with HIV before allowing visitors to work in that country. Where HIV testing is essential, expert counselling on the implications must be given to ensure fully informed consent, and post-test counselling must be available.

Immunization programmes

Where immunization programmes may be required at work, consent can only be regarded as informed if the risks are quantified and communicated. The policy should consider the implications of refusal to be immunized or to seroconvert, and must cover the situation where a worker proves to be a carrier of infection. This will include issues arising from a failure on the worker's part to inform their manager or to comply with reasonable restrictions at work.

Testing for alcohol and drugs

Occupational physicians may be involved in screening and testing for alcohol and drugs. It is important to differentiate between tests for the clinical benefit of the individual and those undertaken primarily to protect the company and third parties.

Physicians should avoid participation in policing procedures wherever possible, as this is likely to compromise their relationships with both workers and management. Tests for alcohol consumption undertaken as part of a company programme need not be performed by physicians or nurses. Breath analysis equipment, made to the appropriate specifications, can be used. Physicians should be involved in setting up such programmes, and should advise on the appropriate action levels for blood alcohol, and ensure that proper respect is given to the rights and dignity of individuals.

Where tests for drugs are instituted as part of company policy, it is important that the purposes and procedures, the criteria for testing, the taking and handling of samples, and the reporting and outcome of results are clearly specified in advance. The Faculty of Occupational Medicine has published detailed guidance.[18] It is important, if medical and nursing staff are involved, that they are properly trained and that their roles are clearly understood by staff and managers. The physician can play a significant role in ensuring that properly informed consent is given to obtaining samples and that, at all stages, ethical practice is allied to carefully defined and controlled procedures.

Medical and nursing staff who are involved in taking and processing biological samples, and in the handling and reporting of results, act as agents for the employer. They must avoid using such occasions to give personal medical advice to individuals. This will reduce the risk of confusion between their role as agents for the employer, and their traditional role as confidential medical advisers.

Business ethics

Business codes

Occupational physicians are expected to abide by the codes of business ethics followed by their employers and contractors. They must ensure that there is no conflict between these obligations and their own, and they must strive to influence company policies in ways that take account of the health of employees and others affected by the organization's activities.

Contracted services

Increasingly, occupational health services are provided by staff who are not directly employed by the organization they serve. The commercial pressures inherent in this type of market can lead to particular ethical difficulties. It is important that occupational physicians abide by sound principles of business ethics in their dealings with client companies and each other, in order to safeguard their own reputations and that of the specialty as a whole. When occupational physicians act as managers, they must also recognize that the ethical standards by which they will be judged will be those standards which would apply to their dealings and relationships with patients.

Advertising

Occupational physicians in the UK, like other doctors, have to be registered with the GMC and abide by its rulings.[4] Similar obligations may exist for medical practice abroad.

In the UK, this limits advertising to the provision of factual information and services. Organizations employing occupational physicians are not restricted in this way, but doctors should dissociate themselves from inappropriate marketing, and ensure that advertising literature does not make claims which are not factual and verifiable.

Competence

Occupational physicians should only accept duties that are within their competence. When tendering for work, they must assess the level of specialist skills required, and refer to a higher level of expertise if that is appropriate.

The term 'occupational physician' is often misused. **Only doctors with postgraduate training in occupational medicine should describe themselves as occupational physicians, and the use of the terms 'consultant' or 'specialist' in occupational medicine within Europe should be reserved for doctors who are eligible for inclusion on the specialist register established under the European Specialist Medical Qualifications Order 1995.**

Competitive tenders

Competition in the provision of occupational health services can be a healthy stimulus towards improving standards. Tendering exercises should be conducted honestly and fairly. Great care must be taken not to damage the reputation of competitors. It is improper either to offer inducements in order to secure business, or to make approaches to the staff of a competitor or existing service provider in order to obtain commercial advantage. Occupational health staff who are employed by an occupational health provider to work with a particular client should not use their position to gain personal advantage by, for example, offering the same service independently at a lower rate, or by disclosing commercially sensitive information to a competitor. Such action constitutes a breach of contract, and could render the individual liable to a claim for damages.

Occupational physicians who act as technical advisers in tender evaluations must not have a commercial relationship with any of the competitors. They should declare any personal or professional interests, and must provide objective advice on the merits of each proposal.

Transfer of services

Services may be transferred from one occupational health provider to another in a variety of circumstances. The abiding principle must be to safeguard the health, safety, and welfare of those to whom the service is being provided. The outgoing provider should make every reasonable effort to facilitate the handover. The cost of special equipment or programmes, which may be the property of the outgoing provider, should be agreed in advance if they are to be handed over. There are a number of legal considerations relating to the transfer of staff from one employer to another. Occupational health records should be transferred if practicable (see above).

Research

The unique environment of the workplace creates a need for special consideration of the ethical issues involved in occupational health research. Such research may involve direct physical contact with individuals, it may relate to medical records, or it may be concerned with the environment. Toxicological studies may be involved, including studies with healthy human volunteers. Frequently the occupational physician is only a link between the researcher and the industry, and may work with staff who have no experience or understanding of research with human subjects or of the ethical constraints required.

The occupational physician will have an important role in communicating with managers and the workforce, especially to ensure informed consent is secured. The research may often be on a small scale, undertaken at short notice and resulting from an incident or illness among the workforce. Even in such studies it is important to ensure that confidentiality is preserved and that there is full consultation. Pressure from the media, from managers, and from the employees to obtain quick answers may not be compatible with scientific needs, and it is important that occupational physicians are prepared for such eventualities.

A clear written protocol must be prepared, addressing the issues involved in the project. Many of these will be similar to those in other medical research. An important principle is that the investigator must not be the sole judge of the adequacy of the protocol, which should be subjected to third party ethical review when human subjects are involved. The Royal College of Physicians of London has recently published guidance on research based on archived information and samples,[19] much of which is very relevant to occupational health research. This emphasizes the need for ethical review to assess the requirement for individual consent.

Occupational physicians who are involved in research should study the ethical requirements carefully. These are summarized in the Faculty of Occupational Medicine guidelines[3] as: careful planning; detailed protocol; full consultation; consent; confidentiality; review during the conduct of the research; and careful, planned handling of results.

Relationships with others

General principles

Occupational physicians have an ethical obligation to put the interests of their patients first. Their obligations to others, including their employers, the workforce as a whole, and the general public, must also be recognized.

Particular attention should be paid to the role of the general practitioner, especially where this concerns treatment and referral, and consent to release clinical information. Occupational physicians in the healthcare sector must be especially careful that the general practitioner is not by-passed.

Other health professionals

Nurses have an important role in occupational health, and physicians must ensure that they understand the ethical requirements for nursing. In many situations the nurse may be the occupational health manager, and that role must be respected.

The occupational physician will work closely with other health and safety professionals such as occupational hygienists and safety officers, as well as with managers and engineers. Exchange of information is important, but scrupulous care must be taken to safeguard confidential medical information.

Managers and workpeople

Managers may not always appreciate the physician's ethical duty to individuals and his independent position on clinical matters. The limits of accountability to managers need to be clarified before difficulties arise. Conflicts of interest between obligations to individuals and to managers or the company can usually be resolved by discussion, but conferring with senior professional colleagues may often assist.

It should be normal practice for occupational physicians to discuss health and safety issues with workpeople or their representatives. A good working relationship with trade unions, while respecting the confidentiality of individuals, will resolve many issues.

The public and the environment

The occupational physician has a duty to society, and occasionally must put the public interest before that of a patient. When safety or public health may be endangered, the physician may, legally and ethically, breach confidentiality. It will be the physician's conscience which will dictate action, but advice from senior colleagues should be sought if possible. Ultimately, physicians may be required to justify their course of action in a court of law.

Selected references

1 *International code of ethics for occupational health professionals*. Singapore: International Commission on Occupational Health, 1992.
2 *Technical and ethical guidelines for workers' health surveillance*. Geneva: International Labour Office, 1997.
3 *Guidance on ethics for occupational physicians*, 5th edn. London: Faculty of Occupational Medicine, 1999.
4 *Good medical practice*. London: General Medical Council, 1998.
5 *Maintaining good medical practice*. London: General Medical Council, 1998.
6 *Medical ethics to-day: its practice and philosophy*. London: British Medical Association, 1993.
7 Lord Woolf. Medics, lawyers and the courts. *J R Coll Physicians Lond* 1997; **31**(6): 686–693.
8 *Confidentiality*. London: General Medical Council, 1995.
9 Beauchamp TL, Childress JF. *Principles of biomedical ethics*, 4th edn. Oxford: Oxford University Press, 1994.
10 Directive 95.46 of the European Parliament and the Council of 24 October 1995 on the protection of individuals with regard to the processing of personal data and on the free movement of such data. *Official J European Communities* L281 1995; **38**, 23 November: 31–55.

11 *Kapfunde* v. *Abbey National and Dr Daniel*. London: Industrial Relations Law Reports 583, 1998.

12 *Genetic screening: ethical issues*. London: Nuffield Council on Bioethics, 1993.

13 Rantanen J. *Conclusions and recommendations of a conference on ethical and social principles in occupational health practices*. Helsinki: Finnish Institute of Occupational Health, 1998.

14 Human Genetics Advisory Commission. *The implications of genetic testing for employment*. London: Department of Trade and Industry, July 1999.

15 *Serious communicable diseases*. London: General Medical Council, 1997.

16 *Protecting healthcare workers and patients from Hepatitis B—Recommendations of the Advisory Group on Hepatitis*. London: Department of Health, 1993.

17 *AIDS/HIV infected healthcare workers: guidance on the management of infected healthcare workers*. London: Department of Health, 1993.

18 *Guidelines on testing for drugs of abuse in the workplace*. London: Faculty of Occupational Medicine, 1994.

19 Royal College of Physicians of London. Research based on archived information and samples. Recommendations from the RCP Committee on Ethical Issues in Medicine. *J R Coll Physicians Lond* 1999; **33**, No 3 (May/June), 264–266.

6

Neurological disorders

R. Willcox and F. B. Gibberd

Neurological disorders cover a wide range of disease processes and functional disabilities. Congenital and acquired disorders that affect the central or peripheral nervous system demonstrate how important an intact system is to the requirements of everyday life and the ability to earn a living.

Disorders of neurophysiology can be divided into those leading to negative symptoms and those leading to positive symptoms.

- **Negative symptoms** arise from a failure of neuronal activity. Such failures may be caused by physical or chemical agents which transiently damage or irreversibly destroy nerve cells or axons. The nuclei of neural cells are irreplaceable and the regeneration which might occur when axons are destroyed rarely leads to full recovery of function.
- **Positive symptoms** arise from excessive neuronal or axonal stimulation. They can also result from malfunction of the inhibitory influences on the system.

Neurological dysfunction needs to be evaluated in terms of the effect it has on the patient's clinical function. As regards capacity for work the precise diagnosis is less important than the functional consequences. Feldman and Pransky[1] divide functional effects into disturbance of awareness; disturbances of posture, balance and gait; extremity pain, numbness and weakness; neurobehavioural impairment; and ophthalmological conditions. These are dealt with from the functional and anatomical points of view in subsequent sections of this chapter.

Size of the problem

Neurological disorders are an important cause of disability in modern western society. Estimates from the British General Household Survey, using self-reporting procedures, suggest that about 6% of the population have a long-standing neurological illness.

It is difficult to make valid comparisons with other major disease groupings, partly because many neurological diseases are age-related. Mortality and morbidity also vary by condition. Diseases which are commonest below 65 years and which have prolonged morbidity have greater relevance to work ability than either rapidly fatal diseases or those whose main clinical impact occurs late in life.

Table 6.1 compares mortality and morbidity rates for some of the more important neurological diseases. (The rates cited are crude and not confined to the working age group, but they provide some indication of the prevalence of the commoner problems.[2]) With the exception of brain tumours and motor neurone disease (MND), the morbidity

Table 6.1   Crude annual mortality and morbidity rates for some neurological disorders per 100 000 population (adapted from Kurtzke, 1985)[2]

	Mortality	Morbidity
Brain neoplasms	4–5	6–16
Multiple sclerosis	0–3	30–300
Parkinson's disease	0.5–3.8	40–190
Motor neurone disease	0.4–1.2	0.4–1.9
Myopathies	0.1–0.5	2–10
Myasthenia	1	0.5–10

rates are an order of magnitude larger than mortality rates. The health impact of the neurological diseases cited in Table 6.1 is small compared to that of cerebrovascular disorders, for which the comparable mortality rates are in the order of 60–600 per 100 000 per year (12% of all deaths), but only about 10% of these deaths occur below the age of 65. Of the 100 000 'first strokes' each year in Britain, a quarter occur in people below the age of 65. The resultant disability is a major drain on health service resources (5.5% of the total). Overall, nervous system diseases take up 9% of all NHS expenditure—exceeded only by circulatory disorders (13%) and mental illness (20%).[3]

Non-occupational versus occupational causes of neurological disease

The non-occupational causes of neurological disease outweigh the occupational causes. Occupational examples of neurological disease arise mainly from peripheral neurotoxins and the neurobehavioural effects of organic solvents.[4] The occupational physician is more often involved with the job adaptation and rehabilitation of patients with neurological disabilities than with eliminating the small number of known occupational neurotoxins from the workplace. Of course, the occupational physician needs to be aware of the possible work-related circumstances that could exacerbate a pre-existing non-occupational neurological disease. The use of organic solvents, therefore, needs to be carefully considered, particularly in patients who already have disturbances of awareness or posture or a neurobehavioural disorder.

Clinical assessment

If a differential diagnosis is not clear after taking a history, then the clinical examination may be equally inconclusive. The history of the illness is of crucial importance, but by the time the occupational physician sees the patient, the diagnosis is likely to have been established. In these circumstances, a more important aspect of the interview is to assess the individual's ability to perform their job, or to return to the job held before the illness began, or to adapt to alternative employment.

In normal subjects, perception and recognition of sensory stimuli are intact; their balance, posture and gait can be maintained; they have good control of delicate motor movement; and have no evidence of loss of control of vasomotor, gastrointestinal, or genitourinary functions.[1] To this catalogue of negative symptoms must be added an absence of any positive symptoms or signs such as involuntary movements, abnormal sensations, or hallucinations.

Disturbances of awareness include alterations in the ability to stay awake. Although classical narcolepsy is rare, sleep apnoea is a common cause of excessive daytime somnolence.[2] Establishing the existence of such a condition can be difficult as patients are frequently unaware of night-time problems. They may contend that night-time sleep is normal—the problem, in their view, is daytime sleepiness! Such individuals are particularly intolerant of rotating shiftwork. In obstructive sleep apnoea sleep disruption is frequent with consequent daytime sleepiness, poor concentration, and impairment of work; it can be a cause of drowsiness when driving. It is commonest in obese middle-aged men. In severe cases continuous positive airways pressure (CPAP) at night can produce alleviation and hence good sleep and improved daytime function.

Disturbances of posture, balance, or gait are usually easy to establish. The patients complain of dizziness, unsteadiness, or spatial disequilibrium and their powers of co-ordination may be impaired. Parkinson's disease is a classic example of this group of disorders. Adjustment of treatment regimes may minimize work problems, but jobs which involve rapid hand co-ordination may be difficult for these patients. Similarly, the limb spasticity associated with demyelinating disorders may prevent fine manual work or even the ability to stand for long periods.

Manual jobs require good muscle power and good peripheral sensation. Lifting or moving objects—particularly if repeated frequently—can be a problem for individuals with peripheral neuropathic disorders. This is especially so if the cause is a radiculopathy, as the repetitive movements may involve vertebral column movement and may exacerbate the original cause of the patient's disability.

Neurobehavioural disorders following head injury, stroke, or encephalitis may range from mild and transient to severe and permanent. Aphasias and apraxias can preclude employment which requires regular communication with other workers. Disturbance of spatial relationships may prevent the patient from driving, and memory disturbances are important for those with intellectually demanding jobs.

Work assessment

Establishing an accurate prognosis is important in neurological conditions. The clinical course may be episodic, transient, progressive or static. Such prognostic considerations are important for the patient's job prospects. Although some diseases such as epilepsy (see Chapter 8) have their own medico-legal implications, most disorders must be dealt with on an *ad hoc* basis. For example, the prognosis of multiple sclerosis is difficult to evaluate—especially at the outset. The disease may never cause more than a transient episode of blurred vision or may progress rapidly and inexorably to quadriparesis. Similarly, cerebrovascular disorders may range from a catastrophic intracerebral bleed to transient ischaemic episodes. Many stroke patients however, recover, at least partially, so it is important, wherever possible, to keep their original job open, albeit in a modified form. Such modifications may be temporary or permanent and will require periodic re-evaluation.

The consequences of neurological dysfunction are different for manual and non-manual workers. Sensory impairment or motor dysfunction (with or without a flaccid or spastic component) makes tasks involving power and/or co-ordination extremely difficult. By contrast, a degree of impairment in intellectual function might not be so serious for the manual worker.

The reverse is often true in non-manual occupations. A stroke patient with a hemiparesis may still be able to undertake a desk-bound job, particularly if the individual is helped to the desk and stays there. Commuting to work may be a bigger problem than the work itself. A stroke patient left with dysarthria or dysphasia will have difficulty with communication, memory recall, and accuracy.

Much can be done to improve the function of the disabled patient by appropriate rehabilitation.[5] Neurological disorders such as demyelinating diseases, extrapyramidal disorders and cerebrovascular accidents can be greatly ameliorated by rehabilitation procedures. However, regrettably, rehabilitation tends to be undervalued and underfunded. When the National Health Service proves inadequate, occupational medical facilities may be able to fill the gap. This can be cost-effective: training employees to a task can be expensive and it may be better to rehabilitate a partially disabled trained worker than to recruit a new one. Neurologically impaired employees should be offered rehabilitation at work. The occupational physician should be actively involved by directly intervening in matching the job to the disabled worker and by advising on reasonable adjustments.

Lay influences on employability

The commitment of the occupational physician to 'do something' for the employee who has developed a neurological disorder can be undermined, curtailed, or even prevented by uninformed lay opinion in the guise of 'management decisions'. Managers should refer all disabled patients to their occupational health adviser. In a well-organized company the health adviser will become aware of such patients as there will be a review procedure triggered by their sick leave. The occupational physician should ensure that managers harbour no misconceptions based on their inadequate lay state of knowledge. Many people, for example, believe that multiple sclerosis (MS) inevitably leads to an incontinent wheelchair-bound existence. Likewise, they often greatly underestimate the improvement in functional ability that can follow a stroke, either from the natural recovery process itself or from the effect of an appropriate rehabilitation programme.

Managers may also be puzzled by the problems of nominal dysphasia, or the variable nature of the disability of Parkinson's disease in a single day. It is the occupational physician's role to explain, to make the relevant clinical assessment, and to advise on the necessary job modifications.

In summary, neurological disease can create a wide variety of disabilities. **The clinical assessment of the symptoms and signs and the review of the patient's work capacity are much more important than the diagnostic label.** In the past the label itself may have been an impediment to future gainful employment through misconceptions about the neurological disability as much as failure to provide energetic and intelligent rehabilitation.

The Disability Discrimination Act 1995 (DDA) requires active, reasonable adjustment and in all these matters the occupational physician plays an important role.

How neurological illnesses influence work

The disability that a patient suffers is dependent on the symptoms and signs that the disease produces and not the disease itself. Injuries, and particularly head injuries, can lead to loss of function anywhere in the nervous system; occupational physicians must be familiar with patients and their work as well as the nature of their disease before they can determine their work capability.

Symptoms related to cranial nerves

Problems relating to the nerves of the eye and ear are considered in Chapters 9 and 10 respectively.

- **Smell**: Dysfunction of the sense of smell most commonly occurs after head injuries. Few jobs require a good sense of smell, but when it is lost there is usually a loss of taste apart from the four primary tastes of sweet, acid (sour), bitter, and salt. Cooks and professional tasters would therefore be handicapped by such a disability. In occupations using noxious substances a sense of smell may help an employee to detect an escape of the dangerous chemical, hence an employee with a loss of smell sensation would be at a greater risk.
- **Lesions of the trigeminal nerve** (v) lesions rarely influence work capacity, but the risk of trauma to the eye should be borne in mind when corneal sensation is lost. Employees working in dusty atmospheres are at risk if there is sensory loss in the ophthalmic division of the trigeminal nerve. In these circumstances there is an even greater need for the employee to wear protective glasses. In contrast, the pain of trigeminal neuralgia can be so great that concentration at work becomes impossible. The condition needs to be distinguished from psychogenic facial pain.
- **Bell's palsy** or **facial palsy** (vii) is common and by itself is not a handicap for most work. It is not painful and usually improves with time. However, it is disfiguring and if the work involves meeting the public it can be embarrassing. The only danger is to the eye. In the early stages, when the eye cannot be closed and the cornea is at risk of becoming dry and ulcerated, it is important to protect the eye. Wearing large protective glasses with side guards helps to protect the eye from wind which can dry the cornea and dust which can irritate it. If necessary a tarsorrhaphy will protect the eye and may even improve the appearance. Fortunately eye closure always recovers, even if the rest of the facial paralysis does not. Bell's palsy and other facial palsies should rarely be a cause of a long-term inability to work.
- **Swallowing and articulation**: (ix, xi, xii) Apart from those who earn their living by talking, such as teachers, broadcasters, or politicians, these problems are associated with social and home handicap far more than difficulty at work. Difficulty with breathing and paralysis of the respiratory muscles are also matters rarely requiring

special consideration at work as the patients so afflicted are usually unable to work. Speech therapists are skilled in re-educating patients to speak and swallow.

Symptoms related to the trunk and limbs

Patients with problems related to their trunk and limbs often find it difficult to describe their symptoms. This makes it difficult to categorize the problem. Often the word 'weakness' is used to describe inco-ordination and sensory symptoms and phrases like 'my hand feels wrong' are used to express weakness when there is no sensory change. The history is particularly important because it allows the patient to describe the problem. Once a patient has been allowed to give the history in their own way, other questions often help to disclose any disability. For example, 'Is there anything you cannot do now that you could do before?', 'Is there anything you would like to do but can't?'. In making an assessment for work the doctor can often be guided by a physiotherapist or occupational therapist. The doctor should explain clearly which problem they would like the therapist to assess. This will then enable them to establish the patient's disabilities and their opinion will be more firmly based.

Weakness can be due to many causes including an upper motor neurone lesion, a lower motor neurone lesion, a neuromuscular junction lesion, a muscle disease (myopathy), or a psychological cause. These causes can usually be distinguished from one another. However, it is hard to distinguish between a lower motor neurone lesion and a muscle disease if there is no sensory loss. The management of the different causes is different and the effects on work capability are different.

Upper motor neurone lesions

In an upper motor neurone lesion spasticity is often a major problem, but the patient's difficulties can often be helped by physiotherapy and rehabilitation. Retraining of movement patterns and posture and control of the trunk allow the central nervous system to adjust to the lesion, so function can be improved. Attempting to make the muscles stronger by using muscle strengthening exercises is usually contra-indicated. Physiotherapy at the place of work is of benefit if the doctor and physiotherapist work together. Small changes in posture at work and external aids can make a big difference to work capacity. The type of rehabilitation needs to be carefully planned, but the outcome is often rewarding. The employee should not expect, or be expected, to have made maximum or full recovery before work is resumed. The rehabilitation process will be helped if the patient can return to the job part-time. The process of going to work and performing a job is part of the rehabilitation and will allow problems to be identified at an early stage. If the patient's intellectual level is preserved employers will often be surprised by the degree of improvement that can occur and the slight extent of any residual disability.

Lower motor neurone lesions

With lower motor neurone diseases the situation is different. Unless there is very severe weakness the decreased tone does not cause a problem and the main difficulty is loss of power. In contrast to upper motor neurone lesions, physiotherapy should be designed to strengthen the appropriate muscles. If there is complete paralysis of a muscle other muscles may be strengthened and trick movements learnt. This will often enable the patient to return to work more quickly. The long-term prognosis depends on the pathology. In acute **Guillain–Barré syndrome** full recovery can occur. In progressive diseases such as MND treatment cannot halt the decline and excessive physiotherapy can lead to exhaustion and a worsening of symptoms. A physiotherapist and an occupational therapist can be helpful in rehabilitation. If there are localized sites of weakness splints may help and aids may allow an employee to work. In more severe cases an environmental control system may allow a severely disabled person to use office equipment and continue at work.[6]

Neuromuscular junction disease

Neuromuscular junction disease is rare and the only one likely to be encountered is **myasthenia gravis**. Patients with this disease find that exercise makes the weakness worse, so muscle strengthening exercises should not be suggested. The disease is difficult to diagnose in its early stages, when it may be misdiagnosed as hysteria if only the limbs are involved. The employee complains first of weakness when asked to do more physical work than usual. Weakness of the eye muscles after repeated movements makes the diagnosis easier but eye symptoms are not always present. If myasthenia is suspected an examination can be carried out before and after exercise, but even then the diagnosis may be difficult unless the edrophonium test is positive and a high acetylcholine receptor antibody titre can be demonstrated in the blood. Edrophonium is a short-acting drug which, when given intravenously, transiently reverses myasthenic weakness. Often the occupational physician will be in a better position to make the diagnosis than the general practitioner.

Muscular dystrophies

Muscle disease is less common than neurological disease. Muscular dystrophies, which are genetic disorders, will rarely become a problem in occupational medicine. The commonest, **Duchenne's dystrophy**, is usually so severe early in life that the patient never works. However, rarer dystrophies can progress very slowly producing increasing disability. The problem at work is usually confined to weakness and therefore with appropriate aids, for travelling to and moving about the workplace the patient can do sedentary work.

With environmental control systems,[6] such as the Possum, it is often possible to set up a workstation which will allow the employee to use a wordprocessor or a telephone, and even initiate simple mechanical tasks. An environmental control system is a computer with links to peripheral equipment, such as doors, telephones, and light switches. From a keyboard the patient can control the equipment; for more seriously disabled patients the keyboard can be simplified or replaced by a joystick which, although slower, needs only small movements, such as can be produced by the lips.[6] There are environmental control co-ordinators based at major rehabilitation units who can advise. The systems are available for home use under the NHS but at work they may allow a disabled person to continue useful work. Their provision would be best made after advice from the co-ordinator and with the help of an occupational therapist. With adequate access even the weakest person can use an electric wheelchair, of which there is a wide range. Specialist help should be sought in choosing the most appropriate one.[7]

Psychological muscle weakness

Weakness due to psychological factors is usually additional to a physical condition, so that the employee is unable to use their remaining potential for activity. If full recovery is to be achieved rehabilitation programmes for such patients should involve a psychological assessment, though not necessarily by a clinical psychologist or psychiatrist. The problem may be only one of confidence, and this could be restored by a skilled physiotherapist or occupational therapist. In these situations a therapist at the place of work is helpful. Specialist help from a psychiatrist or clinical psychologist may be needed. It is sometimes difficult to decide when to ask a psychiatrist because the outcome of rehabilitation cannot be easily assessed in its early stages. However, once it is clear that recovery, using ordinary rehabilitation processes, is not going to be satisfactory for psychological reasons, the help of a psychiatrist or clinical psychologist should be sought without delay.

Tone

Abnormalities of tone rarely occur by themselves. Nevertheless, in patients with long-standing upper motor neurone lesions the increase in tone can be out of proportion to the relatively lesser degree of weakness. In these cases the hypertonia leads to poor posture and clumsiness of movement which often affects the fine movements of the hands or the gait. Patients with these symptoms should not be given muscle strengthening exercises as these would increase their disability. Instead they need help with posture and patterns of movement. It is sometimes felt by employers that giving the patient a lighter or sedentary job might help, but as power may not be a problem a lighter job is not always easier to perform. Instead the patient needs a job which requires less skilful movements. For example, putting in small screws would be more difficult than a heavier, but less precise activity.

In **Parkinson's disease** the increased tone and rigidity is associated with bradykinesia. It is the slowness of movements which is usually the greatest disability. For example, a patient may walk easily for long distances in the open but with great difficulty in a crowded workshop when frequent changes of direction have to be made. The motor skills of patients with Parkinson's disease are considerably impaired. Unfortunately they are not easily helped by physiotherapy because their ability to retain and relearn motor skills is also impaired. Drug treatment is usually more rewarding. If an employee has Parkinson's disease and is unable to do their work in spite of help from the general practitioner and the occupational physician the help of a neurologist must be sought.

Sensory loss

The effects of sensory loss in the limbs can be more disabling than motor lesions, and can be a major handicap to employees. People rarely use their full power and have considerable reserves if they wish to use more force. However, sensation is often used to the full. It is difficult to compensate for even a mild sensory loss in the fingers, and no amount of physiotherapy and training will restore the sensory function. The symptoms and signs, and to an extent the disability, can only become better if the disease improves. Therefore physiotherapy has only a minor role. If the sensory loss involves touch and position sense the therapist can teach the patient about the disability and explain ways of diminishing it by careful use of other sensory organs; for example, using vision when walking rather than relying on the diminished position sense in the legs. A problem that employees are likely to encounter is difficulty with skilled movements of the hands. Using a different type of pen or better lighting or a wordprocessor may help to compensate for the disability.

Loss of sensation

Loss of pain and temperature sensation produces different problems. If touch and position sense are preserved, the patient's skilled use of the hands and walking are unaffected. However, the employee with loss of pain sensation is at risk because the normal protective response of withdrawing from dangerous stimuli is impaired. The employee may be at particular risk when there are hot surfaces or liquids at the place of work, as they may suffer a burn without realizing that they have been in contact with a source of extreme heat. With loss of pain and temperature sensation the patient may remain exposed to a moderate heat source for a long time and so suffer severe injury. Similarly, ill-fitting footwear may not be appreciated, resulting in skin damage. These difficulties occur most frequently in diabetic patients. In more severely disabled employees with a paraplegia the loss of sensation in the buttocks and legs produces a great risk of pressure sores. Proper seating to prevent trauma, both in the wheelchair and at the workstation, is important. Many rehabilitation units have physiotherapists and occupational therapists who specialize in seating appliances.[7]

Ataxia and inco-ordination

The results of ataxia and inco-ordination can be similar to those of peripheral sensory loss, but the disability is likely to be worse because other sensory input, for example vision, cannot be used in compensation. Unless the cause of the ataxia can be corrected, no amount of retraining will help. In these circumstances the environment must be changed if the ataxia is a cause of danger to the employee or if it limits their work. Aids are available for typewriters, wordprocessors, and other equipment which make it easier for such employees to carry out their work.

Loss of sphincter control

Poor sphincter control is a symptom of many neurological diseases. It is a problem at home and at work, and the management in both places is identical. By controlling fluid intake and having easy access to toilets it is usually possible for an employee to remain continent and to cope at work. However, these patients may have other disabilities that limit work effectiveness. During the acute stage of an illness which causes urinary retention or incontinence a catheter may be necessary, but usually the patient learns how to stimulate bladder reflex activity by abdominal pressure or other means and thereby regain control of micturition. This is more likely to be successful with a spinal cord lesion above the conus, and less successful when there is a peripheral nerve lesion. If control cannot be achieved, the use of a catheter with a bag on the leg, or intermittent self-catheterization, will permit employees to continue at work without the embarrassment of urinary incontinence. Faecal incontinence is usually unacceptable, and if it is a risk a careful bowel regime is essential. Laxatives may help to overcome constipation but make incontinence more likely. One method is for the patient to have no laxatives but to have an enema once or twice a week, at a selected convenient time, in the knowledge that they will then have a bowel action and be continent for several days till the next enema. This may possibly entail taking half a day a week off work, but this can be foreseen and planned.

Higher (cerebral) functions

- Many neurological diseases affect **mental functions**, but their influence on work depends very much on the job. A labourer can continue to work with a moderate, or sometimes even a severe intellectual impairment, but an executive cannot. There are no guidelines which can be used generally.
- **Memory loss and dementia** cannot be improved by treatment, but similar effects can arise iatrogenically, and in this latter situation, a reduction in medication may be beneficial. For example, anticonvulsants may impair memory. If the epilepsy is only nocturnal or partial, the epilepsy may be a lesser handicap than drug-induced drowsiness.
- **Presenile dementia, Alzheimer's disease**, is at present untreatable.
- With some neurological diseases **changes in mood** can be so severe as to be a handicap. It is common to develop secondary depression, as the illness tends to be very frustrating. This can be helped by antidepressants, which are best given at night when unwanted effects on mental function will be least. Occasionally, and especially in MS, euphoria may limit an employee's motivation to overcome their disability and to maintain their work potential.
- **Speech disorders**, whether dysphasia or dysarthria, can be helped by speech therapy but it is rare for such a major improvement to occur that it becomes the only therapy needed to enable the employee to return to work. It is often more effective to reduce the importance of speech in the job and to provide aids such as a wordprocessor. Speech aids can be used if the voice is very weak, as can occur in Parkinson's disease, but even then the problem is often the speed of speech as much as the volume. Dysphasia is often associated with dysgraphia, and dysarthria with swallowing problems, and therefore the handicap as a whole needs to be considered when planning therapy with a speech therapist.

Drug management

Patients with neurological disease are often given excessive drug treatment, and this can be a major factor in limiting their ability to work. Therefore, if a patient is unable to work it is important to assess their medication and, if possible, to stop all non-essential treatment that makes work more difficult. Although the long-term prognosis is important there may be occasions when this takes second place to the immediate symptoms. For example, if a patient who is still at work is found to have a cerebral tumour it might be better to maintain them at work leading a relatively normal life rather than submit them to biopsy and intensive therapy, which would curtail their work, in the slight hope of prolonging their life. There are no clear rules or guidelines for assessing the relative importance of present disabilities against future ones, but the work activity of the patient is an important factor which must be considered.

The use of **analgesics** requires as much care as any other medication. Clearly the underlying cause of the pain must be treated, but skill is required in selecting the correct analgesic. Clear advice must be given on how often the drugs should be taken. Some patients want to take them too often, others to take an inadequate dose. Only by discussing the situation with the patient can a correct drug regime be agreed. Any pain which is a disability and prevents efficient working must be controlled with sufficient prophylactic medication. If the employee takes no analgesia while working until pain impedes their work, then they have waited too long. If the pain is continuous or regular then the therapy needs to be taken regularly. The type of analgesia will depend on the cause of the pain; particular causes such as neuralgias may respond to particular therapies, such as carbamazepine.

It is rare for pain alone to prevent an employee working, but it is common for unrelieved pain to reduce the employee's work effectiveness.

Headache is probably the commonest pain which limits work.[8] Organic disease needs to be excluded, especially if the headache is of recent origin, or has changed its character, or if there is no obvious cause. Headaches of many years' duration in the absence of physical signs are rarely due to progressive organic disease. In the older worker temporal arteritis should be considered. The headache may be associated with tension, and treatment with a combination of analgesics and tranquillizers will often help. The analgesia needs to be sufficient to reduce the headache so that it no longer interferes with work and social activities. A small amount of regular analgesia may be more effective than large amounts taken only when the headache has become bad. Tranquillizers can be particularly helpful when taken at night if stress or pain is related to insomnia, which itself may exacerbate headaches. Tranquillizers should be used with caution during the daytime as drowsiness can make driving dangerous and reduce efficiency at work. They are best used for a short course when the patient is going through a limited period of stress because if continued for a long time habituation may result.

If the headaches become frequent the home and work environments must be considered to eliminate avoidable factors. The prevention of eye strain is considered in Chapter 9, pp. 174–175. Smoke, unpleasant smells, and inadequate ventilation make headaches more likely. Migraine is considered on p. 109. Post-traumatic headaches usually decrease over the months following the head injury, but may be prolonged if inadequate measures are taken to control them at the onset or if litigation adds to the stress.

How workplace factors influence neurological function

In considering neurological fitness for work, the most important thing is to review disability in relation to the work demands, and to assess the patient's current status. Nevertheless, it is useful to review specific workplace exposures that can cause or exacerbate neurological disease and which can influence work function. Workplace exposures can be classified as physical, psychological, and chemical. The exposures will be dealt with in turn, distinguishing where necessary between factors which exacerbate pre-existing disease from those which are specific causes of neurological deficit.

Physical agents

Noise

Noise is considered in Chapter 10. Although noise-induced hearing loss is the most obvious problem, other effects such as headaches, diminished ability to concentrate and communicate, and even perceived difficulties with balance can be important, particularly in a patient with imperfect neurological function.

The deafness caused by noise is due to damage to the organ of Corti, in the inner ear, but patients with pre-existing deafness (whether conductive or perceptive) should be protected from further damage. Furthermore, whilst some forms of deafness are ameliorated by the use of hearing aids, noise-induced hearing loss, with its specific effects mainly at 3–6 kHz, is not easily helped.

The problems with communication are two-fold:

- It is difficult to communicate at all at high ambient noise levels and while wearing ear muffs or plugs.
- Some patients may already have a neurological dysfunction which limits communication. This could be a speech defect or a defective ability to interpret speech. Such patients, in particular, should avoid noisy work situations which may worsen their impairment.

Vibration

Vibration is widespread in industry and, often accompanies noise. The health hazards generally occur at vibration frequencies between 1 and 1000 Hz. The vibration may be whole body, as occurs in truck drivers where the vibration is generally at the lower end of the range (1–10 Hz). Hand-transmitted vibration occurs when the worker holds a vibrating tool, such as a chain saw or pneumatic drill, or holds the workpiece to a vibrating machine as in some metal finishing processes. Such vibrations range from 10–1000 Hz.

Little is known about the chronic effects of whole-body vibration (apart from specific influences on body organ resonance and perhaps an association with osteoarticular disorders), but the effects of hand–arm vibration are well recognized and can be disabling. The patient may be unable to undertake fine finger movements and as the vascular component is certainly exacerbated by cold, work is more difficult in the colder months of the year and certain outdoor hobbies may have to be curtailed. Again, a patient who already has a peripheral sensory deficit should be advised to avoid work with exposure to vibration.

Work-related upper limb disorders (WRULDs) are considered in Chapter 14, p. 285.

Temperature

Extremes of temperature may cause a variety of effects but particular interest lies in the influence of temperature on patients with pre-existing neurological disease. At high temperatures the symptoms of MS worsen temporarily but recover when the temperature falls. Such patients should, wherever possible, avoid workplaces where high ambient temperatures are common. However, high temperature does not induce exacerbations of the disease or worsen the prognosis. In contrast, low temperatures, apart from producing a lowered ability for anyone to perform skilled activity, are a particular problem for patients with myotonic disorders especially myotonia congenita.

Light

Poor lighting at work is a particular problem for the visually impaired (Chapter 9). Both poorly lit and dazzlingly bright workplaces may cause headaches. It is thus important that the employee has the correct glasses. Photosensitive epilepsy is considered in Chapter 8. Flashing lights can also precipitate migraine.

Atmospheric pressure

Most of the adverse effects of raised atmospheric pressure in working environments result from the effects of decompression. Neurological damage is associated with the anoxic effect of gas bubbles blocking small blood vessels during the process of decompression following exposure to high pressure. Initial acute symptoms and signs depend on the areas affected but can include sensory and motor dysfunction, dizziness, and headaches leading to convulsions and coma in the worst affected cases. The chronic effects of repeated damage may be extremely difficult to distinguish from other neurological disorders and can, for example, mimic multiple sclerosis, Parkinsonism, or presenile dementia. The commonest source of such exposures is diving, either professionally or for pleasure, and the effects can be disabling and permanent (see also Appendix 4). In general, someone with established neurological disease should avoid exposure to raised pressure (diving and compressed air work) or reduced pressure (flying in non-pressurized aircraft). However, the neurological problems associated with changes in pressure are almost invariably due to inappropriately rapid decompression and so recreational pursuits, if carefully managed, need not be barred.

Psychological factors

Psychiatric disorders are dealt with in Chapter 7, but it should be remembered that a number of adverse psychological effects from work can influence patients with neurological disorders. Apart from stress and boredom there are effects from shiftwork which could either mimic or exacerbate neurological disorders. The main adverse effect of shiftwork is fatigue. Many workers complain of it, and it can result in tiredness or even drowsiness at work with insomnia when attempting to sleep. In practice these symptoms may be more noticeable, in the short term, than the gastrointestinal or cardiovascular effects found in large-scale longitudinal surveys of shiftworkers. The circadian rhythm disruption caused by rotating shiftwork, although measurable, is rarely translated into overt symptoms other than fatigue. For the patient with pre-existing neurological disease this may worsen work performance whatever the nature of the original deficit (motor, sensory, or cerebral function). Obviously a patient with myasthenia or narcolepsy would be particularly affected. The financial pressures to continue shiftwork may be considerable and it must be remembered that some shift patterns (particularly the 10 or 12 hour shift) do provide opportunities for a second job on the days off shifts.

Chemical factors

Neurological damage may sometimes arise from chemical hazards in the workplace. More often non-occupational neurological disorders mimic this appearance. Patients with a non-occupational neurological deficit may also have their symptoms exacerbated by workplace exposure. This is particularly true of organic solvents which are widely used in manufacturing industry, dry-cleaning, degreasing, and paint production and application.

Neurobehavioural disorders and organic solvents

The effects of organic solvents range from mild fatigue to frank psychosis. In view of the vague nature of many of the manifestations, psychometric testing has proved useful for both chemical and epidemiological studies. Nevertheless, there is still considerable controversy over the severity of effects that can arise from workplace exposure. Psychosis, dementia and compensatable disability appear to be frequent in Scandinavian studies but less severe effects have been described in other western countries.

By contrast to organic solvents, the clear cut peripheral neuropathy induced by such chemicals as inorganic lead compounds, *n*-hexane and methyl-*n*-butyl-ketone are relatively easy to evaluate. In these cases, the underlying pathology is either axonal degeneration and/or segmental demyelination. The neuropathy is normally mixed sensorimotor, but inorganic lead is exceptional in causing a pure motor neuropathy.

Other neurological effects

Parkinsonism can be a feature of poisoning by carbon disulfide, manganese and, possibly, carbon monoxide; epilepsy is a feature of toxicity associated with organochlorine pesticides and the organic compounds of tin, mercury, and lead.

Conclusion

It is rare for clinical conditions from neurotoxic causes to cause inability to work. Clearly, adequate protection and regular clinical assessment are important.

Specific diseases

Earlier in this chapter the relation between signs and symptoms of disease and work were considered. Although the signs and symptoms often give a better assessment of work capability than the underlying diagnosis, the latter is important in assessing the prognosis and future work capability. It needs to be known when deciding whether a person should be employed, recommending what adjustment(s) should be made, or recommending retirement on the grounds of ill health. Very often it is not possible with brain disease to decide how much of the employee's disability is physical and how much psychological, and it can even be a disadvantage to attempt to be precise in separating them.

The diseases in the following section are listed in rough order of frequency.

Migraine

Headache is common. In a workplace survey at Cable and Wireless in 1996 involving 1897 employees, 87% had experienced a severe headache in the previous year, 14% of whom had experienced 6 or more. In 73% it had lasted more than 4 hours and Table 6.2 shows their self-perceived limitation of work.

Migraine is common and leads to headache-related sickness absence, but migraine sufferers do not have a higher total sickness rate than other employees.[8,9] However, it is estimated that migraine sufferers are less effective at work, on average, for 20 days per annum. Improved diagnosis and management can lead to improved personal and corporate productivity and recent texts highlight what can be achieved.[10] Migraine is frequently familial and usually starts in childhood, sometimes as bilious attacks with abdominal pain and vomiting. It usually presents with a focal neurological symptom and then progresses to a unilateral headache. It is not uncommon for some of the attacks to occur without the aura or for the aura to occur without the headache. The manifestation of the migraine can change with time so an alteration in the character does not necessarily mean a new pathology. If the attacks occur sometimes on one side and sometimes on the other, even if the attacks on one of the sides are rare, it is most unlikely that the migraine is symptomatic of any underlying localized pathology. However, if all the attacks are on one side then a structural underlying pathology needs to be considered.

If an employee has headaches due to migraine, management should aim at avoidance of precipitants. Many factors, some of which occur at work, can precipitate migraine. It is helpful for the employee to note down activities in the 24 hours before an attack. It may then be easier to identify any precipitating factor. Precipitation of an attack by specific foods is well recognized, but less obvious factors may emerge. Missing meals, alcohol the previous night, or sleeping in late, as well as environmental factors such as temperature and humidity, may be implicated. Occupational health professionals can help to identify the factors and hopefully to remove them. Often patients are reluctant to take sufficient analgesics or seek medical advice if non-prescription medicine is inadequate. When an attack occurs, early treatment with simple analgesic agents is usually sufficient, but for those with more severe symptoms specific treatment with ergotamine or a 5-hydroxytryptamine agonist may be necessary. Sumatriptan, a 5-hydroxytryptamine agonist, is available as an injection and as a tablet for use in the acute attack. Sumatriptan should not be used for prophylaxis. More recently naratriptan and zolmitriptan, new

Table 6.2 How long does a headache limit work? (R. Willcox, 1996, unpublished data)

Answer	Number	%
None	158	22.6
1 hour	146	20.9
1–6 hours	199	28.4
6–24 hours	124	17.7
1–2 days	58	8.3
2–7 days	15	2.1
Total	700	

5-HT agonists, have become available. The many routes of administering ergotamine reflects the variability of response. For those with infrequent but predictable migraine, for example premenstrually, a 2 mg ergotamine suppository, or even a half of one, may prevent the attacks. For those who need rapid relief Lingraine, which can be sucked and absorbed through the buccal mucosa, or an ergotamine inhaler, may work. Ergotamine can have serious side-effects, especially if used frequently, and therefore the prescriptions should be carefully monitored. No acute medication should be used more often than twice a week. Prophylactic options include pizotifen, beta-blockers, and amitryptiline.

More important than the medication itself is the way in which the migraine is handled in the workplace. There is no particular work which is unsuitable for migraine sufferers, but if a patient knows of specific precipitants for migraine these should be avoided or work moved to a more congenial environment. A relatively relaxed attitude by the employer (for example allowing the employee to lie down or rest for a while when the attack starts) and a sympathetic understanding will mean that the employee spends less time off work. Employees will have greater confidence to go to work if they know that an attack at work will be more acceptable—the alternative being to miss work and stay at home. Psychological factors are less important in migraine than in stress and tension headaches.

To be classified under the DDA a condition must be substantial and permanent. Migraine qualifies only rarely, when there needs to be regular preventive medication and no change in the attack pattern is likely. Workplace adjustment might be required in terms of changing lighting or temperature and providing a quiet dark room when a sufferer needs to rest. Migraineurs are likely to be precluded from some safety-critical jobs such as airline pilots and aerial climbers.

Cerebrovascular disease

Cerebrovascular disease can be conveniently divided into two categories, ischaemic and haemorrhagic; the former may lead to infarction. The two may sometimes occur together as haemorrhage can occur into an infarct or the haemorrhage may precipitate arterial spasm and hence ischaemia and an infarct. The method of stroke management depends as much on the clinical state as on the underlying pathology.[11]

Ischaemia

Ischaemic events can be minimal, with only transient numbness or loss of vision and, in themselves, are unlikely to be a handicap at work other than for drivers or work with dangerous machinery. However, transient ischaemic attacks (TIAs) often precede a serious stroke, so the patient should be investigated in order to instigate prophylactic management. Occasionally investigations demonstrate a moderate stenosis of the internal carotid artery without complete occlusion which may be amenable to surgery. If there is no contra-indication, such as hypertension, recurrent TIAs would usually be treated with anticoagulants.

The severity of a cerebral infarct can vary considerably; sometimes there is complete functional recovery; at other times the disability is profound and permanent and incompatible with a return to work. No conclusion about work capability can be made on the diagnosis alone. When the patient is mobile a functional assessment can be made by a physiotherapist or occupational therapist and, with the occupational physician, a policy for future management can be planned. A visit to the workplace by an occupational therapist is helpful in planning return to work or adjustment of work practices.

The time to maximum recovery varies widely, but can be a year or more. However, after about 4 months it is usually possible to give a reliable prognosis as by then the functions which are recovering can clearly be discerned and any function which has not started to recover is unlikely to do so. For example, if a person is unable to walk, even with mechanical aids, by the end of 4 months of therapy it is unlikely that unaided walking will ever be achieved; but if they can walk, say, 200 yards, it is possible that a year later they will be able to walk more than a mile. However, a final prognosis should not be given until the employee has received optimum physiotherapy and rehabilitation. Long-term therapy should concentrate on improving functions. Persisting disabilities may be overcome with mechanical aids or alterations in work practices. Rehabilitation after a cerebral infarct requires considerable skill. If there is any problem the employee should be referred to a rehabilitation specialist even if the disability is not gross. The prognosis for further strokes depends on the underlying pathology. Cardiac factors, blood pressure, and medication can all be important in assessing the prognosis. It would be wrong to prevent a person returning to work just because the employer is concerned that a further episode might occur. Each employee needs to have the prognosis assessed individually and reasonable adjustment made in work practices.

Haemorrhages

With a **haemorrhagic intracerebral stroke** the clinical situation is usually much more serious; most patients become unconscious and death is frequently the outcome. If the cerebral haemorrhage is small some recovery will occur, but because of the cerebral destruction by blood at arterial pressure there is usually a permanent deficit. The rehabilitation process is similar to that in cerebral infarction, except that there is a longer period of acute illness before functional recovery starts.

Decisions about returning to work need not be taken early, especially while improvement is still occurring and there is a reason for optimism. However, once a plateau is reached in the recovery further improvement is unlikely. The prognosis for a further attack depends, as for an infarct, on the underlying cause of the cerebrovascular disease.

If a **subarachnoid haemorrhage** is not severe, bleeding is confined to the subarachnoid space and recovery is complete. In more severe cases there may be cerebral damage, which can be transient or permanent. The rehabilitation process is similar to that of a patient with a cerebral infarct. If the subarachnoid haemorrhage is due to an aneurysm which is treated successfully by surgery then the prognosis is very good and a further haemorrhage is unlikely.

Cerebral tumours

Unlike tumours elsewhere in the body, cerebral tumours do not metastasize outside the central nervous system. The malignancy of a tumour can vary from very benign to rapidly malignant. Most benign tumours can be treated successfully by surgery, some of the malignant ones can be halted by radiotherapy, and a few are amenable to chemotherapy.

After treatment, an assessment of the employee's function and information about the prognosis usually facilitates decisions about work. If function is good, return to work should be automatic but if it is not then the decision to return will rest on two opposing trends:

- the natural improvement that will occur with rehabilitation and recovery from the surgery or other treatment, which is not dissimilar to recovery from a stroke
- the natural history of the tumour, which if malignant or liable to recur, makes the long-term prognosis worse.

In practice information about this is usually available, and the decisions are rarely difficult.

Head injuries

In more severe cases improvement can continue for up to 2 years, but in some cases the injury is so bad and the brain damage so extensive that there is never any possibility of returning to work.[12] However, there are many patients whose injuries are not obviously very severe yet who have difficulty in returning successfully to their previous work.

Many patients with severe head injuries will have other trauma such as fractured limbs, and this hinders recovery. The prognosis is worse when there is associated impairment of vision, hearing, or speech. The prognosis is improved if the previous job remains available and the employer is prepared to make special provisions on return to work.

With concussion multiple minor, or major, injuries occur in the brain with contusion and disruption of cerebral connections. However, the physical signs of organic disease can be minimal. The patient may look normal but feel unwell. A plaster for a simple limb fracture will often prevent a patient turning up for work, but a conscientious employee who has had concussion may seek to return to work too quickly. The plaster encourages sympathy from the employer, but the employee who looks well but complains of a severe headache and cannot concentrate on their work is less well tolerated. The decision when to advise someone with a head injury to return to work[12] can be difficult and it is important that the patient should be given sufficient time to recover. If there are any specific problems the advice and help of an occupational therapist may be needed.

Headaches after brain trauma are common, and are more severe and more frequent if the patient is under stress or working hard. The patient may feel well when resting at home but headaches develop when they have to cope with commuting and the physical and mental demands of their job. It is therefore helpful to allow them to return to work gradually. Returning to work on a Thursday rather than a Monday will mean that after 2 days work they have an opportunity to rest. It is unfortunate and medically illogical that most patients are asked to return to work at the start of a week. In more severe cases a planned return to work with advice from the occupational health service may enable half-day working, say from 10.30 a.m. to 3 p.m., to be considered; or 3 days a week for a few weeks so that in the long term readjustment is more successful.

Symptomatic treatment for post-concussional headaches and other symptoms is important. A small regular dose of an analgesic for a few weeks may be better than waiting for the headache to become severe and then finding that the analgesia does not work. Most patients want to return to work, and with good management this can be achieved successfully.

Unfortunately there are a significant number of patients after head injuries who, without having any demonstrable physical signs, have problems with rehabilitation. This may be because they were encouraged to get back to work too quickly, developed increasing or further symptoms, and lost faith in their ability to recover. Psychological problems are common for many reasons. They can result directly from physical injury to the brain, or arise independently of the trauma. For example, an employee who has been assaulted may suffer from mental trauma as well as the physical trauma and counselling may be necessary. Sometimes the sympathetic encouragement of an employer can help the patient to return to work gradually and so develop confidence, instead of further anxiety. Insomnia is common in this group. Occasionally night sedation is helpful, but should never be allowed to become a habit. More often a tricyclic antidepressant taken only at night will help. The initial dose should be low in order to avoid unwanted effects and then gradually increased if needed.

Patients with neuroses are more difficult to rehabilitate and require a lot of time and effort on the health professionals' part. The neurosis may be fostered by a legal claim for compensation. If the head injury occurred at work this is particularly true and poses unique problems for the occupational physician who has a clinical duty to the patient and an advisory one to the employer. These patients often require specialist help to secure a correct assessment of the problem and appropriate treatment.

Intellectual impairment without other physical signs is not common after head injury, but if suspected and especially if work capability might be affected, it needs to be assessed specifically. Psychometric testing will usually establish the extent of any organic impairment and in association with an occupational therapist's assessment and a knowledge of the work requirement, it may be used to formulate appropriate plans for a return to work. As with other organic lesions of the brain, functional improvement does occur but takes time and, depending on the severity of the injury, may not be complete. For an employee in an executive job it can be counterproductive to return to work too abruptly and a gradual return to work is preferable, taking on only some responsibilities at first and then adding to them. All sedatives and medication which might impair intellectual function or reduce concentration should be stopped unless absolutely necessary. Tranquillizers which might reduce anxiety will only make thought processes slower and can be counterproductive unless taken in the evening for insomnia. Occasionally there is a good indication for medication, for example if there is epilepsy or if depression is reducing intellectual function.

Employees should be advised to do everything they can for themselves to help recovery. This means eating regularly, going to bed at reasonable hours, and adjusting their lifestyle to improve performance. Alcohol should be prohibited until the employee is working to their own satisfaction and their work is acceptable to their employer. Alcohol-related problems[13,14] are not uncommon in patients who have had head injuries (perversely in those who should most avoid alcohol).

Birth injuries and congenital cerebral palsies

In **cerebral palsy** the patient may have no intellectual impairment despite considerable physical disability. Likely success in employment is usually decided long before the patient seeks work. Good training and education allow the child to develop their potential abilities and should result in qualifications for an appropriate job. Minor physical disabilities are rarely a problem except when skilled motor activities are needed. With modern technology there is more need to develop intellectual skills. Many machines can be adapted and driving is usually possible, although this may require special adaptations.

For the employer it is easier to assess the long-term potential of the employee because birth injuries and congenital cerebral palsies are not progressive. With age secondary problems may occur earlier than in the normal population; for example arthritis in a hip is more likely if the gait is affected, but these changes do not develop quickly. At the start of employment it is advisable to have a full medical and functional assessment so that work can be adjusted to allow the employee to use their skills with optimum efficiency. Congenital disease of the spinal cord such as spina bifida is managed in the same way.

Spinal cord

Spinal cord disease secondary to vertebral and disc diseases is considered in Chapter 11. The commonest cause of acute spinal cord lesions is trauma, a significant proportion of which occurs at work. Primary spinal canal tumours are rare and are usually benign, the commonest being neurofibromas. Secondary malignant metastases, especially from the breast and bronchus, are common but are usually associated with advanced disease and management is dictated by the primary neoplasm. The commonest neurological spinal disease is MS.

Multiple sclerosis (MS)

Clinically the diagnosis of MS depends on the demonstration of multiple lesions disseminated in time and space in the central nervous system. Magnetic resonance imaging (MRI) allows lesions to be demonstrated when they are not causing clinical symptoms and hence the diagnosis can be made more easily after a single clinical episode. Evoked potentials can be used to assess the speed of conduction of the nerve impulse within the nervous system. The most commonly used is the visual evoked potential. The response to flashing or other visual stimulation can be recorded in the posterior part of the brain. The response is an assessment of the speed of the nerve impulse from the eye to the visual cortex; when there is demyelination in the optic pathways the response is delayed.

Other evoked potentials, produced by a sound in the ear or stimulation of a limb, can be measured. A delay in response is not proof of MS because other diseases can cause delay, but it can provide evidence of a symptomless lesion and hence demonstrate that there are lesions at more than one site.

A doctor should be cautious before making a diagnosis of MS. In the early stage, the findings may be compatible with various diagnoses and it is often only later that the true diagnosis becomes apparent. Therefore at presentation MS is often a differential, rather than a definitive diagnosis. MS can have a wide range of outcomes. There may be only one clinical episode, with full recovery, and no other trouble throughout life, or it may progress rapidly, or there may be any other gradation in between. The manifestations vary enormously, but they are always due to a lesion of the central nervous system and never the peripheral nervous system. (The optic nerve is a part of the central nervous system and not a peripheral nerve.)

Common manifestations are a single episode of visual deterioration lasting only a few weeks, an area of sensory disturbance in a limb or on the trunk, or an episode of ataxia or sphincter disturbance.

MS usually starts during working age and therefore may develop after an employee has passed a medical examination at the time of initial employment.[17] However, in the era of flexible working practices, pre-employment assessments are likely to increase. Individuals will be covered by the DDA once symptoms interfere with day to day activity.

Some symptoms may influence working ability. Because there is such variation it is impossible to predict the prognosis. On the whole the more frequent the attacks and the less complete the recovery from individual episodes the worse the prognosis. After a single episode with full recovery the prognosis should be hopeful and an employee should be encouraged to return to normal work. If the attacks are infrequent and there is full recovery after each, the amount of time off work over a period of years could be small.[17] No precipitating factors for exacerbations are known and therefore there is no work environment which will alter the prognosis. However, if a patient has not made a full recovery it is possible that certain environments may make the symptoms greater or more obvious. High temperatures are not well tolerated and some patients like to work in slightly colder environments than is usually desired by other employees as this reduces their symptoms. Poor sleep and irregular hours are other factors which may worsen symptoms.

If an employee has established disease then adjustments in work practices may be needed and these will depend on the clinical manifestations and the nature of the work. For those already in work, the majority remain at work for more than 5 years. Attacks of the disease can be acute with good recovery, in which case a limited period of rehabilitation may speed return to work. In more chronic cases regular assessment will be required to decide about physiotherapy or other ongoing help. Urgency of micturition is common but if there is easy access to toilets incontinence is rare. In very severe cases special arrangements may be necessary to enable the use of a wheelchair.

Occasionally, if there is considerable demyelination of the white matter in the brain, there is intellectual deterioration, but usually intellectual function is preserved and this means that if the employee has a sedentary job MS should not occasion medical retirement. Psychological problems do occur in chronic illness and these need to be considered by the employee's medical advisers. Depression is fairly common. Euphoria, best defined in this context as pathological contentment, is often mentioned as a symptom of MS. It is not common but it is more so than in other central nervous system diseases. Patients who are not severely disabled often accept the illness and appear not to be too distressed by their problems. This has advantages for the sufferer as a patient, but not as an employee, as increased commitment is needed to overcome the disability and to continue to cope at work. Euphoria can remove the wish to 'fight' the disability, whereas motivation to work is a very important factor in deciding whether employment can continue. Most patients with continuing symptoms from MS will have attended hospital and their diagnosis and management policy will have been determined. If this has not occurred, referral to a specialist should be made before the employee's future work situation is decided. Recently β-interferon has been used as prophylactic therapy for those with relapsing or remitting MS, but its long-term value is uncertain. It is not a panacea.

Peripheral neuropathy

Neuropathy is a common condition. About 85% of all patients with peripheral neuropathy have diabetes mellitus and the control of the diabetes is the most important factor in the management of the neuropathy. It is necessary for the employee to take particular care of their feet. The second most common cause of peripheral neuropathy is alcohol abuse. In the early stages, alcoholic neuropathy is reversible if the employee ceases taking alcohol and is given vitamin B. Taking vitamin B without stopping alcohol is insufficient, although it may delay the onset, making the neuropathy less easy to reverse when it does occur. Other medical causes of a peripheral neuropathy are relatively rare, but should be sought if no obvious cause is apparent. **Subacute combined degeneration**, due to vitamin B_{12} depletion may come on insidiously, but the neuropathy always responds to vitamin B_{12} injections, although the spinal cord lesion may not.

Hereditary motor and sensory neuropathies, one type of which used to be called **Charcot–Marie–Tooth disease**, can also be insidious, producing gradually increasing disability. A family history makes the diagnosis easier, but as some are due to recessive genes sporadic cases may arise. Usually the signs precede the disability, and poor muscle bulk in the hands or the legs will alert a doctor to the possibility of this diagnosis. The disease is not a reason to cease work and as progression is slow the patient can often continue at work for many years and retire at the normal time. In some severe cases, mechanical aids such as a toe raising splint may increase function.

Peripheral neuropathy is a recognized complication of many toxic chemicals and therefore the onset of a peripheral neuropathy should always alert the doctor to the possibility of toxic chemical exposure at work.

Muscle diseases

Acute muscle disease such as myositis is usually associated with some other disease, on which its prognosis will depend.

Motor neurone disease (MND)

Although rare, MND is an important disease in relation to work. It tends to come on during middle age, before retirement, and progresses relentlessly causing death on average within 3 years of diagnosis. In the early stages it can be difficult to diagnose as the presentation may not be striking. For example, if the condition starts with a weakness in one foot, this may lead to a fall and, perhaps, a sprained ankle and for some time the slow and incomplete recovery may be attributed to trauma or loss of motivation to return to work. However, with time the progression of the disease to other sites makes the diagnosis easier.

Unfortunately no amount of physiotherapy or medication will improve the weakness of MND. In fact excess physiotherapy may exhaust patients, making it harder for them to do their work. Management should be aimed at allowing patients to lead as normal a life as possible. Speech therapy and communication aids are frequently needed as the bulbar muscles are often involved and are usually the major reason for physical deterioration and death. Late in the illness the patient is unable to swallow and will inhale saliva. Unfortunately there is no curative treatment and therefore tracheostomy is rarely justified. Mental ability is unimpaired and with environmental aid systems the patient may be able to manipulate the environment by using a computer-driven motor to open doors, turn on lights, or operate a telephone, as well as being able to use the computer for more ordinary tasks such as writing letters.

Parkinson's disease

Parkinson's disease often starts in the sixth decade, especially if it is idiopathic. Its symptoms and signs were discussed earlier (see p. 102). Cerebrovascular parkinsonism starts later and is usually a part of generalized cerebrovascular disease. There are other less common causes. This means that most Parkinson's disease in the working population is idiopathic. It may very rarely be associated with exposure to manganese, to which the occupational physician should be alert. Drug-induced parkinsonism, from psychotropic drugs, is common. When this occurs it is necessary to review the psychiatric management and if it is deemed important to continue the psychotropic drug, antiparkinsonion therapy may need to be added. The patient may not develop a tremor, although this is often the most striking feature to a lay person. The most disabling feature is the bradykinesia (slowness and poverty of movement). The patient's tremor decreases on voluntary movement and is rarely a disability unless fine movements are needed. However, the bradykinesia makes the employee slower and if there is no tremor colleagues do not realize that the individual has a physical illness.

As Parkinson's disease responds to treatment, an early diagnosis is important. An astute colleague will realize that the employee is not being lazy although they will be slow at dressing, eating. and at everyday tasks as well as being slow at their work. However, some employers mistakenly assume that slowness of movement means slowness of thought, and that a diagnosis of Parkinson's disease is incompatible with further employment. Most patients with Parkinson's disease can stay at work until the usual retirement age. A conscientious employee will often compensate by getting to work early or staying late to refute possible suggestions of laziness. The patient's writing will become smaller (it is often found that their writing was getting smaller long before any other disability was noted). In this respect Parkinson's disease is different from senile or idiopathic tremor in which there is no rigidity and no bradykinesia and the writing does not become smaller though it is spidery and tremulous.

Parkinson's disease responds well to levodopa preparations, Madopar and Sinemet being the two most widely used. Adjusting the dosage to give a good response without unwanted effects may be difficult and much care is required to achieve the optimum dose. This should be kept as small as compatible with good functional improvement. The therapeutic utility of levodopa decreases the longer it is used, so that unwanted effects become worse and its duration of action becomes shorter. Therefore the administration of levodopa should be delayed if the parkinsonism is mild and the employee has no disability. Selegiline, a monoamine oxidase B inhibitor, can enhance the action of levodopa. Antimuscaranic drugs, such as benzhexol, can also be used. Most employees who are able to travel to work and perform their duties satisfactorily will not benefit from physiotherapy, but if the condition is severe, advice from a physiotherapist can often help them to remain at work. When physiotherapy is needed it must be appropriate; muscle strengthening exercises or the methods used to treat strokes are not appropriate. In Parkinson's disease the ability to learn new motor skills is impaired, so inability to execute the physiotherapist's instructions can be a manifestation of the illness and not a failure to co-operate.

Patients with Parkinson's disease have difficulty in performing skilled movements and are particularly bad at developing new skills. However, if the motor skill is a long-standing one, such as playing the piano learned in childhood, it may be retained when other apparently much easier tasks are impossible. Employees with Parkinson's disease should not take early retirement unless the disease makes work impossible as work activities have a therapeutic benefit. Most employees with Parkinson's disease have normal intellectual function, although there is a group, especially the older patients, who do develop intellectual impairment.

Essential (idiopathic or familial) tremor

Benign tremor is common and not associated with bradykinesia or rigidity. It is rarely a disability, except that handwriting may become scrawly. The tremor can be embarrassing and may be mistaken for Parkinson's disease. Reassurance is all that is required, or, rarely a β adrenergic blocking drug.

Alzheimer's disease and dementia

Dementia develops most often after retirement, but when it does occur in someone of working age it is a major problem. Dementia often develops very insidiously. If the employee has been at the same job for many years the dementia may be less obvious. The individual can work relatively well in familiar surroundings at routine tasks but new tasks are difficult. Colleagues will often be aware of the deterioration. Unfortunately there is no treatment and a decision needs to be made about continuing employment. Alcohol is an important factor in exacerbating the dementia, whether it is taken acutely or over a long period.

Rare CNS degenerations such as Creuzfeldt–Jakob disease are usually incompatible with work.

Encephalitis

Encephalitis is relatively rare, and its prognosis and influence on work ability vary. Herpes encephalitis can cause considerable brain damage and these patients may never get back to intellectually demanding occupations. Other, less severe types of encephalitis usually result in full recovery. AIDS encephalitis is a progressive disease which leads to increasing dementia and has a very bad prognosis.

Chronic fatigue syndrome

Chronic fatigue syndrome (CFS) was previously, inappropriately, known as myeloencephalitis (ME). The condition is not well defined although often diagnosed. The symptom complex is best called chronic fatigue syndrome[18] as this highlights the chronic fatigue which is the only certain aspect of the disease. A viral or other illness may precede the syndrome, but this is not invariable and has led to the illness being called postviral fatigue syndrome. There is no evidence of myelitis or encephalitis and no evidence that it is due to a chronic viral infection. For most patients the condition remits spontaneously, but protracted symptoms, in the absence of physical signs, are characteristic and probably due to several factors, both physical and mental.

CFS does not have any explicit diagnostic criteria and there is uncertainty as to whether it is a single clinical entity. Standard laboratory tests are normal. It is important to exclude other illnesses and to formulate a policy for management and rehabilitation which is multidisciplinary, perhaps involving the help of occupational physicians, other physicians, occupational therapists, physiotherapists, or psychiatrists. Following any illness a convalescent phase will arise when exercise and mental and emotional stress are less well tolerated. However, in CFS exercise is important and should be gradually encouraged as resting muscles cannot maintain their strength and endurance.[19] However, excessive exercise leads to increased symptoms. Initially the amount of exercise and mental activity should be small, but gradually increased at a rate which will depend on response. Returning too quickly to a stressful job can lead to poor performance, loss of confidence, and exacerbation of the symptoms. Employees should be encouraged to work themselves back into a job—if a manual worker possibly by starting work on a Thursday or a Friday so that a weekend's rest follows or, if working at a desk, by only doing undemanding work for the first week. People vary in the amount of convalescence needed, and the doctor needs to give individual advice. However, a gradual improvement is to be expected. If symptoms fail to improve or if there has been no definite preceding illness, appropriate specialist advice should be sought. Unfortunately it is not uncommon for CFS patients to fail to recover rapidly enough to return to their normal employment, and, if they do, the adjustment required under the DDA may be neither possible nor reasonable. However, with patience and a firm, encouraging and supportive framework, a gradual return to work should be possible in most cases.

Driving

Decisions on fitness to drive[15,16] can be difficult for patients with head injuries or neurological diseases. The Driving Licence Regulations and the role of the Driving and Vehicle Licensing Agency (DVLA) are discussed in Appendix 1, and the particular problems arising in relation to epilepsy are discussed in Chapter 8. With neurological disease or trauma to the nervous system, the problem is whether the deficit in neurological function is a bar to driving. The doctor should assess the ability of the patient to operate car controls and to respond quickly, accurately, and intelligently to driving conditions. The driving licence states that if a person develops a new medical condition that person must write to inform the Drivers Medical Group, DVLA, Swansea SA99 1TU. The final decision on whether or not a patient should drive lies with the DVLA and ultimately with the courts if a person wishes to challenge the DVLA. The doctor's duty is to advise the patient to inform the DVLA if there is the slightest possibility that driving might be impaired.

In the rare circumstances where the occupational physician judges there to be a significant risk to the public and the patient refuses to inform the DVLA, the physician should consult his professional indemnity association. If the physician has the agreement of his professional indemnity organization he can then write to the DVLA (Appendix 1).

The DVLA will seek further information from the doctor. An occupational physician may have to advise the patient and their employer, for whom the occupational physician is acting, that the patient should not drive until the DVLA has been made aware of the full circumstances to allow driving.

The patient may be able to adapt their car, for example by installing hand controls so that the foot controls are not needed. Adaptations will be considered when deciding whether a licence can be issued or continued. The DVLA may ask doctors with special experience of such cases to assess the patient. A patient who is judged unfit to drive, may, on improvement in their medical condition, reapply to the DVLA.

Employers have a responsibility to ensure that their drivers are medically fit. Generally, if the employee's driving ability is acceptable to the DVLA, when they have all the information, the employee should not be prevented from driving. It is important that the insurance covers disabled drivers. The regulations for large goods vehicles (LGVs) and passenger carrying vehicles (PCVs) are stricter and are discussed in Appendix 1.

Selected references

1 Feldman RG, Pransky GS. Neurological considerations in worker fitness evaluation. In *Occupational medicine: state of the art reviews* **3**(2), 299–308. Philadelphia: Hanley & Belfus, 1988.

2 Kurtzke JF. Neurological system. In *Oxford textbook of public health*, ed. Holland WW, Detels R, Knox G, Breeze E, **4**, 203–249. Oxford: Oxford University Press, 1985.

3 *The health of the nation* (Cmnd 1523). London: HMSO, 1991.

4 Baker, EL. Neurologic and behavioral disorders. In *Occupational Health: recognizing and preventing work-related disease*, ed. Levy BS, Wegman DH, 3rd edn. Boston: Little Brown, 1995.

5 Greenwood R *et al.* (ed.) *Neurological rehabilitation*. Edinburgh: Churchill Livingstone, 1993.

6 Wellings DJ, Unsworth J. Environmental control systems for people with a disability. *BMJ* 1997; **315**: 409–412.

7 *The provision of wheelchairs and special seating. Report of a working group*. London: Royal College of Physicians, April 1995.

8 Cull RE, Wells NEJ, Miocevich ML. The economic cost of migraine. *Br J Med Econ* 1992; **2**: 103–15.

9 Mountstephen AH, Harrison RK. A study of migraine and its effects in a working population. *Occup Med* 1995; **45**: 311–317.

10 MacGregor EA. *Managing migraine in primary care*. Oxford: Blackwell Science, 1999.

11 Tanaka H, Yokoyama T, Cerebrovascular disease. In: *Oxford textbook of public health*, ed. Detels R, Holland WW, McEwen J, Omenn GS, 3rd edn, Vol. 3, pp. 1065–1079. Oxford: Oxford University Press, 1997.

12 Johnson R. Return to work after severe head injury. *Inf'Disabil Stud* 1987; **9**: 49–54.

13 *Alcohol—a balanced view*. London: Royal College of General Practitioners, 1986.

14 *Alcohol and the heart in perspective—sensible limits reaffirmed*. London: Royal College of Physicians, June 1995.

15 Taylor JF (ed.) *Medical aspects of fitness to drive*, 5th edn. London: Medical Commission on Accident Prevention, 1995.

16 *Guide to the current medical standards of fitness to drive*. Cardiff: Driver and Vehicle Licensing Agency, Drivers Medical Group, March 1996.

17 Mitchell JN. Multiple sclerosis and the prospects of employment. *J Soc Occup Med* 1981; **31**: 134–138.

18 *Chronic fatigue syndrome*. London: Royal College of Physicians, October 1996.

19 Fulcher KY, White PD. Randomised controlled trial of graded exercise in patients with chronic fatigue syndrome. *BMJ* 1997; **314**: 1647–1652.

Further reading

Gemne G, Pyykkö I, Taylor W, Pelmear PL. The Stockholm Workshop scale for the classification of cold-induced Raynaud's phenomenon in the hand-arm vibration syndrome (revision of Taylor–Pelmear Scale). *Scand J Work Environ Health* 1987; **13**: 275–277.

Illis LS (ed.) *Neurological rehabilitation*, 2nd edn. Oxford: Blackwell Scientific, 1994.

Newsom-Davis J, Donaghy M. Neurology. In *Oxford textbook of medicine*, 3rd edn, ed. Weatherall DJ, Ledingham JGG, Warrell DA. Oxford: Oxford University Press, 1996.

Romain GC, Neurological and public health. In *Oxford textbook of public health*, 3rd edn, ed. Detels R, Holland WW, McEwen J, Omenn GS, Vol. 3, 1195–1222. Oxford: Oxford University Press, 1997.

Sleep apnoea and related conditions. London: Royal College of Physicians, October 1993.

Stroke: towards better management London: Royal College of Physicians, 1989.

Ward CD (ed). Hither neurology—meeting the challenge of neurological disability. *J Neurol Neurosurg Psychiatry* 1992; **55**(Suppl).

7

Psychiatric disorders

J. Kearns and M. Lipsedge

Recent tragedies in which health professionals have killed, assaulted or maimed patients, have focused attention on the implications of psychiatric abnormality at work.[1] The statutory constraints on professional medical confidentiality were not recognized by those concerned in the hospital, or by those conducting the inquiry. In the Clothier Report, unrealistic expectation that psychiatric screening could have been an effective filter diverted attention from other more important factors contributing to the disaster.

In this chapter, major psychiatric disorders are described briefly in terms that will assist all doctors and employers to exercise their duty of care for all employees, fit or not. In the UK, the vast majority of workplaces have no access to a consultant in occupational medicine who might help to reconcile conflicting needs, most evident when the employee is ill. Moreover, the sophistication of management style and ethos in large companies is not found in the great majority of medium-sized and small companies, though an effective substitute may be the close relationships characteristic of the small group. That being so, general practitioners and consultants in other specialist fields are often the only source of practical guidance about individual fitness for work, or for the promotion of occupational health.

Robust mental health at work is more necessary than ever in today's ever-changing, challenging, even threatening, and competitive climate. The need for both employers and employees to have access to competent expertise in occupational mental health has never been greater.

Mental health and the working environment

A formal postgraduate qualification in occupational medicine will probably have required the specialist to have spent some time in the workplace to gain practical understanding of processes and services, and to experience the physical, chemical, and biological hazards of the working environment. In the UK, the occupational physician who advises an enterprise has statutory responsibility under health and safety legislation for the competence of medical advice given on the establishment, maintenance, and promotion of the physical and mental health of the workforce, and on the means of preventing illness or injury.

A recent study[2] has demonstrated that the psychological environment should now be assessed in the manner accepted as appropriate for physical, chemical and biological hazards under the UK regulations for Control of Substances Hazardous to Health (COSHH). This concept requires an assessment of risks; the determination of means for their control; monitoring the environment to ensure that the controls are effective; and if there is any doubt of the efficacy of control, the conduct of routine biological monitoring. The successful civil action of *Walker* v. *Northumberland County Council*[3] has established that an employer's duty of care includes due regard for mental well-being as well as physical health and safety.

Psychological disabilities extend through a continuum from normality to serious pathology. The familiar features of frank disease may often be heralded by prodromal signs and symptoms. Those working with the individual are more likely than the doctor to notice the earliest signs of persistent behavioural changes. Occupational physicians must be prepared to address such issues of primary prevention by health education and participation in management training. They must assist in the preparation and implementation of policies which enable them to help in the management of individuals. For instance, it is of little use to the victim of bullying to be treated for the resulting psychiatric disturbance, without addressing the root problem.[4] In such a case, the management style may have displayed a poor flow of information; an authoritarian way of resolving conflict; lack of discussion of the group's targets and goals; or lack of autonomy and control of matters which directly affect employees.

Tannenbaum commented in very general terms about a wide range of management styles distributed along a continuum representing a 'mix' of command and consultation, and suggested that the style should be appropriate to the situation.[5]

Perhaps the most direct analogy between the familiar medical processes of diagnosis and treatment, and the lay management approach to problem analysis and decision-making, is to be found in the work of Hertzberg *et al.*[6] who suggest that a number of 'hygiene factors' must be favourable to enable a reasonable degree of individual 'self-fulfilment' which is essential for the organizational health of an effective enterprise (see Table 7.1).

McGregor[7] advocates a participative approach by managers, rather than an autocratic style of command.

Table 7.1 Hygiene factors and motivators[6]

Hygiene factors (which enable motivators to operate)	Motivators (which are to be stimulated and encouraged)
Organizational policy and administration	Achievement
The quality of supervision	Recognition
Relationship with Supervisor	The work itself
Working conditions	Responsibility
Salary	Advancement
Relationship with peers	Personal growth
Personal life	
Status	
Security	

Sickness absence and early retirement on medical grounds

Prevalence

Between 15 and 30% of workers will experience mental health problems each year. Depression alone results in the loss of some 155 million working days per year, amounting to almost 20% of all sickness absence (Royal College of Psychiatrists' Defeat Depression Campaign). Moreover, whatever the reason given, absence may represent withdrawal from a temporarily intolerable working environment.[8] Repeated short periods of absence account for two-thirds of spells of absence from work, and represent a decision not to go to work, as distinct from inability to do so.[9] That understanding was the key to the decision to allow self-certification in the first week of absence attributed to sickness. Repeated short periods are predominantly a problem of human resources management.[10]

Many psychiatric patients 'somatise' their symptoms into physical complaints in the first instance, either because they think that doctors will be more attentive to a physical complaint, or because they regard the signs of overactivity of the autonomic nervous system, such as palpitations or sweating in an anxiety state, as having a physical rather than a psychological basis.

Early retirement

In the early months, the manager looks to the occupational physician for a reasonably firm prediction of the date of return to work, because deputizing arrangements must be made immediately to cover an absent employee. The long-repeated sequence of hopeful reviews, appropriate in a therapeutic environment, is of little help to the employer. As the endpoint of sickness absence management, termination of service on medical grounds may be necessary. References and self-esteem need not be tarnished by any suggestion of a disciplinary offence when service is terminated specifically on grounds of mental ill health. That may be inevitable if there is no prospect of regular and efficient service, as when a psychiatric disorder makes it impossible for the employee to function effectively within, for example, a safety-critical role in an organization. The manager may have no other option for action in such a case. However, it is unethical to recommend an early pension merely as a socially acceptable exit from the organization, particularly if the matter is the subject of a disciplinary enquiry.

The prototypical applicant for long-term permanent health insurance benefit or early retirement on medical grounds is over 50, has become unpopular and unproductive, has outdated technical knowledge his company is 'rationalizing' and there is talk of relocation. Following a recent merger, performance-related pay has been introduced. On the domestic front, the applicant's partner complains of 25 years of neglect. The applicant has mildly elevated blood pressure, irritable bowel syndrome, lumbar backache, 'stress', 'burnout', fatigue, and mild depression and anxiety with occasional panic attacks. The prospect of returning to work makes them feel very anxious but the symptoms are not too severe.

Although such employees feel intensely anxious at the prospect of travelling to work, they are frequently able to make other journeys and indeed, some are able to enjoy long touring holidays overseas. A sort of 'conspiracy' develops in which the employee, supported by their spouse, decides to seek early retirement. This is frequently backed up by the general practitioner who, together with the majority of mental health professionals as their patient's advocates, feel that they have to be protected from the noxious influence of the workplace and the risk of any exacerbation of symptoms.[11] The patient's senior colleagues might also take the view that early retirement is in both the company's and the employee's interests.

In situations such as this, it is vitally important for the occupational physician to adopt a three-pronged approach:

- first, they must ensure that appropriate psychological or psychiatric help has been provided by practitioners who are committed to occupational rehabilitation
- the occupational physician might have to ask management to make adjustments to the patient's workload
- a programme of graded reintroduction to the workplace is essential so that the patient does not feel overwhelmed at the prospect of returning to full-time work in the first instance.

A useful policy is to treat the workplace itself as the most realistic and therefore the most effective rehabilitation workshop, provided the patient's responsibilities and hours at work can be restricted in the first instance and then progressively extended.

Early retirement with a pension is appropriate only if there is a permanent disability. It is in nobody's interest to discourage a recovering patient by implying permanent exclusion from work, if there is hope of eventual recovery. In any circumstance in which an individual poses a serious threat to their own safety, or that of any other employee, contractor, or member of the public, there may be a statutory duty on the patient and the physician to declare that such is the case, on a 'need to know' basis, to enable the employer to meet the personal and corporate statutory duty of care imposed by health and safety legislation.

Finally, in any discussion of early retirement on grounds of physical or mental ill health it is worth recalling the benefits of being employed. It is known that the psychiatric morbidity of housewives is higher than that of employed women.[12] Brown and Harris[13] found that women who have jobs are less vulnerable to depression. This is because of the central role of employment in providing a social network, independence, financial resources and self-esteem.

Management of the mentally sick employee

The absent sick employee should be treated in a supportive and a therapeutic environment. In contrast, work is carried out in a demanding and competitive environment, which can be extremely taxing in both physical and psychological terms. To bridge the gap between the two, when an employee falls ill, many larger organizations will have occupational sick pay schemes, setting out a scale of financial support during defined maximum periods of discretionary company benefits, supplementary to statutory sick pay. These may include arrangements for rehabilitation and redeployment.

Most jobs do not in themselves represent an intolerable psychological burden. Illness is usually the product of several causes. It may be relevant to test for aptitude, but in only a very few extremely demanding jobs is it possible to exclude 'vulnerable' candidates.

Virtually anyone is susceptible to a psychiatric illness, 1 in 6 women or 1 in 9 men being likely to require treatment in a psychiatric unit during their lifetime. The stigma of psychiatric disorder nevertheless persists. Many of those who recover from a psychiatric episode may have benefited from the experience. Many such individuals describe a growth in personal awareness, expressed as 'I would never have believed that that could happen to me', or as 'I know now that I could never have done that job' either because it was beyond their competence, or because they were trying to perform despite inadequate resources. Although they would not have wished it on themselves, they will have had an experience akin to that in the American management training technique of 'sensitivity training', or the 'T-group', intended to give trainees an insight into motivation, job satisfaction, and 'what makes people tick'.

Conversely, people who have recovered from a depressive illness may be left with low residual self-esteem, pessimism, loss of confidence, and a sense of vulnerability and helplessness. They and others who have suffered a serious psychiatric episode, and may have lost their jobs, require special care in their entry or re-entry into a demanding commercial environment. Such a candidate will not be confident. There may be a setback or even intermittent withdrawal from work in the early days of earning a living once more. It is important for the occupational health team to participate in the process in a constructive way. It may be an understandable, but grave, mistake to deny completely an episode of incapacity, physical or mental, because the more serious the episode, the greater the challenge of resuming normal life.

Where there is an occupational physician, rehabilitation of an employee must start at the beginning of the crisis, maintaining contact with the general practitioner throughout, until return to work is contemplated.[14] By the same token, a relationship with the local Disability Employment Adviser (DEA) may enable unemployed candidates who have suffered a psychiatric illness to be helped to seek a new post with an enlightened employer. The Disability Discrimination Act 1995 (DDA) now places such a responsibility on employers. That being so, those caring for the patient may find it easier to declare a significant disability to ensure appropriate placement.

Psychiatric patients as employees

It is well recognized that psychiatric patients often have difficulty obtaining or keeping employment.[15] This is especially true of patients with a history of schizophrenia, which has a lifetime prevalence of about 1%. About one-fifth of patients with schizophrenia make a full recovery; about one-half will have a degree of chronic or recurrent impairment. Nonetheless, many of this group will be able to work at least part-time.[16] Potentially disabling symptoms include auditory hallucinations and paranoid delusions which might cause friction with colleagues, and impaired concentration, lack of drive and motivation, and poor social and self-care skills have an obvious effect on performance and attendance. Most of the research in this field has studied the careers of psychiatric inpatients and there is a paucity of knowledge on the employment and employability of patients with non-psychotic psychiatric conditions. It is known that the return to work of psychiatric patients is significantly correlated with response to supervision, sound relationships, and enthusiasm, and these predict employability.

Enthusiasm is reflected in comments on performance such as 'works continuously, eager to work, looks for more work'. Clearly patients who have been institutionalized for long periods may depend on external supervision to maintain the continuity of their work because they lack the ability to pace their own performance. Social relationships are also a good predictor of the ability to maintain and hold down employment. Those who are 'socially naive', i.e. do not realize the effect of their behaviour on other people or tend to be argumentative, are clearly at a disadvantage in the workplace.[17]

Anthony and Jansen[18] have summarized research which deals with the employability of adults with chronic mental illness. Some of their findings are surprising, and indeed counter-intuitive, but nevertheless of great practical importance: poor predictors of future work performance include the level of psychiatric symptomatology, diagnostic category, and performance on intelligence and aptitude tests. One cannot extrapolate from the ability to function in the community to competence in the workplace, and there is little correlation between symptomatology and most measures of functional ability. Conversely, the best predictors of future work performance are prior employment history and ratings of adjustment skills made in a sheltered job. A significant predictor of future work performance is a person's ability to get along with other people, i.e. to interact appropriately and communicate effectively. Other functional criteria include the ability to concentrate, task-perseverance, and the ability to adapt to stressful circumstances, such as making decisions and achieving a target.

It is therefore important to distinguish between symptoms and functional capacity and to recognize that patients may be able to function competently within the workplace despite persistent psychotic symptoms such as hallucinations. Shepherd[19] has emphasized the potential independence between symptoms and functioning, and the fact that functioning has to be defined in terms of a particular setting rather than generalized across a wide range of different settings.

Floyd[20] has shown that people with mental illness are more likely to remain employed when the job has the following features:

- opportunity to learn on the job
- freedom to organize work
- clear supervision
- a trusting social climate
- working in the company of others rather than in isolation
- the opportunity to evaluate performance in relation to co-workers
- feedback from supervisors.

An accelerated programme of transitional employment, especially for work-experienced clients, produces better rehabilitation results than the traditional approach of very gradually preparing the employee to resume work.[21] It has been suggested that allowing work-experienced clients to remain out of work for too long enhances their fear of failure and allows them to become too dependent on the support system.

Other associated factors which impair effective functioning and the ability of those with chronic mental illness to keep a job include lack of self-esteem and self-confidence which lead to a fear of failure and rejection, pervasive anxiety and difficulties in interpersonal relationships. Training or retraining in critical vocational skills obviously improves the outcome of rehabilitation.

Schizophrenia

The psychoses pose a difficult problem, in that long periods of normal or even exceptional performance can be interspersed with unpredictable marked excursions from normal function and behaviour. The conditions may present with vague signs of abnormality, only sensed by co-workers as being disturbing. That unease may be declared to a superior or to the staff of the occupational health department. There may be a problem in setting up the diagnostic interview when the patient is convinced that there is nothing wrong. The challenge will be to conduct the interview with sufficient expertise to detect diagnostic signs at the earliest stage of the episode, and to put in place the network of professional help. Should sickness absence or the severity of symptoms declare the problem to colleagues at work, they will require some understanding of its implications to them when the patient returns to work. In very general terms, the greater the degree of independent function at work of the patient, the more grave will be the consequence of the onset of schizophrenia. Return to a routine production task under supervision will be much easier to arrange than return to a more senior or highly technical role in which individual judgement is a key component of performance.

In the UK, the DDA expects 'reasonable adjustments' to be made to accommodate those with long-term disability. In managing a psychotic employee, that 'reasonable adjustment' is likely to be inhibiting so that the more severe signs and symptoms of mental illness are prevented or controlled, as a pre-condition to continued employment. As in any condition characterized by lengthy remissions alternating with periods of total disability, the pattern of absence may pose its own problem if it proves impossible to depend on regular attendance.

Depression

Similar comment may be made about chronic or recurrent depression. The great difference is the better prospect of successful treatment. It would not seem appropriate to make a judgement in terms of the DDA for some months after the onset of the condition. The case of *Walker* v. *Northumberland County Council* is particularly relevant, in that a precedent has been set, determining the reasonable steps that an employer must take once the problem has declared itself.

Sheltered work

Ideally, more employees who have had a long period of sickness absence should be rehabilitated by moving through a programme of occupational therapy, sheltered workshops, and occupational retraining units. Unfortunately one or more of the facilities might be unavailable locally. (See also Chapter 4 P. 74).

Long-term antipsychotic medication

The side-effects of medication that can interfere with performance at work can be reduced by careful monitoring and adjustment of dosage or type of medication. Long-acting injectable antipsychotic drugs help to eliminate poor compliance. It is important for patients with a history of psychotic illness to be taught how to identify the early warning signs of a relapse; these are often 'neurotic' symptoms such as anxiety, insomnia, and irritability rather than hallucinations and delusions. It is predictable that a patient with schizophrenia will experience anxiety when starting a new job or returning to their previous job. The multidisciplinary team in collaboration with the occupational health physician and nurse can help to prevent a relapse in this situation by periodic review, temporarily increasing the dose of neuroleptics, and provision of support and advice.

Common non-specific labels used in the workplace

Stress

The word 'stress' is frequently used both in the workplace and in the medical setting as well as in the media. The term is unsatisfactory and ambiguous since it can refer to both an agent and to its effects and consequences. It might be helpful to use the word **stressors** to describe potentially noxious environmental factors and to refer to the effects on the individual as **strains**. A working definition of a stressful situation has been proposed[22] as one in which there is disparity between the demand on the worker and the ability to respond to it, when the individual has little or no control over the situation (Fig. 7.1).

That situation may be actual, or perceived as being so by the individual. Thus a situation at work is potentially stressful when an individual construes it as threatening because they feel they do not have the resources to handle it and are aware that failure to cope could have damaging personal consequences.

Kahn[23] identified three potentially stressful factors in a competitive environment:

- The quantity or quality of the **role load** could be either too great to sustain or too small to stimulate self-fulfilment.
- **Role conflict** could be caused by competition for resources with other members of a team, although all are pursuing a common objective. The demands of home and work might also be difficult to reconcile.
- **Role ambiguity** and insecurity could result from uncertainty about what has to be done, how to do it, for whom and by when.

Confronted by something in the environment which the individual interprets as a threat to themselves or to something they value, the person responds by using a coping strategy which may or may not be effective. Decompensation occurs when individuals consider both their own resources and outside support as inadequate to meet the threat. Psychiatric and psychosomatic disorders, as well as substance abuse, tend to develop in those people whose habitual coping skills are ineffective. A patient who is already suffering from physical symptoms (e.g. chronic fatigue) or psychiatric symptoms (e.g. anxiety), may opt for the ultimately maladaptive coping strategy of achieving the status and short-term privileges of being a patient. Cooper and Payne[24] have characterized work-related stressors as follows:

- **factors intrinsic to the job**, e.g. extremes of humidity and temperature, noise, and shiftwork; dealing with complaints from the public

- **role-related factors**, e.g. managers with conflicting responsibilities to both cut costs and support their staff; role ambiguity etc.
- **interpersonal relationships**, e.g. bullying, poor delegation.

One of the commonest sources of occupational dissatisfaction is the imposition of targets, apparently reasonable at the outset, but proving unattainable owing to unforeseen events outside the control of the subordinate. It is easier to blame the latter than to address the external problem, and even more so the provision of inadequate resources or training when deadlines are missed. In some cases, objectives set by management, for instance those in the recent pensions mis-selling scandal in the insurance industry in the UK, may generate role conflict so severe as to lead to mental illness.

Certain occupations are particularly stressful because of unpleasant physical conditions (e.g. working underground) or because of the need constantly to monitor machines (e.g. in air traffic control). The employee might experience role conflict when they have to switch rapidly from one professional identity to another, e.g. the social worker or probation officer who has to be helpful and supportive but who also has to be, on occasion, authoritarian and judgmental, and inform their superiors or other agencies of unlawful acts or potential hazardous behaviour. Personnel staff who work at the interface of management and work force or head-teachers with competing budgetary, human resources, statutory, disciplinary, pastoral, and pedagogic responsibilities can experience considerable role-conflict.

Worry about change within the organization (e.g. downsizing, mergers, relocation, introduction of new technology) enhances the employee's perception of the job as threatening to their own professional or psychological survival. Furthermore, some aspects of personality can render an individual less capable of coping with occupational stressors. Thus, the type A pattern of behaviour which is characterized by inappropriate competitiveness, sense of time pressure, and ambition and insecurity, tends to be associated with

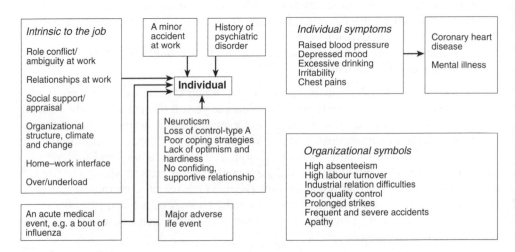

Fig. 7.1 Stressors and strains. Modified from Furham A, *The psychology of behaviour at work,* Psychology Press, 1997.

coronary artery disease,[25] whereas individuals with an external locus of control, i.e. a tendency to doubt one's autonomy, tend to lack resilience.[26]

Burnout

Burnout is a constellation of symptoms characterized by dissatisfaction, disillusionment, negative attitudes to work, loss of idealism and a sense of purpose, as well as emotional exhaustion. Nurses, doctors, teachers, and social workers are professionals commonly manifesting the condition. Other features include 'depersonalization', which is defined as feelings of detachment and callousness towards other people at work, and the loss of a sense of competence and achievement. There is a great deal of overlap between this sense of emotional exhaustion and the symptoms of a depressive illness. However, the feelings of alienation and loss of empathy, and the erosion of a sense of personal achievement and competency, cannot be attributed entirely to a depressive illness. Burnout is covered by ICD*-10 Z73—'problems related to life-management difficulty'. It is not classified as a formal psychiatric disorder in its own right.

Roberts[27] summarized the signs and symptoms of burnout under the headings of changes in behaviour, in feelings, in thinking, and in health. Behavioural changes include attempting to avoid contact with patients, clients, or colleagues, and working harder and later but achieving less. Alterations in feeling include a persistent sense of failure, guilt, and self-blame together with resentment and irritability. Changes in thinking include a cynical and dehumanized attitude to patients and clients, poor concentration, and increasing thoughts of quitting; changes in health include insomnia and weariness. Roberts proposes preventive measures which include encouraging employees to take responsibility for their own experience of stress—'we need to become our own stress-management experts'—and to learn to reset priorities in everyday routines, both at work and at home.

Chronic fatigue syndrome

Chronic fatigue syndrome (CFS) is the diagnostic label applied to patients who have suffered from chronic disabling fatigue for a period longer than 6 months and for which medical assessment and investigation can find no adequate physical explanation. Because there is no pathological evidence of encephalomyelitis in CFS, the term myeloencephalitis (ME) is both misleading and unhelpful.

The Joint Working Group of the Royal Colleges of Physicians, Psychiatrists and General Practitioners[28] concluded that immunotherapy, antiviral agents, vitamin or dietary supplements, magnesium,and evening primrose oil are all ineffective. The Working Group concluded that the most effective treatment is controlled increase in activity by a graded exercise programme combined with cognitive-behaviour therapy. The aim of treatment is gradually and consistently to increase the level and range of both physical and mental activity from the patient's current activity level.[29]

CFS provides a useful example of the interaction between a vulnerable personality, pressure at work, and an episode of physical illness followed by absence from work and, in a significant number of cases, chronic invalidism (Fig. 7.2). The cognitive-behavioural

---

* International Classification of Diseases.

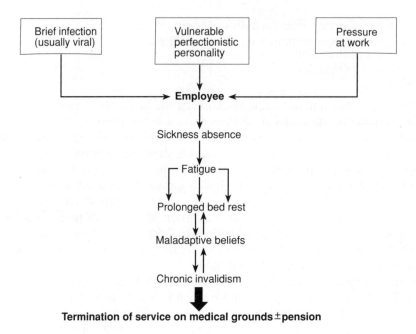

Fig. 7.2 Chronic fatigue syndrome.

model of CFS proposed by Wessely *et al.*[30] has been elaborated[31] to take into account predisposing personality factors.

Psychiatric disorders commonly seen in occupational health

Personality disorder

The most important example of a condition which is defined in actuarial or dimensional rather than categorical terms is personality disorder. Personality disorders are characterized by a constellation of attitudes and antisocial patterns of behaviour which reflect the individual's usual ways of relating to other people and which cause distress to the individual and/or to others. People with these traits tend to lack coping skills and inevitably create difficulties in social and occupational functioning. Habitual maladaptive ways of thinking, feeling, and acting are discernible by the time adolescence is reached and tend to endure throughout adulthood.[32]

In general, employees with a personality disorder include:

- the **paranoid** (0.5–2.5% of the general population)
- the **antisocial**, a pattern of disregard for and violation of the rights of others (3% of men and 1% of women)
- the **emotionally unstable** (2–3%)
- the **histrionic** (2–3%)
- the **obsessional** (1%).

A classification of the most common patterns of maladaption in the workplace has been devised by Neff.[33] These are not pure categories and some people represent mixtures of two or three of them, but it is often useful to juxtapose this taxonomy against the conventional list of personality disorders:

* **low self-esteem, excessive anxiety** in the workplace with undue sensitivity to criticism and a deterioration in performance when closely supervised
* **poor capacity for interpersonal relationships** with irritability, poor self-control, and frequent loss of temper;
* **dependency** with excessive needs for emotional support and supervision
* **failure to internalize the 'work ethic'** with lack of commitment, consistency, responsibility, or ambition.

Depression

Depression is the most commonly encountered psychiatric disorder both in general practice and in the workplace. Its clinical features—emotional, cognitive, and biological—are well known. About 5% of the population will experience an episode of moderate to severe depression at some point in their lives. In one American banking corporation with 18 000 employees, depression accounted for 62% of short-term disability absence associated with a mental health diagnosis. Depressive disorders not only produced longer disability periods than common chronic medical conditions such as low back pain and heart disease, but also showed an exceptionally high rate of relapse within 1 year.[34]

A useful and speedily administered self-rating scale for the detection of depression and anxiety is the Hospital Anxiety and Depression Scale (Box 7.1). This scale, devised by Zigmond and Snaith,[35] comprises 14 items. It was designed specifically for use in non-psychiatric hospital departments. The items on the scale are all concerned with the psychological symptoms of neurosis, thus making it suitable for use in patients with concurrent physical illness and disabilities.

Box 7.1   Hospital Anxiety and Depression Scale (Adapted from Zigmond and Snaith[35])

Name   Date:

This questionnaire will help you to let us know how you are. Read each item and underline the response which comes closest to how you have felt in the last few days. Don't take too long over your replies; your immediate reaction will probably be more accurate than a long thought out response.

	A	D
I feel tense or 'wound up'		
Most of the time	3	
A lot of the time	2	
From time to time, occasionally	1	
Not at all	0	

Box 7.1 contd

	A	D
I feel as if I am slowed down		
Nearly all the time		3
Very often		2
Sometimes		1
Not at all		0
I still enjoy the things I used to enjoy		
Definitely as much		0
Not quite so much		1
Only a little		2
Hardly at all		3
I get a sort of frightened feeling like 'butterflies' in the stomach		
Not at all	0	
Occasionally	1	
Quite often	2	
Very often	3	
I get a sort of frightened feeling as if something awful is about to happen		
Very definitely and quite badly	3	
Yes, but not too badly	2	
A little, but it doesn't worry me	1	
Not at all	0	
I have lost interest in my appearance		
Definitely		3
I don't take so much care as I should		2
I may not take quite as much care		1
I take just as much care as ever		0
I can laugh and see the funny side of things		
As much as I always could		0
Not quite so much now		1
Definitely not so much now		2
Not at all		3
I feel restless as if I have to be on the move		
Very much indeed	3	
Quite a lot	2	
Not very much	1	
Not at all	0	
Worrying thoughts go through my mind		
A great deal of the time	3	
A lot of the time	2	
From time to time but not too often	1	
Only occasionally	0	

	A	D
I look forward with enjoyment to things		
As much as ever I did		0
Rather less than I used to		1
Definitely less than I used to		2
Hardly at all		3
I feel cheerful		
Not at all		3
Not often		2
Sometimes		1
Most of the time		0
I get sudden feelings of panic		
Very often indeed	3	
Quite often	2	
Not very often	1	
Not at all	0	
I can sit at ease and feel relaxed		
Definitely	0	
Usually	1	
Not often	2	
Not at all	3	
I can enjoy a good book or radio or TV programme		
Often		0
Sometimes		1
Not often		2
Very seldom		3

The scores should be concealed from the patient. Column A is the anxiety score and column D the depression score. On both scales scores of 7 or less indicate non-cases, 8–10 doubtful cases and 11 or more are definite cases.

Depression is 2–3 times commoner in women than in men. Most episodes remit within 6 months, although a minority of cases will become chronic, especially if undertreated. A significant number of patients will experience a further episode of depression. Clearly, early intervention and treatment are desirable since it has been established that 80% of patients suffering from depression can be successfully treated with medication, cognitive therapy, or a combination of both. Tricyclic antidepressants can cause drowsiness, tremor and blurred vision but most of the newer antidepressants (SSRIs) are less sedating. Early observation and treatment of behavioural change may pre-empt more severe symptoms.

Most episodes of depression are unipolar, resulting only in a lowering of mood, but there is a lifetime risk of developing mania of 0.6–1%. It is extremely important for patients who have recovered from an episode of depression to continue with an antidepressant at an effective dose for several months which is usually quite compatible with work. Close communication between the occupational physician, the general practitioner, and the consultant psychiatrist is essential in treatment and in the prevention of further episodes, and medical staff at the workplace can help to ensure compliance with therapy.

Recurrent episodes of depression can be prevented by the long-term administration of an antidepressant in the dose which has been shown to be effective in the treatment of the acute episode in any particular case. Recurrent episodes of bipolar affective disorder (i.e. manic depressive disorder) can be prevented or markedly attenuated in perhaps two-thirds of patients by lithium or carbamazepine.

It is important for both physicians and for individual patients to be mindful of the early warning signs of a recurrence of an episode of mood disorder, which might be the presentation of somatic symptoms in depression, or a markedly reduced need for sleep in mania. The occupational hazards associated with an episode of hypomania or mania are predictable from the combination of increased energy and loss of inhibition and self-restraint, and include reckless driving and spending, marked tactlessness if not frank offensiveness in dealing with colleagues and clients, and risk-taking behaviour (alcohol, drugs, and sex).

Employees who have to travel overseas should be warned of the possibility that jetlag or even losing a night's sleep might push a susceptible individual into a hypomanic or manic episode. Discreet discussion of the case between the occupational physician and a sympathetic senior manager should be considered, if the patient agrees. Otherwise, the florid presentation of a crisis to an unprepared manager may prejudice continued employment.

When assessing an individual patient, it is useful to bear in mind three categories of aetiological factors:

- **predisposing factors**, i.e. vulnerability arising from, for example, a genetic loading for bipolar affective disorder or multiple separations and rejections in childhood;
- **precipitating or triggering factors** such as major adverse life events, e.g. bereavement or a teenage child in trouble with the police (paradoxically, bad news such as bereavement can act as a trigger for an episode of hypomania or mania);
- **perpetuating factors** which tend to impede recovery from an episode of mental illness and include a wide range of medical, domestic, social and occupational problems such as chronic physical illness, noise, and intimidation by neighbours.

Patients may remain on sick leave or seek early retirement on medical grounds because of these factors. Although it is now recognized that the underlying biological dysfunction is identical in both 'endogenous' and 'reactive' depression, it is still worth attempting to elicit a history of recent major adverse life events or long-term domestic, family, or social problems. It is also important to exclude an underlying physical disorder such as hypothyroidism and to take into account the possibility that prescribed medication, e.g. methyldopa, calcium antagonists, and corticosteroids, can cause persistent lowering of mood.

Premature reduction of the dose of an antidepressant or cessation of treatment is a very common cause of relapse or recurrence in unipolar depression and it is advisable for patients who have recovered from an episode to continue with an antidepressant at an effective dose for several months at least. Patients who have severe or apparently treat-ment-resistant depression should be referred for a psychiatric opinion. The occupational physician should liaise with both the general practitioner and the consultant psychiatrist to discuss the prevention of further episodes in a patient who has suffered from a severe depression, hypomania, or mania.

'Treatment-resistant' depression is associated with the prescribing of inappropriately low doses of antidepressants or, conversely, non-compliance because of prescribing too high an initial dose rather than progressively achieving a therapeutic level over a period of a couple of weeks. Another cause of failure to respond is too hasty a switch to another antidepressant because of the patient's failure to improve within an unrealisti-cally short space of time. Some depressed patients are inappropriately treated with ben-zodiazepines which can actually make depression worse. Finally, the concomitant use of alcohol will interfere with the effectiveness of antidepressants by hepatic enzyme induc-tion.

The impact of depression on work performance

Depression causes impairment in work performance. Lack of drive, energy, and motiva-tion have an adverse effect on productivity and cause an overall decline in the quantity and quality of work; impairment of concentration is hazardous in employees responsi-ble for driving or operating machinery. In addition to loss of verbal fluency and impaired ability to maintain attention, there is often a difficulty in making decisions and an increase in reaction time. Tricyclic antidepressants may further prolong reaction time and thus add to the hazards of driving, but the SSRI antidepressants are thought to have less adverse effect on psychomotor performance. Patients with chronic depression or who are on therapy for depression may meet the criteria for disability within the mean-ing of the DDA.

Anxiety disorders

The anxiety disorders include generalized anxiety disorder, panic disorder, phobias, obsessive compulsive disorder, and post-traumatic stress disorder.

The symptoms of anxiety can be grouped under two headings:

- cognitive/emotional
- physical.

The anxious patient will be continuously apprehensive, may fear losing control, going insane or having a fatal heart attack, may have an irrational desire to run away, and may feel that they themselves or their surroundings are unreal (depersonalization and dereal-ization). Somatic symptoms of anxiety which are due to overactivity of the sympathetic nervous system (fight-or-flight response) include palpitations, shortness of breath, epi-gastric discomfort ('butterflies in the stomach'), urinary frequency, tension headaches, dizziness and lightheadedness, paraesthesia, shakiness, and sweating.

Generalized anxiety disorder and panic disorder

In **generalized anxiety disorder** the patient worries excessively and unrealistically about not being able to cope, about being criticized, about not functioning properly at work, and about their health. In **panic disorder** the anxiety is not continuously present in a 'free-floating' form but affects the patient in sudden and unexpected bursts. The cognitive model of panic[36] proposes that a vicious circle develops in which a bodily sensation such as palpitations or breathlessness is misinterpreted in a catastrophic fashion as evidence of an imminent heart attack. The patient becomes intensely apprehensive and this in turn causes excessive sympathetic discharge leading to tachycardia which is taken, mistakenly, as further evidence of an incipient heart attack. The cognitive-behavioural therapy of generalized anxiety and panic disorder involves teaching patients how to identify, evaluate, control, and modify their negative danger-related thoughts and associated behaviours. The behavioural approach to phobic disorders is designed to reduce anxiety and avoidance by exposing patients systematically to feared situations.

Agoraphobia

Agoraphobics cannot travel to their place of work; social phobics have difficulties with job interviews and with relating to their colleagues, customers, or clients.

Obsessive–compulsive disorder

This is characterized by repetitive actions such as checking or washing many times over. The condition affects about 2% of the adult population. It has a deleterious effect on productivity. It is also treatable by cognitive-behavioural therapy.

Post-accident psychiatric disorders

These include post-traumatic stress disorder and phobic anxiety states.

The essential feature of **post-traumatic stress disorder** is the development of flashbacks, nightmares and the symptoms of increased arousal following exposure to an extreme traumatic stressor involving direct personal experience of an event that involves threatened death or serious injury. The person's response to the event must include intense fear and helplessness or horror, leading to avoidance of stimuli associated with the trauma and numbing of general responsiveness.

There are few long-term studies of the prognosis in post-traumatic stress disorder but it is recognized that the outcomes may vary. After a follow-up period of 12 months, 10% of nearly 200 road traffic accident victims had post-traumatic stress disorder.[37] A previous history of psychiatric disorder is the most important determinant of vulnerability to psychiatric disturbance after exposure to a traumatic event. Previous traumas also sensitize or predispose the individual to developing post-traumatic stress disorder, as does a positive family history of mental illness.

One electricity company has reduced the incidence of post-traumatic stress disorder and post-incident invalidism by routinely providing employees with an information pack which gives a simple account of acute stress reactions (ICD-10, F43.0) and provides practical advice on how to reduce the impact of witnessing a serious accident or incident (Dr Margaret Samuel, personal communication).

It has been shown that the possibility of financial compensation does not affect the course of post-traumatic stress disorder which has developed following a motor vehicle accident. When patients seeking financial compensation after such an accident were compared with patients who developed post-traumatic stress disorder after an incident where there was no possibility of compensation, there was no significant difference in treatment-compliance and outcome.[38,39] Mendelson[40] found that among groups of patients with a variety of industrial injuries, failure to return to work after legal settlement occurred in 67% after a mean period of 16 months, while Balla and Moratis[41] showed that factors which might contribute to long-term disability after compensation for industrial accidents include dissatisfaction with work as well as heavy physical, repetitive, or dangerous work. This evidence does not support the long held concept of "compensationitis" in which a victim's symptoms are allegedly maintained until compensation is settled (see also Chapter 1, p. 22).

Patients may develop a **phobic anxiety state** *de novo* or as a complication of post-traumatic stress disorder. In phobic anxiety disorder (ICD-10, F40), anxiety is evoked predominantly by certain well-defined situations or objects which are not currently dangerous. It leads to avoidance of certain situations or activities such as driving or being carried as a passenger. There may not be total avoidance and a travel-phobic person may be able to undertake a journey by car at the expense of suffering a significant amount of distress. Phobic anxiety states are eminently treatable by cognitive-behavioural therapy.

Neuropsychological sequelae of head injury

The duration of post-traumatic amnesia, which is defined as the length of time from the head injury itself until the restoration of clear and continuous memory, is the most accurate guide to the severity of a head injury and correlates closely with objective evidence of damage to brain tissue. However, even a minor head injury with a very brief post-traumatic amnesia can lead to significant neuropsychiatric disability. Both in minor head injuries and in acceleration–deceleration cervical sprain injury (so-called **whiplash injury**) the brain is bounced within the rigid cranium. This can cause diffuse damage due to the stretching and tearing of neurones and small vessels within the cerebral substance. Impairment of concentration and memory together with mild depression, emotional instability, lowered tolerance of frustration, sleep disturbance, and loss of sex drive have all been reported in patients who have sustained minor head injuries. Although in the past it was claimed that emotional disturbance and/or motivation for compensation were the primary cause of morbidity from minor head injuries, it is now widely recognized that neuropathological and neurophysiological alterations contribute significantly to the clinical picture.

The view that post-head injury psychological symptoms will remit once the compensation and litigation matters are dealt with is not supported by the scientific literature. In patients with mild head injury several studies have found no association between prolonged psychological consequences and the hope of compensation. By the same token, patients who were seeking compensation for back injuries at work did not describe their pain as more severe than a control series of non-litigants.[40] In fact, malingering or conscious falsification of symptoms for gain in compensation cases has been estimated to occur in less than 5% of cases of chronic low back pain.[42]

Recovery may be slow, and the level of eventual function may not be evident for 2 years. This may pose a difficult management problem, since consistent improvement in the early months suggests eventual recovery may occur long after the usual term of sickness compensation will have expired.

Abnormal illness behaviour, simulation, and malingering

The term 'functional' has had various meanings that have changed over time.[43] Originally, the term meant an alteration in function in the central nervous system. It arose from the condition 'railway spine' in which changes in the working of the central nervous system were thought to have been caused by the vibrations of rail travel. It is now used within psychiatric nosology to differentiate those conditions where brain functions are affected by identifiable organic factors, for example dementia associated with myxoedema, from all other psychiatric conditions whose underlying physical cause has not yet been identified, such as schizophrenia.

By contrast, **functional overlay** refers to those conditions where complaints of pain or the reported degree of disability seem out of proportion to the extent or severity of an underlying organic lesion. The term is thus used as a euphemism expressing disbelief in a physical cause for ostensibly physical symptoms. Synonyms include the pejorative 'supra-tentorial'. The implication is that the patient has symptoms which are being caused or accentuated by 'subconscious factors' or, at worst, the patient is malingering.

Abnormal illness behaviour is the term used to describe the actions of a person whose complaints and symptoms are grossly disproportionate to any possible underlying organic lesion.

Simulated disorders are three forms of abnormal illness behaviour in which physical or psychological conditions are imitated by the patient.

- In **factitious disorder** (ICD-10, F68.1) patients consciously feign the symptoms and signs of disease but have little or no insight into the motives for their behaviour, which are to maintain themselves in the role of an invalid.
- In **dissociative disorder** (ICD-10, F44) patients develop dramatic symptoms of physical or mental illness on the basis of unconscious simulation. Dissociative symptoms tend to mimic the phenomena of neurological and psychiatric disorders to the extent that they reflect the patient's own concept of how such disorders present. These disorders have previously been classified as various types of 'conversion hysteria', but it now seems best to avoid the term 'hysteria' as far as possible, in view of its many and varied meanings.[44] Since the underlying mechanism is assumed to reside within the patient's unconscious, to which we have no direct access, hypotheses based on such mechanisms are not amenable to verification, refutation or authentication.
- The third type of simulated abnormal illness behaviour is **malingering** (ICD-10, Z76.5). This is a form of feigned illness in which subjects are fully aware both that they are simulating the symptoms of disease and also of their motive which, in the context of industrial injury or personal injury litigation, might be financial gain, a quest for early retirement on medical grounds, or avoidance of a disciplinary hearing as recently reported to the Home Affairs Committee.[45]

The presentations of malingering are similar to those of dissociative and factitious disorders and it is generally accepted that it can be very difficult to distinguish between them. To make matters worse, these behaviours and motivations are not mutually exclusive and there can be considerable overlap.

The diagnosis of malingering is an accusation. As it is based on the view that the patient is lying, one should only be prepared to believe such an accusation if this can be unequivocally demonstrated. An example of lying which would support the diagnosis of malingering is the following: if an employee claims to be permanently incapable of carrying a heavy weight this could be convincingly demonstrated to be a conscious fabrication if they were observed carrying furniture.

Some features of the patient's verbal responses during examination can assist in deciding whether or not the patient's own account is reliable. Thus, it is reassuring if the patient readily acknowledges the absence of specific symptoms when asked 'leading questions' or if they spontaneously offer comments to the effect that some symptoms have improved since the accident, because acknowledgement of improvement and denial of specific symptoms are unlikely in patients who are dissimulating or frankly malingering.

Conclusion

The Vauxhall Motors factory at Luton had, at one time, a workshop in which the total requirement for some components and assemblies for cars and lorries was met in a single large workshop. A wide range of specialist consultants from the local hospital attended the site, where production machinery was adapted to provide active and passive productive physiotherapy while the patients recovered. This enabled earlier return to work and the earlier achievement of normal function. Moreover, vehicle engineers designed special splints. For instance, patients with fractures of the fibula and tibia were enabled to return to work in a splint flexible at the knee within weeks, when elsewhere they would have been immobilized for three months.

Psychiatric disability does not lend itself to so radical a resolution, and although there may be local facilities to care for mental dysfunction there are few realistic opportunities to provide such a facility at work. Instead, close relationships between psychiatric departments with local employers may enable capability to be matched with a job opportunity. The better the economic climate, the more feasible such a scheme.

The employee falls ill in a challenging and demanding work environment. It is critical for the general practitioner and the community mental health team to work in open communication with occupational health staff if there are any, or with a senior manager on a 'need to know' basis if there are not. Medical confidentiality must be maintained, but the significance of the clinical condition must be interpreted in lay terms if management is to be able to participate in rehabilitation, helping the individual to function and confront challenge without medical support.

References

1 *Allitt Inquiry: relating to deaths and injuries on the children's ward at Grantham and Kesteven General Hospital during the period February to April 1991.* London: HMSO, 1994.

2 Cox T. *Stress research and stress management: putting theory to work.* London: Health and Safety Executive, 1993.

3   *Walker* v. *Northumberland County Council.* Queen's Bench Division. All England Law Reports
    1ALL ER, 1995.
4   Lipsedge M, Samuel M. ABC of mental health for occupational physicians: anxiety, depres-
    sion, assessment of suicide risk, bullying and occupational health interventions. *Faculty of
    Occupational Medicine Newsletter*, 1998.
5   Tannenbaum R, Weschler IR, Masserik F. *Leadership and management: a behavioural science
    approach.* New York: McGraw-Hill, 1961.
6   Hertzberg F, Mausner B, Snyderman B. *The motivation to work.* New York: Wiley, 1966.
7   McGregor D. *The human side of enterprise.* New York: McGraw-Hill, 1960.
8   Brown JAC. *The social psychology of industry: human relations in the factory.* Harmonsworth:
    Penguin,1954.
9   Ward Gardner A (ed.) *Absence from work attributed to sickness.* Research Symposium, Soc.
    Occupational Medicine, 1966.
10 Kearns JL. *Guidance on employers' Statutory Sick Pay.* London: Society of Occupational
    Medicine, 1982.
11 Lipsedge M. Psychiatric aspects of PHI claims. *Trans Assurance Med Soc* 1991;**19**: 18–35.
12 Gove WR, Geerken MR. The effect of children and employment on the mental health of mar-
    ried men and women. *Social Forces* 1977;**56**: 66–76.
13 Brown GW, Harris T. *Social origins of depression: the study of psychiatric disorder in women.*
    London: Tavistock, 1978.
14 Kearns JL. Return to work. In *Going home*, ed. Simpson JEP, Levitt R. London: Churchill
    Livingstone, 1981.
15 Lipsedge M, Summerfield AB. *The employment rehabilitation needs of the mentally ill.* Final
    report to Manpower Services Commission, February 1987.
16 Turner D, Litchfield P. *Schizophrenia and delusional disorders.* ABC of Mental Health for
    occupational physicians: clinical update series. BMA, London. September 1998.
17 Watts FN. Employment. In *Theory and practice of psychiatric rehabilitation*, ed. Watts FN,
    Bennett DH. New York: John Wiley, 1983.
18 Anthony W, Jansen M. Predicting the vocational capacity of the chronically mentally ill:
    research and implications. *Am Psychol* 1984;**39**: 537–544.
19 Shepherd G. Psychiatric Rehabilitation for the 1990s. In *Theory and practice of psychiatric
    rehabilitation*, ed. Watts FN, Bennett DH. New York: John Wiley, 1983.
20 Floyd M. Employment problems of ex-psychiatric patients. *Employment Gazette*
    1982;**90**,21–27.
21 Bond G, Dinsen J. Accelerating entry into transitional employment in the psychosocial reha-
    bilitation agencies. *Rehabil Psychol* 1986;**31**: 143–155.
22 Caplan RO, Cobb S, French JPR, van Harrison R, Pinneau SR. *Job demands and worker
    health: main effects and occupational differences.* Washington, DC: US Department of Health,
    Education and Welfare, 1975.
23 Kahn RL. Conflict, ambiguity and overload: three elements in job stress. In *Occupational
    stress*, ed. McLean A, Thomas CC. Pub. IL: 1974.
24 Cooper CL, Payne R. *Causes, coping and consequences of stress at work.* Chichester: John Wiley,
    1988.
25 Brand RJ. Coronary-prone behaviour as an independent risk factor for coronary heart dis-
    ease. In *Coronary-prone behaviour*, ed. Dembrosky TM, Weiss SM, Shields JL *et al.* New
    York: Springer-Verlag, 1978.
26 Parkes KP. Locus of control, cognitive appraisal and coping in stressful episodes. *J Pers Soc
    Psychol* 1984;**3**: 655–668.
27 Roberts GA. Prevention of burn-out. *Adv Psychiatr Treatment* 1997;**3**, 282–289.
28 Chronic fatigue syndrome. London: Royal College of Physicians, October 1996.

29 Sharpe M, Hawton K, Simkin, S *et al.* Cognitive behaviour therapy for the chronic fatigue syndrome: a randomised controlled trial. BMJ1996;**312**: 22–26.

30 Wessely S, Butler S, Chalder T, David A. The cognitive behavioural management of the post-viral fatigue syndrome. in *Post-viral fatigue syndrome*, ed. Jenkins R, Mowbray, pp. 305–334. Chichester: John Wiley, 1991.

31 Surawy C, Hackmann A, Hawton K, Sharpe, M. Chronic fatigue syndrome: a cognitive approach. *Behav Res Ther* 1995;**33**: 535–544.

32 Rees L, Lipsedge M, Ball, C (ed.) *Textbook of psychiatry*. London: Arnold, 1997.

33 Neff WS. *Work and human behaviour*, 3rd edn. Hawthorn, NY: Aldine, 1985.

34 Conti DJ, Burton WN The economic impact of depression in a workplace. *J Occup Med* 1994;**36**: 983–988.

35 Zigmond AS, Snaith RP, The hospital anxiety and depression scale. *Acta Psychiatr Scand* 1983;**67**: 361–370.

36 Clark D. A cognitive approach to panic. *Behav Res Ther* 1988;**24**: 461–470.

37 Mayou R, Bryan B, Duthie R. Psychiatric consequences of road traffic accidents. *BMJ* 1993; **307**: 647–51.

38 Bursteine A. Can monetary compensation influence the course of a disorder? *Am J Psychiatr* 1986;**1443**: 112.

39 Bursteine A. Treatment length in post-traumatic stress disorder. *Psychosomatics* 1986;**27**: 632–637.

40 Mendelson G. Persistent work disability following settlement of compensation claims. *Law Inst J (Melbourne)* 1981;**55**: 342–345.

41 Balla JI, Moratis S. Knights in Armour: a follow-up study of injuries after legal settlement. *Med J Aust* 1970;**2**: 355–361.

42 Levitt F, Sweet JJ. Characteristics and frequency of malingering among patients with low back pain. *Pain*, 1986;**25**: 357–364.

43 Trimble M. *Post-traumatic neurosis*. Chichester: John Wiley, 1981.

44 *International statistical classification of diseases and related health problems*, 10th revision (ICD-10). Geneva: World Health Organization, 1992.

45 Scandal of the pensions hole created for police and fire officers. *The Independent* (London), 13 October 1997.

8

Epilepsy

I. Brown and S. D. Shorvon

The World Health Organization's definition of epilepsy is: 'a chronic brain disorder of various aetiologies characterized by recurrent seizures due to excessive discharge of cerebral neurones'.[1] In practice, the diagnosis of epilepsy is applied to a person who has a persisting tendency to recurrent epileptic seizures. Neither single nor occasional epileptic seizures, febrile seizures, nor acute symptomatic seizures (those occurring during an acute illness) are usually classified as epilepsy. A single unprovoked seizure is not considered sufficient evidence to justify a diagnosis of epilepsy, unless other evidence of a tendency to recurrence is found (e.g. EEG evidence of epilepsy or a structural lesion on neuroimaging). Epilepsy can cause medical, psychological, and social problems, each of which can have an important impact on everyday life. It is a common condition which affects large numbers of working people. In about one-third, epilepsy is the only handicap, and in the others there are additional neurological, intellectual, or psychological problems.

Classification of epilepsy

Epileptic seizures can take highly variable forms, of which the well-known grand mal (tonic–clonic) convulsion is only one example. Thus, epilepsy is commonly classified according to seizure type.[2] Seizures are divided into two main categories:

*   In **generalized seizures**, initial epileptic discharges involve widespread areas of both cerebral hemispheres simultaneously. Generalized seizures are subdivided into
    *   tonic-clonic seizures
    *   absence seizures (petit mal)
    *   myoclonic seizures
    *   tonic seizures
    *   atonic seizures.

Each differs in clinical form, but consciousness is lost in all.

*   In **partial seizures**, which focus in a small area of the cerebral cortex, the clinical features vary greatly, reflecting the function of that part of the brain involved in the epileptic discharge. Partial seizures are subdivided into three main types:
    *   simple partial seizures in which there is no alteration of consciousness
    *   complex partial seizures in which consciousness is lost or impaired
    *   secondarily generalized seizures in which the epileptic discharge starts focally and then spreads triggering a generalized convulsion.

Prevalence and incidence

There are practical problems in establishing the prevalence and incidence of epilepsy.

- The condition is episodic. Between attacks the patient may be perfectly normal, with normal findings on investigation. Thus, the diagnosis is essentially clinical, relying heavily on an eye-witness account of the attacks.
- Many other conditions occur in which consciousness may be transiently impaired and which may be confused with epilepsy.
- The condition may go unreported, for several reasons. The patient may be unaware of the nature of the attacks, and so does not seek medical help. Patients with mild epilepsy, or partial seizures, in particular, may not consult a doctor, and may be overlooked in surveys.
- The term 'epilepsy' needs to be clearly defined in such studies. The question arises of whether to include single seizures, as does the issue of whether people who have been seizure-free for several years still have epilepsy. Febrile convulsions, which affect up to 3% of all healthy children between the ages of 18 months and 5 years, are usually excluded from population statistics.

Even using the most restricted definition, epilepsy is a common condition. A recent British study of treated epilepsy showed an incidence rate of 80.9 (95% confidence interval 76.9—84.7) per 100 000 per year. The incidence rate is higher in childhood and late life.[3] Throughout working life, from the ages of 16 to 65 years, first seizures occur at a rate of approximately 40 cases per 100 000 people per year. The cumulative incidence of epilepsy, i.e. the risk of having a seizure at some point in life, has been estimated to lie between 2 and 5%.[4]

The prevalence of active epilepsy has usually been found to be 5–10 cases per 1000 people, depending on the definition and methods of investigation; epilepsy is thus amongst the most common of serious medical conditions.[3,4] Its prevalence is approximately similar at all ages after early childhood, and it affects all races and classes. The majority of patients suffer tonic–clonic (grand mal) seizures, either generalized or secondarily generalized. A recent British-based population prospective study (the National General Practice Study of Epilepsy, NGPSE), has provided comprehensive data on the characteristics of epilepsy in an unselected population.[5,6] In this investigation, 62% of patients had tonic–clonic seizures (grand mal seizures, either primary or secondarily generalized), 11% complex partial seizures, and 12% mixed partial seizure types; other seizure types were uncommon. A similar breakdown of seizure types has been recorded in other community-based studies. The frequency of seizures between affected individuals is highly variable. About one-third of cases suffer seizures less than once a year, and about 20% more than once a week.

Causes of epilepsy

Studies have shown that a cause can be confidently established only in a minority of new cases of epilepsy (20–40%). The likelihood of establishing the underlying aetiology in a given patient is dependent on the extent of investigation. The wider use of magnetic

resonance imaging (MRI) will greatly increase the pick-up rate of previously unde-
tectable underlying structural cerebral disorders, especially of the developmental type.
The cause of epilepsy varies with age of onset. Thus, epilepsy developing in young adults
is most frequently due to alcohol or cerebral tumour, and, in late adult life, to cerebrovascular disease, when a cause is found. Box 8.1 is a list of the most common causes
of epileptic seizures in adults.

Box 8.1   Common causes of adult onset epileptic seizures
- Genetic propensity
- Developmental anomalies (especially neuronal migrational defects)
- Head trauma (and neurosurgery)
- Structural cerebral lesion (e.g. tumour, haemorrhage, arteriovenous malformation)
- Cerebrovascular diseases (e.g. infarction, hypertensive vascular disease)
- CNS infection (e.g. meningitis, encephalitis, abscess)
- Degenerative disorders (e.g. Alzheimer's disease)
- Systemic diseases (e.g. renal, hepatic, haematological)
- Birth trauma
- Congenital/developmental disorders (e.g. cortical dysplasia)
- Toxic/iatrogenic (e.g. alcohol, psychotropic drugs, drug abuse)
- Metabolic disorders (e.g. hypercalcaemia, inappropriate antidiuretic hormone secretion)
- Drug withdrawal (e.g. psychotropic drugs)

Toxic causes of epilepsy are rare. Seizures may very occasionally occur as a result
of lead encephalopathy, almost always in children. Seizures have occurred in employees overexposed during the manufacture of chlorinated hydrocarbons, and ingestion
of or gross overexposure to organochlorine insecticides has resulted in status epilepti-
cus.[7] EEG abnormalities of epileptic type have been recorded in the absence of any
clinical abnormality in workers exposed to methylene chloride, methyl bromide, carbon disulfide, benzene, and styrene, although the significance of these observations is
uncertain.

Recurrence of seizures

Usually, a person who has suffered a single seizure is not regarded as having epilepsy.
Estimates of the risk of a second attack after a first have varied from 27 to 80%, the variation reflecting selection bias in the study population. The NGPSE was used to calculate
recurrence rates by actuarial analysis in 564 unselected patients with newly presenting
non-febrile seizures.[6] Overall, 67% of patients had a recurrence within 12 months of a
first attack and 78% had a recurrence within 36 months. Seizures associated with a neurological deficit presumed to be present at birth had a 100% rate of relapse within the
first 12 months, whereas seizures associated with a lesion acquired postnatally carried a
risk of relapse of 75% by 12 months, and 85% by 36 months. Seizures occurring with an

acute insult to the brain carried a risk of relapse of 40% by 12 months, and 46% by 36 months.

It is well known that the risk of seizure recurrence is much higher in the first weeks or months after an initial attack, and the hazard rates for recurrent seizures in the NGPSE were 3.3% for the first 6 month period after the first attack, 0.7% each week for the next 6 month period, and 0.4% each week for the following 12 months. The longer the time period which passes without a second seizure, the less is the overall risk of subsequent recurrence, a fact which is often of great importance in resolving issues concerned with safety at work.

Chances of remission

Although there is a high risk of recurrence after a first attack, most people developing epilepsy become seizure-free.[6,8] A simple comparison of prevalence and cumulative incidence rates shows that seizures cease in the great majority of patients.[8] Similarly, hospital-based studies of initial therapy in newly diagnosed patients show that seizures are rapidly controlled in about 60–70% of patients.[9] Population-based studies have also revealed that, 10 years after diagnosis, about 65% of epileptic patients were in remission from seizures (defined as a 5 year period without attacks), and by 15 years from diagnosis, about 75% were in remission. Most patients who enter remission do so in the first 2 years after diagnosis. As time elapses without seizure control, the prospect of entering subsequent remission decreases markedly. In one British study, a patient whose epilepsy was still active after 5 years had only a 1 in 3 chance of being in remission (fit-free for 2 years) over the next 5 years; and a 38% chance over the next 10 years. This contrasts with patients who were seizure-free at 5 years, of whom 100% and 95% were in remission 5 and 10 years later.

About 20–30% of patients will continue to have seizures, regardless of treatment, and

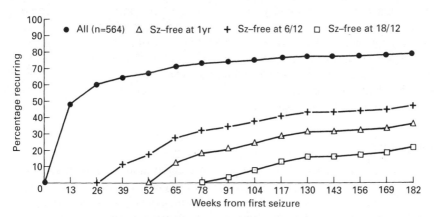

Fig. 8.1 Actuarial percentage recurrence rates after a first seizure for those still free of recurrence at 6, 12, and 18 months, and for all patients. Three-year recurrence rates for all patients was 78%, which fell to 44% if a second seizure had not occurred within the first 6 months, and to 32% and 17% for those seizure-free for 12 and 18 months, respectively.[6]

suffer from chronic epilepsy. The good outcome in patients with newly diagnosed epilepsy is in sharp contrast to the subsequent prognosis for patients with chronic established epilepsy, only a minority of whom can expect to become seizure-free. Factors indicative of a poor prognosis include:

- a long duration of uncontrolled epilepsy;
- a combination of different seizure types;
- frequent seizures;
- partial epilepsy;
- structural cerebral disorder;
- mental handicap or the presence of associated neurological or psychiatric deficits.

Benign Rolandic epilepsy occurs in adolescence and does not usually recur after the initial manifestation. From an employment point of view it is important that these young people are not labelled epileptic.

Prevention of epilepsy in the workplace

Primary prevention

The prevention of head injuries is the most important preventive measure and is fundamental to safety at work, in the home, and on the road. Epilepsy does not follow a trivial head injury; however, if the head injury is associated with a depressed fracture (especially if the dura is torn), an intracranial haematoma, or focal neurological signs, then there is a significant risk of later epilepsy.[10]

The wearing of seat belts by all motorists and the introduction of a comfortable and strong safety helmet when appropriate are the obvious first preventive measures. (Paradoxically this reverses the usual order of safety steps in occupational health and makes personal protection top of the list.) Making the working environment safe should be the first step, but often the unpredictability of events makes this impossible. It should be compulsory that safety helmets are worn at all times in areas specified by the works safety officer or safety committee. As a second step, the workforce should be made aware of areas where other employees are operating above, so that these can be avoided if possible. A safety helmet will not protect an individual from serious head injury if anything heavy is dropped from a great height. If work has to be performed underneath such a hazard, steel netting should be rigged to catch anything that falls.

Secondary prevention

Patients who have had a penetrating head injury, or a cerebral abscess, have such a significant risk of seizures in the next 2 years that there are good arguments for arranging work for them during this period, as for someone who has already had a seizure, including a ban on driving. Although it is customary to give prophylactic anticonvulsants after a head injury liable to be followed by epilepsy, controlled trials have yet to show any advantage.[11] The other main preventive measure is the avoidance of precipitating factors. Some of these are discussed below.

Shiftwork

Seizures are common just before and just after waking, especially in primary generalized epilepsy, and so it might be supposed that the introduction of a shift system into the work programme of a person with well-controlled epilepsy would predispose them to an increased frequency of seizures. Documentary evidence of a change in seizure frequency has not been established. This may be due to people with epilepsy electing to avoid shiftwork, as indicated by Dasgupta *et al.*[12] Many people with well-controlled epilepsy, however, can work on rotating shifts without problems.

Night work may be an exception. Patterns of sleep are disturbed by night work and to a lesser extent by other types of shiftwork. Night workers sleep for shorter periods during their working week and sleep longer on rest days, to make up the deficit.[13] Sleep deprivation is an important precipitant of seizures for some individuals, and is best avoided by those with epilepsy.

Stress

An association between stress and seizure frequency has often been reported anecdotally. Changes in brain arousal lead to changes in excitability and this may affect neuronal discharges, particularly of those neurones that surround an epileptic focus.[14] Is there any scientific evidence to support this association? Substantial numbers of patients report that the frequency of their seizures increases if they are exposed to stress, but stress itself may also be associated with other seizure-provoking factors such as alcohol and sleep deprivation and there may be reporting bias, as people search for an explanation for the build-up of their seizures.

Paradoxically, inactivity and drowsiness may also be related to an increase in seizure frequency. The possibility that stress and its associated factors may affect seizure control should be considered when employees with epilepsy are moved to different areas of responsibility.

Photosensitivity and visual display equipment

Photosensitivity epilepsy is rare in adults and usually associated with primary generalized epilepsy. It may need to be considered where a light source flickers. The overall prevalence is 1 in 10 000 but it is twice as common in women; 90% of patients have suffered their first convulsion due to photosensitivity before the age of 22 years.[15] Photosensitivity may be increased following deprivation of sleep. Spontaneous seizures may occur in photosensitive subjects.

The diagnosis of photosensitive epilepsy is supported by performing an EEG recording with photic stimulation and eliciting a photoconvulsive response. This is usually a generalized discharge of spike wave activity elicited by the flickering stimulus, persisting after the stimulus has ceased. False positive tests can also arise: some individuals have a paroxysmal EEG response to photic stimulation, without any evidence of having had a seizure.[15]

Television is a common precipitant of photosensitive epilepsy. The provocative stimulus is the pattern of interlacing lines formed by the flying spot from the electron gun.

Proximity to the screen appears to be an important factor, as this enables the viewer to discriminate the line pattern. Background illumination is another factor. Flickering sunlight (e.g. through the leaves of a tree), faulty and flickering artificial lights, and glare are also occasional precipitants. Swimming in bright sunlight may constitute some risk because of glare and flicker patterns on the water surface. Helicopter rotor blades and aeroplane propellers may also provoke episodes.

The use of a visual display unit (VDU) in employment constitutes a much smaller risk than that incurred while viewing television. The majority of VDUs have relatively slow phosphors in the tubes to reduce apparent flicker, and, in addition, they usually do not use an interlaced line pattern.

The probability of a first convulsion being induced by a VDU is exceedingly small and, even in the established photosensitive subject, seizures are unlikely to occur. It is therefore essential that a known sufferer of epilepsy is not disadvantaged in any way when applying for work which involves the use of a VDU. Regrettably this is still a common reason for job refusal, although it cannot be justified on the grounds of risk.

The Civil Aviation Authority (CAA) has recognized the special risks that may be associated with flying, especially from the slow flicker that is visible through helicopter blades. The CAA has always performed an EEG investigation as part of its routine medical screen on helicopter pilots applying for commercial licences. This is now required in the UK for professional fixed-wing aircraft pilots following the harmonization of aviation medical standards throughout the European Union and another 12 states (known collectively as the Joint Aviation Authorities, JAA). Introduced on 1 July 1999, it is now a mandatory investigation on all professional pilots on initial examination. No requirement exists for the investigation to be repeated routinely, and none is proposed, other than when indicated clinically.

Interestingly, medical assessors in the UK used to undertake EEG investigation as part of their routine medical screen on all applicants for professional fixed-wing aircraft pilots, but after many years of data collection the risk and cost–benefit analyses showed that this was not helpful. Although the UK has largely influenced the European harmonization process it was unable to avoid the re-introduction of this test.

Other types of reflex epilepsy

Although reflex epilepsy may occasionally be induced by reading, concentrating, being suddenly startled, or hearing music or bells, this is rare.

Alcohol and drugs

Alcohol consumed as beer appears to be a potent precipitant of seizures, especially if large volumes are consumed. This may be due to the moderate overhydration that occurs and a similar mechanism is possibly at work just before menstruation (although hormonal factors also contribute here).

A number of drugs have been incriminated as epileptogenic agents. By far the most common are the tricyclic antidepressants. Others include isoniazid, bronchodilators such as theophylline and terbutaline, and antipsychotic drugs such as haloperidol and chlorpromazine.

Fluctuating serum levels of anticonvulsant drugs, which may arise from poor compliance, interactions with other drugs, **or sudden withdrawal** may also result in a seizure.

What to do if a seizure occurs

If a seizure is likely to occur at work, supervisors and workplace colleagues should be warned and instructed in appropriate first-aid measures. Convulsive seizures are almost always short-lived and do not require immediate medical treatment. The person should be made as comfortable as possible preferably lying down (eased to the floor if seated); the head should be cushioned and any tight clothing or neckwear loosened. The patient should remain attended until recovery is complete. During the attack, the patient should not be moved, unless they are in a dangerous place—in a road, by a fire or hot radiator, at the top of stairs, or by the edge of water, for instance. No attempt should be made to open the mouth or force anything between the teeth. After the seizure has subsided, the person should be rolled on to their side, making sure that the airway is cleared of any obstruction, such as dentures or vomit, and that there are no injuries which may require medical attention. When the patient recovers consciousness, there is often a short period of confusion and distress. The person should be comforted, reassured and allowed to rest. **An ambulance or hospital treatment is not required unless there is a serious injury, or the seizure has lasted more than 10 minutes; or the person has had a series of seizures without recovering consciousness between them; or the seizure has features which differ significantly from the patient's usual form.**

Responsibility of the physician in the workplace

The first task is to establish without doubt that a seizure has occurred. The employee should attend the occupational health department as soon as possible and remain off work in the interim period. A detailed history of the event should be obtained and information sought from the patient and any reliable witness to try and establish the nature of the attack. Interviewing work colleagues and relatives who witnessed the event can be extremely useful, as the subject usually remembers very little beyond the first few seconds. It is very unwise to rely solely on written reports and second-hand information. Relevant points about family history and consumption of drugs or alcohol should also be obtained. The patient should be fully examined, as a seizure may occasionally be the first symptom of a serious systemic illness such as meningitis, or of a structural cerebral lesion: detailed medical assessment is always necessary (but see Box 8.2).

Not all episodes of unconsciousness are epileptic seizures: other possible diagnoses include syncope, drug overdose, paroxysmal cardiac arrhythmia, transient cerebral ischaemia (TIA), and simulated attacks.

Prolonged cerebral anoxia due to syncope may produce some twitching and even incontinence, although a generalized seizure is unusual. The focal ischaemia of a TIA

Box 8.2   Confidentiality

Permission to contact both the family doctor and any hospital consultant should be obtained from the patient. It is often useful to contact these physicians informally and discuss the situation that has arisen. This should be followed by a formal letter giving a concise account of events and the examination findings, and requesting any further relevant information.

---

does not usually involve loss of consciousness and often causes neurologically negative features, such as aphasia, and only rarely produces a convulsion. The possibility of a simulated attack may need to be considered.

Once it has been established as far as possible that a single, unprovoked, convulsion has taken place at work, the following procedure should be adopted:

1   The medical notes must state clearly the course of events and that a single seizure has taken place.

2   Management should be contacted and given clear and concise recommendations, in writing, regarding placement of the employee. Such written recommendations should be constructed with the agreement of the employee and should not breach codes of medical confidentiality. Some employees prefer to inform their immediate supervisor that they suffer from epilepsy and that this is well controlled with medication; it is worth discussing the possibility of such disclosure, which is usually agreed to by the patient.

3   The occupational physician and occupational health nurse must become familiar with any anticonvulsant prescribed and have a sound knowledge of both unwanted and toxic effects.

4   Consideration should be given to sensible employment restrictions (see below).

Consideration of potential new employees

The most significant factor in recruiting a new employee is how well qualified that individual is for the job. It would be unrealistic to state that all jobs are suitable for a candidate with epilepsy, but it is reasonable to state that the majority of jobs are suitable. Individual cases should be considered on their merits and the reader is strongly recommended to consult the training manual prepared by the International Bureau for Epilepsy (IBE).[16] This gives some excellent practical advice, provides an assessment questionnaire and illustrates some typical cases with vocational scenarios.

In December 1996 the provisions of the Disability Discrimination Act 1995 (DDA) came into force. This legislation is intended to protect disabled people, and people who have been disabled, from discrimination in the field of employment. An impairment is still relevant in the Act even if it is medically controlled and therefore epilepsy falls within the Act. However, precedence is given to the Health and Safety at Work etc. 1974 (HSAWA) when safety issues arise. In the case of epilepsy, the decision must be based on **risk assessment and medical evidence** and never on prejudice or assumption (the decision may have to be defended in court). It is essential that sufficient thought is given to the possibility of making 'reasonable adjustments to the workplace'. With epilepsy, this is nearly always possible except where there is a statutory bar (e.g. the driving of large goods vehicles). Often a safe place of work can be found for any employee, unless the hazard and risk is an integral part of the job (e.g. working as a steeplejack or on an oil rig). Similarly, provided that driving is only a small component of the job (less than 15%), an employee should not be refused employment if they do not hold a valid driving licence.

In summary, therefore, when considering the placement of an applicant with epilepsy the most important consideration is risk and methods of risk reduction or elimination. Every case will need to be assessed on its merits by a suitably qualified team after examination of the medical and occupational evidence. This action will protect both the applicant and the employer.

Sensible restrictions on the work of people with epilepsy

Proposed restrictions must be discussed fully with the employee and with management. Clear written instructions should be given to management regarding placement, responsibilities, and review. Confidentiality must not be breached (see above). Restrictions should be no more than necessary on common-sense grounds, as would apply equally to any individual subject to sudden and unexpected lapses in consciousness or concentration, however infrequent.

In the US it is illegal to deny employment to an otherwise qualified applicant because of disability, provided the disability does not impair health and safety standards at the workplace. However, this begs the question 'for what type of work is someone with epilepsy qualified?' The Epilepsy Foundation of America (EFA) has developed a comprehensive interview guide summarized by Masland.[17] The guide helps to define the important characteristics of a person's epilepsy, and draws attention to both advantageous and disadvantageous features. A consistent warning of attacks is certainly an advantageous feature, but this is unusual. Conversely, sudden loss of consciousness without warning must be considered disadvantageous. The frequency of attacks is another important consideration and the success rate in placing people with epilepsy is far greater if they have fewer than six seizures per year.

In general, minor attacks are less disruptive than major ones, but periods of automatism (performance of acts without conscious will) may upset colleagues. Other particularly disadvantageous characteristics are prolonged periods of postictal confusion, and sudden akinetic attacks where the possibility of serious injury is increased.

It is impossible to provide dogmatic advice as the circumstances in individuals and industries vary a great deal. Sensible restrictions, however, include avoidance of the following:

- climbing and working unprotected at heights
- driving or operating motorized vehicles
- working around unguarded machinery
- working near fire or water
- working for long periods in an isolated situation.

Hand-held powered tools may be a hazard if they can be fixed in the 'on' position.

There are certain jobs with special hazards where the risk of even one seizure may give rise to catastrophic consequences. These jobs fall into two groups:

- The first of these is mainly in transport, and includes vocational drivers, train drivers, drivers of large container-terminal vehicles, crane operators, aircraft pilots, seamen, and commercial divers.
- The second group are jobs that include work at unprotected heights, e.g. scaffolders, steeplejacks, and firemen; work on main-line railways; with high-voltage electricity, hot metal, or dangerous unguarded machinery or near open tanks of chemical fluids (see Box 8.3).

Box 8.3   Examples of jobs with special risks for seizure-prone workers (from Espir and Floyd 1986[18])
- Vocational drivers, (i.e. of large goods and public service vehicles, and taxis)
- Drivers of trains, cranes, straddle carriers
- Aircraft pilots, seamen, coastguards
- Work at unprotected heights, (e.g. scaffolders, steeplejacks, and firemen)
- Work with high-voltage electricity
- Work with dangerous unguarded machinery (e.g. chain saws)
- Work with valuable fragile objects and equipment
- Work near tanks of water or chemical fluids

The working environment and any equipment to be used by the employee with epilepsy should always be inspected by the occupational physician. The safety officer and the employee's immediate supervisor should be involved in any decisions.

It is important to remind the employee that contravention of agreed restrictions may endanger not only their own life, but also those of their colleagues and friends. The employee should also be reminded that it may be impossible to make any insurance claim for financial compensation for personal injuries should an accident occur as a result of evasion of agreed restrictions.

Lifting of restrictions

A policy should be established for terminating any restriction on work practices. This policy should be made known to the affected employee and not altered unless circumstances are exceptional. There is little place for partial lifting of restrictions: the employee is either considered safe or not. If a work restriction is removed after a period of freedom from seizures, the employee should be instructed to report any further attack to the occupational health staff or to a personnel officer or manager. If anticonvulsant medication is stopped or changed, consideration should be given to close monitoring at work for a period, or to the temporary re-introduction of restrictions.

It may be found that following the introduction of medication, control is still poor with an unacceptable rate of seizure recurrence. It is important that every effort is made to improve control before the individual is rejected or restrictions imposed for employment or promotion. Perhaps there are specific precipitating factors that can easily be avoided, e.g. alcohol. It is important to consider whether or not an appropriate anticonvulsant has been chosen, and whether adequate blood levels have been achieved (see p. 501).

Perhaps the employee forgets to take their medication or decides not to take it? Is there a correctable reason? All these possibilities should be explored and the occupational physician or occupational health nurse should co-ordinate their efforts with the family doctor and hospital consultant.

There should be a planned timescale for the review of restrictions. An explicit date should be offered, as this will confirm that the employee's future is considered to be important and that they are still a valuable member of the workforce. In this respect it seems reasonable to follow, for employment purposes, those guidelines issued by the Department of Transport for ordinary driving licences (see Appendix 1). An employee who is safe to drive a machine as dangerous as a car should be safe to undertake virtually all industrial duties. Jobs with special hazards are listed in Box 8.3. After an initial seizure, the Department of Transport advises that a subject may not drive a car for 1 year, and it seems reasonable to follow the same practice for restrictions relating to physical safety in industry.

Effect of anti-epileptic drugs on work performance

A clear distinction must be made between chronic side-effects and acute toxic effects of drugs. The latter occur when doses are too high, are rapidly reversible, and can be prevented easily by medical intervention. The chronic side-effects of anti-epileptic drugs are, unfortunately, less easy to control, and may be an unavoidable penalty of effective long-term drug therapy. However, these should be slight, and should not prove a major handicap in the working environment; indeed, the drug should seldom be prescribed if serious toxic effects are experienced. Minor effects on concentration, speed of reaction, and cognitive performance should not be allowed to cause significant impairment. Some anti-epileptic drugs have a sedative effect or can cause depression or irritability, but again this should not be of a degree which interferes with daily activity. In most patients with epilepsy, monotherapy in conventional dosage ensures seizure control, and in this situation no side-effects should be expected. In patients with uncontrolled epilepsy, however, drug treatment often needs to be more complex, and minor side-effects are acceptable. The balance between efficacy and toxicity depends on individual factors and it is difficult to generalize. An appropriate level of toxicity for one person may be unacceptable to another. In patients with mental impairment and cerebral damage causing epilepsy, side-effects are more common and more severe; most such individuals will be in a sheltered working environment, where some degree of drug-related impairment of work performance should be expected. Drug level monitoring provides a guide to appropriate dosing and a check on compliance.

The occupational physician should work closely with the neurologist so that they both understand what is happening to the patient. The occupational physician must understand the clinical situation as well as the work situation. The occupational physician and the neurologist must liaise closely to determine whether the patient's drug regime is appropriate for their particular employment or whether it could be modified or changed to better meet particular employment requirements. Being made aware of the latter by the occupational physician, the neurologist may be able to exploit new therapeutic opportunities.

Special work problems

Disclosure of epilepsy to employers

In an ideal world, individuals with epilepsy would freely disclose how their seizures affect them, and how often and when they occur, and information would exist on their medication and likely prognosis. The occupational physician could then, from their own knowledge of the work processes at the factory or office, advise employment in a sector which maximized the employee's production and opportunities for promotion, and minimized any risk to them or to their colleagues.

Only about a third of the working population have even a nominal contact with an occupational physician, however, so the situation is less than ideal. People with epilepsy are aware that they are at a competitive disadvantage and that their choice of vocation is limited. Their opportunities for mobility and promotion within a company may also be limited. They may suspect that they will not be allowed to join the pension fund. Finally, they may have to face the condescension and scrutiny of their fellow workers.

It is not surprising that the presence of epilepsy is often concealed from employers. A survey of people in London with epilepsy[19] showed that over half of those who had had two or more full-time jobs after the onset of epilepsy had never disclosed their epilepsy to their employer, and only 1 in 10 had always revealed it. If seizures were infrequent, or usually nocturnal, such that the applicant considered that they had a good chance of getting away with concealment, then the employer was virtually never informed. Among those who declared their condition two variables correlated with failure to gain employment: frequent seizures, and lack of any special skill.

This state of affairs will be improved only slowly by educational programmes. Another possible way forward includes a clearer definition of jobs that can be done by people with epilepsy. Such a definition has been considered and published by the International Bureau for Epilepsy (IBE)[20] which considered that the vast majority of jobs are suitable for people with epilepsy, especially where the person possessed the right qualifications and experience. **Blanket prohibitions should be avoided** and the organization of work practices should be examined to reduce potential risk to an acceptable level.

Accident and absence records of those with epilepsy

It is widely held that people with epilepsy are more accident-prone and have worse attendance records than other workers. However, this view is not substantiated by the small available literature. Many studies must be biased, as workers with epilepsy tend to get placed in inherently less risky work. The most significant study of work performance which attempted to eliminate this bias was conducted by the US Department of Labor more than 45 years ago. A statistical comparison was made of 10 groups with different disabilities, including people with epilepsy, with matched unimpaired controls in the same jobs. Within the epilepsy group, no differences were found in absenteeism, but their incidence of work injuries was slightly higher. The differences noted in accident rates were not, however, statistically significant. The general conclusion of this study was that people with epilepsy perform as well as matched unimpaired workers in the same jobs in manufacturing industries.

In a small study in 1960 Udell demonstrated that discriminatory practices against the recruitment of people with epilepsy are unwarranted, if based on the notion that as a group they have high accident rates, poor absence records, and low production efficiency. However, any applicant with epilepsy must be appraised individually with regard to the degree of seizure control, and any other associated handicap. Employers should have a receptive policy for recruitment and job security. This may encourage employees to admit the problem, and allow industry an opportunity to appraise their abilities and place them most appropriately.

The more recent study of epilepsy in British Steel[12] generally supported these findings. There was no significant difference between epilepsy and control groups with regard to overall sickness absence, accident records, and five different aspects of job performance. Work performance, however was significantly reduced in people with epilepsy who also had an associated personality disorder. The British Steel study emphasized that, although some degree of selection has to be applied when employing people with epilepsy, the overall performance of those with epilepsy compares well with that of their colleagues.

The major task, however, is not to prove that performance at work is satisfactory, but to challenge and change the often firmly held and deeply entrenched prejudices of employers.

Current employment practices

An informal survey (Ian Brown, unpublished data, 1996) of current attitudes and practices with respect to epilepsy within the previously nationalized industries, armed forces, teaching profession, National Health Service, and Civil Service, revealed an interesting dual approach adopted by most occupational health departments. There was often a carefully worded and apparently inflexible statement of corporate policy, yet many occupational physicians adopted a more sympathetic approach. This was usually only obvious, however, if the physician was contacted personally. Such manoeuvres were only found in doctors who worked in industries and services that had flexibility to relocate affected workers.

The armed forces were found to be the least flexible. In the case of new entrants, proven cases of epilepsy are not accepted for service and those who had suffered a single seizure less than 4 years before entry, are also rejected. For serving personnel, a single seizure after entry necessitates full examination of the individual, restricted activities, and observation for a period of 18 months. Full reinstatement is awarded only after assessment by a senior consultant. Aircrew who have suffered a single seizure after entry are grounded permanently, and servicemen who suffer more than one seizure will be considered for discharge on grounds of disability. The armed forces also employ a large number of civilians and the policy for these individuals is more flexible than for servicemen. For civilians the most significant factor is how well qualified an individual is for a particular job and if that job is safe or can be safely adapted to accommodate a person with a history of epilepsy.

Epilepsy is also a contra-indication for employment in the police force. The police expect all their officers to be fit for all duties. Officers who develop epilepsy during service are usually retired, but only after careful individual assessment (personal communication to I.B.).

Many of the large and often previously nationalized industries follow similar codes of practice and are able to pursue a more sympathetic and accommodating approach. Epilepsy declared at the pre-employment stage may be a contra-indication to employment, but is not an absolute bar. The discretion of the examining physician may allow for some compromise if the applicant has a special skill or quality to offer, and if the job is suitable. Epilepsy developing in service can often be accommodated if the employee is willing to be relocated, but this may involve some loss of earnings and status. If unacceptable, retirement on grounds of ill health is usually offered.

The Department of Education and Employment has a flexible policy for the employment of school teachers with epilepsy and allows its locally appointed part-time medical officers to use reasonable discretion. Difficult cases are referred to the Department's medical advisers, and each is judged on its own merits.

The National Health Service (NHS) has made considerable progress over the last decade but still has no national guidelines. This is by virtue of the numerous separate employers which collectively form the entity of the NHS. Virtually all trusts and health authorities have an occupational health service and many have the benefit of a consultant adviser in the specialty. Guidelines on occupational health issues, as they may affect NHS employees have been constructed by the Association of National Health Occupational Physicians (ANHOPS), and these include guidance on epilepsy. The guidelines state that all individuals must be assessed on their merits. They emphasize that the epilepsy should be well controlled and that the care of the patient must never be compromised.

The Civil Service has an open and documented policy on the recruitment and employment of people with epilepsy. The health standard for appointment in the Civil Service requires that a candidate's health is such as to qualify that person for the position sought, and that the person is likely to give regular and efficient service for at least 5 years or for the period of any shorter appointment. The Civil Service Occupational Health Service stresses that epilepsy *per se* is not a bar to holding any established appointment, apart from those posts with special hazards.

Getting employers to understand about epilepsy

Many of those with epilepsy are unemployed. Even if employed, many workers with epilepsy are still frequently denied promotion because of their disability or because of misconceptions about it. In a survey of employers in the US[21] it was found that few would employ people known to them to have had a generalized seizure within the previous year. In this study, Hicks and Hicks recorded a consistent reason given for the failure to offer people with epilepsy employment, that 'they create safety problems for themselves and other workers'. Such reasoning has not varied for more than two decades. These authors pointed out that this assumption is misconceived, and not supported by published data. An encouraging feature of this study was evidence of a positive change in attitude. Although the cause remains uncertain, changes in the law in the US and the continued efforts of public and private agencies may well be responsible.

To improve employers' understanding, regular informal health education seminars could take place at work. A well thought out programme that involves the personnel department, occupational health team, and interested union representatives may prevent some problems occurring. Topics such as epilepsy, stress, or alcohol abuse should be discussed openly, with the benefit of expert advice being immediately available. The occupational physician or occupational health nurse can play a major role in informal health education and in changing attitudes. Health education is concerned not only with the prevention of disease, but in the understanding of disease in others. Problems such as epilepsy are often shrouded in mystery, or considered as too unsavoury to discuss in detail. For such a common complaint, with a prevalence of about 5–10 per 1000 of the population, the ignorance still demonstrated is astonishing. Many employees, both on the shop floor and in management, consider that someone with epilepsy also has some degree of mental handicap combined with a lesser or greater physical infirmity. Certainly such problems may co-exist, but they are the exception. It is of paramount importance that health professionals should dispel myths and bring a sense of proportion to the issue.

The hard work of agencies such as the British Epilepsy Association (BEA), the National Society for Epilepsy (NSE), and the Employment Medical Advisory Service (EMAS) has done much to inform employers. Misconceptions about epilepsy are slowly disappearing and attitudes changing.

Opportunities for sheltered work

Most people with epilepsy are capable of normal employment without need for supervision or major restrictions. A minority will have additional handicaps and may only be able to work in a sheltered environment. Poorly controlled seizures, physical disability, low intelligence, and poor social adaptive skills will pose additional problems. The following specialized facilities are available in the UK for people with epilepsy.

Medical services

The NHS provides medical services for people with epilepsy through its general practitioner and hospital services. Most patients will be seen in neurology, paediatric or mental handicap clinics, and the great majority of people with epilepsy are satisfactorily managed in this way. Residential care, where needed, is usually provided by the social services departments, as part of their community care responsibilities. In addition, there are, however, epilepsy charities, residential centres and special assessment centres which cater for the particular needs of patients with epilepsy, as outlined below.

Epilepsy charities

National Society for Epilepsy

The NSE was founded in 1892, and is the oldest epilepsy charity of its type in the world, and the largest epilepsy charity in the UK. Its aims are:

- To provide services for people with epilepsy nationally. This includes NHS out-patient and in-patient assessment services (in association with the National Hospital for Neurology and Neurosurgery), residential care, medium-term in-patient rehabil-itation, community nurse services, and a network of community support groups.
- To provide educational services for the general public, employers, the media, and the medical and paramedical professions. These are provided via a telephone helpline, study days, lectures, and written and visual material.
- To carry out medical research, in conjunction with the Institute of Neurology, Uni-versity College London.

British Epilepsy Association

The BEA is an epilepsy charity which provides a telephone helpline to the general pub-lic and a system of lay self-help groups. Its activities are particularly aimed at modifying regressive attitudes to epilepsy, and to providing social support. It also provides written and visual information on epilepsy.

Residential centres and schools for epilepsy

In the UK, there are a number of special schools and centres for epilepsy, the largest of which are the Chalfont Centre (National Society for Epilepsy, Chalfont St Peter), the David Lewis Centre, and St Piers Lingfield. These provide residential care for people with epilepsy, usually associated with other handicaps, with a condition so severe that independent life in the community is not possible. Some include provision for sheltered employment or daily activities, in which residents perform useful and satisfying jobs. The financial support is usually provided through local authority grants, health service grants, or private or charitable funds.

Special medical assessment centres

There are three NHS special assessment centres in the UK. These provide short-term medical and social in-patient assessment for people with severe or complicated epilepsy, funded through the NHS. The largest is at the Chalfont Centre for Epilepsy, run jointly by the NSE and the National Hospital for Neurology and Neurosurgery. The paediatric special centre is run from the Park Hospital in Oxford. The other centre is at Bootham Park Hospital in York. Referral to any of the centres is through the normal medical channels, usually from general practitioners, paediatricians or neurologists. The centres admit patients from anywhere in the UK. (For full addresses, see Appendix 7).

Relationship between the occupational physician, consultant neurologist, and general practitioner

Recommendations received from the neurologist may differ from those acceptable to the occupational physician, who must consider the best interests of the patient in their par-ticular working environment. The family doctor, who may have cogent views and is likely to have closer knowledge of the patient, can liaise with both these two specialists. It is advantageous if all the physicians involved work together to avoid conflicting advice.

In companies with an occupational health service, an employee with epilepsy should be encouraged to contact the nurse and discuss problems as they arise. The nursing service at work is often readily accessible to the employee and has a special role in counselling and health education. Confidential notes should be kept and the case discussed with the occupational physician at the earliest opportunity. Any employees with epilepsy should be reviewed regularly by the occupational health service.

Existing legislation and guidelines for employment

For a more detailed discussion of legal aspects, see Chapter 2 and also Carter.[22]

HSAWA makes no reference to the disabled, and applies to all employees regardless of their health. The dual responsibility of employer and employee to safeguard health and safety is entirely reasonable, but may create problems. Many people with epilepsy do not disclose it to an employer for fear of losing their job, or not being offered one.[19] Under these circumstances the employee with epilepsy may contravene Section 7 of the HSAWA, if they knowingly accept a job that poses unacceptable risks. An employer may legally refuse to employ an applicant for a job on any grounds except those of sex and race without necessarily giving reasons for the decisions. The law relating to discrimination does protect disabled applicants (see below and Chapter 3) and became law in 1995 as the DDA. Part II of the Act introduces a general principle of non-discrimination into employment. A special legal duty is imposed on the employer to make reasonable adjustments to working arrangements to safely accommodate the disabled person. It may be genuinely impossible for employers to make such arrangements, or the costs to do so may be prohibitive. Under these circumstances and quite uniquely (as compared to other discrimination legislation) the Act allows the employer to discriminate where the discrimination can be justified by reasons that are 'material to the circumstances of the particular case and substantial'.

Someone who suffers from epilepsy will be covered by the DDA because they suffer from a substantial, long-term impairment, which may affect day to day activities. Furthermore, the fact that epilepsy may be controlled by medication does not deny the person protection. The Act clearly states that

an impairment which would be likely to have a substantial adverse effect on the ability of the person concerned to carry out normal day to day activities, but for the fact that measures are being taken to treat or correct it, is to be treated as having that effect.

It goes on to state that 'measures include, in particular, medical treatment'.

Employers therefore must be prepared to make reasonable adjustments to accommodate a person with epilepsy. A typical and common example might be an applicant for a job who is unable to presently hold a group I driving licence because of a recent convulsion. The job applied for requires the applicant to hold a group I driving licence but the driving component of the job is only about 10% of the duties. Under these circumstances it would be reasonable for the employer to provide an alternative means of transport for the employee. If the driving component was a substantial part of the job then it would not be reasonable for the employer to provide an alternative means of transport.

What are the legal implications if a worker develops epilepsy while in service? The DDA applies equally to employees in service with the same provisions as stated above. All employees are also covered by the Employment Protection (Consolidation) Act 1978; as amended this Act protects against unfair dismissal, and, from 1 October 1999, protection is conferred after 1 year's continuous employment. It is possible to avoid its provisions by offering a temporary or probationary contract, but this can only be for a limited period.

Is dismissal on medical grounds unfair? The Employment Relations Act 1999 has increased maximum compensation for unfair dismissal from £12 000 to £50 000. This is more likely to be a deterrent to the unscrupulous employer. The employer may be obliged to justify their decision to an industrial tribunal on at least one of five fair reasons for dismissal. Three of these are pertinent to this Chapter:

* Is the employee capable of performing their duties safely and efficiently?
* Has it become impossible for the employee to continue to work without contravening a statutory duty or restriction?
* Is it extremely difficult or financially prohibitive for the employer to make reasonable adjustment to working arrangements which would allow the employee to be safely accommodated (DDA 1995)?

The third reason was upheld in a recent industrial tribunal and is a good example of the employer justifying impracticability (*Smith* v. *Carpets International UK plc*, 11 September 1997, case no. 1800507/97). Mr Smith, an employee with a history of epilepsy. was employed as a warehouseman in 1994. He had not suffered a seizure for 9 years and the company's occupational physician considered his condition to be well controlled. No restrictions were therefore imposed. Mr Smith regrettably suffered further convulsions and the doctor therefore considered it was dangerous for him to work in the warehouse because of the heavy machinery and forklift truck work. From a risk assessment it was concluded that no adjustments could be made to the job. An offer of alternative work was not accepted by Mr Smith as it would have been less well paid. The case went to an industrial tribunal and the employer's case was upheld as the case had been appropriately assessed and reasonable investigations had taken place to examine what adjustments could be made to accommodate Mr Smith. Alternative work was offered and the employer was not expected to totally reorganize the way in which the warehouse carried out its work.

Incapability, illegality, and impracticability are all fair grounds for dismissal. The industrial tribunal makes the final decision, subject to an appeal to the employment appeal tribunal, but will require that the employer has discussed their state of health with the employee (if possible), made absolutely sure that the employee is incapable of doing the job in question, that an alternative job is not available, and the present job cannot be suitably adapted or adjusted.

Some employers are under the misconception that an applicant with a history of epilepsy will not be accepted into the pension fund. This is generally untrue, but the pension scheme assessors will consider all cases on their merits and very occasionally certain restrictions are placed on individuals joining with specific medical problems. Life cover or ill health retirement provision may be reduced if the risk is considered very significant but this will only be in relation to an accident or disability occurring in direct relation to the specific disability described. In the majority of cases there is no restriction and occupational pension schemes are far more liberal than independent life assurance schemes.

No special insurance arrangements are necessary for a worker with epilepsy. The employer's liability insurance covers everyone in the workplace—provided the employer has taken the disability into account when allocating the individual to a particular job. Failure to disclose epilepsy will render the employer's insurance invalid and should an accident occur as a direct result of the condition, it is unlikely that a claim for compensation will be met.

To summarize the legal position, the employee with epilepsy is protected by the same legislation and should enjoy the same pension rights as any other employee. They can be dismissed from employment if the disability seriously interferes with their capability to perform their duties satisfactorily. Dismissal can also take place if the employee's medical condition contravenes statutory regulations governing the job.[22]

The Driving Licence Regulations and their effects

The licensing for driving is one of the few areas in which there is legislation related to epilepsy (see also Appendix 1). Regulation is deemed necessary because of the higher than normal incidence of road traffic accidents (and accidental deaths) in drivers suffering from epilepsy and known to have collapsed at the wheel. Ideally legislation should balance the excess risks of driving against the social and psychological disadvantage to the individual of prohibiting driving. In the UK, it is the licensing authority (DVLA) and not the sufferer's personal medical advisers, which makes the decision to allow or bar licensing. The regulations are based, where possible, on research into the risks of seizure recurrence in different clinical circumstances. Licensing is divided into two groups, with more stringent conditions applied to group 2 licences because more time is spent driving and the consequences of accidents are often more serious.

- **Group 1 licences** (those for motorcars and motorcycles). An applicant for a licence who suffers from epilepsy shall satisfy the following conditions:
  - He shall have been free of any epileptic attack during the period of one year immediately preceding the date when the licence is granted; or
  - In the case of an applicant who has epileptic attack(s) only whilst asleep, shall have demonstrated a sleep-only pattern for three years or more, without attacks whilst awake.
  - The driving of a vehicle will not be likely to endanger the public.

The special regulations with regard to sleep and epilepsy are designed so as not to prejudice the small subgroup of epilepsy-sufferers whose attacks are confined to sleep and therefore who will not constitute a danger to driving. The third condition is concerned with situations such as those where drug therapy or associated neurological or neuro-psychiatric conditions may compromise road safety.

- **Group 2 licences** (those for large goods vehicles and passenger carrying vehicles, i.e. vehicles over 7.5 tonnes, or 9 seats or more for hire or reward). An applicant for a licence shall satisfy the following conditions:
  - No epileptic attacks shall have occurred in the preceding 10 years.
  - The applicant shall have taken no anti-epileptic drug treatment in the preceding 10 years.
  - There will be no continuing liability to epileptic seizures.

The purpose of the third condition is to exclude people from driving (whether or not epileptic seizures have actually occurred in the past) who have a potentially epileptogenic cerebral lesion, or who have had a craniotomy or complicated head injury, for example.

With all driver licensing, single seizures and mild seizures are subject to the same regulation. If a seizure is considered to be 'provoked' by an exceptional condition which will not recur, driving may be allowed once the provoking factor has been successfully or appropriately treated or removed, and provided that a 'continuing liability' to seizures is not also present. For group 1 licence holders treatment status is not a legal consideration, but it is recommended that driving be suspended from the commencement of drug reduction and for 6 months after drug withdrawal.

Van, crane, and minibus drivers will need to be found alternative employment within the company, as will those whose job also involves driving. The safety of forklift truck drivers will depend on individual circumstances.

For advice on driving with other neurological disorders and after head injuries, see Chapter 6 and Appendix 1.

Conclusions and recommendations

Many people do not disclose a past or present medical history of epileptic seizures when applying for a job, or during a routine examination at the workplace.[19] This may well cause major problems for the individual and the employer and, on occasions, inadvertently contravene HSAWA or invalidate insurance cover. However, the DDA now confers some protection on those with epilepsy. The unenlightened attitudes of some employers have led to secrecy or denial by those affected. The possibility of dangerous situations arising at work, or dismissal without recourse to appeal may be the outcome. A competent occupational health service, trusted by both shop-floor and management, can be invaluable in resolving conflicts and giving advice.

Responsibility for the employment and placement of a person with epilepsy rests with the employer, and they should have appropriate medical advice. Each case must be judged on its merits in the light of all available information. Any attempt to advise managers without a sound and complete understanding of the requirements of the job is unfair to both the employee and the employer. Every employee with epilepsy must be regularly reviewed. The development of good rapport and mutual trust will encourage employees to report any changes in their condition or medication and discuss any anxieties that have arisen.

A sensible approach by managers, with access to medical advice, should help the individual to come to terms with their condition, appreciate the reasons for any restrictions, and understand that decisions taken on the basis of such medical advice are in their best interests. The employer should drop old prejudices in favour of current knowledge about epilepsy. This will only occur when all those concerned with epilepsy undertake the responsibility of educating employers, the general public, and perhaps some members of the medical profession.

Selected references

1 Hopkins A, Shorvon S. Definitions and epidemiology of epilepsy. In *Epilepsy*, ed. Hopkins A, Shorvon S, Cascino G, 2nd edn, pp. 1–24. London: Chapman & Hall, 1995.

2 Dreifuss FE. The different types of epileptic seizures, and the international classification of epileptic seizures and of the epilepsies. In *Epilepsy*, ed. Hopkins A, pp. 83–113. London: Chapman & Hall, 1987.

3 Wallace H, Shorvon S, Tallis R. Age-specific incidence and prevalence rates of treated epilepsy in an unselected population of 2,052,922 and age-specific fertility rates of women with epilepsy. *Lancet* 1998; **352**: 1970–1973.

4 Sander JWAS, Shorvon SD. Incidence and prevalence studies in epilepsy and their methodological problems: a review. *J Neurol Neurosurg Psychiatry* 1987; **50**: 829–839.

5 Sander JWAS, Hart YM, Johnson AL, Shorvon SD (for the NGPSE). National general practice study of epilepsy: newly diagnosed epileptic seizures in a general population. *Lancet* 1990; **336**: 1267–1271.

6 Hart YM, Sander JWAS, Johnson AL, Shorvon SD (for the NGPSE). National general practice study of epilepsy: recurrence after a first seizure. *Lancet* 1990; **336**: 1271–1274.

7 Davies JE *et al.* Lindane poisonings. *Arch Dermatol* 1983; **119**: 142–144.

8 Shorvon SD. The temporal aspects of prognosis in epilepsy. *J Neurol Neurosurg Psychiatry* 1984; **47**: 1157–1165.

9 Goodridge DMG, Shorvon SD. Epilepsy in a population of 6000. *BMJ* 1983; **287**: 641–647.

10 Jennett WB. *Epilepsy after non-missile head injuries*, 2nd edn. London: Heinemann, 1975.

11 Jennett WB. Epilepsy after head injury and intracranial surgery. In *Epilepsy*, ed. Hopkins A, pp. 399–409. London: Chapman & Hall, 1987.

12 Dasgupta AK, Saunders M, Dick DJ. Epilepsy in the British Steel Corporation: an evaluation of sickness, accident and work records. *Br J Indust Med* 1982; **39**: 146–148.

13 Wilkinson RT. Hours of work and the 24 hour cycle of rest and activity. In *Psychology at work*, ed. Warr PB, pp. 31–54. Harmondsworth: Penguin, 1971.

14 Betts T. Epilepsy and stress. *BMJ* 1992; **305**: 378–379.

15 Jeavons PM, Harding GFA. *Photosensitive epilepsy: a review of the literature and a study of 460 patients*. Clinics in Developmental Medicine. Spastics International Publications, No. 56. London: Heinemann, 1975.

16 Troxell J, Thorbecke R. *Vocational scenarios: a training manual on epilepsy and employment.* Second Employment Commission of the International Bureau for Epilepsy. Heemstede, The Netherlands: International Bureau for Epilepsy, April 1992.

17 Masland, RL. Employability, Part VIII. Social aspects. In *Research progress in epilepsy*, ed. Rose C, pp. 527–532. London: Pitman, 1983.

18 Espir M, Floyd M. Epilepsy and recruitment. In *Epilepsy and employment*, ed. Edwards F, Espir M, Oxley J, pp. 39–46. London: Royal Society of Medicine,1986.

19 Scambler G, Hopkins AP. Social class, epileptic activity and disadvantage at work. *J Epidemiol Community Health* 1980; **34**: 129–133.

20   Employment Commission of the International Bureau for Epilepsy. Employing people with epilepsy. Principles for good practice. *Epilepsia* 1989; **30**(4): 411–412.

21   Hicks RA, Hicks MJ. The attitudes of major companies towards the employment of epileptics: an assessment of 2 decades of change. *Am Correct Ther J* 1978; **32**: 180–182

22   Carter T. Health and safety at work: implications of current legislation. In *Epilepsy and employment*, ed. Edwards F, Espir M, Oxley J, pp. 9–17. London: Royal Society of Medicine, 1986.

9

Vision and eye disorders

P. A. M. Diamond and G. Munton

Vision is necessary for most types of work, although there are some jobs such as keyboard work which can be performed with a low degree of visual acuity and even with total blindness, if a voice operated computer is an option, or Braille. A consideration of visual acuity is of primary importance when deciding whether on ocular grounds any particular work can be undertaken. The extent of the visual fields, problems of binocularity and double vision and the integrity of colour vision may also influence decisions about suitable work. Visual parameters may determine whether the Disability Discrimination Act 1995[1] (DDA) will apply to some types of work. The use of spectacles and contact lenses may improve visual acuity, and if correction enables work to be undertaken satisfactorily, there is no disability within the meaning of the Act. There are, however, some occupations where neither of these aids can be used. Some of these occupations are excluded from the legislation, and in some there may be justification on grounds of health and safety or to comply with road transport regulations, but in all other circumstances alternative work may have to be sought. The eye should always be guarded against damage from the work process with appropriate eye protection and visual equipment.

Prevalence of ocular defects

In both sexes a wide range of visual acuity may be encountered at any age, though serious defects are commoner in later life. Other ophthalmic defects, such as monocularity, visual field defects, and imbalance of the eyes, also occur in both sexes and throughout life. Ocular injuries in particular may cause serious visual defects.

It is estimated that there are 181 958 people in the British Isles who are registered as blind and 133 823 who are registered as partially sighted (Royal National Institute for the Blind, 1996).

Clinical aspects affecting work capacity

There are varying degrees of visual defect. Some people on the register of blind people have no sight, but the register contains others, for instance those with macular disease or advanced glaucoma, who have enough vision to walk about independently, even though they experience some difficulty and are unable to read, or recognize others at a distance.[2] Certain types of work can only be undertaken by those with normal visual function, but people with poor vision, or even none, will often be able to do some work. A period of training may be required when visual function has been damaged but thereafter there is no reason why the standard of work should not be satisfactory and done at home if necessary, without interruption.

People with defective vision which cannot be improved with spectacles may be helped by low vision aids. The simplest of these is a hand-held magnifying glass of about 12 dioptres which helps a person with low visual acuity to read, but this is an inefficient method. Desk or chest-mounted magnifiers free the hands for some tasks. Some low vision aids are small telescopes, with compound lenses fitted into spectacle frames, and these can improve near or distant vision. Such aids provide considerable magnification, but the associated reduction in visual field is a disadvantage. They may, however, enable people with severely defective vision not amounting to blindness to carry on with some close work. Recent advances in electronic scanning and machine vision with visual display on voice output enable the visually handicapped to acquire information, and even to inspect engineered parts. Voice-operated wordprocessors may allow even the totally blind to engage in detailed business and scientific correspondence. Audible output micrometers and gauges have a valuable role and can enhance the work prospects of workers with quite severe visual handicaps. These examples illustrate how reasonable adjustments can be used to meet the requirements of the DDA.

Blindness

The definition of a blind person, for registration purposes, is one in whom there is insufficient sight to carry out work for which sight is essential; for practical purposes this is considered to be a corrected visual acuity of 3/60 or less in each eye. This is an inability to read the top letter of the standard sight testing chart at a distance greater than 3 metres. Severe visual field defects, even in the presence of good visual acuity, may be sufficient to prevent independent activity in daily life.

Blind people receive instruction through the Royal National Institute for the Blind (RNIB). Braille or Moon and keyboard skills are taught, together with instruction in how to walk about independently using a stick, usually white, which denotes a significant visual handicap. The long-cane technique, and devices using ultrasound, allow even more independence. Further improvement may derive from electronic global positioning indicators, though at present programmes for the visually handicapped are at an early trial stage of development. Training in personal life skills is undertaken soon after the sight is damaged. Blindness associated with deafness causes additional problems.

Blindness has many causes. Congenital defects and trauma are the usual causes in the young, whereas acquired defects such as cataract, glaucoma, macular degeneration and diabetic retinopathy damage sight in older age groups. Increasingly the results of trauma can be treated to prevent loss of sight. Cataract can be surgically treated in almost all people, sometimes as day cases. The newer surgical methods afford a higher success rate and result in better spatial co-ordination. It is essential that glaucoma is treated in its early stages to limit further damage. Macular degeneration, which damages central vision, is fairly common in the elderly and is in many cases untreatable. Some cases can be halted by laser treatment, but the condition cannot be cured. Diabetes is the commonest cause of blindness in the western world and accounts for 7–8% of all registrations.

Visual field defects

Many conditions cause visual field defects. Vascular lesions of the nervous system can result in hemianopia (loss of half the visual field) and may be bilateral, complete, or partial. Homonymous hemianopia causes some difficulty in walking, and especially in crossing roads, since the same side of the vision is absent in each eye. A complete quadrant homonymous defect, upper or lower, is a bar to driving, since traffic information and hazards exist in both upper and lower areas of field.[3,4] Bitemporal hemianopia occurs in disease of the pituitary gland and usually results in defective vision on both sides while the vision straight ahead is usually satisfactory. Sometimes, however, it may result in intractable diplopia. Bitemporal hemianopia precludes the driving of any vehicle and also the performance of any work where safety would be compromised by lateral field loss. In retinitis pigmentosa, or pigmentary degeneration of the retina, the entire peripheral field of vision may be lost so that only the 5–10° of central vision persists. This is commonly known as **tunnel vision**, and causes considerable, often progressive, disability. Additionally, night vision may be severely compromised. Hence this condition should be considered to be a bar to all driving. It also affects the capacity to do many other tasks safely and effectively. A similar condition occurs in advanced chronic simple glaucoma (see below), and should be similarly regarded.

Special work problems

The main difficulty for those who have defective vision is that they are more likely to have accidents, particularly in hazardous situations. People with defective vision, restricted visual fields, or imbalance of the eyes with resulting diplopia should not work at heights, for example, on ladders, gantries or scaffolding, where they will fall if they overstep the boundaries, and they should not work in the vicinity of moving machinery where they might also suffer injury. People with seriously defective visual function are barred from driving vehicles not only on the public highway, but also as heavy plant operators on construction sites and industrial and other locations. They should not operate cranes, hoists, or forklift trucks. They cannot usually be employed in the armed services, the police, or the emergency services, although there may be some jobs, such as radio-telephone operators, which may be suitable.

It is particularly important that young people with visual problems should receive informed advice about a suitable career after their visual state has been assessed. Blind and partially sighted registration may expedite access to advice via the associated social workers and careers officers. It is essential that their career prospects should be considered in the light of visual prognosis. Candidates for the armed services, the police force, aircrew (see Appendix 2), and seafarers (see Appendix 3) undergo full medical examination on entry, and careful examinations are undertaken for train and bus drivers. Normal vision and ocular function are required in all people who will work in transport or in occupations where driving is an essential component, and it is necessary that they can be given reasonable assurance that their ocular function (with correction, if necessary and if allowed) will remain at a satisfactory level for their expected work-span; for instance, the fire services require a test for latent hypermetropia.

Normal vision

The majority of the population has normal vision, meaning that the visual acuity is normal (6/6 in each eye), with or without correction; the visual fields are full, the balance between the two eyes is normal, and colour perception is satisfactory. Such people can in general undertake any occupation, though the wearing of contact lenses or spectacles may, exceptionally, result in some difficulty. Special visual standards are required for aircraft pilots (see Appendix 2), for seafarers (see Appendix 3), and for drivers of trains and public carriage and large goods vehicles. Officers in the police force and members of the fire and rescue services must also have a high standard of visual acuity. People who wear breathing apparatus must not wear spectacles, as these may prevent a gas-tight fit and can allow the ingress of toxic fumes and gases. Members of the armed services are required to achieve defined visual standards which differ according to the duties to be undertaken.

All workers in occupations with rigorous visual requirements must have regular examinations to ensure that they have not fallen below the necessary standards. Serious visual defects, such as the loss of an eye, may indicate the need for alternative employment.

Intermediate vision

The intermediate vision group comprises those who have defective sight (less than 6/6, corrected, in each eye) but who are not in the blind or partially sighted categories. Many can achieve satisfactory visual acuity with spectacles or contact lenses, but others have some degree of subnormal vision even with optical help. Some have mild defects of visual fields, ocular muscle balance, or colour vision. People in this group are ocularly fit for all occupations except those requiring the highest visual standards. They can undertake clerical work, most manufacturing and servicing tasks, information technology (IT) and most professional occupations, (exceptions include pilots and microsurgeons), and are usually fit to drive private cars. Those with marked defects of the visual fields (see above) must be regarded as at risk of injury if they work at heights or among moving machinery. Crane operators, forklift truck drivers, and drivers of electric trucks within stores or on work sites all require good peripheral vision both for driving itself and for the control and manipulation of the loads they carry. Difficulty with the task may indicate the need for further visual investigation. There is little evidence that stereopsis is essential for distance tasks. If there is any doubt, full orthoptic investigation should be requested, via the ophthalmic services. Uncontrolled double vision should disqualify from work in all hazardous situations, and from driving. In less exacting tasks the disability can be overcome by retraining and covering one eye.

Aphakia and pseudophakia

In aphakia the lens of the eye is absent, usually as the result of a cataract operation to remove an opaque lens. Such cataracts are commonly of the senile type but they can occur after trauma or as a secondary consequence of some eye diseases. Removal of the lens alters the optical properties of that eye so that in most cases satisfactory vision can be obtained only by the use of strong convex spectacle lenses. These magnify the image seen in the operated eye, so that if only one eye has been operated on, fusion of the images of the two eyes is not possible and double vision may result. People who are aphakic in one eye and who have no implanted lens or contact lens are functionally monocular. Even in bilateral aphakia the spectacle optics may produce severe spherical aberration, so that linear objects are curved and visual space is distorted, which can make walking difficult. Additionally, the optical defect causes the 'jack-in-the-box' phenomenon, where peripheral objects (such as a pedestrian crossing the path) disappear at the outer lens zone, and reappear in the central zone magnified and with alarming suddenness. All these problems (unilateral aphakia, spherical aberration, and 'jack-in-the-box') can now be overcome very successfully by the use of a contact lens or by an intraocular lens implant at the time of operation (pseudophakia).

Monocularity

An eye may have to be removed because of injury, because of severe and continuous pain, or as the result of malignancy. Damage to the vascular supply of an eye by embolism or thrombosis may cause loss of vision, as will an unoperated cataract and the chronic inflammation of uveitis in some patients. Monocular vision results not only from the removal of an eye but in circumstances where the vision in one eye is very defective.

Monocular vision causes difficulty in the estimation of distance, although this improves with learning. People who are monocular are at increased risk if they work in hazardous jobs, such as on scaffolding or moving machinery. They are excluded from work as pilots of ships and as drivers of trains, large goods vehicles (LGV), and passenger carrying vehicles (PCV).[5] A minimal level of binocularity is required for all new entrants requiring LGV and PCV licences. LGV and PCV drivers who become monocular are required to surrender their licences, although such drivers who have had cataract surgery with an intraocular implant or contact lens are allowed to continue after a period of adaptation, provided they fulfil the necessary minimum binocular visual standard and are subject to annual checks.[6]

Injuries

Sharp and blunt trauma can cause perforating injuries to the globe. Injury commonly occurs from the use of a hammer and chisel, and other percussive machine tools. When the intraocular foreign body is a chip of metal from the hammer, which is usually made of hard but brittle steel, damage to the lens and retina is a common result. Heavy blows on the eye with a blunt object may rupture the eyeball, necessitating major surgical repair or its removal. Lesser blows, as from a fist, may cause a traumatic cataract or retinal haemorrhage and detachment. These do not usually necessitate or need removal of the eye, but a cataract may require removal of the lens (see Aphakia, above).

Eye protection

Eyes should always be protected from high-velocity particles, dust, irritant fumes, gases, radiation, and chemical splashing. Safety spectacles, or goggles where a complete seal is required, can be supplied with correcting lenses manufactured from toughened glass or plastic to British Standard specification.[7] Spectacles cannot be worn satisfactorily under goggles or breathing apparatus. Protection is particularly important where there is effective vision in only one eye, since this is uniquely valuable, and monocular workers must be warned especially about ocular hazards in the workplace. Monocular vision, however, has a considerable effect on employer liability and a skilled craftsman who loses the sight in one eye may need to be moved to a less hazardous occupation. People who have a squint in early life may have an amblyopic or lazy eye which renders them virtually monocular. Such people, together with the monocular group, should be advised not to enter occupations which may involve an increased risk to the remaining eye.

Conditions causing sudden variation of vision

Sudden variation of vision is unusual but may cause difficulty, especially in exacting work. It may occur in migraine, sometimes associated with positive scotomata, fortification spectra or sensations of flashes of light. Spasm of the central vessels of the retina may cause blurred vision, which is usually transitory. Blood sugar variations in diabetics who are unstable or undergoing stabilization, and medication which affects accommodation are among the commonest causes of altered focus. The onset of cataract or glaucoma may cause similar variation.

Colour perception

Defective colour vision is inherited in the majority of cases, occurring in 8.0% of men and about 0.2% of women. There are different types of defect, but for practical purposes the problem is identification of red and green. Acquired defects are rare, but do exist, and may be permanent. They may be temporary in various ocular diseases such as tobacco amblyopia, toxic amblyopia due to medication, and lens opacities. Where good colour perception is required for safety reasons, therefore, periodic re-examination is warranted. Prolonged work with display screen equipment (DSE) may produce a perceived transient colour shift, which is complementary to the colour of the screen. Workers using high-powered lasers may also experience a permanent shift in colour sensitivity.

Only a very small proportion of occupations require perfect colour discrimination; a few others present some difficulties but are not necessarily precluded. Pre-employment rejection of those with defective colour vision will eliminate up to 8.0% of male applicants, depending on the tests used. Colour vision assessment is only necessary if normal colour vision is essential for the job in question. Further investigations to diagnose the type and severity of the colour defect are best left to specialists.

Methods of colour vision testing

Conditions for all tests are exacting, and findings will be useless if these are not followed. Equipment must be clean, and colour plates should not be left on the window sill to collect dust and fade in the sun. The most practical acceptable ambient illumination is ordinary daylight through a north-aspect window. There are significant variations in the wavelength mix of lighting by filament bulbs, fluorescent lamps, and discharge 'energy saving' lights. Artificial illumination standards must be precise, and variations in the colour of light are not acceptable. Subjects should wear corrective lenses (not tinted) if necessary, to enable them to define the characters. There needs to be a good understanding between the tester and subject as the procedures are complex. It is not unknown for pre-employment applicants to memorize the characters and plate numbers, and rapid random replies should be sought.

Pseudoisochromatic tests, such as the Ishihara plates or the City University test, are the most common methods of assessment. Matching tests are the oldest type of colour vision examination. The Holmgren wool test, which requires the subject to match colours of various skeins of wool, was used in the railway industry until other more sophisticated techniques were developed. Modern matching tests, such as the Farnsworth–Munsell 100 Hue test, detect more subtle defects. Lantern tests rely on transmitted light through filters. Ambient illumination is less critical, and lanterns more easily simulate the signals that are used for navigation and transport purposes. Often they use only the relevant signal colours, but they may include any colours in the range. Well-known lanterns are the Giles–Archer, Holmes–Wright, and Edridge–Green. Practice and custom usually decree which test is used in any occupation or industry: for instance, the railway industry currently uses the Edridge–Green lantern as an ancillary test to the Ishihara plates. The anomaloscope is a highly specialized diagnostic instrument which has no place in occupational screening procedures. There are promising new developments in computer-generated (visual display) methods of testing colour thresholds.

It should be noted that although colour contrast and discrimination can be aided by specially tinted (usually deep red, e.g. x-chroma and chromas) contact lenses, which produce pseudo colour vision, these devices are unsuitable for use in safety-critical tasks that require accurate colour perception. Nor should they be worn during screening tests. A good comprehensive review of tests for colour vision with recommended lighting standards, etc. can be found in *Defective Colour Vision* by Fletcher and Voke.[8]

Occupations requiring normal colour perception

These fall into three categories which are described below.

Transport, navigation, the armed services

For these occupations the need is to interpret colour signals without error, both in operating tasks and in the installation, maintenance, and testing of these signals. There is usually no positional reference, and the signal may be at a great distance and weather conditions adverse, with fog, rain, or bright sunshine. Testing procedures have evolved because accidents on the railways and in navigation were attributed to incorrect colour perception. Driving on the road, however, does not require accurate colour perception because road traffic signals can be interpreted by the relative position of the lights. These are of a standard high intensity, but other red and amber lights of low intensity may be difficult to distinguish. There is no statistical evidence that drivers with defective colour perception have more traffic accidents than those with normal vision[9], probably because they learn to compensate for their defect and become more vigilant. Drivers of passenger carrying and large goods vehicles, for example, undergo intensive training.

Occupations using colour coding for safety and technical purposes

Colour differentiation is used for hazard warning systems, cables and wiring, coding of pipes, etc. In the concept of British Standard colour coding,[10] those with defective colour vision have not been sufficiently considered. Coding may have to be done under dirty and poorly lit conditions by people who are not aware that they have a problem. The best solution is a practical test, e.g. wiring or gas cylinder codes. Other features which augment the safety of colour coding such as the pin index used with medical gas cylinders are useful. Chemical analysis and medical diagnosis (clinical and technical) may present difficulties, such as with urinalysis and, indeed, with colour vision screening itself. These problems may be reduced by screening at school so that appropriate career advice can be offered to the very small number of affected children who are unable to follow these colour critical occupations.

Occupations commercially dependent on sophisticated colour selection

Examples range from fruit picking to ticket collection, but mainly arise in the dyeing, textiles, paper, and printing industries. Employers in these industries may not consider formal colour vision screening necessary until an expensive mistake has been made. Trade tests are useful, and for some less exacting tasks colour filters may help, by producing pseudo colour vision, (see above). Coloured pens can be labelled; this helped a clerk to avoid writing in green on accounts sheets, the colour reserved exclusively for audit checks within the firm. With more artistic vocations, there will be a degree of self-selection.

Visual fatigue at work

Visual fatigue does not ordinarily occur in people who have normal vision and satisfactory balance between the two eyes, given adequate levels of illumination. A person will seek relief from any exacting visual task by changing focus to infinity or looking out of a window. This can be assisted by altering the desk position or with the help of a picture or mirror.

Display screen equipment

Rapid expansion in the use of DSE has aroused concern about the ability of the eyes to cope.[11,12] There is no evidence that working with DSE can harm eyesight. Partially sighted people need not be excluded from this type of work, if adjustments can be made, as required by the DDA, such as enlarged text on the display screen or the provision of voice activation systems. The Disablement Employment Adviser (DEA), who can be contacted at the Employment Services' Job Centres, can provide low-vision aids if they are necessary for a particular job.

Headaches attributed to eyestrain usually arise because of ergonomic problems, that result in awkward posture and muscular strain. Equipment should be properly maintained to avoid flicker, glare and reflection, and there should be sufficient flexibility in positioning of screen, keyboard, and source documents to enable the operator to adjust the workstation to meet their particular visual requirements.[11] Middle-aged and elderly people may experience difficulty because their ordinary reading glasses do not correct their sight at the distance required for DSE work. They may be more comfortable with glasses designed for work use, with focus adjusted to the screen distance. Bifocal and var-ifocal spectacles may not be as convenient; difficulties in locating the correct near or intermediate focal zone of the lenses may exacerbate neck strain. Excessive heat gener-ated by electronic equipment in a confined or overcrowded space with inadequate venti-lation may exacerbate dryness or soreness of the eyes. The EC Directive[12] entitles 'users' (generally people who use a screen for several hours a day) to be tested periodically. This can be achieved by software tests used on the DSE and the results can be collated for the employer in the computer (i.e. VueTest, Keeler Ltd, Windsor, Berks and others. See Appendix 7). These use software generated on screen test types of varying sizes. A polar-ized screen overlay and cross-polarized goggles are used to isolate the view of each eye to parts of the screen. Horizontal and vertical line displays can be moved by the arrow keys on the keyboard to measure ocular muscle imbalance at the screen distance. Thus the test is interactive with the software and results can be printed out or stored. Failure on these tests may indicate a full optometric review. The regulation makes the employer responsible for provision of an optical correction necessary for the DSE task at the appropriate working distance, usually 50–60 centimetres.

Limitations of spectacles and contact lenses at work

Some circumstances can pose problems for people who have to wear spectacles or contact lenses at work. Protective clothing, such as safety helmets, welding visors, and ear defend-ers can make spectacle-wearing and even the use of contact lenses uncomfortable. In such cases goggles incorporating correcting lenses should be provided. Spectacles with flat tem-ple pieces improve compatibility with certain items of personal protection, such as ear-muffs or respirators, but when worn with self-contained positive pressure breathing apparatus may still allow ingress of toxic fumes. Recently in some essential services, including the fire service, rail and air transport, a few potential recruits have had corneal refractive surgery such as photorefractive keratectomy (PRK) or laser *in situ* keratomileu-sis (LASIK) to overcome their need for contact lenses or spectacles and in the hope of thereby qualifying themselves. However, because of a risk of increased disability from glare and reduced contrast sensitivity following these procedures, the Royal College of Opthalmologists (Visual Standards Sub-Committee) has recommended that applicants from these services be individually assessed and counselled by an opthalmologist.[13]

The wearing of tinted spectacles or lenses reduces visibility, especially in dull weather and at night. Reactive lenses do not change sufficiently quickly to cope with sudden changes of illumination such as driving through road tunnels, or passing headlights, and their use should be limited. Drivers may have to perform exacting manoeuvres such as reversing, even when spectacles have become dislodged by accident. For this reason large goods and passenger carrying vehicle drivers must have an unaided visual acuity in each eye of at least 3/60. For further details on visual standards and driving, particularly voca-tional driving, see Munton.[5]

Contact lenses may be useful in occupations where spectacles may become misted, in aphakia, and where distortion occurs when looking through the marginal parts of the spectacle lenses. Although hard acrylic contact lenses are still widely in use, particularly the micro-lens type, there is a trend towards soft water-permeable and highly oxygen-permeable contact lenses, both hard and soft. Some of these lenses allow longer periods of wear but the soft lenses are less applicable where there is high astigmatism of the cornea, as the contact lens may mould to the astigmatism. Contact lenses help in aphakia where they overcome the magnification problem of aphakic glasses. Recently, intraocular lenses and small incision surgery have largely overcome this problem and that of surgically-induced astigmatism. Some dusty occupations generate particles that may get trapped under contact lenses and cause irritation. Usually the particle cannot be removed without removing the lens, and headache or conjunctivitis may persist. This is a hazard in dirty and dusty environments, such as railway track work, mining, and work with rescue teams, and requires constant vigilance.

In high-speed lathe and machine work, where a slurry of oil/water emulsion may be used to cool the cutting tools, a fine aerosol of the slurry can be deposited on the contact lenses. These aerosols can contain large numbers of bacteria with infective risk particularly to wearers of soft water-permeable contact lenses. Examples of such occupations are aluminium spinning and optical surface finishers.

Ultraviolet and infrared rays are partly filtered by contact lenses. **People who wear contact lenses at work must be identified because there are certain occupations in which they should not work**, for example, rescue services and mining, and in some cases protective measures may be required. There has been a recurrent and unsubstantiated myth that contact lenses can be welded to the cornea by ultraviolet exposure in occupations such as arc welding. This does not occur, but the ultraviolet component of electric arc welding can cause corneal epithelial loss, with or without contact lens wear.[14]

Cosmetic considerations are the motivating factor for many people who wear contact lenses, but there is also no doubt that contact lenses give better optical correction where myopia exceeds 5 dioptres. They are also useful in irregular astigmatism. Oxygen is absorbed by the cornea, and those contact lenses which are not gas permeable may inhibit this absorption with resulting discomfort, and long-term limbal neovascularization. Soft contact lenses may absorb fumes and this can cause irritation. Working in extreme cold, as in cold stores, and sometimes in air conditioning, can cause discomfort in people who wear soft contact lenses.

Contact lenses may therefore be helpful at work, but there are certain disadvantages which must be considered. Individual tolerance is variable and is affected by sensitivity to lens care solutions, by photophobia, and by personal lens hygiene. Carrying a spare pair of spectacles may be essential in some occupations, such as offshore work. PRK and LASIK can be of value to those who need but cannot cope with contact lenses, but these procedures carry some potential disadvantages, as described above.[13]

Conditions of work which may be detrimental to vision

Contrary to popular opinion, the intensive use of the eyes either for distance vision or close work does not result in damage to the vision of healthy eyes.

The presence of dust may cause irritation and diminished corneal sensation may sometimes occur in workers in dusty occupations. This may be reduced by wearing protective goggles. Diminished corneal sensitization and corneal vascularization may be sight threatening in some cases and can indicate a need for a change of occupation. Corneal ulcers have many causes. They are usually treatable but tend to recur and this may restrict affected workers in dusty atmospheres.

Workers under constant fluorescent lighting may complain of some discomfort, but there is no evidence that this illumination damages the sight. Flicker is a more severe problem which can be avoided by timely replacement of tubes or by the use of electronic high-frequency fluorescent lighting which avoids both flicker and stroboscopic effects. (The stroboscopic effect may cause moving machinery to appear stationary.) The use of tinted spectacles may minimize the symptoms.

Non-ionizing radiation

Ultraviolet light may cause superficial corneal lesions associated with gross discomfort, and workers who are exposed to this form of radiation should wear appropriate goggles to BSI specifications. Similar corneal lesions may occur with electric arcs from short circuits, arc lights, and welding. Welding goggles must be adapted to the type of welding as wavelength emission peaks vary between standard electric arc and inert gas (argon or carbon dioxide, 'MIG') welding. Infrared rays can cause lens opacity. Heat, from furnaces and in the glass-blowing industry, can also cause lens opacity and it is essential that ocular protection by filtered goggles or visors is provided. High-output pulsed and cutting laser devices pose a specific hazard for workers.[15] Protective goggles should be worn that are designed specifically for the laser types in use. These will ensure that the appropriate wavelengths of radiation are absorbed. The working head of the laser should also be enclosed. The goggles should be checked regularly for wear or damage, and must not bleach or shatter under high laser irradiation. Bleaching could otherwise allow a sudden and unpredictable transmission of high laser irradiation through to the eye with consequent hazard. The side shields are as important as the lens filters in such goggles. Stringent safety precautions should always be enforced and practised in work with lasers or with microwaves. Periodic clinical eye examinations are recommended to screen for corneal, iris, lens, and retinal damage; see Fig. 9.1.

Ionizing radiation

Ionizing radiation resulting from exposure to radionuclides and X-rays can cause cataract, and workers in radiology departments should always be provided with leaded glass eye protection or remain behind a leaded glass screen when there is a possibility of exposure.

Ocular problems in older workers

It is inevitable that some older workers will suffer a degree of visual disability, but the extent of disability in any individual cannot be foreseen. Cataract, macular degeneration,

DATE: ....

NAME OF WORKER: ....

ADDRESS: ....

TYPE OF WORK AND EXTENT
OF EXPOSURE TO LASER:

TYPE OF LASER:

WAVE LENGTH(S) n.m.

PROBABLE POWER LEVEL OF LASER:

LASER ENCLOSED/NOT ENCLOSED:

PROTECTIVE GOGGLES WORN:

HISTORY OF ANY LASER ACCIDENTS:
(i.e. specular reflections etc.)

WORKING ON THE RAW BEAM: YES/NO

EXPOSURE TO FOCAL/DIFFUSE:
OUTPUT OF THE BEAM

PREVIOUS HISTORY OF LASER WORK ELSEWHERE
OR WITH OTHER TYPES OF LASER:

VISUAL ACUITY: Corrected   Right ....   Left ....
                    Uncorrected   Right ....   Left ....

ISHIHARA:

RED AMSLER CHART: REDUCED AMSLER CHART:

FUNDUS WITH/WITHOUT MYDRIASIS:

PHOTOGRAPH TAKEN:

OCULAR MEDIA (SLIT LAMP ETC.):

PRESENCE OF ANY LASER ATTRIBUTABLE LESIONS:

ASSESSMENT OF LIKELY RISK:

SUGGESTED TIME OF FURTHER REVIEW:

Fig. 9.1 Pro-forma for ophthalmic examination of laser workers.

and glaucoma may occur in later life without any indication of these conditions being present in earlier years. If visual acuity is reduced as a result of these diseases, treatment must be undertaken according to the current clinical findings. Cataract can be treated surgically sometimes as a day case, and this may enable patients to continue at work. Early macular degeneration can sometimes be controlled by laser therapy. In some people, premature retirement may become necessary. Experience may compensate for the disability and it is not always appropriate to apply the same strict visual standards to older employees. The DDA will require adjustment or offer of alternative work for some of these people. Good illumination is necessary for the maximum degree of close work by older people; intermediate range spectacles may be required. For demanding work a period of adaptation may be necessary for bifocal or varifocal glasses, and after cataract surgery where there can be altered refractive status.

Anaesthetic cornea

The cornea is normally a very sensitive part of the eyeball and, with the corneal reflex, reacts immediately to injury and to the presence of a foreign body. Corneal sensitivity declines in later life but the cornea still reacts even to minor trauma. Injury or disease of the trigeminal nerve can cause complete corneal anaesthesia. This usually requires treatment by tarsorrhaphy which effectively produces monocular vision with all its consequences (see above). More recently, the use of a bandage soft contact lens instead of tarsorrhaphy has enabled binocular vision to be retained. Bandage lenses are very thin, soft, and highly permeable large contact lenses having an optic centre comparable with corneal size and an outer 'haptic', non-optical, scleral supporting zone. They are used both as a mechanical cover and occasionally as a slow release store for antibiotics and other drugs.

Some common eye diseases and their effects

A number of common eye diseases cause difficulty at work.

Conjunctivitis

Conjunctivitis is characterized by discomfort rather than pain, and by a discharge from the eyes which may be mucopurulent and contagious. It rapidly yields to treatment with antibiotic drops. Conjunctivitis may be associated with ulceration of the cornea and with inflammation of the eyelid margins (blepharitis). This latter condition is the result of inflammation of the glands at the margin of the eyelids and responds to the same treatment. Watering of the eyes due to obstruction of the nasolacrimal ducts may cause annoyance at work but can usually be treated by simple surgery requiring little time off work.

Uveitis

Uveitis is an inflammation of the uveal tract. A part or the whole of the uvea, which is responsible for the nourishment and focusing of the eye, may be affected. It occurs in all states of severity from the mild form, causing only a slight blurring of vision, to the acute state where there is severe pain and serious visual defect. The condition usually responds to treatment with local or systemic steroid preparations but a long period of therapy may be necessary and uveitis can be a recurrent condition. It is sometimes associated with secondary glaucoma, complicated cataract, and rarely with the loss of sight of the eye. It may occasionally cause severe disablement and inability to continue in employment. Early treatment is therefore important. Ophthalmic herpes zoster may cause uveitis, but this can usually be treated and does not usually recur thereafter.

Glaucoma

In glaucoma the pressure in the eyeball is higher than normal. It occurs in two common forms.

- **Acute glaucoma** causes sudden severe pain and visual defect, and may be preceded by premonitory attacks with brow ache and haloes round lights at night. When treated immediately the long-term results are good.
- **Chronic glaucoma**, which usually occurs in later life, may cause a serious degree of visual defect with contracture of the visual fields and resulting inability to continue at work. Because of its insidious onset, it is often unnoticed until advanced. Regular eye tests and tonometry are useful aids to detection in the over 55s.

Myopia

Myopia, or short-sightedness, is characterized by difficulty with distant vision. It can be overcome by wearing spectacles or contact lenses. Most short-sighted people have minor degrees of myopia and are not seriously disabled. However, a minority of myopic people have such a gross error that, even with optical correction, useful vision is not possible. Occupations where spectacles or contact lenses cannot be worn are unsuitable for such people. Several new types of treatment are emerging to remodel the cornea, for example radial keratotomy (RK) and Excimer laser PRK.[16] PRK is possible for refractive errors up to –6 or –8 dioptres, and to a large extent has superseded RK. For larger errors, LASIK has less postoperative pain but is more interventional.

Retinal separation (detachment)

Detachment of the retina is not uncommon, particularly in association with high degrees of myopia such as 12 dioptres or more and after ocular trauma. It should be treated as a surgical emergency and in most cases good vision is restored. The prognosis depends on the amount of retina which separates and whether or not the macula is detached. Detachment of the macula results in diminution of vision to about 6/60 even if the retina is reattached. Patients whose retina cannot be reattached with surgery will lose all vision in that eye. Patients whose retina has been reattached should subsequently avoid heavy manual work and some sports, such as boxing or squash.

Conclusion

To determine fitness for work it is important to assess visual function adequately. Where there is doubt, specialist advice should be sought. There are many occupations which require very high standards of visual performance, but defective ocular function does not necessarily prevent people from working in the majority of other occupations; adjustments are available in many cases, and will usually be required under the DDA. Career guidance should ensure that young people do not embark on unsuitable careers, where an uncorrectable or progressive disability will restrict future advancement.

Selected references

1　*Disability Discrimination Act 1995: guidance notes and code of practice.* London: HMSO, 1996.
2　*Notes for guidance. Record of examination to certify a person as blind or partially sighted.* BD8. London: HMSO, 1990.
3　Munton CGF. The development of visual standards in the UK. In *Vision in vehicles*, ed. Gale AG *et al.*, **IV**, 17–25. Amsterdam: North-Holland, 1993.
4　Drivers Fields Agreed. College News. *Q Bull Coll Ophthalmologists, London,* Spring 1991; p6.
5　Munton CGF. Vision. In *Medical aspects of fitness to drive*, ed. Taylor JF, 5th edn. London: Medical Commission on Accident Prevention, 1995.
6　Commission of the European Communities. *Proposals for a council directive on the driving licence.* COM (88) 705 Final, 1989.
7　*Specification for eye protectors in industrial and non-industrial users. BS2092.* London: British Standards Institution, 1983.
8　Fletcher R, Voke J. *Defective colour vision, fundamentals, diagnosis and management.* Hilger: Bristol, 1985.
9　Norman LG. Medical aspects of road safety. *Lancet* 1960; **i**: 989–994, 1039–1045.
10　*Specification for identification of pipelines and services. BS 1710.* London: British Standards Institution, 1984.
11　Health and Safety Executive. *Visual display units.* London: HMSO, 1992.
12　Commission of the European Communities. *Council directive on the minimum safety and health requirement for working with display screen equipment.* 90/270 EEC Article 9, 1990.
13　*Excimer laser photo-ablative surgery: best clinical practice guidelines.* London: Royal College of Ophthalmologists, 1998.
14　Smokerings. Editorials, *Model Engineer*, August and November 1989.
15　*Radiation safety of laser products and systems. BS4803.* London: British Standards Institution, 1983.
16　Marshall J, Trokel S, Rothery S, Kruger RR. Long-term healing of the central cornea after photo-refractive keratectomy using an excimer laser. *Ophthalmology* 1988; **95**(10): 1411–1421.

10

Hearing and vestibular disorders

C. M. Jones and K. B. Hughes

Hearing

Disorders of the ear such as hearing difficulty, tinnitus, ear discharge, associated skin conditions of the outer ear, problems associated with barometric pressure changes, and disturbances of balance can affect fitness for work in a variety of ways.

Hearing difficulty

A hearing difficulty may be associated with hearing disorders which have been present since birth or acquired diseases of the middle ear, but in other cases the cause is unclear. The affected person may be unaware that anything is wrong; for example, in noise-induced hearing loss where the deterioration progresses gradually over a period of time before the impairment becomes evident. In the majority of jobs, hearing problems do not affect ability to work but there are some tasks where hearing loss is not compatible with employment because of a need for good communication, where the safety of the sufferer or others may be compromised, or where there are exceptionally high levels of responsibility, such as radio operators and civil airline pilots. There are also situations where further noise exposure risks aggravating an existing impairment. Fitness for employment in these situations depends on the degree of disability as compared with the auditory demands of the job. In severe or profound hearing loss, especially if congenital, speech production may also be impaired, and in jobs that require vocal communication, fitness for work may be adversely affected.

Hearing is vital for normal social and working communication. In contrast to a blind person whose disability is evident, however, the person with defective hearing has a hidden disability. A hearing aid, even if visibly worn, is usually regarded not as a sign of a disability but as an appliance that restores normal hearing; however, this is not so for the majority of hearing aid wearers. The consequence may be that when a hearing-impaired person fails to comprehend, they may be regarded as incompetent or mentally backward, and may be shunned because of the embarrassment and the effort involved in communication.

These attitudes extend to the employment of hearing-impaired people. The deaf, hard of hearing, and those with ear disorders need be excluded only from a minority of jobs.

Tinnitus

Tinnitus is usually associated with a hearing disorder and is present in approximately half of those with substantial hearing difficulties. Although the impairment of hearing is usually the more significant factor in assessing fitness for work, tinnitus may be associated with psychological upsets which may include tiredness and irritability due to insomnia. These can be severe and incapacitating and can impair performance at work in jobs that are heavily dependent on interpersonal skills. In addition, exacerbation of a troublesome tinnitus from whatever cause, by exposure to noise at work, even when wearing hearing protectors, will occasionally preclude further employment in a noisy environment. Such exacerbations are usually, but not always, temporary.

Ear discharge

An ear discharge most commonly arises from a bacterial or fungal infection of the middle or external ear, but some forms of otitis externa are more akin to an eczematous dermatitis. Fitness for work can be affected by considerations of appearance, hygiene, or ability to use hearing protectors or telephonic equipment.

A predisposition to eczematous reactions of the canal skin aggravated by certain working conditions, particularly where there is the additional problem of wearing hearing protectors, may lead a patient who is otherwise fit to move from that particular environment.

Hygiene considerations preclude work as a food handler at all stages, from processing raw food products to food retailing or catering. Active or recurrent ear infections should be regarded as unacceptable in these industries. Where hearing protection has to be worn, it is sometimes possible to prevent skin problems by using ear-muffs in preference to ear-plugs, but ear-muffs worn in certain environments cause considerable sweating and can exacerbate the skin condition.

Conditions of the outer ear may also lead to conductive hearing losses. Infections of the middle ear can cause both conductive and sensorineural hearing loss.

Barometric problems

Chronic or recurrent eustachian tube insufficiency, or middle ear disease, bar people from certain occupations, notably in flying, diving, and working in compressed air (see also Appendices 2 and 4).

Balance disorders

Disturbances of balance are covered later in this chapter, but the possibility of their association with ear disorders, hearing defects, or tinnitus needs to be kept in mind when assessing an individual's fitness for work, particularly where safety is a factor.

Prevalence

There are no reliable figures concerning the extent of deafness in the UK. In April 1992, the Employment Service Register of Disabled Persons between 16 and 64 years of age indicated that approximately 8% of the registered disabled population, about 0.1% of the total population in this age group, were registered because of hearing impairment. The extent to which this is an underestimate is indicated by data from the National Study of Hearing (NSH), a nationwide epidemiological study in the UK. The prevalence of stated degrees of impairment ('hearing loss') as a function of age is given in Table 10.1. It should be noted that a 25 dB average hearing threshold level (HTL) in the better ear is just outside what is conventionally regarded as the range of normal hearing, though many do suffer from problems in some circumstances from less than this; an HTL of 35 dB is the usual level at which otologists start to consider the prescription of a hearing aid or surgery where the condition is amenable to surgery. An HTL of 45 dB can definitely be considered a degree of handicap in most patients and an HTL of 65 dB represents a severe handicap.[1,2]

Pure tone audiometric thresholds, however, are not a guaranteed guide to handicap and disability as handicap is very much a subjective condition. In addition, hearing performance will be different in conductive and sensorineural deafness in different individuals. Nevertheless, audiometric tests are repeatable and accurate and provide the only reliable means of assessing an employee's apparent hearing ability.

Box 10.1 Some definitions

Pure tone audiometry measures the hearing threshold level (HTL) at each of a range of test frequencies in each ear. The physical unit of measurement is decibels (hearing level), abbreviated to 'dB HL', except that the 'HL' should be omitted when the statement refers to HTL. The reference zero for dB HL is based on a standardized biological baseline of normal hearing in young persons, which varies with test frequency and with type of earphone and measuring coupler used for calibration and is covered by an ISO standard.

The unit 'dB SPL' (sound pressure level) or 'dB(lin)' relates to an absolute physical measure of sound pressure of 20 mPa. The unit 'dB(A)' refers to the SPL after application of standardized A-weighting filters to reduce the influence of low-frequency and very high-frequency components of a sound, thus giving a better representation of its potential to cause hearing damage, speech interference, reduced work performance, and annoyance.

Data on the proportions of people experiencing various degrees of hearing difficulty, and ear discharge, are also available from the NSH and are shown in Table 10.2. It can be seen that hearing difficulties are common in the population at all ages and in both sexes, a factor which has to be taken into account in considering fitness for work.

Clinical aspects affecting work capacity

Loss of hearing will seldom lead to a period off work. The impact is related more to working efficiency, the employee's health, and the safety of others. Tinnitus, on the other hand, quite often results in absences from work, as do infections of the ear and, in

Table 10.1 Percentage of people in six age groups whose hearing threshold levels (averaged over 0.5, 1, 2, and 4 kHz) were at or over 25, 45, and 65 dB HL in the better ear[3]

Age group	Percentage at or exceeding		
	25 dB HL	45 dB HL	65 dB HL
17–30	1.8	0.2	<0.1
31–40	2.8	1.1	0.7
41–50	8.2	1.7	0.3
51–60	18.9	4.0	0.9
61–70	36.8	7.4	2.3
71–80	60.2	17.6	4.0
Overall	16.1	3.9	1.1

Table 10.2 Frequency of hearing difficulty and of ear disorder by age and sex[3] (percentages with sizes of samples shown in brackets)

	Age group (years) and sex					
	17–24		25–44		45–64	
	M	F	M	F	M	F
Difficulty in hearing						
(better ear)	(1980)	(2157)	(4038)	(4300)	(3734)	(4161)
None	97	98	96	97	86	92
Slight	2	2	4	2	11	5
Moderate	0.4	0.1	0.5	0.4	2	2
Great	0.1	0.2	0.1	0.2	0.6	0.7
Cannot hear at all	0.1	0.0	0.1	0.2	0.2	0.5
Difficult to hear in a quiet room						
Normal voice	(1674)	(1881)	(3291)	(3512)	(2937)	(3178)
	1	2	2	2	7	5
Loud voice	(1664)	(1842)	(3457)	(3255)	(2837)	(3051)
	1	1	1	1	3	3
Very difficult to hear in noise	(2859)	(3052)	(6030)	(6430)	(5709)	(6346)
	12	15	20	19	36	27
Discharging ear (ever)	(2584)	(2761)	(5347)	(5762)	(5043)	(5617)
	13	15	15	17	18	16
Hearing aid (ever)	(2603)	(2774)	(5396)	(5827)	(5113)	(5722)
	0.6	0.6	0.7	1	3	3
Registered disabled	(295)	(341)	(748)	(778)	(778)	(894)
(hearing impaired)	0.3	0.3	0.0	0.3	0.6	0.3

particular of the ear canal skin and the pinna, particularly where they are aggravated by working conditions.

Working efficiency and safety

There are few jobs in industry where perfect hearing is essential. With the requirements of the Disability Discrimination Act 1995 (DDA) that employers make 'reasonable adjustment to the workplace' the number of jobs that cannot be done, even by people with a total or profound hearing impairment, should be reduced even further. For the majority of jobs it is sufficient that the applicant (wearing a hearing aid if appropriate) can communicate in the normal working environment. Hence no special tests are needed for pre-employment assessment unless the work environment will expose them to further risk of hearing loss.

Where auditory requirements are more stringent the needs for hearing, particularly the safety aspects, should be considered carefully to identify the real requirements of the job and to consider possibilities for counteracting the effect of any hearing impairment. The increased use of other senses by the deaf and hearing impaired, including the ability to lip read, may not be appreciated by the employer.

Occasionally, in some quiet work environments or where there is contact with the general public, it is essential to hear voices which may be quiet, or spoken from a distance. For these, a simple clinical test for the hearing of speech (aided, if appropriate) is sufficient, for example. voice tests carefully performed to a defined protocol (see p. 199), though this should not override the practical 'on the job' test. Correct identification of speech in a background of noise may be needed. Here, the relative levels of speech and noise (the signal-to-noise or S/N ratio) are critical, together with the individual's ability to detect one sound in the presence of another (frequency resolution) or immediately preceding or following another sound (temporal resolution). A practical test of hearing in the workplace is probably the most appropriate way to check the disabling effects of these and other forms of hearing dysfunction.

Most conductive hearing losses are due to middle-ear disorders and result only (or mainly) in loss of auditory sensitivity. Sensorineural hearing losses arising from cochlear damage (e.g. by noise exposure or associated with ageing) can impair both frequency and temporal resolution as well as causing a loss of sensitivity.

Some jobs have highly specific auditory requirements, for example the need to hear weak pure tones over a range of possible frequencies in radio operating, or to detect changes in pitch or to identify the character of echoes in sonar operating. For jobs of this nature, audiometry may have a place in the initial screening, but a practical test with particular listening tasks is more appropriate. This is especially true with a trained operator, as experience and skill in the job usually outweighs any potential disadvantage suggested by some arbitrary auditory test which is unrelated to the task.

Many people believe that musicians need to have very good hearing, but there are famous examples to show that this is not necessarily so. The interactions between the type of music and instruments played and the nature and degree of hearing disorders are so varied and complex that audiometric fitness standards cannot be specified. For these types of work, a practical test with a particular listening task is more appropriate.

A more common requirement that may affect employment is the need to hear warning signals and to detect the direction of their source. These sounds often occur against a noisy background, and their detection is dependent primarily on the S/N ratio. Sensorineural hearing losses may make the task markedly more difficult, but the same is not true of conductive losses.

Communication difficulties arising from hearing protection

Ear-muffs or ear-plugs have to be worn in noisy occupations in order to protect against occupational deafness. Currently, in the UK ear defenders have to be worn at EP,d of 90 dBA but this mandatory standard only protects approximately 89% of the population. The remainder suffer a degree of increased susceptibility. The proposed EU Physical Agents Directive could reduce the standard to 85 dBA. Although hearing protection will reduce both signal and noise equally, it may also reduce the intrusiveness or attention-demanding properties of abnormal machinery sounds and warning signals. This is due to a combination of factors including a general reduction in their apparent loudness (particularly in hearing-impaired people); an alteration of the spectrum of the noise reaching the ear with increased masking of high-frequency signals by low-frequency components; and an impaired ability to identify the direction of sound.

The solution is to increase the S/N ratio of the warning signals to at least 15 dB above its masked threshold,[4,5] and perhaps also to alter the frequency spectrum of the warning signals. The 'design window' approach of Coleman and colleagues[6] would seem at present to provide the most useful set of guidelines. In situations where more than one auditory signal occurs, the signals can have standardized, distinctive patterns to assist in recognition. In many cases the auditory signals should be supplemented by visual signals. Modifications to warning or communication systems may qualify for financial support from the Employment Service (Chapter 4), if carried out for the safety of hearing-impaired people.

The problem of hearing protection is often made worse by the tendency to provide 'best protection' and the tendency to try and standardize on the least number of protection devices. The requirements of the individual need to be taken into account when fitting hearing protection. The examiner should also bear in mind that existing conductive hearing loss is not an effective protection against sensorineural deafness from occupational noise.[7] The inability to hear changes in sounds made by machinery has often been used as a reason for not wearing hearing protection, but usually wearers can adapt to cope with any qualitative or quantitative differences. For the person with hearing impairment, however, unless changes are made to warning sounds, the use of hearing protection may make it impossible for them to be heard. For example, warning sounds need to be separated by a combination of frequency and spatial resolution from the background sound against which they operate.

In general, hearing protectors should provide adequate attenuation. Excessive attenuation, however, can lead to social isolation as well as problems with warning signals. It is important that those choosing the type of hearing protector should be aware that the manufacturers' figures are derived from standardized laboratory tests. They do not necessarily reflect the attenuation achieved in use and often, especially in the case of ear-plugs, significantly overestimate it. Two European Coal and Steel Community (ECSC) research projects suggest that, whilst the mean minus 1 standard deviation (SD) is acceptable for normal ear-muffs, those that are helmet attached afford around 5 dB less protection than expected. The importance of training in the use of ear-plugs cannot be overemphasized. The National Institute of Occupational Safety and Health (NIOSH) also suggest de-rating noise reduction ratio (NRR) figures for hearing protectors in a similar way. Although some protectors have been developed to assist the hearing of speech and/or warning signals, they have inherent limitations. Amplitude-sensitive ear-plugs can protect against occasional explosive noises while interfering minimally with verbal communication, during quiet intervals, but this situation is not often encountered in industry. Malleable ear-plugs may not be fully effective at noise levels above 95 dBA and others at even lower levels. Noise attenuation communication headsets can be helpful, but may have reduced attenuation properties and tend to be heavy and bulky. If cords are needed for signal-source connections, they are cumbersome; if cordless, using magnetic induction or radio systems, they are expensive and somewhat delicate.

Rehabilitation

Hearing aids improve hearing sensitivity, provided that there is some residual hearing to improve. However, they do not compensate for the reduction in the frequency and the temporal resolving difficulties associated with sensorineural hearing loss, which is the most common form of hearing disorder in the general population, and many hearing aids prescribed for noise-induced hearing loss remain unused. They can also add their own distortions in greater or lesser degree. Thus, the benefit they provide is limited. Because of this, the fairest way to judge the capability of a person wearing a hearing aid is to test hearing ability under actual working conditions, including, if appropriate, ability to lip read in the intended working environment.

Most occupations are compatible with the wearing of a hearing aid. However, only certain hearing aids are safe for use in coal-mines or other places where there may be flammable atmospheres. Only particular models are safe; these change from time to time so it is important to check with the suppliers. If in doubt, the Medical Devices Agency of the Department of Health should be contacted (for full details of address, see Appendix 7). If the employee is dependent on a hearing aid, the safety implications in the event of a possible failure of the aid should be considered. Of more concern is a dependence on hearing aids where noise levels are too high for any form of aid to provide adequate protection. On the other hand, communication in such conditions even for those with normal hearing often depends largely on lip reading and hand signals, at which hearing-impaired people are better skilled.

Special work problems, restrictions, or needs

Defective hearing and accidents

It seems likely that noise sometimes contributes to accidents from failure to hear warning signals. Nevertheless, serious accidents due to deafness or noise interference appear to be uncommon. In a lifestyle survey conducted by the Trent Regional Health Authority in 1992, there were over 6000 respondents to a postal questionnaire who were under the age of 50 years. Fifty-one of these possessed hearing aids: these people's reports indicated a sixfold increase in odds for accidental injury at work, but no increase in the home or on the road, as compared with those without hearing aids.[6]

Unsuitable work for people with hearing defects

Questions of capability arise particularly in jobs in which the actual task is an auditory one and where accurate hearing of speech and/or of other auditory signals is important. Exceptions can be made, particularly where the hearing-impaired person is already trained and experienced, or where there is some special connection with defective hearing, e.g. teachers of the deaf, and social workers for the deaf. Major factors in defining acceptability include the degree of expected responsibility for others and the extent to which the impairment may undermine the public's confidence. These factors cannot be quantified. Each employer should consider carefully, in each case, whether or not it is essential to exclude people with defective hearing from certain jobs. For further information on the impact of defective hearing on employability and the means of reducing its effect at work the reader should consult Kettle and Massie[1] and the *Deaf and hearing impaired* booklet (EPWD 20) issued by the Employment Service.[2]

Legislation and guidelines for employment

Noise

The main employment problem related to hearing and the ear is that of noise exposure and the inherent risk of irreversible sensory deafness.

General legal background

In 1981, the Health and Safety Commission (HSC) reported that in British manufacturing industry alone about 600 000 individuals worked in noise levels exceeding an equivalent continuous sound level of 90 dBA, and over 2 million more were exposed to levels over 80 dBA. This followed two earlier publications, the Department of Employment's voluntary code of practice on noise in 1972 and the Health and Safety Executive's (HSE) discussion document on industrial audiometry in 1979. The Noise at Work Regulations 1989 are concerned with protection from noise exposure. Limited hearing conservation measures are now required for equivalent continuous sound levels in excess of 85 dBA; above 90 dBA a comprehensive programme is required, led by engineering control with ear protection as the lower priority. Some employers have chosen to ignore the concept of two 'action levels' and elected to introduce all of the requirements at the 85 dBA action level (anticipating that further reductions are likely to occur in the future). These regulations permit the granting of exemptions from the requirement to use hearing protectors if their use increases the overall risk to the health and safety of the workers concerned, but they do not include any guidelines on the employment needs of hearing-impaired people.

HSE's guidance note *A guide to audiometric testing programmes*[8] does, however, give advice of a general nature. It suggests consideration of the following questions:

- Is the hearing condition stable or unstable?
- Will it be aggravated by further exposure to noise?
- What is the extent of the established hearing loss?
- Will the person use a hearing aid and will it be safe to do so at work?
- Are there any specific hearing requirements for the job in question?

It advises that, in view of the stability of noise-induced hearing loss, continuing exposure 'will usually be acceptable where adequate hearing protection is used and where residual hearing ability is not so poor as to make the risk of further hearing loss unacceptable'. According to the guidance, even if a doctor advises against continuing employment, if there is no risk to others, then employees should be permitted to continue in the same job with the employer's agreement (it would be prudent to record this agreement).

The guidance recognizes that there will be a 'few employees who have responsibility for the safety of others and who need to communicate easily and to hear auditory warning signals where 'severe hearing loss' (undefined) will cause difficulties. It suggests that this requirement is **made clear at the time of recruitment** and that assessment based on the average hearing threshold above the speech frequencies 'or those of particular warning sounds may be helpful'.

The need to carry out audiometric testing is not, however, explicitly required by statute, but is implicit in Regulation 5 of the Management of Health and Safety at Work Regulations 1992 which requires the provision of appropriate health surveillance in relation to any risk to health and safety. The leaflet *Health surveillance in noisy industries* (INDG 193 : HSE 1995) confirms that employers should 'normally provide hearing checks when noise levels reach or exceed 90 dBA'.

The next legislation likely to concern noise exposure at work is the EC's proposed Physical Agents Directive. If this is implemented it may lead to a further reduction in action levels.

The extent of the problem

It is difficult to obtain an accurate assessment of the prevalence of noise-induced hearing loss in industry as comprehensive figures are not available.

The HSC's Annual Report for 1995–96 gives figures for those qualifying for benefits for occupational deafness. In April 1995 an estimated 14 200 people were receiving benefit, 99% of whom were male. The annual numbers newly qualifying for benefit have declined steadily from 1170 in 1989 to 763 in 1995. Qualification for payment requires at least 50 dB of hearing loss, averaged across 1, 2, and 3 kHz (though handicap is calculated from 30 dB). The records of audiological examinations also showed that there were 1200 claimants annually with hearing loss between 35 and 49 dB. The point is made that '50 dB or more of hearing loss represents a substantial impairment'—a sentiment few would disagree with.

The threshold for payment by the insurance companies however is as low as a disability of 10 dB—a level which some would not consider to be a handicap—and it is understandable that most claims for noise-related compensation are made by this route. These claims represent the largest group for disease-related claims for the employers' liability insurance companies. The Association of British Insurers (ABI) represents around 440 insurance companies and accounts for over 95% of the business of UK insurance companies. In its publication *Occupational disease enquiry—1995*[9] they published the number and percentage of claims for various occupational diseases. Those relating to occupational deafness are presented in Table 10.3. A possible reduction can be seen in recent years.

Table 10.3 Deafness claims to ABI members from 1991 to 1995 inclusive

Year	All claims No.	Deafness claims No.	% of total
1991	57 653	46 583	80.8
1992	65 007	52 785	81.2
1993	68 671	56 722	82.6
1994	51 857	40 344	77.8
1995	43 312	34 043	78.6
Total	285 500	230 477	80.4

Data on the annual frequency for the North East region

The annual number of deafness claims since 1981 is available from the Iron Trades Insurance Group which covers the heavy industrial area of South Yorkshire and the North East. These are shown in Fig. 10.1 along with their total claims figures. Here a clear downward trend can be seen starting from the high plateau lasting from 1989 to 1992. In the period 1981–96 two-thirds (144 439) of the claims were for deafness, which is a lower percentage than received by the ABI. In the same period there were 144 270 settlements. The pattern of claims in other areas may be different, reflecting local patterns of employment and awareness.

Further information on the extent of the problem can be obtained from *Self-reported work-related illness in 1995 (results from a household survey)*[10] which included questions about self-reported work-related illnesses. Ninety-nine subjects among a sample of about 40 000 respondents reported deafness, tinnitus, or other ear conditions caused or made worse by work. This translated into a national estimate of 170 000 affected individuals and a rate per 10 000 among men of 14 for 16–44 year olds, 120 for 45–64 year olds and 220 for 65–74 year olds. Most respondents (97%) reported their illness was due to noise, including 23% with exposure to blasts or gunfire.

Inevitably some of the above figures represent a historical situation and the number of sufferers that are still employed is not known. The extent of the deafness is also not quantified, but in community terms a significant burden of disability and handicap appears likely.

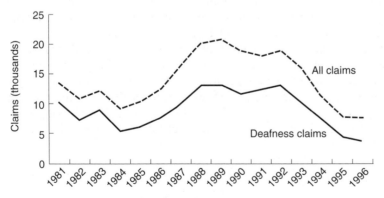

Fig. 10.1 Claims received by the iron trades insurance group for the north east region 1981–96

Current situation in industry

Until the mid-1980s, the greater part of industry was apathetic towards hearing conservation. Effective programmes were limited largely to those organizations with comprehensive occupational health services (around 15% of firms). However, the situation has improved considerably since then. This progress can be ascribed to the Noise at Work Regulations 1989 and enforcement by UK Health and Safety Inspectorates, but also to fear of civil litigation. In one major manufacturing industry, over a recent 10 year period, the cost of settlement of claims related to noise damage exceeded the costs of accident claims.

An attempt to quantify the size of the problem of noise exposure is made in the Self-Reported Working Conditions Survey 1995 sponsored by HSE.[11] In this survey 2230 workers who were employed in full-time or part-time jobs were interviewed: 41% of men and 32% of women experienced noise levels which required them to raise their voices, and 11% of men and 6% of women experienced ringing in their ears and temporary deafness after work. In the case of men, 6% experienced it every week, as did 3% of women. The male dominated manual occupations showed significantly higher than average rates, notably metal processing (27%), repetitive assembly and inspection (24%), and other transport and machinery operatives (23%).

If hearing impairment does not involve substantial and unpreventable risks to the health and safety of the individuals concerned or others, there is seldom any convincing reason for excluding individuals from employment in high levels of noise, but the employer should provide them with properly selected and fitted hearing protectors and adequate training on how to use them and also keep them fully informed of the importance of wearing them and when to do so.

The employer has a greater duty of care where an individual has only one functional ear (Chapter 2, p. 28), the other ear being totally or severely impaired. This is a not uncommon condition in the general population. The person is not always aware of it, sometimes even if the asymmetry is gross, and especially if it has been present since childhood. Such individuals may therefore have to be excluded from jobs where there is an inherent and not always preventable risk of damage to the remaining ear. In some working environments, good directional hearing ability or ability to understand speech in a noisy environment may be particularly important, and those with marked asymmetry of hearing may not be able to cope in these situations. Great care is also needed in considering whether or not to employ people with severely impaired hearing in conditions where there is a substantial risk of damage to the eyes.

Tinnitus can also present particular problems. It is often exacerbated by noise and/or stress at work, being much reduced during weekends or holidays. Hearing protection is advisable for people with troublesome tinnitus when the noise level rises above approximately 80 dBA even for short periods. Davis and Roberts[12] have demonstrated a significant association between tinnitus and accident reporting, most closely related to the degree of hearing impairment and age (those aged over 50 appeared to be at particular risk).

Medico-legal considerations

One of the arguments sometimes advanced for pre-employment audiometry and assessment of aural status is that it may safeguard against civil claims when damage actually predates the employment. A questions then arises regarding the wisdom in medico-legal terms of employing, in noisy surroundings, the considerable number of people who have been revealed by audiometry to have some degree of hearing impairment (Table 10.1) or who have evidence of ear disease. However, the medico-legal risk is very slight providing that the assessment is followed by appropriate and properly conducted hearing conservation measures, including documented explanation to the employee about the hazards to hearing, the implications of hearing loss, and the means of preventing it. The presence of pre-existing hearing impairment *per se*, or ear disease, is not a valid bar to employment. Similar considerations apply to the use of serial monitoring audiometry and the action to be taken when hearing deterioration is detected.

Assessment of fitness for work

In the absence of guidelines, the position varies across industry. Many employers, particularly small firms, recruit staff without any medical screening. Conversely, there are some employers who reject applicants if their pre-employment audiogram demonstrates a dip at or around 4 kHz. This policy is very difficult to justify now that the DDA and the Noise at Work Regulations are in force. This is particularly relevant since many employees with hearing damage are bringing particular skills to a noisy occupation and are otherwise well qualified for the job in prospect. The majority of employers who perform audiometry do so for three purposes:

- to establish a baseline for the individual, particularly if they are to work in a noisy environment
- as a means of monitoring change in their employees' hearing so that appropriate steps can be taken to prevent any further deterioration
- as part of an ongoing process of education.

In practice, very few cases are identified in industry where the hearing loss causes a severe enough disability to preclude employment.

Serial audiometry

Periodic audiometric testing is generally considered to be a necessary part of a comprehensive hearing conservation programme. It should be conducted annually for 2 years after the baseline pre-employment audiogram so that those particularly vulnerable to noise-induced hearing loss are detected early on, and thereafter every 3 years.

The main use of serial audiometry is to detect deterioration in the hearing status of individuals or groups; also as an aid to their effective counselling. Safety indications for redeployment are restricted to those situations where hearing impairment puts the individual, the working group, or the plant at risk. Such instances are rarely encountered in general industry. Each case has to be assessed in the light of the particular job content and working conditions in order to reach an equitable decision.

HSE's Guidance Note MS 26, *A Guide to audiometric testing programmes* (1995)[8], provides reference information.

Specific employment regulations and standards

Where there are particular demands on hearing in relation to occupation, organizations often develop their own internal standards. Examples are given below. In some cases there are detailed and particular regulations. More often, the decision is left to the occupational physician or the personnel officer, and the requirement is simply that of fitness for the job, informally and intuitively assessed.

Flying (civil)

The detailed requirements for professional pilots, engineers, and air traffic controllers are given in Appendix 2. Professional pilots rarely lose their licences because of hearing loss since the aircraft radios and intercom systems function rather like hearing aids, amplifying the speech signal as required. A history of vertigo, however, does present a more serious risk (see p. 207).

The Civil Aviation Authority (CAA)'s hearing standards for professional pilots are given in Table 10.4. These are unchanged by European harmonization throughout the 29 states comprising the Joint Aviation Authorities (JAA) (15 EU states and 14 other member states) which became effective in July 1999.

For private pilots (class 2) certification, the hearing is tested by conversational speech at 2 metres with the candidate's back to the examiner, as long as the individual does not apply for an instrument rating. If an instrument rating is being sought, then the standards apply as for class 1.

Although hearing standards are described for the four frequencies in the table below, the JAA requirements call for pure tone audiometry to cover the eight frequencies normally tested (250, 500, 1000, 2000, 3000, 4000, 6000, and 8000 Hz).

Hearing will be tested audiometrically every 5 years up to the age of 40, and thereafter every 2 years.

Armed services

Medical fitness is expressed in terms of the PULHEEMS system (see Chapter 1), in which 'H' refers to the hearing acuity. Each quality is judged on a scale 1–8, where 1 is exceptionally good and 8 is unfit for service. The fitness standard (PULHEEM grade) tends to be stricter for recruits than for personnel already serving. The general entry standard is H2, but for aircrew it is H1, as defined by audiometry (Table 10.5).

Table 10.4 Hearing standards of the UK CAA for pilot licences: class 1 (professional pilot) medical certification

Hz	Initial (dbAs)	Renewal (dbAs)
500	20	35
1000	20	35
2000	20	35
3000	35	50

Table 10.5 Audiometric standards in the armed services

PULHEEMS	Sum of HTLs (dB)		General description
H grade	0.5, 1, and 2 kHz	3, 4, and 6 kHz	
H1	Not >45	Not >45	Good hearing
H2	Not >84	Not >123	Acceptable practical hearing for service purposes
H3	Not >150	Not >210	Impaired hearing; usually unfit for entry
H4–H8	>150	>210	Very poor hearing; several restrictions on employability of serving personnel

The assessment is recorded as a two-digit number under H, the first digit for the right ear, the second for the left. The higher digit, representing the worse ear, will determine the individual's overall hearing category. The Royal Navy has a more stringent definition of H1, and certain branches within each service have particular requirements.

Police

The tests performed and their interpretation vary from one police force to another. In Nottinghamshire, for example, the screening test for hearing is based on pure tone audiometry, with a preliminary upper HTL limit for new recruits of 30 dB in each ear and at each test frequency in the range 250 Hz–8 kHz. This limit is only for general guidance, however, and, subject to specialist ENT advice, may be relaxed in particular cases, especially for older recruits who may have worked previously in noisy occupations. There is also periodic audiometric screening of serving officers who are headphone users or those who sometimes work in noisy environments, for example firearms instructors, and motorcycle traffic officers. The maximum acceptable HTL for such people is 40 dB, again with flexibility in its application to individual cases.

Fire service

In 1970 the Home Office issued guidance on entry and periodic medical examinations in the fire service (Godber Report[13]). Baseline assessment was advocated as well as 3 yearly assessments in the over 40s. The basic criterion was defined in a general way, typical of many occupations: that no one should engage in duties (operational firefighting in this case) who was not fit for those duties. Although the definition is circular, it has the merits of flexibility, adaptability, and relevance.

The Godber Report was superseded in 1989 by the Report of the Joint Working Party of the Home Office on Medical Standards and Firefighters. With respect to hearing it commented:

It is essential that firefighters should be able to hear instructions and signals, and good hearing is necessary. The whisper test combined with otoscopic examination and tuning fork tests can be used but audiometry is more accurate. A portable audiometer with ear-muffs, used in a quiet room, would give sufficiently accurate readings capable of detecting significant hearing loss which could then be more fully assessed at an audiological clinic.

Merchant navy

The General Council of British Shipping provides an audiometric testing service for shipping companies, but the required standards of fitness vary according to individual company policy (see Appendix 3). Impaired hearing sufficient to interfere with communication often leads to classification as 'permanently unfit'. A unilateral hearing defect is considered in relation to the particular job. Hearing aids are allowable in certain trades provided the aided hearing is sufficient for communication and safety: they are not allowed for engine-room, electrical, and radio personnel.

Railway companies

Railtrack has issued guidelines on medical examinations and standards, but discretion is allowed in individual cases in respect of voice tests and, in the case of train drivers, a practical hearing test is carried out under operational conditions according to a defined protocol. With pure tone audiometry there are stricter standards for new entrants than for periodic reviews of employees. For example, for entry to train crew and safety grades the HTLs must not exceed 20 dB averaged over 0.5, 1, and 2 kHz or 25 dB at 4 kHz, whereas this is relaxed to 30 dB at the periodic reviews carried out at ages 25, 30, 35, 40, 45, 50, 55, 57, 60, 62, 63, and 64 years. It is considered unsafe to employ a worker who is dependent on a hearing aid to undertake footplate duties on main lines, or in any grade which involves working on operating track.

British Steel

One of the major risks encountered in heavy manufacturing companies, such as British Steel, is the potential to cause hearing damage. Such companies have often responded by implementing a comprehensive hearing conservation programme encompassing noise surveys and the identification of noise-hazard areas, engineering control measures, education and training, in addition to screening audiometry, and the provision of personal protection. Audiometry is performed on all new employees to establish a baseline and is mandatory at 3 yearly intervals for those employees working in noisy areas. Very few employees have been found to have hearing loss severe enough to act as a bar to employment. The basic criterion for auditory fitness is the ability to perform the job safely and competently. Each case is considered individually, and no specific hearing standards have been laid down.

Driving

Defective hearing may result in failure to hear a warning sound and thus lead to an accident. However, profoundly deaf people do not need to notify the DVLA until they are 70 years of age and they are only likely to be refused a licence if they are totally unable to communicate in an emergency.[14] The same criteria apply for large goods (LGVs) and passenger carrying vehicles (PCVs). Defective hearing need not be declared in an application for a driving licence, or at onset of the condition in the case of the holder of a current ordinary driving licence, unless it is indicative of some other disorder liable to affect fitness to drive in which case that disorder must be notified to the Licensing Centre at Swansea.

The EC Directive on driver licensing states: 'driving licences shall not be issued to, or renewed for applicants or drivers in group 2 if their hearing is so deficient that it inter-feres with the proper discharge of their duties' (personal comunication, J. Taylor, previ-ous Chief Medical Officer, Department of Transport).

See Appendix 1 for further details.

Diving

Divers should be able to clear their ears in order to equalize the pressure across the tym-panic membrane and to cope with the changing barometric pressures when diving. Com-plications of otitis media such as glue ear, deafness, perforation, and persistent discharge debar diving under UK Regulatory Standards. The presence of a mastoid cavity is also a reason for restriction. The following points should be covered during an assessment of otological fitness:

* The external auditory meati should appear normal. If wax is present, it is not neces-sary to disturb it unless it is excessive or obstructing the canal. Acute or chronic oti-tis externa is a bar to diving until resolved. Exostoses are not harmful unless the canal is occluded, when the diver should be referred for their removal.
* The ear-drum should be inspected: well-healed scars are acceptable. New entrants must demonstrate the ability to clear their ears. A similar requirement exists after infection or barotrauma.
* The diver should be able to hear and understand normal levels of conversation.
* Audiometric examination should be carried out at each annual examination, using equipment covering the frequencies 250 Hz–8 kHz and according to the recognized procedure. Particular attention should be given to divers who have only unilateral hearing, and the risks of further hearing damage should be discussed with the diver.

See Appendix 4 for futher details.

Further education

Some universities specialize in providing supplementary education for particular types of disability (Chapter 4, p. 78), such as Durham, in the case of the hearing disabled; many other colleges of further education provide technical courses to prepare deaf students for jobs that do not require interpersonal communication. In order to teach deaf and hard-of-hearing students, and to overcome poor room acoustics in lectures, supplementary aids may be needed, such as a microphone and an induction loop, a radio or infrared transmission system. An audiological assessment prior to admission, or assessment by an educationalist with relevant experience, is valuable.

Conclusions and recommendations

Normal hearing is difficult to define, as the definition is essentially arbitrary and age dependent. Wide individual variation exists in the degree of perceived handicap arising from a given measurable level of hearing disability. Moreover, the effect of a disability in the context of fitness for work depends greatly on the particular job requirements and working environment. These difficulties have to be seen in relation to the quite high prevalence of measurable hearing impairments (Table 10.1) and of reported hearing dif-ficulties (Table 10.2) in the general adult population.

Totally normal hearing, implying a stringent audiometric definition, is truly necessary only in very few jobs. But there are a number of occupations in which more than a minor impairment or disability, or having monaural hearing, is not acceptable for a variety of reasons. These include high levels of responsibility to others, need for efficient and easy communication, particular listening tasks, and safety with respect to hearing warning signals, especially when having to wear hearing protectors. The hearing requirements of each job have to be considered carefully when setting standards for entry or for continued employment, but care is needed to counteract prejudice against employing hard-of-hearing or deaf people. The problems that their hearing difficulties cause can be much less than are widely imagined, and can often be reduced or abolished by suitable modifications in equipment and/or in work and safety procedures.

For the majority of jobs, actual tests of hearing are unnecessary, other than a simple observation of the applicant's or employee's hearing ability at interview. (Where appropriate an interviewee can be allowed to wear a hearing aid or to lip read.) Ideally this should be coupled with some form of health declaration and a statement of disability. For those already employed, there may also be evidence regarding the importance or otherwise of any problems due to hearing difficulties that may have occurred with the particular employee and job.

Where the job requires a more definite degree of hearing ability, a test of ability to hear speech would probably be sufficient in most cases. Such tests are discussed in the next section. The choice depends on the nature and environment of the work, particularly whether or not there is need to hear speech against a background of noise. Audiometry is less relevant as a test of the ability to communicate, as it is relatively costly, and also poses problems of interpretation and management. It is probably best reserved for those in whom particularly good hearing is required and for circumstances where a baseline or criterion is required for medico-legal reasons, or for periodic monitoring in support of a hearing conservation programme.

Tests of hearing for assessment of fitness for work

Various hearing tests may be used to assess auditory fitness. Those outlined below should meet most situations. In selecting a test, it is advisable first to define clearly the objective of the test and to agree this with the involved parties. It should then be a relatively simple matter to choose the most suitable tests. The final selection may be influenced by financial, administrative, and space considerations, and by the acoustics of the proposed test environment.

Tests of hearing speech in a quiet background: voice tests

Free-field live-voice testing, widely used in clinical and occupational assessment of hearing ability, gives both a quantative method of assessing hearing and one which has obvious practical relevance. It requires no instrumentation. It has, however, fallen into some disrepute in recent decades due to inadequate test protocols, calibration, and interpretative criteria, as well as appearing to be overtaken in accuracy by audiometry.

The principal deficiencies in live-voice tests have been:

1 substantial inter-examiner and intra-examiner variability in voice levels and clarity

2 a tendency to raise the voice level when the ambient noise level rises, or

3 when distance from the subject increases

4 lack of a standard technique or a sufficiently detailed test protocol

5 too much ambient noise

6 test space too small, or

7 too narrow and reverberant.

A major contribution to restoring confidence in voice tests has been made by Browning *et al.*[15] They showed that deficiency 1 need not be a cause of major concern given suitable interpretative criteria, and deficiencies 3, 6, and 7 can be obviated by using the near field only. They further argued that deficiency 2 is rarely a problem and 5 should not be for most medical examination rooms. They also showed how the non-test ear can be efficiently, easily, and inexpensively masked. As a consequence, it is hoped that the recommendations below will meet the remaining need for a detailed protocol for conducting and interpreting the tests.

Test protocol for voice tests

The examiner sits or stands in front of the subject, leaving a nominal distance of 60 cm between the examiner's mouth and the subject's ears, and speaks the test material clearly in a whispered voice after full expiration (WV), conversational voice (CV), or loud voice (LV). The test material consists of trios of sounds: a numeral, a letter, a numeral (e.g. 5 B 6). Different combinations of numerals and letters must be used in each trio. Two trios are used for each type of voice. The subject is considered to have passed that voice test when they have repeated correctly at least three of the possible total of six numerals and letters. If fewer than three are repeated correctly, the next (louder) type of voice is used, and so on. When required, masking of the non-test ear is accomplished by pressing a finger on the tragus of the non-test ear and moving the skin over the cartilage to and fro, thus producing a continuous noise in the ear.

The hearing requirements of the job will define the other test details as follows:

- whether each ear is to be tested separately with masking of the non-test ear in order to detect monaural disorders, or whether the ears are to be tested together
- whether the subject's hearing aid may be worn, which in turn depends on whether it is possible and permissible at work
- whether the subject can make use of lip reading (told to watch the examiner's face) or not (told to shut their eyes), which also depends on whether lip reading is always or normally possible at work.

The correspondence of such voice tests to the audiometric thresholds of the large number of clinical patients included in their study, both retrospectively and prospectively were given.[15] For test distances nominally at 60 cm and for hearing by a single ear without hearing aid or lip reading, they established the approximate equivalents shown in Table 10.6, which include the effects of inter-clinician variability in voice levels.

Table 10.6 Relationship between voice test results and pure tone HTLs (after Browning *et al.*[15])

Grade	Voice test result	Approximate equivalent HTL (0.5, 1, and 2 kHz average)
1	Pass WV	<30 dB
2	Fail WV, pass CV	20–60 dB
3	Fail CV, pass LV	>45 dB, >60 dB

WV, whispered voice after full expiration; CV, conversational voice; LV, loud voice.

Since voice levels can vary considerably between examiners and also between occasions within the same examiner, the best practice would require assessors to calibrate their own voice levels and clarity for the test materials and in the test environment, both initially and at intervals. They can then be compared with, or adjusted to, the mean voice sound pressure levels. These were 57, 71, and 91 dB(A) for WV, CV, and LV, respectively when measured at a distance of 60 cm from the clinician's mouth with a sound-level meter set to the fast response. For such self-calibration of voice levels an inexpensive non-precision sound-level meter is adequate.

Where the test is conducted binaurally, with or without a hearing aid, and with or without help from lip reading, the result of the voice tests can be expressed in functional terms equivalent as above to unaided monaural listening. Grade 1 hearing would be quite adequate for nearly all jobs; grade 2 for all jobs, other than those in which there is an operational or safety requirement for good hearing *per se* or possibly when wearing ear protection and/or working in noise. Grade 3 applicants should be carefully considered in relation to the actual hearing requirements of the jobs concerned and not be excluded unnecessarily.

Finally, it is recommended that where audiometry is to be carried out, this should not replace voice tests but supplement them. For each subject, the results of voice tests can provide a very useful check on the apparent hearing ability as measured with an audiometer; and they also give information on another often more relevant dimension of hearing ability.

Test of ability to understand speech in noise

In noisy conditions, someone with a substantial loss of hearing sensitivity only (such as caused by conductive hearing loss) would not be disadvantaged relative to people with normal hearing and even at some advantage, as they often hear better in noise than in quiet, an observation resulting from the fact that those with normal hearing raise their voice levels in noise. This well-known diagnostic feature (paracusis Willisii) suggests that the patient's hearing loss is probably of the conductive type.

By contrast, people with sensorineural hearing loss have particular difficulty in hearing in a background of noise. Lip reading and signing help but cannot always be relied on, although workers in high levels of noise tend to learn from experience how to make maximal use of their hearing. These factors, together with a wide range of individual variability in the relationship between hearing sensitivity (as measured by voice tests or pure tone audiometry) and ability to identify correctly speech sounds in noise, may make it desirable to have a test of the latter. Ideally, this should be based on representative samples of the speech expected, or with the communication equipment likely to be used, and in the actual noise background. Unfortunately, this is usually impracticable.

A general purpose test of hearing speech in noise would have rather limited face validity, and no such test is available in standard clinical use. Thus it may be better, and certainly much simpler, to use the sort of voice and whisper tests outlined above. These can be interpreted more stringently and appropriately. Alternatively, if the auditory requirement is very exacting, a practical test of hearing ability may be arranged in the actual working environment and with the sort of sounds that need to be heard.

Pure tone audiometry

In the present context, the purposes of audiometry are to obtain a frequency-specific and a more precise and diagnostic measurement of hearing ability than is provided by speech tests, although its results will usually have less practical relevance to defining fitness for work than voice tests. It also has many disadvantages, needing costly and carefully calibrated equipment, trained operators, and (for low frequencies) particularly good acoustic conditions. Tests of the latter will require an acoustic booth which takes up more space and is heavy and expensive. Recommended techniques and maximum ambient noise levels for audiometry have been defined in international and national[16] standards. Despite the basic precision of the stimulus and measurement technique in audiometry, its sources of imprecision are often overlooked. Not everyone performs well at audiometry and it is not always easy to detect poor performers. There is a considerable degree of test–retest variability, which may be due to several factors. Substantial uncertainties in interpretation of audiograms may lead also to misjudgements of work fitness. Audiometry is a double-edged tool and one not to be employed without careful consideration.

Further guidance on industrial audiometry equipment and techniques and interpretation of results is available from two booklets specially written for the purpose.[17,18] A third source provides a useful description of a standardized technique for manually performed audiometry.[19] However, automatic self-recording audiometry is preferred to manual audiometry in industry, particularly when large numbers have to be tested or the audiometrician's skill is uncertain.

Balance

A study of the mechanisms of balance is a delight to physiologists who appreciate the sophistication of the systems involved. To physicians facing patients, often anxious and unsure, the complaint of 'dizziness' induces a feeling of dismay as they grapple with imprecisions in the history and try to relate it to pathology. Often their own lack of knowledge transmits itself and destroys the confidence between patient and doctor which is so important.

Gowers, in 1893, defined vertigo as 'any sense of movement either in the individual himself or in external objects that involves a defect, real or seeming, in the equilibrium of the body'. More succinctly, vertigo is a hallucination of movement.

The sophisticated system developed in humans to maintain equilibrium involves integration of sensory information from the visual senses, the vestibular apparatus, and the proprioceptive systems, especially those in the neck and limbs. This information is integrated with activity arising in the cortex, cerebellum, and extrapyramidal systems. Output is via the cortical awareness of position and movement, control of oculomotor activity, and control of posture and motor skills (see Fig. 10.2).

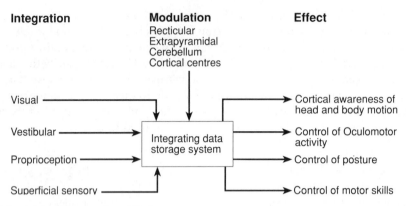

Fig. 10.2   Maintainance of equilibrium

Pathology affecting any of these systems, together with the pervasive influences of cardiovascular, endocrine, and intrinsic neurological disease, can affect this integrated system and lead to disequilibrium. In attempting to understand the pathology, physicians must focus on the symptom complex and history, for investigations are rarely definitive and often, at best, only a guide.

The difficulty is compounded by any psychological reaction on the patient's part, and the possibility that the patient may be intentionally or unintentionally influencing their environment. It is important therefore that the occupational physician understands the physiology of balance and the pathophysiology of imbalance in order to make a proper judgement on the employment role. The first concern of the occupational physician is to ensure the safety of the individual and other workers; but they will also need to consider the risk and the effects of future sickness absence, particularly where the employee is part of a team.

Principal disorders

'Dizziness' and 'giddiness' are terms that describe a wide variety of experiences. They may result from disorders of the vestibular, neurological, ophthalmic, cardiovascular, or musculo-skeletal systems, or they may be of psychological origin, or some combination of these. Their cause, and even the likely system of origin, is often difficult or impossible to define. Distinction between central vascular and general neurological (including psychological and vasovagal) disorders is often arbitrary, or unwarranted when both forms of disorder are present (as quite often occurs). On the other hand, differentiation between peripheral (end-organ and eighth cranial nerve) and central neural origin is usually possible and helps to define the type of disorder, its likely prognosis, and appropriate management.

Two important aspects of vestibular physiology explain most of the features of peripheral vestibular disorders.

*   The vestibular end-organs have a basal rate of nerve discharge and can be stimulated to increase or decrease their rate of firing. The end-organs of the semicircular canals on the two sides of the head are paired, and the afferent inputs to the central nervous system from each side act in opposition. Most, but probably not all, disorders of the

peripheral vestibular system cause a reduction in the resting rate in the corresponding part of the eighth cranial nerve. In such cases, the left–right imbalance so caused results in the eyes and body being reflexly deviated towards the side of the lesion. This is often reported as a sense of falling, or imbalance, to that side. The slow phase of nystagmus is also observed in this direction. The vertigo (or sense of rotation) and the fast phase of nystagmus localize to the opposite direction (the unaffected side) in such a case.

- The central vestibular system has a marked ability to compensate for chronic imbalance in the neural tonus between the two sides, and to habituate or adapt to frequently repeated or constant stimulation. Such habituation enables the acute disturbance of a severe unilateral vestibular failure to become self-limiting, especially in young patients. Over a few weeks, the sufferer passes from a state of intolerable vertigo with nausea and vomiting at rest, through to vertigo only on movement and, finally to momentary vertigo on major rotational movement of the head or body. **If symptoms of dizziness last continuously for longer than 2–3 weeks, the cause is rarely vestibular.**
- Compensation for chronic imbalance in neural tonus is achieved more easily in the younger patient. Labyrinthine sedatives are useful in the acute phase, to overcome the unpleasantness of the initial nausea and vomiting, but thereafter the key to rehabilitation is active provocational exercises such as those devised by Cawthorne and Cooksey.[20] Overprotection should be avoided. A confident and positive attitude in the attending physician will aid recovery and dispel ideas of early retirement on medical grounds.

Stimulation by sound

The cochlea responds readily to faint acoustic stimuli and yet is susceptible to damage by sustained excessive noise levels. In contrast, the vestibular apparatus, whose perilymph and endolymph are in direct continuity with the corresponding fluids in the cochlea, is less liable to injury. The explanation lies in the cochlea's microstructure which is so uniquely responsive to mechano-acoustic stimulation. On the other hand, the organization of the vestibular labyrinth is such that the cupulae or maculae are much less likely to respond to rapid to-and-fro stimulation arising from sound at ordinary levels. Nevertheless, the human vestibular system does respond to acoustic stimulation to some extent.

Even in health, very high noise levels—at and above 135 dB sound pressure level (SPL), e.g. those very close to powerful jet engines running at high power—can cause vertigo, nausea, and other unpleasant symptoms, such as fluttering of the cheeks, chest, and abdomen, and heating of hairy surfaces and skin folds. The saccule may also function as a receptor for low-frequency acoustic signals.

When a pathological disorder of the internal ear is present, however, levels of sound in the region of 110–120 dB SPL may cause a form of vertigo. This is known clinically as the Tullio effect. The 'sono-ocular' test takes advantage of this: if such stimuli cause nystagmus in the absence of visual fixation, this is taken as evidence of internal-ear pathology. The mechanism is uncertain. Its importance in the industrial context is that industrial noise seldom stimulates giddiness unless there is some pre-existing disorder of the internal ear.

The potentially damaging effects of noise exposure on the cochlea are now well recognized. Noise-induced damage to the vestibular part of the internal ear is less well documented, although evidence relating to this is accumulating.[21] Noise-induced vestibular disorders exist, but further epidemiological and clinical research is required to determine whether or not these (apart from the Tullio phenomenon) can be produced by the noise levels in industry. However, it should not be assumed automatically, even when vestibular and cochlear disorders co-exist, that the occurrence of the former implies disease of constitutional origin. Not only is it perfectly possible for coincident vestibular and cochlear disorders to have different aetiologies, it seems possible that the vestibular disorder itself might sometimes be due to damage by noise.[21]

Understandably, employers are anxious about employing people who suffer from dizziness. Their prejudice is often heightened by the inherent difficulty of ruling out psychological illness and uncertainties about prognosis.

Prevalence

Two community surveys, conducted in the 1950s, in the Vale of Glamorgan and in Annandale (Dumfries and Galloway) suggest that dizziness and giddiness are very common:[22] 23% of a random sample of men and women had experienced the symptom at some time (Table 10.7). Episodes were mostly transient, but in 3% vertigo symptoms lasted for a year or longer.

Hinchcliffe considered that this was largely due to endolymphatic hydrops but that in about one-third of these (1%) a diagnosis of Ménière's disorder seemed probable. He suggested that most cases, especially episodes of transient vertigo in the elderly, may have been arteriosclerotic in origin. He surmised further that the bulk of vertiginous histories, especially the episodes of transient vertigo, may have been arteriosclerotic in origin in the older individuals, but not in the younger ones.

The National Study of Hearing

In a postal questionnaire to a random sample of adults from the electoral register, a question was posed on vestibular-type disorders: 'Have you ever suffered from attacks of giddiness, dizziness, unsteadiness, or light-headedness?' Forty-one per cent of respondents

Table 10.7 Prevalence of history (past or present) of dizziness or giddiness according to age (after Hinchcliffe[22])

Age group	History of dizziness or giddiness (percentage of each age group)
18–24	17
25–34	20
35–44	19
45–54	23
55–64	35
65–74	29

reported experiencing these symptoms, women more commonly than men. A feature of this and the Hinchcliffe studies was the lack of age dependence in the prevalence of dizziness. This might be an artefact, due to faulty recall or stoicism in older respondents, because several other studies have shown a considerably increased prevalence of vertigo-like symptoms after retirement age.

A further questionnaire was sent to a subset of 1720 people in the NSH study who had symptoms. Only 657 (38%) responded, so important response biases may have been introduced. Only 13% of these respondents said their dizzy symptoms caused moderate or severe restriction of their current activities. In the context of fitness for work, this suggests that perhaps 2–5% of people of working age experience at some time a disturbance of their working ability from this cause.

The episodes reported were transient (a few seconds) in 55% of the respondents, and fairly infrequent (less than once a month) in 43%. Responders were asked about associations with other factors. These included physical events such as transport (10% of people); faints or near-faints (23%); physical strain (32%); or psychological factors such as heights (29%); open spaces (5%); enclosed spaces (15%); mental strain (30%); strong emotion (21%); anxiety (37%); and tiredness (46%). Episodes were sometimes brought on by getting up from a bed or chair (53% of people); straightening up after bending down (62%); looking down or bending down (41%); and looking around or making a sudden turn (51%).

Clinical aspects affecting work capacity

Relation to fitness for particular types of work

There are two main concerns in fitness assessment:

- that acute disorienting episodes which come on without warning may cause a danger to the worker or to others;
- that recurrent attacks may result in unpredictable absences from work.

Disorders of balance may sometimes lead to premature retirement, especially when the effects are recurrent or prolonged and there seems no reasonable prospect of an acceptable degree of recovery or rehabilitation. Only rarely does the acute, unexpected disorientation lead to serious accidental injury or death.

In some cases, however, dizziness is a manifestation of a more serious underlying disorder, such as cardiovascular disease, cerebral tumour, or multiple sclerosis, which itself may have serious implications for work ability and life expectancy.

Treatment and rehabilitation

In the acute phase, the management of vestibular symptoms should be based on vestibular suppressive drugs; in the chronic phase Cawthorne and Cooksey's[20] head and balance exercises are more effective. Dizziness may nevertheless lead to prolonged or frequent absences from work. Additionally, sedative side-effects may occur with many of the vestibular suppressive drugs, such as cinnarizine and prochlorperazine. This is especially true of drugs used to prevent motion sickness, such as hyoscine, and those with antihistamine-like properties, e.g. meclozine, dimenhydrinate, and promethazine. Treatment with these drugs may impair work efficiency and safety, and especially safety to drive.

They also interact with alcohol. Treatment of unsteadiness in older people with phenothiazines, such as prochlorperazine, tends to aggravate postural hypotension and to cause parkinsonism. Because of these side-effects, vestibular suppressive drugs should be phased out as soon as possible and replaced by a programme of vestibular rehabilitation.

Special work problems, restrictions, or needs

The problems of recurrent or prolonged periods of illness and the side-effects of treatment have been mentioned above. They are not specific to any particular job, but there are certain work tasks in which an acute attack of vertigo or imbalance could prove extremely dangerous. These are outlined below.

Work on or near potentially hazardous machinery

The risk will depend on the size, nature, and power of the machine, and the extent to which its dangerous parts are shielded. Each case has to be weighed individually. Factors to be considered include the ways in which the disorder affects the person and whether they are likely to experience warning symptoms of an impending attack and to be able to take appropriate avoiding action.

Other potentially dangerous situations

Working with molten metal, caustic acids, or alkalis, and working in isolation or near deep water, is also potentially dangerous. Much the same considerations apply as with work near moving machinery. Some patients' attacks may be related to, or induced by work at heights.

Work in moving environments

The likelihood of motion sickness is increased by most forms of vestibular disorder. Preventive drugs may be used, but due consideration must be given to the risk of side-effects that undermine work safety and efficiency. Probably the best solution, if possible, is to give the affected worker a conditional trial in the environment in question.

Diving

Chronic or recurrent vestibular disturbances are usually a bar to diving, especially scuba diving (see Appendix 4). This is because spatial orientation depends on three main factors: vestibular function, pressure sense, and visual cues. Underwater surroundings may be dark or murky, reducing or removing the visual input; there is also a much reduced pressure sense even when the diver is on the bottom, as the human being then has a similar specific gravity to that of the environment. Orientation thus depends heavily on the vestibular system; if this is deficient a very dangerous situation can easily arise.

Jobs with high levels of responsibility for the safety of others

Sudden onset of acute vestibular impairment while in control of a vehicle can give the operator a false impression that the vehicle has veered from its correct direction. This may lead to unnecessary corrective action and cause an accident. Acute vertigo may also cause a reflex response which causes the driver to misdirect the vehicle. People subject to vestibular or similar disturbances should not drive on-road vehicles, off-road vehicles, boats, or planes until they are fully recovered and have had no attacks for at least a year.

Existing legislation and guidelines for employment

Medical assessment

Unlike hearing, vestibular function cannot be measured quickly and easily. Therefore, vestibular function tests have not been standardized for use in occupational assessments. Testing is generally limited to simple clinical manoeuvres such as the Romberg test or heel–toe walking in a straight line, and inspection of the eyes for nystagmus. These procedures can only detect substantial disturbances of balance, or nystagmus due to central, or to recent and severe peripheral, vestibular disorders. Usually most reliance is placed on the history of severity, duration, frequency, nature, and effects of vestibular episodes.

Special restrictions

Driving

The DVLA must be informed by a licence holder or applicant with this disability (see also Appendix 1). People who are liable to sudden disabling attacks of giddiness or fainting are banned from holding a motor vehicle driving licence. In the case of attacks of vertebrobasilar artery insufficiency, a person is advised to stop driving and report the condition. After a first episode, the ordinary driving licence is usually revoked for at least 3 months. Recurrent cases may be reviewed when satisfactory control of symptoms is achieved. A licence may be restored for 1, 2, or 3 years, and permanently if there have been no symptoms for 4 years. The same policy is adopted for Ménière's disorder, vestibulopathies, and positional vertigo. Normally, any person with a persisting vestibular disorder, Méniere's disease, positional vertigo, or a single transient ischaemic episode is regarded as unfit to drive vocationally (passenger carrying vehicles, large goods vehicles, and taxis).

Flying

The determining factors in fitness assessment are whether the licence holder may become incapacitated while in control of an aircraft and whether they can function effectively. Clearly, vertigo or imbalance arising from Ménière's disorder, vestibulopathies, or positional vertigo would not be compatible with flying. More borderline or uncertain conditions do occur, and in these cases, fitness decisions are made by the Civil Aviation Authority following an examination by a doctor specially qualified in aviation medicine (see also Appendix 2).

Merchant navy

Ménière's disease is the only vestibular disorder specified in the Department of Transport regulations on medical fitness of seafarers: it implies permanent unfitness, as do transient ischaemic attacks, which often present as episodes of dizziness (see also Appendix 3).

Diving

Fitness to dive is covered by statutory medical standards. With few exceptions, disorders of balance constitute an absolute bar to working as a commercial diver (see also Appendix 4).

Armed forces

The degree to which a vestibular disorder will affect the physical (P) assessment in the

PULHEEMS system depends on its nature, severity, and effects. The interpretation of the P assessment in terms of fitness for service depends on the particular branch of service, and is closely related to the actual requirements of the job and the limitations which physical disorders would place on its performance.

Police, fire, and other public services
In general, there are no specific regulations. Certification of fitness depends on a non-specialist medical opinion on the likelihood of incapacity during operational duties. For firefighters, who may work up ladders or in conditions of minimal visibility, a more stringent criterion needs to be applied. The Home Office guidelines of 1970 specified that 'evidence of labyrinthine disturbance, a history of vertigo or any condition which would impair a candidate's sense of balance' would render a recruit unsuitable for employment in firefighting.

General industry
Where pre-employment screening is performed, unless there is a specialized need, enquiry tends to be limited to the general question: 'Do you suffer from fits, faints, blackouts, or dizzy attacks?' The data from the NSH imply that such symptoms rarely interfere with work (see pp. 184–185). Where the severity is sufficient to cause problems, the potential employer tends to err on the side of caution, sometimes to the detriment of the individual. Occupational physicians tend to be more liberal. This unsatisfactory situation arises from the difficulties in diagnosis and uncertainties in prognosis mentioned earlier.

Similar problems are encountered during employment. If an employee develops disabling vertigo, the employer must review the safety of the individual and the group with whom they work. Restrictions on driving, work at heights, or near moving machinery are commonly imposed. These, and the uncertainties regarding regular attendance at work, raise questions of employability. In such cases, as much information as possible should be obtained on the aetiology, treatment, and prognosis and weighed against the job requirements before taking any final decision.

Conclusions and recommendations

Disturbances of equilibrium are common in men and women of all ages. Mostly these are transient and inconsequential. Confidence in the attending physician, sympathy from the occupational medical services, and a positive attitude to rehabilitation, using provocational exercises rather than trying to sedate the vestibular system with drugs, are the key to a successful and early return to work.

Few causes of disequilibrium have substantial implications for fitness at work, although absences from work can arise and can be recurrent. Except in classical cases these disorders are difficult to diagnose and to assess.

Real work limitations may arise if there is a liability to acute episodes of vertigo or imbalance, especially if these are unpredictable. Restrictions have to be imposed where the work is near unguarded, moving machinery or at heights, involving driving or exposure to motion (as in ships), or where the job has a high level of responsibility, or where there is a potential risk of injury to others. Episodes like these are incompatible with diving, flying, or work in safety-critical situations.

Selected references

1 Kettle M, Massie B. (ed.). *Employers' guide to disabilities*, 2nd edn, 19–23. Cambridge: Wood-head-Faulkner, 1986.

2 *Deaf and hearing impaired.* Booklet EPWD20. Sheffield: Employment Service, 1988.

3 Davis AC. The prevalence of hearing impairment and reported hearing disability among adults in Great Britain. *Int J Epidemiol* 1989; **18**: 911–917.

4 Acton WI, Wilkins PA. Can noise cause accidents? *Occup Health Saf* 1982; **12**: 14–16.

5 Wilkins PA. The role of acoustical characteristics in the perception of warning sounds and the effects of wearing hearing protection. *J Sound Vib* 1982; **100**: 181–190.

6 Coleman, G.J. *et al. Communications in noisy environments.* Report TM/84/1. Edinburgh: Institute of Occupational Medicine, 1984.

7 Alberti PW, Hyde ML, Symons BA, Milles RB. The effect of prolonged exposure to industrial noise on otosclerosis. *Laryngoscope* 1980; **90**: 407–413.

8 *A guide to audiometric testing programmes.* Guidance note. Sheffield: Health and Safety Executive, 1995.

9 *Occupational disease enquiry 1995.* London: Association of British Insurers, 1996.

10 Jones JR, Hodgson JT, Clegg TA, Elliott RC. *Self-reported work-related illness in 1995. Results from a household survey.* London: HMSO, 1998.

11 Health and Safety Statistics 1996/7. Sheffield: HSE Books.

12 Davis A, Roberts H. In *Proceedings of the fifth international tinnitus seminar 1995*, ed. Reich GE, Vernon JA. Portland, Oregon: American Tinnitus Association, 1996.

13 Godber Sir G (Chief Medical Officer of the Home Office). *Report of the committee to review the medical standards for the fire service.* London: Home Office, 1970

14 *At a glance guide to the current medical standards of fitness to drive.* Swansea: DVLA, 1998.

15 Browning GG, Swan IRC, Chew KK. Clinical role of informal tests of hearing. *J Laryngol Otol* 1989; **103**: 7–11.

16 *Pure tone air conduction threshold audiometry for hearing conservation purposes. BS 6655.* London: British Standards Institution, 1986.

17 Bryan ME, Tempest W. *Industrial audiometry.* London: Werth, 1976.

18 Bryan ME, Tempest W. *Examples of industrial audiograms.* London: Werth, 1978.

19 Recommended procedures for pure-tone audiometry using a manually operated instrument (Joint recommendations by the British Society of Audiology and the British Association of Otolaryngologists). *Br J Audiol* 1981; **15**: 213–216; *J Laryngol Otol* 1981; **95**: 757–761.

20 Cooksey FS. Rehabilitation in vestibular injuries. *Proc R Soc Med* **39**: 273–278. 1946

21 Hinchcliffe R, Coles RRA, King PF. Occupational noise-induced vestibular malfunction? *Br J Indust Med* 1992; **49**: 63–65.

22 Hinchcliffe R. Prevalence of the commoner ear, nose and throat, conditions in the adult rural population of Great Britain: a study by direct examination of two random samples. *Br J Prev Soc Med* 1961; **15**: 128–140.

11

Spinal disorders

E. Macdonald and I. Haslock

Back pain is the largest single cause of time lost from work, and low back pain will affect about 70% of the working population at some time during their working life. There are few tests which are of use in predicting who is going to get pain in any particular working environment, and so pre-employment screening is of limited value.

Although back pain can occur spontaneously, it is more common in occupations that involve heavy manual work. Most individuals with short-term pain in the back can be successfully rehabilitated to their normal work, but the outlook is much worse for those with chronic pain. The emphasis should therefore be placed on prevention, by a combination of improving workplace design, setting up good work practices, and providing adequate training for the worker. When back pain does occur it must be treated promptly to prevent chronicity.

The vertebral column is the jointed bony core of the spine. It allows movement in addition to providing strength and rigidity. The jointed bony structures are supported by muscles which provide strength with flexibility. Extra strength is provided at the thoracic and lumbar levels by the muscles of the chest and abdomen. The constant demands made on the spine in nearly all activities lead to recognizable changes. The changes, that result from normal wear and repair are often termed 'spondylosis' and can be seen on a radiograph. This condition is generally asymptomatic but when use is excessive or injudicious, symptoms may result.

The symptoms have several cardinal characteristics. The most common is pain. This is generally intermittent, related to movement, and clearly emanates from the spine. The pain usually arises from the joints themselves, when it is often axial; it may derive from the dural covering of the nerve roots and be proximally referred, or it may arise from true nerve root irritation or damage, when it is often distal and shows classical neurological features. Similarly, the abnormal signs may be related to the joints—asymmetrical production of pain or restriction of movement; dural pain on nerve root stretching, or nerve root pain with reflex weakness, or sensory changes.

By contrast, a minority of spinal disorders are congenital, inflammatory, or neoplastic. Inflammatory disorders may be idiopathic (e.g. ankylosing spondylitis) or infective, and neoplastic disorders in the spine generally arise from secondary deposits. In these patients pain will be constant and progressive, and restriction of movement symmetrical, increasing to complete rigidity.

Disorders of the spine are very common and their occupational significance is frequently an issue for individuals, their medical advisers, and employers. Despite the fall in numbers employed in manual industries, low back and neck pain appear increasingly to cause absence from work. Low back pain is the major cause of retirement through ill health in many industries, ranging from mining to healthcare, and has a huge personal and social cost. Conversely, the employment opportunities for those with inflammatory back disorders such as ankylosing spondylitis are now greater, given the growth in the service and retail sectors and the use of information technology.

Prevalence and morbidity

Between 70 and 80% of the population will experience low back pain at some time, causing absence from work, but most of these episodes will be self-limiting and of short duration—albeit with a tendency to recur. Low back pain of acute onset tends to improve spontaneously and the recovery rate in a cohort of back pain sufferers has a half-life of about 10 days (i.e. half the sufferers will be better in 10 days), whatever the treatments delivered and the skills of the therapists.

Over the past 40 years there has been an enormous growth in certified incapacity due to back pain. This growth has occurred in many developed countries. The British experience is summarized in Fig. 11.1.[1]

In 1993, approximately 150 million days of total working capacity were lost due to back pain. In 1994, the estimated annual cost of back pain, including loss of production and NHS costs, ranged between £3.5 billion and £6.9 billion.[2] Diagnoses of spondylosis and allied disorders and intervertebral disc disorders accounted for about 50% of the total. There was little difference in the prevalence of back pain in different occupational groups. Low back pain is most prevalent in the fifth decade. The accuracy and relevance of precise diagnosis is questionable, but within this total, about 50% of low back pain is attributed to prolapsed intervertebral disc.[3]

About 16% of all adults will consult their general practitioners with back pain each year, and estimates of the lifetime consultation rate with general practitioners for back pain range between 26 and 40%. A population-based survey of back pain showed that the severity of symptoms reported by those who attended their general practitioner was no greater than the severity in those who did not consult.[4] It appears, even at this early stage of interaction with the health service, that other factors are influencing the lifestyle decisions regarding back pain. Of those consulting their general practitioner, about 30% will be referred to a physiotherapist, osteopath, or hospital doctor, and about 20–25% of all new out-patient orthopaedic appointments are for back pain. About 50% of the average hospital physiotherapy treatments are for spinal conditions. About one-third of those referred to hospital with a disc problem will have operative treatment.

Clinical aspects affecting work capacity

A recent major review has pointed out that back pain and sciatica have affected humans throughout recorded history and that these symptoms are now no more frequent and no more severe than they have always been.[4] Yet the tendency to report incapacity and to seek medical care has been growing. Hence this growth would appear to be due to psychosocial factors. In the past, few people became chronically disabled. Furthermore, the 'medicalization' of back pain, theories about the ruptured intervertebral disc, the lack of clarity of information for patients, the lack of precision in diagnosis by doctors, and the

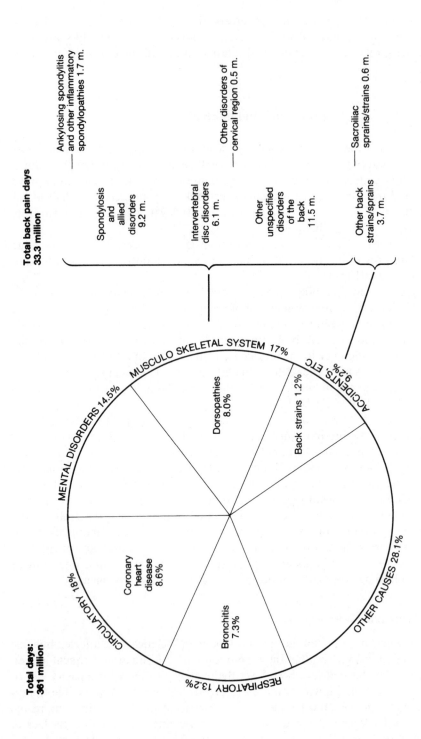

Fig. 11.1 Estimated impact of back pain over the course of a 12 month period (days of certified incapacity for work, England, Wales and Scotland 1982–3)[2]

ready certification of patients complaining of low back pain, which may be a symptom of other forms of distress, have compounded the problem.

Neck pain

A population study has shown a lifetime prevalence of chronic neck pain of 71%, with 41% reporting neck pain in the previous month.[5]

Most people over the age of 40 will have some spinal radiographic changes. These include narrowing of one or more intervertebral disc spaces in the middle or lower cervical regions, often with osteophytic outgrowths. The apophyseal and neurocentral joints are also affected. However, there is a poor correlation with symptoms and many people remain symptom-free. Radiology is of value in assessment and in investigating injury, possible infection, or malignancy. Its value as a guide to prognosis, treatment, or fitness for work is debatable.

Symptoms

Pain is the most common symptom of orthopaedic neck disorders, but deformity (torticollis) or neurological patterns of complaint may dominate. The intermittent nature of symptoms and their provocation by posture are important and reassuring features. In many patients a history of an unaccustomed activity or an injury (e.g. whiplash) may be elicited. After road traffic accidents prolonged symptoms are common (although this does not occur in countries where there is no compensation for whiplash injuries.) If sustained at work, the problem is often more persistent. Most pathology is in the low cervical spine (C6–7), but the symptoms of pain are often referred away from the actual site of injury. The pain may be entirely local, or referred to the occiput, towards the shoulders, or to the interscapular region. Restriction of movement is usually asymmetrical. The delineation between articular and dural pain is often unclear, but true nerve root pain is usually more distal by virtue of the sclerotomes supplied from the lower cervical levels which are usually involved.

Signs

Physical examination should start with observation of posture and any deformities and swellings. The range of neck movements should be examined in the three standard planes: flexion–extension, lateral flexion, and rotation. Next, shoulder movements should be examined partly to check for shoulder pathology but also to look for dural tension signs, and this should be followed by a neurological examination of the arms. In addition, a history of bladder or bowel symptoms should be sought, and the long tracts and plantar responses examined.

Treatment

The basic treatment for a condition due to injury or wear and tear is rest. This rarely needs to be complete (i.e. bed rest), and frequently a restricting collar is helpful. Collars need to be carefully fitted so as to achieve at least a 70% reduction in neck movement, as opposed to merely providing warmth and draught-proofing (comforting though this may be). Non-steroidal anti-inflammatory drugs (NSAIDs) may help the minor inflammatory component of the disorder, and do have a modest analgesic action. Muscle relaxants are often used. There is some evidence that treatment by physiotherapists or osteopaths can hasten recovery from individual episodes, and prophylactic advice is important in preventing a recurrence.

Occupational factors

The symptoms and degree of disability vary considerably. The provoking occupational factors are not well understood, but disability is more frequent in jobs where there is restricted headroom, work in awkward and confined places, work requiring the head and neck to be held in a constant position, and strenuous work using the arms. All of these may aggravate neck stiffness, pain in the neck and arms, and paraesthesiae. Prolonged working with the arms above the head may also precipitate shoulder and arm pain.

After an exacerbation, it is wise initially to avoid tasks which involve heavy carrying (e.g. certainly not more than 20 kg, and often less), lifting, shovelling, manual loading and unloading, the use of heavy vibratory tools, and working with the arms elevated and the neck extended. Attention should be paid to the ergonomics of display screen equipment, workstations, seating, and the organization of clerical work. Clerical workers can be helped by having raised and tilted work surfaces, so that flexion of the neck for long periods is avoided. Document holders should be supplied for workers who have to refer to documents while working with display screen equipment.

Those with persisting neck stiffness may not be fit for their jobs if these require a full, free range of neck movement, as in driving a motor vehicle, crane, or forklift truck. However, symptoms usually improve in most cases and so occupational restrictions should be reviewed and lifted as soon as possible.

Ankylosing spondylitis

Ankylosing spondylitis is an important cause of chronic pain and disability in young adults. It affects men and women in the ratio of 4 : 1, and women are less severely affected. The overall prevalence is about 1% but many will remain undiagnosed. Six per cent of cases will have a family history. The age of presentation is usually between 18 and 30 years. It may present atypically, in association with Reiter's syndrome, psoriasis, and chronic inflammatory bowel disorders. There is a close relationship to the HLA B27 tissue antigen.

In many cases the disease will remain mild and will have little impact on functional ability and will not cause absence from work.

Symptoms

The condition classically starts as a disease of the sacroiliac joints with back, buttock, or posterior thigh pain, and often morning stiffness. It may be unilateral, bilateral, or alternating from side to side. In the more severely affected patient, there will be widespread inflammatory change spreading up the spinal joints, causing virtually complete spinal fusion in those most affected. In some patients a severe kyphosis and general ill health may occur, and the disease is occasionally complicated by amyloid deposits. The two main pillars of treatment are NSAIDs and exercises. Although formal treatment by physiotherapists is invaluable in the management of ankylosing spondylitis, educating the patient in a life-long self-management regime of exercises and postural awareness is the most important part of disease management.

Occupational prognosis

Work is beneficial for people with ankylosing spondylitis, as increased activity reduces discomfort and the risk of permanent deformation. Eighty per cent of people with the disease can work full-time and heavy manual work is not contra-indicated, although only about 10% will tend to remain in such work, and most are employed in sedentary, professional, or light manual work.

In one series,[6] after 30 years of ankylosing spondylitis 31% were still working at their original jobs and 22% had changed to lighter work. However, even in the armed forces, 70% were able to follow a full service career. The majority will cope with work for at least 20 years and only minimal work adjustments are required. The prognosis is less good in those with severe hip involvement, or fixed and extreme flexion of the thoracic spine, or in the few people who develop a severe peripheral polyarthritis.

The specific limitations at work are usually related to joint stiffness, and thus individuals without free neck movements and all-round vision may be unsuitable for some tasks such as driving cranes, large goods vehicles, passenger carrying vehicles, or forklift trucks. Work requiring agility or working in confined spaces may be contra-indicated, but any restrictions should be recommended only on an individual basis. Workers who have prolonged periods of relative immobility, such as those using computers, will benefit from short break-periods in which they can carry out a few simple exercises for their back and neck. Patients fare better if they are kept under regular review, if their symptoms are adequately treated, and if they participate in regular physiotherapy classes, and remain physically active. The National Ankylosing Spondylitis Society (see Appendix 7 for address) has local branches and self-help groups and provides information and support. Some regional centres are still able to arrange short courses of in-patient treatment for groups of patients, with considerable benefit. Where workplace physiotherapy is available this should be used on a routine basis to maintain maximal function.

Low back pain

Low back pain is generally defined as pain between the lower rib border and the inferior gluteal fold in the region of the lumbosacral spine. It is generally intermittent. In most patients it arises from a mechanical disorder of the lower lumbar joints, most often at the L4–5 and/or L5–S1 levels. Occasionally it may be referred from a neoplastic or vascular lesion in the abdomen or retroperitoneum. Other lumbar pathology, such as inflammation or neoplasm, will produce more relentless features. Cauda equina claudication may result from narrowing of the lumbar canal and gives rise to leg pain or weakness on exercise. Some important clinical features that suggest serious pathology are listed in Box 11.1.

Low back pain is a symptom rather than a diagnosis, is remarkably common, often poorly understood in individual cases, and causes much morbidity. Twenty-three per cent of patients who consult their general practitioners during a year seek advice on

---

Box 11.1   Clinical indicators of potentially serious spinal pathology
Age of onset under 20 or over 55

- Non-mechanical pain (i.e. pain unaffected by movement)
- Thoracic pain
- Past history of carcinoma, steroids, HIV
- Unwell, with weight loss
- Widespread neurological signs
- Structural deformity

---

rheumatic complaints, and of these, back troubles account for 27% of the caseload. However, this does not reflect the true size of the problem, as half of the patients attending osteopaths will do so for back pain and one-third of these will not have attended their own doctor.

In the workplace, absenteeism attributed to back pain is common in all occupations. In mining it accounts for 12–18% of all certificated absence. About 50% of nurses will experience back discomfort in a year, and back pain is very prevalent in manual workers, drivers, helicopter pilots, and many other groups. Office workers experience almost as much back pain as manual workers, although their associated sickness absence is far less.

In considering the fitness for work of back pain sufferers a number of aspects must be weighed including the physiological cause of the back pain, the occupational and individual risk factors, and an appreciation of the ergonomics of the workplace and the task requirements.

Symptoms

Pain is the dominant feature. It is generally centred on the low lumbar spine, especially when arising from the intervertebral joints themselves. Classically it is intermittent and related to movement. Irritation of nearby dural coverings or nerve root sheaths may produce chronic referred pain. This is felt in the buttocks or thighs but sometimes radiates up the spine. Symptoms that truly arise from the nerve roots are more severe and more distal (as the L5 or S1 roots are usually involved), and are more closely related to changing cerebrospinal fluid (CSF) pressure—as in coughing or straining. In these patients there may be bladder and bowel symptoms.

Signs

Initially one should look for postural or fixed deformity. Paraspinal muscle prominence due to spasm is common, as is loss of the expected lordosis. Local tenderness is commonly present. Movements should be examined in the two main planes: flexion–extension and lateral flexion. In these mechanical disorders, restriction of movement is classically asymmetrical. Signs of dural tension are elicited by checking the straight-leg-raise and the femoral nerve stretch tests, which relate to the L5 and L3–L4 nerve roots respectively. Restriction of movement, or production of pain, is sought. Finally, a standard neurological examination should be conducted from L1–S4 with particular attention to checking the L5 dermatome (which has no reflex) and the saddle area for anaesthesia.

Computed tomography (CT) scanning and magnetic resonance imaging (MRI) define the dimensions of the spinal canal and may confirm the presence of a discrete lesion. However, MRI, in particular, may reveal apparent pathology in clinically unaffected discs, and even the most sophisticated imaging techniques are only of value within the context of a careful clinical evaluation of the patient.

Management

Until recently the perceived wisdom for treatment of back pain placed a strong emphasis on rest. It is now recognized that this prolonged recovery times from acute episodes and engendered unrealistic expectations of complete pain relief, and this has been one of the major causes of subsequent chronicity. Thus a careful history and physical examination is required to determine if the problem is musculoskeletal and to exclude abdominal, gynaecological, or renal pathology. The diagnostic triage for musculoskeletal back pain requires determination of whether the back pain is:

- simple, due to mechanical strain or dysfunction
- nerve root pain, due to disc prolapse spinal stenosis or spondylosis
- serious spinal pathology, due to tumour, infection, metabolic or other disorders.

These determine the further management of the patient.

The modern, more dynamic, approach to treatment requires both re-education of doctors' attitudes to this symptom and, crucially, of patients' expectations regarding its management. The current approach of early diagnostic triage requires doctors to be confident in their clinical assessment of the patient and positive in their approach to early mobilization and rapid return to activities.[4] Patients will be familiar with the 'if it hurts, rest it' approach to management, and the new strategy must be carefully explained. In a society that increasingly demands a painless transaction from cradle to grave, the message that some discomfort is inevitable and must be tolerated is often poorly received.

Once the diagnosis of simple low back pain has been made, the aims of treatment are to minimize immobility and maximize function. This will require confident reassurance that an active treatment programme is both appropriate and safe. Rest should be restricted to 2–3 days at most. In order to facilitate this, adequate analgesia is necessary. This will normally be achieved by adequate oral doses of NSAIDs or plain analgesics, but intramuscular NSAIDs, occasionally supplemented with the muscle-relaxant effect of diazepam, or an intramuscular injection of an opiate, may be required. Pain relief is an essential prerequisite to restoring full mobility, so an aggressive analgesic policy is essential.

It may also be helpful to provide the patient with a copy of *The back book* at this early stage of treatment, as this underlines the principles of modern treatment and its use has been shown to aid the active management process.[7]

Patients with simple low back pain should be encouraged to remain active. If symptoms last more than a few days, manipulation, graduated active exercise, and physical activity can help to modify pain and will speed recovery. In such patients activity is not harmful, and early return to work should be encouraged provided that work can be modified if needed or that appropriate redeployment is possible. It is clear that the psychosocial management is as important as the medical management. The longer people are off work the less is their likelihood of returning to work[2] (see Fig. 11.2) and maintaining individuals in employment or an active life is likely to reduce the overall morbidity.

Many accessory treatments are available for particularly painful aspects of the syndrome.[8,9] Manipulation has been shown to hasten the relief of pain when the patient has marked asymmetry of spinal restriction, and particularly if there is a dural tension abnormality, e.g. restricted straight-leg raise. Traction is probably helpful when root pain is a prominent feature. When root features are severe and a root lesion is detectable, then epidural anaesthetic-steroid injections can hasten relief. When these accessory treatments are required, it is essential that they are provided rapidly. There is little point in stressing the need for rapid action to the patients if they are then faced with a wait of weeks or even months before treatment can be given.

Frequently, patients go directly to osteopaths or chiropractors. These practitioners are often skilled and highly trained in the art of manipulation and may hasten relief when the underlying pathology is not too severe. Acupuncture is sometimes helpful in relieving pain, and transcutaneous electrical nerve stimulation (TENS) machines have an established, but not universal, role. There is rarely a need for surgery but this should be considered when a grossly unstable joint can be shown to be causing pain. A fusion is then indicated. More often, sciatica can be shown to arise from nerve root pressure secondary to disc prolapse. The offending disc protrusion can then be removed by surgery or by chemonucleolysis. Advances in surgical technique, such as minidiscectomy, mean

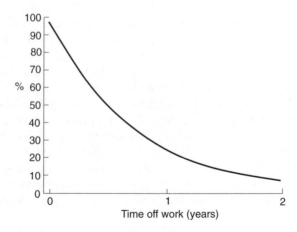

Fig. 11.2 Probability of return to work.

that surgery can be carried out with only a single night in hospital or even on a day-patient basis. This enables the impetus to recovery to be maintained.

A significant proportion of patients with back pain threaten to develop a chronicity in their symptoms which is not easily explicable on a physical basis. For these patients a longer period of rehabilitation treatment may be useful. Indeed, it may be the only alternative that is available to seeking fringe methods of relief, such as osteopathy, chiropractice, and acupuncture. The conventional treatments used involve a blend of psychiatry, physical methods, occupational therapy, and exercises. At one extreme might be the patient whose problem is thought to be due to a mixture of pain leading to weakness and symptoms of mild depression, and at the other, a patient who is clearly clinically depressed. This leads to diminished motivation, weakness, and pain. The former may be helped by a physical approach such as isometric exercises, hydrotherapy, and an exercise regime, the latter by a method based mainly on psychotherapy and drugs.[10] The role of back schools is controversial but the formation of small groups who are taught the principles of back care, isometric exercises, and avoidance of harmful stress is popular. The principles are both physically and psychologically sound and assessment to establish their value should be encouraged.

When chronic back pain does occur it is essential that rehabilitation is based on a biopsychosocial model which takes an holistic view of the people concerned and their interaction with their environment, both at home and in the workplace. (Box 11.2) Two large studies show the importance of 'non-medical' factors in back pain.

In a 4 year study of 3000 blue-collar workers undertaken at the Boeing Corporation, 180 variables were assessed. This showed no correlation between sickness loss for back pain and commonly perceived 'causes' such as workload, physical fitness, muscle control, mobility, age, and sex, but did show a correlation with previously reported back pain, smoking, abnormal personality, job satisfaction, and the relationship with fellow workers and supervisors.[11] Deyo and Diehl[12] undertook a detailed analysis of 179 patients with low back pain, and found that the strongest predictors of future function, employment, and medical utilization were the three variables education, previous episodes of back pain, and 'always feel sick'. These three items created a scale, defining subgroups with threefold differences in outcomes, with 35% good outcomes in the worst group (left school at earliest opportunity + previous back pain + 'always feel sick') compared with 93% in the best group (higher education, first episode, do not 'always feel sick'). An inception cohort in general practice showed a similar preponderance of social rather than physical factors, with sociodemographic and job-related characteristics being the most sensitive predictors of return to work.[13]

Special work problems

Accidents

Low back pain is frequently attributed to an accident at work. Studies in various occupational groups have shown, with surprising consistency, that although accident rates vary, about 20–25% of 'accidents' affect the back, and of these manual handling (e.g. lifting, loading, or carrying) is a factor in about 50–60% of cases. However, a detailed analysis[15] of 236 back injuries showed that in 48% the back pain arose spontaneously and was not

Box 11.2 Biopsychosocial model of low back disability[14]

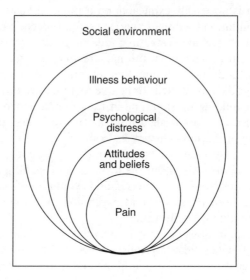

An overview of biopsychosocial assessment
Bio
- Review diagnostic triage
  - nerve root problem
  - serious spinal pathology
- ESR and plain radiograph

Psycho
- Attitude and beliefs about back pain
  - fear avoidance beliefs about activity and work
  - personal responsibility for pain and rehabilitation
- Psychological distress and depressive symptoms
- Illness behaviour

Social
- Family
  - attitudes and beliefs about the problem
  - reinforcement of disability behaviour
- Work
  - physical demands of job
  - job satisfaction
  - other health problems causing time off or job loss
  - non-health problems causing time off or job loss

attributable to an accident at all. The precipitating causes in the remainder were slipping and stumbling on rough or unstable surfaces and loss of balance in 75%, a sudden unexpected load in 12%, and blows to the back in 7%.

Manual handling

Jobs that involve a lot of heavy lifting are associated with an increased risk of back pain. Those who lift infrequently are at greater risk than those who perform a moderate amount of lifting regularly—probably because of a training effect. Thus, back pain occurs frequently in the sedentary worker after weekend gardening or other unaccustomed physical activity.

The size and shape of the load is important—a 10 kg block of lead is much safer to handle than a 10 kg box of feathers. The presence or absence of handles matters too.

Body space

Work in restricted headroom or confined environments, particularly work involving manual handling, greatly reduces a worker's safe lifting capacity, and a 3% reduction in headroom has been shown to reduce the maximum lifting capacity of the individual by 50%.[14] Other physical constraints can prevent the use of safe handling techniques.

Driving

Professional drivers, lorry drivers, and salesmen who drive over 24 000 miles (38 000 km) a year have an increased risk of low back pain,[16] possibly because of a combination of vibration, prolonged sitting, and the task of loading and unloading. Vibration in other environments is an established risk factor.

Personal risk factors

A number of personal risk factors have been defined which have relevance in the occupational setting.[17] Men are more likely to experience disc protrusion than women, but during pregnancy women are particularly at risk of back pain because of their lax ligaments. Height and weight are important. One study of a large group of military recruits who were followed up over 20 years showed that those with both height above 182 cm and a weight over 82 kg were more likely to experience back problems.[18] Back pain generally starts between the ages of 20 and 40 years and its prevalence increases with age. Disc lesions are most common between the ages of 35 and 59 years. Absence from work attributed to back problems increases with age. Fitness is inversely related to the risk of back injury, as is muscle strength. The amount of space available in the spinal canal for the nerves is a factor and so measurement of spinal canal diameter could be useful, if it were less expensive to make. Smoking is definitely associated with the occurrence of low back pain although whether this is because of an association with other adverse lifestyle behaviours (e.g. smokers are generally less fit and active), or whether it is due to smoking alone (e.g. a vascular effect or due to coughing) is still debatable.

Prevention of low back pain

Much effort has been invested by industry and by researchers in the pursuit of effective strategies to prevent low back pain at work. On the basis of the morbidity statistics, it would not be unreasonable to conclude that these have failed. However, there have been some examples of a reduction of back pain problems in industry. Usually these have involved a multifaceted approach, including good early effective treatment and rehabilitation, good ergonomic design of workplaces, and appropriate attention to selection and training.[17] Recently a review has shown that training in manual handling appears to have little effect, but programmes designed to improve the fitness of the workers did reduce the number of back injuries.[8] Programmes aimed at maintaining the general well-being and fitness and strength of employees, if appropriately designed, may reduce the prevalence and incidence of back pain in an occupational setting.

Existing legislation and guidelines for employment

Recognition of the potential risks of manual handling has led to much legislation. The Factories Act 1961 states that 'a person shall not be employed to lift, carry or move, any load so heavy as to be likely to cause injury to him'. Specific regulations apply to some industries including the woollen and worsted textiles, jute, pottery, agriculture, and construction industries. Some of these have proposed specific weight limits and in 1967 the International Labour Conference adopted the International Labour Organization (ILO) Convention 127 recommending a maximum permissible weight to be lifted by one person (male) of 55 kg, with smaller limits for women and young people. This recommendation was not ratified by the UK and many other countries.

In recent years the legislation has been more general than specific. The Health and Safety at Work, etc. Act 1974 requires all employers to provide and maintain a system of work that is safe and without risks to the health of all their employees, 'so far as is reasonably practicable'.

Further directives on health and safety have emanated from the European Union, including one on manual handling. This has led to the Manual Handling of Loads Operations Regulations 1992, which requires employers to minimize manual lifting, to establish a process to assess the risks in any manual handling task, to control or minimize those risks, to provide information and training to employees, and to regularly review the arrangements.

This approach is preferable to the imposition of arbitrary limits, although some organizations establish their own. Thus, one information technology company has established a limit for a one-person lift of 55 lb (25 kg), and a major pharmaceutical company has a limit of 30 kg, whereas a cement manufacturer may expect employees to handle 50 kg bags all day. Clearly, arbitrary limits would be impracticable in mining, nursing, and construction work. Given the significant risk which can arise from certain tasks with very much smaller loads, the general approach of assessing and controlling the risk associated with each task, is preferable.

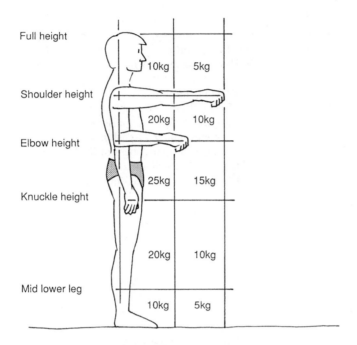

Fig. 11.3 Lifting and lowering heights and distances from the body.[19]

However, useful recommendations have resulted from medical research. The guidelines to the Manual Handling Regulations[19] include a chart showing the weights which may be lifted at different heights and distances from the body (see Fig. 11.3).

In *Force limits in manual work*, Davis and Stubbs[20] took the same approach, publishing sets of diagrams indicating acceptable loads at different distances from the erect trunk. These were based on studies of intra-abdominal pressure during lifting and on earlier work which showed that lifts that caused intra-abdominal pressures to rise above 90 mmHg were associated with an increased risk of back injury.

However, these guidelines are based on laboratory studies of healthy volunteers, and can only be extrapolated to workplaces with caution. Because of their inadequacies the risk assessment approach, which is the basis of most current legislation, is preferred.

Risk assessment

To assess the risks of any particular activity the individuals must be considered in the context of the task and the working environment. In some occupations, such as dock work or community nursing, some aspects of the working environment may be outside the control of the employer. In most working situations however, the potential hazards can be identified and control measures established. The factors to be considered in performing an assessment are given in Table 11.1.

Table 11.1   Task assessment

The tasks	Do they involve:
	• Holding loads away from the trunk?
	• Twisting or stooping?
	• Reaching upwards?
	• Moving the load vertically a long way?
	• Carrying the load long distances?
	• Strenuous pulling or pushing?
	• Unpredictable movement of loads?
	• Repetitive handling?
	• Insufficient rest or recovery?
	• A work rate imposed by a process?
	• Lifting patients?
The loads	Are they:
	• Heavy, bulky, unwieldy?
	• Difficult to grasp?
	• Unstable/unpredictable?
	• Intrinsically harmful e.g. sharp/hot?
The working environment	Are there:
	• Constraints on posture?
	• Poor floors?
	• Variations in floor levels?
	• Hot/cold/humid conditions?
	• Strong air movements?
	• Poor lighting conditions?
Individual capability	Does the job:
	• Require unusual capability?
	• Endanger those with a health problem (e.g. spinal disorders)?
	• Endanger those who are pregnant?
	• Call for special information/training?
	• Require special clothing?
Instruction and training	Does the job include:
	• Use of mechanical aids?
	• Principles of good task design?
	• Good handling methods?

Reducing risks at work

The priority in the prevention of back pain at work must always be to remove or minimize the hazard, by changing work practices, providing lifting aids, or simply modifying the layout of the workplace. Most risks can be reduced by simple and inexpensive changes. If this is not possible, the use of mechanical aids, such as levers, barrows, and trolleys, will reduce the demands of the job. Forklift trucks may be required. Simple rollers and conveyors can assist loading and unloading. Consideration should be given to reducing the size of the load; and any load which is either large, or heavy (e.g. over 20 kg), should preferably have handles.

Loads should not be stored above shoulder height, as the biomechanical stresses of lifting to this height are considerable, and reduce by about 75% what would be a 'safe' load at lower levels. Whenever possible, heavy loads that have to be handled should not be stored below knee height. Loads that are held at arms length increase back strain by fivefold, compared with those held against the body, and frequent lifting reduces the 'safe' load to about 25% of the acceptable maximum lift for any single operation. Reasonable space in which to work is essential and many accidents occur in situations where the worker has restricted room to stand or move.

A particular hazard to the spine is the lift while bending and twisting. This can provoke rupture of an annulus even with light loads; for example, reaching down to pick up a bottle of milk, or reaching down and to the side to lift while seated without moving from the chair. Other common hazardous tasks include lifting loads into or out of the boot of a car, or out of high-sided boxes, bins, or stillages.

Seating

It is likely that tasks that involve little manual handling adversely affect the back if they involve poor seating postures, or standing and leaning over a work surface for long periods. Elevating the work surface, or the item of interest (the ideal height for a work surface when standing is 8 cm below the elbows), providing a stool or appropriate seating, and encouraging frequent changes in posture, are all beneficial. The Display Screen Regulations 1992 address the importance of correct seating at workstations (see Fig. 11.4) and detailed guidance is available.[21]

Badly designed chairs can contribute to the onset of back pain and aggravate preexisting complaints. If workers have to sit for prolonged periods their seats should be adjustable for height and back support. The seat should allow the worker to rest the feet on the floor, and if not, as with workers of short stature, a footrest should be provided.

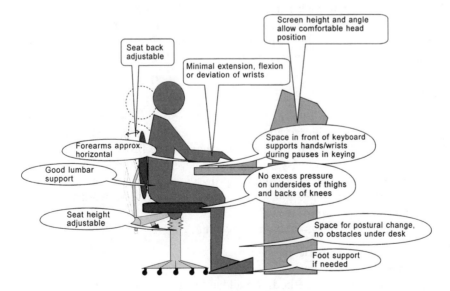

Fig. 11.4 Correct sitting position at a display screen workstation.

The seating should be firm and the back support appropriately curved to support the lumbar spine.

The seat should normally be horizontal but with a forward tilting ability so that back pain sufferers can be helped by tilting the seat forward so that the front edge is about 10–15° below the horizontal. The extreme version of this is the Scandinavian 'kneeling chair', which can provide relief to some back sufferers by increasing the pelvic–femoral angle. However, a simple back support fitted to a chair can often improve comfort. The doctor should resist making firm recommendations about alternative seating for a back sufferer, as no one chair is suitable for all, and simple remedies should be tried first. Seats with arm rests are preferable to ones without.

The classical luxurious 'director's chair' is often the least ergonomically appropriate. Many unsatisfactory chairs can be improved by the provision of a simple ergonomically designed back support such as the 'Backfriend' available from Medesign Ltd (see Appendix 7 for the full address).

Sedentary workers should be encouraged to move around, stretch, and do simple exercises, and the Japanese tradition of group exercise in the workplace may have some physiological merit.

Driving

As mentioned earlier, driving is a risk factor for back pain, and particularly affects those travelling long distances, who are often driving company cars.

The choice of company car is normally influenced more by issues of image and self-esteem than by practical considerations. Thus, the older or very tall employee, or the back pain sufferer, may choose a car completely unsuitable for their condition. Ample headroom, easy access, and good adjustable seating should be of primary importance in the choice of car. Power steering and automatic transmission can help some people with cervicobrachial pain, low back pain, or sciatica. Vibration is often considered to cause back pain and insufficient attention has been paid to reducing the vibration levels, particularly in commercial vehicles. In particular, the frequencies produced in lorry seats are often near to the resonant frequency of the spine, a factor that may predispose to injury.

Training

There is a clear need to educate the worker in safe working practices, safe manual handling techniques, and self-preservation. However, training cannot compensate for poor workplace and task design, and these should be addressed first. All too often the provision of training is seen as an easy option by employers who think that the purchase of an off-the-shelf package, or video, and the provision of a short training session is sufficient to discharge their obligations. Failure to address adverse workplace conditions often renders training completely ineffective.

Successful training requires taking into account:

*   the specific task to be performed
*   the established work practices
*   the perception that new methods are difficult or time-consuming
*   the poorly understood mechanisms of injury

- the weight, shape, and general handling properties of the material/articles
- how any improved job methods might be constrained by poor workplace layout and job design.

Training on the job with a more experienced colleague is rarely adequate, as bad habits have often been acquired and are passed on. Although education and training are widely used to prevent low back pain, there is no clear evidence that they are effective.[16]

The number of proffered training methods is almost as large as the number of trainers, and there is little evidence that any specific lifting technique is better than any other. The traditional technique—with a straight back, feet apart, and flexed knees—imposes less stress on the lumbar spine than lifting with a bent back (this has been confirmed by studies of intradiscal pressure). Avoidance of the turning and twisting lift, by turning with the feet rather than twisting with the trunk, also has a good anatomical and pathological rationale. Large loads, such as oil drums and people, require entirely different techniques of lifting, and training needs to be tailored to the task. In providing training it helps to follow an eight-point plan:

- analyse the job
- identify the risks
- identify unsatisfactory postures
- identify the desired procedures and methods
- provide training
- ensure there is supervision and support
- refresh training regularly
- audit the process.

New employees require more time for training and should not be expected to perform at high work rates initially, but allowed to build up work speed gradually, especially if the task is repetitive. Frequent review of techniques and re-training when necessary should be an established part of a prevention programme. A single session of training in manual handling techniques can be likened to a single golf lesson: the former is as unlikely to aid safe lifting as the latter is to impart the perfect swing!

Fitness for work

Pre-employment screening

Self-selection usually ensures that people with serious pre-existing back complaints do not take up heavy manual work. Additional measures such as pre-employment screening, whether by questionnaire or examination, are of little value and should only be considered in special circumstances such as work in some types of heavy industry, the fire and rescue services, or as required by law in industries such as coal-mining.

Although many large organizations have an occupational health nurse or doctor, it is regrettable that most industries do not have regular access to occupational medical advice. In these circumstances the recruiting officer, manager, or foreman may depend on the opinions and advice of the local general practitioners. However, it is preferable to establish contact with a local group occupational health service, or a local occupational health nurse or doctor, who can provide more authoritative advice. Generally, doctors tend to err on the side of caution, which is often a mistake: many heavy manual workers have been told at some time in the past that they would never be fit for the task they now happily perform!

In assessing fitness for lifting and manual handling the minimum information required is as follows:

- A **detailed medical history**: Has the recruit had any major illness, injury, or occupation likely to reduce their ability to undertake such work?
- The **occupational history**: What previous manual work has the applicant performed successfully? Has there been a back injury or prolonged or recurrent absence from work attributed to back pain?
- Does the individual appear fit to do the job on offer?

In general, a recruit who has a normal range of movement of the spine and limbs, an absence of significant musculoskeletal deformity, and no other abnormalities, should be fit for manual activities.

Guidance note MS20 from the Health and Safety Executive deals with pre-employment screening, and indicates that refusal of employment on health grounds should only be on the basis of defined job specific criteria.[22]

Specific screening tests

A number of biological variables that may affect lifting capacity can be usefully measured.

Strength is obviously important and strength testing may sometimes be valuable. Chaffin *et al.*[23] showed that **isometric testing** can be useful in predicting future back injuries, and that these were less common if an individual's maximum strength exceeded the largest force they had to exert at work by a wide margin. More recently, **dynamic strength tests** have been developed, and these are thought to replicate the work task more accurately. However, strength testing is prone to inaccuracy, and sophisticated equipment is necessary to perform testing adequately. Recent research has shown an association between chronicity of back pain and poor spinal muscular fitness, so it is possible that objective assessment in this area may be more important in the future.

Height and weight are also important and have some weak predictive power, but recent studies have confirmed that there is no justification for excluding tall men from heavy manual tasks.[24]

Studies of the relationship between spinal canal diameter and back pain have shown that people with narrower spinal canals are more prone to back pain and have longer associated absence. However, the measurement of canal diameter is difficult and prone to inaccuracy except by MRI scanning which is expensive. Because of this, it is not a strong enough predictor to help in the occupational setting.

Many years ago, diagnostic radiographs were often undertaken in the belief that these were predictive and that individuals with radiographic abnormalities should be excluded from manual work. However, numerous studies have confirmed that radiographs do not predict who will get back pain at work, and the radiation hazard is now considered unjustifiable.[25] There is no longer any place for the use of spinal radiography as a pre-employment screening test to exclude potential back problems.

Personality tests have been used to investigate chronic back pain sufferers, but are notoriously unreliable, and have no place in pre-employment testing in relation to back pain.

Screening after sickness absence

Careful management, both medically and generally, is required for the employee returning to work after back or sciatic pain or other illness affecting manual handling ability. Absence may be self- or doctor-certified, and with each the significance of any disability is equally liable to miscalculation. At one extreme the absence may be spurious; at the other, the individual may be trying to return to work too early for financial or other reasons. **The general practitioner or hospital doctor is unlikely to be familiar with the physical requirements of the patient's job, and the decision to return to work will often be made on subjective information from the patient.**

Many employers contribute to the unnecessary prolongation of absence by adopting an inflexible approach to fitness—that the worker is either fully fit or fully unfit. Medical advisers should try to influence this attitude by communicating with the employer at an early stage when they feel that the patient is capable of lighter work. If the functional restriction is temporary, some employers can be persuaded to make an accommodation and provide alternative work.

If the back problem has been caused by work, this should also be brought to the employer's attention so that the workplace can be assessed and preventive action taken. The following signs and symptoms are useful in the prediction of recurrence of back pain in those returning to work after an episode: [26]

- from the history
  - two or more previous attacks
  - a fall on the buttocks or back as the cause of injury
  - sickness absence of 5 weeks or more in the present illness episode
    residual pain in the leg on return to work
- from the examination
  - restriction of pain-free straight-leg raising to 45° or less
  - pain or weakness on resisted hip flexion
  - inability to sit up from lying flat
  - back pain on lumbar extension
- general
  - poor physical fitness
  - self-rated health poor
  - heavy smoking
  - psychological distress and depressive symptoms
  - disproportionate illness behaviour
  - low job satisfaction
  - personal problems (alcohol, marital, financial, etc.)
  - adversarial medico–legal proceedings.

If any of these features are present, the patient should be employed initially on lighter work or be considered for further rehabilitation. (For a further review of this subject see Troup and Edwards.[27])

Rehabilitation back to work after the development of a spinal problem or any of the previously listed signs and symptoms of discomfort will now need to take account of the Disbaility Discrimination Act 1995 (DDA). Under the terms of the Act, disability is defined as a physical (or mental) impairment with a substantial and long-term (over 12 months) adverse effect on a person's ability to carry out normal day to day activities. Impairment also covers physical, mental, and sensory ones, and people who have a disability within the definition are protected from discrimination against them in the workplace even if they have since recovered.

A substantial adverse effect is interpreted as meaning a limitation going beyond the 'normal differences in ability which might exist among people' (from the Approved Code of Practice—ACOP—of the DDA).[28] Such a disability might thus prevent the employee from 'rendering regular and efficient service' in their job. But under the DDA it must now be the employer's duty to make reasonable adjustments to the work site or to the job to assist in rehabilitating the disabled employee back to work. The exact nature of what may constitute reasonable adjustments to a workstation or work process will clearly be different according to individual cases and until a body of case law is produced, it will need to be arrived at by bench marking of best practice.

Employers may have to make one or several of the following adjustments for people with spinal disorders:

- alter premises
- allocate some duties to another employee
- transfer the person to fill an existing vacancy
- alter working hours
- transfer the person to another place of work
- allow absences during working hours for rehabilitation, assessment, or treatment
- supply additional training
- acquire or make alterations to equipment
- alter instructions in reference manuals
- modify procedures for testing or assessment
- provide supervision

Employers do not have to make changes if:

- the disabled person experiences only a minor disadvantage
- they do not know that a person has a disability (and it is reasonable that they do not know)
- the change required to overcome the disadvantage is not reasonable.

Reasonable changes can cover physical features in or giving access to premises, and also arrangements regarding recruitment, working terms and conditions, transfers, training, and other benefits.

The guidelines to the DDA stress that the reasonableness or otherwise of changes will include:

- how much an alteration will improve the situation for the disabled employee or applicant
- how easy it is to make the change

- the cost of the measure
- the employer's resources
- financial help or other help that may be available.

Spinal cord injuries

The incidence of spinal cord injuries in Britain is about 3 per 100 000 of the population. Motor vehicle accidents account for 50% of cases. Spinal cord injury occurs most often in teenagers and young adults at the beginning of their careers.

The functional independence which may be achieved in the end depends ultimately on the level and completeness of the lesion and the adequacy of training (see Table 11.2). Excluding those with a high cord lesion, paraplegics should be able to lead an independent life, though this is only achieved by rehabilitation in a special unit where there is rigorous training in self-care and no concessions to dependence or invalidism.

Spinal cord injury is not simply a malady of the spine—physical, psychological, and social adjustment continue indefinitely. Paraplegics are likely to stay in the spinal injury centre for 4–6 months and quadriplegics about 8 months.

Quadriplegics are liable to:

- orthostatic hypotension
- autonomic hyper-reflexia with increased sympathetic activity usually provoked by

Table 11.2 Functional expectations at different levels of spinal injury

Level of injury	Functional expectation
Above C5	Totally dependent: special respiratory equipment is required; speech is restrained; a powered wheelchair may be controlled by head or mouth micro-switches
C5	Some assistance is needed in all activities.
C6	Can propel a manual wheelchair with difficulty; a powered wheelchair is needed on slopes; sometimes driving is possible; in men, bladder drainage is to a leg bag after bladder outlet surgery
C7–T1	Can be completely independent with a wheelchair. May achieve bladder evacuation by reflex bladder contraction; bowel evacuation is by suppository and rectal stimulation
T2–T6	Fully independent with a wheelchair.
T7–T12	Fully independent with a wheelchair; can 'walk' wearing orthoses to brace the lower trunk and legs, but not far
L1–L3	Can walk using knee–ankle–foot orthoses and crutches
L4–S1	Can walk using ankle–foot orthoses and two sticks or crutches; bladder is emptied by straining and applying suprapubic pressure; lower bowel is emptied by straining or manual removal of faeces
S2–S4	Only urinary control is difficult

overdistension of a viscus causing hypertension, severe headache, flushing, goose-flesh, and sweating
- thromboembolism
- spasticity
- impaired respiratory function.

All patients with spinal injuries lose control of the bladder and bowels, have impaired genital function, and are liable to pressure sores and successive emotional reactions of shock, denial, depression, and hostility before gradual acceptance. After spinal injury, capacity for physical work is low at first. Endurance and muscle strength are regained by physical training. Subsequently, medical complications and social isolation are lessened. The goals of rehabilitation may not be reached for several years. Return to work may be delayed by psychological, physical, environmental, and opportunity constraints, and by claims for compensation. Vocational counsellors in the spinal injury centres work closely with the Disability Employment Adviser (DEA), previous employer, training services, and institutions for further education. Rehabilitation must include the acquisition of new skills. Open employment may prove difficult for many people with spinal injuries, especially quadriplegics, who may consider sheltered employment where productivity is geared to new capabilities. Rather than severity of disability, the best predictors of successful occupational resettlement, in rank order, are:

- previous employment status and ability
- previous attitudes towards work
- maturity
- verbal ability.

If attention is paid to removing the architectural barriers to employment and maintaining a positive attitude throughout, many should be able to return to useful employment.

In assessing paraplegics who depend on wheelchairs, their ability to propel, open, go through and close doors, go up and down ramps, transfer from wheelchair to lavatory, chair, or bed must be ascertained. Their independence in dressing and the time taken to prepare for work in the morning should be measured.

Again the DDA is clear about reasonable adjustments that will require to be made in such cases, but the specific changes that will be deemed reasonable will depend on individual circumstances, with benchmarking of best practice the best guide.

In any situation, the occupational physician will require to be deeply involved in advising managers and the disabled employee on details of adjustments that would be deemed reasonable as a function of practicability; significance of the benefit to the disabled employee; and lasting nature of the disability. The ACOP[28] and also the guidance booklet on employment[29] will be of assistance.

There is a requirement under the DDA to make reasonable adjustments to the job to prevent or reduce any adverse effects of the job on the person's disability. There is a requirement for a period of rehabilitation back to work (gradual return to work), with assessment of the employee's progress and further reasonable adjustments if necessary. It is unlikely to be reasonable for an employer to have to make an adjustment involving little benefit to the employee. It would be reasonable to transfer the employee to fill an existing vacancy, even one involving retraining, if they cannot work in the same place and there is no reasonable adjustment which would enable the employee to continue doing the current job.

Conclusions and recommendations

Disorders of the spine are many and varied, and continue to present an enormous challenge to the individual sufferers, their medical advisers, and employers. The treatment of the degenerative conditions is largely symptomatic, and the emphasis must be on support to the individual to help improve symptoms and psychological well-being until remission which usually occurs. For more enduring conditions rehabilitation is vital and employers should be encouraged to accommodate the disabled worker in the knowledge that the 'rehabilitation of work' may be more effective than occasional visits to physiotherapy departments, and will often speed recovery and return to normal function. Given the frequency of spinal problems in the working population, employers must take particular care to ensure compliance with the DDA when recruiting or undertaking pre-placement assessments of individuals with spinal disability. The reasonable adjustments which the Act requires for individuals are in general, merely good practice within the various strategies available to prevent disability within the able-bodied.

Selected references

1 Wells, N. *Back pain*. Studies of current health problems No 78. London: Office of Health Economics, 1985.
2 Clinical Standard Advisory Group. *Back pain*. London: HMSO, 1994
3 Lawrence JS. Disc degeneration, its frequency and relationship to symptoms. *Ann Rheum Dis* 1969; **28**: 121–138.
4 *Clinical guidelines for the management of acute low back pain*. London: Royal College of General Practitioners, 1996.
5 Makela M, Helliovara M, Sievers K, Impivaara O, Knekt P, Aromaa A. Prevalence, determinants and consequences of chronic neck pain in Finland. *Am J Epidemiol* 1991; **134**: 1356–1367.
6 Wynn Parry CB. Management of ankylosing spondylitis. *Proc R Soc Med* 1965; **59**: 619.
7 Burton K, Cantrell T, Klaber Moffett J, Main C, Roland M, Waddell G. *The back book*. London: HMSO, 1996.
8 Poppel MN, Van Koes BW, Smid T, Bouter LM. A systematic review of controlled clinical trials on the prevention of back pain in industry. *Occup Environ Med* 1997; **54**: 841–847.
9 Mathews JA *et al.* Back pain and sciatica. Controlled trials of manipulation, traction, sclerosant and epidural injections. *Br J Rheumatol* 1987; **26**: 416–423.
10 Franks A. Low back pain. *BMJ* 1993; **306**: 901–909.
11 Bigos SJ, Baltie MC, Spengler DM *et al.* A prospective study of work perceptions and psychosocial factors affecting the repeat of back injury. *Spine* 1991; **16**: 1–6.
12 Deyo RA, Diehl AK. Psychosocial predictors of disability in patients with low back pain. *J Rheumatol* 1988; **15**: 1557–1564.
13 Coste J, Delecoeuillerie G, de Lara A Cohen, Le Parc JM, Paolaggi JB. Clinical cause and prognostic factors in acute low back pain: an inception cohort study in primary care practice. *BMJ* 1994; **308**: 577–580.

14 *Clinical Standards Advisory Group Report* (Back pain: Report of a CSAG Committee on back pain, 1994. HMSO).
15 Manning DP, Mitchell RG, Blanchfield PL. Body movements and events contributing to accidental and non-accidental back injuries. *Spine* 1984; **9**: 734–739.
16 Graveling RA. The prevention of back pain from manual handling. *Ann Occup Hyg* 1991; 14: 427–432.
17 Porter RW. *Management of back pain*. Edinburgh: Churchill Livingstone, 1986.
18 Hubrec A, Nashbold BS. Epidemiology of lumbar disc lesions in the military in World War II. *Am J Epidemiol* 1975; 102: 366–376.
19 *Manual handling. Guidance on the manual handling operations regulations*. Sheffield: HSE Books, 1992.
20 Davis PR, Stubbs DA. *Force limits in manual work*. Guildford: Science and Technology Press, 1980.
21 *Display screen equipment. Guidance on regulations*. Sheffield: Health and Safety Executive, 1992.
22 *Pre-employment health screening*. Health and Safety Executive Guidance Note MS20. London: HMSO, 1982
23 Chaffin DB, Herrin GD, Keyserling WM. Pre-employment strength testing—an updated position. *J Occup Med* 1978; **20**: 403–408.
24 Walsh K, Cruddas M, Coggon D. Interaction of height and mechanical loading of the spine in the development of low back pain. *Scand J Work Environ Health* 1991; **17**: 420–424.
25 Rowe ML. Are routine spine films on workers in industry cost or risk benefit effective? *J Occup Med* 1982; **24**: 41–43.
26 Lloyd DCEF, Troup JDG. Recurrent back pain and its prediction. *J Soc Occup Med* 1983; **33**: 66–74.
27 Troup JDG, Edwards FC. *Manual handling and lifting. An information and literature review with special reference to the back*. London: HMSO, 1985.
28 *Disability Discrimination Act 1995 Code of Practice*. Department of Education and Employment. London: HMSO, 1996.
29 *The Disability Discrimination Act: employment* (DL70). London: HMSO, October 1996.*

* Available from DDA information line 0345 622633.

12

Orthopaedics

A. Ross and I. Nugent

Musculoskeletal disorders are among the commonest reasons for attendance at general practitioner and accident and emergency services. These disorders can have a significant impact on the workplace, employment, and productivity but their correct diagnosis and early treatment can reduce morbidity and facilitate an early return to work. The commoner musculoskeletal disorders are discussed in this chapter, along with guidelines on their diagnosis, management, and prognosis.

Most morbidity in the working population arises from acute soft tissue or bony injury, but, with age, joint problems contribute increasingly. Congenital limb anomalies and acquired limb deficiencies are also discussed as well as genetic abnormalities and inherited conditions which affect the musculoskeletal system. As professional sport and leisure activities become more popular, a bigger population is seeking rapid access to diagnostic and treatment services: acute injuries are discussed in the chapter on trauma (Chapter 13), but the more chronic sequelae are included here. The demands on physicians to return athletes to the arena quickly without compromising future health and performance are increasing.

The Disability Discrimination Act 1995 (DDA) places a responsibility on employees and employers to evaluate the impact of physical health on safety and performance at work. Some occupations, such as the armed forces and rescue services, although excluded from the DDA, require high levels of physical fitness for safe working practices. The role of the occupational physician is to assess the nature of the disability and how it affects functional activity in the occupation in question, and to give advice on possible adaptations. Management will then need to decide if such adaptations are feasible. They may also need encouragement to employ those with unsightly deformities. Advice should also be given on how financial assistance may be obtained from the Department for Education and Employment (DfEE) for adaptations to the workplace, or to provide additional equipment to help a disabled person cope with the job successfully. Some of the conditions considered in this chapter are also referred to in Chapter 14 (Rheumatological disorders).

Arthritis

Osteoarthritis

By the age of 50, 80% of the population have radiographic evidence of osteoarthritis (OA) in the hip, knee, or elbow. General 'wear and tear' is still considered an important aetiological factor. The knee and hip joints are most commonly affected and there appears to be a genetic predisposition to arthritis affecting the fingers, posterior spinal facet joints, and knees. Generally OA deteriorates with time, but the rate at which this happens is variable. Stiffness and deformity follow insidiously, with swelling which may be due to synovitis, effusion, or osteophyte formation. Radiological changes often lag behind pathological features and there is little correlation between the clinical status and the radiological appearance. The characteristic radiological features are narrowing of the joint space, formation of osteophytes at the articular margins, sclerosis, and cyst formation. Simple analgesics are appropriate for mild disease, with the addition of non-steroidal anti-inflammatory drugs (NSAIDs) as necessary. NSAIDs inhibit prostaglandin synthesis and 70% of patients will respond to them in the early stages of disease. Femoral head collapse has been reported with the use of NSAIDs but appears to be a rare idiosyncratic reaction. Intra-articular injection of local anaesthetic and steroid tends to provide short-term relief and physiotherapy including heat, cold, short-wave diathermy, and ultrasound may lead to symptomatic improvement. Surgery is required when function and symptoms cannot be supported by these measures.

Adaptations such as powered appliances or high stools may be made to the workplace to relieve the need for prolonged standing. Pain, often common 24–36 hours after excessive exertion, may be the limiting factor especially in physically demanding occupations. Following a minor injury, persisting symptoms may suggest the presence of underlying arthritis and the occupational physician may have to decide whether it is reasonable for an employee to continue in a demanding physical role. An employee who is severely restricted due to arthritis may be able to continue in their occupation after a joint replacement. Occupational physicians will need to work closely with general practitioners, orthopaedic surgeons, and employers in such circumstances to ensure a satisfactory outcome.

Rheumatoid arthritis

Rheumatoid arthritis (RA) is the commonest form of chronic inflammatory joint disease. Typically it is a symmetrical, erosive, deforming, polyarthritis affecting both small and large peripheral joints. The course of the disease is often prolonged with exacerbations and remissions. The prevalence is approximately 1% and it is commoner in women (3 : 1), typically beginning in the third to fifth decade. The cause of rheumatoid arthritis is obscure, but there appears to be a multifactorial genetic predisposition. The onset is usually insidious with joint pain, stiffness, and symmetrical swelling of peripheral joints. Typically, the small joints of the fingers and toes are the first to be affected. The articular manifestations of RA are described in detail in Chapter 13. In many occupations employment is still entirely possible despite this condition; in others, modifications can be made to allow the employee to stay at work. However, heavy manual jobs and those requiring repetitive movements of affected joints are best avoided.

Juvenile chronic arthritis

Juvenile chronic arthritis (JCA) is a heterogeneous group of inflammatory joint diseases in young people characterized by chronic joint inflammation resulting in muscle weakness and osteoporosis. Partial involvement of the epiphysis may cause asymmetrical overgrowth and deformity and may cause limb length inequality. Pauciarticular onset (involvement of up to four joints) is the commonest presentation (70%), and this has a good prognosis (70% will be in remission with little functional disability after 15 years follow-up). Resulting minor disability rarely requires surgery but occasionally major joint replacement is needed in the young adult. Polyarticular disease (five or more joints within the first 3 months of onset) occurs in 20% of cases. The majority of patients are seronegative for IgM rheumatoid factor and these patients respond well to early treatment. Seropositive disease resembles adult rheumatoid arthritis and commonly presents in girls approaching the menarche. It affects the hands and feet initially and later involves the larger joints. It tends to persist into adult life and is often referred to as **juvenile rheumatoid arthritis** (JRA). This variety often causes growth impairment and major joint destruction requiring multiple surgical procedures in late adolescent years and young adult life. Children who have suffered from this condition need careful career advice. It is important that they work within their strengths and capabilities and do not enter employment which would further stress already compromised joints. There are specific clinical problems related to each joint. These are principally due to growth disturbance, contracture and joint destruction and will be considered in later sections.

Arthritis of the hip

Pain from an arthritic hip is normally felt in the groin or in the region of the greater trochanter and radiates down the front of the thigh to the knee. Osteoarthritis of the hip occurs in up to 40% of the population over 60 years. Osteoarthritis in all joints in the age group under 65 years (i.e. the working population) has a prevalence of 94/1000 and an incidence of 50/1000. Arthritis of the hip, knee, and spine are by far the commonest clinical presentations. In rheumatoid arthritis the hip is involved radiographically in 33% within 5 years of onset, rising to 50% at 8 years. Problems in the hip joint in adolescence and young adulthood also follow congenital dysplasia or dislocation, Perthes' disease, slipped upper femoral epiphysis, or infection.

Hip arthroplasty is indicated in patients with incapacitating pain which is refractory to conservative treatment. Most hip replacements undertaken have both components cemented to bone but sometimes, in younger individuals, uncemented prostheses are used. The latter facilitate future revision operations and require a postoperative period of non-weight-bearing and so have a longer initial recovery time. The improved success rate of total hip replacement as a result of advances in surgical techniques and materials has increased the frequency of joint replacement in the younger patient. Men and women of working age regularly undergo hip replacements, and this has a significant effect on their ability to return to work and the jobs they may do.

Total hip replacement significantly relieves pain and increases range of motion. Recovery from surgery depends on the original severity of the symptoms and the aetiology of the arthritis. Typically 6–8 weeks will elapse before driving can be recommended and 3–4 months before any manual work can be resumed. Total hip replacement allows an otherwise active healthy individual to return to a light manual job. Heavy arduous work is likely to cause premature failure of the prosthesis and individuals need to be counselled to avoid this. Working where safety could be jeopardized if a hip replacement subluxes or dislocates (such as working at heights or at sea) may be inappropriate, and placement should be considered carefully.

The occupational physician should carry out a risk assessment, taking account of the demands of the job and the mobility of the employee. It is important that employees with joint replacements are not allowed to undertake roles which may put a strain on the joint and disadvantage them in later life, but this may be hard to accept when a successful joint replacement has relieved their symptoms.

In many posts return to work will be possible, but in those where mobility and agility are essential the occupational physician should defer final assessment until the outcome of surgery is apparent. Risk assessment is more meaningful at this stage. It may be possible to adapt the job but, if not, a relocation or retirement may be necessary.

Complications of joint replacement are infrequent but do occur. Failure due to aseptic loosening occurs at a rate of 1–2% per year. Infection occurs in 1–2% of arthroplasties and is particularly associated with diabetes, rheumatoid arthritis, immunosuppression, and alcoholism. Deep venous thrombosis (DVT) after hip replacement occurs in 40–80% of people, pulmonary embolism (PE) in 1–10%, and fatal PE in 1% if preventive measures are not used.

Arthritis of the knee

Arthritis of the knee commonly presents with pain on weight-bearing which radiates from the knee down the anterior aspect of the tibia. Night pain is less common than in hip disease. Examination reveals an antalgic gait, swelling, and a restricted range of movement. Genu varum deformity is commoner in osteoarthritis and genu valgum in rheumatoid arthritis. Symptoms from early disease may be controlled by NSAIDs, quadriceps exercises, ultrasound, and ice. Knee bracing may control instability. Arthroscopic washout, resection of unstable meniscal fragments, and debridement of the knee may produce improvement in symptoms for up to 5 years in 60% of cases.

Total knee replacement is less common in the working population than is hip replacement, but its frequency is increasing. Total knee replacement has a 10 year success rate of over 90% in osteoarthritic patients over 60 years of age. The revision rate by 10 years is 3%. Rates for the survival of total condylar knees of 90% at 15 years and 97% at 10 years have been reported. The initial recovery time from surgery tends to be slightly longer than for hips, but the later restrictions and limitations are similar. Employees should not be expected to be involved in manual lifting and physical activity. Work involving walking on uneven surfaces may be difficult, as will prolonged standing. Jobs that involve sitting for part of the time and standing at other times are ideal.

Arthritis of the shoulder

The arthritic shoulder is much rarer than the arthritic hip or knee and is usually secondary to chronic destructive inflammatory disease or local trauma. Unilateral shoulder arthritis can often be managed symptomatically. Profound functional disability occurs when the condition becomes bilateral. Primary osteoarthritis of the glenohumeral joint is rare but does occur. Degenerative arthritis is usually secondary to trauma (e.g. following intra-articular fracture), or to a long-standing rotator cuff injury. It is most common in those engaged in heavy manual work and in divers and compressed air workers who suffer aseptic bone necrosis. It presents most commonly between the ages of 50 and 60 with a history of painful arc syndrome and a decreased global range of movement. The glenohumeral joint is commonly involved in rheumatoid arthritis usually bilaterally. Synovitis of the rotator cuff may produce impingement, and tenosynovitis around the long head of biceps may lead to its rupture. Most shoulder arthritis can be controlled with simple analgesics and NSAIDs. Physiotherapy may maintain or restore the range of movement.

In rheumatoid arthritis, aspiration of a tense joint effusion and intra-articular corticosteroid injection may control the symptoms. Arthroscopy with joint debridement, shoulder decompression, removal of loose bodies, and limited synovectomy may all give symptomatic relief. In young patients, excision of osteophytes and acromioplasty (partial excision of the acromion to reduce impingement with the humerus) may defer more radical surgery. When symptoms persist despite this, total shoulder arthroplasty (replacement of the humeral head and glenoid) may be necessary. The best functional results of total shoulder replacement are obtained in patients with osteoarthritis, as the rotator cuff is usually intact and bone quality is good. These patients may regain a good range of movement as well as obtaining relief of pain.

Arthritis of the shoulder causes problems in occupations which require full mobility of the upper limbs. Carers often present with injuries of which resolution is prolonged by the presence of arthritis. Occupations which involve work above shoulder height, especially if lifting is involved, are going to be affected by loss of mobility and pain in the shoulder. Driving, especially driving HGVs, may be difficult even with power steering, and chronic problems are a contra-indication to holding such a licence. The occupational physician will have to carry out risk assessments when lifting is inevitable, e.g. in mechanics and paramedics, but such posts are likely to be considered unsafe in those with arthritis of the shoulder. Adaptations under the DDA may be very difficult if not impossible to recommend unless mechanical aids can be introduced.

Arthritis of the ankle

Primary osteoarthritis of the ankle is rare. Secondary osteoarthritis occurs most commonly after ankle fracture, ligamentous instability, or inflammatory arthritis. Despite being the most frequently injured weight-bearing joint, the ankle is least likely to suffer degenerative joint disease. Osteoarthritis after displaced ankle fractures occurs in 20–40% of patients, the frequency depending on the severity of the injury and the accuracy of its reduction. Physiotherapy is likely to give only temporary relief in established arthritis but may improve the instability. Shoe inserts and insoles can correct minor varus and valgus deformities, and boots with ankle supports may help with instability. Degenerative arthritis accompanied by lateral instability may be improved by lateral ligament reconstruction. Arthrodesis is indicated in isolated ankle joint osteoarthritis or in rheumatoid arthritis with unilateral ankle involvement. The role of arthroscopy is well defined for the removal of loose bodies, but its role in the symptomatic relief of arthritis is less clear. Ankle joint replacement is not commonly performed, but has a role in specific circumstances. Ankle arthrodesis provides good pain relief and little effect on physical mobility or agility, and is often the preferred procedure. Arthrodesis of the ankle joint itself produces minimal loss of function and limitations are likely to be minor. However, triple arthrodesis of the hindfoot is different and leads to a degree of loss of inversion and eversion which will affect balancing. People who have had a triple arthrodesis may therefore have difficulty walking over rough ground, so farmers, foresters, and construction workers may not be able to work satisfactorily. Those who need to climb ladders may jeopardize their safety. Occupations which demand mobility or involve long hours of standing are likely to be difficult in people with arthritis of the ankles. Adaptations to the job may be possible, but where agility and pain free movement are needed relocation or retirement may be the only practical solution.

Driving need not be affected as adaptations such as automatic transmission or hand controls can be established. The Disability Employment Adviser (DEA) may well be able to help with a grant for such alterations in a car which is vital for employment.

Arthritis of the elbow

The elbow joint is involved in approximately half those with rheumatoid arthritis, in whom it is often disabling. Osteoarthritis of the elbow is usually the result of trauma. Arthroscopy may aid diagnosis and allows the removal of loose bodies. Joint replacement may produce satisfactory results in 90% of rheumatoid patients at 5 years, but only 75% in young patients with osteoarthritis. Occupations requiring full mobility of the upper limbs especially involving lifting are not suitable for those with this condition. Work involving long hours on keyboards is also likely to be difficult unless the keyboard can be placed well back on the desk and the elbows supported by the desk in a relaxed position. Heavy fire doors in the working environment may cause considerable problems to those with arthritis of the elbow and other upper limb joints.

Arthritis of the wrist

Arthritis of the wrist may be primary (idiopathic) or secondary to fractures of the scaphoid or distal radius, or scapholunate dissociation (severe wrist ligament injury). A trial of non-surgical treatment is indicated in most patients. Steroid injections, NSAIDs, and splintage may be of benefit. Arthroscopy may be indicated to assess the state of the joint surfaces, to remove loose bodies, or to biopsy the synovium. Proximal row carpectomy relieves pain in approximately 90% of patients. It must be undertaken before degenerative change occurs in the midcarpal joints. It is indicated in those for whom residual mobility is important, but in manual labourers an arthrodesis is a better option. If surgical treatment is not possible any occupations requiring repetitive movements at the wrist, especially lifting or forced pronation or supination, may be impossible. Milder forms of arthritis may be helped by splints, especially before operative treatment becomes necessary. A voice-activated computer may help keyboard operators with chronic wrist problems. Occupations requiring a powerful grip, e.g. the fire service, are very likely to be adversely affected if pain is a prominent feature.

Arthroscopy

Arthroscopy has revolutionized the management of many joint conditions. Advances in technology have allowed clear visualization of joints and manipulation of intra-articular structures. Surgery can be performed with minimal morbidity, usually as a day-case procedure and often under local anaesthesia. The techniques pioneered in the knee are now employed in many joints. Certain procedures which were previously impossible or technically demanding can now be undertaken (e.g. repair of a posterior meniscal tear). Indications for arthroscopy include synovial biopsy, removal of loose bodies, excision of osteophytes, irrigation of septic arthritis, drilling, or shaving within the joint (e.g. osteochondritis dissecans, chondromalacia patellae), and synovectomy.

The knee is the joint most commonly arthroscoped. Procedures include meniscectomy, meniscal repair, loose body removal, and cruciate ligament repair. The commonest arthroscopic procedure is meniscectomy. Postoperatively patients describe the knee as sore for a few days but it is not normally a painful procedure. Simple analgesia for 2–3 days is generally sufficient. Patients should be encouraged to walk as soon as recovery from the anaesthetic allows. Prolonged sitting on long car or air journeys is discouraged to reduce the risk of DVT. Regular specific exercises must be performed to maintain muscle strength and range of motion. Patients may drive when able to walk comfortably unaided or using a single stick: generally this point is reached 5–6 days after surgery. Long journeys within 2 weeks of the arthroscopy should be discouraged. Most people should be advised to return to work after about 2 weeks provided that short car or rail journeys are possible and the job does not require more than simple desk work. If a job involves heavy activity or repetitive climbing (including stairs) then 3 weeks may be required. For heavy manual labour, working at height using ladders, or kneeling or squatting, 4 weeks may be needed. Sports should be avoided for at least a month after surgery. Individual adjustments may be required, depending on specific details of any injury and its duration. Generally speaking sport should not be restarted until the joint is free of swelling, the wounds have healed, and the leg is strong enough to exercise on comfortably.

Ankle arthroscopy is used for treatment of articular and ligamentous pathology. Acute or recurrent ankle sprains may produce osteochondral fractures, loose bodies, or adhesions which can all be managed by arthroscopy. Ankle arthritis and bony spurs caused by repetitive injury are amenable to arthroscopic debridement. Ankle arthrodesis is now being performed arthroscopically.

Shoulder surgery is increasingly being performed arthroscopically. The use of lasers to perform shoulder stabilization and intra-articular burrs for subacromial decompression have reduced morbidity and allowed such operations to be done as day-cases. Elbow and wrist arthroscopy both have an increasing role in treating arthritic and traumatic conditions.

There is now such a wide variation of procedures performed on different joints through the arthroscope that advice on returning to work varies considerably. Recovery time depends entirely on the complexity of the procedure undertaken and the necessity for non-weightbearing, splintage, etc. rather than wound healing. Each case must be assessed on an individual basis.

Complications of arthroscopy are rare (around 1%) and are usually minor but can include haemarthrosis, infection, and thrombo-embolic disease.

Shoulder

Impingement syndromes

Shoulder impingement can be diagnosed when a patient has a positive impingement sign (pain on passive elevation) and a positive impingement test (disappearance of the pain following intrabursal injection of local anaesthetic). Subacromial impingement results in a painful arc of movement in active and passive forward flexion and abduction. Classically, the rotator cuff is impinged between 60° and 120° of abduction. Acute primary injury in young athletic individuals causes oedema and haemorrhage. There is diffuse pain located over the deltoid, local tenderness over the greater tuberosity, muscle spasm, and limitation of movement. The impingement sign and test are positive. A chronic impingement syndrome may occur over 40 years of age with progressive persistent disability. In addition, symptoms often include locking and pain at night. Frequently there is either a rotator cuff tear or biceps tendon rupture and secondary bone changes.

Subcoracoid impingement occurs in younger patients with an intact rotator cuff. The symptoms are more anterior and impingement occurs with the arm in flexion and internal rotation. Soft tissue impingement occurs between the lesser tuberosity and the coracoid/coracohumeral ligament complex. This presents in gymnasts, javelin throwers, swimmers, and tennis players. It may also occur after fractures or scarring after an anterior dislocation.

Non-surgical treatment of impingement syndromes consists of steroid or NSAID injection with local anaesthetic into the subacromial bursa, physiotherapy, and occasionally splintage. Surgical treatment may involve repair of the rotator cuff tear, excision of calcific deposits, decompression acromioplasty or arthroscopic decompression. Chronic impingement may lead on to rotator cuff rupture, adhesive fibrosis (frozen shoulder), or degenerative arthrosis.

Rotator cuff injuries

The rotator cuff consists of the tendons of supraspinatus, infraspinatus, teres minor, and subscapularis blended with the fibrous capsule to form a hood over the gleno-humeral joint. The actions of these muscles combine during elevation of the arm to draw the humeral head inwards and downwards, thereby stabilizing it in the glenoid fossa. The rotator cuff mechanism is susceptible to degenerative disease, trauma, and inflammation which, singly or in combination, may cause it to rupture. Rotator cuff rupture occurs more commonly in men (10 : 1) and more often in the dominant shoulder. Rupture can be complete or partial. When the patient elevates the arm there is a characteristic reversal of the scapulohumeral rhythm, seen as a hunching of the shoulder at the start of abduction. There is an inability to hold the arm in mid abduction, but there is retention of a good range of passive movement. Ninety per cent of patients with rotator cuff tears recover without surgery. Non-operative treatment is directed towards the relief of pain, stiffness, muscle spasm, and muscle atrophy. Physiotherapy, NSAIDs, subacromial injections of local anaesthetic, and steroids can all be used to good effect. The acute episode usually settles within 2–3 months after appropriate treatment. Operative treatment is indicated early for acute injuries in active individuals.

The extent of limitation of function depends whether the rupture is partial or complete. Both will result in a degree of pain and loss of power in the arm. Lifting of any load, especially above shoulder height, is therefore likely to be considerably limited.

Shoulder instability

Acute anterior dislocation is the commonest shoulder dislocation and accounts for 98% of all cases. The humeral head usually dislocates in response to forced external rotation in an abducted extended position. Recurrent dislocations occur in 90% of patients who have their first traumatic dislocation under the age of 20 years; in 60% who dislocate for the first time between the ages of 20 and 40; and in only 10% who dislocate over the age of 40 years. Men are four times more likely to redislocate than women. All patients presenting with a recurrent dislocation should undergo a supervised rehabilitation programme. No further treatment may be needed if modification of work or recreational activities can be achieved. A full assessment should be undertaken before anyone with a history of shoulder instability is employed in an occupation which involves lifting, restraining or pulling activities.

In the shoulder, disorders of the periarticular soft tissues are more common than arthritic conditions, and account for up to 95% of all shoulder pain. Abnormalities of the rotator cuff tendons are the commonest and most important intrinsic cause of **painful shoulder syndromes.** They are often associated with mechanical derangement related to degenerative change, or with an inflammatory arthropathy. Extrinsic causes of shoulder pain such as cervical nerve root or diaphragmatic irritation, myocardial disease, and thoracic outlet syndrome should be excluded.

Calcific tendonitis may present in two ways. The **acute** syndrome occurs as a sudden attack, often at night without any clear precipitating factor, and is resistant to analgesics. Early aspiration of the calcific liquid deposit with infiltration of local anaesthetic and steroid may be the only way to relieve symptoms. The subacute syndrome comes on over several months with features of impingement but with an overlying element of pain at rest. Calcification occurs 1–2 cm medial to the insertion of the supraspinatus on the humerus and can be identified on a plain shoulder radiograph. Open surgical incision of chronic calcinosis is sometimes indicated.

Frozen shoulder is a relatively common problem, first described by Codman in 1934; it exists in the presence of a normal radiograph. Its cause is unknown and it can only be diagnosed when other intrinsic and extrinsic causes of pain have been excluded. Symptoms include diffuse pain (often at rest) which is worse at night. There is progressive restriction of active and passive movement, particularly external rotation (adhesive capsulitis). Initial treatment is with analgesics and frequent physiotherapy. With intractable cases manipulation under anaesthetic with steroid injection or occasionally shoulder arthroscopy, to divide adhesions, is necessary.

Frozen shoulder can cause considerable problems in occupations where full use of the upper limbs is essential. Most cases respond eventually to treatment but an employee may be unable to carry out their full duties for some 12–18 months and employers will need to be persuaded that in most cases there is likely to be a good outcome. If the employee is involved in repetitive work, in particular involving lifting, it may not be possible for the patient to return to full duties after recovery.

Biceps tenosynovitis is most commonly a secondary phenomenon but is primary in 5–10%. It is usually due to overuse or direct injury sustained at work or sport. Occasionally it is due to a congenitally shallow bicipital groove or to a tight transverse humeral ligament. Treatment with an injection of an anti-inflammatory drug is helpful but direct injection of steroid into the tendon must be avoided as this can cause later rupture. Arthroscopic decompression is sometimes required.

Subacromial bursitis is commonly secondary to a degenerative or inflammatory process but can occur primarily after acute or repetitive trauma. It presents as a subacromial 'painful arc syndrome' between 60° and 120° of abduction. Treatment with physiotherapy, management of any primary inflammatory condition, and local injections are often successful, but surgical decompression may be necessary.

Careful evaluation of the work processes is essential to make sure work is not the cause of such problems. Repetitive movements of the upper arm or handling or lifting of patients, as carried out by nurses or other carers, can result in biceps tenosynovitis or subacromial bursitis. Recurrent attacks in such employees may mean alternative roles may have to be considered. Working with arms at, or above, shoulder height, especially lifting even small objects, may exacerbate the problems and adaptations may have to be made if successful treatment is not to be undone on return to work.

Wrist pain

Wrist pain may arise from the joint itself or from any of the structures around it. The pain is usually the result of trauma, inflammation or degeneration, i.e. tenosynovitis, carpal instability, rheumatoid arthritis, or wrist osteoarthritis.

Persistent pain following an injury may be due to ligamentous instability or secondary arthritis after an intra-articular fracture. Scaphoid fracture, which is the second commonest 'wrist fracture' after the distal radius, may lead to chronic pain if non-union occurs. Fractures occur most often in young adult men, and a proportion remain undetected. Ununited fractures may initially become asymptomatic but most will develop wrist arthritis within 10 years. Symptomatic arthritis causes stiffness and weakness and in an occupation where this becomes restrictive, some form of wrist arthrodesis may be necessary.

Other causes of wrist symptoms with medically definable signs and symptoms may require surgical treatment. The commonest problems arise from ganglia, which present as swellings at the wrist. On the palmar aspect, they usually lie lateral to the flexor carpi radialis tendon and close to the radial artery. On the dorsum, they arise either from the scapholunate joint or from the midcarpal joint. Many remain asymptomatic and require no treatment but others may require excision. There is a 10% recurrence rate following surgery.

Hand

Dupuytren's disease is a common condition characterized by contractures of the palmar and digital fascia. It is twice as common in men, and the incidence rises with age. It is associated with diabetes, alcoholism, and epilepsy treated with phenytoin or phenobarbitone. It is no more common among smokers. A history of trauma is not infrequently elicited, but it is uncertain whether blunt trauma and manual work are causative. It is likely that genetic predisposition is important and that the other factors determine the age of onset. The digits most frequently involved are the ring and little fingers, followed by the middle finger and thumb. The earliest sign of palmar disease is nodule formation when overlying skin blanches on full extension of the hand. Splintage may delay progression of the disease but will not reverse it. Surgery should be considered when deformities become fixed and the hand can no longer be placed flat on a table. In employees whose work depends on fully working hands and fingers, early treatment of Dupuytren's disease may be essential. Surgery is performed under general or regional anaesthetic and the involved fascia is excised from the palm and fingers. With more severe contractures skin grafting is often necessary. After correction of digital contractures, splintage in plaster for at least a week is recommended. Thereafter, a thermoplastic splint may be worn between periods of exercise, and later only at night. In severe disease long-term dexterity may be compromised following surgery, and following skin grafting manual workers may need to protect the palm by wearing gloves.

Lower limb

Knee

Chronic knee instability may occur as a result of undiagnosed acute injury, inadequate treatment, or repeated trauma. Stability depends on the cruciate ligaments and collateral ligaments and the extrinsic muscles. Clinical examination, often under general anaesthetic, is essential. Arthroscopy can assess the state of the articular surfaces and menisci and may confirm cruciate ligament injuries. Magnetic resonance imaging (MRI) can be used as a non-invasive method for assessing these structures. Physiotherapy and exercises to strengthen the quadriceps, hamstrings, and gastrocnemius muscles may overcome a functional instability. If the knee recovers dynamic stability, surgery may be unnecessary. Instability associated with sport or certain occupations may be controlled by bracing.

Surgical reconstruction may be undertaken in intractable cases in those involved in high-level sport or when extreme physical fitness is required in the occupation, e.g. fire service or armed forces. Intra-articular procedures using bone–tendon–bone patellar tendon graft are currently popular. After reconstruction physical work may not be possible for 3–6 months and return to sport or full work for 6–9 months. The occupational physician will have therefore to warn management of a prolonged period of rehabilitation. Although results are likely to be favourable they cannot be guaranteed. Untreated chronic knee instability may progress and cause meniscal degeneration, meniscal tears and subsequent early degenerative change. It is not currently known how reconstruction affects this cycle.

Ankle

The commonest ankle complaint is pain following ankle sprain. Recurrent instability of the ankle usually occurs after repeated acute inversion injuries. The three parts of the lateral collateral ligament are partially or completely torn and heal in a lengthened position, resulting in lateral joint laxity. This commonly affects the anterior talofibular and calcaneofibular parts, allowing anterior subluxation of the talus in the ankle mortice (anterior draw sign of the ankle). It has been suggested that repeated 'going over on the ankle' may be due to proprioceptor damage in the ligament rather than laxity. Isolated injuries of the medial collateral ligament are much less common and chronic instability is rare. Medial ligament injuries tend to occur in conjunction with ankle fractures. There is no reliable information about the incidence of ankle ligament injuries, the incidence of instability, or the risk of developing arthritis after ligamentous injury. The risk of developing instability is related to the severity of the initial injury and to the method and duration of treatment. Risk assessment of the situation after a full examination of the employee is the only way forward after such injuries. Any occupation demanding stability of the ankles may be affected by such injuries. Scaffolders, those involved in ladder work and working at heights, as well as those involved in lifting and carrying, especially over uneven surfaces, are likely to be affected.

MRI is increasingly used in diagnosing the extent and precise location of ligamentous disruption. Minor degrees of laxity without subluxation may be treated with ice, ultrasound, and 'wobble-board' exercises which are thought to improve proprioception. Shoes with a lateral float on the heel may be of help. If disability is related only to certain sporting activities, a lateral supporting ankle orthosis may be worn. Chronic conditions involving weakness, paralysis, or arthritis may require a calliper. Operative repair of acutely torn ligaments may be advisable in athletes. After early immobilization in plaster, mobilization in supportive orthoses is recommended. Adhesions are common after acute injury and may cause continuing disability unless appropriate rehabilitation is undertaken. Surgical reconstruction may be appropriate for chronic instability with disabling symptoms and positive MRI evidence. Surgical reconstruction may achieve stability at the expense of reduced inversion range and eversion power but this does not significantly affect normal function.

The occupational implications of such surgery will depend on the exact nature of the operation and the subsequent restriction in movement. In some cases driving and in other cases prolonged standing may be impaired.

Foot

Painful afflictions of the foot frequently cause morbidity in the general population. Although some conditions can be attributed to particular professions, they may be exacerbated by many activities. Considering the frequency of foot disorders, there are surprisingly few medico-legal claims for 'lower limb repetitive strain' or 'work-related lower limb disorder'.

Hallux rigidus is a painful limitation of movement of the metatarsophalangeal joint (MTP) of the big toe. The condition probably starts with repeated trauma to the big toe in adolescence. This produces a chondral defect on the metatarsal head between the apex of the dome and the dorsal margin of the articular surface. As the hallux is extended, abutment of the proximal phalanx against the defect causes pain. Later, osteophytes appear on the dorsal articular margin and form a mechanical block to extension. Further progression results in the characteristic radiographic appearances of osteoarthritis.

Hallux rigidus presents in early to middle adult life when patients are physically active. Exercise exacerbates the symptoms and the desire to exercise must be taken into consideration when planning treatment. The ridge of the dorsal osteophyte can be a source of irritation in footwear. High heels and flexible-soled shoes also increase pain. NSAIDs and a change to rigid-soled footwear may alleviate symptoms.

Excision of the dorsal osteophyte (cheilectomy) sufficient to allow 70° of passive dorsiflexion at surgery produces good results unless osteoarthritis of the joint is advanced. Arthrodesis is recommended in active younger individuals who do not wish to wear high-heeled shoes. After 10 years, 90% of patients report excellent results. The toe should be arthrodesed in approximately 15–20° of valgus and in 10–15° extension. Replacement of the first MTP joint with a prosthetic replacement produces satisfactory results in 80% of cases when fusion is inappropriate.

Hallux valgus is a very common condition consisting of excessive lateral deviation of the big toe at the first metatarsophalangeal joint and medial deviation of the first metatarsal. There is resultant prominence of the bone and soft tissues on the medial side of the first metatarsal head. The first MTP joint may be subluxated or dislocated. The treatment of hallux valgus is controversial. In younger people with relatively normal anatomy but a prominent bunion, existing footwear should be modified. If symptoms persist, a simple bunionectomy may be indicated. In more severe deformity a realignment osteotomy of the first metatarsal bone and soft tissue correction may be indicated. Following surgery 6–8 weeks will be necessary before return to work if this involves a great deal of standing or walking, and up to 3 months if heavy manual labour is involved. In older individuals or those with degenerative change, a Keller's procedure (excision of the basal one-third of the proximal phalanx with trimming of the medial osteophyte) may be the procedure of choice. Overall, the results of 90% of these operations are satisfactory.

Problems of the lesser toes are common and in the majority of cases the aetiology is unknown. A hammer toe occurs with hyper-extension of the MTP joint accompanied by flexion at the proximal interphalangeal (PIP) joint with the distal interphalangeal (DIP) joint in neutral alignment. Callosities develop on the dorsum of the PIP joint and on the weight-bearing tip of the toe just distal to the nail. A claw toe occurs where there is hyperextension of the MTP joint accompanied by flexion deformity of both the PIP and DIP joints. Both claw and hammer toe deformities may follow a synovitis of the MTP joint whether the cause is idiopathic, traumatic or arthritic. Dorsal subluxation of the proximal phalanx occurs first and may be influenced by longitudinal crowding of the toes in the shoe. The severity of the patient's symptoms determines the need for treatment. Examination of the foot will indicate whether the deformity is flexible or fixed. Any underlying neurological cause should be identified. If foot ulceration or a mallet deformity is present, the patient should be investigated for the presence of diabetes.

In cases of mild deformity, the patient may only require advice about footwear and stretching of the shoes to prevent areas of pressure. Strapping deformities is no longer recommended, but chiropody may be helpful. Surgery is sometimes needed: the options include proximal hemiphalangectomy, arthrodesis or excision arthroplasty of the PIP joint if there is troublesome contracture.

Metatarsalgia is pain arising from the metatarsal heads. Any condition which causes dorsal subluxation and clawing of the toes may cause the transfer of load from the toes to the metatarsal heads and consequent pain. Painful metatarsal heads may also occur from Freiberg's infraction, which is a condition most commonly occurring in the second and third decades. It is an example of an osteochondrosis in which avascular necrosis of the second, or rarely the third, metatarsal head occurs. The characteristic clinical features are pain on weight-bearing, swelling due to synovitis, and limitation of extension of the toe. Rarefaction is seen on the dorsal side of the head on early radiographs. Later, fragmentation and broadening of the head occur with thickening of the metatarsal shaft due to increased metatarsal load-bearing. These must be differentiated from a stress (march) fracture or Morton's metatarsalgia caused by an interdigital neuroma. Morton's metatarsalgia mainly affects middle-aged women and the condition is usually unilateral (85%). Patients complain of intermittent shooting pains or a constant ache in the region of the metatarsal heads which is worsened by walking and relieved by rest or removal of their footwear. There is frequently tenderness in the third web space and a palpable click on squeezing the metatarsal heads. If the neuroma is large the toes may be spread. Subjective numbness in the distribution of the common digital nerve is a frequent complaint but there is often no objective sensory loss. Dorsal or plantar excision is usually followed by good relief of symptoms. Metatarsalgia can be a significant disability in workers who stand or walk for long periods.

Deformities of the feet may mean that the protective footwear now mandatory in many occupations cannot be worn comfortably. Equally so, it is often difficult to wear rigid footwear immediately after foot operations and adaptations may have to be allowed on a temporary basis after a suitable risk assessment.

In employees experiencing foot pain, the use of a high stool or chair may relieve the need for excessive standing, but work patterns may need temporary reorganization to reduce excessive walking. After operations feet are often painful because of the weight-bearing function and mobility of these areas. Adequate analgesia is important and both employees and employers may need to be reassured as such operations often take considerable time for complete recovery.

Neuromuscular disorders

Neuromuscular disorders and their orthopaedic sequelae may be caused by disease of the upper motor neurone (e.g. cerebral palsy), the lower motor neurone (e.g. poliomyelitis), or muscle. Problems arise because of instability from muscle weakness or joint abnormality and from deformity due to relative shortening of soft tissues, muscle imbalance, and impairment of co-ordination.

Poliomyelitis is a very common cause of disability worldwide, but is relatively uncommon in western Europe. There is an enormous variation in the extent and severity of weakness or deformity and, as with cerebral palsy, surgical and non-surgical treatments have to be tailored to individual problems. Surgery is sometimes needed to correct deformity (e.g. release of contractures, tendon transfer, arthrodesis) or manage secondary complications of paralysis (e.g. arthritis). Although many people with limbs that have been markedly affected by polio are able to work for many years, premature retirement may have to be considered, especially from jobs which have been physically demanding. The requirements of the DDA will prevail and relocation, or job adaptations, should be considered before putting up a case for retirement.

Arthrogryposis multiplex congenita is a rare condition and is probably an intrauterine neuropathy. This causes fibrous contractures of joints and muscle and is characterized by severe joint stiffness and weakness. Knee deformities, clubfoot, and hip dislocation are common in early childhood. In severe cases life expectancy is reduced but in those surviving to working age there will be a major limitation in mobility although intelligence is normal. Often individuals require multiple surgical procedures to reduce contracture and to improve posture.

Peripheral nerve entrapment

Peripheral nerve entrapment may result from compression, distraction, angulation, or friction-producing symptoms and/or signs in a specific nerve distribution. The commonest is **median nerve compression—carpal tunnel syndrome** (see Chapter 14, p. 283).

Ulnar nerve entrapment at the elbow is the second commonest site for nerve entrapment in the upper limb. The patient describes numbness and tingling in the ulnar nerve distribution, followed by pain in the elbow and forearm which may disturb sleep. Motor signs include weakness of pinch with a positive Froment's sign (flexion of the terminal phalanx of the thumb occurs when adduction is attempted), weakness of grip due to paresis of flexor digitorum profundus to the ring and little fingers, small muscle wasting, and varying degrees of ulnar claw hand. If surgery is indicated, the choice lies between simple release, medial epicondylectomy, and anterior transposition of the nerve.

Ulnar nerve entrapment can also occur more distally where the nerve enters the hand through Guyon's canal. The commonest causes are a ganglion from one of the carpal joints or an occupational injury.

Radial nerve entrapment is rare. **Radial tunnel syndrome** (resistant tennis elbow) causes pain over the interosseous nerve which should be distinguished from the lateral epicondylar pain of tennis elbow.

Brachial plexus lesions may be traumatic lesions, either from injury at birth or later by traction, penetration, irradiation, compression (including thoracic outlet syndrome), or neoplasia. The brachial plexus is formed by the convergence of the anterior rami of C5, C6, C7, C8, and T1. In the anterior triangle of the neck, behind the clavicle and into the axilla, nerve fibres interweave to form the trunks, the cords, and ultimately the radial, median, and ulnar nerves. Major brachial plexus palsies are rare but when they occur are devastating to limb function. In civilian life most palsies are caused by motorcycle accidents, but they may be caused by penetrating wounds, traction to the limb during falls, or sport. Most clinicians classify injuries as either upper plexus injuries (Erb's) or lower plexus injuries (Klumpke's). There are three degrees of severity of plexus injury which affect the likelihood of recovery:

• neuropraxis (traction of nerve without loss of continuity)
• rupture of the nerve or nerve root distal to the dorsal root ganglion (DRG)
• avulsion of the nerve root proximal to the DRG.

Neuropraxias can recover spontaneously but may take up to 2 years for functional recovery. Rupture distal to the DRG may recover after surgical repair or nerve grafting but recovery is never complete. Avulsed nerve roots never recover and the only chance of any functional recovery is with salvage surgery either involving stabilizing joint arthrode-sis or tendon transfer. In permanent palsy there is severe weakness, numbness, and often unremitting pain. Pain is not helped by the usual analgesics but may be helped by car-bamazepine, or transcutaneous nerve stimulation (TENS).

The majority of individuals affected by this condition are young men and if the dom-inant limb is involved this has a devastating effect on the ability to work. Such injuries are likely to be incompatible with occupations demanding safe lifting and handling. This requires appraisal of all aspects of the job and the workplace and will often require retraining and relearning of basic skills. Initial prolonged absence from work will need considerable patience from patient, colleagues, and employer, but with appropriate input and modification to the workplace many can return to full useful employment.

Peripheral nerve entrapment in the lower limb is rare. Idiopathic entrapment of the common peroneal nerve may occur in the fibular tunnel. Most are neuropraxias from acute trauma or compression which result in a foot drop with inversion. Tarsal tunnel syndrome is due to entrapment of the distal part of the posterior tibial nerve at the level of the medial malleolus. Patients complain of pain in the foot in one or more distribu-tions of the three terminal branches of the posterior tibial nerve. It may wake them from sleep and is worse after activity. There is local tenderness and a positive Tinel sign behind the medial malleolus.

Non-operative treatment relies on avoidance of repetitive movements, splintage, local injection of anaesthetic or steroid, physiotherapy, and short courses of diuretics. During treatment, climbing ladders and stairs, repeated use of foot pedals, and driving are best avoided.

Surgical decompression relieves the pressure on the nerve by removing the anatomical structure causing compression.

Congenital limb deformities

A clear distinction must be made between genetic abnormalities and congenital defor-mities. The former can produce the latter, but most congenital deformities do not have a genetic predisposition. Congenital limb deformities causing major functional disability are rare, but minor deformities are relatively common. As a rule, the more proximal the deformity, the rarer and the more significant it is. Deformity may be classified as either the failure of **formation** of parts (transverse or longitudinal) or the failure of **separation or differentiation** of parts. Transverse failure of formations present as congenital ampu-tations. Longitudinal failures (e.g. thalidomide) produce conditions such as radial club hand, cleft hand, or fibular hemimelia.

Commoner conditions such as duplications (e.g. polydactyly), hypoplasias, and hyper-plasias are less serious. Surgery to improve function and not just appearance may include joint fusions, digit transplantation, limb shortening/lengthening, or even amputation. The commonest deformities presenting at birth to an orthopaedic surgeon are clubfoot (congenital talipes equinovarus, CTEV) and developmental dysplasia of the hip (DDH, previously called CDH). The majority of patients with CTEV and DDH are treated suc-cessfully in childhood and rarely have problems at work.

Some genetic abnormalities produce orthopaedic conditions which may influence normal day to day activities. A number of autosomal dominantly inherited conditions are of interest including **osteogenesis imperfecta tarda** (the adult form of brittle bone disease), **classic dwarfism** (achondroplasia), and **neurofibromatosis**. Adults with achondroplasia can often cope well in the workplace provided they choose their jobs carefully and the workplace is ergonomically adapted. **Osteogenesis imperfecta** (OI) is an abnormality in the structure of collagen. This can either cause death *in utero*, severe deformity, and growth retardation, or only minor bone fragility. A previous orthopaedic history will define an individual's suitability for particular employment so that avoidance of certain physical activities may be planned. Severe growth retardation can occur with this condition, and allowances in the workplace may be needed to accommodate those of marked short stature. However, the nature of the work must also be carefully considered. Any job requiring strong repetitive or forceful movements of the skeleton would be unsuitable. If aids can be reasonably provided to alleviate such situations then their procurement may be necessary to fulfil the requirements of the DDA.

Leg length inequality

Leg length inequality (LLI) may be due to an abnormally short or abnormally long limb. Any significant inequality in leg length is likely to interfere with a person's ability to cope with a physically demanding occupation. A short leg may be due to a congenitally short femur or tibia, congenital hemiatrophy, fracture malunion or growth plate injury. A long leg may be due to a congenital long limb in association with vascular anomalies or neurofibromatosis. Infection may destroy an epiphysis, causing shortening, or conversely, may cause overgrowth due to chronic osteomyelitis. LLI of less than 1.5 cm requires no corrective treatment. LLI of between 1.5 and 3 cm in an adult should be managed with a raised shoe. Discrepancies of more than 3 cm are not usually treated with a shoe raise, owing to its bulk and unacceptable cosmetic appearance. LLI of more than 4 cm leads to marked asymmetry of spinal rotation. It is generally accepted that discrepancies over 2.5 cm can give rise to problems in the spine. Leg length discrepancies of this magnitude may be treated by lengthening the short limb or shortening the longer limb. In general, an average or tall individual with less than 5 cm discrepancy should undergo shortening of the opposite leg, as this involves less morbidity. The safe limit for lengthening is approximately 15% of the original bone length. Discrepancies greater than this are not correctable by one procedure and may require a combination of leg lengthening and contralateral leg shortening, or more than one lengthening procedure.

Amputations and prosthetics

Between 5000 and 6000 new amputees are seen in limb-fitting centres in England each year. The commonest reason for amputation is vascular insufficiency (54%) followed by diabetes (20%), trauma (11%), embolism (4%), and malignancy (4%).

Upper limb amputations usually occur in younger patients as a result of trauma. Amputation in the upper limb can be devastating, usually more so than a loss of the corresponding part of the lower limb.

The most effective upper limb device is still the split hook, but technology is rapidly advancing. Artificial hands tend to be passive devices used for cosmetic purposes. Mechanical hands are bulky and heavy. 'Phantom limb' is present in all amputees to some degree but disappears more quickly in younger patients. Loss of a hand in an occupation requiring repetitive fine movements is likely to demand a change of occupation. Alternative jobs are possible but support of the employee may be critical, especially when the job involves contact with members of the public when the individual may feel awkward or embarrassed.

Consideration of the job situation must be given to making sure that the remaining limb is not placed at risk. Under the DDA it is likely that attempts must be made to mechanize the job to allow the individual to continue if at all possible. Voice-activated software would be beneficial in a visual display unit (VDU) worker to make sure the remaining limb was not overworked. Dictating machines may be a substitute when the ability to write easily is lost because of a limb amputation and adaptations to telephones in the office situation may allow a 'hands off' approach.

Many occupations can be resumed following an **amputation of a lower limb**, but work in any of the emergency services, or jobs requiring climbing, ladder work, or scaffolding, are obviously excluded. An individual assessment of each case is essential. In below-knee amputations 75% of patients will walk with a prosthesis but with a 10–40% increase in energy expenditure. With an above knee only 20% are able to work because of the increased (65%) energy expenditure, although this is age related. Energy-storing feet and hydraulic joints allow efficient effective leg prostheses (see also Chapter 13, Trauma, p. 262 and p. 271).

Careful examination of the workplace is essential to determine what part of a particular job can still be managed effectively. It is likely that most office-based and manufacturing jobs can still be done, providing adaptations in the workplace allow easy access and ergonomic adaptations are made to accommodate a wheelchair if necessary. Particularly in above-knee amputations in older people, the use of an electric wheelchair may facilitate movement about the workplace which would not be possible if long distances have to be walked. Employees who need to drive may have their vehicles adapted to hand controls.

History has shown that the capabilities of those who have had amputations vary considerably and adaptations of the working conditions may well allow the individual to continue in their employment. In the foot, toe and ray amputations do not usually cause problems except in the case of the big toe and first ray. Through-ankle amputation provides better function than amputations through the foot.

Individual assessment of the disability produced by a foot problem is necessary. Job adaptation may be necessary prior to, or during recovery from the operation. High stools allowing employees who normally stand to take the weight off their feet may be useful, and temporary reduction in walking duties may be necessary. An assessment of alternative footwear may be necessary to facilitate an early return to work. However, where safety boots are essential such adaptations may be unwise.

Bone and joint infection

Septic arthritis

Septic arthritis is a rare conditon, which occurs by haematogenous spread, penetrating injury, or spread from neighbouring osteomyelitis. Staphylococcus aureus is the most frequent infecting organism; streptococci and coliforms account for most of the rest. In adults there is frequently an overlying wound or distal portal of entry, but this may be absent in the immunocompromised host. Previous arthritis is a predisposing factor. The classical signs are fever, erythema, effusion, and severely restricted range of movement. Treatment consists of joint drainage, antibiotics, and splintage. Prompt diagnosis and treatment are vital to avoid permanent cartilage damage. **Tuberculous arthritis** is occasionally seen in Europe, and this should not be forgotten when individuals travel widely during their working life. With a septic arthritis a monoarticular arthritis is the rule. The order of frequency is hip, knee, ankle, sacro-iliac joint, wrist, and shoulder. A synovectomy can be considered in those with pronounced synovitis and an abscess may require drainage.

Acute infection of bone

Acute infection of bone occurs directly by contamination of an open wound (exogenous) or indirectly by haematogenous spread. The commonest causative organism is *Staphylococcus aureus* (80%). Osteomyelitis may become chronic as the result of inadequate treatment, a highly virulent organism, or impaired host resistance. Open fractures or penetrating injuries to bone may be complicated by osteomyelitis. Antibiotics are used immediately the diagnosis is suspected. Initial 'best guess' choice of antibiotic can be altered if blood cultures or pus allow specific organisms to be cultured. Open drainage is advised if there is swelling suggestive of an abscess or a sequestrum is identified. Splintage relieves pain and aids healing.

Hand infections

Infections of the hand usually follow an open injury and rarely occur by haematogenous spread from a distant focus. The commonest infecting organisms are *Staphylococcus aureus* (50–80%), streptococcal species, and coliform bacilli, but after an open wound any organism may be present. A human bite sustained from a punch injury may be contaminated by *Eikenella corrodens* (and may be associated with an osteochondral fracture in up to 60% of cases). *Bacteroides* and *Pasteurella multocida* are frequently isolated from animal bites. Infection of the nail fold (paronychia) often follows a minor penetrating injury. A chronic paronychia occurs in people whose occupation involves sustained immersion of the hand in water and is characterized by an inflamed eponychium with loss of the cuticle. Occupational infections include orf (sheep workers), erysipeloid (meat workers), pilonidal sinus (hairdressers), and infections with *Mycobacterium marinum* (swimming pool attendants). In cases of unusual tenosynovitis, consider the possibility of tuberculosis or *Mycobacterium kansaii*.

Infections of bone are likely to cause problems at work, mainly related to the time that is needed for a cure to be achieved. In rare cases persistence of a discharging sinus may make employment inappropriate in a hospital setting or where control of infection is vital.

Musculoskeletal tuberculosis

Skeletal tuberculosis is caused by infection with *Mycobacterium tuberculosis* in the majority of cases, with *Mycobacterium bovis* and the rarer mycobacteria accounting for the rest. The incidence of tuberculosis is decreasing in the western world, but not in Africa and Asia where there are 400 new cases per 100 000 population per year and one-tenth of all those infected have musculoskeletal tuberculosis. Involvement of the spine occurs in 50% of those with disease of the musculoskeletal system. In tuberculous osteomyelitis any long bone may be affected. There are various regimes of chemotherapy using combinations of rifampicin, isoniazid, and pyrazinamide. Surgery is rarely required.

The length of time required for treatment to be effective especially in those with physically demanding jobs is likely to be a problem in most occupational situations. Whether any return to such posts is possible, or wise, depends on the site of infection and the stability of the bones and joints involved.

Further reading

1   *Disability Discrimination Act 1995.* Department of Education and Employment. London: HMSO.
2   *Management of Health and Safety at Work Regulations 1992.* London: HMSO.
3   Sheppeard H, Bulgen D, Ward DJ. Rheumatoid arthritis—returning patients to work. *Rheum Rehab* 1981; **20**: 160–163.
4   Symmons D, Bankhead C. *Health care needs assessment for musculoskeletal diseases.* University of Manchester: Arthritis Research Council Epidemiology Research Unit, 1994.
5   Health and Safety Executive. *Work related upper limb disorders. A guide to prevention.* London: HMSO, 1990.
6   Barton NJ, Hooper G, Noble J, Steel MW. Occupational causes of disorders in the upper limb. *BMJ* 1992; **304**: 309–311.
7   Millender LH, Tromanhauser SG, Gaynor S. Occupational disorder management. *Orthop Clin North Am* 1996; **24**, 4.
8   Nugent IM, Ivory JP, Ross AC. *Key topics in orthopaedic surgery.* Oxford: Bios, 1995.

13

Trauma

D. Snashall and B. Povlsen

Trauma is the commonest cause of death in people under 40. Limb injuries are the commonest, head and visceral injuries are the most lethal. This chapter will deal with the effects of direct trauma to limbs, thorax and abdomen. The effects of major trauma to the head are dealt with in Chapter 6 (Neurological disorders) and injury to the spinal cord is dealt with in Chapter 11 (Spinal disorders). Lower limb amputations and prostheses are also covered in Chapter 12 (Orthopaedics).

Traumatic injuries

In the industrialized world most severe injuries arise from road traffic accidents, which claim approximately 1 in 10000 lives each year. Most deaths occur within the first hour following the injury, before the patient arrives at a hospital, and brain or chest/cardiovascular injuries are the commonest causes. With improved emergency treatment at the roadside, more and more severely injured patients now reach hospital alive. Early treatment of visceral injuries and cardiorespiratory complications is ideal, with definitive treatment of musculoskeletal injuries delayed until after the patient's condition has been stabilized.

Mechanical trauma

Skin and subcutaneous tissue

Skin and the underlying fatty tissue (subcutaneous tissue) can be damaged by direct laceration (puncture, tear, or shear), by thermal injury (hot or cold) and by electrical injury. Puncture or clean sharp cuts of the skin are usually treated by primary repair following adequate cleansing and debridement. Unless there is an underlying medical condition or infection (e.g. caused by biting), repair will take place quite rapidly after opposition of the tissue edges. Sutures or steristrips can be removed after about 10 days and minimal time need be lost from work. Patients who work with food should not be allowed back to work until all wounds are healed and normal hand hygiene precautions are possible. Wet work should similarly be avoided. More extensive damage, where large areas of skin are lost, may require covering with skin grafts. These may be split skin grafts or full thickness skin grafts, depending on the depth of the injury. Special areas such as the palm of the hand and fingers may present recurrent problems, even though initial healing was successful, when the grafted or healed tissue provides inferior mechanical strength compared to the original cover—a problem sometimes for heavy tool handlers. This can lead to time off work due to secondary infections and may require later secondary surgery involving reconstruction with full thickness tissue from other parts of the body.

Muscle

Muscle may be directly severed, severely bruised, or crushed, or may be damaged indirectly as a result of trauma to the nerves or blood vessels supplying it. In cases of muscle laceration, it may be possible to restore function by direct suture, providing the blood supply is adequate. In cases of severe bruising or contusion, the muscle compartment may need to be decompressed or the muscle partly removed. Where a group of muscles is profoundly damaged, it may be possible to restore function by transferring another group of muscles into the same compartment.

The rotator cuff of the shoulder represents the most frequently damaged functional muscle unit that requires repair. This vulnerable structure runs in a bony tunnel between the humeral head and the acromion. Injuries to the shoulder therefore quite often lead to injuries of the rotator cuff resulting in muscle rupture causing persistent pain and weakness and a reduced range of motion in the shoulder. This may require surgical intervention and lead to permanent inability to lift heavy weights. (See also Chapter 12 p. 242).

Tendons

The commonest tendon injuries arise from sharp injuries to the hands. The appropriate treatment depends on whether injury is to the extensor or to the flexor tendons. Extensor tendon injuries can be treated successfully with simple repair and immobilization for approximately 4 weeks, after which an equivalent rehabilitation period will lead to an acceptable functional outcome. Injuries to the flexor tendons of the fingers require skilled surgical repair and then postoperative rehabilitation by a dedicated hand therapist. A specially designed brace is used which passively flexes the fingers by means of a pulley but allows the patient to actively extend the fingers. Such a device will be necessary for 8–10 weeks before the patient is allowed to start active flexion exercises. Full rehabilitation may take up to 3 months after the initial repair. When flexor tendon repair has been delayed, a two-stage repair may be needed using spare tendons from other parts of the body after an initial operation has created a tunnel within which the grafted tendon can slide.

Ligaments

The commonest ligamentous injuries are about the ankle; next, the knee. The commonest injuries to the knee are to the medial and lateral collateral ligaments. A more serious injury is to the anterior cruciate ligament which occurs when torsion of the body takes place with the lower leg secured, or vice versa. Two typical examples are the footballer who twists his knee or the skier who crashes. There may be a loud crack, immediate swelling, and severe pain. The injury causes instability of the knee which may lead to secondary meniscal tears. Anterior cruciate ligaments are seldom repaired or reconstructed in adults over 30 unless they are engaged in contact sports at a professional or semi-professional level, as rehabilitation after reconstruction can sometimes take up to a year. In the older age groups building up muscle strength around the knee and using stabilizing knee braces has just as good an effect but with significantly reduced rehabilitation time. No firm guidelines can be given regarding whether patients can work while on waiting lists for surgery to meniscal tears or cruciate ligament injuries. However, patients who for safety reasons require full use of their knees such as scaffolders, construction workers, and steeplejacks, or those who need to work on uneven ground, such as farmers, foresters, or emergency workers, should be directed towards less physically demanding work until surgery has been carried out. The same restrictions apply to carers who have to lift and support others. Office workers may return to work about 2 weeks after arthroscopic surgery for meniscal tears. Individuals who have physical jobs may not be able to return to work until normal muscle strength around the knee is re-established, particularly if they have been off work for a long time and developed significant muscle atrophy. With patients who have had surgery for reconstruction of ligaments a return to high physical activity may take up to a year and they will normally be required to wear a brace or plaster for 6–12 weeks after the operation.

A common site of ligamentous injury in the hand is the ulnar collateral ligament of the thumb (gamekeeper's or skier's thumb). This occurs when the ligament is stressed and subsequently ruptured due to radiovalgus trauma to the metacarpophalangeal joint. If it is completely unstable it is advisable to explore the injury and if necessary effect a repair. Postoperative rehabilitation requires 6 weeks in plaster followed by subsequent rehabilitation which can normally be carried out by the patient himself. Depending on the dominant side, lighter work tasks can be carried out even in the immediate postoperative period and also during rehabilitation depending on the requisite grip strength in the affected hand.

Cartilage

There are three types of cartilage: hyaline, elastic, and fibro-cartilage. Hyaline cartilage, which consists mainly of mucopolysaccharides, is the most common. Hyaline cartilage persists in adult life not only on the articular surfaces of joints, where it covers the opposing bone edges, but also in the supporting framework of the nose, larynx, trachea, and bronchi. Because of the mucopolysaccharides, hyaline cartilage has a very high content of water which acts as a sponge, transforming the cartilage into a buffer, and acting as a barrier to mechanical trauma. However, if damaged, it is replaced not by new hyaline cartilage but by fibro-cartilage which does not have the same mucopolysaccharide content and is therefore not able to re-establish the same good mechanical shock-absorbing qualities. This is the reason why, after joint trauma, although no injuries may be discerned initially, the joint may develop osteoarthritic changes later when the original cartilage is replaced with a less mechanically favourable type.

Blood vessels

Localized damage to blood vessels is sometimes amenable to direct repair by vascular surgery or micro-surgery. More extensive damage may be overcome by the use of bypass grafts, though not commonly, because such damage is likely to co-exist with other tissue, nerve, and bone injuries as well as with soft tissue which leads to cover problems. If severe trauma is sustained to the blood vessels, resulting in complete disruption of the blood supply to the distal limb, amputation may be required; however, most amputations following trauma are due to bone and soft tissue loss.

Nerves

The best-known classifications of nerve injuries are those of Seddon and, later, Sunderland (1951). However, these classifications do not cover ischaemic, thermal, electrical, or chemical lesions. Neither do they incorporate the important factors of viability or contamination of the surrounding tissue. For practical purposes the functional description by Seddon is the more useful.

Seddon classification

- Following mild compression injuries **neuropraxia** can occur which causes a local conduction block but no injury to the axon and will lead to almost complete restoration of function.
- If a more severe crush injury has occurred the continuity of the axon may be broken but with the immediate surrounding tissue of each nerve fibre left intact. This injury type (**axonotomy**) will lead to functional recovery as the neurone re-enters the remaining sheath after regeneration and thus will not benefit from surgical intervention. However, the functional outcome will frequently be related to the distance that the nerve cell has to cover before it reinnervates its target area. With an average growth rate of approximately 1 millimetre per day, irreversible atrophic changes may have taken place in the target organ even though the nerve itself has regenerated almost completely. The functional outcome may be minimal if, for instance, the muscles have completely wasted during such a prolonged regeneration time. Transcutaneous electrical nerve stimulation (TENS) in order to combat the muscular atrophy occurring during denervation during prolonged regeneration times has been used experimentally.
- If the entire nerve has been divided (**neurotmesis**) little if any spontaneous regeneration will occur since the distal and proximal stumps tend to move apart due to their inherent elasticity, creating a gap. Surgical repair is therefore required in order to ensure, at least the possibility of regeneration. The speed at which a nerve regenerates and grows towards its target area is considered to be the same following crush or transection and suture. However, functional outcome following crush injury is far superior to that which can be created by surgical repair, even with the most advanced techniques.

Sunderland classification

Sunderland's classification has five grades.

- **First-degree injury** corresponds to Seddon's neuropraxia.
- **Second-degree injury** corresponds to axonotomy.

Sunderland divided Seddon's neurotmesis into subgroups, depending on the continuity or discontinuity of individual connective tissue components:

- In a **third-degree injury** both axons and endoneural tubes have been divided, but the perineurium remains intact. This injury may be seen following severe compression or traction trauma and is sometimes accompanied by intrafascicular bleeding, oedema, and ischaemia.
- In a **fourth-degree injury** the axons, the endoneural tubes, and the perineurium have all been divided, but the epineurium is preserved.
- In a **fifth-degree injury** the entire nerve trunk has been divided.

Functional outcome

Several factors affect the functional outcome following a nerve injury. The best outcome is following a simple neuropraxia where the nerve fibre itself is not divided, or a crush injury which does not require surgical intervention. The least successful is any nerve injury which requires surgical intervention. The other important factor is the distance from the injured nerve to the target organ. Little if any function can be re-established following 2 years' lack of nerve supply. As the distance, in a mature adult, from the cervical spinal cord to the hand is in the region of 80 centimetres, with a regeneration growth of 1 millimetre per day the nerve-damaged hand is on the borderline as far as eventual function is concerned. Thus a significant delay in carrying out a surgical procedure may prevent a useful functional outcome even though the nerve eventually reaches the target organ. It is important therefore to establish as early as possible whether an injury has caused nerve damage requiring surgical intervention. **If surgery is necessary, it should be carried out as soon as possible.**

Age has been cited as an important factor for establishing good functional outcome following injury, but it is not clear whether this is a matter of age or size (and therefore a matter of growth distance). Experiments have not shown that young animals have superior regeneration to older ones under controlled conditions.

Hand injuries

Most nerve injuries are to the hand and therefore most often affect sensory nerves. When dealing with sensory nerves it is important to remember that the most significant disability following such injuries is not the loss of sensation but the neurogenic pain that such nerve lesions can cause. Two types of neurogenic disturbance can occur following such injuries.

- The best-known is **post-traumatic neuroma** which normally occurs when the nerve has been completely transected and the proximal stump of the nerve has separated from the distal end. This prevents the growing axons from reaching the distal stump and they form a neuroma. Even small neuromas in the upper limb can cause significant pain and functional disability. It is important therefore that such nerve injuries are explored if possible and repair effected, as this significantly reduces the chance of post-traumatic neuroma formation. If a neuroma has formed, desensitization carried out by a specialist hand therapist can in some cases reduce discomfort. Utensils or tools with special handles which reduce direct compression of the neuroma can sometimes be useful. However, in most cases where a significant neuroma has formed the best method of treatment is excision and grafting of the nerve if the distal end can be located. If that is not the case then transfer of the neuroma to a location which is less likely to be exposed to direct compression can help reduce the functional disability.

- A less common problem is **post-traumatic Raynaud's syndrome** which can occur after either crush or transection injuries. This often leads to cold intolerance which, particularly for individuals who normally work in low temperatures or wet climates, may prove to be severely disabling. There is no proven treatment for this disorder but sympathetic blockade can be attempted using oral medication. Guanethidine blockade, sympathetic stellate blockade, or transthoracic sympathectomy in well-selected patients can improve their work ability although some form of persistent disability is always found.

Specific nerve injuries
(see also Chapter 12)

Brachial plexus injuries

Injuries occur in two main situations:

- Traction injuries sustained at birth. These are most frequently unilateral and fortunately tend to recover spontaneously during the first month of life. However, if permanent disability ensues, tendon transfers are preferred to nerve repair in the very young, though some centres have now started to reassess this approach.
- Later in life—particularly in the late teens—as a result of motor cycle accidents where the driver is thrown off the motor bike and sustains traction injuries on hitting the ground. Such injuries are more commonly observed now, as more motor cyclists avoid fatal head injuries by using helmets. The trend is to treat them as early as possible. Even avulsed roots can be reimplanted into the spinal cord with some functional regeneration. Brachial plexus injuries causing persistent functional disability of the hand are best treated by tendon transfers.

Peripheral nerve injuries

The axillary nerve, which innervates the important deltoid muscle, is vulnerable to traction injury during dislocation of the shoulder. This injury is usually relatively benign enabling regeneration and reasonably good functional recovery. It is best treated conservatively.

More common are injuries to the **median and ulnar nerves**. The median nerve is damaged by lacerations around the wrist, either self-inflicted as part of a suicide attempt or accidental when the patient smashes a window. Less often the ulnar nerve is injured, usually around the elbow where it runs superficially. Because this site is remote from the hand, the functional outcome following ulnar nerve injuries is often poor. However, some improvement can be achieved if the repair is carried out by expert surgeons. The ulnar nerve has a major role in the innervation of the intrinsic muscles of the hand, and the motor problems that arise in the absence of recovery cause more handicap than the sensory loss.

For both the ulnar and median nerves two types of deficit result—motor and sensory. Resultant motor dysfunction is the more sensitive to the level of the laceration. Median and indeed ulnar nerve lacerations cause similar sensory dysfunctions as the major sensory target is distal to the division of the main nerve trunk. If the ulnar nerve is divided above the elbow there will be weakness in both flexion and extension of particularly the ulnar half of the hand. If, however, the injury is at wrist level normal flexion is likely to persist but the patient will be unable to straighten the fingers. Median nerve injuries at elbow level and above will result in poor flexion of the thumb and first and second fingers, but also an inability to oppose the thumb to the other fingers of the hand. If the injury is more distal the motor dysfunction will be the same but will pose, at this level, a more significant functional disability than an ulnar nerve lesion, preventing in many cases the patient from properly gripping a pen, hammer, etc.

Median nerve laceration around the wrist is extremely disabling, particularly if the dominant hand is injured, as the patient is initially left without any sensory innervation in the most important part of the fingers. The median nerve also innervates the muscles around the thumb which enable the thumb to be brought into opposition and act as a post for the rest of the fingers. If this motor function is lost and not restored in any other way the functional deficit will be similar to the disability seen following an amputation. The lack of motor function in the thumb can, however, be compensated for if the more proximally innervated muscles of the forearm are intact as tendon transfers can be carried out especially if the ulnar nerve is intact. However, sensory deficit in the hand cannot be made up and the best option is to carry out meticulous repair of the median nerve to gain optimal sensory reinnervation. Hand rehabilitation following nerve damage is to a great extent preventive as nerve regeneration cannot be enhanced but, owing to long regeneration times, significant permanent contractures can develop which can prevent the patient from using the hand even after complete successful nerve regeneration has taken place. It is therefore important that during rehabilitation all joints in the affected extremity are treated regularly by a hand therapist. Between exercises a special splint may have to be worn ensuring the joints are placed in the most appropriate position to prevent contractures. After regeneration has taken place it may be necessary for the patient to be given a specific exercise programme in order to rebuild the strength of the affected muscles. As function has been impaired or is absent it generally takes twice as long for strength to return. Although partial sensation may have returned to the hand the input is not of the same quality as before the injury because the individual nerve cells do not grow back in exactly the same order as previously. If patients have had major sensory nerves repaired then sensory re-education may be necessary.

Limb reimplantation

Limb reimplantation is, for practical purposes only, carried out on upper extremities—usually only around the wrist and more distally. Muscles in the extremities suffer permanent damage if they are deprived of their circulation for more than 6 hours. It is possible to reimplant a whole leg and achieve survival of structures such as bone and skin, but if the muscles do not function such reimplantations often cause more disability than amputation which leaves a stump that may be fashioned for a useful prosthesis. As a result of these considerations, only whole-hand reimplantation is commonly attempted today. The intrinsic muscles of the hand may not work, but because of the function of the extrinsic long tendons and a hope of functional sensation in the hand, useful results can be achieved despite complete loss of the intrinsic muscles. Single-finger reimplantation is no longer advocated except when the thumb is involved. The reason for this is that reimplanted digits often lose their full range of movement and normal sensation. As, to all intents and purposes, a three-finger grip only is required, such patients will often avoid using such a disabled finger. Patients who have had reimplantation of a single finger have worse function than those who have had an immediate functional filling of the amputation stump. In addition rehabilitation following finger reimplantation can, due to prolonged healing problems and loss of sensation, be very long whereas revision of an amputation may enable a heavy labourer to return to work within a month with good permanent functional ability. Single-finger amputation (either right or left) should not prevent an individual returning to work. However, many-finger amputations lead to problems of post-traumatic cold intolerance which, apart from the milder degrees, does not seem to improve with time. This can also be the case even if the finger has been successfully reimplanted; quite often patients who have experienced significant limb injuries suffer as much from pain and cold intolerance as they do from actual loss of function as a result of reduced mobility in the extremity. Obviously if an individual requires, for their particular occupation, to use all five fingers of both hands, or needs normal mobility of all fingers, then such injuries can prove extremely limiting. With dominant hand injuries younger adults seem to be surprisingly able to compensate by increasingly using the non-dominant hand if only one hand is required. If both hands are required at normal strength and range of motion, such compensation cannot take place.

Upper-limb prosthesis

There are fewer than 100 upper-limb amputations per year in the UK. These amputations are carried out because of malignancy or severe trauma. A third group needing upper-limb prostheses may be children with congenital loss of whole or part of the upper extremity. Children will generally have the best foundation for useful function of their upper-limb prosthesis as they may from an early age develop the ability to use an advanced neurocutaneous electrically operated prosthesis. Such prostheses are also available for adults, but are not so successful.

The function that patients may be able to achieve with prostheses varies greatly: at one extreme is the patient who never accepts psychologically the loss of a limb and, as a result, rejects the whole concept of using a functional prosthesis and even sometimes a cosmetic prosthesis. Often, at the other extreme are younger and otherwise fully fit individuals who are able to learn how a myoelectric prosthesis works and are able to operate it with such accuracy that even complex activities can be achieved, e.g. lifting up a child using a normal hand and a myoelectric upper limb prosthesis.

Fractures

Fractures can arise from traumatic injury to healthy bone, repetitive strain to healthy bone, or during normal use of a pathologically weakened bone. Treatment depends on the nature and site of the injury.

Stress fractures

Stress fractures as a result of repetitive strain occur in sites where there is an altered blood supply, and healing may be prolonged because the body's normal healing response and the formation of callus is reduced.

Stress fractures are rare but can occur at sites repeatedly subjected to bending or twisting forces. One is the 'march fracture', so named because it occurs in soldiers, and affects the metatarsal neck. Stress fracture can occur in the navicular bone. Stress fractures of the medial malleoli are seen most frequently in runners. These injuries present with a constant ache in the foot or ankle and the fractures are often not seen on plain radiographs. The diagnosis may be made with an isotope bone scan or MRI scan. Stress fractures of the patella have been described in athletes participating in jumping sports, and similarly stress fractures of the neck of the femur are sometimes seen in young, vigorous people who run or march for long distances. Stress fractures of the upper extremity are most frequently described in the hook of the hamate in individuals who use hammers or clubs. This presents with a dull ache and an ulnar nerve neuritis may develop.

Apart from fractures of the femoral neck, stress fractures do not require surgical treatment. However, owing to the nature of the fracture they often heal very slowly and slower than an acute undisplaced fracture in the same location, i.e. the period of rest and rehabilitation usually has to be longer.

Traumatic fractures

The three most common fractures in individuals of working age are to the forearm, the femur, and the lower leg.

The first two often occur with low-energy impact. The third, of the tibia and fibula, affects either the mid-shaft as a result of a road traffic accident, or the ankle as a result of a less violent accident. Fractures of the tibia and ankle can either be treated surgically or by immobilization depending on the inherent stability of the fracture and joint congruity.

The most common fracture in the western world is that of the distal end of the radius (the Colles fracture). It is commonly treated by manipulation under local anaesthesia and a plaster cast for 4–6 weeks. However, more and more attention is being given to these fractures and they are increasingly treated by external or internal fixation in order to prevent redisplacement. During plaster immobilization it may be possible to use the fingers for light activities such as office work, etc., but not for activities requiring heavy lifting or special hand hygiene. Patients are often left with significant stiffness in the wrist which may disappear if there are no other injuries to the carpal joints and the fracture has united in a good anatomical position. However, **malunion** in a grossly deformed position or concomitant injuries to the wrist can cause chronic problems which may lead later to a need for wrist fusion in order to restore a hand which is still strong but pain-free.

The second most common fracture is of the neck of the femur which can be intra- or extra-capsular. In elderly patients intra-capsular fractures are treated with immediate hemi or total hip replacement but in individuals below the age of 50 reduction of the fracture and internal fixation may be attempted. These patients may not be fully weight bearing for at least 6 weeks. There is a risk of between 10–50% of developing avascular necrosis of the femoral head (depending on displacement) and this may require later total hip replacement. Those patients who have received a hemi or total hip replacement will have a rapid rehabilitation if they are otherwise medically fit and normally expect to leave hospital within 2 weeks. At that stage they should be partially weight bearing and have a rehabilitation programme similar to those who have had a total hip replacement for osteoarthritis.

The third most frequent fracture is to the ankle which, if minimally displaced, can be treated in plaster of Paris for about 6 weeks if no other complication has occurred, but during this time the patient will be non-weight-bearing. After the plaster is removed the ankle is usually stiff but the patient can be allowed to weight-bear if the fracture has clinically healed. They will, however, require significant time before being fully able to balance on the ankle. This may take from 3 to 6 months after the initial injury and obviously this will have particular relevance to individuals in dangerous and active industries such as construction workers. Others who have to stand or whose legs are immobilized for long periods (e.g. lorry drivers) may suffer from swelling and discomfort around the ankle. Patients who have had an uncomplicated fracture of the ankle are quite often fully mobile 3 months later, but patients who have had significant contusions to the soft tissue or to the articular surfaces may develop permanent swelling, stiffness and pain. For patients who fracture the midshaft of the tibia, uncomplicated cases take about 3–6 months to fully heal but with tibial nailing, which provides a rigid fixation of the fracture, it may be possible for the patient to walk with the aid of crutches within a week of the injury. In patients with mid-shaft femoral fractures the healing time is often between 6–12 months but if treated with intramedullary nailing they may, in favourable situations, be able to fully weight-bear within the week following the injury even though the fracture is still uniting. If infection occurs it may lead to non-union and long-delayed recovery.

Fracture of the scaphoid is common and is conventionally treated with a special below- elbow cast for 6 weeks initially but sometimes requires immobilization for up to 12 weeks. It is possible to work with such a cast if duties are light especially if the fracture is in the non-dominant wrist. However, as the thumb and wrist are completely immobilized there is significant functional restriction of the hand. Most patients after a conservatively treated scaphoid fracture, will be able to return to their full previous occupation. However, this depends on the specific requirements of the job, especially the range of movement required. Frequently, associated injuries to the rest of the carpus are sustained, most commonly ligamentous injuries which may have been ignored initially but pose problems later. If the fracture is very displaced or does not unite within 6–12 weeks a surgical procedure with internal screw fixation is necessary. In such a situation the patient will be able to resume light activities without plaster support 4–6 weeks after surgery, but heavy work should not be commenced until complete healing has taken place, as development of avascular necrosis may lead to osteoarthritis in the wrist and permanent functional disability. The outcome relates to whether the fracture heals and whether the adjacent joint function is affected.

Non-Union of fractures

It is unusual to see non-union of fractures of the upper extremity except for the scaphoid, and very severe proximal humeral fractures. As a result fractures of the upper extremity are nearly always treated conservatively with immobilization. However, problems can arise owing to loss of joint function following immobilization while the fracture heals. Sometimes these problems are lasting and lead to secondary reconstructive surgery to improve joint mobility and function.

If the fracture does not heal, disability can develop due to pain or instability. It is also possible to develop symptomless non-union, albeit rare. Most cases require reconstructive surgery to ensure that healing takes place. If a patient develops chronic non-union caused by infection or a severely impaired blood supply, then the situation may not be resolvable and permanent disability will ensue. If non-union or malunion persists for more than 1 year, resulting in a substantial impairment in the performance of day to day activities, these patients will fall within the definition of the DDA.

Fractures to the lower extremity around the ankle joint rarely lead to non-union or avascular necrosis, but may lead to stiffness and loss of function following immobilization, particularly if joint congruity has not been restored to normal. This may lead to slow progress with rehabilitation and later osteoarthritis in the affected joint.

Fractures around the hip joint have a high incidence of non-union and avascular necrosis. As a result, fractures of the femoral neck in the older patient are usually treated with a prosthesis with or without cement fixation. The procedure is in many ways similar to total hip replacement (Chapter 12). If the fracture is more distal, e.g. in the pertrochanteric region, an open reduction and fixation with a plate and screws is often carried out. In ideal circumstances full weight-bearing is allowed the following day and the patient can often be discharged from hospital within a week. More distal fractures can sometimes be treated with intramedullary nailing which enables the patient to weight-bear immediately.

Increasingly, fractures, particularly those of the lower extremities, are treated by internal or external fixation. The benefits of early mobilization after internal or external fixation greatly outweigh the remote risk of bone infection.

Burns

Burns injuries may occur in isolation or in combination with mechanical injuries or electrical injuries. The patient with extensive burns suffers a combination of neurogenic shock caused by pain and hypovolaemic shock caused by fluid loss through the burned area or second-phase oedema. The amount of fluid loss is directly proportional to the percentage of skin area burned and the depth of the burn. These injuries require specialized treatment.

Another type of injury arises from high-voltage electrical currents. These may appear trivial when first assessed, but can kill after a delay. The delayed progressive oedema of peripheral nerves, and in particular an effect on the heart's conduction system, can lead to cardiac arrest several hours after the apparent escape from serious trauma. In the absence of this complication and provided that a large amount of soft tissue has not been electrically coagulated, recovery is complete, and fairly rapid.

In many cases electric shocks from the domestic supply (240 V) cause no thermal damage to skin or deeper tissues and have no more than a possible transient effect on the cardiorespiratory system. In these cases recovery is immediate and without sequelae.

Minor head injuries

Head injuries occur in approximately 300 per 100 000 of the population every year in England and Wales. They can be divided into mild, moderate, and severe categories on the basis of the Glasgow Coma Scale (GCS), which incorporates factors such as the period of unconsciousness, post-traumatic amnesia, and the presence or absence of a skull fracture or intracranial mass. More than 90% of cases are patients with mild head injuries. These patients have a GCS of 13[*] or greater in the emergency department, a loss of consciousness of less than 15 minutes, post-traumatic amnesia of less than 1 hour, and no evidence of either a skull fracture or intracranial mass.

In the moderate and severe categories patients are more likely to have associated injuries and to have obvious somatic, cognitive, and affective deficits which require treatment before a return to work can be contemplated. Many patients will require the ongoing help and advice of their family practitioner and some will require the help of neuropsychologists, occupational and speech therapists, physiotherapists, social workers, and psychiatrists.

Patients with isolated minor head injuries are not so obviously in need of formal therapy before their return to work, but between one-third and one-half develop a troublesome array of somatic and psychological symptoms over the ensuing weeks or months (see also Chapter 6, p.112). Somatic symptoms include headache, dizziness, fatigue, and intolerance of noise and bright light. Psychological symptoms can be both cognitive (e.g. poor memory and concentration) and affective (e.g. depression, anxiety, emotional lability and irritability.) The majority of patients recover fully within a few months, but a significant minority are still symptomatic 6–12 months later. This grouping of symptoms is described under the umbrella term **postconcussion syndrome**. Cognitive deficits such as memory and concentration difficulties may disrupt the progression of career or education. Affective deficits such as anxiety and depression may cause domestic changes, ranging from an overprotective family reinforcing the patient's sick role, to marital disharmony and breakdown. Entering into litigation over the original injury can lead to conflict and further emotional upset with pressure to demonstrate persistence of symptoms. Directing blame at those felt to be responsible for the injury has also been found to be related to the frequency of symptoms.

Any of these complaints can lead to difficulties at work or in returning to work. This can result in repeated visits to the general practitioner, accident and emergency, or occupational health departments. Clinical examination is usually normal and the available investigations add little to the diagnosis. An understanding of the aetiology of such symptoms, and an ability to recognize factors influencing morbidity, are necessary to optimize initial management and minimize chronic sequelae.

It was originally thought that patients with postconcussion syndrome were suffering

---

[*] The higher the number the less severe the head injury.

from an 'accident neurosis' initiated and perpetuated by litigious attempts to obtain compensation for their injury. This theory has since been questioned and it is now thought that physical and psychosocial factors are more important in both causing and perpetuating the syndrome. Pretraumatic, peritraumatic, and post-traumatic factors may all contribute to the aetiology.

- **Pretraumatic factors** include age and sex, with older patients and women more likely to develop problems. Pre-existing problems such as alcohol abuse or psychiatric illness appear to induce a state of vulnerability, as do domestic and financial stressors. Susceptibility to the syndrome is also induced by recent adverse life events and ongoing social difficulties, and accidents are more likely to happen at a time when the patient is already coping with other sources of 'social stress'.
- Contributing **peritraumatic factors** include direct brain injury and attendant psychological trauma. The patient may experience extremes of fear, anger, or resentment at the time of injury which are felt again during the anxiety and depression of the ongoing syndrome. Iatrogenic factors may compound the situation and the response of the treating physician to the patient can have lasting effects on outcome. Acceptance of the patient's symptoms and reassurance about the outcome may help to foster recovery.
- In the **post-traumatic phase** psychosocial factors come into play. The patient may have to deal with the physical and psychological effects of other injuries sustained. Cognitive and emotional difficulties can adversely affect performance at work. Patients may develop postconcussional behaviour patterns such as arguementativeness, sloth, and overdependence on analgesia and sedatives. These may in fact be passive coping mechanisms developed unintentionally by the patient.

The course of the condition is variable, with patients appearing to fall into one of three groups:

- in the commonest (**acute**) group, patients are relatively symptom-free by 6 weeks after injury
- the **chronic** group still have symptoms 6–12 months after injury
- in the **symptom exacerbation** group, patients initially recover within 6 weeks but then relapse 6–12 months after injury.

Advances in neuroimaging allow for objective evidence of brain damage to be detected in patients with postconcussion syndrome. CT has revolutionized the detection of secondary brain injury (e.g. cerebral oedema, extradural haemorrhage), although it provides little evidence of primary brain damage (e.g. cerebral contusions, diffuse axonal injury). MRI is more sensitive in detecting subtle primary lesions, and can be used to identify the cause of the patient's symptoms.

Electroencephalography (EEG) and auditory brainstem responses (ABR) have also been used to confirm an organic basis for the syndrome. ABR changes appear to reflect the initial severity of injury and the chronicity of symptoms, whereas EEG changes reflect the intensity of symptoms.

Failure to recognize the presence of the syndrome and advise the patient appropriately can lead to unnecessary emotional distress and aggravate symptoms. This may lead in turn to prolongation of the illness and increased time off work. Early clinical intervention is recommended with provision of information, assessment for the presence of neurobehavioural deficits, and advice on a graded return to work and activities. Follow-up examination is advised a month after injury, probably by the patient's general practitioner. In difficult cases referral to a neuropsychiatrist or neuropsychologist may be required for out-patient cognitive-behavioural therapy, supportive counselling, and further follow-up. MRI detection of subtle lesions may help to explain the patient's symptoms, and ameliorate the emotional distress associated with uncertainty. If medication is required, antidepressants have been found to be the most useful. Occasionally the neuropsychiatric effects of minor head injury lead to permanent disability to the extent of having a significant deleterious effect on the patient's life. Work may be impossible, especially if the individual had a job requiring exceptional mental skills. Rehabilitation into a more physical job may be possible.

Thorax

The thorax is a bony cage comprising the breastbone, the ribs, and the spine; it protects vital organs, principally the heart and lungs.

Fractures of the ribs are usually caused by direct impact, such as a fall against a hard surface, and produce severe pain made worse by deep breathing. Complications occur if a fragment of a rib is displaced so that it pierces the underlying lung, causing the lung to collapse (**pneumothorax**) with or without associated bleeding (**haemothorax**). However, individuals with pre-existing chest disease will be more susceptible to pneumonia even after an undisplaced fracture, because the pain will inhibit normal chest movement. Any lung complications will require specific treatment, but simple undisplaced rib fractures will heal spontaneously.

Fractures of the sternum may occur from direct injury from the front, or vertical compression of the chest with simultaneous fracture of the thoracic spine. In the latter case, the main problem is the spinal fracture and the sternal fracture rarely requires specific treatment. When the sternum is pushed inwards it can cause direct pressure on the heart and lungs, and may need to be restored to its original position surgically.

The term **stove-in chest** is used when multiple injuries cause a complete segment of the thorax to become detached and 'flail'. This serious injury requires prompt treatment to save life because the underlying heart and lungs are compromised. The flail segment may be controlled by use of a ventilator, but if this is not possible, surgical fixation will be required.

Abdomen

The abdomen contains vital organs which can be damaged by direct trauma. Severe crush injuries cause rupture or tearing. Loss of blood may cause collapse (hypovolaemic shock) and extravasation of urine or faeces can cause infection and peritonitis. Certain organs, such as the spleen, are sometimes removed after severe injury. When the bowel or bladder is injured, temporary diversions such as colostomy or ureterostomy may be required, which can be reversed later.

The lower part of the abdomen is protected by the bones of the pelvis, which meet at the front in the symphysis pubis and attach to the spine at the back. An isolated fracture of the pelvis seldom causes any problem as there is unlikely to be any significant displacement. When the pelvis is fractured in two places, there is a possibility of displacement and injury to underlying structures. The most common complications are rupture of the urethra or bladder, and occasionally damage to one of the arteries of the leg. If the fracture passes through the roof of the hip joint (acetabulum) it can cause roughening of the joint surface and predispose to later development of osteoarthrosis of the hip.

Most abdominal and thoracic injuries require surgical exploration with prolonged convalescence depending on the precise nature of the damage and the remaining functional disability. Time off work, is, therefore, likely to be prolonged and, if recovery is incomplete, it may not be possible for an employee to return to work, especially to a manual job. **Each case needs individual assessment by an occupational physician but some patients will suffer permanent disability and impairment.**

The degree of disability must take into account travel to work as well as the workplace where adjustments may be necessary.

Amputations and congenital limb deficiencies

The last national statistics for amputations were for 1997/98. A National Amputee Database has now been established. These statistics reflect only patients being referred to the Prosthetic Centres in England and therefore do not give the full incidence of new amputations. The figures, however, allow some points to be drawn. In 1997/98, 4837 patients were seen for the first time. Lower-limb amputations are more frequent than upper-limb amputations, the ratio in 1997/98 being 18:1. The causes of lower and upper limb amputations are quite different and are shown for 1997/98 in Table 13.1. Limb deficiencies, or congenital growth anomalies, form a very small percentage of the whole. They may present as a transverse deficiency (such as an amputation) or a longitudinal deficiency, which usually presents as a shortened limb with or without an abnormal hand or foot.

In 1988, the overall ratio of male to female amputees was 1.04 : 1 and this has shown no significant change over recent years. Only 21.3% of patients are in the 20–60 year age group (working age), 60.3% being between 60 and 79 and 16.2% over 80.

Functionally, the effect of an amputation is on mobility for lower-limb amputees and dexterity for upper-limb amputees. The extent of disturbance of function depends mainly on the level of amputation; the more proximal, the greater the disturbance.

Table 13.1 Amputation by cause 1997/98 (Amputee statistical database for the United Kingdom 1997/98).

Upper limb	Number (%)	Lower limb	Number (%)
Trauma	93 (37)	Dysvascularity	2238 (49)
Neoplasia	26 (10)	Trauma	329 (7)
Dysvascularity	8 (3)	Infection	141 (3)
Infection	4 (1.6)	Neurological disorder	154 (3)
Neurological disorder	1 (0.4)	Neoplasia	123 (3)
Other causes	34 (13)	Other causes	407 (9)
No cause provided	87 (35)	No cause provided	1192 (26)
Total	**253 (100)**	**Total**	**4584 (100)**

However, it is worth noting that although one cannot walk without two legs, it is perfectly possible to do most activities with only one arm. As a rough guide, lower-limb amputees will need 6 months before returning to work and upper-limb amputees 3 months, although if the dominant arm was amputated rehabilitation may take longer.

Complications of amputation

Complications of amputation can be divided into immediate and late (see Table 13.2). Each of these complications can not only delay return to work, but can limit working effectiveness or lead to further absence, with associated social and psychological problems.

In lower-limb amputees there is an increased incidence of premature degenerative change in the joints of the contralateral limb, the knee more than the hip. In upper-limb amputees there appears to be an increased incidence of shoulder and neck problems.

In addition to these medical complications there is the inconvenience of relying on a mechanical device which itself requires maintenance and repair to provide reliable

Table 13.2 Complications of amputation and their management

Complication	Treatment
Immediate	
1. Delayed healing	
Infection	Antibiotics
Ischaemia	Vasodilators
	Angioplasty
	Sympathectomy
	Higher amputation
2. Postoperative oedema	Stump elevation
	Exercises
	Elasticated stump sock
	Mobilization on an early walking aid
3. Phantom pain	Massage
	Analgesics
	Antidepressants
	Carbamazepine/other anticonvulsants
	Anticoagulants
	Behaviour modification
Late	
4. Late changes in stump volume	Adjust or refit socket
5. Stump abrasions	Adjust socket
6. Infected epidermoid cysts	Socket fit
	Stump hygiene
	Surgical excision
7. Neuromata	Adjust socket
	Neurectomy
8. Stress on other parts of the body	

service. Individuals may require time off during working hours to attend for appointments.

Prosthetic services

In 1984 a working party was set up under the chairmanship of Professor Ian McColl to review the artificial limb and appliance centre services. Its report[6] was published in 1986 and, as a result, an interim authority, the Disablement Services Authority (DSA) was established. This authority was operational from 1 July 1987 to 31 March 1991, at which point the services were transferred to the National Health Service. Prosthetic services became part of rehabilitation medicine and are now provided by consultants in the specialty. Several new prosthetic centres were set up during the time of the DSA to make the service more accessible. New prosthetic companies were established with emphasis on local manufacture and the ability to provide all limb systems. Wheelchair services were, in the main, devolved to district clinics run by occupational therapists, providing assessments for more routine types of wheelchairs. In most regions, specialized wheelchair assessments are still available at the regional centres, most usually for those clients requiring complex or 'specialized' seating.

Rehabilitation

Rehabilitation of the amputee requires multidisciplinary teamwork. Ideally, the team (surgeon, nurses, physiotherapist, occupational therapist, and rehabilitation physician) should assess the individual preoperatively. The technique of amputation is critical, as satisfactory fitting of a prosthesis starts with the surgeon's fashioning of the stump, which must be viewed as an 'organ of locomotion'. Postoperatively the amputee will work on general muscle strength and specific stump exercises and be assisted in restoring independence in daily activities. Walking, using an early walking aid under the supervision of the physiotherapist, commences 5–7 days after amputation. The amputee is usually referred for prosthetic fitting about 3 weeks after the amputation. Rehabilitation continues following discharge from hospital, until the amputee has achieved maximum functional independence, and in the case of those of working age, has returned to suitable employment (see below).

Prosthetics

The prosthetist is the person who tailors the fit of the artificial limb or prosthesis to the individual. This is a highly skilled job and requires knowledge of traditional materials, such as leather, metal, and wood as well as an increasing range of modern synthetics such as plastics, silicone, and carbon fibre. Prosthetic joints are becoming more sophisticated; for example energy-storing feet, which incorporate elastic materials which mimic normal gait more closely, and microprocessor-controlled knee units (which automatically control the rate of swing of the calf in relation to the speed of the gait).

Upperlimb prostheses can be purely cosmetic, body-powered, or externally powered. Body-powered limbs can be adapted to a wide range of functions and very fine movements can be achieved. Servo-assisted mechanisms can augment weak muscles. Myoelectric prostheses, which are triggered by signals from muscle groups in the residual limb, are increasingly available. At present they still tend to be much heavier than body-powered limbs, are less reliable and offer relatively crude hand movement. In complex congenital deficiencies such as those in thalidomide patients, individually designed prostheses may be required.

Special work problems

A number of general and specific points should be borne in mind when advising both amputee and employer about working conditions. In general, employers should be made aware that a patient has an artificial limb. It is particularly important that adequate washing facilities can allow the amputee to attend to the limb and stump in reasonable privacy.

Lowerlimb amputees should avoid working at heights, climbing ladders, and habitually walking over uneven ground. Generally, the more proximal the amputation the more limited the mobility. Lower limb amputees may not be able to stand all day, but equally it is inadvisable to sit all day without periodically getting up and moving around. Bilateral lowerlimb amputees may need to use a wheelchair if they have stump or prosthetic problems. These employees, therefore, require wheelchair-accessible premises (see below). In the case of upperlimb amputation, there is little or no restriction on the clerical worker and manual workers can adapt remarkably well, with self-evident limitations. A full assessment by an occupational physician, including an employment evaluation, should always be performed before giving a definite opinion.

Use of walking aids and wheelchairs

Individuals who return to work using sticks or crutches experience particular difficulty with heavy spring-loaded doors (e.g. fire doors) and steps and stairs. The latter need to have at least one handrail to ensure safety. People using a walking frame generally find steps or stairs impossible to negotiate unless the depth of step accommodates the frame as well as the individual.

Individuals who require a wheelchair need suitable ramps over all steps and sills. Doorways and corridors need to be of suitable width to allow easy movement with adequate turning space. Particular attention must be given to toilet facilities. If the person has to work on more than one floor, then the use of lifts will be needed, with controls placed at an accessible height. Attention may also be required to desk heights, access to filing cabinets, and other working surfaces or furniture.

Conclusions

Despite increasing efforts to improve safety on the road, and legislation on safety at work, traumatic injuries still continue to have an impact on the working population. The majority of individuals, however, eventually return to work functionally intact.

Further reading

1 Apley AG, Solomon L. *Apley's system of orthopaedics and fractures*, 7th edn. Oxford: Butterworth–Heineman, 1993.

2 Cranshaw AH (ed.) *Campbell's operative orthopaedics*, 8th edn. St Louis: Mosby yearbook, 1991.

3 Doberman RH (ed.) *Operative nerve repair and reconstruction*. Philadelphia: J P Lippincott, 1991.

4 Green DP (ed.) *Operative hand surgery*, 3rd edn. New York: Churchill Livingstone, 1993.

5 Department of Health. *On the state of the public health for the year 1988*. London: HMSO, 1989.

6 *Review of artificial limb and appliance centre services. The report of an independent working party under the chairmanship of Professor Ian McColl*. London: Crown Publishers, 1986.

7 Ham R, Cotton L. Limb amputation—from aetiology to rehabilitation. In: *Therapy in practice*, Vol 23. London: Chapman & Hall, 1991.

8 Teasdale G, Jennett B. Glasgow Coma Scale: Assessment of coma and impaired consciousness. A practical scale. *Lancet* July 13 1974; 81–84.

14

Rheumatological disorders

C. English and H. A. Bird

Over 150 diseases can affect the musculoskeletal system. The vast majority are not caused by work, although work may become more difficult as a result of some.

In this chapter we consider mainly the commoner conditions:

- inflammatory polyarthritides, degenerative joint diseases and some rarer conditions
- conditions affecting mainly muscles, tendons, connective and soft tissue including work-related upper limb disorders (WRULDs), previously known as repetitive strain injuries (RSI).

A patient may have more than one of these disorders, particularly in the upper limbs, and their interaction with the workplace may produce complex problems.

Some of the conditions considered in this chapter are also referred to in Chapter 12 (Orthopaedics) and spinal disorders are covered in Chapter 11.

Rheumatoid arthritis

Rheumatoid arthritis (RA) is the commonest of the three major inflammatory diseases; its current prevalence in the UK is around 1–2%. In a small number of subjects this disease will therefore complicate any musculoskeletal problems acquired at work. RA affects women 2–3 times as often as men and usually starts in the metacarpophalangeal joints of the hands with local involvement of the wrists. The disease is normally easily identifiable from circulating rheumatoid factors in the blood and the presence of a particular type of erosion on radiographs. Diagnostic confusion is unusual but may occur in the early stages before the specific blood and radiographic tests become positive. At this stage RA may also affect tendons, though it would still normally be distinguishable from tenosynovitis by its bilateral nature and by its systemic symptoms including tiredness and malaise. Current theories on pathogenesis involve an as yet unidentified antigen, perhaps infective, superimposed on a genetic predisposition. RA is, therefore, not caused by work, though mechanical aspects are also important as potentially aggravating factors. If a unilateral stroke is superimposed on RA, the affected and less mobile side ultimately displays less joint damage. Whether this results from local neurological influences or is a direct mechanical effect is uncertain, but suggests a potentially damaging interaction between inflammatory arthritis and mechanical joint loading.

Juvenile RA and adult Still's disease are separate conditions characterized by seronegativity and a different anatomical distribution of joint involvement. In particular the mandible is involved, to produce a receding chin.

RA can cause substantial joint deformity, with consequences for hand function.

Careful occupational therapy and ergonomic assessment is required for rheumatoid patients in the workplace so that their capabilities can be matched to suitable jobs. However, it is surprising how intricate movement can still be accomplished even with the most severely affected hands, particularly if thumb–finger grip is preserved. More widespread involvement, particularly of the lower limb, may necessitate substantial changes in working practices.

Prognosis should be guarded. At present there is controversy over whether RA shortens life expectancy (by perhaps about 10 years). In severe forms there is substantial morbidity with associated infections. The work record may be at risk, although many patients are surprisingly resilient, retaining a will and motivation to work if at all possible.

A variety of prognostic markers have been suggested for use when the condition first presents. The most useful indicators of a poor prognosis are a strong positive rheumatoid factor and the early presence of bone erosions. Multiple joint involvement and extra-articular features, older age at onset, and a lower level of formal education are all bad prognostic features.

Treatment is based on the principles that apply generally to arthritis, described later in this chapter. In addition, intra-articular and intramuscular steroid injections, and specific disease-modifying drugs for the control of RA all play a part, though management of the latter drugs normally requires hospital supervision. Replacement surgery is also available and is particularly successful for the hip, knees, and finger joints although technically it is not as easy as in osteoarthritis because of the bone friability associated with rheumatoid disease.

When considering the recruitment of an individual with known RA, a detailed history of the symptoms, the individual's physical limitations, and a careful functional assessment are essential. Although few employers may be willing to recruit an individual with aggressive disease, significant function limitations and an uncertain future, they must consider each case in the light of the requirements of the Disability Discrimination Act 1995 (DDA). Recommendations include the avoidance of work activity that would place affected joints under significant mechanical strain, due either to force, repetitive movements or adverse postures. Indoor work requiring skill, rather than strength, is to be preferred.

If, as is more common, the symptoms first manifest themselves when an individual is in established employment, it may be necessary to consider ergonomic adjustments or the provision of handling aids if hand function is impaired. In extreme cases, relocation or retraining for less physically arduous tasks may help an individual to remain at work. Expert advice can be obtained from officers of the local Placing, Assessment and Counselling Team (PACT) or National Health Service occupational therapy department on writing aids, electrically operated devices or specialised hand-held tools.

Seronegative spondarthritis

This group of disorders comprises ankylosing spondylitis, psoriatic arthritis, colitic arthritis, Crohn's arthritis, and Reiter's disease and can be separated genetically, clinically and serologically from RA. There is greater family clustering associated with the inheritance of the HLA-B27 antigen and rheumatoid factor is invariably negative (hence the term 'seronegative'). Initial involvement in the arm is most common at the interphalangeal joints of the fingers. In the lower limb the knee and ankle are affected and the sacroiliac joints in ankylosing spondylitis. These conditions are more likely to involve the enthesis (i.e. the site where the tendon is anchored to the bone) than in RA, often mimicking tennis elbow (lateral epicondylitis). They also sometimes improve with exercise, whereas RA is more likely to respond to rest.

In general the prognosis is better than RA, though vision can deteriorate significantly if there is substantial uveitis. Treatment is similar to that of RA, though the spinal involvement is more refractory to drug treatment, particularly requiring intensive physiotherapy to keep the spine mobile and to prevent ankylosis. Some disease-modifying drugs are effective but not as many as in RA.

Ankylosing spondylitis

Work is beneficial for people with ankylosing spondylitis as activity reduces discomfort and the risk of spinal deformity. For many, the symptoms of the condition remain mild enabling them to work full-time and not causing absence. Although heavy physical work is not contra-indicated, those employed in less physically onerous or sedentary work are likely to require minimal work adjustments. Functional limitations are usually secondary to joint stiffness, particularly if free neck movements are essential for driving forklift trucks, passenger carrying vehicles, large goods vehicles, etc. Work requiring considerable spinal flexibility, such as work in confined spaces, may be contra-indicated. The maintenance of maximum spinal function is to be encouraged and regular physiotherapy classes are likely to help in preventing flexion deformities of the spine in the long-term.

Psoriatic arthritis

Frequent time off work rarely occurs in psoriatic arthritis, as the symptoms usually respond to appropriate treatment with NSAIDs and treatment of the underlying skin condition. Where frequent severe exacerbations affect the joints of the feet, relocation to sedentary work may help but, for the majority, significant task and work modifications are unlikely to be required.

Connective tissue disorders

This third group of inflammatory conditions is less likely to involve the joints than the two described above, though arthritis may occur.

The cause of these various disorders is uncertain. Infective agents have been sought but not found. Prognosis depends mainly on whether there is renal involvement (and in the case of lupus, central nervous system involvement). If the kidneys are spared, prognosis is relatively good with a near normal life expectancy, though pregnancy may be complicated by other abnormalities, for example the antiphospholipid antibody syndrome which is associated with arterial and venous thrombosis and recurrent spontaneous abortions and, when it occurs during pregnancy, with premature fetal death, especially in mid-pregnancy.

Systemic lupus erythematosus

The commonest disease in this group in the UK is systemic lupus erythematosus (SLE). Women are affected more frequently than men. Pain may occur in almost any joint, but often in the hands, and is associated with a photosensitive skin rash and Raynaud's phenomenon. At a later stage almost any other joint may become involved.

The prevalence of SLE, worldwide, averages 20–25 per 100 000 population (0.02%). The highest prevalence is in the West Indies and California, and women in their reproductive years account for 90% of patients.

Where the disease is mild, work modifications are unlikely to be required but in more severe cases, the systemic effects of the condition cause extreme fatigue and may require a change to less onerous, more sedentary work.

In extreme cases, with widespread organ involvement, long-term immunosuppressive treatment may be needed. If so, employment exposing the individual to infection, e.g. hospital work or primary school teaching, may be inappropriate, and the opportunity for relocation and retraining could enable the individual to remain in active employment.

Polymyalgia rheumatica

Polymyalgia rheumatica, a condition of the elderly and of uncertain aetiology, characterized by bilateral shoulder girdle stiffness and pelvic girdle stiffness, is closely associated with cranial arteritis which can cause visual symptoms leading to blindness. Because the disease normally occurs over the age of 60 years and is exceptionally rare below the age of 50 years, it is only occasionally encountered in the workplace. When treated with high doses of steroids it has a good prognosis.

Osteoarthritis

The heterogeneous group of conditions that share common pathological features of osteoarthritis (OA), in particular focal loss of the articular cartilage, is the subject of increasing interest as more predisposing causes are identified. This leads to a basic classification of primary (idiopathic or generalized) OA for which no obvious cause exists, and an expanding group of conditions that comprise secondary OA due to specific anatomical, inflammatory, or metabolic abnormalities.

- **Generalized (idiopathic) OA** affects many joints. Its frequency increases with age. Postmenopausal women are particularly vulnerable. The condition is invariably constitutional, an appropriate genetic background and perhaps hormonal factors all contributing to its causation. Sites commonly involved in the hand include the terminal interphalangeal joints where characteristic Heberden's nodes are found, and the base of the thumb. The presence of the disease at this latter site causes particular problems with workers who need regular fine apposition of the thumb as part of their job. Some argue that this condition is a natural consequence of ageing. Osteoarthritic hand involvement, for example, is found in 75% of women between the ages of 60 and 70 and in many of these it is relatively symptom-free.

- **Secondary OA** is usually localized to a single joint or group of joints unless it is secondary to a widespread metabolic abnormality in the body, either biochemical (such as ochronosis) or hormonal (such as acromegaly). A previous orthopaedic condition (such as Perthes' disease) may exist and this is more typical in the leg than the arm. Extreme hyperlaxity (suppleness) of the thumb base may accelerate damage at this joint. A fracture line into the joint cavity with resultant incongruity of the joint surfaces, the operation of menisectomy, or injuries that damage ligaments causing joint instability, predispose to OA. Although the influence of major trauma of this sort is undisputed, the evidence that repetitive impulse loading (as in regular jogging or in the use of vibratory power tools) predisposes to OA is much more contentious. Many other factors impinge, among them being obesity.

Although diagnosis is ultimately made on radiographic change (or less certainly on clinical history if radiographic change has not yet occurred) support for the diagnosis may also come from negative blood tests. These include a normal erythrocyte sedimentation rate (ESR), normal plasma viscosity, normal C-reactive protein, a negative rheumatoid factor, and a negative antinuclear factor.

Generalized OA presents in postmenopausal women or men over the age of 50. Secondary OA may present earlier, depending on the cause. Often there is a direct correlation between the severity of symptoms and radiographic changes. Typical symptoms are pain, and sometimes swelling, around affected joints, particularly with exercise and sometimes after immobility. The course of the condition varies according to the cause and classification. Prognosis varies but is normally much better than for inflammatory polyarthritides, particularly with the advent of large joint replacement surgery which is technically easier in OA than in RA because of the good bone stock found in the former condition.

Management and the prevention of functional limitations require a strategy to maintain flexibility of affected joints and mobility, the strengthening of adjacent muscles, and the avoidance of secondary postural strains including those due to obesity. Work that facilitates movement and encourages flexibility of the affected joints, thus avoiding stiffness, is likely to be of benefit provided the tasks are not too physically onerous.

An ergonomic workplace assessment may be of benefit in assessing postural strains and giving appropriate preventive guidance. Where hand joints are affected, the provision of writing aids, the use of a dictaphone, voice-activated control systems for computer work, or grasping aids may be of benefit. Where there are significant symptoms in the knee joints, mobility will be restricted and standing should be avoided, together with work activities requiring climbing, walking over rough ground, kneeling, or crouching.

Gout

Gout, an arthritis characterized by joint inflammation provoked by the release of uric acid crystals in the joint, must be distinguished from benign symptomless hyperuricaemia, a condition associated with hypertension, which is found in a small proportion of the population. The big toe is the joint most frequently affected by gout, and after that the knee. Tophaceous deposits may be found, particularly on the ear.

Attacks tend to be acute and are nowadays treated effectively by high doses of non-steroidal anti-infammatory drugs (NSAID)s. If attacks become more frequent, serum uric acid is particularly high or there is renal deposition of uric acid, long-term prophylactic treatment, normally with allopurinol, is indicated. Severe tophaceous gout affecting many joints is rarely seen nowadays. The condition therefore rarely interferes with employment.

Paget's disease

Paget's disease is an ill-understood metabolic condition of bone, normally affecting elderly men. Osteoclast-mediated bone resorption with subsequent compensatory over-production of new bone causes the architecture to become distorted, and local pain occurs. The aetiology is ill understood. Symptoms are often localized but the disease can affect any part of the body. Occasionally it is widespread, ultimately leading to bony deformity.

Pain is controlled by analgesics and usually this suffices. If pain persists or if the alkaline phosphatase is unacceptably high, treatment with diphosphonates or calcitonin is recommended. Occasionally the disease mutates into an osteosarcoma.

The disease rarely proves troublesome in the workplace as it predominantly affects elderly people and adequate treatment is now available.

Algodystrophy

Algodystrophy, also known as Sudek's algodystrophy or reflex sympathetic dystrophy (RSD), may complicate WRULDs. Traditionally, an acute painful swollen extremity follows trauma, infection, or a burn. The complete florid form is virtually unmistakable and the trauma, infection, or burn that precedes it may or may not result from the workplace. The difficulty arises with incomplete or atypical forms of the syndrome. All are characterized by loss of bone density, most accurately imaged with bone scintigraphy. This most commonly follows an acute event such as a Colles' fracture, myocardial ischaemia, or acute hemiplegia. However, the trauma may be relatively mild, provoking claims for compensation. The rest that is often recommended to remedy RSD, particularly if enforced by immobilization of the affected limb in a plaster of Paris case, may also provoke similar symptoms. Pain tends to be localized to the bone and the bone is tender on palpation, sometimes to an exquisite degree. When the changes have been induced by work or trauma they are usually unilateral. Bilateral loss of bone density on radiography is more likely to suggest idiopathic osteoporosis, an affliction of elderly people.

Treatment requires adequate pain relief, wrist splintage to maintain good posture, and a graded exercise programme to maintain muscle tone and power and prevent further disability. Work adaptations may be needed following an ergonomic assessment, to facilitate the maintenance of neutral wrist and forearm postures; and the introduction of variety to the range of work tasks undertaken may prove of benefit. The provision of writing aids, power-operated staplers and hole punchers, or modification of handheld tools requiring less application of force should be considered, when appropriate.

Hypermobility syndrome

The range of movement at a given joint varies from individual to individual. There are several reasons for this. The precise contour of the cartilaginous articulating surfaces varies between individuals, a shallow joint socket allowing a greater range of movement than a deep one. The chemical structure of the inherited collagen that gives stability to the joint capsule and surrounding tissues also varies between individuals and may be further modified by stretching. Neuromuscular tone also varies, and can be influenced by training. As a result some people inherit very supple joints and others very stiff joints. Joints stiffen with age as collagen structure alters to render it more stable.

Because joints that are unduly supple require greater effort to control them, it can be postulated that patients with joint hypermobility may require greater muscular effort to perform a given task than their normal counterparts, with consequent earlier fatigue.

Joint hypermobility also predisposes to injury—the unstable joint may be unco-ordinated and easily damaged. Minor injury probably predisposes to a traumatic synovitis that can mimic RA and even tenosynovitis. This has implications for differential diagnosis. Careful pre-placement assessment of patients with hypermobile joints will ensure that their employment will not lead to unnecessary injury.

Fibromyalgia

Until recently fibromyalgia was the non-specific rheumatological diagnosis by exclusion for which occupational predisposing factors could not be identified. Recently there have been attempts to formulate more precise diagnostic criteria based on the supposition that this widespread and diffuse musculoskeletal syndrome, with no evidence of synovitis or joint damage and no clear abnormalities on physical examination other than discrete tender areas in muscle on palpation, may be a pain-amplification syndrome. Since 90% of patients have an age range of onset between 30 and 50 years, and the majority are female, hormonal factors may contribute. The pain and discomfort are widespread, with almost any joint in the body affected, and this has considerable consequences in the workplace. Associated features include fatigue, sleep disturbance, headaches, and irritable bowel syndrome. Investigations are invariably normal and the history of chronic fatigue syndrome, a diffuse condition in which tiredness predominates over pain, is regarded by some as being almost indistinguishable.

Compensation neurosis

Psychosocial factors are an inevitable influence in claims for compensation for any reason. Sometimes these feature so prominently in a case that the neurosis dominates any physical condition. Although the greater prevalence of many such conditions in women is traditionally ascribed to hormonal factors, economic circumstances in certain societies may render women more in need of compensation than men. Certain risk-associated jobs may largely be restricted to women, others to men. It is possible that individuals with more fortunate financial circumstances may leave the workplace at the first onset of symptoms rather than remaining until the later development of the condition restricts any further employment.

Against this background, prevalence rates for putative industrial injuries vary from 5% to 60%, implying that factors other than purely mechanical ones may contribute. A relative paucity of occupational disorders amongst the self-employed, to whom compensation would not normally be available, speaks for itself. Inevitably some subjects will overplay their symptoms, if only subconsciously, leading to the diagnosis of 'compensation neurosis'. When the need to obtain compensation becomes paramount, presentation of the history may become more histrionic, symptoms much more widespread, and the link between ergonomic factors and involvement of the appropriate muscle groups completely blurred.

Rarer arthritides

Many other conditions exist, some inherited and others acquired, sometimes through infection. If a single joint only is involved, e.g. perhaps tuberculous arthritis of the wrist, an employee may be tempted, quite understandably, to attribute its occurrence to the workplace if by chance the condition occurs at the joint that is most frequently used. Clearly in this example the cause is independent, though work will certainly be rendered difficult until the condition is diagnosed and adequately treated.

Disorders of the upper limb

Cervical spondylosis

Cervical spondylosis causes symptoms of local neck pain with restriction of movement, may be associated with distressing headaches and episodes of dizziness, and may cause referred pain in the upper limb or interscapular region. It is usually degenerative in aetiology, the frequency of cervical spondylosis increasing in all populations with age. In one study[1] the condition was identified on radiographic examination in 60% of women and 80% of men at the age of 49 years and in 95% of both sexes by the age of 90, but there was a poor correlation between radiographic changes and symptoms. Degeneration is maximal in the discs and the apophyseal synovial joints of the middle lower cervical region. Dislocation of the disc leads to instability with pressure on nerve roots causing neurological symptoms in the arms. Degeneration may progress at different rates in different people. The inherited shape of the spinal canal is also important in determining the likelihood of disc prolapse. Local mechanical factors predispose to symptoms, either exacerbation of pain (which may result from pressure of the disc on the ligaments of the spine) or neurological symptoms in the upper limb due to nerve root irritation or compression, including pain and paraesthesiae.

Symptoms may be induced by poor posture or by faulty movements of the neck. Conservative treatment focused on rest, intermittent use of a restrictive collar and adequate analgesic and NSAIDs normally suffices and surgery is only rarely required. Epidemiological studies[2] suggest that at any one time 9% of men and 12% of women over the age of 15 years will claim to have neck pain. The lowest prevalence of symptoms is found in sedentary office workers and the highest where work requires strenuous use of the arms. Workers on assembly lines seem to be particularly at risk. Many patients with proven radiological cervical spondylosis remain asymptomatic, so proof of an association with work can be contentious if the ergonomic history is not clear-cut. Only a small minority of subjects will demonstrate undoubted 'porter's neck'—so called because bags of meal weighing 90 kg loaded on to a porter's head are unequivocally linked to radiological changes, including disc compression in the spine. Where a link is demonstrated between symptoms and the workplace, appropriate ergonomic and postural advice will prove to be essential in preventing a recurrence, but non-occupational causes of exacerbation of cervical spondylosis will also need to be excluded.

The frequency and severity of symptoms and degree of functional limitation vary considerably and the severity of changes on cervical spine radiographs are not a reliable guide to prognosis and fitness for work. Occupational factors may precipitate symptoms, particularly if work requires the head and neck to be held in a constant or constrained posture or there is strenuous physical effort of the shoulder girdle muscles as in heavy lifting, carrying or labouring tasks, including the use of vibratory tools. Working with the arms elevated above shoulder height or frequently extending the neck to look upwards should be avoided. For sedentary desk-oriented work, attention should be paid to seating, spinal posture, and the ergonomic layout on the desk, particularly if display screen equipment (DSE) is used. All commonly used articles should be within easy arm's reach, L-shaped workstations being provided where necessary to increase the readily accessible work surface area. The availability of desk lecterns will help to avoid prolonged periods of neck flexion, and placing document holders adjacent to DSE will encourage an upright neck posture. For the majority, the symptoms associated with acute exacerbations improve and permanent occupational restrictions are unlikely. Where permanent restriction of neck movement becomes established, driving motor vehicles or forklift trucks, or similar activities, may no longer be possible.

Epicondylitis of the elbow

Lateral epicondylitis (**tennis elbow**) and medial epicondylitis (**golfer's elbow**) are the commonest soft tissue lesions at the elbow. Both need to be distinguished from other causes of elbow pain such as osteoarthritis, olecranon bursitis, or biceps tendinitis. A careful clinical examination is essential. In epicondylitis there is exquisite point tenderness at the enthesis, lateral or medial, that can be accentuated by resisted activity of the muscles attached to that site, as in the resisted wrist extension test or the forced elbow extension test.

Although the diagnosis is usually clear-cut, the aetiology is less certain. At some time 1–3% of the population may be affected by epicondylitis,[2,3] involvement of the lateral epicondyle being much more common than that of the medial. A sporting cause is relatively rare. It is most often found in non-athletes and not necessarily manual workers. Local trauma may play a part as in an acute wrenching injury, though this is more likely to aggravate established epicondylitis in the older patient. Ageing is associated with anatomical alteration at the enthesis including changes in collagen content and increasing lipids that may predispose to injury. Repeated pronation and supination of the forearm, which may be an integral part of some jobs, will certainly aggravate the condition. Whether symptoms can arise *ab initio* from this action is more contentious. Even allowing for a clustering of the condition in families and a tendency for those individuals affected to have widespread soft tissue lesions at other sites, not necessarily all simultaneously, the balance of probability is that this lesion can be induced at the workplace, particularly if the ergonomic insult corresponds with the use of the forearm muscles and, in turn, the enthesis affected.

The use of power tools, such as saws, jack hammers, etc., may cause tennis elbow and although it is generally rare in athletes it does occur frequently in professional tennis players.

The condition is considered self-limiting, some patients improving with or without treatment within 1 year, but a majority still having symptoms after 1 year, particularly if they have persevered with the activity that caused it.[4] Recurrence does appear to be more common in manual workers and attributable to repeated grasping or lifting activity. Treatment, most commonly by intralesional steroid injection and advice to avoid aggravating activities, tends to be more ineffective in those who do not take a break from work or avoid its aggravating activities. Postural and ergonomic adjustments, task modification, or job rotation may need to be considered to prevent recurrence.

Local steroid injections may remedy epicondylitis and local tenosynovitis, particularly in the early stages. Hydrocortisone or prednisolone are to be preferred for injections close to tendons; the more potent triamcinolone with its potential side-effects including local tissue necrosis should be reserved for intra-articular injections in skilled hands. Later, if tethering of tenosynovitis has occurred or if epicondylitis becomes chronic, surgery may be preferred.

Carpal tunnel syndrome

Carpal tunnel syndrome is compression of the median nerve on the flexor aspect of the wrist in the carpal tunnel. Once this compression has occurred, whatever the reason, symptoms will result. These normally comprise paraesthesiae in the area of the median nerve distribution in the hand, often worse at night and aggravated by certain positions or by repetitive work, particularly stamping movements. Diagnosis will need to be confirmed by nerve conduction studies. Local space-occupying lesions such as a ganglion, haemangioma, or lipoma occasionally cause this condition, and a more generalized swelling of adjacent tendons in their sheaths, as occurs in early RA, can also predispose. The condition, which may be uni- or bilateral, is more common in women, and in certain metabolic and endocrine diseases such as diabetes and myxoedema. Where no predisposing cause is discovered the term **idiopathic carpal tunnel syndrome** is used.

A causal link with occupation remains unproven, though carpal tunnel syndrome in vibration-exposed workers is a prescribed disease, but with refined diagnostic techniques and more sensitive ergonomic analysis the balance of probability is now shifting to the acceptance that this can be a work-associated condition. It is seen less frequently in patients who do not use their hands substantially, and occurs more often in the dominant hand. Workers using a keyboard seem to be particularly susceptible, though adequately controlled epidemiological studies to identify the precise causal factors are awaited. Musicians and meat cutters who may need to keep the wrist in a flexed position for long periods are particularly susceptible. A stamping or punching action involving the wrist also by predisposes, presumably by regular direct compression.

By analogy with the cervical spine, an inappropriate occupation superimposed on an inherited or acquired propensity for the condition may combine to cross a threshold allowing it to occur. Symptoms are undoubtedly intensified by occasions that involve persistent flexion and extension of the wrist, not necessarily confined to the workplace, and also simple activities such as grasping a steering wheel or holding a book.

The injection of steroids may relieve symptoms temporarily but it is often associated with relapse. The elimination of possible work-associated causes will require alterations to ensure good wrist and forearm posture, the avoidance of prolonged wrist flexion, direct pressure over the carpal tunnel and the avoidance of vibratory handheld tools. Attention to the above factors may in itself result in resolution of symptoms. If not, the use of a wrist splint may also prove of benefit, as may a local steroid injection, but where delayed nerve conduction is confirmed by electromyogram (EMG) studies, surgical decompression of the carpal tunnel as a day-case procedure will be required, including removal of local space occupying lesions if present. Resolution of symptoms is to be expected enabling a return to unrestricted work activity.

Tenosynovitis

The term tenosynovitis describes the inflammation of a tendon and tendon sheath at the wrist or hand causing swelling and localized pain that is aggravated by movement. This can be confirmed on clinical examination when there is local swelling, actually of the tendon sheath rather than the tendon itself, which is painful on palpation, sometimes with crepitus or triggering and occasionally with tethering if the condition is chronic. The treatment is avoidance of the cause or aggravating movements with anti-inflammatory agents topically, orally or by intrasynovial injection of corticosteroids and local anaesthetic. If surgery is required to relieve tethering, histopathological confirmation of the condition can be obtained. The distinctive nature of this condition has long been recognized in the UK as industrial disease A8. When it can be established that the inflammation was caused by manual labour, Industrial Injury Benefit can be claimed under the Social Security (Industrial Injuries) (Prescribed Diseases) Amendment Regulations 1991.

The term **de Quervain's tenosynovitis** is restricted to tenosynovitis of the abductor pollicis longus and extensor pollicis brevis, both tendons to the thumb. Since repetitive movement of the tendon in its sheath is a prime causal requirement and the feature most distinctively lost when the condition is present, the ergonomic case for this being an occupationally-related injury is extremely strong. It is commoner in women than men, perhaps suggesting a hormonal influence (unless women are more likely to be ascribed repetitive tasks in the workplace), and the condition, like frozen shoulder, may be more frequently seen in association with certain diseases. However, a good working history and a positive Finkelstein's test (when ulnar deviation of the wrist with the fingers flexed over the thumb placed in the palm stretches the tendon and reproduces pain over the distal radius and radial side of the wrist) normally leaves no doubt as to the diagnosis and causation. Medical treatment as above is appropriate but surgical release may be required.

Trigger finger or **trigger thumb (stenosing digital tenosynovitis)** implies tenosynovitis of one of the flexor tendons to the finger or thumb. This characteristically occurs with repetitive gripping activities that increase pull and friction on the flexor tendons. Although it can be associated with other conditions (including rheumatoid arthritis, diabetes mellitus, sarcoidosis, and hyperthyroidism) a clear ergonomic history normally correlates with the anatomical abnormalities. In common with other forms of tenosynovitis, rest is beneficial and too early a return to the workplace retards the resolution of the condition. In the prevention of recurrence of symptoms, a postural and ergonomic assessment should be undertaken and, where required, alterations made to upper-limb movements, work practices or workplace design. Modifications to handheld tools may also prove beneficial and, where groups of workers are similarly affected, automation of a process may be indicated.

Work-related upper-limb disorder

The term WRULD covers the non-specific and most contentious of the putative occupationally-related upper limb disorders which may also include such conditions as carpal tunnel syndrome and tenosynovitis. The older term 'repetitive strain injury' (RSI) has justifiably fallen into misuse since the term 'injury', not always true, implies fault.

Although historical nomenclature can be confusing, it seems likely that a syndrome similar to WRULD has been present for centuries. Before the industrial revolution symptoms occurred in agricultural workers. These were perhaps most pronounced in the afflictions experienced by fish workers who, prior to the advent of refrigeration, had to work fast to fillet and prepare the catch before it decayed. Clerk's palsy, described 275 years ago, may have been a white-collar equivalent, and epidemics of 'writer's cramp' described amongst male clerks in the British civil service in the 1830s were then attributed to the introduction of the steel nib—long before the advent of the computer. Interestingly, at a time when only 4–10% of telegraphic staff in the USA were describing 'cramp symptoms', Britain experienced a simultaneous epidemic with up to 60% of a comparable workforce describing symptoms within a period of 4 years.[5] By implication, local psychosocial factors are also important. The most recently reported epidemic has been in Australia in 1985.[6] The growth of the Australian epidemic coincided with the introduction of a work compensation system that allowed lump sum payments for work-related disease. Once the emphasis had been removed from the term 'injury' and the criteria for qualification for compensation made more stringent, the epidemic quietly faded away.

The cause of WRULD, assuming it to exist, is not clear. Studies from Australia[7] purporting to show histological abnormalities in affected muscles of patients complaining of pain due to chronic overuse have no control comparisons. Others have sought to explain the condition in terms of a pain-amplification problem.[8] There remain no clear diagnostic criteria based on symptoms, clinical findings, or tests. There may be overlap with conditions presumed to be predominantly neurological such as focal dystonia and 'writer's cramp', the predominant condition for category A4 (cramp of the hand or forearm) of the work-related conditions that may qualify for industrial injury disablement benefit in the UK. Condition A8, more clearly defined as tenosynovitis, is also clear-cut as a separate entity. It remains to be established whether the symptoms may sometimes form the prodromal phase of a forearm tenosynovitis.

Certain features may occur in the history. There is reasonable agreement on the importance of a change in technique or working practice in initiating symptoms, or sometimes the total amount of a repetitive task can exceed a certain threshold, as when management requires a production line conveyor to be driven faster than it was before. There is agreement that symptoms are initially relieved by a short period of rest, perhaps just overnight, though as symptoms become more chronic not even the weekend or the 2–3 week annual holiday will suffice. Symptoms are variously described as aching, soreness, or tingling. Frequently, symptoms are localized to a particular part of the musculoskeletal apparatus, normally that required for the particular ergonomic task in question. Sometimes they may be more widespread which can cause confusion. The wrist, forearm, and elbow areas are most typically involved at the onset. There may be disturbance of sleep patterns, and generalized fatigue is common.

There are few consistent diagnostic clinical signs. These authors' studies have demonstrated that a reduction in grip strength, when measured by a sphygmomanometer bag inflated to 30 mmHg, is helpful. Others have found an alteration in pain threshold when measured by an algometer. There may be involuntary contraction of muscles and sometimes vasomotor changes, particularly prominent in workers in refrigerating plants.

In investigating the patient it is advisable, having taken a detailed history, first to arrange baseline investigations to exclude conditions such as RA and then, on clinical grounds, to exclude other conditions which may contribute to symptoms. These include cervical spondylosis, frozen shoulder, epicondylitis, and Sudeck's algodystrophy. Often a proportion of symptoms may be attributed to one of these causes. Should they all be absent, non-specific WRULD may be considered a clinical diagnosis by exclusion. An assessment of the patient's psychosocial circumstances may also be helpful. Treatment should include a full explanation of the uncertainties of the diagnosis and reassurance as to a likely favourable outcome if aggravating movements and activities are avoided.

Analgesic and anti-inflammatory medication may prove of some benefit. A workplace postural and ergonomic assessment should be undertaken and modifications introduced where appropriate. Where several individuals have similar complaints, other possible factors also need to be considered including work rate, method of pay, excessive noise, heat or cold or other factors which might increase levels of anxiety and muscular tension when at work. Individuals should be reviewed until resolution of their symptoms and, should this not occur, relocation might need to be considered.

A recent judgement by Judge Prosser,[9] who found against the existence of this condition, may have performed a good service, not only in discouraging people from seeking unreasonable damages in the courts but in highlighting the dichotomy in populations in which prevalences varying from 5% to 60% can be alleged for the same condition. The view that WRULD has 'no place in the medical books' does not, however, accord with the two most recent major seminal textbooks of rheumatology,[10,11] both of which now devote specific sections to this condition. Perhaps the more benign view of a judge , who recently awarded a record settlement to a typist who developed this condition is equally admissible (Personal Communication). He commented that medical evidence on the subject 'would be worthy of medieval theology'. His apt statement 'while I do not rule out the existence of some wider diffuse condition, I do not find it proved to exist' acts both as a concise summary and indictment of current medical understanding (and dispute) on the condition.

Whatever the legal viewpoint, the Health and Safety Executive recognizes the existence of this condition by producing published guidelines[12] for its prevention that employers are now well advised to follow.

Psychosocial factors often predominate. Our own research on production line workers in a biscuit factory, which demonstrated that impaired grip strength was really the only definite physical sign, also showed that psychosocial factors may play a major role.

Prevention concentrates on ensuring that all repetitive actions are performed in the position and style of maximum ergonomic advantage. Job rotation is also important as are adequate periods of rest. Workers should be advised to report to the occupational health department for diagnosis, counselling and medical attention if symptoms of WRULD are noted which, in the early stages are likely to be reversible if adequate precautions are taken.

Conclusions

Some common principles apply in the treatment and management of many of the conditions described above. This section includes aspects of self-management of these conditions for both employers and employees.

Many rheumatic conditions respond to rest. At the workplace this may comprise avoidance of the precipitating action or dilution of the action in the first instance. Changes in technique, posture, or equipment often alleviate symptoms. If not, attention should be directed to appropriate 'pacing' of the workload. For example, if 2.5 hours at a keyboard or on a production line cause symptoms, the maximum duration of working at any one time should be restricted to a lesser period (say 2 hours). The 8-hour day becomes correspondingly extended with half-hour breaks between each 2-hour working period.

If such attention to technique fails to remedy the situation, the total time spent at the workplace may have to be reduced. Ultimately a period of complete rest, perhaps of 1–2 weeks' duration, may be required with a cautious reintroduction to work. Splinting may help up to a point, particularly to stabilize movement of a joint at the workplace, but complete immobilization of part of a limb in a plaster of Paris case may cause disuse osteoporosis with worsening of symptoms and is generally to be avoided other than for brief periods of 10–14 days.

The patient can self-medicate by purchasing either paracetamol, which is a pure analgesic, or ibuprofen, which is an anti-inflammatory drug in oral or topical form. The general practitioner may prescribe from a much wider range of analgesics or NSAIDs. Practitioners are also empowered to prescribe these drugs in doses higher than those recommended on the packets purchased over the counter. Drugs of short half-life can be taken on an 'as required' basis a little before the circumstances that cause discomfort. If these circumstances persist throughout the day, a drug of longer half-life that is suitable for once daily dosing without any fall in blood concentration might be preferred.

An ergonomic assessment at the workplace is often valuable. Where direct access to professional advice from an occupational health department, an ergonomist or occupational therapist is not available, the Disability Employment Advisor (DEA) at the local

Job Centre should be contacted and will provide such a service through the Access to Work scheme.

If individuals are overweight, additional strain is placed on joints. When lower-limb problems predominate, employees should be encouraged to diet to reach the optimum weight for their height.

A variety of physiotherapy techniques are available. These include short-wave diathermy, ultrasound, exercises and hydrotherapy, amongst others. Relaxation techniques and acupuncture are gaining popularity. Physiotherapists may advise on the use of appliances that reduce pain such as a TENS machine.

Employees often resort to fringe medicine, consulting chiropractors, acupuncturists, reflexologists, and others. Chiropractic may be particularly helpful for degenerative conditions of the spine, providing there is no inflammatory component. Otherwise, controlled clinical trials for efficacy of these attentions are often lacking, with the implication that improvement often depends on a brisk placebo response. Nevertheless, if the procedures allow patients to escape the side-effects of drugs, particularly NSAIDs, they should not be denigrated.

Selected references

1 Schmorl G, Junghanns H. *The human spine in health and disease* (trans. EF Besemann). New York: Grune and Stratton, 1971.

2 Allender E. Prevalence, incidence and remission rates of some common rheumatic diseases or syndromes. *Scand J Rheumatol* 1974; 3: 145–153.

3 Kivi P. The aetiology and conservative treatment of humeral epicondylitis. *Scand J Rehab Med* 1982; **15**: 37–41.

4 Binder AI, Hazelman B. Lateral humeral epicondylitis - a study of the natural history and the effect on conservative therapy. *Br J Rheumatol* 1983; **20**: 73–76.

5 *Great Britain and Ireland Post Office Departmental Committee on Telegraphists Cramp Report.* London: HMSO, 1911.

6 Hocking B. Epidemiological aspects of 'repetitive strain injury'. Telecom Australia. *Med J Aust* 1987; **147**: 218–222.

7 Dennett X, Fry HJH. Overuse syndrome: a muscle biopsy study. *Lancet* 1988; **339**: 905–908.

8 Kellgren JH. Observations on referred pain arising from muscle. *Clin Sci* 1938; **3**: 174–190.

9 *Industrial Relations Law Report:* IRL.R 571 1993.

10 Klippel JH, Dieppe PA (ed.) *Rheumatology*, 2nd edn. St Louis: Mosby, 1998.

11 Maddison PJ, Isenberg DA, Woo P, Glass DN (Ed) *Oxford Textbook of Rheumatology*, 2nd. Ed. Vol 2: Oxford Medical Publications, 1998.

12 Health and Safety Executive. *Upper limb disorders: assessing the risks.* Sheffield: HSE Books, 1994.

15

Gastrointestinal and liver disorders

C. Astbury and R. J. Wyke

The gastrointestinal tract and liver are subject to many disease processes, several of which can affect employment and result in large numbers of consultations with general practitioners, referral to hospital specialists, and hospital admissions. The annual financial burden of gastrointestinal disease in 1995–96 was estimated at £10.26 billion of which £7.2 billion was attributed to sickness absence and £3.06 billion to National Health Service (NHS) costs. Long-term sickness absence from gastrointestinal diseases has been estimated to cost £0.89 billion and short-term sickness absence £1.7 billion (Dr G. Lewinson, personal communication). The latter probably represents 0.8–1.4 days lost per employee per year for blue-collar and white-collar workers respectively. In the UK, of the 455 000 people absent from work each day due to sickness, 91 000 (20%) attribute it to gastrointestinal causes, although what proportion of these represent specific gastrointestinal disease is not known. Despite this, there have been very few studies of the influence of diseases of the gastrointestinal tract or liver on work.

Conditions likely to cause employment problems, or risks to individuals and the public, are:

- gastro-oesophageal reflux and hiatus hernia
- peptic ulceration
- acute and chronic liver disease
- inflammatory bowel disease
- ileostomy and colostomy
- gastroenteritis and infestations of the gut
- functional disorders (non-ulcer dyspepsia, irritable bowel syndrome)
- coeliac disease
- chronic pancreatitis.

Conditions likely to meet the definition under the Disability Discrimiation Act 1995 (DDA) are discussed in the appropriate sections below.

Oesophageal reflux and hiatus hernia

The prevalence of gastroesophageal reflux is difficult to assess because of the lack of an accepted definition and a gold standard.[1] Based on the occurrence of symptoms of gastroesophageal reflux and antacid consumption, the prevalence has been calculated at 10% for Scandinavian and American adults. With appropriate positioning during a barium meal, most people over 40 can be shown radiographically to have a hiatus hernia. Only a small number of these patients have symptoms and the precise relation between hiatus hernia and reflux is not clear. Chronic gastroesophageal reflux results in oesophagitis which may be complicated by haematemesis or oesophageal stricture formation. Both these complications tend to occur in the elderly. Dilatation for the latter condition is required in about 1% of all cases; mortality for this procedure is extremely low.

Oesophageal reflux and heartburn are made worse by bending, especially when this is accompanied by heavy lifting. Symptoms often improve with simple measures such as stopping smoking, weight reduction, wearing looser clothes, and antacid therapy. The use of acid suppressing drugs—H2 antagonists and, especially, more powerful proton pump inhibitors (e.g. omeprazole) improves symptoms of reflux and heals oesophagitis. Long-term use may be necessary to enable work to be continued. Patients with severe persistent reflux may develop oesophagitis and oesophageal strictures which, if symptomatic, may require dilation under sedation or, in extreme cases, surgery. Surgery is also undertaken to control severe persistent reflux in severely incapacitated cases, unresponsive to intensive medical therapy. Time off work will depend on the type of work and incision used although laparascopic hiatus hernia repair has resulted in a shorter convalescence and is discussed in Chapter 22.

Special work problems

The following types of work may produce symptoms of reflux in some individuals with these conditions:

- frequent bending
- lifting and carrying heavy or awkward loads
- pulling and pushing of heavy loads
- work involving stooping, crouching, or working in confined spaces, e.g. maintenance fitters, plumbers.

Although the effects of increases in intra-abdominal pressure and stooping can be reduced by safe lifting techniques or modification of manual handling and other work tasks, the effect on symptoms is variable and each case should be assessed on an individual basis. This may need to be taken into account under 'individual factors' as part of a manual handling risk assessment. Provision of a lifting aid may eliminate altogether the lifting component of a task.

Peptic ulceration

Prevalence and incidence

Peptic ulceration is the most important organic gastrointestinal disease in many western countries, affecting at some time approximately 10% of all adult men. During the 1970s there was a fall in hospital admissions and in deaths from peptic ulcer, both of which occur mainly in the elderly patient. The reasons for this change are not clear but it may be due to the influence of modern treatment. Although declining, the resultant sickness absence, morbidity, and mortality are still substantial. In 1991/92, 2.7 million days of sickness/invalidity in England and Wales were attributed to ulcers of the stomach and duodenum; unfortunately, such information may not be based on accurate diagnoses and could include functional disorders of the gut. The risk of developing peptic ulceration is greater for people in jobs with a high level of physical activity than for those undertaking sedentary work and is more prevalent in the north of England and Scotland.[2]

The prevalence of peptic ulcers is difficult to establish as the only accurate way, in life, would be to perform endoscopy or barium meals on a representative sample of the whole population. Data from 13 000 autopsies in Leeds, reported in 1960, showed that 13% of men and 5% of women over the age of 35 suffered from duodenal ulceration, and 3.9% and 2.9% respectively from gastric ulceration. Doll and Avery-Jones' survey of factory workers in London (1951) showed that 5.8% of men and 1.9% of women aged 15—64 had peptic ulceration.[3] A study of a static population in Aberdeen (1968) showed that 8% of men aged 15–64 years had peptic ulcers.

The annual incidence rates for gastric ulcer are 42 per 100 000 in men and 45 per 100 000 in women, while duodenal ulcer occurs in 180 and 85 per 100 000 respectively.[4] There is a tendency for the incidence of peptic ulcers to increase with age. During this century the incidence of gastric ulcer has declined and that of duodenal ulcer has risen.

The incidence of perforation of a gastric ulcer has decreased; this now occurs chiefly in the elderly, and may be associated with smoking and ingestion of non-steroidal anti-inflammatory drugs (NSAIDs) which also result in gastrointestinal bleeding.

Mortality

During the past 30 years there has been a decline in mortality from peptic ulceration among younger people. In 1995 in England and Wales there were 905 deaths from peptic ulcer among people aged 15–64 years. Most deaths occurred in patients aged over 45 years There were more deaths among men than women, with a ratio of 1.3 : 1 for gastric ulcers, and 1.7 : 1 for duodenal ulcers. Although deaths are related to bleeding or perforation, more than half occur after surgery, especially in the elderly patient with intercurrent illness.[5]

Clinical aspects of peptic ulceration affecting work

The most common complaint of patients with peptic ulceration is epigastric pain: less common are vomiting (more frequent with duodenal or pyloric ulceration), gastrointestinal bleeding, and perforation. Gastric and duodenal ulcers cannot be distinguished from the history alone and so endoscopic or barium meal radiography examination is necessary to establish the diagnosis. In patients with gastric ulcer, endoscopy has the advantage of enabling cytology and histological specimens to be obtained to exclude malignancy. Only a few hours off work is required for a barium meal radiographic examination, or for endoscopy performed without sedation (with an analgesic throat spray). When endoscopy is performed with sedation, normal work can usually be resumed the next day.

The clinical course of duodenal ulceration is one of spontaneous relapses and remissions which can vary from a single episode to a progressive disease with few remissions and major complications. The latter include haemorrhage, perforation, or pyloric stenosis, which occur in 1% per year of patients followed, and are commoner in the elderly. The clinical course of gastric ulceration tends to be more continuous and is more often associated with weight loss.

Work may be affected by episodes of abdominal pain, consequent loss of sleep, vomiting, and anaemia. The use of H2 antagonists and the newer gastric proton pump inhibitors (such as omeprazole) heal up to 97% of duodenal and 89% of gastric ulcers by 8 weeks and should avoid loss of time from work. A course of medical treatment relieves symptoms and heals ulceration, but does not prevent further ulceration. Ulcers recur in 80% of treated patients within 1 year, mainly in the first 6 months, and 25% of these ulcers are asymptomatic.

The recognition that most peptic ulcers, in patients not receiving NSAIDs or steroids, are related to the presence in their stomach of infection with *Helicobacter pylori* has revolutionized management and changed the natural history of the disease.[6] Successful eradication of the infection with a combination of an ulcer-healing drug and antibiotics results in healing of 90% of ulcers with a very low (less than 10%) relapse rate. Successful eradication should be confirmed either by repeat gastroscopy and gastric biopsy or by a non-invasive urea breath test. Both techniques must be performed with the patient off proton pump inhibitors for at least 4 weeks. Serology can remain positive for some years after eradication and so should not be used to assess its permanence. Thus the majority of patients can be cured and many of the traditional dietary and occupational restrictions no longer apply. This leaves a small group of patients with ulcers in whom infection with *H. pylori* is resistant to antibiotic treatment or who are taking NSAIDs, corticosteroids, or anticoagulants, or with other chronic medical conditions that might predispose to peptic ulceration. For these patients long-term drug therapy with an H2 receptor antagonist or gastric proton pump inhibitor is the best management.

Surgery is very seldom performed for peptic ulcers. However it is indicated for gastric ulcers which have been shown, endoscopically, to have failed to heal with intensive medical treatment, including eradication of infection with *H. pylori* if present, as there is always the fear of undiagnosed malignancy.

Surgery is also necessary for the small proportion of patients with duodenal ulcers who develop complications, are non-compliant or have symptomatic ulcers unresponsive to medical treatment including eradication of *H. pylori*. Surgical treatment (Chapter 22, p. 441) may require 6–12 weeks absence from work, depending on the type of operation and the work. The most widely used operation is proximal gastric vagotomy or truncal vagotomy and drainage, with a mortality of 0.5% or less and an ulcer recurrence of under 5%.[5] In comparison, partial gastrectomy has a mortality of 3% and a similar recurrence rate.[5] Long-term complications occur in 3% of patients after proximal gastric vagotomy, compared to 14% for patients treated by partial gastrectomy in whom the dumping syndrome and intractable diarrhoea after eating can have very serious consequences for work. Patients may benefit from eating small dry meals and avoiding drinks containing carbohydrate. Other long-term complications, especially of partial gastrectomy, include anaemia, osteomalacia, and, with increasing time, a low risk of carcinoma of the gastric remnant.[5]

Predisposing factors

The most important predisposing factor for peptic ulceration is infection in the stomach with *H. pylori*. Ingestion of aspirin, NSAIDs (see above), and corticosteroids in high doses are generally accepted clinically as predisposing to the complications of peptic ulcer and dyspepsia, but evidence for causing ulceration is not conclusive. Patients with chronic renal failure on dialysis or following transplantation, however, have an increased frequency of peptic ulceration and there is probably an association with hepatic cirrhosis and hyperparathyroidism. Smoking increases the risk of perforation and patients with peptic ulcer should be advised to stop smoking.

Special work problems

Generally, patients with peptic ulceration can pursue any type of work. There is no clear relation between peptic ulceration and stress, but some patients experience exacerbations of symptoms during periods of stress and some, in stressful occupations, may require long-term maintenance drug treatment or even surgery. Men with peptic ulcers tend to perceive stressful life events more negatively and may exhibit more emotional distress in the form of anxiety.

Shiftwork

Although there has been a steady increase in the number of people working shifts, such work probably does not cause peptic ulcers although it may exacerbate symptoms in certain individuals. Furthermore, although many shiftworkers report gastrointestinal disturbances, fewer than the expected number of deaths from gastrointestinal complaints are observed among shiftworkers when compared with national rates. Perhaps shiftworkers are a self-selected group and people with significant gastrointestinal problems, which tend to deteriorate with disturbed routine, seek different work.

Sometimes people are forced to work shifts, temporarily as part of in-service training, or owing to unforeseen circumstances. The financial rewards for working unsocial hours may also encourage an employee with an exacerbation of peptic ulceration to continue working shifts. Where peptic ulceration arises in a shiftworker, medical treatment including eradication of infection with *H. pylori* must be pursued. Only in extremely resistant cases should it be necessary to discontinue shiftwork.

Work in remote areas

If infection with *H. pylori* has been confirmed to be eradicated (see earlier section, Clinical aspects of peptic ulceration affecting work) there should be no bar to patients with peptic ulcers working in remote places, e.g. at sea or offshore. Patients in whom infection was not present in the stomach, or for whom eradication has failed, should be considered for maintenance treatment while working in remote areas. (See Appendices 3 and 4 for details of the Merchant Shipping Regulations and guidance for offshore workers and divers).

Acute liver disease[7]

Acute viral hepatitis

There were 1146 cases of hepatitis A and 908 cases of acute hepatitis B notified in England and Wales in 1998.[8] Figures for acute Hepatitis C, as distinct from those who have antibody to the virus alone, are not available but are certainly smaller than for acute hepatitis B.

There is confusion among lay people and some doctors regarding modes of transmission and the relative risks presented by patients with different types of hepatitis. In addition there is a lack of understanding of the interpretation of serological tests for hepatitis B which can result in people being regarded incorrectly as infectious.

Hepatitis A (infectious hepatitis)

Hepatitis A is caused by an enterovirus (HAV) transmitted by the faecal–oral route and affects chiefly children, with only 20% of cases in patients over 16 years of age.

Prevalence

Children in institutions and adults in communities with poor sanitation, as in developing countries, are at highest risk. Although the prevalence is generally decreasing worldwide there was actually an increase in the UK from 3.65 cases per 100 000 in 1987 to 14.4 in 1990. In 1997 there were 1837 notified cases of hepatitis A in the UK. Serological evidence of previous infection is found in 45% of adults, and increases with age from less than 20% in people under 30 to nearly 60% in those over 45. Most seropositive individuals do not give a history of jaundice. Sporadic cases and epidemics are caused by eating virus-containing shellfish or cold food (particularly dairy products) contaminated by food handlers during the prodrome of acute or anicteric hepatitis.

Clinical aspects affecting work

Hepatitis is anicteric in 50% of cases and has an excellent prognosis with a mortality of less than 0.15%, no progression to chronic liver disease, and no carrier state.

The incubation period is 21–40 days and the patient is infectious while virus is in the stools, i.e. from 2–3 weeks before until not more than 8 days after jaundice is apparent (Fig. 15.1). Hence the period of maximal infectivity occurs before the patient is symptomatic. Patients feel unwell during the prodrome but often improve with the onset of jaundice. Lethargy may continue for 6 weeks or for as long as 3 months. Diagnosis is based on the detection in the serum of the IgM antibody to hepatitis A. The presence of the IgG type of antibody indicates either previous exposure to HAV or passive immunity from immune serum globulin or blood transfusion.

Special work problems

With the exception of food handlers, patients can resume or continue all forms of work as soon as they feel fit.

Food handlers must stay off work until jaundice has disappeared, or for 1 week after the onset of jaundice, whichever is the longer. Those with anicteric hepatitis should remain off work for 1 week after serum transaminases have reached a peak. It must be recognized that the patient will have been infectious during the asymptomatic phase, and special efforts should be made to monitor other staff to detect contact cases. Ideally staff should report even minor indispositions, so that liver function tests and IgM hepatitis A serology can be checked on anyone with suspicious symptoms. This surveillance should be continued for 10 weeks after the index case is diagnosed. It is unnecessary to give

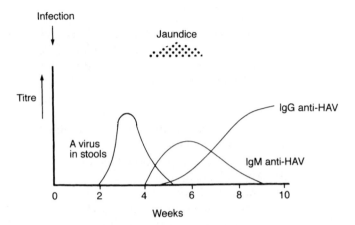

Fig. 15.1 Sequential appearance and disappearance of hepatitis A virus in stool and antibody (IgM and IgG anti-HAV) in the serum of a patient with acute hepatitis A. The infectious period (excretion of virus) is normally before the development of jaundice.

unaffected staff immune globulin since this may attenuate symptoms without preventing virus excretion.

Prevention of hepatitis A infection[9]

Active immunization with hepatitis A vaccine, two doses intramuscularly 2–4 weeks apart induces seroconversion in 90–95% of recipients. It is recommended for frequent travellers to areas of high or moderate HAV endemicity or for those staying for more than 3 months. The only occupational group for whom routine immunization is recommended are laboratory workers working with the virus. Serological evidence of previous infection (IgG HAV) should be checked before immunizations. Immunization for health-care workers and those working in residential institutions and with young children is not routinely recommended but may be considered as a control measure in the case of local community outbreaks. There is a potential risk for sanitation workers exposed to untreated sewage, and immunization should be considered as part of the control measures required under the Control of Substances Hazardous to Health Regulations 1994.

Hepatitis B (serum hepatitis)[7]

Hepatitis B results from the transfer of the hepatitis virus (HBV) in blood, blood products, or body fluids and secretions from an infected to a susceptible individual. Transmission by blood transfusion is extremely rare in this country, but drug addiction, tattooing, body piercing, acupuncture, dental treatment, and homosexual practices are well-recognized means of transmission.

Horizontal transmission from person to person may result from sexual contact or sharing the same razor blade, toothbrush, or syringe. Vertical transmission from mother to child is particularly important in highly endemic areas such as the Far East. If the mother is a carrier of hepatitis B or suffers acute hepatitis during the third trimester, infection of the newborn infant is likely.

Prevalence

The number of notified cases of acute hepatitis B in the UK has fallen from more than 1500 in 1986 to 908 in 1998.[8] Few cases occur in children and the elderly, with 50% of cases aged 15–34 years. The prevalence of acute hepatitis B in adults aged 15–65 years has been calculated at 6 per 100 000 for men and 2 per 100 000 for women.

Mortality

Mortality from acute hepatitis B among adults aged 15–64 is about 0.6% for men and 0.3% for women, and tends to increase with age.

In the UK, approximately 3% of the normal population have serological markers of previous exposure to HBV. Approximately 10% of patients, mainly men, progress to the carrier state with persisting hepatitis B viraemia. Worldwide, however, there are estimated to be 350 million carriers, varying from less than 0.15% of the UK population to 15% in the Far East. The risk of becoming a carrier is highest after hepatitis in neonates.

Clinical aspects affecting work capacity

Acute hepatitis B has an incubation period of 3–6 months, with maximum infectivity during the late incubation and prodromal periods (Fig 15.2). Clinical illness tends to be more severe than in hepatitis A, but over half of the infections are mild and often anicteric. In addition to the normal features of hepatitis an urticarial rash and arthropathy, part of a serum-sickness-like syndrome, are occasionally seen.

Serological markers of HBV indicate the stage of infection and the degree of infectivity. Serological findings in a typical case of acute type B hepatitis and progression to chronic infection are shown in Figs 15.2 and 15.3. The presence in patients' serum of hepatitis B surface (Australia) antigen (HBsAg) should be followed by clinical

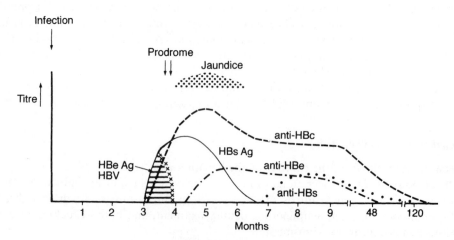

Fig. 15.2 Relation of serological markers and symptoms of hepatitis to infection with hepatitis B in an uncomplicated acute case. The period of maximum infectivity (shaded area) during which hepatitis B, viral DNA, and HbE antigen are found in the serum is mainly immediately before jaundice develops. Note clearance of surface (HbsAG) and e antigens with formation of antibodies (anti-HBe and anti-HBs).

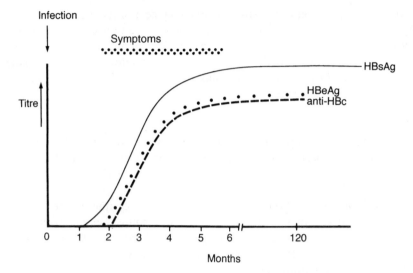

Fig. 15.3 Development of a hepatitis B carrier after acute hepatitis B. Note persistence in a very high titre of surface (HBsAg) and e antigens, and antibody to core (anti-HBc); also absence of antibodies to hepatitis B surface (anti-HBs) and e (anti-HBe) antigens.

examination for features of acute or chronic liver disease and further tests for other serological markers of hepatitis B. The presence of hepatitis B surface antibody (Anti-HBS) indicates previous contact with the HBV or vaccination with development of immunity, but the patient is not infectious. High titres of the IgM antibody to core (IgM anti-HBc) denote an acute type B viral hepatitis (Fig 15.2). The finding of hepatitis e antigen correlates with a high degree of infectivity, while antibody to e shows seroconversion with a low degree of infectivity. From a practical point of view the patient with a resolving acute hepatitis is not infectious once hepatitis B surface antigen (HBsAg) is no longer detectable in the blood.

Chronic carriers are those patients who fail to clear the surface antigen from the blood 6 months after acute hepatitis B (Fig 15.3) and can be subdivided into:

- **Simple carriers**: Blood contains hepatitis B surface antigen in low titre and antibody to hepatitis e, but hepatitis B virus and DNA polymerase activity are absent. Such cases have a low infectivity.
- **Super carriers**: Blood contains high titre of hepatitis B surface antigen *and* e antigen. DNA polymerase activity, and hepatitis B viral DNA are present and the patient is highly infectious.

Prognosis of carriers

Most carriers are in good health and able to work normally but should be referred to a hepatologist. The 'healthy' carriers who are diagnosed by chance will tend to be HBeAg negative and have a near normal liver biopsy, with fewer than 2% developing chronic active hepatitis or cirrhosis. By contrast, in the person who becomes a carrier after a clinical attack of hepatitis B there is a 70% chance of histological evidence of chronic liver disease, mainly chronic persistent hepatitis, and 10% chance of cirrhosis. Such cases tend to be HbeAg positive; in the long term they may seroconvert and liver diseases improve, but cases with persistent infection have a high risk of developing cirrhosis and hepato-cellular carcinoma, which has a bad prognosis. Strenuous efforts are being made to develop treatments for chronic carriers to make them clear the virus by means of immunotherapy and antiviral agents.

Time off work

During the acute phase the symptomatic patient will not feel well enough to work and usually rests at home for a period which is normally about twice the time of bed rest.

Risk of spread of infection

There is no evidence of transmission of hepatitis B by casual contact in the workplace, or from contaminated food, water, airborne, or faecal–oral routes. Spread of infection is likely only through intimate contact with the patient's blood, or body secretions, as occurs during normal sexual intercourse and some homosexual activities. Infection may also occur through needlestick injuries.

Prevention of hepatitis B[10]

Passive immunity can be provided by hepatitis B hyperimmune serum globulin but is only of value if administered prophylactically or within 48 hours of exposure to infection (0.06 mg/kg intramuscularly). Such treatment is indicated only for victims of parenteral (needlestick or mucous membrane contamination) exposure to HBsAg-positive blood or body fluids, babies born to HbsAg-positive mothers, and sexual contacts of acute sufferers. Active hepatitis B immunization should be started at the same time as passive immunization.

Active immunization can be achieved by hepatitis B vaccine, three doses over 6 months. The vaccine should be given to people who are exposed regularly to, or at increased risk of contracting, hepatitis B; in particular certain healthcare personnel (Box 15.1). However, immunization of people at risk is not necessary if their serum contains antibody to hepatitis B surface (anti-HBs) or core (anti-HBc) antigen. Overall, approximately 10% of individuals fail to produce a response to the vaccine with hepatitis B surface antibody (anti HBs) levels of >10 iu/ml, so the antibody response should be checked 2–4 months after completion of the primary course. Booster doses should be considered 5 years after completion of the primary course and if accidental or occupational exposure to the virus occurs. The vaccine must be administered into the deltoid muscle and not into the buttocks as there is less subcutaneous fat and a higher antibody response is obtained. These measures cannot be regarded as a substitute for safe work practices.

Special work problems of the hepatitis B carrier

The hepatitis B carrier is usually in good health and should not be treated as a hepatitis leper or barred from any type of work (except certain procedures undertaken in health-care work) provided that simple measures are taken. The only risk to others is from accidental inoculation of blood or body fluids and this is unlikely to occur in the work situation except in situations where first aid is administered. Carriers must appreciate the importance of covering cuts and abrasions.

Box 15.1   General indications for vaccination against hepatitis B

- Healthcare staff including medical students
- Surgical and dental staff and dental students
- Hospital and laboratory staff in regular contact with blood or needles
- Necropsy staff
- Direct carers of hepatitis B carriers, including genitourinary, endoscopy, and accident and emergency staff
- Staff in oncology, haemodialysis, haemophilia, and liver units
- Staff providing maintenance treatment with blood or blood products
- Blood transfusion service staff
- Accidental exposure to hepatitis B material
- Staff on secondment to areas of the world with a high prevalence of hepatitis B
- Patients
  - first entrants to residential care for mentally handicapped
  - on maintenance haemodialysis or with chronic renal failure before dialysis or transplantation
  - requiring multiple blood transfusions or injections of blood products—e.g. haemophilia
  - natural or acquired immune deficiency
- Contacts of patients with hepatitis B
  - sexual partners of patients with acute hepatitis B or carriers
  - other family members in close contact
  - infants born to women with acute hepatitis B or who are hepatitis B carriers, especially those with e antigen
- Other staff
  - ambulance and rescue services
  - staff at reception centres for people from high endemic areas (e.g. SE Asia)
- Others at risk
  - promiscuous homosexuals or prostitutes (male or female)
  - intravenous drug abusers
- Lower risk
  - long-term men prisoners
  - staff of custodial institutions
  - some police personnel
- People living in intermediate and high prevalence areas
  - women
  - infants
  - children
  - susceptible individuals

In general, people in low-risk careers or those in administrative posts, out-patient sections, and those working in the community will not require vaccination.

Concern is sometimes expressed over the action to be taken if carriers cut themselves. Like any normal individual, they should dress the wound and clean up any spilt blood from the object or area thoroughly with a solution of household bleach to kill the virus and then apply warm soapy water and wipe again with bleach. Food contaminated with blood as a result of the accident should be discarded for both hygienic and aesthetic reasons. With these provisos, the carrier can continue to work in all jobs including food handling, catering, hairdressing, and teaching but should, of course, not act as a blood donor. Carriers should not be barred from using office equipment, toilets, showers, or eating facilities.

First aid

First aid personnel should be reassured that the risk of contracting the disease during normal first aid procedures is minutely small, providing standard good cross-infection control procedures are followed for all casualties. First aiders should be trained in the safe handling of body fluids, including the use of household bleach to disinfect contaminated surfaces, and in the safe disposal of clinical waste. Disposable gloves should be provided for use in situations where contamination with blood or body fluids may occur.

Hepatitis B and healthcare workers

The specific problem of healthcare workers is addressed in Department of Health Guidelines.[10,11] Healthcare workers who are hepatitis B e antigen positive are restricted from performing exposure-prone procedures, which are defined as those where there is a risk that injury to the worker may bring the patient's open tissues into contact with the worker's blood. Such procedures include those where the worker's gloved hands may be in contact with sharp instruments, needle tips, and sharp tissues (spicules of bone or teeth) inside an open body cavity, wound, or confined anatomical space where the hands or fingertips may not be completely visible at all times.[11] These include most surgical procedures and dentistry. Currently healthcare workers who are hepatitis B surface antigen positive but e antigen negative are not restricted unless they have been associated with transmission of infection to a patient. The guidance is under continuing review and, in future, additional tests of infectivity may be required. Occupational physicians should discuss individual cases with the Expert Advisory Panel listed in the guidelines. (See also p. 476.)

Non-A–non-B hepatitis and hepatitis C[7]

Acute hepatitis without serological markers of hepatitis A, hepatitis B, hepatitis *delta* virus, cytomegalovirus, or Epstein–Barr virus has been termed non-A–non-B hepatitis of which 50% is hepatitis C. Such cases are responsible for 15% of sporadic hepatitis in England and Wales and 90% of post-transfusion-related hepatitis. Hepatitis C is responsible for 95% of hepatitis occurring after transfusion of blood products. Blood donors in the UK are routinely screened for antibody to hepatitis C which is present in less than 0.1% of samples. The currently available serological tests for hepatitis C do not always indicate an infectious state and there is probably no risk to people in normal social activities and work contact with a serologically positive individual, so no particular restrictions are required; but these individuals should not donate blood. Epidemiologically hepatitis C resembles hepatitis B with an incubation period of about 5–12 weeks. The hepatitis is usually mild and frequently subclinical but progression to chronic liver disease, including cirrhosis, occurs in 25% of cases over 10–20 years. As with cases of hepatitis C, cases of non-A–non-B hepatitis pose no threat to others in the course of normal social and work activities so no restrictions are necessary except on blood donation.

There are currently no specific guidelines restricting the practice of healthcare workers who are hepatitis C positive, but they should be restricted in the same way as those with hepatitis B.

Chronic liver disease[7]

Cirrhosis

Cirrhosis results from chronic liver injury as a result of which inflammation and necrosis of liver cells leads to fibrosis and nodule formation. Alcohol is the commonest cause of cirrhosis, but it will be seen from Box 15.2 that not all cirrhotics are alcoholics. The important sequelae of cirrhosis are hepatocellular failure and portal hypertension. These cause serious complications including the development of ascites, encephalopathy, jaundice, gastrointestinal bleeding from oesophageal varices, and malnutrition. Any of these complications can have serious implications for work. This section deals with the problems of patients with cirrhosis, in particular the alcoholic type of cirrhosis.

Box 15.2   Some common causes of cirrhosis

- Alcohol
- Viral hepatitis type B, C, D, or non-A–non-B
- Chronic active (lupoid) hepatitis
- Metabolic, e.g. haemochromatosis
- Wilson's disease
- α_1-antitrypsin deficiency
- Drugs, e.g. methotrexate
- Hepatic venous outflow obstruction
- Budd–Chiari syndrome
- Chronic cholestasis, e.g. primary biliary cirrhosis
- Cryptogenic

Prevalence

The prevalence of cirrhosis in the UK is 15 per 100 000. 60% is due to alcohol, 30% is cryptogenic, and 6% results from chronic active hepatitis. The mean age of diagnosis of alcoholic cirrhosis is 47 years in women and 52 years in men.

Alcoholism continues to be a serious problem, with 2 million people in Britain experiencing symptoms of alcohol dependence (male to female ratio 3 : 1). The 1993 Health Survey of England considered that 9% of men and 5% of women who drank more than occasionally could be regarded as 'problem drinkers'. The definition of 'problem drinker' was that they had experienced two or more problems from psychological or physical dependence on alcohol. The peak age for problem drinking was 25–34 years for both sexes.[12]

In England and Wales 28% of men and 12% of women drink at or above the recommended sensible limits (21 and 14 units of alcohol per week respectively).[13] In 1995 the Department of Health caused some confusion by suggesting that the limits might be increased moderately, but this did not meet with the agreement of the main medical and scientific bodies who continue to recommend that 21 and 14 units of alcohol per week are the respective sensible drinking limits for men and women.

Alcoholic liver disease has been increasing in women, who develop it at an earlier age than men and have a worse prognosis.

Prognosis

There were 2200 deaths from alcoholic liver disease and cirrhosis among people aged 15–64 years in England and Wales in 1995, with a ratio of 1.7 : 1 men to women. In the most acute form of liver injury, alcohol causes acute alcoholic hepatitis which is a pre-cirrhotic condition. The overall 5 year survival depends on the severity of the liver inflammation and on whether the patient stops drinking: for those who stop drinking it is 74%, compared to 34% for those who continue. Prognosis is worst for women and patients with bleeding oesophageal varices, and best for cases with well-compensated liver disease.

Clinical aspects affecting work

The time off work required for treatment depends on the severity of the liver disease, ranging from none to several months for severe hepatic decompensation such as occurs in alcoholic hepatitis. Follow-up is likely to vary according to whether the patient is attending an alcohol-dependency clinic or medical out-patients. In the extreme case of a patient at work but undergoing endoscopic sclerotherapy to obliterate oesophageal varices, appointments, often with overnight stay, may be necessary every 2–3 weeks for up to 6 months. Such treatment reduces the risk of bleeding and may improve prognosis.

The effect of chronic liver disease, regardless of the aetiology, depends on the degree of hepatic decompensation, in particular on hepatic encephalopathy, ascites, and gastrointestinal bleeding.

Hepatic encephalopathy

Mental impairment, reduced physical fitness, and tremor may all reduce work capacity. The development of hepatic (portal-systemic) encephalopathy is usually a feature of severe liver disease or a complication of the now unfashionable operation of portacaval shunt. Some patients with cirrhosis but without clinical features of encephalopathy have impairment of psychomotor function on testing sufficient to disrupt their everyday life and even render them unfit to drive. This condition has been termed **latent encephalopathy.** Encephalopathy can be chronic or intermittent and precipitated by a number of causes including a high protein meal, infection, drugs, or bleeding into the gut. Some patients are very susceptible to meals high in animal protein and have to take a special diet and/or lactulose to alter the bowel flora.

Ascites

The presence of ascites may limit physical performance, both by virtue of the mechanical effect of the large volume of fluid (up to 30 litres) and the associated malnutrition.

Fortunately, ascites can usually be controlled with diuretics or paracentesis and hence problems with work can be avoided.

Bleeding from oesophageal varices. The prognosis of patients with bleeding from oesophageal varices depends on the severity of the underlying liver disease and on further episodes of bleeding. Recurrence of bleeding occurs in 60% of patients within 1 year.

Varices secondary to extrahepatic portal venous obstruction. Oesophageal varices also occur in patients without cirrhosis, in whom obstruction, for example from thrombosis to the portal venous system, results in portal hypertension. Such patients commonly present as children with variceal bleeding which can recur during childhood but becomes less frequent after puberty. They have an excellent prognosis, unlike patients with portal hypertension secondary to cirrhosis.

Associated conditions
Other conditions associated with cirrhosis include diabetes mellitus (which is 2–4 times commoner than in the normal population), malnutrition, and peptic ulceration (although this association has been challenged by some). Bone disease, especially affecting the back, is a problem for patients with chronic cholestasis, such as from primary biliary cirrhosis. They may also be troubled by pruritis which can be so distressing and intractable that it may cause suicide. In those with alcoholic liver disease, other systemic effects of alcohol (such as on the central nervous system including acute withdrawal; peripheral neuropathy; cerebrovascular accident; or cardiomyopathy) may all impair or prevent work.

Special work problems
Ideally, patients with complications of cirrhosis, that is ascites, encephalopathy, or bleeding from oesophageal varices, should have been managed by a specialist before resuming work. Although alcohol addiction and dependency are excluded from the definition of impairment under the DDA, the complications arising from alcoholism especially ascites and hepatic encephalopathy, will require individual assessment.

Certain occupations are particularly associated with the risks of alcoholism. They include those working in the manufacture, distribution, and sale of alcohol; commercial travellers; seamen and those in the armed forces; and journalists, doctors, and entertainers. To employ someone with an alcohol problem in one of these jobs is inadvisable. Whether alcohol is a problem to the individual can be assessed quickly by the use of four 'CAGE' questions (Box 15.3; see also Chapter 25).

Box 15.3   CAGE questions[14]
1. Have you ever felt you ought to **C**ut down your drinking?
2. Have people **A**nnoyed you by criticizing your drinking?
3. Have you ever felt bad or **G**uilty about your drinking?
4. Have you ever had a drink first thing in the morning (an '**E**ye opener') to get rid of a hangover?

Two or more positive replies are said to identify problem drinkers.

Overt encephalopathy is uncommon but such patients may be a hazard to themselves and others and should not be relied on for jobs requiring a high degree of vigilance, including driving. The presence of latent encephalopathy is more difficult to identify but may have equally serious consequences for work. Individual suitability for driving duties should be discussed with the medical branch of the Driver and Vehicle Licensing Authority (DVLA) (see Appendix 1). Patients who have been dependent on alcohol are barred from holding a vocational licence until they can demonstrate evidence of uninterrupted absence of dependency and misuse for 3 years. Confirmation of satisfactory liver enzyme tests and mean corpuscular volume as well as examination by a consultant with a special interest in alcohol abuse is required.

There is no evidence that bleeding from oesophageal varices is precipitated by particular occupational activities. Patients who have suffered episodes of bleeding from varices will normally have undergone sclerotherapy to obliterate the varices by the time they resume work. If treatment has not been completed or undertaken, it is prudent for them to avoid jobs involving heavy lifting as the associated increase in intra-abdominal pressure might rupture a varix. It is also advisable for them to avoid contact sports.

Once sclerosis of the varices is completed there is no reason why their work should be restricted, although it would be unwise to travel to remote places where medical services are limited. Patients with ascites may experience difficulty with strenuous work, especially lifting, or with bending and stooping.

Handling of hepatotoxic substances by patients with liver disease

Many substances, including drugs and certain chemicals, particularly solvents which are found in workplaces and are hepatic enzyme inducers, are known to cause liver damage, but by far the most important environmental hepatotoxin is alcohol. Data on these substances are derived from the accidental or deliberate exposure of animals or humans with normal liver function to toxic substances. For obvious ethical reasons, there are virtually no data on the effect of these toxins on patients with liver diseases. Unfortunately, even a knowledge of the mode of action of these substances and the potential influence of liver disease cannot predict accurately the outcome of exposure on the individual patient with hepatic disease.

Hepatotoxic substances exert their effect in one of two ways:

- by the action of a toxic metabolite, produced by the microsomal enzymes in the liver, which binds to liver macromolecules and results in the necrosis of the cell
- by immunological action the metabolite binds to the liver cell and results in a change of antigenicity of the cell membrane with destruction of the cell by the immune system.

Susceptibility to liver damage depends on whether the rate at which the toxic metabolite is formed is greater than the rate of the detoxification, usually by conjugation with compounds such as glutathione. Once the stores of these protective compounds are exhausted, liver necrosis follows. Chronic exposure to certain substances, such as anticonvulsants, results in induction of the liver microsomal enzymes with increased production of hepatotoxic metabolites. But, paradoxically, these enzyme inducers may stimulate other pathways for the production of non-toxic metabolites. Although alcohol elevates the levels of hepatic enzymes, the effect on the handling of hepatotoxins is variable and inconsistent. Thus, chronic alcohol exposure can potentiate the toxic effect of paracetamol, whereas acute exposure protects against paracetamol damage but potentiates carbon tetrachloride hepatotoxicity. It is impossible to predict the result of exposure to hepatotoxic agents of a patient with a normal liver who is also taking an enzyme-inducing agent.

Influence of liver disease

There are great variations in the metabolism of toxic substances by patients with liver disease. These are related not only to the severity of the liver disease but also to genetic and environmental factors which result in changes in the activity of liver enzymes. The reduced hepatic mass may result in reduced conversion of the substance to a toxic metabolite and so protect against damage. But protective co-factors and detoxifying enzymes are likely to be reduced and will tend to potentiate liver damage. The outcome of exposure depends on the relative balance between these two effects of the liver disease.

Guidelines for the employment of workers handling hepatotoxins

The previous paragraphs show the unpredictability of hepatotoxins in patients with liver disease and explain the need for restricting the exposure of such people to these substances.

Patients with chronic liver disease or active acute liver disease should not work or be exposed to hepatotoxins, but there are exceptions such as those who have had hepatitis A; resolved acute viral hepatitis B, or hepatitis C in whom liver function tests and liver histology have returned to normal; and patients with gallstones unless they are jaundiced or have developed secondary biliary cirrhosis which is very rare. All people working with hepatotoxic agents should avoid alcohol and enzyme-inducing agents such as anticonvulsants, in particular phenobarbitone and phenytoin.

Inflammatory bowel disease[15]

The most common types of inflammatory bowel disease in the UK are ulcerative colitis and Crohn's disease, both of which are of unknown aetiology. In ulcerative colitis inflammation is limited to the mucosa of the colon, whereas in Crohn's disease the whole of the gastrointestinal tract from the lips to the anus may be affected by transmural inflammation. Both diseases are characterized primarily by diarrhoea, but abdominal pain and the formation of abscesses, gut perforation, and fistulae are features of Crohn's disease.

Inflammatory bowel disease and employment

Inflammatory bowel disease remains poorly understood by employers and doctors, many of whom remember from their student days the sight of a young patient with extensive, progressive, and disabling Crohn's disease. Such cases are the exception rather than the rule, and most patients with controlled inflammatory bowel disease lead a normal life and work with little sickness absence. Nevertheless, unnecessary concern is expressed over their employment, especially of those with stomas, and employers must learn that most will make perfectly satisfactory employees capable of most occupations, although exacerbations of their chronic condition may require them to have more periods of sickness absence than non-affected employees.

Prevalence and incidence

The prevalence of these diseases varies in different parts of the UK. A survey from Oxford between 1951 and 1960 estimated that there were 80 cases of ulcerative colitis and 9 of Crohn's disease per 100 000 population, with an annual incidence of 6.5 and 1.8 per 100 000 population respectively. Crohn's disease is becoming more common, due in part to increased familiarity with the condition: recent estimates suggest there are 40 000 people in the UK with Crohn's disease and 3000 new cases are diagnosed each year.

Men and women are equally affected by Crohn's disease, while ulcerative colitis is more common in women. Both diseases can start at any age with a peak from 15 to 40 years and a secondary peak at 55.

Mortality and morbidity of inflammatory bowel disease

Both types of disease are associated with diarrhoea which can result in intermittent or persistent morbidity the incidence of which is difficult to estimate accurately. The occasional patient experiences one isolated episode only; conversely, a fulminating presentation may require early emergency surgery.

Ulcerative colitis

Patients with ulcerative proctitis have a normal life expectancy but may have considerable urgency of defecation and diarrhoea. Sometimes such distal disease may spread to the whole colon. Patients with more extensive ulcerative colitis have an increased mortality during the first year after diagnosis, but after this mortality is the same as for the general population. Surgery is necessary for patients who fail to respond to medical treatment and is likely in 1 in 50 patients within 5 years of the onset of proctitis, 1 in 20 with left-sided colitis and 1 in 3 with total colitis. The most common type of surgery is panproctocolectomy with creation of an ileostomy, which has a mortality of less than 1% in experienced hands. Such patients have a normal life expectancy with only minor limitations of their work. An alternative to an ileostomy, for patients with ulcerative colitis but not Crohn's disease, may be the creation of an ileoanal anastomosis with a pouch. The advantage is that patients do not require a stoma but usually have to have their bowels open approximately 3 times a day. The surgical morbidity tends to be higher than for the creation of a stoma and more than one operation is required with consequent loss of time from work. Patients with total colitis of more than 10 years duration, especially those in whom disease commenced before the age of 20, have an increased risk of carcinoma of the colon and prophylactic colectomy may be advisable.

Crohn's disease

Morbidity

The transmural inflammation of the bowel can result in thickening, obstruction, and perforation of the bowel wall, with liability to fistulae or abscess formation. Such complications can cause major morbidity requiring surgery or may be relatively asymptomatic. The natural history of the disease is not related to the age of onset but depends on the extent and site of the lesions. Thus, disease limited to the terminal ileum has a better prognosis than diffuse inflammation of the small bowel. Disease of the colon and rectum will result in distressing symptoms of diarrhoea and urgency, while small bowel disease can have a profound nutritional effect. Exacerbations of the disease occur at variable intervals after presentation, with 70% of patients experiencing relapse within 5 years.

Mortality

The risk of dying does not increase with duration of disease and is highest for patients whose disease began before the age of 40. Late mortality is only slightly in excess of that expected, with deaths related to complications of surgery and the development of carcinoma of the bowel.

Clinical aspects of inflammatory bowel disease affecting work

The main problems for patients, irrespective of the type of inflammatory bowel disease, are frequency and urgency of defecation, general fatigue, and less commonly, arthritis. In line with the DDA, functional capacity assessment (FCA) may be necessary for such patients. Urgency is related to inflammation and reduced capacity of the rectum and is as major a problem for someone with proctitis as it is with inflammation involving the whole colon. The urgency and resultant incontinence are very disabling and cause serious restrictions to a patient's life and work. The National Association for Colitis and Crohn's Disease (see Appendix 7) issues members with a 'Can't Wait' card which can be presented in shops and places displaying the NACC logo, to help gain access to a toilet.

Most patients with a mild attack of inflammatory bowel disease without constitutional upset can be treated as out-patients and usually without loss of time from work. Treatment of moderate or severe attacks generally requires rest in bed, or in hospital if there is constitutional upset. Time off work for relapses treated medically varies from 2 weeks to 2 months.

Other conditions associated with inflammatory bowel disease

- **Arthritis**, which occurs in 10% of patients with ulcerative colitis and in 20% with Crohn's disease, tends to be mild and to affect the lower limbs and is associated with active bowel disease.
- **Sacroiliitis** occurs in 15% of patients with inflammatory bowel disease but is usually not severe and seldom progresses to involve the lumbar and thoracic spine. Unlike peripheral arthritis, sacroiliitis is not related to the extent or severity of underlying

bowel disease and can antedate the onset of the latter. These problems may cause some limitation of activity and may need to be assessed on a individual basis (see also Chapters 11 and 14).

- **Iritis** is an uncommon (0.5–3%) but serious complication of inflammatory bowel disease, causing painful blurred vision and headaches. It is usually associated with exacerbations of disease and with other extra-intestinal manifestations, such as arthritis and erythema nodosum. Steroid therapy may be required, but colectomy does not always result in resolution.
- **Skin problems**, the most severe of which are pyoderma gangrenosum and erythema nodosum, occur in up to 9% of patients, mainly those with ulcerative colitis. Lesions tend to occur on the legs, are associated with active bowel disease in the case of erythema nodosum, and often require steroid therapy.

Side-effects of medical treatment

Systemic steroids are seldom used long-term in the management of patients with inflammatory bowel disease, with the exception of a small number of cases with extensive Crohn's disease of the small bowel. Large doses used in an acute severe attack can cause greater side-effects than in a normal person, owing to the low serum albumin. **Salazopyrine**, used to reduce the frequency and severity of relapse in ulcerative colitis, can cause distressing headaches and rashes, but side-effects are less frequent with the more commonly used preparations containing only 5-aminosalicylic acid.

Surgical treatment

Surgical treatment is necessary for patients with ulcerative colitis who fail to respond to aggressive medical treatment or who are at risk of developing carcinoma of the colon. For Crohn's disease, surgery is indicated for the relief of mechanical problems such as strictures or fistulae, or for resection of severely diseased segments of bowel which fail to respond to intensive medical therapy.

Time off work for bowel surgery

Time off work depends on the type of operation and ranges from 2 weeks for a minor procedure to up to 6 months for panproctocolectomy and ileostomy. Employers should be encouraged to be supportive of patients during this time, as ultimate return to work can be expected. Surgical treatment, especially the formation of an ileostomy, usually restores the patient's general health to normal with greater energy, fewer problems with work, and less sickness absence. It is often only after surgery that everyone appreciates just how debilitating the inflammatory bowel disease has been. An ileostomy may require surgical refashioning, especially during the first year after its creation, but thereafter it should be relatively trouble-free. The formation of a pouch and ileoanal anastomosis is more complex and more time off work is necessary.

Patients with ulcerative colitis are usually restored to normal health once the colon has been removed. Crohn's disease, however, is frequently characterized by recurrence of disease despite surgical resection. Thus, 55% of cases develop recurrent disease 10 years after resection of affected bowel. The patient with Crohn's disease affecting long segments of small bowel can be a particular problem, as surgical resection is undesirable. Such cases are uncommon and may require long-term corticosteroid therapy.

Special work problems

Despite the potential for ill health, most patients with chronic inflammatory bowel disease are able to continue to work. One survey found 70% of out-patients to be working with good continuity of employment, over a 6 year period of follow-up. Sickness absence was not high, with 70% of patients having lost no time off work in the preceding year. Irrespective of the type of inflammatory bowel disease, patients with an ileostomy took less sickness absence and experienced fewer problems at work, than those without.[16]

Changes of work due to health and surgery[16]

Premature retirement on account of ill health is necessary for a few patients (4%) often due to associated conditions (arthritis) rather than to the inflammatory bowel disease itself or surgery. About 50% of patients may find it necessary to change their employment due to their health and about 10% have to modify their work. After surgery many patients are able to resume work often after long periods of sickness absence. Time off work after surgery tends to be longer for patients who undergo panproctocolectomy or ileoanal anastomosis with a pouch than for segmental resections or ileorectal anastomosis. These differences are in part related to the delayed healing of the perineal wound of panproctocolectomy and the more complex nature of the surgery necessary for the creation of a pouch.

Unsuitable work for patients with inflammatory bowel disease

Most work is suitable for patients with inflammatory bowel disease. Some patients, however, do experience more problems with their disease during periods of increased stress. The following may need to be considered in relation to the DDA.

The main problems patients experience with work are frequent bowel action, general fatigue, arthritis, and leakage from their stomas. Frequent bowel action may present problems for workers with limited access to toilets. These include people working out of doors; with restricted toilet access; with restricted mobility due to wearing protective clothing; with severe arthritis; production-line workers, especially on paced work. Hence it may be important to consider the siting of work to provide easy and adequate toilet access.

Shiftwork may be a problem to some patients, especially those with active or severe disease. Patients are often the best judge of what work is suitable for them.

Food handling and preparation

Once inflammatory bowel disease has been diagnosed and an infectious cause for the diarrhoea excluded, there is no reason why the patient should not work as a food handler, providing that the normal standards of personal hygiene expected of such a worker are satisfied. Although such patients may always have loose stools, they are usually able to recognize any changes from their normal pattern which would indicate a superimposed gastroenteritis. If this happens the patient should be investigated in the usual way.

Special facilities

The only provision needed for patients with inflammatory bowel disease is unrestricted access to adequate toilet and washing facilities, which should include privacy for those with an ileostomy.

Ileostomy or colostomy

Ileostomies and colostomies are created either as permanent stomas, or temporarily to enable an acute bowel problem to resolve following which the normal route for bowel function is re-established. Such patients have to adjust to their new body image and functions but are generally able to lead a full and normal life. Unfortunately, some of them experience problems and discrimination in obtaining or continuing work, in part due to prejudice and ignorance by both employers and doctors.

In the UK there are around 15 000 people with a permanent ileostomy and about 1700 new stomas are created each year. The majority of ileostomies are created in young people for inflammatory bowel disease. In comparison, there are probably 30 000 people in England and Wales with a permanent colostomy. About 6500 new permanent and 5000 temporary colostomies are created each year. They tend to be older (peak age incidence 65 years) with a male to female ratio of 1.1 : 1; 60% of these stomata are created for cancer of the colon or rectum.

Clinical aspects affecting work capacity

The capacity of someone with a stoma to work will depend both on the reason for surgery and on the individual's general health after convalescence. Hence, the patient with ulcerative colitis who has had an ileostomy created as part of a colectomy should be returned to full fitness with a near normal life expectancy, but the prospects of a patient with a colostomy for carcinoma of the colon may be less favourable.

Time off work for creation of the stoma is generally 3–4 months, but in the case of a permanent stoma very little further surgery is usually necessary. Complications include electrolyte imbalance, dehydration, and intestinal obstruction, and, in the long-term, an increased risk of biliary and renal stones.

A survey of 1033 members of the Ileostomy Association of Great Britain and Ireland found 79% of women and 96% of men to be working after their operation. Of these, 6% began work for the first time after the operation. Continuity of employment was good.[17]

Special work problems[18]

Although people with an ileostomy or colostomy can be found performing almost every type of work including deep-sea diving (but see Appendix 4), certain jobs are more likely to cause problems. Excessive stooping or bending, especially if accompanied by heavy lifting or carrying loads close to the abdominal wall, and working in a very confined space, may result in leakage from the appliance or injury to the stoma. Modern appliances and a better understanding of optimum siting of the stoma have resulted in appliances that are less vulnerable. Work in the emergency services, which generally combines the problems of heavy lifting close to the body with the use of restrictive clothing, tends to be difficult for the person with a stoma, although there are a few patients working in this capacity. Miners with stomas who work at the coal face find the hot, dirty, sweaty environment combined with the heavy work and the poor toilet facilities unsuitable.

Food handling

The bacterial content of ileostomy effluent is one-twentieth that of normal faeces. Hence, provided the patient has good personal hygiene, the risk of spread of infection should be no greater than in a normal person, and possibly less; in these circumstances a patient with an ileostomy should not be barred from working as a food handler. Colostomy effluent has a bacterial content more akin to normal faeces. Patients with colostomies tend to be older, and are sometimes less dexterous, and so the question of food handling is more contentious, but again a decision should depend on the level of personal hygiene.

Hot environments

Dehydration is a potential problem for anyone with an ileostomy as the stoma results in loss of water and salt such that the total body water is reduced by 10% and salt by 7%, compared to a normal person. People with an ileostomy are thus more susceptible to dehydration when in extremely hot environments or during periods of gastrointestinal upset. Work in hot environments is not contra-indicated, provided that fluid and salt intake are maintained. Patients visiting the tropics should be instructed on the use of oral rehydration solutions.

Work in remote places

Concern has been expressed over someone with an ileostomy working in very remote places with limited medical and surgical back-up in case of emergency. Each case should be considered on its merits. Factors to be considered are the reason for the ileostomy, any previous problems, and the length of time since the stoma was created. For example, a person with an ileostomy as part of a panproctocolectomy for ulcerative colitis will not suffer further problems from the colitis, whereas patients with Crohn's disease may still develop recurrent disease. The need for further surgery to the stoma, regardless of the type of underlying bowel disease, tends to be greatest during the first year after its formation (see also Appendix 4).

Handling of hazardous substances

The handling of toxic chemicals and/or pathogenic material should not be a risk to people with an ileostomy provided that they maintain normal safety standards and safe working practices.

Air travel

Air travel results in reduced ambient pressure. Gas in the bag expands and unless vented can burst the appliance. People with a stoma should wear an appliance with a flatus valve and avoid aerated drinks before and during the flight.

Special facilities

The patient with a stoma needs good toilet and washing facilities with privacy so that the appliance can be changed or leakage cleaned up. If a medical department is readily available, staff will help with this and any other problems.

Gastroenteritis and infestations of the gut

Gastrointestinal infections can result in diarrhoea and ill health which may impair work capacity, but the main concern is the risk of spread of infection, in particular by food handlers. Fortunately, most of the infections encountered in this country are self-limiting but travellers from abroad may contract more serious chronic infection.

For guidance on the prevention of specific infections, the report *The prevention of human transmission of gastrointestinal infections, infestations, and bacterial intoxications*[19] should be consulted. Because the risk of contamination of the environment and of hands is greatest with liquid stools, all cases of gastroenteritis should be regarded as potentially infectious and should be excluded from work until the person is free from diarrhoea and vomiting. This is particularly important for:

• food handlers
• staff of healthcare facilities in direct contact with susceptible patients or their food
• people who may find it difficult to implement good hygiene standards either because of physical/mental limitations or restricted access to washing/toilet facilities.

Each case must be assessed on an individual basis.

Because of limited space we have dealt only with the most common infections and with those of particular consequence to the occupational physician. They are viruses; campylobacter enteritis; salmonella infections; giardiasis; cryptosporidiosis; staphylococcus aureus and amoebiasis.

Viral gastroenteritis

Viruses probably cause more gastroenteritis than bacteria, but only a small number of cases are confirmed owing to the difficult identification techniques required. In 1991, viruses accounted for 16 000 cases of gastroenteritis of which 13 000 were due to rotaviruses chiefly in children.

Norwalk viruses are probably responsible for 40% of outbreaks of epidemic gastroenteritis. Outbreaks particularly affect families, schools, recreation camps, and cruise ships. Transmission is by eating contaminated food, contact with vomit, or faecal–oral routes. Prevention of infection is difficult as transmission of the virus by aerosol or ingestion of contaminated food occurs during the short incubation period and acute stages of the illness.

The patient should stay off work until asymptomatic and, in the case of food handlers, for 48 hours after recovery.

Campylobacter enteritis[20]

Campylobacter (jejuni and intestinalis) enteritis is now the most common cause of gastroenteritis in adults in Britain and has increased from 32 600 cases in 1991 to 50 247 in 1997. Infection is more common in the summer months.

The most common source of infection is eating inadequately cooked poultry, or food contaminated from poultry by poor kitchen hygiene. After 3–5 days' incubation period, a prodrome is followed by a systemic upset, with abdominal pain and diarrhoea. Mortality is extremely low, occurring mainly in the young or elderly. Infection is usually self-limiting, although patients may excrete the organism in the stool for up to 5 weeks. Treatment of severe or persistent infection with erythromycin or ciprofloxacin has become a more common practice although the true place for this approach is still not clear. Reduced excretion of organisms from treated cases may reduce the risk of transmission of infection.

Person to person transmission is only a problem between young children and siblings to parents. Thus, there is no significant occupational health hazard and even food handlers can resume work once fit.

Salmonella infections

In 1997, 31 353 cases of *Salmonella* enteritis were notified and between 1992 and 1994 *Salmonellae* were responsible for more than a half of 640 outbreaks of food poisoning, with July being the peak month.[21]

Although there are more than 1700 types of *Salmonellae*, from a practical point of view, only a relatively small number cause human disease. *Salmonella typhi* and *S. paratyphi* A, B, and C are primarily human pathogens causing enteric fever. Other *Salmonellae* are primarily animal pathogens but may cause illness in humans. Most infections are caused by a small number of different serotypes. The source of most *Salmonella* infection is poultry and agricultural animals, or food contaminated during preparation. Person to person spread can occur in closed communities. Watery diarrhoea occurs 12–72 hours after infection, accompanied by abdominal pain, vomiting, and fever. The illness lasts a few days and is usually self-limiting, but in 1–2% of cases septicaemia results in dissemination of infection to other sites, for example chest and bone.

Patients who are frail, taking immunosuppressive drugs, or who have undergone gastric surgery, and those with achlorhydria or on antacid therapy, seem to have an increased susceptibility to infection. Fatalities are rare but occur in the young or elderly. Antibiotics are indicated for the patients with septicaemia or focal sepsis. Adults excrete the organism for 4–8 weeks, but can resume work once fit, except for being food handlers and water workers. Treatment with the fluoroquinolones (ciprofloxacin) clears infection in 50–70% of cases.

Salmonella typhi and paratyphi

Salmonella typhoid and **paratyphoid** are uncommon gastrointestinal infections in the UK, and are usually acquired in countries with poor sanitation. Despite widespread recognition by the layman these infections are of little importance to the occupational physician except in the context of food handlers (see p. 315).

Immunization

Immunization against *S. typhi*[9] should be considered for travellers to endemic areas and laboratory staff who may handle *S. typhi*. There are now three different types of typhoid vaccine but none provide 100% protection and travellers to endemic areas should still observe scrupulous attention to personal, food, and water hygiene.

Giardiasis[22]

The protozoan *Giardia lamblia* is common all over the world and is endemic in several developing countries. The prevalence in the UK is 5–16%.

In the UK, there were 5300 cases of infection with *Giardia lamblia* in 1997. Infection results from ingestion of mature cysts and although most subjects remain asymptomatic some people, after an incubation period of generally 6–15 (but occasionally up to 75) days, develop diarrhoea often with malabsorption. Many patients have non-specific abdominal and general symptoms even after infection has cleared. Excretion of cysts in the faeces is a potential source of infection, especially for food handlers, although the risk for asymptomatic carriers is probably low. Treatment with metronidazole or tinidazole results in a cure in 90% of cases. Some cases prove particularly difficult to treat, raising the question of reinfection particularly in an endemic area.

Cryptosporidiosis[23]

Cryptosporidium, an intestinal parasitic protozoan, is responsible for 2% of cases of infectious diarrhoea.

In 1997 there were 4300 cases of cryptosporidiosis in the UK. Although it chiefly affects children and the immunocompromised, there is increasing isolation of this organism from immunocompetent adults. A quarter of cases probably arise from drinking raw milk or close contact with farm animals; the remainder are probably water-borne or spread from person to person, and outbreaks are common.

After an incubation period of 3–8 days the acute presentation of abdominal cramps and watery diarrhoea lasts 7 days. Severe cases with fever and vomiting occur in 10% of cases, especially young men. Some people may have infection with both *Cryptosporidium* and *Campylobacter*. In immunocompetent individuals infection usually resolves in 1–3 weeks and asymptomatic carriers are uncommon.

Staphylococcus aureus

Infected food handlers do not normally play a significant role in bacterial food poisoning, except for *S. aureus*. This organism may be found in septic lesions and as a commensal in the nose and on the skin. If transferred to food that is not at adequately low storage temperature, the organism will multiply, producing an enterotoxin that is not inactivated by further cooking. If ingested, it will lead to an abrupt onset of severe nausea, vomiting, abdominal cramps, and diarrhoea. The incubation period is short, usually 2–4 hours, and the duration of the illness is less than 48 hours. Deaths are usually rare.

Amoebiasis and the gay bowel syndrome

Amoebiasis is generally transmitted by ingestion of contaminated food or water, and is principally a problem of underdeveloped countries with poor sanitation. While the highest incidence is still in South America and southern Asia, in the US and Europe amoebiasis has become more common as a sexually transmitted disease, mainly among male homosexuals. Such patients may also be infected with one or more other enteric organisms including *Giardia lamblia, Campylobacter, Salmonellae,* and *Shigellae,* a condition termed the gay bowel syndrome. Cysts of *Entamoeba histolytica* are endemic among homosexual men, being excreted by 4% of those attending clinics for sexually transmitted diseases in the UK. As patients are usually asymptomatic and the amoebae of nonpathogenic types, the value of treatment is controversial. The risk of spread of infection during everyday contact, rather than sexual contact, is low. However, there is evidence from the US of transmission among homosexuals of *Shigella* dysentery and isolated cases of *Salmonella typhi* probably by oral–anal contact. The acquired immune deficiency syndrome (AIDS) is discussed in Chapter 24.

Food handlers[24]

The growth of ready prepared foods and more facilities for eating out mean that food poisoning can affect all sections of the population with serious and even fatal consequences, especially in the very young or weakened individual. In spite of increased legislation, inspection and education, the notification of food poisonings reported to the Registrar General (Office for National Statistics) have increased steadily from 82 041 in 1995 to 93 901 in 1997.

Raw meat and poultry, eggs, and raw milk are commonly contaminated with food poisoning organisms. The majority of food-borne infections emanate from the failure to follow good food preparation or manufacturing practices such as proper temperature control for cooking and storage of food, cross-contamination from raw to cooked foods, and inadequate or inappropriate reheating of cooked foods.

Infected food handlers account for only a small proportion of food poisoning outbreaks.[21]

Definition of a food handler

A food handler is defined as a person **employed directly in the production and preparation of foodstuffs including the manufacturing, catering, and retail industries**. Those undertaking maintenance work or repairing equipment in food handling areas, enforcement officers, and visitors to food handling areas should also meet the same health and hygiene standards as those involved directly in food handling.

People who handle only prewrapped, canned, or bottled food or those involved in primary agriculture or harvesting processes are not considered as food handlers.

Food safety

The selling and processing of food is covered by the Food Safety (General Food Hygiene) Regulations 1995. Department of Health guidance on food handlers' fitness to work[24] was produced in 1995 to assist food businesses to meet their obligations under the regulations and to guide health professionals advising on a person's suitability to work as a food handler.

Symptomless contacts of cases of food-borne disease

Typhoid fever will have to be investigated by a Consultant in Communicable Disease Control (CCDC) in conjunction with the Local Environmental Health Department, the Public Health Laboratory Service, or a consultant microbiologist. Laboratories isolating *Salmonellae* usually inform the CCDC who will issue an exclusion order if the individual is a food handler.[19]

For all other conditions there is no need to investigate unless the contacts develop symptoms. Advice should be given daily to all food handlers to report any symptoms promptly, and to practise a good standard of personal hygiene.

Selection of food handlers

On recruitment prospective employees should be requested to complete a specific questionnaire to determine whether there are any impediments to work as a food handler. Any positive responses should be followed up with medical enquiry and/or examination before employment commences. Stool examinations are not required routinely but should be undertaken if there is a history of illness which could be due to, or a history of contact with, enteric fever.

Impediments to work as a food handler[19,24]

The single most important impediment to working as a food handler is a lack of understanding and awareness of the principles of hygiene.

The following conditions should normally exclude an individual from working as a food handler:

- history of paratyphoid or typhoid disease until six consecutive negative stool samples
- history of recurrent attacks of gastroenteritis, unless a carrier state has been excluded by bacteriological tests
- history and presence of persistent and recurring staphylococcal or streptococcal infections on the skin
- chronic infections of the ears, eyes, nose or throat and gums
- poor oral hygiene.

There is no evidence that chest and upper respiratory tract infections pose a risk of food contamination but there may be aesthetic reasons for excluding employees with conditions resulting in chronic coughing or frequent sneezing;

Medical certification

There are a number of specific regulations which apply to suppliers and manufacturers of products of animal origin, such as dairies, meat processors, and wholesale fish suppliers. These regulations require medical certification of prospective employees to ensure there is no impediment to their employment as food handlers.

Prevention of microbiological contamination of food

Food handlers should be trained in the safe handling of food, have a good understanding of the principles of food hygiene, and be aware of their obligation to report to management any infectious conditions which might arise during their employment.

The most commonly reported conditions which have implications for food handlers are diarrhoea and vomiting. It is important for employees to understand that diarrhoea implies a **change** in bowel habit as some non-infectious bowel conditions (inflammatory bowel diseases) may result in the passage of frequent loose stools.

Food handlers who develop symptoms of gastrointestinal infection should report immediately to management and leave the food handling area. Cases will need to be managed on an individual basis[19] with medical investigation, stool sampling, treatment, and referral to the local CCDC depending on the nature, duration and severity of symptoms and on the number of workers affected.

Following illness due to any of the common causes of gastrointestinal infection food handlers can return to work if:

* there has been no vomiting for 48 hours once any treatment has ceased
* the bowel habit has returned to normal for 48 hours either spontaneously or following cessation of treatment with anti-diarrhoeal drugs
* good hygiene practice is strictly observed.

Gastrointestinal infections requiring special consideration include enteric fever (*Salmonella typhi* and *Salmonella paratyphi* A, B or C), verocytoxin producing *Escherichia coli* and hepatitis A.[19]

Functional disorders

Non-ulcer dyspepsia

The widespread use of endoscopy and double-contrast barium-meal radiography has revealed that many people with dyspepsia do not have peptic ulceration. Most of these patients are aged between 20 and 40 years, with a predominance of men. A survey from Sweden estimated that patients with non-ulcer dyspepsia suffered 2.6 times more sickness absence than the general population. Their condition also results in substantial numbers of both in- and out-patient consultations, and inappropriate use of anti-ulcer medication. The role of infection in the stomach with *H. pylori* is unclear. Eradication of *H. pylori* is not recommended at present for patients with non-ulcer dyspepsia. Although some patients improve after eradication, others, particularly those with symptoms of gastroesophageal reflux, may be worse. For some patients improvement in dyspepsia may be a placebo response and there may be an element of psychological dependence. Dyspepsia is more likely to be due to other causes, such as the irritable bowel syndrome and/or gastrooesophageal reflux, but in a quarter of cases no explanation can be found.

Irritable bowel syndrome[25]

Irritable bowel syndrome (IBS, spastic colon) is a disorder of unknown aetiology characterized by abdominal pain, distension, and bowel upset (diarrhoea, passage of mucus per rectum, and/or constipation) in the absence of demonstrable organic disease (see Table 15.1). It is the most common disorder of the gastrointestinal tract, affecting one-third of the general population, yet only 20% of sufferers seek medical advice. Many doctors do not appreciate the diverse clinical features of the condition which may result in inappropriate treatment for dyspepsia, and some patients with severe pain may even have a normal appendix or gallbladder removed without relief of symptoms (Table 15.1). In two-thirds of patients, the onset of symptoms is preceded by an anxiety-provoking life situation or an episode of psychiatric illness, such as depression. It seems likely that the syndrome is a normal somatic response to stress rather than a disease.

Prevalence

Although only the more severe or chronic cases tend to be referred to a specialist, these account for approximately 50% of gastroenterology out-patient work. There are twice as many women as men amongst those referred.

The onset of symptoms is generally from late adolescence to the late 30s, and is slightly later in men. The syndrome is rare in the over 60s and should only be diagnosed after other causes of gastrointestinal upset have been excluded, especially in the older patient.

The most incapacitating symptoms are diarrhoea and abdominal pain and bloating, which are usually intermittent but can have a profound effect on capacity to work. Data on sickness absence are not available.

The response to treatment, especially of those seeking specialist advice, is often transient and variable, with 25% deriving no benefit or even deteriorating. For some patients with food intolerance dietary manipulation can prove beneficial, but for many this is short-lived. There is a move to subdivide patients into one of three groups according to whether their predominant symptom is diarrhoea, constipation, or pain.

• In the case of **diarrhoea-predominant** IBS, symptomatic treatment with loperamide or the bile acid binding drug cholestyramine may be helpful.

Table 15.1 Clinical features of irritable bowel syndrome

Symptom	% affected
Abdominal pain, often left lower quadrant	98
Disordered bowel habit	80
Weight usually steady or increasing	80
Flatus-distension	65
Nausea with occasional vomiting	50
Dyspepsia (and occasional dysphagia)	25–50
Previous 'normal' appendicectomy	33
Cancer phobia	<50
Urinary symptoms—frequency and dysuria	20
Gynaecological symptoms	
Dysmenorrhoea	90
Dyspareunia	33

- **Constipation-predominant** IBS may benefit from increased fibre intake, sometimes plus an osmotic laxative (lactulose). The prokinetic drug cisapride acts on the myenteric plexus and increases small bowel and colonic transit.
- Patients with **pain-predominant** IBS may benefit from the gut-selective agent cimetropium bromide or antidepressants which act by relieving coexisting depression, or via their central analgesic effect.

Severe chronic cases may be helped by learning self-hypnosis. Reassurance and explanation of the nature of the condition and its relation to stress can be helpful.

The majority of patients manage to work unaffected by the condition, but for a small number work may be severely affected by severe or chronic diarrhoea and/or abdominal pain. For patients with frequent bowel action, toilet access can be a problem. Avoidance of excessive stress may be helpful for some patients, although as a group they will tend to worry excessively.

Coeliac disease

Coeliac disease is due to an allergy to gluten in wheat and results in atrophy of the small bowel mucosa, especially the jejunum. The prevalence varies widely from 1 : 100 in Galway, Ireland, to around 1 : 300 in England and Wales. Confirmation of the diagnosis depends on histological examination of the small bowel (duodenum or jejunum). Most patients present in childhood with failure to grow and/or diarrhoea, but a small number present as adults. Exclusion of gluten from the diet usually results in complete restoration of normal health. Relapse of symptoms usually occurs only if gluten is inadvertently or deliberately introduced into the diet. Thus, the only restriction for employment of someone with coeliac disease is if they have to consume gluten-containing food as part of their work (i.e. food taster). Travel is not usually a problem provided that gluten-containing foods are avoided.

Chronic pancreatitis

Chronic pancreatitis is a rare disorder characterized by chronic severe epigastric pain, steatorrhoea, and diabetes due to damage to the islets of Langerhans. Alcohol abuse is a common cause and this problem has obvious consequences for work. The chronic pain may be so severe as to require opiate analgesia or even pain control by nerve block. Fortunately, with time the condition tends to burn out. There are no special restrictions for work apart from those related to coexistent diabetes mellitus and/or alcoholism (Chapters 16 and 25).

Summary

Diseases of the gastrointestinal tract are seldom a hazard to others, but if they are not managed correctly they can impair ability to cope with work. Modern drug therapy and, or simple adaptations to work, especially for patients with gastroesophageal reflux, should enable them to work productively. New drug regimens to eradicate infection in the stomach with *H. pylori* can cure peptic ulceration and reduce morbidity.

Once recovered from the acute phase, patients with viral hepatitis A should be able to resume work without restrictions. A small proportion of patients with hepatitis B may progress to chronic ill health but spread of infection results only from intimate contact which should not occur in the normal workplace. Complications of chronic liver disease especially hepatic encephalopathy, ascites, and gastrointestinal bleeding may seriously impair ability to work and usually have a poor prognosis.

Exacerbations of inflammatory bowel disease may result in impaired quality of life but employment record and continuity of work is usually good, so that employers should be encouraged to adopt an optimistic outlook. Surgery for ulcerative colitis dramatically improves health and newer techniques avoid a permanent stoma. The possession of a stoma should not bar patients from most types of work and does not pose a risk of spread of infection provided good standards of hygiene are practised.

Gastroenteritis generally causes more inconvenience than risk and newer drugs show promise in reducing infectivity and speeding resolution. There is still need for the careful medical management of infected food handlers.

Functional bowel disorders are extremely common but have a good prognosis and may indicate a reaction to psychological stresses and life events.

Selected references

1 Bouchier IAD, Allan RN, Hodgson HJF, Keighley MRB (ed.). *Gastroenterology: clinical science and practice*, 2nd edn. London: W B Saunders, 1993.

2 Katchinski BD, Logan RFA, Edmond M, Langman MJS. Physical activity at work and duodenal ulcer risk. *Gut* 1991; **32**: 983–986.

3 Doll R, Avery Jones F. *Occupational factors in the aetiology of gastric ulcer and duodenal ulcer*. MRC Special Report Series 276. London: HMSO, 1951.

4 Langman MJS. *The epidemiology of chronic digestive diseases*, London: Edward Arnold, 1979, pp. 9–39.

5 McCloy R, Nair R. Surgery for acid suppression in the 1990s. *Baillières Clin Gastroenterol* 1993; **7**: 129–148.

6 McColl KE. *Helicobacter pylori*: clinical aspects. *J Infect* 1997; **34**: 7–13.

7 Sherlock S, Dooley J. *Diseases of the liver and biliary system*, 10th edn. Oxford: Blackwell, 1997.

8 *Comm Dis Rep CDR wkly* 1999; **9**(3): 19.

9 *Immunisation against infectious disease. Bicentenary edition*. Department of Health, Welsh Office, and Scottish Home and Health Department. London: HMSO, 1996.

10 *Protecting health care workers and patients from hepatitis B. Recommendations of the Advisory Group on Hepatitis*. London: UK Health Departments, August 1993.

11 *Guidance for clinical health care workers: Protection against infection with blood borne viruses. Recommendations of the Expert Advisory Group on AIDS and the Advisory Group on Hepatitis*. London: UK Health Departments, 1998.

12 *Alcohol as a medical and social problem*. London: Institute of Alcohol Studies, 1997.

13 Royal College of Physicians. *A great and growing evil*. London: Tavistock, 1987.

14 Mayfield D, McLeod G, Hall P. The CAGE questionnaire: validation of a new alcoholism screening instrument. *Am J Psychiatry* 1974; **131**: 1121–1123.

15 Allan RN, Keighley MRB, Rhodes Jonathan M, Alexander-Williams J, Fazio VW, Hanauer SB. *Inflammatory bowel diseases*, 3rd edn. Edinburgh: Churchill Livingstone, 1997.

16 Wyke RJ, Edwards FC, Allan RN. Employment problems and prospects for patients with inflammatory bowel disease. *Gut* 1988: **29**; 1229–1235.

17 Whates PD, Irving M. Return to work following ileostomy. *Br J Surg* 1984; **71**: 619–622.

18 Wyke RJ, Aw TC, Allan RN, Harrington JM. Employment prospects for patients with intestinal stomas: the attitude of occupational physicians. *J Soc Occup. Med* 1989: **39**; 19–24.

19 Working party of the PHLS Salmonella subcommittee. The prevention of human transmission of gastrointestinal infections, infestations, and bacterial intoxications. A guide for public health physicians and environmental health officers in England and Wales. *Commun Dis Rep Rev* 1995; **5**(11): R158–R172.

20 Pearson AD, Healing TD. The surveillance and control of Campylobacter infection. *Commun Dis Rep CDR Rev* 1992; **2**(12): R133–R139.

21 Ryan MJ, Wall PG, Gilbert RJ, Griffin M, Rowe B. Risk factors for outbreaks of infectious intestinal disease linked to domestic catering. *Commun Dis Rep Rev* 1996; **6**(13): R179–R183.

22 Farthing MJ. Giardiasis. *Gastroenterol Clin North Am* 1996; **25**: 493–515.

23 Casemore DP. Human cryptosporidiosis. In: *Recent advances in infection,* ed. Reeves DS, Geddes AM, Vol 3, pp. 209–236. Edinburgh: Churchill Livingstone, 1989.

24 *Food handlers fitness to work. Guidance for food businesses enforcement officers and health professionals.* London: Department of Health, 1995.

25 Camilleri M, Choi M-G. Review article: irritable bowel syndrome. *Aliment Pharmacol Ther* 1997; **11**: 3–15.

16

Diabetes mellitus and other endocrine disorders

E. Waclawski and G. Gill

Diabetes

Classification

For practical clinical purposes there are two types of diabetes:

- **Insulin-dependent diabetes mellitus (IDDM), or type I diabetes**: The cause is not known but it may result from viral damage to pancreatic islet beta cells in genetically susceptible individuals. Autoimmunity may also play a part, and islet cell antibodies can be demonstrated in most type I patients. It can occur at any age, although the vast majority of those diagnosed with diabetes under 30 years of age are of this type.
- **Non-insulin-dependent diabetes mellitus (NIDDM), or type II diabetes** has a strong genetic component but the cause in most cases is not known. It affects predominantly those over 30 years of age and is strongly associated with obesity. Prevalence is also raised in the elderly, and some ethnic minorities—notably Asian immigrants. Approximately three-quarters of diabetic patients are of this type.

Diabetes and employment

Despite recent advances in the control of diabetes the condition remains poorly understood and is sometimes feared by employers and even by their medical advisers.[1] As a result, significant numbers of people with diabetes encounter largely unjustifiable difficulties in finding and keeping work because of their condition. There is a paucity of published scientific data on the work experience of diabetic people in general, or in particular situations (for example shiftwork), but their underrepresentation in the workforce[2] in some studies indicates that there may be prejudice against their employment, or that they do not always declare their diabetes to their employer or occupational health service. Another study has shown employment rates for young diabetic school leavers equivalent to non-diabetic rates.[3]

The risk of hypoglycaemia and visual impairment may legitimately debar those with poorly controlled type I diabetes from jobs where safety is an important factor, but people with diabetes are not invalids and most can work normally and should not be discriminated against in job selection. The British Diabetic Association (BDA) has published a *Diabetes employment handbook*[4] and patient information leaflet,[5] which are comprehensive and useful guides to the employment implications of diabetes in a wide range of occupations. Publications such as these help employers to familiarize themselves with the condition and to recognize that the work record of those with diabetes is good and that they make perfectly satisfactory employees.

Diabetes is normally treated by dietary advice and insulin for type I diabetes and dietary advice with or without the addition of oral hypoglycaemic agents or insulin for in type II diabetes. The Disability Discrimination Act 1995 (DDA) provides that where an impairment is being treated or corrected the impairment is considered as having the effect it would have without the measures in question. This applies even if the measures result in the effects of the impairment being completely under control or not at all apparent. In addition the Act provides for a person with a progressive condition to be regarded as having an impairment which has a substantial adverse effect on their ability to carry out normal day to day activities before it actually does so. Where a person has a progressive condition, they will be treated as having an impairment which has a substantial adverse effect from the moment any impairment resulting from that condition first has some effect on their ability to carry out normal day to day activities. Diabetes should therefore be regarded as a disability within the meaning of the Act, as treatment for type I diabetes has to be ignored in considering the impairment that exists. For type II diabetes the matter may be different, as people with this type of diabetes may be asymptomatic and have no complications. Where complications such as retinopathy exist, and such complications can be found at initial presentation in some cases, they will be covered by the Act as they display evidence of a progressive condition.

Prevalence, morbidity, and mortality

Epidemiology

Type I diabetes has an incidence of about 10–30 per 100 000 head of population per year.[6] Rates vary greatly geographically (being higher in northern countries e.g. Finland, Scotland), and the incidence appears to be increasing, particularly in young children.[7] Type II diabetes makes up 70–80% of the total diabetic population. Its prevalence is rapidly increasing worldwide, due to factors such as obesity, migration, and the adoption of western habits. In the UK, current prevalence rates are about 2–3%, with higher rates in areas with large ethnic communities or elderly populations.[8]

Morbidity and mortality

The scale of the morbidity of diabetes cannot be estimated accurately, although it is said to be the commonest cause of blindness in the working age-group. Coronary heart disease is increased by a factor of 2–3; diabetes is the second leading cause of fatal kidney disease and a diabetic patient is many times more likely to need an amputation.[9] It should be emphasized, however, that only a minority of people with diabetes develop disabling complications.

Recent studies of sickness absence and diabetes indicate that rates are higher than in the non-diabetic population.[10–14] Prolonged absence is mainly associated with a minority of diabetic employees who have complications of the disease. Life expectancy is reduced in all age-groups, mainly as a result of renal failure and vascular disease. There is great variation, however, and many diabetic people live for 40 years or more after the onset of the disease without developing serious complications. There is also evidence that the outlook of diabetes, particularly type I diabetes, has improved considerably in the last 10–15 years.[15] Traditional mortality figures are often based on actuarial studies which are now very dated.

The prevalence of diabetes and its complications as a cause of ill health retirement is still greater than would be expected, indicating that increased morbidity is still present in the working population. However, improved methods of control of diabetes and more effective treatment for end-stage renal failure have improved the prognosis.

Clinical aspects affecting work capacity

Management of Type 1 diabetes

There are a large number of insulin regimens, varying from once a day injections of long-acting insulin (perhaps with short-acting insulin) to three injections of short-acting insulin with an intermediate-acting type given late in the evening. These can be given by conventional syringe or by injector pen. A single injection is effective in only a minority of cases, and is now rarely used. Short-acting with intermediate-acting insulin given twice daily is a popular regimen. For those with a variable lifestyle, multiple injection treatment (MIT)—as above—with a pen-injector is often acceptable and effective. The use of flexible regimens with MIT and pen-injectors is now relatively common and allows for greater variation in the timing of meals, and a better quality of life. Such systems can also facilitate shiftwork, particularly if the person is educated to vary insulin doses and diet according to the varying pattern of work.[16] Continuous subcutaneous insulin infusion by electronically-controlled pump has not proved as successful as first hoped: this treatment involves the permanent wearing of a pump, which though miniaturized, is still an impediment. There is also a possibility of failure with a rapid deterioration of diabetic control.

The major guideline for insulin treatment is that any method which works should be continued; there is no merit in making changes for their own sake. The objectives are always that the patient should feel well, hypoglycaemia should be uncommon, mild, and preceded by warning, and blood glucose control should be acceptable—in that order.

Insulin was originally extracted from animal pancreas, at first cattle and later pigs. In the last 10–15 years it has been made by genetic engineering; most insulin made this way is now identical to the human insulin molecule, and is termed 'human insulin'. There are minor chemical differences between the different species of insulin, but their actions are essentially the same. Bovine insulin (which is now little used) is slightly less potent than porcine and human insulin (perhaps because beef insulin is more frequently associated with insulin antibody production). Pork and human insulin however are of similar potency. Claims that human insulin may be particularly associated with hypoglycaemia and/or hypoglycaemia unawareness have not been substantiated. Nevertheless, most diabetologists believe that if patients prefer a particular insulin species, then they should be allowed to use this.

A new 'designer' insulin, Insulin Lispro, has recently been introduced. This is human insulin with a minor amino acid sequence change. Its absorption characteristics are closer to human pancreatic insulin production after food. Though this insulin does not improve overall glycaemic control, it can be given with meals, rather than before, and is less likely to cause postprandial hypoglycaemia.[17]

It is hardly ever possible to achieve consistently normal blood glucose levels in type I diabetes throughout the 24 hours, and attempts to do so will lead to frequent hypoglycaemia. There is nearly always considerable variation in results due to differences in food or exercise, and the inherent imperfections of current insulin treatment and delivery systems. Self-blood glucose testing is an important advance, but it can have the drawback of undermining confidence and producing worry unless it is seen in context, and is combined with an appropriate education programme.

Management of type II diabetes

Type II diabetes is managed with diet alone, diet and oral hypoglycaemic agents (OHAs), or diet and insulin. Patients are frequently obese and the main objective of diet is to reduce body weight, principally by controlling fat intake, although excessive intake of refined carbohydrates is not advisable. High fibre intake seems to be beneficial for all types of diabetes, as fibre delays carbohydrate absorption and reduces blood glucose excursions. Oral hypoglycaemic drugs are of three types:

- **Biguanides**, for example metformin. Biguanides appear to act by reducing glucose absorption from the gut, reducing glucose release from the liver, and enhancing glucose uptake by the tissues. Metformin is the only member of this class of drugs available in most countries (including the UK). Metformin is of moderate potency, does not cause hypoglycaemia, but is prone to be associated with gastrointestinal upsets (notably diarrhoea). Metformin also has slight weight-losing properties, and is indicated mainly for obese type II diabetes.
- **Sulfonylureas**, for example glibenclamide, gliclazide, chlorpropamide, tolbutamide and glipizide. The sulfonylureas act mainly by stimulating pancreatic insulin release. They may be relatively powerful, and can cause hypoglycaemia, especially after unaccustomed exercise, high alcohol consumption, and/or inadequate food intake. This appears to be less common with shorter-acting sulfonylureas, such as tolbutamide, glipizide or gliclazide; but is more common with glibenclamide and chlorpropamide. Sulfonylureas may also be associated with weight gain. This class of drugs is predominantly indicated for type II diabetic patients of normal weight.
- **Glucosidase inhibitors** are a new class of OHAs; the only one currently available is acarbose. This drug partially inhibits the enzymes that control carbohydrate absorption from the gut. Acarbose is not associated with hypoglycaemia or weight gain, but diarrhoea and flatulence (due to undigested carbohydrate) are common side-effects which often limit the drug's usefulness.

Newer concepts of control

With the realization that careful control of diabetes can reduce the risk of long-term complications (at least in type 1 diabetes),[18] increasing emphasis is now placed on achieving not only clinical well-being but also optimal blood glucose levels. Self-monitoring of blood glucose has largely replaced urine testing, especially in younger insulin-treated patients. The main advantages of blood testing are that it more accurately reflects current diabetic control and is not retrospective, nor subject to variations in the renal threshold for glucose. Self-monitoring of blood glucose gives information on low values, as well as high, and can thus give warning of impending hypoglycaemia. It is also more acceptable to many patients. Blood glucose strips are now included in the drug tariff in the UK and are readily available. Careful regulation of insulin dosage together with blood glucose monitoring, reduces the risk of hypoglycaemia and enables individuals to cope more easily with variations in daily work patterns. Blood glucose testing is a vital part of management for insulin-treated patients who might otherwise experience difficulty in coping with certain types of employment (for example those involving shiftwork).

Special work problems caused by diabetes

Work record of people with diabetes

There have been considerable changes in recent years concerning employment and diabetes. Previously there was both fear and mistrust between employer and potential employee with diabetes. These attitudes were largely due to ignorance, but there is now more general awareness of diabetes. The result has been wholly beneficial; employers are much less likely to operate overall bans for diabetic job applicants, and diabetic employees are better able to manage their condition and less inclined to conceal their diabetes.

Occupations closed to those with insulin-treated diabetes are usually those in which hypoglycaemia could be highly dangerous, e.g. airline pilots or large goods vehicle (LGV) drivers. The risk here comes not from the diabetes itself but from its treatment. It has also traditionally been considered unwise for insulin-taking diabetic people to work in potentially hazardous environments e.g. with moving machinery, in foundries, on scaffolding, and fighting fires. But even here there is room for latitude. Much depends on the exact nature of the work, control of the diabetes (in particular the frequency and warnings of hypoglycaemia), and the good sense of the patient.

The situation with UK firefighting in particular is of interest. In common with other emergency and armed services, applicants with existing type I diabetes are not accepted for employment in the fire service. Those who develop insulin-requiring diabetes while in service, however, are now assessed on an individual basis. Criteria such as those mentioned above are used, and considered jointly by an occupational physician and a diabetologist. This situation seems sensible as it takes into account the great variability of control, education, and motivation amongst those with insulin-treated diabetes, as well as the potential for employment-related risk assessment. This approach may be applicable to other potentially dangerous occupations, and has led the British Diabetic Association (BDA) to publish guidelines for such employment (see p. 329).[19]

Restrictions on the employment of those with diabetes treated without insulin are much less stringent. Although hypoglycaemic episodes can occur with sulfonylurea tablets (and may be serious and prolonged), they are less common. If the physician is satisfied with treatment over a period of time, and especially if the patients monitor their own blood glucose levels, the risk of hypoglycaemia is remote and will rarely be a bar to employment. There are exceptions, for example in aircrew and train drivers. Treatment with metformin or acarbose does not carry hypoglycaemic risk (unless combined with insulin or sulfonylureas, when they may potentiate the hypoglycaemic actions of these agents).

The suitability of a diabetic person for employment also depends of course on their general health. In the case of diabetes this means freedom from sight-threatening retinopathy, severe peripheral or autonomic neuropathy, advanced ischaemic heart disease, serious renal failure, or disabling cerebrovascular or peripheral vascular disease.

With the improved general knowledge of diabetes, and more positive attitudes to the disease (as well as its improved management in recent years), the work performance of most people with diabetes is very good and their rate of unemployment is no worse than for other people.[3] However, they are likely to have about 1.5–2 times as much time off work, although in well-controlled cases the excess is small or nil.[10–14] This is especially true of those on diet and/or OHAs. Good medical treatment and good liaison between physician and occupational health staff are important in controlling diabetes and minimizing its effects. Treatment has improved greatly in recent times, and with better self-monitoring of blood glucose and newer types of insulin and treatment regimens, the trend is likely to continue.

Working patterns and diabetic treatment

Generally there is no reason why a diabetic person on insulin should not undertake shiftwork, though diabetic workers do experience more problems with shiftwork than non-diabetic workers.[11] Most sensible and well-motivated diabetic shiftworkers can rapidly learn how to adjust their treatment, especially if they are measuring their own blood glucose levels and using MIT techniques. Thus, shiftwork should not be an automatic bar. One recent development in shift patterns may complicate matters: this is the introduction of shorter shift cycles in which day, evening, and night shifts may follow each other at 2-day intervals. This may test the ingenuity of the most intelligent insulin-dependent diabetic worker. These problems can occur in different types and grades of employment, for example supervisors and managers may also be required to undertake such shiftwork or work irregular hours.

Acute complications of diabetes

'Diabetic coma' is an inexact and outmoded term, and should not be used. There are two acute diabetic complications which can cause coma—or more likely, clouded consciousness.

* **Diabetic ketoacidosis** may occur if there is serious loss of control of diabetes, resulting in hyperglycaemia, dehydration, and acidosis due to the accumulation of ketones. Ketoacidosis occurs only in type I diabetes. The onset is gradual and it is not a cause of sudden collapse at work. It only rarely leads to significant sickness absence.
* **Hypoglycaemia** can occur when treatment is with insulin, or more rarely, with sulfonylurea tablets. It may cause confusion and clouded or lost consciousness, and so is a much more serious problem from the work standpoint. Most insulin-treated diabetics receive ample warning of impending hypoglycaemia (e.g. sweating, nausea, palpitations, etc.), take preventive steps (i.e. take glucose) and experience neither loss of control nor unconsciousness. In some, however, hypoglycaemia can develop suddenly and without warning. This is why many employers have reservations about people with diabetes on insulin working in potentially hazardous situations. The majority however very rarely experience serious hypoglycaemia and the risks have been exaggerated. Nonetheless, it is a factor which has to be considered by employers and occupational physicians when deciding on the placement of those with insulin-treated diabetes at work. It may be important for some to have regular breaks

when they can carry out blood tests, consume snacks, or take insulin. As yet there has been no formal study of the impact of hypoglycaemia at work. Improvements in treatment regimens and education may have reduced hypoglycaemic problems at work. Preliminary evidence suggests that when hypoglycaemia occurs, it is usually outside working hours.[20]

As mentioned, sulfonylureas are much less likely to cause serious hypoglycaemia than insulin, and there are relatively few jobs barred to those on these drugs. The guiding principle must always be to assess the risk of hypoglycaemia, and whether or not its development might put the diabetic employee or others at risk. Unfortunately, many occupational guidelines do not recognize the different modes of action of oral hypo-glycaemic agents, and 'tablets' are considered as carrying identical risk profiles. This is not the case, as metformin and acarbose do not cause hypoglycaemia.

Chronic complications of diabetes

A relatively small proportion of people with diabetes develop significant long-term complications, usually after many years of type I diabetes, though complications can exist at the time of diagnosis in type II diabetes. From the employment viewpoint the most important are

- **retinopathy**, which can lead to visual impairment and blindness
- **neuropathy**, either sensory or autonomic (which may cause postural hypotension)
- **nephropathy**, which can lead to renal failure
- **foot ulceration**, which occasionally necessitates amputation.

There is an increased risk of coronary artery disease, stroke, and peripheral vascular disease. Treatment may occasionally cause problems: for example, 'pan-retinal photo-coagulation', sometimes used in the treatment of retinopathy, may cause significant diminution in peripheral visual fields and affect the ability to hold a driving licence. However, it must be emphasized that few working-aged people with diabetes develop such severe disabling complications. Individuals who hold driving licences and develop significant complications should be advised to notify the licensing authorities; often they will still be able to continue driving.

Pension schemes

Difficulty in arranging associated life insurance is sometimes cited as a reason for not employing those with diabetes. This is not usually a problem in medium or larger-sized organizations, where group life insurance schemes can include diabetic employees without requiring any medical evidence or additional premium. Problems may arise in smaller firms where employees have to be assessed individually, or in larger organizations where the salary of a highly paid executive may rise above the 'free cover level' and attract additional premiums. The attitude of different insurance companies to diabetes can vary considerably.[21] If a diabetic person is penalized by a particular insurance company or scheme, and this is a major obstacle to employment, then there should be an option available to arrange separate cover with another company, if necessary paying additional insurance premiums. In this context private pension plans are now commonly used by employees, whether with or without diabetes. The BDA can give useful advice on insurance matters.

Advisory services

The diabetes specialist, general practitioner, and occupational health services should be able to give advice in cases of employment difficulty. The diabetes specialist or family practitioner can provide detailed medical information, and the occupational physician is best placed to assess the suitability for a particular occupation. For especially difficult decisions, the combined opinions of specialists in diabetes and occupational health are particularly useful.

Disability Employment Advisers based at Department of Education and Employment Job Centres can advise and help anyone with diabetes and disabilities affecting their work to find or keep suitable employment. Careers officers and teachers should also be able to advise diabetic school leavers. The BDA's *Employment Handbook* is a comprehensive source of information.[4]

Guidelines for employment

Guidance for employers and occupational health services is published both by the BDA[4,5,10] and the American Diabetes Association.[22] The current situation can be summarized as follows:

- **People with diabetes treated with diet alone** should be able to undertake virtually any occupation providing they are not suffering from significant and disabling complications of the disease.
- **People with diabetes treated with diet and OHAs** can undertake most occupations subject to being free from disabling complications. However, currently they are not recruited to the armed forces or emergency services (fire service, police force, and ambulance service). They are also not usually permitted to work in air traffic control, pilot transport aeroplanes, or work on off-shore oil platforms. The criteria relating to mainline train driving have recently been relaxed. This occupation is now open to diabetic applicants and employees on OHAs provided they are well controlled, under regular specialist supervision, monitor their blood glucose levels, do not suffer from any significant complications, and do not experience hypoglycaemia. Vocational drivers with diabetes which is well controlled by diet alone or with oral agents are usually allowed to continue driving LGVs and passenger carrying vehicles (PCVs), subject to not suffering from any significant complications. Merchant seafarers (see Appendix 3) and deep-sea fishermen are allowed to remain at sea, subject to regular medical reviews. As mentioned, almost all employment regulations for those on OHAs do not differentiate between the type of drug used and therefore fail to differentiate between the risk of sulfonylurea-induced hypoglycaemia and the safety of metformin and acarbose.
- **People with diabetes treated with insulin** should not work in situations where sudden attacks of hypoglycaemia are a significant risk, and a likely source of danger to themselves or others. For this reason they are usually not permitted to drive LGVs or PCVs, enter the armed forces or emergency services, fly aeroplanes, drive trains, or

continue as seafarers or divers. It may be undesirable for them to work in some other very hazardous surroundings. They may also be barred from certain occupations such as railway signal operators because of the possible risks to the safety of others.

Guidelines on recruiting insulin-treated diabetic applicants to occupations are usually fairly clear but the situation is often unclear when someone develops insulin-requiring diabetes during employment. The example of firefighters has already been mentioned; and the approach of individual assessment is increasingly being applied elsewhere (e.g. police and armed forces). However, though employment may be continued, the nature of the job may alter; for example, in the police force newly diagnosed diabetic personnel on insulin treatment may not necessarily lose their jobs, but there will be restrictions (e.g. driving at high speed and membership of armed response units will not be allowed).

Finally, the BDA Working Party on Driving and Employment has produced the guidelines in Box 16.1 for the employment of insulin-treated diabetic people in potentially hazardous occupations. These suggest the factors to be considered when an 'individual consideration' policy is adopted, and they provide a sensible framework for the safe employment of insulin-treated diabetic people.

Box 16.1   Diabetes and potentially hazardous occupations
1. People should be physically and mentally fit in accordance with non-diabetic standards.
2. Diabetes should be under regular (at least annual) specialist review.
3. Diabetes should be under stable control.
4. People should self-monitor their blood glucose, and be well educated and motivated in diabetes self-care.
5. There should be no disabling hypoglycaemia and normal awareness of individual hypoglycaemic symptoms.
6. There should be no advanced retinopathy or nephropathy, nor severe symptomatic peripheral or autonomic nerve damage.
7. There should be no significant coronary heart disease, peripheral vascular disease, or cerebrovascular disease.
8. Suitability for employment should be re-assessed annually by both an occupational physician and diabetes specialist; and should be based on the criteria outlined above.

(after ref. 19)

Conclusions and recommendations

A few studies of employment and diabetes in the UK[6,7,10] indicate some increase in sickness absence. Further research is required on the impact of hypoglycaemia at work. Information is also needed on the impact of particular work activities on diabetic control, especially shiftwork and vocational driving. Because of the paucity of definitive information, the advice given to diabetic workers is often arbitrary, and employment decisions are taken with little supporting evidence. Physicians should take care to inform employers and potential employers factually about diabetes and to dispel any prejudice that might exist.

The introduction of blood glucose self-testing and modern systems of treatment have enabled those with diabetes to cope more easily with irregular work patterns. Careers officers and teachers need to know more about diabetes, so that they can give school-leavers accurate advice and enable them to make sensible career plans. A sustained effort is required to educate employers and to persuade them to take a more objective view of diabetic workers.

Some pension schemes still exclude those with diabetes and this is a frequent cause of employment difficulties. Many insurance companies now take a more liberal view, so individuals should be able to make their own pension arrangements if rejected by a group scheme. Employers should be encouraged to allow more flexible pension arrangements, which should reduce the occurrence of this distressing problem.

It is essential that each individual case be assessed on its own merits with full consultation between all medical advisers. Diabetes *per se* should not limit employment prospects, since the majority of diabetics have few, if any, problems arising from the condition, and make perfectly satisfactory employees in a wide variety of occupations.

Endocrine disorders

There appears to be less information available on the effects of work on other endocrine disorders. Absence of a specific hormone would result in illness which would require to be permanently controlled by therapy. Some of these disorders if untreated, such as hypothyroidism and hypoadrenalism would have a significant effect on day to day activities, so they would be classed as disabilities under the DDA. Endocrine disorders which result in overactivity may be treated by drugs, surgery, and radionuclides. Long-term problems with day to day activities may therefore be removed, though if there is a likelihood of recurrence (such as with pituitary tumours in the past) this would lead to a classification as a disability under the DDA.

Thyroid disease

Thyroid over- or underactivity is fully treatable and should have little or no long-term employment effects.

Hypothyroidism

In adult life, hypothyroidism (primary, or secondary to hypopituitarism) is usually insidious and can easily be missed. Increasingly with frequent 'routine' thyroid function testing, hypothyroidism is diagnosed early. Untreated thyroid deficiency in a baby can cause lasting damage if not diagnosed and treated, but this will not concern employment.

In untreated hypothyroidism, performance at work is likely to be affected. Poor memory and concentration and slowing of mental and physical activity are likely to lead to a decline in efficiency, both physical and mental. Treatment with thyroxine is simple and effective, and needs to be continued indefinitely. A patient with well-controlled hypothyroidism can lead a normal life in all respects.

Hyperthyroidism

Thyroid overactivity (thyrotoxicosis) presents classically with agitation, tremor, sensitivity to heat, tachycardia, and loss of weight. The diagnosis is not usually difficult, though it must be differentiated from acute and chronic anxiety states. In some cases however, especially in older patients, thyrotoxicosis may present non-specifically, or as sinus tachycardia or atrial fibrillation. If the diagnosis is still not made the patient may develop severe heart failure.

Treatment with drugs, partial thyroidectomy or radioiodine is effective. There should be no long-term employment problems.

Pituitary disease

Growth hormone deficiency in childhood can be effectively treated with replacement therapy, which is now produced using recombinant DNA techniques (somatropin). The academic achievements of individuals are no different from siblings, or the general population.[23-25] However, their later employment prospects appear to be less favourable with studies suggesting that fewer are in employment, and they have a lower professional scale and lower income than siblings.[23,25] The reasons for this are unclear but do not appear to be related to treatment. Adults with growth hormone deficiency have decreased psychological well-being and the numbers receiving a disablement pension tend to be higher than expected.[26] Pituitary hormonal disorders can result from pituitary adenomas. If very large and extending supratentorially, they can affect the visual fields (classically a bitemporal hemianopia) which may affect ability to drive or work near moving machinery, for example. Formal perimetry can help to define the extent of the problem and whether it will result in a restriction from specific duties.

Hypoadrenalism

Underactivity of the adrenal glands (Addison's disease) may be due to primary adrenal disorders (usually autoimmune destruction), or to pituitary underfunction, leading to reduced ACTH secretion. The result is reduced adrenal cortisol secretion leading to symptoms and clinical features such as postural dizziness, increased pigmentation, and even hypoglycaemia. Once diagnosed however, treatment with hydrocortisone replacement is straightforward and there are no long-term health or employment implications.

Insulinoma

Finally, this rare but important endocrine syndrome should be mentioned. An insulinoma is a tumour of the pancreatic beta cells leading to autonomous insulin overproduction, and consequent unpredictable hypoglycaemia. This of course has serious implications for employment and driving, particularly as the patient is unable to prevent hypoglycaemic attacks. The condition is cured by removal of the tumour. However, in some cases localization of the tumour is difficult, or the patient may be too old for surgery. In these cases, a combination of dietary advice and the drug diazoxide is used.

Selected references

1 Lister J. The employment of diabetics. *BMJ* 1983; **287**: 1087–1088.
2 Waclawski ER. Employment and diabetes: a survey of the prevalence of diabetic workers known by occupational physicians, and the restrictions placed on diabetic workers in employment. *Diabet Med* 1989; **6**: 16–19.
3 Ardran M, MacFarlane I, Robinson C. Educational achievements, employment and social class of insulin-dependent diabetics: a survey of a young adult clinic in Liverpool. *Diabet Med* 1987; **4**: 546–548.
4 *Diabetes employment handbook*. London: British Diabetic Association, 1997.
5 *Diabetes and employment*. London: British Diabetic Association, 1997.
6 Karvonen M, Tuomilehto J, Libman I, LaPorte R. A review of the recent epidemiological data on the world-wide incidence of Type 1 (insulin-dependent) diabetes mellitus. *Diabetologia* 1993; **36**: 883–892.
7 Metcalfe MA, Baum JD. Incidence of insulin-dependent diabetes in children under 15 years of age in the British Isles during 1988. *BMJ* 1991; **302**: 443–447.
8 Zimmet P, McCarthy D. The NIDDM epidemic: global estimates and projections—a look into the crystal ball. *IDF Bull* 1995; **40**: 8–16.
9 Morrish NJ, Stevens LK, Fuller JH, Keen H, Jarrett RJ. Incidence of macrovascular disease in diabetes mellitus: the London cohort of the WHO Multinational Study of Vascular Disease in Diabetics. *Diabetologia* 1991; **34**: 584–589.
10 Waclawski ER. Diabetes and employment. MFOM thesis, Faculty of Occupational Medicine, Royal College of Physicians, 1989.
11 Robinson N, Yateman NA, Protopapa LE, Bush L. Employment problems and diabetes. *Diabet Med* 1990; **7**: 16–22.
12 Griffiths RD, Moses RG. Diabetes in the workplace. Employment experience of young people with diabetes mellitus. *Med J Aust* 1993; **158**: 169–171.
13 Poole CJ, Gibbons D, Calvert IA. Sickness absence in diabetic employees at a large engineering factory. *Occup Envir Med* 1994; **51**: 299–301.
14 Waclawski ER. Sickness absence among insulin-treated diabetic employees. *Diabet Med* 1990;**7**: 41–44.
15 Sarter G, Nystrom L, Dahlquist G. The Swedish Childhood Diabetes Study: a seven-fold decrease in short-term mortality? Diabet Med 1991; **8**: 18–21.
16 Robinson N, Stevens LK, Protopapa LE. Education and employment for young people with diabetes. *Diabet Med* 1993; **10**: 983–989.
17 Barnett AH, Owens DR. Insulin analogues. *Lancet* 1997; **349**: 47–51.
18 Diabetes Control and Complications Trial Research Group. The effect of intensive treatment of diabetes on the development and progression of long-term complications in insulin-dependent diabetes mellitus. *New Engl J Med* 1993; **329**: 977–986.
19 *Diabetes and potentially hazardous occupations*. London: British Diabetic Association, 1996.
20 Beck J, Miller BG, Frier BM, Grant J, Waclawski ER. *A pilot study of the frequency of hypoglycaemic episodes in people with insulin-treated diabetes and the relationship of hypoglycaemia to employment*. Report No. TM/96/10. Edinburgh: Institute of Occupational Medicine, 1997.
21 Jones KE, Gill GV. Insurance company attitudes to diabetes. *Prac Diabetes* 1989; **6**: 230–231.
22 American Diabetes Association. Hypoglycemia and employment/licensure. *Diabetes Care* 1997;**20**(suppl 1): S59.
23 Dean HJ, McTaggart TL, Fish DG, Friesen HG. The educational, vocational and marital status of growth hormone deficient adults treated with growth hormone during childhood. *Am J Dis Child* 1985; **139**: 1105–1110.

24   Mitchell CM, Joyce S, Johanson AJ *et al.* A retrospective evaluation of psychological impact of long-term growth hormone therapy. *Clin Pediatr* 1986; **25**: 17–23.
25   Dutch Growth Hormone Working Group. Riksken B, van Busschbach J, le Cessie S, Manten W, Sperman TR, Grobbee R. Impaired social status of growth hormone deficient adults as compared to controls with short or normal stature. *Clin Endocrinol* 1995; **43**: 205–211.
26   Rosen T, Wiren L, Wihelmsen L, Wiklund I, Bengtsson BA. Decreased psychological well-being in adult patients with growth hormone deficiency. *Clin Endocrinol* 1994; **40**: 111–116.

17

Haematological disorders

A. L. Fingret and P. M. Emerson

In the context of employment, haematological problems arise either as the result of inci-dental findings during routine health screening procedures in industry or during the course of specific investigations of ill health by general practitioners or hospital consul-tants. Screening procedures in industry may be required statutorily because of exposure to toxic substances or ionizing radiation, but many large industries also have well-estab-lished policies for routine health screening of staff.

Haematological disorders are common and it is beyond the scope of this chapter to encompass the full range. Some conditions, e.g. pernicious anaemia, are easily diag-nosed, treatable, and curable, and these will not be described as they have little relevance to fitness to work. We have concentrated on conditions of a subacute or chronic nature where work performance, types of employment, or absenteeism are a problem, with spe-cial reference to up-to-date therapy and advances in treatment. The conditions covered in this chapter include iron deficiency, polycythaemia, the significance of a high mean corpuscular volume (MCV), the platelet count, malignant haematological disorders, the haemoglobinopathies, inherited coagulation disorders, and anticoagulant control.

Before proceeding to specific conditions, a general word on anaemic patients is rele-vant. Chronically anaemic patients may remain asymptomatic even with extremely low haemoglobin levels, particularly in the case of some of the congenital anaemias where a compensatory right shift in the oxygen dissociation curve allows patients with very low haemoglobin levels to have functional haemoglobins of several grams higher. For this reason it is absolutely essential to assess every patient individually with regard to employ-ment—a low haemoglobin detected in an asymptomatic patient as part of a routine screening procedure clearly requires investigation, but is not *per se* a contra-indication to employment.

Iron deficiency[1]

About 3% of adult men and 14% of postmenopausal women are anaemic. Iron defi-ciency should be considered not as a diagnosis but rather as a marker of an underlying disorder; certainly, treatment with iron is not sufficient and the cause should be sought assiduously. These causes are not listed as they are well known, but it should be noted that dietary lack (except in physiological states of increased need such as pregnancy), is an unlikely explanation given the high-quality foods now available, which are often for-tified with iron. The most likely cause of iron deficiency in a previously healthy individ-ual is occult bleeding from the gastrointestinal tract from such lesions as hiatus hernia, peptic ulceration, carcinoma of the colon, diverticulitis, and angiodysplasia. Aspirin and non-steroidal anti-inflammatory drugs (NSAIDs) may also cause gastrointestinal bleeding because of gastric irritation and their effect on platelet function.

Iron deficiency may be detected as part of a routine screen in an individual who feels perfectly fit, but adequate investigation is still required. Patients who present to their doctor with symptoms of iron deficiency which are non-specific, i.e. lethargy, easy fatigue, mild dyspnoea on effort, are often quite severely anaemic and it is not unusual for the haemoglobin to fall to below 9.0 g/dl (in men) or 7.0 g/dl (in women) before help is sought. Iron therapy can be started immediately while other investigations are in progress but should be continued long enough (at least 3 months) to replenish the depleted body stores after the haemoglobin has risen to normal (men 13.0–18.0 g/dl; women 11.5-16.0 g/dl). It is difficult to assess how much iron deficiency affects work capacity, but it should be remembered that iron is an essential cellular component of all tissues of the body in addition to haemopoeisis. There are often no symptoms at rest but these may occur during periods of demanding physical work and more severely anaemic patients will almost certainly show reduced tolerance on exercise testing. In countries where iron deficiency is common it has been shown that work capacity and productivity are sub-maximal. Finally it should be remembered that individuals with α or β thalassaemia trait may have low red cell indices, MCV and mean corpuscular haemoglobin (MCH) owing to the lack of the globin content of haemoglobin. Although these patients are usually iron replete they can suffer from associated iron deficiency and this possibility should be considered in a previously healthy individual who becomes symptomatic.

Polycythaemia[2]

Abnormally high haemoglobin levels give rise to problems which are potentially more hazardous than an equivalent fall in haemoglobin. The blood viscosity rises sharply when the haematocrit is above 0.50 and transient ischaemic attacks, visual disturbances, peripheral vascular disease, and other manifestations of ischaemia may occur at values above 0.55. Thus, the polycythaemic patient is more likely to have accidents at work or put colleagues at risk than a moderately anaemic one. The upper limits of normal for adult men and women are haematocrits of 0.54 and 0.47 respectively (Hb 19.0 g/dl and 16.0 g/dl).

Polycythaemia is classified as primary—**polycythaemia rubra vera** (PRV) or primary proliferative polycythaemia—or secondary, the latter being far more common. Polycythaemia rubra vera is a clonal myeloproliferative disorder in which the red-cell mass is increased and which requires therapy to keep the haematocrit and platelet count, which is frequently raised, within the normal range. Treatment is essential (the median survival time in untreated patients is less than 18 months) and is either by regular venesection, oral chemotherapy or occasionally the intravenous injection of radioactive phosphorus (P^{32}). Patients can continue in full-time work and the condition runs a protracted course, the median survival being over 10 years. Time off work for attendance at hospital outpatients is variable but averages about once per month.

The condition usually terminates with bone marrow failure and patients enter a final stage where treatment is no longer necessary and they may become transfusion dependent. Increasing splenomegaly is common and transformation to acute leukaemia occurs in a small proportion of cases. Obviously patients will be incapacitated during this final stage.

Secondary polycythaemia, in which there is also an absolute increase in the red-cell mass, is associated with conditions in which there is either a reduction in arterial oxygen, inappropriate secretion of erythropoietin, or rarely an abnormal haemoglobin. Treatment consists of removing the underlying causes and venesection to reduce the haematocrit to a safe level. Work limitation will depend on the severity of the causative condition (e.g. cyanotic heart disease or chronic obstructive airways disease). It should be stressed that patients presenting with either primary or secondary polycythaemia are at high risk from thromboembolic complications and no time should be lost in referring the patient to an appropriate specialist. Occasionally a high haemoglobin is found in normal individuals who have returned from working abroad at high altitude: they require no special treatment as the haematocrit rapidly returns to normal.

Particular attention should be paid to what is now termed apparent or relative polycythaemia. Other terms used for this condition are Geisbock's syndrome, stress-, spurious-, or pseudo-polycythaemia. These individuals have a high haemoglobin and haematocrit but although the red-cell mass is normal the total plasma volume is reduced 12.5% below average. The condition is much commoner in men, with a maximum prevalence in the 40–70 year age group. The cause is not known; contributory factors may be hypertension, smoking, diuretics, alcohol, and obesity but treatment or an improvement in lifestyle is not always followed by a fall in haematocrit. Suggestions that the condition is due to stress, inappropriate secretion of antidiuretic hormone, sleep hypoxia, or low aldosterone levels have not been confirmed. Arterial hypoxaemia is found in about one-fifth of patients but the extent of any possible vascular complications is debatable. It is very important to differentiate this condition from true polycythaemia as there are obvious life insurance implications.

High mean cell volume[3]

The MCV is available as part of the routine blood profile but the normal range varies slightly with the type of equipment used. Generally speaking, however, a patient's red cells can be said to be macrocytic if the value exceeds 100 fl. As with iron deficiency and polycythaemia, abnormal values may be picked up on a routine blood count and discretion as to when to investigate must be left with the physician, as it is not unusual to find a raised MCV in the presence of a normal haemoglobin. Having excluded the well-known causes, such as B_{12} and folate deficiency, the commonest cause is excessive alcohol intake. Alcohol causes many haematological problems, ranging from the complications of liver disease, such as bleeding from varices, coagulation disturbances, hypersplenism, and dietary folate deficiency, to an effect on the bone marrow itself. Alcohol is a tissue toxin and there is considerable evidence for a direct suppressive effect on all aspects of haemopoeisis. This is probably the cause of the macrocytosis in excessive drinkers, who are otherwise healthy, as the index rapidly returns to normal on alcohol withdrawal. Physicians encountering a raised MCV as an isolated finding should take a detailed history of alcohol intake from the patient, especially if work performance is in doubt and appropriate help should be offered if needed. A persistently raised MCV suggests permanent liver damage or continued drinking. (Alcohol is also discussed in Chapters 15 and 25.)

In patients with no history of excessive alcohol intake, macrocytic red cells may be due to myxoedema or myelodysplastic conditions. The latter are preleukaemic states but the time to evolution of the terminal phase varies from months to years depending on the chromosomal abnormality and is usually preceded by a period of cytopenia of varying severity. Specialized investigations are required to confirm the diagnosis.

Low platelet count

One of the problems which is continually encountered by the haematologist is the patient, usually with refractory idiopathic thrombocytopenic purpura (ITP), who runs a persistently low platelet count. These patients are often young and may be concerned about the nature of their employment. Generally speaking, patients with a count of $>100 \times 10^9$/l will be symptom free and not bleed excessively following trauma; between 50 and 100×10^9/l there may be haemorrhagic manifestations following trauma but otherwise few problems. The patient with a count persistently below this level and certainly below 25×10^9/l may suffer from spontaneous bleeding, usually purpuric, the major risk to life being intracranial haemorrhage although this is a rare complication. This group is at risk and employment involving heavy manual work is best avoided and should be replaced by more sedentary occupations. It should be stressed, however, that some patients with counts in the $25–50 \times 10^9$/l range rarely bleed or even bruise easily and few restrictions on employment are necessary in such patients. There is a saying that the patient and not the platelet count should be treated.

Splenectomy

A proportion of patients with chronic idiopathic thrombocytopenic purpura may be receiving steroid or immunosuppressive therapy or have been subjected to splenectomy in the past. The latter group are prone to the development of overwhelming and potentially fatal bacterial infections, especially from the pneumococci, and there should be no delay in referring the patient to hospital if this is suspected. It is recommended that all splenectomized patients be vaccinated against the influenza virus and against pneumococcus, meningococcus, and *Haemophilus influenzae*. In addition younger patients should receive twice daily prophylactic penicillin and adults prophylaxis for 2 years postoperatively. A card should always be carried stating the nature of the condition and when and where the operation was performed. Special warnings should be given to people travelling abroad, as malarial infections are of increased severity. Few occupations are barred, including healthcare, but veterinary practice or dog handling is not recommended as fatalities have occurred from infections by the *capnocytophanga canimorsus* bacteria following dog bites.

Malignant disease[4,5]

Incidence and meaning of remission

Table 17.1 shows the incidence of haematological malignant disease in the 16–64 age group. These conditions are rare when compared with other forms of malignant disease and until 30 years ago their often rapidly fatal outcome precluded any consideration of return to work. However, the discovery of effective chemotherapeutic agents in the 1950s and 1960s, together with improvements in supportive care and successful bone marrow transplantation, has led to an increase in remission rates and length of survival and to the possibility of a cure in some conditions. The definition of remission is of considerable importance concerning fitness to work. Generally speaking, a patient can be said to be in complete remission if no signs of active disease can be detected clinically or in the laboratory, i.e. the patient feels well, has no organomegaly, a normal bone marrow and cerebrospinal fluid, and a blood count within the normal range except when suppressed by chemotherapy.

During complete remission there is no reason why a patient should not return to almost any type of previous employment and many do, but, especially with acute leukaemias and some lymphomas, there is a period of absence from work during induction of remission. It is current clinical practice for a patient to be informed of the nature of their condition and the objectives of treatment and given some idea of prognosis. Medical practitioners can be extremely helpful during this period by reassuring both patient and employer that the aim is to return the patient to normal life and to full-time employment as soon as possible.

Aim of treatment and general effects of chemotherapy

The aim of treatment is to destroy as many abnormal cells as possible by the use of chemotherapeutic agents without permanently damaging the bone marrow or other tissues. Treatment is mainly by cytotoxic drugs but radiotherapy may be given as the treatment of choice or as an additional form of therapy. All chemotherapeutic agents have side-effects and are frequently used in combination, thus compounding these effects. The

Table 17.1 Reported cases of haematological malignant disease in the population of working age (16–64) in England and Wales in 1991[6]

Type	Number (both sexes)
All leukaemias	1433
Myeloid leukaemias	839
Lymphoid leukaemias	512
Other leukaemias	82
All lymphomas	3257
Hodgkin's disease	790
Non-Hodgkin's lymphoma	2467
Multiple myeloma	647

drugs are not specific for tumour cells and some damage to normal tissues is inevitable with effective therapeutic dosages. Different drug combinations are used for the different conditions and a detailed description is beyond the scope of this chapter. Broadly speaking the more acute or high grade the malignancy the more likely the patient is to receive combination chemotherapy with up to four or more drugs.

Acute myeloid leukaemia

In the age group 15–65 years, acute myeloid leukaemia (AML) and its variants are approximately twice as common as acute lymphoblastic leukaemia (ALL). The majority of patients in the UK are entered into one of the Medical Research Council's trials of therapy. Treatment can be divided into four phases:

- induction of remission
- consolidation of remission
- a period of observation off treatment
- bone marrow transplantation.

The patient is likely to be in hospital during the initial induction and intermittently during the consolidation period; these two phases together can last anything up to 6 months or longer, but a patient who feels well enough should be encouraged to return to part-time or even full-time work. From the patient's point of view the most distressing side-effects of chemotherapy are nausea and vomiting, which may be prostrating, but good drugs are now available which can control all but the worst affected. It is useful to give the patient, the family doctor, and the occupational physician a schedule of treatment so that times off work can be anticipated. Absence from work may also occur owing to intercurrent infections as a result of immunosuppression, or the need for blood transfusion; these can be minimized by arranging blood transfusion and chemotherapy over weekends. Patients who are immunosuppressed should not work in areas where the risk of infection cannot be eliminated. There are a number of work environments where the occupational physician will need to assess the risk, including certain types of health-care work and work peripheral to healthcare such as hospital laundries and mortuaries; other areas of concern are sewage treatment works and animal processing plants.

With modern treatment patients in the relevant age group have an 80% chance of attaining full remission and a 50% chance of being alive at the end of 5 years.

Acute lymphoblastic leukaemia

ALL is the most common leukaemia in childhood but constitutes only 20% of adult acute leukaemia. In adults, the disease does not carry the excellent prognosis of childhood leukaemia, where a cure (i.e. 5 year survival after stopping treatment) can be expected in 75% of cases. Adults have lower remission rates and shorter survival times. The complete remission rate for all adult cases is about 70% and the median survival time, without bone marrow transplantation, is 3 years from diagnosis. Intensive induction and post-remission consolidation necessitates frequent hospital attendance but many patients return to work early in the course of their disease. Maintenance therapy lasts for about 2 years and is almost entirely given on an out-patient basis.

Chronic lymphatic leukaemia

Chronic lymphatic leukaemia (CLL) is a disease of the middle-aged and elderly and is often diagnosed incidentally during routine screening. These individuals feel fit and may not need therapy for many years; once assessment has shown that the disease is not progressing, all that is required is a blood count at regular intervals. Progressive disease as diagnosed by commencement of symptoms, anaemia or thrombocytopenia, and increase in size of lymph nodes or spleen, requires therapy. This may range from gentle oral therapy with chlorambucil and prednisolone to more aggressive combined chemotherapy. Whatever the treatment, the main problems are recurrent infections, usually respiratory in nature, which require early antibiotic therapy and are often prolonged because of the associated immunosuppression.

It is of considerable importance to recognize the relatively benign nature of the condition in many individuals, particularly in terms of employment, pension schemes, and life insurance. At one time it was thought that younger patients had a more aggressive form of the disease, but this is not the case as the mean (50%) survival for patients aged under 55 years at the time of diagnosis is 12 years. Death is likely to occur from the same medical conditions as in the general population. Attempts have been made to stage the disease but the most important poor prognostic signs are anaemia (Hb < 10 g/dl) and/or thrombocytopenia (platelet count $< 100 \times 10^9$/l) at presentation and the rate of doubling of the white cell count when the survival time may be as low as 2 years. The nature of the lymphocytye cell-surface markers is also of prognostic significance.

Chronic myeloid leukaemia

Chronic myeloid leukaemia (CML) may also be diagnosed during routine screening, either as a result of a blood count or the presence of splenomegaly. Once diagnosed, therapy should be commenced immediately. The condition has been designated a preleukaemic state by some authors, as progression to an accelerated phase and untimely transformation into an acute leukaemia (blast-cell crisis) is the usual course of the disease. The condition is due to a mutation in a pluripotential stem cell and the blast-cell crisis may be either myeloid or lymphoblastic in nature. During the chronic phase the disease is usually treated by oral chemotherapy with hydroxyurea, busulphan, and/or interferon. The majority of patients continue in full-time work during this period which lasts on average under 4 years but occasional patients may live as long as 10 years. However, interferon has severe side-effects in some patients which may limit attendance at work. Bone marrow transplantation is the treatment of choice if a donor is available and offers the only chance of a cure. Once patients enter the accelerated phase, anaemia, thrombocytopenia, and increasing splenomegaly present problems requiring regular supportive therapy and lost time from work is inevitable. Once acute transformation has occurred the prognosis is poor. Patients are treated with a regime according to the type of transformation, the median survival for patients in lymphoblastic transformation being 12 months, compared with 2 months for those with myeloid markers.

Hodgkin's disease

Hodgkin's disease (HD) has proved one of the most rewarding conditions to treat: 80% of all patients can be expected to obtain a complete remission and of these approximately 65% will remain disease-free at 10 years. The condition is staged I to IV prior to treatment, the higher numbers designating more widespread disease. Prognosis depends on histology, the extent of disease at presentation, and the presence of non-specific symptoms such as weight loss and night sweats. Recurrent disease still remains a problem but the best series show a median survival of >5 years from the time of relapse. Patients with stage I and some with stage II disease are treated by radiotherapy alone, but the remainder are given combination chemotherapy at monthly intervals and treatment usually lasts 6–9 months. Patients are usually well enough to work throughout, apart from during courses of chemotherapy. It is important that occupational physicians and employers are aware of the excellent prognosis.

Non-Hodgkin's lymphoma

The ability to give accurate statistics regarding remission rates and survival in non-Hodgkin's lymphoma has been bedevilled by the number of histological classifications and until recent years by the lack of properly controlled clinical trials. However, the modern use of a wide panel of monoclonal markers has lead to better diagnosis of the various cell types involved and inevitably to improvement in treatment and survival. Lymphomas may occur at almost any site and many are highly sensitive to irradiation and chemotherapy. The simplest classification for the purposes of this chapter is to divide them into low-grade and high-grade lymphomas. The treatment and prognosis vary with each group and it is important to stress that there is now a possibility of cure of some cases within each group. As with Hodgkin's disease, the lymphomas are staged clinically from I to IV and approximately 40% of all cases are low-grade tumours. The latter have a longer clinical course and occur in the older age groups. Stage I and II tumours are usually treated with radiotherapy and stage III and IV by chemotherapy, often with a single agent. Few patients in this group are cured but long remission rates have occurred. The median time to relapse is approximately four years and the survival time is 7–10 years in most series. When relapse occurs it is often due to transformation to a more aggressive form of lymphoma.

High-grade tumours are more aggressive, affect younger patients and early spread to the bone marrow, central nervous system, and other organs is common. These patients are always treated with multiple drug regimes whenever possible. The prognosis is poor but cures are possible. Unfortunately, bone marrow transplantation has not been as effective as with the leukaemias. Treatment usually lasts 6–12 months and it is unusual for patients to return to work during this period.

Multiple myeloma

Although multiple myeloma affects mainly the middle-aged and elderly, there are over 600 cases per annum in those of working age. Response to chemotherapy has not been as satisfactory as in other forms of leukaemia and lymphoma, and life expectancy has not been greatly improved. Complete remissions are unusual, and a greater than 75% reduction in tumour burden is classed as a good response. The main clinical problems are bone pain, infection, and bone marrow suppression, either due to the disease or as a result of treatment. Poor prognostic indicators are a presenting pancytopenia and renal failure which cannot be reversed by rehydration. The severity of the condition varies greatly between individuals; some patients lead a relatively normal life for many months or even years and are capable of full-time work. Treatment varies according to the severity of the disease and the age of the patient, and ranges from single-agent oral chemotherapy to intensive multiple drug regimes and autologous bone marrow transplantation. Intractable bone pain, which is a major problem, can often be relieved by radiotherapy. The median survival in most large studies has been less than 3 years from diagnosis.

General comments on malignant disease

It must be stressed that haematological malignancies are unlike many other forms of disseminated neoplasia in that the patient in complete remission is clinically disease free and it is unusual for there to be a slowly progressive downhill course preceding relapse, which is often of sudden onset. There is little literature about patients' attitudes to their disease and their employment prospects; however, the majority feel capable of working and most return to their previous jobs within a year of diagnosis even if they are receiving chemotherapy. After an initial period of intensive treatment the average time lost from work is less than 4 weeks per year. Negative attitudes of employers who are uninformed about modern therapy can be a problem, and the support of the physician in encouraging patients to return to work is very important: patients place great reliance on this advice, as optimistic outlooks improve shattered morale and self-esteem. Practical advice on life insurance, pension prospects, and estates is also extremely helpful as individuals often feel greatly relieved if they have settled their affairs even if the prognosis is good. Close communication between all doctors involved in the patient's care (at work, hospital, and family practice) is necessary and every effort should be made to organize treatment in such a way as to minimize interruption of the normal working routine.

Another problem which concerns the occupational physician is whether and when to immunize. Patients on chemotherapy and for a period following cessation of treatment should not receive live vaccines but immunization with other agents can be given although the ability to mount an immune response may be sub-optimal. Finally, it should be remembered that chemotherapy may result in sterility in both men and women; sperm and ova storage should now be offered to all patients.

Thalassaemia and the haemoglobinopathies[7,8]

Of the many currently described variants of haemoglobin production and structure, only two present problems which are likely to be encountered by prospective employers and their occupational health services.

Thalassaemia major

In thalassaemia major there is insufficient production of adult haemoglobin because of the inability to manufacture the β chains of the haemoglobin A molecule. It is inherited as an autosomal recessive disorder, i.e. both parents are carriers and there is a 1:4 chance that a child will be affected. There are over 400 patients in the UK of whom 60% are over the age of 16, most being the offspring of immigrants from Mediterranean and Asian countries. Antenatal diagnosis early in pregnancy followed by abortion has led to a substantial reduction in the number of younger patients. Affected individuals present in the first year and require regular transfusions to maintain their haemoglobin level; these repeated transfusions produce massive iron overload which ultimately affects vital organs producing cardiac, hepatic and endocrine failure. The introduction of intensive iron chelation by the administration of desferrioxamine on 5 days of each week has extended the lifespan of patients and the majority now reach adult life though their ultimate life expectancy is still reduced. The need for regular transfusion at monthly or 6 weekly intervals necessitates some absence from work, but many centres arrange treatment over weekends so that time lost is minimal. Most British thalassaemia patients have not encountered major difficulties in obtaining employment, although most are employed below their potential because of previous loss of schooling. Bone marrow transplantation is curative but the procedure carries considerable morbidity and an appreciable mortality.

Thalassaemia trait

As mentioned on p. 336, affected individuals show a blood picture resembling iron deficiency. It is of considerable importance that these patients are not disadvantaged or advised wrongly about their work prospects, as the vast majority are symptom-free, healthy individuals.

Sickle-cell disease

Sickle-cell disease has arisen as a clinical problem in the UK in the past 30 years, mainly as a result of the large influx of immigrants of African ancestry. It is estimated that there are currently at least 5000 sufferers in the UK. Like thalassaemia major, it is inherited as an autosomal condition: heterozygotes are symptom-free but homozygous patients present with a severe and potentially crippling and life-threatening condition. Affected individuals have a point mutation resulting in the substitution of valine for glutamic acid on the β chain of haemoglobin A. The resulting haemoglobin S polymerizes under conditions of lower oxygen tension into rigid units which deform the red cell and produce the classical sickle or holly-leaf cell which can be seen microscopically. These abnormal cells give rise to the clinical effects, namely chronic anaemia (Hb 7.0–9.0 g/dl) due to haemolysis, painful episodic crises from stasis and infarction in small vessels, aplastic crises due to intercurrent viral infections, and sequestration crises when there is massive pooling of blood in the spleen in infants and more rarely in the liver in older patients. These latter three events should be treated as acute medical emergencies and the patient should be referred to hospital immediately if symptoms arise at work.

The frequency of sickle-cell trait in the UK is about 8% among the Afro-Caribbean community; approximately 1:600 births in this population group produce a homozygous individual. Antenatal screening is routine in this country and parents can be counselled about the possibility of producing an affected child. It is extremely important to differentiate between heterozygote carriers and patients with sickle-cell disease, as the former should be treated no differently from other members of the community with the exception that work in environments with risks of low oxygen tension is best avoided. Flying, diving, and compressed air work would be examples.

Patients with sickle-cell disease should be given professional advice when selecting a working environment and as they are functionally asplenic, because of repeated infarction of the spleen, they should be given the same prophylaxis against infections as described earlier (p. 338). Because of the factors mentioned in the introduction they tolerate their anaemia remarkably well, and a low haemoglobin level is not a contraindication to employment. Factors which may have an adverse effect on their condition are hypoxia, acidosis, extremes of temperature, dehydration, and changes of atmospheric pressure. There is no reason, however, why most forms of employment should not be undertaken, including outside and relatively heavy work. Modern airlines have cabin pressures adjusted such that travel is safe, but sufferers should not be accepted as flight crew. It is of considerable importance to note that a few patients with sickle-cell disease are remarkably free from any form of complication and they should be assessed separately. Specialist advice should be sought in these cases as it is possible to differentiate them from the others by laboratory testing.

There is little information about the employment prospects of patients with sickle-cell disease. Advances in supportive care rather than specific prevention of sickling, which is still a major therapeutic problem, have allowed many patients with sickle-cell disease to reach adult life and enter the job market. The possibility of frequent absence due to intercurrent illness and the environmental restrictions described above has prejudiced employment. However, individuals suffering from genetic disorders that interfere with their ability to undertake normal day to day activities are now protected by the Disability Discrimination Act 1995 (DDA). This requires employers to make reasonable adjustments to accommodate the individual's particular needs.

Glucose-6-phosphate dehydrogenase deficiency

Glucose-6-phosphate dehydrogenase deficiency is a sex-linked condition present in the same ethnic groups as haemoglobin S and thalassaemia, and affecting approximately the same number of people. Most sufferers are entirely symptom-free and are unaware that they have the condition. Once diagnosed they should carry a list of drugs to be avoided, because most problems arise as a result of haemolysis due to the ingestion of oxidative agents. The drugs considered unsafe are listed in the *British national formulary*.[9] From the point of view of employment these individuals should be advised not to work in chemical plants manufacturing naphthalene or trinitrotoluene. If there is a history of favism, agricultural work involving broad bean cultivation or processing should be avoided; otherwise there should be no problems with employment.

As in all these inherited conditions genetic counselling is essential, especially in pregnancy, and patients should carry a card stating the diagnosis and a list of drugs to be avoided.

Coagulation disorders

Haemophilia A and B[10]

There are approximately 5000 individuals with haemophilia A and 1000 with haemophilia B (Christmas disease) in the UK; these two disorders are discussed together as their clinical presentation and treatment are similar. Both are sex-linked disorders and female homozygotes are extremely rare (estimated 1 per 50 million population) so, in practice, all patients are male. The condition varies in severity from mild cases who may not be diagnosed until adult life, to very severely affected individuals who require regular replacement therapy. The severity of the condition tends to run true in families and is assessed by measuring the blood coagulant activity of either factor VIII or factor IX. Haemophiliacs are classed as severe (factor VIII:C $<$ 1 iu/dl) moderate (1–5 iu/dl) or mild ($>$5 iu/dl). The clinical presentation varies according to the level of activity, the most severely affected individuals suffering repeated haemorrhages into joints, deep tissues, and occasionally externally. These episodic bleeds can cause severe arthroses and contractures which, before the advent of modern treatment, led to crippling disability early in life. Mildly affected haemophiliacs, with factor VIII:C levels of $>$5iu/dl, escape these deformities and tend to bleed only after accidental trauma, surgery, or dental extraction.

Modern therapy has greatly improved the prognosis with regard to mobility, motivation, education, employment, social activities, and life expectancy. Treatment consists of replacing the missing factor by intravenous injection as necessary, a procedure which takes about 15 minutes. There are designated Haemophilia Centres throughout the UK where programmes of replacement therapy are arranged to suit individuals. Home therapy, whereby patients are instructed to inject themselves with factor VIII, has been of major benefit in limiting the severity of bleeds and reducing travelling and waiting time at hospital. Other problems related to haemophilia are associated with chronic pain (there is a relatively high degree of drug dependency), unavoidable absence from school, college or work, and the psychological aspects of suffering from an inherited and potentially crippling condition.

The occupations which haemophiliacs can be expected to follow vary according to the severity of the condition. There are no limitations in obtaining driving licences unless debarred by associated medical conditions. Haemophiliacs are not accepted into the armed forces, nor usually allowed to fly passenger aircraft. In one instance a patient with a factor VIIIC value of 2 iu/dl, who had previously flown in Australia, was accepted as a commercial airline pilot in the UK but could not take up the position as insurance cover was refused (personal communication). Apart from these, no occupations are unsuitable for mildly affected individuals but severely affected patients are best suited to sedentary jobs, such as office or clerical work, and heavy manual labour should be avoided. However, there is no fixed rule as some haemophiliacs with extremely low coagulant activity seldom bleed, whereas some patients classed as moderately affected may suffer repeated haemorrhages. In the 1980s about 50% of severely affected haemophiliacs contracted AIDS but this has now been superseded by the high incidence of hepatitis C and at least 95% of all patients treated with coagulation factor concentrate are affected. This obviously has implications for employment (see Chapter 15, p. 300) and life assurance.

One of the major problems encountered is a lack of suitable facilities for self-treatment at work. Many patients leave a refrigerated pack at their place of work (there is remarkable self-perception of early bleeds by haemophiliacs), but in those places without a first-aid room the treatment may have to be administered in unsuitable surroundings such as kitchens, washrooms, or offices. Treatment kits should never be stored alongside food. Bleeds at work result mainly from accidental impact injuries rather than from heavy work or machinery. The occupational physician has a vital role to play both in assessing suitable work for the haemophiliac and in making suitable arrangements for self-treatment; also in counselling employers about haemophilia and correcting many misconceptions. There is, for example, a common misconception that haemophiliacs are liable to bleed severely from a simple pinprick, which is nonsense.

Employment prospects for haemophiliacs have improved dramatically in the last two decades, following the introduction of self-administration of factor VIII. The actual employment record for younger haemophiliacs is extremely good and approximates to that of the general population and to that in other developed countries. A major problem facing haemophiliacs is whether to tell prospective employers of their condition as many feel that there is a general lack of awareness about the dramatic improvement in quality of life and treatment; but where employers are told they are generally sympathetic and helpful. Haemophiliacs experience problems with life insurance and there is usually a loading of the premium. Advice on insurance and pension schemes is available from the Haemophilia Society (see Appendix 7 for address). As a genetic disorder resulting in disability, haemophilia brings sufferers under the protection of the DDA. Advice can be obtained from the Disability Employment Adviser in the local employment service on how best to accommodate individual requirements, if the employee has no access to an occupational health service.

Anticoagulant therapy

The exact number of patients on long-term anticoagulant therapy in the UK is unknown but the number is substantial: it has been estimated that up to 10 million coagulation control tests are performed per annum. The major problems encountered are with dose control as response to therapy varies with changes in diet, alcohol intake, intercurrent illness, and changes in other medication. It is essential that the doctor responsible for prescribing anticoagulants is informed of any alteration to other therapy, as many drugs potentiate and some inhibit the action of anticoagulants. A full list is available in the *British National Formulary*.[9] Patients are encouraged to continue in their present employment and no occupations are barred except those needing strenuous physical work. However, in practice the patient's lifestyle may already have changed as a result of the underlying condition necessitating anticoagulant therapy.

Selected references

1   Herbert V. Iron disorders can mimic anything so always test for them. *Blood Rev* 1992; **6**: 125–132.
2   Landaw SA. Polycythaemia vera and other polycythaemic states. *Clin Lab Med* 1990; **10**: 857–871.
3   Pohorecky LA. Stress and alcohol interaction: an update of human research. *Alcohol Clin Exp Res* 1991; **15**: 438–59.
4   Hoffbrand AV, Lewis SM. *Postgraduate haematology.* Oxford: Heinemann, 1989.
5   Altmaier EM, Gingrich RD, Fyfe, MA. Two year adjustment of bone marrow transplant. *Bone Marrow Transplant* 1991; **7**: 311–366.
6   *Cancer statistics registration.* Series MBI, No. 19. London: HMSO, 1997.
7   Weatherall DJ, Clegg JB. *The thalassaemia syndromes.* Oxford: Blackwell, 1989.
8   Serjeant G. *Sickle-cell disease.* Oxford: Oxford University Press, 1989.
9   *British national formulary.* Published biannually by the British Medical Association and the Royal Pharmaceutical Society of Great Britain.
10 Bloom AL. Progress in the clinical management of haemophiliacs. *Thromb Haemost* 1991; **66**: 166–177.

Further reading

Evans G. What are the occupational implications of thalassaemia? *Occup Med* **49**, *117–118.*

18

Cardiovascular disorders

P. J. Baxter and M. C. Petch

Cardiovascular disorders affect fitness to work in two ways. First, an individual may suffer from symptoms on effort which limit working capacity. Such disability is quantifiable and can often be alleviated by effective treatment, e.g. coronary artery bypass grafting (CABG). The second and much more difficult problem is the risk of sudden incapacity. This may take the form of a simple faint; loss of vision through systemic embolism; a ruptured aortic aneurysm; Stokes–Adams attack; or sudden cardiac death as a result of ventricular fibrillation. Assessment of this risk and its effect on the individual and colleagues at work has been the focus of considerable discussion in recent years and forms a recurrent theme throughout this chapter. Although the risk of instantaneous incapacity is very small, the consequences can be disastrous and are generally remembered indefinitely: the most notorious example is the London bus driver who fainted at the wheel when approaching a bus stop, with the result that several people in the bus queue were killed. Regulatory medicine has to strike a difficult balance between restricting the liberty of the individual, and protecting that individual and others from the effects of sudden incapacity.

Limitation of working capacity and the risk of sudden incapacity can both be well-judged in populations by specialist opinion, aided by the results of non-invasive tests such as echocardiography and exercise testing. Unfortunately, however, disease progression can be unpredictable, and individuals judged to be at low risk from further cardiovascular events may nevertheless suffer incapacity. This difference between the individual and the population is not well understood by employers and employees and can be a source of misunderstanding and confusion.

A further source of confusion is the profound psychological disturbance that may follow the development of cardiovascular disease. The victim is typically an overweight, smoking, male manual worker in his forties, who has always enjoyed robust good health. A heart attack proves devastating and he never returns to work despite prompt treatment, a full cardiac recovery, and the demonstration of only modest coronary disease. Atypical chest pains and tightness, shortness of breath, dizzy spells, loss of fitness, fatigue, and depression persist despite attempts at rehabilitation, reassurance, and treatment that often includes myocardial revascularization. Such individuals deserve sympathy and support. Management is, however, extraordinarily difficult and retirement on grounds of psychological ill health may be the only option.

Clinical aspects affecting work capacity

Coronary heart disease

Epidemiology

The greatest scourge affecting the working population is undoubtedly coronary heart disease (CHD). In developed countries, about one-quarter of all deaths are due to CHD. In England and Wales in 1994 there were 135 440 deaths and 304 078 hospital discharges with a diagnosis of CHD.[1] The Royal College of General Practitioners' third national study confirmed the high level of morbidity.[2] Epidemiological surveys such as the British Regional Heart Study may overestimate the prevalence of CHD, but by using a questionnaire, physical examination, and electrocardiogram, the prevalence was estimated at 24.7% of men aged 40–59 years.[3] The Whitehall study showed that the incidence was higher in social classes 4 and 5 as compared with classes 1, 2, and 3.[4]

Some CHD is preventable; employers have a duty to support and reinforce community measures by discouraging smoking, encouraging healthy activities during rest and recreational hours, and providing a healthy diet at work. Some victims of CHD die suddenly and unpredictably from ventricular fibrillation. In the WHO Tower Hamlets study[5] 40% of heart attacks (defined as myocardial infarction or sudden death from CHD) were fatal and 60% of deaths occurred within 1 hour of the onset of any symptoms. This fact has been reinforced by more recent studies, is widely recognized, and has naturally affected employers' attitudes towards employees known to be, or suspected of, suffering from CHD. Heart attacks tend to occur more frequently in the morning, or towards the beginning of shiftwork, as compared with other times of the day.[6] Their onset may be associated with unaccustomed vigorous effort.[7]

Clinical features

CHD usually presents as chest pain, either myocardial infarction or angina; it may also present with symptoms resulting from arrhythmia (including sudden death), or heart failure, or be detected incidentally by electrocardiography. Anyone with chest pain who is suspected of suffering from myocardial infarction should be taken urgently to the nearest coronary care unit as prompt treatment can save lives. After recovery the risk of further cardiac events (i.e. sudden death, recurrent myocardial infarction or need for interventional treatment) is assessed by the combination of clinical features and simple investigations (see below). The likelihood of returning to work after a cardiac event is affected by a variety of physical, psychological, and social factors.[8]

Medical management strategies

Lifestyle management and drug therapy have transformed the management of all manifestations of CHD. Prognosis after myocardial infarction is improved by thrombolysis and subsequent treatment with aspirin. Myocardial ischaemia may be alleviated by nitrates, β-adrenergic antagonists, and calcium antagonists. The symptoms and survival of patients with heart failure is improved by diuretics and angiotensin-converting enzyme (ACE) inhibitors. Statins improve prognosis and reduce the risk of subsequent events in all groups of patients with CHD. These and other cardiovascular drugs are generally well tolerated and seem remarkably free from long-term side-effects. Many owe their efficacy to their vasodilating action; hence hypotension and faintness are possible complications.

Angioplasty

Coronary angioplasty is nowadays straightforward, safe, and effective in relieving angina. Plain old balloon angioplasty (POBA) is bedevilled by a high recurrence rate—approximately one-third of patients will experience a recurrence of cardiac pain within 4 months. The procedure is therefore commonly accompanied by the implantation of a metal mesh or stent which is delivered on the balloon in a collapsed state down the artery and subsequently deployed at high pressure (e.g. 14 atmospheres) into the arterial wall. The angiographic results are truly remarkable and recurrent symptoms are less usual, although the precise incidence with this technology is not yet known. Complex, distal, and multiple stenoses can be tackled. Groin haematomas are an unusual but well-recognized complication. Return to work within 1 week is commonplace. Angioplasty does not improve long-term survival of patients with CHD.

Coronary artery bypass grafting

CABG is more complex than angioplasty but is also remarkably safe, with most centres reporting mortality rates of around 1% for elective operations. Recovery is rapid and most patients resume work within 2–3 months of surgery. Most patients are relieved of their angina. Patients who are able to work before surgery should generally be able to work afterwards, and restrictions that may have been appropriate previously should no longer be relevant. Similarly, many who could not work before surgery because of their disability should be able to do so afterwards. Unfortunately, cardiac surgery is a rather dramatic event that may prompt overprotective attitudes among family members, friends, employers, or even medical advisers. Many individuals who could and should return to work fail to do so for this reason, rather than because of continuing incapacity. No special restrictions are usually necessary after return to work. Coronary graft stenosis and occlusion, however, leads to a recurrence of angina at a rate of about 4% per annum. This is generally less severe than previously but will affect long-term occupational planning. CABG for left main stem or three-vessel disease will improve prognosis. Unfortunately waiting times, both for coronary arteriography and bypass surgery, are such that many patients do not return to work. One study showed that of those who had lost more than 6 months' work before operation, fewer (only 35%) returned to work compared with those who had lost less than 6 months.[9]

Rehabilitation programmes are now well-established in many hospitals. These enable many patients to make a full physical and psychological recovery following a cardiac event such as myocardial infarction or CABG.

Assessment

The risk of sudden disability and death through ventricular fibrillation is the major factor affecting work capacity amongst victims of CHD. The risk is greatest in the early days following a myocardial infarct and in those with most myocardial damage. The extent of ventricular damage may be judged by the presence of heart failure, gallop rhythm, and estimation of left ventricular function using simple imaging techniques such as echocardiography and radionuclide ventriculography. The presence of residual areas of myocardial ischaemia is the second determinant of prognosis in the longer term and is a manifestation of more extensive coronary disease. This may be judged by a recurrence of cardiac pain or the development of angina pectoris, which may be confirmed by exercise testing. An exercise test may also reveal cardiovascular incapacity in other ways: exhaustion, inappropriate heart rate and blood pressure responses, arrhythmia, and electrocardiographic change, especially ST segment shift.

In practice, the exercise test in combination with an experienced clinical opinion, has superseded the coronary angiogram in assessing fitness for work. This is reflected in the DVLA guidance material relating to vocational drivers (see Appendix to this chapter). Individuals who are free of symptoms and signs of cardiac dysfunction, and who can achieve a good workload with no symptoms or other adverse features, have a very low risk of further cardiac events. This applies particularly to younger individuals whose employers need have little hesitation in taking them back to work.

An ability to reach stage 4 of the Bruce protocol on a treadmill is judged to place an individual at such low risk of further cardiac events that vocational driving may be permitted (see Appendix to this chapter). The DVLA guidelines, which are the result of careful deliberation by an Honorary Medical Advisory Panel, are now being applied more widely to other groups of workers whose occupation may involve an element of risk to themselves or others should the individual employee affected suffer cardiovascular collapse. Most employees, however, are not required to demonstrate such high levels of cardiovascular fitness and lower levels would be acceptable for those in more sedentary and low-risk occupations.

Subjects with continuing severe disability, sinister arrhythmias, or poor left ventricular function should generally be advised to retire. This also applies to other individuals with progressive cardiac disorders, e.g. dilated cardiomyopathy. In contrast, subjects with good ventricular function, a stable cardiac rhythm, and minimal disability will usually fare well and should be encouraged to work.

Following myocardial infarction, assessment of prognosis along the lines outlined above is recommended: those with no complications and good exercise tolerance may return to work in 4–6 weeks. A few will take longer. Patients with CHD and persistent angina despite medical treatment should be assessed with a view to myocardial revascularization.

Return to work

In all cases, when work is resumed, the levels and duration of activity should be increased progressively; returning to work implies a level of sustained activity well above that achieved by most who are recovering at home or who are undertaking hospital rehabilitation programmes.

Psychological difficulties may be experienced even by those with no signs of cardiac damage. Anxieties of both the patient and partner have been shown to affect the ability of men surviving myocardial infarction to return to work; half may have some anxiety or depression and, of those, half may have severe symptoms persisting, if untreated, a year later.[10]

In general, physical activity is good for the heart. The degree of physical activity must take into account patients' previous fitness and the results of exercise testing, etc. Patients with stable angina pectoris can safely work within their limitations of fitness but should not be put in situations where their angina may be readily provoked. Although it may be possible to be dogmatic in giving advice about physical work, guidance about the psychological stresses associated with managerial duties must be individually tailored.[11] Personality does have a small influence on survival after myocardial infarction.

The existence of patterns of coronary-prone behaviour is well-embedded in western business culture. The results of epidemiological and clinical studies have been conflicting; the idea that psychological stress has a role in the aetiology of coronary heart disease is nevertheless a persistent one and owes much to the work of Friedman and his colleagues who suggested that modification of hectic work patterns marked by long hours, competitiveness, time urgency, and aggression (so-called type A behaviour) as part of other stress reduction measures may be beneficial.[11]

Psychological stress at work from jobs with high demands and low control has been linked to a higher risk of coronary heart disease in some studies.[12–14] The risk of acute myocardial infarction has been shown in Japan to be increased in jobs with very long work hours.[15] Everyday mental stress associated with high levels of tension, sadness, and frustration may trigger myocardial ischaemia.[16] Programmes of psychosocial rehabilitation or teaching of stress management techniques may be helpful in assisting the return to work of vulnerable patients.[16]

Not everyone will be able to go back to their own work after a coronary event. In light engineering it has been observed that after one year about half those returning were fully fit, requiring no job change.[8] The remainder had some limitation of fitness; half required a job change. About one-tenth of all those returning to work had severe limitations of fitness requiring a change of work. Work that involves responding to emergency calls may place unacceptable demands on the cardiovascular system, and such duties should be avoided. Heavy physical work, the need to climb up and down stairs, rapid and tight pacing of repetitive operations, such as component assembly, technical skill, and the stress of responsibility are all relevant.

Tiredness is often burdensome initially, but usually resolves over the subsequent days or weeks. Although in most situations a full working day is expected from the day of restarting, it may be helpful to arrange temporary shorter hours, perhaps curtailing both ends of the day, so as to avoid rush-hour travelling. This recommendation can usually be accomplished by a defined time through which the hours can be extended towards the full working day. By defining this time period, the perceived stress on colleagues and working arrangements is notably less than leaving the period open-ended.

The stress of managing or supervising may be underappreciated, and consideration should be given to the time necessary to catch up with events that the employee will have missed while away, and to allow a gradual resumption of responsibilities. The requirements of overtime work, meetings that occur early or late in the day, and the managerial responsibility that may be exercised all demand understanding. For some, shortening the hours of work temporarily signals to the organization that the employee is not yet fully recovered, and perhaps encourages those who have been managing in the employee's absence to continue to do so for a further period of time.

Psychological stress may arise from a variety of circumstances peculiar to the patient, their relatives, friends (and others), or their particular working circumstances. These factors are usually the source of discouragement and may delay recovery. In the present climate of employment many individuals will take the opportunity to cease work and hope to obtain favourable financial terms; many will be disappointed.

Risks of sudden incapacity

In some jobs sudden incapacity would be disastrous and the likelihood of a further sudden illness such as a ventricular arrhythmia needs careful assessment. Airline pilots, mainline train drivers, and those at sea in merchant shipping, are rarely allowed to resume their former employment after the development of cardiovascular disease. This may also apply to policemen, fire service officers, and others on active duty. Formerly, vocational drivers, i.e. those holding large goods vehicle (LGV) and passenger carrying vehicle (PCV) licences, rarely regained their licences following the development of heart disease and then only after extensive testing including angiography. This situation has now changed, partly because of our better understanding of the natural history of CHD, our ability to identify those at high risk, and because of the availability of more effective treatments. Those groups of workers at low risk of cardiovascular collapse can be identified by a combination of clinical factors and 'non-invasive' testing as outlined in the Appendix to this chapter.

Screening

Those groups at high risk of collapse can be identified once their disease has declared itself, but silent coronary disease is extremely common. Coronary angiograms in patients being investigated before heart valve replacement for example, have revealed coronary arterial disease in approximately one-third.[17]

Many cardiac events will therefore occur in those who appear to be fit—approximately one-quarter in studies of the causes of road traffic accidents for example. These may well be sudden and cannot be predicted. One solution to this problem is to attempt to screen employees for 'silent' myocardial ischaemia. This may be justifiable in certain groups of individuals and has been adopted by the US Air Force, for example. The usual screening measures are a clinical examination and an exercise test. Exercise-induced electrocardiographic ST segment change in an asymptomatic individual has a variety of causes: using the criterion of 1 mm ST segment depression, about one-third will turn out to have coronary disease on angiography.[18] Screening for asymptomatic CHD in this way cannot therefore be routinely recommended because of the high prevalence of false positive results. Simple clinical features such as age, male sex, history of chest pain, smoking habit, or a strong family history of premature CHD, are better at predicting risks in apparently asymptomatic individuals. If there is a strong clinical suspicion of CHD and an accurate diagnosis is essential, then coronary angiography should be undertaken. This policy, however, would only be justifiable in those with very high-risk occupations. In the past, myocardial perfusion imaging using thallium has been recommended for this group of individuals, but the improved safety and ease of coronary angiography, coupled with the significant number of inconclusive results from myocardial scintigraphy,[19] makes angiography preferable.

Congenital and valvular heart disease

Congenital heart disease

Congenital defects will generally be detected in childhood, and individuals with such defects should seek cardiological advice before entering employment. Employers should not be deterred from taking on young people who have undergone cardiac surgery in childhood for the correction of congenital defects, as many lead a normal life and are capable of full-time employment.

Acquired valvular disease

Acquired disease, usually degenerative aortic stenosis or mitral regurgitation, is most commonly seen nowadays in those beyond working age, but the condition of **mitral valve prolapse** deserves emphasis because it affects some 2% of the population and is generally benign; it often presents as an auscultatory finding at a pre-employment medical examination, may be associated with electrocardiographic change, and may sometimes lead to a false diagnosis of significant heart disease.

Valvular surgery

The safety and excellent results of valvular surgery have led to the practice of early operation, before left ventricular function declines. Many mitral valves can be repaired nowadays, leading to full functional recovery and freedom from medication. The use of catheter techniques is growing; percutaneous balloon valvotomy is now the treatment of choice for pulmonary stenosis in children and for rheumatic mitral stenosis; clam shell devices for closing atrial septal defects are now widely available.

Following replacement of the aortic or mitral valves by mechanical or biological prostheses, patients generally recover rapidly and resume work fully within 2–3 months after the operation. Those with mechanical valves need to take anticoagulants indefinitely and are thus at slightly increased risk from bleeding, serious bleeding occurring at a rate of some 2% per annum in most series (see also Chapter 22, Surgery). Sudden failure of mechanical valves is extremely uncommon. Biological valves undergo slow deterioration and do fail suddenly, some years after implantation. For this reason they are rarely used in people of working age.

Cardiac arrhythmias

Transient cardiac arrhythmias (e.g. extrasystoles) are extremely common and do not usually indicate heart disease. They may be provoked by a variety of substances, including alcohol and coffee. Assessment by a cardiologist is recommended for those with persisting symptoms. A few individuals will suffer recurrent arrhythmias. The commonest is atrial fibrillation, which affects 2% of the population at some time in their lives and tends to be paroxysmal in individuals of working age. Drug treatment is sometimes required and, for some, an opportunity to withdraw from work and rest for a short period may be necessary. For others with supraventricular tachycardia, curative treatment is now available in the form of catheter ablation of the accessory electrical pathway which subserves the re-entrant tachycardia.

The prognosis for individuals with more serious arrhythmias occurring in the context of heart muscle disease is determined by the underlying cardiac pathology, which is often myocardial scarring as a result of CHD or cardiomyopathy. Continued employment for these individuals is usually inadvisable. **Complete heart block** generally requires permanent pacing (see below) but first- and second-degree block may be incidental findings in otherwise healthy people and require no further action.

Syncope

Syncope requires specialist evaluation including a neurological review if appropriate. Following unexplained syncope, provocation testing and investigation for arrhythmia must be implemented. If the results are satisfactory, return to work is recommended including (re-)licensing for vocational drivers after 3 months. Careful follow-up is mandatory.

Pacemakers and implantable devices

Pacemakers

The presence of an implanted cardiac pacemaker to maintain regular heart action is entirely compatible with normal or even strenuous exercise. The underlying heart condition for which the pacemaker was implanted may, however, impose its own restrictions.

The indications for cardiac pacing are widening as the efficacy of this form of treatment improves; modern pacemaker technology allows pacing of atria and ventricles, variation in the output of the generator, facilities for telemetry, etc.

Virtually all pacemakers have the capacity to sense and be inhibited by the patient's own heart rhythm. Somatic muscle action potentials, e.g. pectoralis major, can occasionally interfere with the pacemaker, causing temporary cessation of pacing which may induce faintness. Usually the interference will be brief and the pacemaker will revert to a fixed-rate mode which will prevent symptoms.

In theory, cardiac pacemakers are vulnerable to extraneous electrical interference but in practice most pacemakers have good discrimination.

Implantable cardioverter defibrillators

The implantable cardioverter defibrillator (ICD) is now the preferred treatment for individuals with ventricular tachycardia and/or fibrillation whose arrhythmia is refractory to drugs or myocardial revascularization. Generally the individual will have experienced at least one cardiac arrest. The device is implanted by a cardiologist under local anaesthetic but is tested under general anaesthetic. Both ventricular tachycardia and fibrillation can be detected and treated, the former by antitachycardia pacing and the latter by a DC shock. In either case transient impairment of consciousness is possible and hence certain jobs, e.g. vocational driving, are not permitted. To date approximately 2500 have been implanted in the UK.

Hypertension

Untreated hypertension carries the risk of sudden disability from heart attack or stroke; discovery of this condition may thus require stopping some employment where a serious accident risk exists. For **controlled hypertension** the risks must be carefully assessed in the context of the individual's work. When considering the need to continue in employment, well-controlled hypertension may be risk-free, especially if control is by diet only or with small doses of a mild diuretic. Control with more powerful drugs may carry the risk of side-effects, such as hypotension with resultant giddiness and fatigue, and limited effort tolerance. Central nervous system side-effects may affect judgement and the performance of skilled tasks. But modern antihypertensive therapy with β-adrenergic and calcium antagonists, diuretics, and ACE inhibitors is remarkably free from side-effects.

Patients with controlled hypertension can expect to manage most varieties of working activity. Frequent postural changes occasionally prove troublesome due to altered central and peripheral vascular responses. Very heavy physical work and exposure to very hot conditions with high humidity may result in postural hypotension. Such work should not be attempted if these ill effects might prove dangerous either to health or because of the associated risk of accidents. Provided blood pressure can be maintained under satisfactory control and it is checked regularly, HGV and PSV driving is allowed.

Other circulatory disorders

- **Peripheral vascular disease** may cause intermittent claudication which limits the patient's mobility. Medical treatment is relatively unsatisfactory, although surgical treatment may be very successful. The prognosis depends on any associated coronary disease.
- The presence of an **aortic aneurysm** also indicates arterial disease and a liability to vascular catastrophe.

These groups of patients should be carefully assessed, both clinically and by non-invasive investigations, with particular attention being paid to the likelihood of cardiac involvement.

- **Raynaud's phenomenon**, on the other hand, is a benign, albeit distressing, complaint. Underlying disorders, such as collagen disease, should be excluded. Sufferers should work in a warm environment and be allowed to wear gloves and heated socks if indicated. They should also be advised not to enter employment that involves exposure to hand-transmitted vibration (e.g. work with chain saws or pneumatic hammers).

- **Vibration-induced white finger (VWF)** is Raynaud's phenomenon secondary to work involving the use of hand-held vibratory tools. Workers with significant occupational exposures should be under a programme of health surveillance to detect new and worsening symptoms, and to offer advice on career placement. The HSE and the Faculty of Occupational Medicine advise that this should be tailored to the severity of disease: continuing exposure may be possible in early cases of VWF, but avoidance is recommended if disease is more advanced or progressive.[19,20]

Where a worker suffers from either Raynaud's phenomenon or VWF a review of control measures should be promoted to determine whether levels of exposure to transmitted vibration could be limited at source (e.g. by redesign of the tools or processes).

- **Varicose veins** of the legs may cause problems; accidental injury may lead to severe blood loss, and protection is essential. Work routines involving standing still are difficult to cope with, but some walking is helpful. Sitting for long uninterrupted periods may aggravate ankle swelling and, if the hip and knee are awkwardly flexed, there could be some risk of vascular thrombosis.

Cerebrovascular disease may produce disturbances of consciousness and other neurological effects (see Chapter 6).

Special work problems and restrictions

For most forms of heart disease the general rule is that activities causing no undue symptoms can be undertaken safely. Artificial restrictions are, therefore, unnecessary.

Lifting weights

The limits of weights that can safely be lifted regularly in manufacturing industries have been reduced in recent years and can usefully be considered on the scale indicated by the US Department of Labor 1981[22] (see also Chapter 1). Only the very fit and confident might reasonably attempt heavy work, such as lifting 50–100 lb (23–45 kg). Many employees may quite comfortably manage medium work, such as lifting 25–50 lb (11–23 kg) perhaps at the rate of once a minute, providing they do not have any other physical limitations. The presence of support for the weights and keeping them at waist height eases the strain considerably, and if the task only requires the weights to be slid along benches or roller tracks, then the effective strain will be reduced by some 50%. Those with moderate to severe restriction may need to be confined to a maximum of 10 lb (4.5 kg) or an equivalent degree of force on levers, turning wheels, and similar machine controls. In any work organization there may be a few jobs requiring lightweight detailed work or simple checking which are suitable for those who are quite severely disabled. Some patients have sufficient skills to learn inspection tasks which may be physically much less stressful. Other opportunities may be found in material and production control, progress chasing, recording, indexing, etc., which may allow continued work in fairly heavy industries.

Physical effort requirements well above normal, such as work in foundries and forges, may well be reasons for barring such employment in patients with heart disease, especially those with symptoms of shortness of breath or angina.

Rapid and tightly controlled pacing of work, such as on assembly lines, has not been shown to be a precipitating factor for myocardial infarction and should not inhibit a normal return to work after a heart attack. If employees were managing satisfactorily before their infarction they may well manage afterwards if they are not severely disabled by shortness of breath or angina. Returning to their own work, where social support is provided by former rather than new colleagues, may be less of a problem than trying a new task.

Management roles and shiftwork

The desirability of returning to familiar work also applies to shift workers and to those in supervisory and management work who have to cope with responsibility. If all has been well before the illness, returning to the same job may be the least stressful option. Permanent night working can be easier if it has been managed well previously. At night, organizations tend to function more routinely with less interference from peripheral parts of the undertaking. The co-operation amongst members of a team may well be higher and productivity can appear better. Those who have shortness of breath or angina find it an advantage to be able to rise from their bed during the day when the weather may be warm, or at least the house warm, to have some contact with their family, and to travel to and from work in quieter times than their day-shift colleagues. New work can bring new situations, different personalities, different tasks, and different sorts of components, all of which can be difficult to cope with even without heart disease. But working reduced hours on a temporary basis may be all that is required.

Working time regulations

Health assessments are required under these regulations if the individual is a night worker and suffers from a medical condition which may be made worse by night work. Some heart and circulatory disorders, particularly those which affect physical stamina, will come into this category. The worker may need to be transferred to the day shift if the assessment so indicates.

Toxic substances

Work involving exposure to certain hazardous substances may aggravate pre-existing coronary heart disease and careful consideration should be given to patients who are returning to jobs involving exposure to chemical vapours and fumes. **Methylene chloride**, a main ingredient of many commonly used paint removers, is rapidly metabolized to carbon monoxide in the body and in poorly ventilated work areas, blood levels of carboxyhaemoglobin can become elevated enough to precipitate angina or even myocardial infarction. A blood carboxyhaemoglobin level of 2–4% has been shown to be associated with impairment of cardiovascular function in patients with angina pectoris. The WHO[23] recommends a maximum carboxyhaemoglobin level of 5% for healthy industrial workers and a maximum of 2.5% for susceptible people in the general population exposed to ambient air pollution; this level may also be applied to workers whose jobs entail specific exposure to **carbon monoxide**, e.g. car park attendants, furnace workers, etc. There is a good correlation between carbon monoxide levels in the air and blood carboxyhaemoglobin, in accordance with the Coburn equation, and the WHO guideline level of 2.5% implies an 8-hour occupational exposure average, well below the current occupational exposure standard of 50 ppm.

In fact, to ensure that the 2.5% carboxyhaemoglobin level is not exceeded, the ambient carbon monoxide concentration should not be higher than 10 ppm over an 8-hour working day: equivalent to exposure to the current occupational exposure standard (50 ppm) for no more than 30 minutes. Occupational exposure to **carbon disulfide** in the viscose rayon manufacturing industry is a recognized causal factor of coronary heart disease, but the mechanism remains unclear. Reports of sudden death from angina are well-recognized in dynamite workers, particularly after a period of 36–72 hours away from work and following re-exposure, an effect almost certainly related to direct action of nitroglycerine on the blood vessels of the heart or peripheral circulation. People with clinical evidence of coronary heart disease should avoid occupational exposure to these substances.

Solvents such as **trichloroethylene** or **1,1,1-trichloroethane** may sensitize the myocardium to the action of endogenous catecholamines resulting in ventricular fibrillation and sudden death in workers receiving heavy exposure in poorly ventilated workplaces.[24] **Chlorofluorocarbons** (CFCs) were widely used as propellants in aerosol cans and as refrigerants—CFC-113 has been implicated in sudden cardiac deaths and CFC-22 has been reported to cause arrhythmias in laboratory workers using an aerosol preparation. Certain industrial workers will need proper assessment of their workplace by an occupational physician together with an occupational hygienist, so that they can be advised on their suitability for work handling chlorinated hydrocarbon solvents or involving exposure to gases.

There are no formal medical requirements for workers who have to enter confined spaces where there may be hazards of oxygen deficiency or a build-up of toxic gases. People with heart disease or severe hypertension may need to be excluded. Certain occupations may require the use of special breathing apparatus, either routinely (e.g. asbestos removal workers), or in emergencies (e.g. water workers handling chlorine cylinders). The additional cardiorespiratory effort required while wearing a respirator, combined with the general physical exertion, usually means that people with a previous history of CHD need to be excluded from such work.

Hot conditions

Working in hot conditions may prove difficult for some patients with heart disease. High ambient temperatures or significant heat radiation from hot surfaces or liquid metal, added to the physical strain of heavy work, will produce quite profound vasodilatation of the vessels in muscle and skin. Compensatory vascular and cardiac reactions to maintain central blood pressure may be inadequate and lead to reduced cerebral or coronary artery blood flow. The resulting weakness or giddiness could prove dangerous. Since many cardioactive drugs have vasodilating and negative inotropic actions, some reduction in dosage may be necessary in such circumstances.

Cold conditions

Cold is a notorious trigger of myocardial ischaemia and caution must therefore be exercised for individuals who suffer from CHD. Impaired circulation to the limbs will result in an increased risk of claudication, risk of damage to skin (frostbite), and poor recovery from accidental injury to skin and deeper structures.

Cuts and bruises from accidental contact with furniture, machinery, etc., or from dropped objects, may not heal at all well in the presence of circulatory restriction, and there could be a risk of the onset of gangrene and the subsequent need for disabling operations. Limbs at risk need adequate protection continuously while at work.

Driving

Ordinary driving may be resumed 1 month after a cardiac event, provided that the driver does not suffer from angina which may be provoked at the wheel. **Vocational driving** may be permitted at 6 weeks, subject to a satisfactory outcome from non-invasive testing (see the Appendix to this chapter. Ordinary driving licence holders do not need to notify the DVLA, Swansea, if they have made a good recovery and have no continuing disability, but vocational drivers must notify the DVLA. Insurance companies vary in their requirements but most policies are temporarily invalidated by illness.

Electromagnetic fields

Industrial electrical sources such as arc welding, faulty domestic equipment, engines, anti-theft devices, airport weapon detectors, radar and citizen's band radio, can all potentially affect pacemakers but, in general, the patient has to be very close to the power source before any interference can be demonstrated, and the pacemaker abnormality is confined to one or two missed beats or reversion to the fixed mode. The number of documented cases of interference in the UK is fewer than three a year.[25,26]

If pacemaker patients are expected to work in the vicinity of high-energy electric or magnetic fields capable of producing signals at a rate and pattern similar to a QRS complex (e.g. on some electrical generating and transmission equipment and welding), formal testing is recommended. The cardiac centre responsible for implanting the pacemaker will usually provide a technical service for this purpose, thus enabling the risk of interference to be defined precisely. Nuclear magnetic resonance (NMR) imaging machines may be found in certain chemical laboratories and hospital radiology departments. Patients with pacemakers should not be subjected to NMR imaging and they are generally advised to avoid work which may bring them into close contact with strong magnetic fields. A pacemaker patient who experiences untoward symptoms while near electrical apparatus should move away.

In the event of collapse the patient should be moved but other causes for the collapse should also be sought. Pacemaker patients carry cards which identify the type of pacemaker, the supervising cardiac centre, etc. Further advice is readily available from the British Pacing and Electrophysiology Group (see Appendix 7 for the address).

Patients with an ICD commonly have severe underlying heart disease and may well not be able to work. But if they can work then this should be in a safe electromagnetic environment. There has been one report of a patient who collapsed in the vicinity of an electronic anti-theft surveillance system in a bookstore and who was shown to have ICD malfunction.[27]

There has been considerable interest in the possibility that mobile telephones might interfere with pacemakers and ICDs. Studies have shown that this is a theoretical possibility and that re-programming of a pacemaker can be achieved under exceptional circumstances if the telephone is held close (less than 20 cm) to the pacemaker. In practice no clinically significant interference has yet been reported, but individuals are advised to use the hand and ear furthest from the pacemaker and not to 'dial' with the telephone near to the pacemaker.

Travel

Following a cardiac event such as myocardial infarction, individuals should convalesce at home and should not travel until they have been assessed by their physician at 4–6 weeks. Those with no evidence of continuing myocardial ischaemia or cardiac pump failure can then travel freely within the UK for pleasure, e.g. holidays. Business and overseas travel is more problematic because the physical and psychological demands are greater. Additional difficulties for the overseas traveller include the uncertain provision of coronary care facilities in some countries and the justifiable reluctance of insurance companies to provide health cover. Such travel is best deferred until 3 months have elapsed and any necessary further investigations and treatment have been carried out to ensure cardiovascular fitness.

Overseas travel need not be prohibited even for those with continuing cardiovascular problems. Utilizing the airport services for disabled travellers can ease a passenger through check-in, customs, passport control, and security at major airports. Modern aircraft can be very comfortable. The cabins are kept at a pressure equivalent to 6000 feet (2000 metres) so that those with angina are not likely to experience an attack. Most developed countries have a coronary care service at least as good as that in the UK. Businessmen with continuing cardiac disorders may therefore fly to Europe and North America with very little risk. But flights in unpressurized aircraft, work in undeveloped countries or in remote areas of the world, and work in a hostile environment (both climatic and political) is best avoided. Aircrew are subject to CAA guidelines whose advice should always be sought (See also Appendices 2, and 5).

Travel at high altitude will exacerbate symptoms in those who already experience symptoms at sea level, but asymptomatic individuals with coronary heart disease are unlikely to be at special risk. Cardiac deaths are uncommon in trekkers or workers at high altitude (8000–15 000 feet, 2440–4570 metres); most are screened to some degree beforehand.

Seafarers

The Merchant Shipping (Medical Examination) Regulations state that any manifestation of ischaemic heart disease renders the individual permanently unfit to return to sea. This regulation has been in force since 1983 and applies to all those seafarers who serve in UK registered vessels of 1600 tons and over (a small coaster upwards). The reasons for this draconian policy are as follows:

- Any manifestation of coronary heart disease exposes the individual to an increased risk of a further coronary event. Admittedly, 'low-risk' cases can be identified, but any increase in risk is unacceptable at sea.
- Seafarers are exposed to environmental hazards. Even an apparently easy and short ferry trip can go wrong and the seafarer may be required to undertake vigorous physical effort in adverse circumstances, a well-recognized trigger for a heart attack.
- The seafarer is denied rapid access to coronary care facilities. This also has medico-legal implications; a seafarer who is allowed to return to work and who then suffers a myocardial infarction can argue that they should not have been allowed to return to sea if there was any risk of this occurrence. Dramatic rescues by helicopter from vessels, as depicted in television drama, are not generally safe or feasible.
- Any incapacity of a seafarer has an adverse effect on the efficiency and safety of the vessel. The staffing levels on many large ships nowadays are low, perhaps 10–12 people on a super-tanker. The incapacity of one seafarer may impose a considerable

additional burden on the others. Putting into port to land the victim of a heart attack and take on an extra crew member is not usually an option. (See also Appendix 3.)

Disability

Significant cardiovascular disorders are likely to last at least 12 months, and even for the rest of the life of the person affected, and so will come under the DDA. An assessment of the job and its attendant risks for the new or existing employee will be needed and this task should be undertaken by the organization's occupational health service. A certain amount of job restructuring may be recommended to the employer to limit the number of extra hours worked and/or some of the aspects that may be especially stressful to the employee. In practice, individuals who develop symptoms of angina or suffer arrhythmias at work are unlikely to be willing to continue with the occupation, and it is best to consider medical retirement unless more suitable and congenial work can be found. For most jobs, asymptomatic individuals, e.g. those who have made a good recovery from a myocardial infarction or who have had straightforward CABG, need not be on any restrictions and should be encouraged to lead as normal a life as possible, even though they may come within the DDA definition of disability.

Selected references

1 *Coronary heart disease statistics*. London: British Heart Foundation, 1997.
2 *Morbidity statistics from general practice 1981–2*. Royal College of General Practitioners Third National Study. London: HMSO, 1986.
3 Shaper AG, Cook DG, Walker M, Macfarlane, PW. Prevalence of ischaemic heart disease in middle-aged British men. *Br Heart J* 1984; **51**: 595–605.
4 Rose G, Marmot MG. Social class and coronary heart disease. *Br Heart J* 1981; **45**: 13–19.
5 Tunstall-Pedoe H, Clayton D, Morris JN, Brigden W, MacDonald I. Coronary heart attack in East London. *Lancet* 1975; **2**: 833–838.
6 Muller JE *et al*. Circadian variation in the frequency of onset of myocardial infarction. *New Engl J Med* 1985; **313**: 1315–1322.
7 Mittleman MA, Maclure M, Tofler GH, Sherwood JB, Goldberg RJ, Muller, JE. Triggering of acute myocardial infarction by heavy physical exertion. *New Engl J Med* 1993; **329**: 1677–1683.
8 Nagle R, Gangola R, Picton-Robinson I. Factors influencing return to work after myocardial infarction. *Lancet* 1971; **12**: 454–6.
9 Clark DB, Edwards FC, Williams, WG. Cardiac surgery and return to work in the West Midlands. In: *Cardiac rehabilitation,* pp. 61–70. Proceedings of the Society of Occupational Medicine Research Panel Symposium, London, 1983.
10 Cay, EL. The influence of psychological problems in returning to work after a myocardial infarction. In: *Cardiac rehabilitation,* pp. 42–60. Proceedings of the Society of Occupational Medicine Research Panel Symposium, London, 1983
11 Friedman M, Thorensen CE, Gill, JJ. Alteration of type A behaviour and its effect on cardiac recurrence in post myocardial infarction patients. Summary results of the recurrent coronary prevention project. *Am Heart J* 1986; **112**: 653–655.
12 Everson SA, Lynch JW, Chesney MA *et al.* Interaction of workplace demands and cardio-

vascular reactivity in progression of carotid atherosclerosis: population based study. *BMJ* 1997; **314**: 553–558.

13 Bosma H, Marmot MG, Hemingway H, Nicholson AC, Brunner E, Stansfield SA. Low job control and risk of coronary heart disease in Whitehall II (Prospective Cohort Study). *BMJ* 1997; **314**: 558–565.

14 Marmot MG, Bosma H, Hemingway H, Brunner E, Stansfield S. Contribution of job control and other risk factors to social variations in coronary heart disease incidence. *Lancet* 1997; **350**: 235–239.

15 Sokejima S, Kagamimori S. Working hours as a risk factor for acute myocardial infarction in Japan: case control study. *BMJ* 1998; **317**: 775–779.

16 Gullette ECD, Blumental JA, Babyak M *et al.* Effects of mental stress on myocardial ischaemia during daily life. *JAMA* 1997; **277**: 1521–1526.

17 Enriques-Sarano M, Klodus F, Garratt KN, Bailey KR, Tajik AJ, Holmes DR. Secular trends in coronary atherosclerosis—analysis in patients with valvular regurgitation. *New Engl J Med* 1996; **335**: 316–322.

18 Froelicher VF *et al.* Angiographic findings in asymptomatic aircrew with electrocardiographic abnormalities. *Am J Cardiol* 1977; **39**: 31–38.

19 Faculty of Occupational Medicine of the Royal College of Physicians (1993). *Hand-transmitted vibration:clinical effects and pathophysiology, Part 1: Report of a working party,* London:RCP.

20 Health and Safety Executive (1994) *Hand-arm vibration.* HS(G)88; London: HMSO.

21 Schwartz RS, Jackson WG, Celio PV, Richardson LA, Hickman JR. Accuracy of exercise Th[201] myocardial scintigraphy in asymptomatic young men. *Circulation* 1993; **87**: 165–172.

22 US Department of Labor. *Selected characteristics of occupations defined in the Dictionary of Occupational Titles.* Washington, DC: US Government Printing Office, 1981.

23 *Carbon monoxide.* Environmental health criteria, No. 13. Geneva: World Health Organization, 1979.

24 Boon NA. Solvent abuse of the heart (editorial). *Br Med J* 1987; **294**: 722.

25 Gold RG. Interference to cardiac pacemakers—how often is it a problem? *Prescribers J* 1984; **24**: 115–123.

26 Sowton E. Environmental hazards and pacemaker patients. *J R Coll Physicians Lond* 1982; **16**: 159–164.

27 Santucci PA, Haw J, Trohman RG, Pinski SL. Interference with an implantable defibrillator by an electronic anti-theft surveillance device. *New Engl J Med* 1998; **339**: 1371–1374.

27 *At a glance guide to the current medical standards of fitness to drive.* Swansea: Driver and Vehicle Licencing Agency, March 1998.

Appendix: DVLA guidelines

The table and notes below set out the DVLA guidelines to the entitlements to driving in respect of cardiovascular fitness requirements (revised 1998). See also Ref.28.

The left-hand column of the table lists the conditions that should prompt consideration of driving entitlement. The middle and right-hand columns list the precise requirements that prompt withdrawal of that entitlement (in **bold type**), and the requirements that enable the driver to regain entitlement (in *italics*). Group 1 are ordinary driving licences (car and motor bicycle) and group 2 are vocational licences (LGV, PCV).

Medication (groups 1 and 2)

If drug treatment for any cardiovascular condition is required then any adverse effect which may affect driver performance will disqualify.

Licence duration (group 2 only)

An applicant or driver who has, after cardiac assessment, been permitted to hold either an LGV or PCV licence will usually be issued with a short-term licence (maximum duration 3 years) renewable on receipt of satisfactory medical reports.

Exercise testing

Exercise evaluation shall be performed on a bicycle or treadmill. Drivers should be able to complete three stages of the Bruce protocol or equivalent safely, without anti-anginal medication for 48 hours and should remain free from signs of cardiovascular dysfunction, viz. angina pectoris, syncope, hypotension, sustained ventricular tachycardia, and/or electrocardiographic ST segment shift which accredited medical opinion interprets as being indicative of myocardial ischaemia (usually >2 mm horizontal or down-sloping). In the presence of established coronary heart disease exercise evaluation shall be required at regular intervals not to exceed 3 years.

If the cause of the chest pain is in doubt, an exercise test should be carried out as above. Those with a locomotor disorder who cannot comply will require specialist cardiological opinion

Coronary angiography

In coronary heart disease angiography is not required for (re-)licensing purposes. If angiography has been undertaken, (re-)licensing will not normally be permitted if the left ventricular ejection fraction is equal to or <0.40 on contrast angiography, or if there is significant proximal, unrelieved coronary arterial stenosis (left main and proximal left anterior descending equal to or >30% or proximal >50% elsewhere unless subtending a completed infarction).

Table 18.1 DVLA guidlines to the entitlements to driving in respect of cardiovascular fitness requirements (revised 1998)

Cardiovascular disorders	Group 1 entitlement	Group 2 entitlement
Angina (stable/unstable)	***Driving must cease when symptoms occur at rest or at the wheel.*** *Driving may recommence when satisfactory symptom control is achieved.* *DVLA need not be notified.*	***Refusal or revocation with continuing symptoms (treated and/or untreated).*** *Re-licensing may be permitted when free from angina for at least 6 weeks, provided that the exercise test requirements can be met and there is no other disqualifying condition.*
Mycocardial infarction (CABG)	***Driving must cease for at least 4 weeks.*** *Driving may recommence thereafter provided there is no other disqualifying condition.* *DVLA need not be notified.*	***Disqualifies from driving for at least six weeks.*** *Re-licensing may be permitted thereafter provided that the exercise test requirements can be met and there is no other disqualifying condition.*
Angioplasty	***Driving must cease for at least one week.*** *Driving may recommence provided no other disqualifying condition.* *DVLA need not be notified.*	
Peripheral vascular disease	*Driving may continue unless another disqualifying condition.* *DVLA need not be notified.*	*Re-licensing may be permitted provided there is no symptomatic myocardial ischaemia, the exercise test requirements can be met and there is no other disqualifying condition.* *When exercise testing <u>cannot</u> be completed to the required level, Specialist cardiological opinion may be required.*
Hypertension	*Driving may continue <u>unless</u> treatment causes unacceptable side effects.* *DVLA need not be notified.*	***Disqualifies from driving if resting BP consistently 180 mmHg systolic or more and/or 100 mmHg diastolic or more.*** *Re-licensing may be permitted when controlled and treatment does not cause side effects which may interfere with driving.*
Aortic Aneurysm (including Marfan's Syndrome)	***Driving may continue unless other disqualifying condition.*** *DVLA need not be notified.*	***Disqualifies from driving if the aortic transverse diameter is >5.0 cm.*** *Re-licensing may be permitted following satisfactory repair unless there is another disqualifying condition.*

Table 18.1 *Continued*

Cardiovascular disorders	Group 1 entitlement	Group 2 entitlement
Arrhythmia Sinoatrial disease Significant atrio-ventricular conduction defect Atrial flutter/fibrillation Narrow or broad complex tachycardia *See also pacemaker and ICD section* NB: transient arrhythmias occurring during the acute phase only of a myocardial infarction or CABG do not require assessment under this section.	*Driving must cease following incapacity due to an arrhythmia.* *Driving may be permitted when underlying cause has been identified and controlled for at least 4 weeks* *DVLA need not be notified unless there are distracting/disabling symptoms.*	*Disqualifies from driving if the arrhythmia has caused or is likely to cause incapacity (including systemic embolism)** *Driving may be permitted when arrhythmia controlled for at least 3 months provided that the LV ejection fraction is >0.4, the exercise test requirements can be met and there is no other disqualifying condition.* ** See Valve Section*
Pacemaker implant	*Driving must cease for 1 week. Driving may be permitted thereafter provided no other disqualifying condition. License shall be subject to review at least every 3 years.*	*Disqualifies from driving for 6 weeks.* *Re-licensing may be permitted thereafter unless there is no other disqualifying condition.*
Successful catheter ablation	*Driving must cease for 1 week. Driving may be permitted thereafter provided no other disqualifying condition. DVLA need not be notified.*	*Disqualifies from driving for 6 weeks.* *Re-licensing may be permitted thereafter unless there is no other disqualifying condition.*
ICD implant	*Driving may occur when the following criteria can be met:* *(1) The device must have been implanted for at least 6 months and shall not have discharged during the past 6 months (except during formal clinical testing).* *(2) Any previous discharge must not have been accompanied by incapacity.* *(3) The device is subject to regular review with interrogation.* *(4) A period of 1 month off driving must elapse following any revision of the device (generator or electrode) or alteration of anti-arrhythmic drug treatment.* *(5) There is no other disqualifying condition.* *The license shall be subject to annual review.*	*Permanently bars*

Table 18.1   *Continued*

Cardiovascular disorders	Group 1 entitlement	Group 2 entitlement
Atrial defibrillator (patient activated)	*Driving may continue provided no other disqualifying condition.*	*Re-licensing may be permitted provided the arrhythmia section is met and there is no other disqualifying condition.*
Hypertrophic cardiomyopathy (HCM) *(See also Pacemaker arrhythmia and ICD sections).*	*Driving may continue provided no other disqualifying condition.* *DVLA need not be notified.*	***Disqualifies from driving if symptomatic.*** *Re-licensing may be permitted provided that the following criteria can be met and there is no other disqualifying condition:* *(1) He/she is asymptomatic.* *(2) There is no family history of sudden cardiomyopathic death.* *(3) The cardiologist can confirm that the HCM is anatomically mild.* *(4) No serious abnormality of heart rhythm disturbance has been demonstrated, i.e. ventricular tachyarrhythmia excluding isolated VPBs.* *(5) Hypotension does not occur during exercise testing.*
Dilated cardiomyopathy *(See also Pacemaker ICD and arrhythmia sections).*	*Driving may continue provided no other disqualifying condition.* *DVLA need not be notified.*	***Disqualifies from driving if symptomatic.*** *Re-licensing may be permitted provided that there is no other disqualifying condition.*
Heart failure	*Driving may continue provided there are no other disqualifying symptoms and no other disqualifying condition.* *DVLA need not be notified.*	***Disqualifies from driving if symptomatic.*** *Re-licensing may be permitted provided that the LV ejection fraction as measured by contrast angiography (or equivalent) is >0.4, the exercise test requirements can be met and there is no other disqualifying condition.*

Table 18.1 *Continued*

Cardiovascular disorders	Group 1 entitlement	Group 2 entitlement
Heart and/or lung transplant	*Driving may continue provided no other disqualifying condition.* *DVLA need not be notified.*	**Disqualifies from driving if symptomatic.** *Re-licensing may be permitted provided that there is no other disqualifying condition.*
Heart valve disease (to include surgery, i.e. replacement and/or repair)	*Driving may continue provided no other disqualifying condition.* *DVLA need not be notified.*	**Disqualifies from driving:** **(1) whilst symptomatic.** **(2) For 12 months after cerebral embolism <u>prior</u> to anticoagulant therapy.** **(3) <u>Permanently</u> after systemic embolism whilst on anticoagulant therapy.** *Re-licensing may be permitted provided that there is no other disqualifying condition.*
Congenital heart disease	*Driving may continue provided there is no other disqualifying condition. DVLA need not be notified.* **NB: Arrhythmogenic right ventricular dysplasia and licensing fitness will be considered on an individual basis.**	**Disqualifies from driving when complex or severe disorder(s) is(are) present.*** *Those with minor disease and others who have had successful repair of defects or relief of valvular problems, fistulae etc may be licensed provided that there is no other disqualifying condition.* * *Further details available from DVLA on request.*
Syncope	**Driving must cease whilst symptoms persist.** *Driving may recommence once cause identified and symptoms controlled.*	**Disqualifies from driving following single or recurrent episodes.** **Unexplained syncope requires Specialist evaluation to include:** **(1) Provocation testing.** **(2) Investigation for arrhythmia.** **(3) Neurological review if appropriate.** *Re-licensing may be permitted 3/12 after the event provided that the results are satisfactory.*

Table 18.1 *Continued*

ECG abnormality		
ECG abnormality Suspected myocardial infarction left bundle branch block	*Driving may continue unless another disqualifying condition.*	*Re-licensing may be permitted provided that there is no other disqualifying condition and the exercise test requirements can be met.*
Pre-excitation		*May be ignored UNLESS associated with an arrhythmia (see Arrhythmia Section) or other disqualifying condition.*

19

Respiratory disorders

K. Palmer and S. Pearson

Respiratory illnesses commonly cause sickness absence, unemployment, visits to the general practitioner's surgery, disability, and handicap. Collectively these disorders cause the loss of 14% of available working days (approximately 38 million days lost per year) in men and 11% of work days in women (5 million days lost per year). In the 16–64 year old population, they account for about 18% of general practitioner consultations, 10% of all hospital admissions, and 3–9% of all deaths. Ten per cent of working-aged men and 5% of working-aged women receive invalidity benefit because they are too disabled by respiratory diseases to work.

Disease of the respiratory system may be caused, and pre-existing disease may be exacerbated by the occupational environment. More commonly respiratory disease limits work capacity and the ability to undertake a particular job. Finally, respiratory fitness in safety-critical jobs can have implications for colleagues at work and the public as well as for the affected individual. Within this broad picture, different clinical illnesses pose different problems. For example, acute respiratory illness commonly causes short-term sickness absence, whereas chronic respiratory disease has greater significance in long-term sickness absence and work limitation; and the fitness implications of respiratory sensitization at work are very different from non-specific asthma aggravated by workplace irritants.

Occupational causes of respiratory disease represent a small proportion of the total burden, except in some specialized work settings where particular exposures predominate and give rise to particular disease excesses. The corollary is that the common fitness decisions on placement, return to work, and rehabilitation more often involve non-occupational illnesses than occupational ones. By contrast, statutory programmes of health surveillance revolve around specific occupational risks (such as spray painting with isocyanates) and specific occupational health outcomes (such as occupational asthma).

In assessing the individual it is important to remember that respiratory problems are often aggravated by other illnesses, particularly disorders of the cardiovascular and musculoskeletal systems.

Methods of assessing respiratory disability

General considerations

Respiratory fitness needs to be assessed in the context of the intended employment and its particular elements and demands. However, a number of general questions will influence the decision-making:

- Does the combination of work and respiratory fitness result in an immediate fore-seeable risk to the individual's health and safety, or that of others?
- May future standards of health and safety be compromised?
- If so, how great are the risks likely to be?
- Is the work in the safety-critical category, where the worker has substantial responsibility for the safety of colleagues or members of the public?
- Can the work be discharged effectively, and can reasonable levels of attendance be anticipated?
- Are there special considerations in placement, health review or workplace adaptation?
- Are particular policies required in selection, control, and monitoring?
- Are there legal standards or other codes of good practice that need to be observed?

These questions are not particular to respiratory fitness assessments, but quite commonly occur in people with respiratory illness, e.g.:

- the importance of aerobic capacity in the emergency rescue worker or the manual labourer
- the risk posed to members of the public by tuberculosis in a healthcare worker, or pneumothorax in an airline pilot
- the potential for life-threatening asthma following occupational sensitization.

Physicians in the UK have responsibilities under the Health and Safety at Work etc. Act 1974 (HSAWA) to place people in safe employment and under the Disability Discrimination Act 1995 (DDA) to ensure that disabled workers are not discriminated against unfairly on health grounds. The dual requirements of these two Acts challenge physicians to weigh matters carefully. They need, for example, to consider the likely duration of illness and its prognosis in the individual; the weight of evidence for incapacity on the one hand and risk on the other; and the scope for reasonable accommodation by the employer. These points are touched on elsewhere, but here we emphasize the complexities in making blanket judgements in respiratory fitness assessment:

- Many aspects of lung function can be objectively measured, but except at extreme departures, a poor correlation exists between measurements and disabling symptoms (motivation may perhaps be more important).
- Assessment of workplace demands and risks may be limited in scope or in their relevance to individual circumstances.
- Many conditions improve given sufficient time, appropriate treatment, proper environmental control, or work modification.

Fitness assessment should embrace these issues. An employer's failure to control potentially modifiable respiratory hazards (dusts, fumes, etc.) may be construed not only as a failure of control under regulation 6 of the Control of Substances Hazardous to Health Regulations 1994 (COSHH), but a failure to make a reasonable accommodation under the DDA.

Some organizations and public services apply predefined fitness standards; many others conduct routine measures of respiratory function and apply predetermined protocols and decision algorithms. These aid fitness assessment, but it should be noted that the status of these procedures under the DDA and their inter-relation with health and safety legislation, has not yet been adequately tested in the law courts.

Measurements of lung function

Respiratory disease produces impairment in lung function and this, if severe enough, will interfere with the ability to perform some work tasks. Whether a given level of lung function impairment causes work difficulty depends on the nature of the job and the presence or absence of co-existing disease. The duration, intensity and pattern of work, the environmental conditions (such as temperature, humidity, dust, and fume content), and the attitude and personality of the individual all play a part. Pulmonary function testing is, therefore, only one component in the process of assessing fitness for work.

In an occupational setting lung function tests are used routinely in one of two ways:

- as a single set of measurements performed at a point in time (typically the pre-employment assessment, or during or following illness), to assess lung function in relation to accepted norms
- as serial measurements over time, to monitor disease control or progression, or detect adverse occupational effects at an early stage.

The diagnostic value of the testing is probably higher when used in the second way.

Standard lung function tests are conveniently classified into measurements of airway function, measurements of static lung volume and measurements of gas exchange. Measurements of airway function (spirometry and peak expiratory flow) should be routinely available in occupational health care and can be augmented, under medical supervision, by tests of response to bronchodilator medication; the other tests, as well as measurements of bronchial responsiveness to inhaled histamine or methacholine, require specialist facilities and are generally employed in secondary care investigation and research settings.

Spirometry

Spirometry is performed by taking a maximal inspiration and then blowing as hard as possible into the machine, and continuing to blow until the lungs are empty. The volume of gas expired is plotted against time to produce a spirogram (see Fig. 19.1). The trace should be a smooth curve and there should be good reproducibility between successive measurements with superimposition of traces. The volume of gas expired in the first second (FEV_1) is a measure of the speed of airflow. The total volume expired is the forced vital capacity (FVC). The absolute values obtained depend on age, height, sex, and racial origin and values need to be compared with appropriate predicted normal values.

A number of basic points of technique need to be observed to minimize measurement errors.[1] Spirometry equipment needs to be calibrated at regular intervals and checked for leaks, wear and tear, and blockages. Spuriously low results can occur if inspiration is incomplete, if partial leakage occurs around the mouthpiece or in the tubing, or if expiratory effort is submaximal. The FVC is commonly underestimated because the blow is finished early; this is apparent in tracings that fail to attain a plateau. Variable effort is indicated by wobbly curves and poor reproducibility. Subjects should be encouraged to repeat the procedure until three acceptable curves are achieved; the best two FVCs

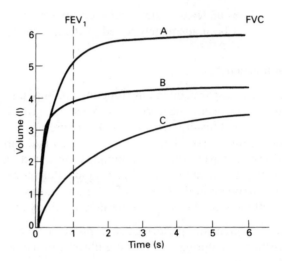

Fig. 19.1 Spirograms illustrating obstructive and restrictive patterns of abnormal ventilation: A, normal spirogram; B, restrictive deficit; C, obstructive deficit.

should be within 5% or 0.1 litre of each another. The documented values should be the highest values from any of the three chosen curves. Benchmark standards and a more detailed account of these techniques have been provided by the British Thoracic Society and Association of Respiratory Technicians and Physiologists,[2] and by the American Thoracic Society.[3] Other factors that need to be considered include variation between observers and between machines, recent infections, irritant exposures, and exercise.

Sometimes, despite encouragement and multiple attempts, subjects are unable to produce acceptable tracings. This commonly results from an inability to master the technique but there is evidence that, in some of these cases, so-called 'test failure' is a marker of incipient health problems.

Two main patterns of ventilatory abnormality can generally be defined-namely obstructive and restrictive. Obstruction arises in asthma and in chronic obstructive pulmonary disease (COPD) and tends to produce a diminution in FEV_1 greater than that in FVC. The ratio of FEV_1 to FVC should normally be greater than 0.7 (70%), but in airflow obstruction lower values arise. Restrictive lung changes are caused by diffuse inflammatory and fibrotic diseases of the lung parenchyma such as fibrosing alveolitis and asbestosis; and in this case FEV_1 is reduced, but so too is FVC, so that the ratio of FEV_1 to FVC is preserved (and often increased).

When interpreting lung function tests, however, it needs to be remembered that the range of normal values is generally large, two standard deviations being approximately 20% of the average value. This means, on the one hand, that a healthy individual can appear to have deficient lung function simply because they lie in the lower tail of the normal Gaussian distribution; and, on the other hand, that an individual with impaired lung function can still remain within the normal range of values. In the latter case, if the individual has moved from the top of the predicted normal range for a particular parameter to the bottom, the fall represents 40% of the population mean. Hence serial patterns are more informative than a single snapshot. Furthermore the pattern of a number of different measurements should be considered rather than one single index of lung function. For example, in chronic airflow limitation the FEV_1 will be reduced but this will also be associated with a reduction in $FEV_1/FVC\%$ and an increase in residual volume (RV) and functional residual capacity (FRC). This pattern of results would indicate significant airflow limitation for that individual even if FEV_1 remained within the normal range for the population.

Measurements of airflow such as FEV_1 and peak expiratory flow (PEF) are influenced most by disease in the larger airways where most of the resistance to flow lies. The cross-sectional area of the bronchial tree increases approximately exponentially with distance from the trachea as the bronchi divide and resistance to flow falls concomitantly. Narrowing in the peripheral airways of less than 2 mm in diameter has little effect on FEV_1 and PEF unless the damage is extensive. This means that early disease in small airways, such as that caused by smoking and toxic fume damage, is poorly reflected in these measurements.

Most modern spirometers will also present the information in the form of an expiratory flow–volume curve, plotting flow against volume expired between maximal inspiration (total lung capacity or TLC) and maximal expiration (RV). From these curves additional information such as flow at 25% or 75% FVC may be obtained. Flows towards the expiratory end of the flow–volume curve represent flow in smaller airways but accuracy of measurement, reproducibility, and reference ranges are all less precise for these low flows than they are for FEV_1 so these tests are not generally helpful in assessing fitness for work.

Peak expiratory flow

The PEF measures the highest flow recorded during a forced expiratory manoeuvre and is measured with a peak flow meter. The subject is asked to perform a short, sharp, hard blow into the meter. It is usual to take the best of three attempts, if the readings are reproducible. As with simple spirometry a number of errors are possible, particularly variable subject effort, errors in reading PEFs and transcribing them to a diary, and incomplete returns. A great deal of instruction and encouragement is required to obtain adequate data. Self-treatment with bronchodilators and corticosteroids may affect the record but the influence of the first of these factors can be minimized by recording PEFs before drug delivery. Upper respiratory tract infections can cause large (20%) falls in PEF for a week or more making interpretation difficult.

PEF measurements are usually made serially over time, and used in one of two ways:

• to assess the degree of control achieved in patients with established asthma
• to look for work-related changes in situations where occupational asthma is suspected (the later section on asthma describes this last application more fully).

Other tests

Measurements of **static lung volumes**, such as TLC and RV, involve advanced techniques including helium (or other inert gas) dilution and body plethysmography; they require a specialized pulmonary function laboratory and skilled technicians, but may be useful in clarifying diagnoses. Thus, in airflow obstruction, all static lung volumes are increased but the increase in RV is proportionately greater than in TLC because of gas trapping; while in restrictive lung disease, such as pulmonary fibrosis, all lung volumes are reduced.

Measurements of **gas exchange** such as oxygen consumption (V_{O_2}) during incremental exercise, carbon dioxide production (V_{CO_2}), and arterial blood gases, are useful in assessing disability, especially in those with interstitial lung disease or emphysema. However, the findings reflect total cardiorespiratory function as well as peripheral muscle deconditioning, require a sophisticated laboratory and are time-consuming to perform. Carbon monoxide diffusion, expressed as transfer factor (T_{LCO}) or gas transfer coefficient (K_{CO}), measures the uptake of carbon monoxide from the lung to the blood. Carbon monoxide is of similar molecular weight to oxygen and is bound to haemoglobin, so its uptake provides a measure of oxygen diffusion. It is reduced in interstitial lung disease and in emphysema but it is also affected by other factors such as smoking habits, haemoglobin levels and resting cardiac output. Again its measurement requires a dedicated lung function laboratory and skilled technicians. In the clinical setting the portable pulse oximeter provides a simple inexpensive guide to diffusion and can be used to detect desaturation of haemoglobin at rest and during exercise in patients with pulmonary fibrosis or COPD.

Several other tests are used as adjuncts to diagnosis. Asthma in an occupational setting is sometimes investigated by **serology**, **skin prick tests,** or **bronchial provocation challenge**. Immunological responsiveness (sensitization) to workplace agents may be detected by the identification of specific IgE antibodies using radioallergosorbent tests (RAST) or enzyme-linked immunosorbent assays (ELISA); or in response to a specific challenge to the skin or airways. The usefulness of these investigations varies from one agent to another. They also depend on identification of the suspected agent and, in the case of skin prick and provocation tests, may depend on obtaining a correct formulation of the material or achieving a representative challenge. The subject is more fully discussed later (see Asthma, below).

Screening questionnaires

In occupational health practice, screening questionnaires are widely used to assess respiratory fitness. This is particularly true prior to certain job placements and periodically in certain jobs that may affect respiratory health.

The best known respiratory questionnaire is the MRC standardized questionnaire on respiratory symptoms.[4] This was devised for the epidemiological investigation of chronic bronchitis but has since been adapted in a variety of ways to assess respiratory symptoms and risk factors in working groups. The original questions on sputum production had a high sensitivity and specificity in relation to measured sputum production but these questions are of limited interest today. Several other versions have been tried including the European Coal and Steel Community (ECSC) questionnaire, the American Thoracic Society and the Division of Lung Disease (ATS-DLD-78) questionnaire and the International Union Against Tuberculosis and Lung Disease (IUATLD) questionnaire. (For sample questions, and an assessment of their validity, see Toren *et al.*[5]). Venables *et al.*[6] have proposed a simple nine-item panel of questions for use in asthma epidemiology that correlates well with tests of bronchial hyperresponsiveness, and a simple extension to cover work-related symptoms (Table 19.1).

Table 19.1 Screening questions used in the epidemiological investigation of asthma (adapted from Venables *et al.*[6] with permission).

Current health (during the last 4 weeks)	
If you run, or climb stairs fast do you ever:	
cough?	Yes/No
wheeze?	Yes/No
get tight in the chest?	Yes/No
Is your sleep ever broken by:	
wheeze?	Yes/No
difficulty with breathing?	Yes/No
Do you ever wake up in the morning (or from your sleep if a shiftworker) with:	
wheeze?	Yes/No
difficulty with breathing?	Yes/No
Do you ever wheeze:	
if you are in a smoky room?	Yes/No
if you are in a very dusty place?	Yes/No

Answers of 'yes' to three of the nine questions correspond to a sensitivity of 91% and a specificity of 96% for current bronchial hyper-responsiveness

Work limitation arises most commonly from the sensation of breathlessness and for monitoring and documentary purposes this can be graded on a clinical scale such as the one proposed by the MRC (Box 19.1).

Box 19.1   The MRC breathlessness scale
1   Troublesome shortness of breath when hurrying on level ground or walking up a slight hill
2   Short of breath when walking with other people of own age on level ground
3   Have to stop for breath when walking at own pace on level ground

---

Chest radiography

Chest radiography plays an important role in monitoring patients exposed to fibrogenic dusts such as asbestos, silica, and coal dust. It is a requirement, on entering employment for the first time, and at regular intervals, in certain professions such as airline pilots and commercial divers. It is also valuable in the assessment of workers exposed to tuberculosis who develop persistent respiratory symptoms. Some of these aspects of surveillance and fitness assessment are more fully described in later sections.

However, the routine application of chest radiography in many other traditional situations has fallen into disfavour. For example, it is no longer considered helpful in routine surveillance of asymptomatic healthcare workers with potential tuberculosis exposure; likewise, the yield in asymptomatic workers who work with lung carcinogens is considered too low to justify the cost or radiation risk. Indeed, for the common round of health problems (upper respiratory tract infections, asthma, and COPD), decisions on fitness for work seldom rest on the outcome of radiography.

In the detection of pleural and interstitial lung disease more information is obtained by CT scanning than radiography, but the procedure is expensive, and its routine application for screening cannot presently be justified. It is also quite difficult, at present, to interpret the findings of a sensitive technique that frequently reveals changes in asymptomatic individuals.

Clinical conditions and capacity for work

Asthma

Asthma has a prevalence in the adult population of about 5%. It is a condition of variable airflow limitation associated with bronchial hyper-responsiveness and symptoms of cough, breathlessness, and tightness of the chest. The predominant physical sign is wheeze. Onset in childhood or early adult life is frequently associated with the syndrome of atopy, characterized by elevated IgE antibody levels, positive skin prick tests to common inhaled antigens, and an increased incidence of eczema and allergic rhinitis. Childhood symptoms often remit in early adult life but frequently recur in middle age. Onset in middle life is not usually associated with manifestations of atopy, and the condition tends to be more persistent and more likely to progress in severity with time.

There are some difficulties in defining asthma. Wheeze is a highly prevalent symptom in the community and many people with occasional wheeze do not have asthma. Conversely, subjects with bronchoconstriction do not recognize the symptom as often as might be supposed. A further difficulty arises in distinguishing between chronic asthma and COPD as there may be overlap between the classical features of asthma (such as wheeze and reversibility) and those of COPD (sputum, dyspnoea, and irreversible airflow obstruction). It is important, therefore, for doctors making a fitness assessment to decide whether the diagnosis is truly asthma and whether some response to treatment is likely. A more detailed history, including smoking habits, periodicity and remission of symptoms, and precipitating factors is essential. Ideally this should be supported by diurnal measurements of PEF and evidence of responsiveness to bronchodilators. Simple screening questions and a single measurement of lung function may prove misleading. The most usual pattern on spirometry is to observe an obstructive deficit (low FEV_1 with a normal FEV_1/FVC % ratio) but these measurements, though highly specific, have a relatively low sensitivity[7] in a disorder characterized by variable airflow limitation. Another common mistake is to confuse asthma with recurrent chest infection, especially in those who smoke. One unfortunate consequence of this mislabelling is to undertreat asthma and thereby limit employment opportunities.

In the worker with established asthma, fitness and placement judgements may hinge on a number of important questions.

How severe is the condition?

Hyper-responsive airways represent a biological continuum. Asthma varies from mild disease with intermittent symptoms, through mild-to-moderate persistent disease requiring regular prophylactic treatment, to severe disease requiring regular high-dose inhaled steroids, or more rarely, continuous oral steroids. It is difficult to estimate how often disease falls into the different categories of severity, but it is widely considered that most asthma is relatively mild and amenable to treatment. In employment terms asthma accounts for 2% of all lost working days in men and these typically fall in the winter months when viral respiratory infections are more prevalent.

In the common situation where asthma is mild, infrequent, or amenable to simple treatment, job placement decisions are straightforward. Adequate control may require only occasional use of a bronchodilator at times of unusual exertion or intercurrent infection. The anticipatory use of an inhaler (before exertion and in the early stages of respiratory infection) will further ameliorate any problem, though short-term work modification may be helpful and brief spells of sickness absence can arise (on average around 1–2 weeks a year). Under these circumstances the label 'asthmatic' may be unhelpful, leading simply to misinformed and prejudicial decisions on work fitness. Disease at the moderate to severe end of the spectrum poses more concern. At the extreme end brittle asthma may be severe and life-threatening. A particular worry arises if the workplace is far removed from medical care facilities and emergency transfer is expensive, disruptive, or technically difficult.

A broad indication of disease activity can be gained from the frequency of bronchodilator use and the degree of sleep disturbance. In more severe disease it is essential to know whether, or how often, a patient has been admitted to hospital with asthma; whether or not they have ever required ventilation because of asthma; or received emergency intravenous therapy; or take regularly prescribed oral steroid medication. A number of guidelines on assessing disease severity have been produced by specialist societies such as the British Thoracic Society. The American Thoracic Society has proposed some guidelines for assessing residual disability in controlled asthma. These relate to the degree of reversibility of airways obstruction or hyper-responsiveness and the minimum drug dose required to maintain asthma control.[8]

An alternative approach, particularly in physically demanding jobs, is to measure changes in lung function during representative work tasks. Exercise tests are not specific enough to be used routinely in pre-placement screening, but in subjects with active troublesome disease a fall in FEV_1 >15% may be a useful indicator of current work handicap.

Are there any work factors that are liable to aggravate constitutional asthma?

Asthmatic airways are hyper-responsive to a wide range of non-specific irritants that are commonly encountered at work as well as many highly prevalent environmental allergens. Extremes of temperature and humidity, irritant dusts and fumes, pollens, and house dust mites may all provoke or aggravate constitutional asthma, as may work stress, heavy physical exertion, and exposure to animals in stables, kennels, and laboratories. This can pose temporary or enduring employment problems to asthmatics in a wide range of occupations from cold-store workers in refrigeration plants through to outdoor workers in construction and farming. In practice, however, it is not easy to predict the sensitivity of a sufferer to irritant conditions. The degree of susceptibility to different irritant stimuli varies considerably between individuals: for example, airways that bronchoconstrict in response to cold air may be less sensitive to dusts and vice versa. In general, individuals with severe disease tend to be most vulnerable to irritant conditions, but not to the point where generalized judgements can be applied. Thus, severe asthmatics with a significant component of fixed airways obstruction may be less susceptible to nonspecific irritants than those with severe labile asthma.

Can the principal aggravating factors be removed or limited?

For example:

- Can irritant fumes or dusts be better controlled by exhaust ventilation or different work practices?
- Can less irritating materials be used?
- Can the process be enclosed?
- Can respiratory protection be used to limit exposure?
- If physical exertion is a limiting factor, can the effort of the work be reduced (e.g. by providing a lifting aid)?

These are areas in which occupational health practitioners need to be particularly influential.

Has the best treatment been offered, or could disease control be improved?

There is a growing appreciation that asthma tends to be undertreated, and that insufficient use is made of long-term prophylactic treatment, especially inhaled corticosteroids. Regular use of inhaled steroids has been shown to have a beneficial effect on attack frequency, sleep disturbance, hospital admission rates, and absenteeism and, recently, consensus guidelines have emerged on the optimum management of adult asthma.[9] The well-educated patient should be able to self-monitor, self-medicate, and self-refer. Deteriorating serial peak flow and worsening nocturnal symptoms should trigger an increase in medication and early medical attendance; in brittle asthma a home supply of oral steroids has enabled earlier treatment in those most in need and has transformed employment prospects in some subjects. A number of rule-based guidelines have now been published and evaluated[10,11] and it is important, before reaching irrevocable placement decisions, to determine whether better control is possible.

Might the patient have occupational (sensitization) asthma?

It is important to consider occupational asthma when asthma begins or recurs in adulthood. The possibility is suggested if symptoms are worse at work, or on work days, better when away from work (at weekends and on holiday), and deteriorate on return to work. A similar picture can arise from a non-specific response to irritant conditions, as described above, and the distinction between these possibilities is important. The reason is that **occupational asthma** may result in severe bronchospasm and sensitized workers may react to amounts of material so tiny that workplace controls cannot be guaranteed to afford reliable protection. By contrast, it is more realistic to achieve the control measures that ease the problems of **aggravated asthma,** so the prospects for continued healthy employment are correspondingly brighter.

In practice it may be difficult to distinguish between the two diagnoses: irritant industrial exposures often co-exist with the presence of a workplace sensitizer and workers with pre-existing asthma are not immune to occupational sensitization. A separate diagnostic problem arises in sensitized workers who manifest late asthmatic reactions rather than immediate ones. Symptoms often arise at night-time and thereby mimic the pattern of constitutional asthma.

FEV_1 is an insensitive indicator of occupational asthma and alternative investigations are required to secure a diagnosis. Agents that cause occupational asthma can be classified broadly into those that sensitize by the induction of specific IgE antibodies (e.g. laboratory animal proteins, platinum salts, and halogenated anhydrides) and those such as isocyanates, western red cedar, and colophony that sensitize by other poorly understood means and have mute or inconsistent antibody responses. Hence, for some causes of occupational asthma the detection of specific IgE antibodies may serve as an indicator of sensitization as may a positive skin prick test. These tests can be specific and relatively sensitive for some agents and can be used in case investigation. (The predictive value of a test depends not only on its sensitivity and specificity, but also on the prevalence of the disorder in the population tested so they tend to be less helpful in screening.) However, corroborative evidence is generally required before making placement decisions.

If the patient is still exposed, and fit for further exposure, the standard investigative tool is serial measurement of PEF.[12] A pattern is sought of exaggerated PEF variability and a fall in mean PEF level around times of exposure. Normally, several readings a day (at work and away from it) will be required over a 3–4 week period. Care is needed in the execution and interpretation of the test and the variability of occupational asthma needs to be differentiated from normal diurnal changes in PEF and other determinants of airways responsiveness (exercise, treatment, infection, etc.). The record must cover a period in which the potential for exposure exists and this may require some planning if exposures are intermittent or infrequent. It is important to keep to the same pattern of measurement at work and on rest days.

Different PEF patterns can arise in affected workers, dependent on their response and recovery times. An immediate response and a short recovery interval will generate obvious PEF dips related in time to work but late responses will produce dips at home and those that occur at night can readily be confused with constitutional asthma. Slower recovery times may result in a day on day decline in the working week with recovery at weekends. If recovery is protracted ordinary work breaks may be insufficient for recovery and a week on week decline ensues leading to a nadir of persistently low values. Recovery may take weeks or months away from exposure, a pattern readily misdiagnosed as COPD, especially in smokers. Diagnosis has traditionally been based on the relatively subjective approach of pattern recognition by an experienced physician, but rule-based quantitative approaches have been suggested and computerized diagnostic algorithms are currently being tested (see Bright and Burge[13] for a full discussion).

The 'gold standard' for diagnosis is a bronchial provocation challenge test (BPT) or an inhalation challenge test with the suspected sensitizer: a simulated industrial exposure conducted under controlled conditions with FEV_1 and responsiveness to histamine or methacholine measured serially. A late response, in particular, is taken as evidence of an allergic response; bronchial hyper-reactivity can also be demonstrated for 2–3 days after the challenge. The procedure entails some risk of severe bronchospasm and needs to be undertaken in a specialist hospital unit. The patient has to be admitted prior to the procedure, to ensure an adequate (exposure-free) baseline, and kept in for a day or so afterwards to measure late responsiveness. Because of its risk and cost BPT is usually reserved for special circumstances which include the investigation of mixed exposures and novel agents and situations of significant diagnostic uncertainty. Although it is often assumed that BPT is always correct, false negatives can arise if testing is conducted with the wrong material or too low an exposure.

Occupational asthma is important and comparatively common; over 400 causal agents have been identified and around 1000 new cases are diagnosed annually by UK specialists. It can result in acute severe bronchospasm in the workplace and chronic ill health during employment. For some sensitizing agents such as isocyanates, non-specific bronchial hyper-responsiveness is known to persist for several years after leaving employment. Early re-deployment may mitigate against the risk of continuing symptoms and thus improve the long-term prognosis. In the UK, the COSHH regulations therefore require health surveillance programmes to be conducted where there is a reasonable risk of occupational asthma. Guidance on the ingredients of suitable programmes has been provided by the Health and Safety Executive (HSE). Periodic symptom enquiries, measurements of lung function, and review of sickness absence reports are advised, the exact schedule being based on an assessment of risk.[14]

The strong presumption is that those with occupational asthma should be redeployed and removed from further exposure to the sensitizing agent that caused their asthma. The American Thoracic Society suggests that such subjects should be regarded as fully and permanently debarred from jobs that give rise to further exposure to the causal agent,[7] but some doctors perceive a difficulty for employees who develop mild occupational asthma with normal pulmonary function when exposures are low or occasional. The pressure to continue in work (and preserve earning power) has to be balanced against the longer term risks of deterioration, chronicity of symptoms, and fixed airflow limitation. There is a commonly held view that differences exist between sensitizers in their potency to sensitize, and in the severity and persistence of the symptoms they provoke. Isocyanate asthma, for example, may be induced by minute concentrations and may result in severe asthmatic attacks at work. The symptoms are also known to persist after exposure ceases, albeit with some improvement. More than half of those affected by small molecule asthma remain symptomatic after 2 years away from work, and in this group the disorder is usually permanent. Asthma resulting from sensitization to large molecules, such as flour dust, by contrast, is often milder with a better prognosis. With respiratory protection, modification of their job to reduce exposure, and effective treatment, many bakery workers have continued to work successfully. Other sensitized workers have also continued in employment wearing higher level respiratory protection. Under these circumstances close medical supervision is essential and the ever-present risk of control failures should be borne in mind. Every effort should be made to explore work and process modifications that minimize the risk. Ideally patients should withdraw permanently from further exposure.

Some authorities have recommended pre-employment policies that restrict the employment of workers perceived to be at greater risk of occupational asthma. Atopic individuals appear to be at increased risk from some agents that induce specific IgE such as animal proteins, whereas smokers are at a greater risk of asthma from platinum salts, phthalic anhydride, green coffee bean, snow crab, and ispaghula. For other agents, such as isocyanates and red cedar, lower risks have been described in atopics and smokers; and, in general, these risk factors are so common as to form a poor basis for health-based pre-placement selection. However, prudence would dictate that symptomatic asthmatics should not be newly employed in environments known to contain respiratory sensitizers since supervening occupational asthma will be more difficult to detect than in normal people and may be more troublesome.

Chronic obstructive pulmonary disease

COPD is common, affecting 5–8% of men and rather fewer women. Smoking leads to a syndrome of chronic mucus production with goblet cell hyperplasia (simple chronic bronchitis) and also to a condition of chronic airflow limitation with airways narrowing and emphysema. It appears that exposure to industrial dust and fumes may contribute to both syndromes, although smoking tobacco is a more important cause.

The principal symptoms in COPD are cough, sputum, and breathlessness on effort. Frequently, however, as the symptoms and signs are not very specific, detection of airflow limitation is delayed until disease is more advanced and some authorities have advocated annual spirometry to aid earlier detection in smokers and in people with recurrent respiratory symptoms or a family history of premature lung disease.

In assessing the fitness of a person with COPD for employment, a number of matters need to be considered and these broadly parallel those described earlier for asthma.

Is the problem primarily one of mucus hypersecretion or of airflow limitation?

Mucus hypersecretion by itself does not limit capacity to work and, in the absence of airflow limitation, simple chronic bronchitis is compatible with a wide range of normal employment. Infective exacerbations and sickness absence may be more frequent, although a programme of winter influenza vaccinations may reduce them. In these circumstances a medical label may be unhelpful and prejudicial to employment prospects. Frequently, however, mucus hypersecretion coexists with airflow limitation which can be a real cause of disability.

If airflow limitation is present, how severe is it and what is its functional effect?

Emphysema is defined in pathological terms but in life its presence can be presumed when there is an obstructive pattern on spirometry with evidence of increased static lung volumes (TLC), gas trapping (disproportionate increase in RV with reduced RV/TLC ratio) and impaired gas transfer (TLCO). Although FEV_1 may be normal despite significant small airways disease there is a broad correlation in COPD between FEV_1 and breathlessness and it provides a better guide to disability than PEF. People with FEV_1 values of less than 60% of predicted tend to show moderate disability whereas those below 40% of predicted tend to display severe disability. Ventilatory failure (hypercapnia) is unusual if the FEV_1 is more than 1.5 litres. Measurements of lung function and maximum oxygen uptake (VO$_2$ max) should, in principle, provide a fair guide to work capability in patients with airflow limitation and two broad approaches have been adopted towards the objective assessment of impairment:

- banding spirometry findings according to their likely relation to representative activities of daily living (Table 19.2 describes the European Respiratory Society guidelines on classifying impairment[15])
- comparing the measured V_{O_2} max with the approximate energy demands of a range of common occupations and occupational activities (using a scheme such as that in Table 19.3, or the US Department of Labor's job by job analysis of work demands[16]).

Unfortunately, the energy demands of work vary from one time to another as the component activities of a task vary; individuals also vary in their oxygen requirements for a

Table 19.2   Categories of respiratory impairment according to the European Respiratory Society[15]

Impairment	FEV$_1$	FVC	FEV$_1$/FVC	DLCO
None (normal)[a]	± 1.64 SD	± 1.64 SD	± 1.64 SD	± 1.64 SD
Slight	Not normal but >60%	Not normal but >60%	Not normal but >60%	Not normal but >60%
Moderate	40–59%	50–59%	40–59%	40–59%
Severe	<40%	<50%	<40%	<40%

All values represent percentage of predicted. SD, standard deviation.
[a] The American Thoracic Society criteria[3] are similar except that normal is >80% (or >75% for FEV$_1$).

Table 19.3   The energy cost of some occupational and reference activities

Activity	Cal/ml	Mets[a]	Activity	Cal/ml	Mets[a]
Rest	1.0	1.0	Bricklaying	4.0	3.5
Sitting	1.2	1.0	Plastering	4.1	3.5
Standing	1.4	1.0	Ploughing (tractor)	4.2	3.5
Watch repair	1.6	1.5	Wheeling barrow (115 lb, 2.5 mph)	5.0	4.0
Sweeping floor	1.6	1.5	Carpentry	6.8	5.5
Machine sewing	1.8	1.8	Tree felling	8.0	6.5
Armature winding	2.2	2.0	Shovelling	8.5	7.0
Playing piano	2.5	2.0	Ascending stairs (27 ft/min, 17 lb load)	9.0	7.5
Radio assembly	2.7	2.5			
Planing	9.1	7.5			
Driving car	2.8	2.5	Ascending stairs (54 ft/min, 22 lb load)	16.2	13.5
Making beds	3.9	3.0			

Adapted from Rusk HA (ed.) *Rehabilitation medicine* St Louis, CV Mosby 1977 (with permission).
* Met = Metabolic equivalent. One Met = 3.5 ml/kg/min oxygen consumed (or the amount of basal oxygen consumption at rest).

given task because of personal and job-related factors (e.g. differences in their metabolic efficiency and different working methods); and finally resting lung function tests explain only a small part of the variance in $\dot{V}o_2$ max.[17] The subjective appreciation of breathlessness usually proves to be the limiting factor. Hence, 'objective' measurements of disability provide no more than a rough guide to work capacity.[18] Crudely speaking, those with 'slight' impairment (Table 19.2) can manage most ordinary work, whereas those with 'moderate' impairment fail to meet the physical demands of many jobs, and those with 'severe' impairment do not cope in most jobs. However, given wide individual variation and scope for job modification, fitness decisions still depend on subjective medical judgements.

Has the best treatment been offered, or could disease control be improved?

In individuals with airflow limitation due to COPD there is scope for therapeutic improvement but the scope is much less than for asthma. Inhaled β-agonists are less effective and need to be used in doses that often provoke tremors. Anticholinergic agents, such as ipratropium bromide, may be more effective and in disease of moderate severity either or both may be employed on a regular basis. Bronchodilators may improve breathlessness and exercise tolerance, even in the absence of measurable bronchodilation.

The inflammation of COPD tends to be less responsive to steroids, with only about 10% of patients deriving real benefit. Response to treatment can be tested objectively by prescribing 30 mg of oral prednisolone daily for 3 weeks and conducting follow-up spirometry. In all patients with moderate or severe disease consideration should be given to such a therapeutic trial. In those who show an improvement (e.g. $\geqslant 20\%$ increase in FEV_1), inhaled steroids can be continued as maintenance therapy and oral steroids offered during acute exacerbations.

The role of mucolytics and nebulized saline in COPD are less well defined. Theophyllines have only a modest bronchodilatory effect, but may modify small airways function and gas trapping. Beneficial effects on exercise tolerance have been reported but not consistently. Plasma theophylline levels should be monitored in users, in view of the narrow therapeutic range of these drugs and their propensity to cause side-effects and drug interactions.

Graded exercise programmes appear to increase exercise tolerance in some patients, although this occurs in the absence of any clear physiological improvement and may arise simply through an improved sense of well-being. However, work activity can be increased safely and beneficially within the limits of airflow limitation. Exercise needs to be regular and frequent and the benefit is lost within 6–8 weeks if the programme lapses.

It is very important to encourage COPD sufferers to stop smoking. In people with smoking-induced COPD the rate of decline in FEV_1 is increased from an average value of 20–30 ml per year seen in non-smokers to a value of around 60–80 ml per year. In smokers with moderate impairment of lung function the rate of loss of function returns to normal on smoking cessation, but the benefit in severe COPD and in industrial disease is less certain. Thus, an important preventive role for an occupational health service is to educate and to provide support for employees who attempt to stop smoking, especially in those with COPD.

Finally, intercurrent infections require prompt treatment to prevent acute deterioration and chronic airways damage. Consensus guidelines on disease management have now begun to emerge, including one excellent review by the British Thoracic Society.[19]

Are there any work factors that are liable to aggravate COPD?

In workers who develop troublesome progressive airflow limitation, continuing employment may still be possible in more sedentary work or under a modified work schedule. Exercise physiology experiments on leg effort and degree of dyspnoea have shown that a doubling of work intensity causes a fourfold increase in effort and dyspnoea whereas a doubling in the duration of work causes only a 30% increase: thus one possible strategy may be less arduous work spread over a longer time period. Better process control (dust and fume control at source, assisted mechanical lifting, etc.) may also extend the range of employment possibilities and these measures should all be considered before declaring the worker unfit.

Are there special work problems for COPD sufferers?

The wearing of respiratory protective equipment (RPE) may increase the effort of work. Some RPE, such as self-contained breathing apparatus (SCBA), can be bulky, heavy, or awkward. Other RPE systems, such as canister respirators and half-face masks, increase the work of breathing, requiring the wearer to inspire air against the resistance of a filter. It may be possible to provide a filter-free 'active' system in which air-fed respirators blow a stream of fresh air across the face behind a visor, the positive pressure generated preventing the ingress of hazardous fumes, but even these require extra weight to be carried around during physical activity; and the choice of system may be dictated by the circumstances – for example the need to attain very high degrees of protection may necessitate SCBA and work in oxygen-deficient atmospheres may necessitate the carriage of gas cylinders. Fitness decisions need to be made in the light of residual lung capacity, the work in question, and the options for process control over and above RPE use.

The presence of emphysema, particularly bullous disease, increases the risk of spontaneous pneumothorax and is thus a bar to employment in certain occupations that involve changes in barometric pressure such as flying and diving (see Appendices 2 and 4, respectively).

Interstitial lung disease

The important diseases in this group include interstitial fibrosis, chronic pulmonary sarcoidosis, and extrinsic allergic alveolitis. In functional terms these conditions reduce pulmonary compliance, reduce static lung volumes, and impair gas transfer. $FEV_1/FVC\%$ is usually preserved but airflow limitation may be present in addition to fibrosis. These conditions are all associated with radiological abnormalities but high-resolution CT scanning is more sensitive than plain radiography in assessing the extent and progress of disease.

Pulmonary fibrosis may be cryptogenic, secondary to other clinical disorders such as rheumatoid arthritis, systemic sclerosis, inflammatory bowel disease, sarcoidosis, and chronic allergic alveolitis, or due to occupational contact with fibrogenic dusts. A number of professional groups, including miners and quarrymen, stone dressers, foundry fettlers, and construction workers are at special risk although this fact may go unrecognized.

Established fibrosis from whatever cause frequently progresses, although the rate of progression can be very variable. In the case of fibrogenic dust disease progression may occur despite removal from the industry, although early identification and withdrawal from exposure may result in a better long-term outcome. It therefore seems prudent to identify this disorder at an early stage and to recommend avoidance of further exposure. Unfortunately, there are no unique symptoms or signs, and disease onset is insidious (over a decade or longer). Gradually progressive dyspnoea may be erroneously attributed to simple ageing, particularly when the potential for exposure is overlooked. A programme of regular surveillance in high risk professions obviates this problem. In Britain there is a legal requirement to conduct health surveillance in asbestos workers under certain conditions,[20] and the surveillance programme and the physician need to be approved by the HSE.

Tests of pulmonary function are not diagnostically specific, so plain radiography provides the mainstay of screening programmes. Radiography is considered to be about 80% sensitive in asbestosis and silicosis, and other diagnostic methods such as high-resolution CT may one day be used in preference.

Table 19.4 details two model surveillance programmes advocated by the World Health Organization.[21] These include radiography, symptom enquiry, and spirometry. In the UK guidance has been provided by HSE, although this is somewhat different in its content. In the case of crystalline silica exposure the HSE advocates surveillance in employees who are regularly exposed to levels exceeding 0.1 mg m^{-3} 8-h TWA[22] (generally in quarrying, certain heavy clay activities, and the refactory and foundry industries). A 2-yearly programme of chest radiography and respiratory questioning is suggested but spirometry is not advocated on a serial basis. According to the HSE the number of respiratory

Table 19.4 WHO recommendations for health screening of workers exposed to asbestos or silica

Agent	Surveillance procedure	Interval/frequency[a]
Silica (crystalline quartz) dust exposure	Chest radiograph	At baseline, after 2–3 years of exposure, then every 2–5 years
	Spirometry + symptom questionnaire	At baseline, then annually, or at the same frequency as chest radiograph
Asbestos exposure	Chest radiograph	At baseline, then: – every 3–5 years if less than 10 years since first exposed – every 1–2 years if longer than 10 years but less than 20 years – annually if longer than 20 years since first exposure
	Spirometry + symptom questionnaire + physical examination	Annually, or at the same frequency as the chest radiograph

[a] In both cases, surveillance should be life-long.

(Adapted with permission from: Wagner GR. Asbestosis and silicosis. *Lancet* 1997; 349: 1311–15. © The Lancet Ltd[21]) episodes should be determined by questioning and perusal of sickness absence records and evidence sought of any serial trends that may suggest disease onset. Pre-employment assessment should identify those more vulnerable to respiratory infection (those with COPD and asthma, for example), and should include enquiry about current symptoms, chest radiography, and baseline spirometry. Old tuberculosis may become reactivated in silica-exposed workers, so a history of earlier respiratory tuberculosis should also be sought. For health surveillance in asbestos workers HSE provides guidance for its Appointed Doctors.

Radiographs may be scored against a standard set of ILO films, based on the presence, profusion, size, and shape of opacities.[23] In coal worker's pneumoconiosis category 1 changes can occur without evidence of impaired lung function. Such workers can continue to work under surveillance. Category 2 change and above is associated with increasing impairment of lung function and warrants removal from contact with fibrogenic dust, as does simple silicosis and asbestosis.

Fibrotic lung disease is irreversible and presently untreatable. Oral corticosteroids and other forms of immunosuppression, such as cyclophosphamide or azathioprine, have been tried but the results are disappointing.

The principal disability is breathlessness on effort which is often accompanied by significant falls in arterial oxygen levels. Spirometry and measurements of Vo_2 max and arterial Po_2 in representative exercise provide a basis for fitness assessment; the general considerations are the same as those for COPD with airflow limitation. Affected workers may remain gainfully employed in less manual work but disability tends to progress with time and a periodic medical review is appropriate. All forms of pulmonary fibrosis are probably associated with an increased risk of bronchogenic carcinoma.

Sarcoidosis is a rare condition of uncertain aetiology, characterized by the prescence of non-caseating epitheloid granulomata. Pulmonary involvement may take one of three forms: bihilar lymphadenopathy (in association with erythema nodosum), parenchymal lung infiltrates, and lung fibrosis. The first of these has no important effect on lung function and it regresses over a few months. The second pattern is typically self-limiting, but may be progressive, and require long-term treatment with steroids. Any restrictive effects are usually slight in comparison with the appearance of the chest radiograph, and so do not prevent most normal work. However, chronic parenchymal involvement with fibrosis, can cause a severe restrictive defect and impairment of transfer factor which seriously limits exercise tolerance. Fibrosis is irreversible. Work capacity depends on the residual lung function, but modified or light duties may be warranted in the few workers so affected.

Extrinsic allergic alveolitis (EAA) is a hypersensitivity pneumonitis provoked principally by occupational allergens, such as mouldy hay and bird excreta. In its acute form it produces a mild systemic flu-like illness with fever, aches and pains, malaise and dry cough, and respiratory crackles. Symptoms develop within a few hours of exposure. Mild attacks resolve spontaneously but severe attacks may require corticosteroid therapy. The condition is self-limiting if contact with the offending protein ceases or if adequate respiratory protection is provided. However, chronic exposure can cause pulmonary fibrosis and permanent respiratory disability. Established fibrosis is unresponsive to treatment so regular surveillance (radiography and lung function testing) is appropriate for those with continuing potential for exposure.

Respiratory infections

Acute upper respiratory tract infections

Infections of the upper respiratory tract are very common. Occupational environments which are enclosed with little natural ventilation favour the spread of prevalent respiratory infections, particularly viral ones. These contribute importantly to short-term sickness absence but are self-limiting and pose no special difficulties in fitness assessment.

More serious are a range of viral upper respiratory tract infections that may be complicated by chest problems or protracted debility. **Influenza** is a highly infectious condition that involves a longer period of sickness and a greater risk of complicating illness (tracheobronchitis, pneumonia, exacerbated COPD). Some occupational groups, such as healthcare workers and teachers, are at particular risk, and may benefit from prophylaxis with influenza vaccine; so may those with pre-existing lung diseases such as asthma and COPD.

Glandular fever and the other infectious mononucleoses are relatively common in young adults, and cause a protracted period of illness and work difficulty. A severe tonsillitis occurs, often associated with palatal petechiae, cervical lymphadenopathy, and a palpable spleen. The diagnosis is confirmed by the finding of atypical mononuclear cells on the blood film. In glandular fever the Paul–Bunnell test is positive in about 60% of patients during the first week of illness and abnormal liver function tests occur in 50% of the cases.

Although these diseases are self-limiting it is not uncommon to feel tired and fatigued for 3–6 months after the acute stage of illness. Sufferers who lack their normal stamina are often signed off as unfit to attend work although a modified work programme with phased rehabilitation is a more constructive approach. Ideally this would encourage the sufferer to work normal duties, but only for a part of the week to begin with, the hours gradually increasing as stamina assumes more normal levels.

Some respiratory infections may be occupationally acquired—for example Q fever in slaughterhouse workers and veterinary surgeons and legionella pneumonia in industries using humidification and water cooling plants, but these are uncommon occurrences. Occasionally respiratory infection may be transmitted from workers to members of the public as well, the most important example being tuberculosis in healthcare workers.

Tuberculosis

Tuberculosis is a respiratory infection spread by infected droplets from person to person. In the UK, since 1950, the number of new cases notified has fallen tenfold from around 50 000 per year to 5000 per year, but there is now good evidence that this decline has ceased. Around 9 million new cases occur each year worldwide, 95% of which arise in low-income countries. Migrants from these countries bring with them an increased risk of tuberculosis. In England and Wales the 1993 MRC survey showed an incidence of 4.3/100 000 per year for white people, but the rate was 27 times higher in people from India and more than 30 times greater in people from Africa. In countries with a high prevalence of tuberculosis the advent of HIV disease is promoting tuberculosis in people of working age. The same effect is apparent in the HIV-positive population of New York, but it has yet to be seen in the UK where the reservoir of tuberculous infection is mainly in elderly people at low risk of HIV infection.

Cross-infectivity in tuberculosis arises principally in the close domestic contacts of patients with smear-positive sputum. The British Thoracic and Tuberculosis Association survey[24] found that around 9–13% of close contacts of smear-positive index cases developed disease. In casual contacts the risk was 0.3%, and in close contacts of smear-negative index cases only 0.5% of non-Asian and 2.8% of Asian subjects developed tuberculosis. The risk of cross-infection with non-respiratory tuberculosis is very low. The principal risk, therefore, lies with close contacts of smear-positive cases. In an occupational setting each case needs to be assessed individually in the light of the clinical details of the index case and the working environment. In the UK cases of tuberculosis are statutorily notifiable to the Public Health Service, which will institute screening of people at risk, usually via the local chest diseases department.

Figure 19.2 summarizes the guidelines of the Joint Tuberculosis Committee of the British Thoracic Society (1994) on pre-employment screening for healthcare workers.[25] Doctors, nurses, physiotherapists, postmortem technicians, laboratory workers, and others at risk of contact should be assessed and protected as necessary. Students, locums, agency staff, and contract ancillary workers may easily be overlooked and should be included in assessment procedures, as should laboratory technicians in commercial and private research facilities.

At the pre-employment stage details should be sought of any symptoms suggestive of tuberculosis and of previous BCG vaccination or the presence of a BCG scar. A tuberculin test, preferably the Heaf test, is only necessary in new employees without a BCG scar. If the tuberculin test proves negative, or Heaf grade 1, a BCG vaccination should be offered and the scar re-examined after a few weeks for evidence of a reaction. In British studies vaccination has been shown to reduce the risk of active tuberculosis by 70–80%. Quite often, a strongly positive tuberculin test arises. Formerly this was taken to be suggestive of current infection and further investigation (chest radiography) ensued; recent evidence suggests this is unnecessary in the absence of symptoms. An exception may be made for individuals with strongly positive reactions who come from tuberculosis-endemic areas.

BCG vaccination is contra-indicated in HIV-positive individuals, and HIV-positive healthcare workers should not be employed in areas where there is a risk of contracting active tuberculosis.

During employment routine periodic chest radiography is neither necessary nor effective in screening. Awareness and early reporting of suspicious symptoms is the mainstay of detection.

If a worker contracts tuberculosis treatment will initially comprise at least three first-line drugs (isoniazid, rifampicin, and pyrazinamide), with the addition of a fourth drug (usually ethambutol) if the possibility of drug resistance is considered significant. Treatment should be supervised by a physician (usually a chest physician) experienced in the management of tuberculosis. Providing sensitivity results are available, continuation therapy can be reduced to isoniazid and rifampicin after 2 months of treatment and then needs to be maintained for a further 4 months. In fully sensitive infections, the majority in the UK, the patient is non-infectious after 2 weeks of treatment and it is not usually necessary to restrict work after 2–3 weeks of treatment. Caution may be appropriate,

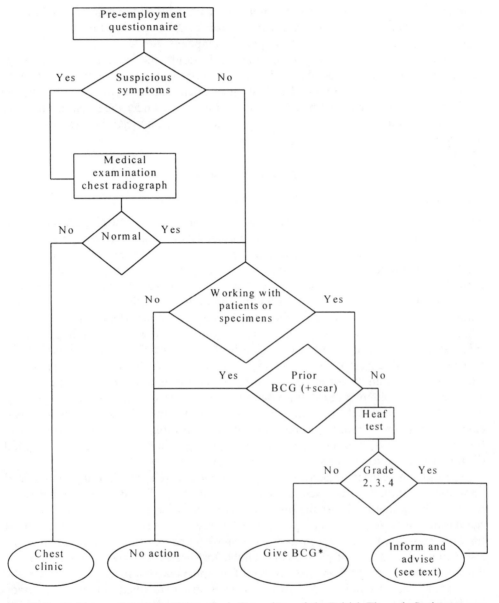

Fig. 19.2 Guidance of the Joint Tuberculosis Committee of the British Thoracic Society on protection of healthcare workers (reproduced with permission of the BMJ Publishing Group)[25].

however, where there is reason to suspect drug resistance and in healthcare workers who deal with vulnerable patient groups, such as the immunosuppressed and young children. An infectious risk should be assumed until drug sensitivities are shown or the sputum is known to be negative on culture. Drug resistance should be suspected in patients who have relapsed from earlier treatment and those who come from areas where drug resistance is common (e.g. Africa, the Indian subcontinent, and certain parts of the US such as New York). HIV infection is a risk factor for drug-resistant tuberculosis. Problems may also arise in patients who are poorly compliant with treatment.

In cases where compliance with treatment is in doubt the administration of drugs under supervision may be necessary (directly observed short-course treatment or DOTS) to prevent the risk of developing drug resistance. Such treatment could be given by the staff of the occupational health service provided it is done under the supervision of the local expert in tuberculosis control, usually the consultant physician in chest diseases or infectious diseases.

Neoplastic disease

Lung cancer

The most important aetiological risk factor for lung cancer is smoking. A number of occupational risk factors are also well recognized, asbestos exposure being numerically the most important. In asbestos-induced lung cancer the risks multiply with those of smoking. Occupationally-related lung cancers may also arise in the extraction of chromium from its ore, the manufacture of chromates, nickel refining, and exposure to polycyclic aromatic hydrocarbons, cadmium compounds, arsenic (in mining, smelting, and pesticide production), and bis-chloromethyl and chloromethyl methyl ethers.

Different histological types of lung cancer vary in their growth rate. In the absence of treatment, a patient with adenocarcinoma is likely to survive for about 2 years from the time of diagnosis, a patient with a squamous cell tumour for about 1 year, and a patient with a small-cell tumour for about 4 months. Small-cell tumours metastasize early and are rarely amenable to surgical cure; but 85% respond to combination chemotherapy. The median survival is thus extended to about 8 months in patients with extensive disease and to about 14 months in patients with limited disease; but a minority survive longer (10% for 2 years, 4% for 5 years). During this period patients often enjoy a good quality of life, and can sometimes continue in light work.

For other lung cancers (adenocarcinoma, squamous carcinoma, and undifferentiated tumours), chemotherapy is much less successful and the preferred treatment is surgical resection. Radiotherapy is usually used as an adjunct to surgery, or for the palliation of specific problems such as haemoptysis and localized bone pain. Unfortunately, most tumours present when advanced and other smoking-related lung disease often limits resectability. About 25% of patients are suitable for surgery. Of these about a third survive for 5 years – 65–85% in the absence of lymph node, chest wall, and metastatic involvement, but around 25–35% when there is ipsilateral mediastinal lymph node involvement. The 30-day operative mortality is about 6% for pneumonectomy and 3% for lobectomy. Patients below retirement age who undergo successful resection may well be able to return to work, although the choice of employment will depend on the physical demands of the job and the residual lung function after resection.

Mesothelioma

Mesothelioma is a rare tumour in the absence of asbestos exposure. It is a malignant condition affecting the pleura or, less frequently the peritoneum. The tumour arises after a long latent period—rarely less than 20 years from first exposure, and typically 35–40 years; this means that cases tend to arise after retirement.

The incidence of the tumour is rising in the UK, reflecting a greater use of asbestos during, and after the Second World War. In 1984 there were 534 new cases in men and 84 new cases in women, but by 1991 the annual total had risen to 1009. A gradient of risk exists for different fibre types; it is greatest for crocidolite (blue asbestos) and least for chrysotile, with amosite occupying an intermediate position.

Mesothelioma often presents with chest wall pain, breathlessness, and pleural effusion. It progresses mainly by local invasion although distant metastases can sometimes occur. Involvement of the chest wall, diaphragm, mediastinum, and neck root is common and results in local pain, restricted chest movement, dysphagia, obstruction of the great veins, and pericardial involvement. The condition is incurable and most patients die within 2 years of presentation. It is rare for a patient with mesothelioma to be able to continue for long in active employment.

Other diseases of the pleura

One of the commonest manifestations of pleural disease is **pleural effusion**. Effusions that result from inflammatory processes are exudates with a high protein content (>30 g/litre). Underlying causes include infection, collagen vascular disease, malignancy, and pulmonary infarction. The effusions from pleural malignancy, pulmonary infarction, and asbestotic pleurisy may be bloodstained. Effusions of low protein content (transudates) may arise in cardiac failure and low-protein states such as nephrotic syndrome and cirrhosis of the liver.

Fitness decisions require accurate information on the cause of the effusion and its prognosis. Investigation by aspiration, examination, and culture of the fluid, and closed pleural biopsy normally enable the various possibilities to be distinguished, but otherwise thoracoscopy with biopsy or open pleural biopsy is necessary.

When inflammatory effusions resolve, they frequently leave behind an area of pleural thickening and adhesions that obliterate the pleural space. If extensive this thickening can restrict lung movement and produce chest discomfort and breathlessness on exertion.

At work, asbestos exposure frequently causes pleural plaques, which are circumscribed areas of thickening on the parietal pleura which may gradually calcify. They are composed of areas of hyaline fibrosis, a few millimetres up to 1 centimetre in thickness. Plaques are discovered radiographically and seldom become evident within 15 years of first exposure, but they do not obliterate the pleural space and produce no impairment of lung function or other disability. Their presence does not correlate well with that of pulmonary fibrosis (asbestosis), nor do they predicate the occurrence of mesothelioma, which is related to levels of exposure but no more common in those who develop plaques than in those who do not. They tend to be discovered accidentally and do not require work restriction or redeployment.

Asbestos exposure sometimes leads to pleurisy and haemorrhagic exudative pleural effusion. Effusion may also be discovered as an incidental radiographic finding. The majority occur 10–15 years after first exposure. They may persist for several months, recur after drainage, or affect both sides in sequence over a year or two. Biopsy simply shows non-specific pleural inflammation. These pleural effusions may lead on to adhesions and diffuse pleural thickening. This latter condition, if extensive enough, produces restriction of lung expansion, dyspnoea and work limitation. Bilateral diaphragmatic thickening is therefore a prescribed disease. There is no evidence that simple pleural plaques progress to diffuse pleural thickening which is a different entity.

Smoking

Smoking is a major cause of respiratory disability, being the principal cause of both COPD and lung cancer. These two diseases together account for the majority of deaths from respiratory disease. The heavier the smoking, the greater the risk. It is clearly good preventive practice to offer help and support to those who want to stop smoking and to make the workforce generally aware of the risks. The benefits of stopping smoking in COPD have already been discussed.

Smoking at work has major health implications for smokers but also some consequences for their colleagues. Patients with lung disease, especially asthma, are vulnerable to the irritant effects of a smoke-filled environment and there is growing evidence that passive smoking is harmful: the children of smoking parents are more vulnerable to respiratory infections than those of non-smoking parents; the non-smoking wives of male smokers have higher risks of lung cancer than the wives of non-smokers; and the US Environmental Protection Agency has concluded that environmental tobacco smoke (ETS) is a carcinogen that accounts for some 2000 deaths per year in non-smokers in the US. Although the health effects of ETS are small compared to those of active smoking, the large number of people exposed makes ETS an important public health problem. Responsible employers should therefore establish non-smoking policies in the workplace.

Special work problems and restrictions

Sometimes work is conducted in adverse environments, or in safety-critical roles characterized by a requirement for high standards of respiratory fitness. Such is the case in airline pilots and cabin crew, commercial and military divers, caisson workers, and members of the armed forces, police, and rescue services. A number of these work activities involve changes in gas pressure and composition and the use of breathing apparatus to extend the range of hostile environments in which work can be conducted; and all require a general level of fitness that transcends simple good respiratory health.

The fitness standards required of pilots and commercial divers, and the physiological demands of their work, are more fully described in Appendices 2 and 4 respectively, but reference is made here to some of the respiratory aspects of the work.

Flying and diving result in ambient gas pressure changes that pose major respiratory problems. The lung walls rupture at transmural pressures of about one-tenth of an atmosphere (10 kPa), the muscles of the chest tire within minutes if transmural pressures exceed 5 kPa, and the airways become easily irritated by changes in pressure and humidity. The fall in ambient pressure encountered in aeroplane ascent may thus result in pneumothorax, if gas trapping occurs in the chest, as might arise in bullous disease, asthma, or recent chest trauma. Similarly, ascent from a commercial or military dive may result in trapped gas at higher than ambient pressure seeking a means of escape and causing pulmonary barotrauma or decompression sickness. Pneumothorax, peribronchial rupture, mediastinal emphysema, and gas emboli are all well-recognized outcomes.

Related problems arise from altered oxygen tensions. The lowered partial pressure of oxygen (Pao_2) at elevated altitudes may aggravate hypoxia in aircrew with existing airways disease; and, in fighter pilots, the problem may be exacerbated by physiological shunting in the dependent parts of the lung during high-G turns.

High standards of respiratory fitness are required in these categories of work from the viewpoint of personal safety and well-being, and, especially in the case of aircrew, because of their responsibility for expensive equipment and other peoples' lives. In new entrants, a history of spontaneous pneumothorax, asthma, or obstructive respiratory disease is normally a bar to employment, as are most radiographic abnormalities.

In established workers who develop chest disease the criteria are slightly less stringent: it may, for example, be possible for well-controlled asthmatics, or patients with a pleurectomy or pleurodesis, to continue as members of an aircrew. The standards are set down respectively by the Civil Aviation Authority and armed services for flight fitness, and HSE, in the UK, for fitness to dive.[26] In each of these cases regular assessment is required by approved medical assessors followed by certification of continuing fitness. Assessments include a number of subsidiary investigations, such as an annual chest radiograph in divers, as well as a detailed appraisal of other health issues as described in Appendices 2 and 4.

Intercurrent respiratory illness is a temporary bar to diving and flying. Failure to equilibrate pressures across the eustachian tube in catarrhal illness and air trapping in the sinuses can cause decompression trauma, so diving and flying are best avoided until natural recovery has occurred. Professional divers who have recently surfaced (decompressed) sometimes wish then to fly: this may represent a further extreme of decompression and they should be advised to refrain from flying until 24 hours has elapsed.

Recommended minimum fitness standards for workers in the UK **armed services** are laid down in a Joint Services System of Medical Classification (JSP 346). New applicants with active tuberculosis, chronic bronchitis, or bronchiectasis are normally rejected but if disease appears for the first time in service, the worker is individually assessed. Current asthma, or recurrent wheeze requiring recent treatment (within the past 4 years), is treated similarly; those with a more distant history are tested for exercise-induced decrements of FEV_1. The occurrence of pneumothorax requires individual assessment and depends on the nature of the work and the success or otherwise of surgical treatment.

The armed services use the PULHEEMS system to rank fitness for a number of physical and mental attributes against an eight-point scale of descriptors. Respiratory fitness is not separately identified in the rubric, although the P scale (physical fitness) encompasses cardiorespiratory fitness. There may be some differences between services and between jobs. For example, the fitness standards for RAF air-flight crew are more stringent than for ground personnel, such as engineers and technicians. However, for many jobs the minimum standard (fit with training for heavy manual work, including lifting and climbing, but not to endure severe or prolonged strain) precludes those with significant chest disease.

UK regulations require **fire service workers** to have their FEV_1 and FVC measured by a doctor, and to have their aerobic capacity (Vo_2 max) measured in a step test prior to employment. The regulations stipulate that a duly qualified medical practitioner must be satisfied that these measurements are compatible with the fitness requirements of firefighting, but refers to these only in general terms. Guidance by the Home Office, however, recommends a Vo_2 max standard of 45 ml $kg^{-1}min^{-1}$ for recruit firefighters and various age-related values for serving firefighters. The guidance further recommends regular fitness (Vo_2 max) assessments and a 3 yearly health surveillance programme that involves measurement of height, weight, pulse, blood pressure, and visual acuity, as well as FEV_1 and FVC but the performance standard for spirometry is not specified. To assist Fire Service Medical Advisers with the interpretation and application of these rules, the Association of Local Authority Medical Advisers (ALAMA) has produced consultative guidance on respiratory fitness for firefighters[27] and this provides the basis of the further details that follow.

Firefighters are required to operate in very adverse environments, to wear breathing apparatus, and to perform physically arduous tasks. Intercurrent illnesses provide no more than a temporary bar to active duties, but conditions with airflow limitation may jeopardize employment prospects. Rescue workers may encounter irritant or sensitizing fumes and many products of combustion; some of these will exacerbate asthma, and some, including products of PVC combustion, may incite new asthma (reactive airways dysfunction syndrome or RADS). Active asthma on application often leads to rejection. If there is a prior history, or disease develops during employment, the circumstances should be individually assessed but recurrent, severe or refractory symptoms may lead to medical retirement as may poor performance on spirometry (<2 SD of predicted). Established COPD of more than slight severity (as defined by the European Respiratory Society: $FEV_1/FVC\%$ <60%), and chronic restrictive lung disease are considered incompatible with active firefighting duties at the recruitment stage and their development during employment generally leads to early retirement. The occurrence of pneumothorax should trigger individual review, but a successful pleurodesis may enable active duties to continue. Finally, the development of lung cancer would lead to rejection or retirement but a successfully resected benign tumour is not a definite bar.

The Disability Discrimination Act (DDA) and respiratory illness

'Disability' in the DDA is defined as a more than trivial impairment of everyday activities such as mobility, likely to last a year or more. COPD with moderate or severe impairment of lung function (Table 19.2), fibrotic lung diseases that have the same functional consequences, and severe steroid-dependent asthma are all likely to fulfil these criteria. Terminal lung cancer and mesothelioma also qualify. In such cases, the onus is to make reasonable workplace changes to accommodate or limit impairment. Some of the means (control of aggravating occupational factors, provision of aids, optimum treatment etc.) have been described where relevant. Ultimately, however, the onus extends to rescheduling, reallocating or sharing work duties, redeployment and acceptance of part-time working (see also Chapter 4). Vocational rehabilitation services may also assist in terms of functional assessments and access to work schemes for those with disabling respiratory illness (p. 66 *et seq*).

Selected references

1 Cotes JE, Chinn DJ, Reed JW. Lung function testing: methods and reference values for forced expiratory volume and transfer factor. *Occup Environ Med* 1997;**54**: 457–465.

2 British Thoracic Society and the Association of Respiratory Technicians and Physiologists. Guidelines for the measurement of respiratory function. *Resp Med* 1994;**88**: 165–194.

3 American Thoracic Society. Standardization of spirometry: 1994 update. *Am J Respir Crit Care Med* 1995;**152**: 1107–1136.

4 *Questionnaires on respiratory symptoms*. London: Medical Research Council, 1976.

5 Toren K, Brisman J, Jarvholm B. Asthma and asthma-like symptoms in adults assessed by questionnaires: A literature review. *Chest* 1993;**104**: 600–608.

6 Venables KM, Farrer N, Sharp L, Graneek BJ, Newman Taylor AJ. Respiratory symptoms questionnaire for asthma epidemiology: validity and reproducibility. *Thorax* 1993;**48**: 214–219.

7 Stenton SC, Beach JR, Avery AJ, Hendrick DJ. The value of questionnaires and spirometry in asthma surveillance programmes in the workplace. *Occup Med* 1993;**43**: 203–206.

8 American Thoracic Society. Guidelines for the evaluation of impairment/disability in patients with asthma. *Am Rev Respir Dis* 1993;**147**: 1056–1061.

9 British Thoracic Society, Research Unit of the Royal College of Physicians, King's Fund Centre, National Asthma Campaign. Guidelines for the management of asthma in adults. I. Chronic persistent asthma. *BMJ* 1990;**301**: 651–654.

10 Jones KP, Mullee MA, Middleton M, Chapman E, Holgate ST, British Thoracic Society Research Committee. Peak flow based asthma self-management: a randomised controlled study in general practice. *Thorax* 1995;**50**: 851–857.

11 Beasley R, Cushley M, Holgate ST. A self-management plan in treatment of adult asthma. *Thorax* 1989;**44**: 200–204.

12 Burge PS. Single and serial measurements of lung function in the diagnosis of occupational asthma. *Eur J Respir Dis* 1982;**63**: 47–59.

13 Bright P, Burge PS. The diagnosis of occupational asthma from serial measurements of lung function at and away from work. *Thorax* 1996;**51**: 857–863.

14 Health and Safety Executive. *Medical Aspects of Occupational Asthma*. London: HMSO, 1991.

15 Siafakas NM, Vermiere P, Pride NB *et al.* Optimal assessment and management of chronic obstructive pulmonary disease (COPD). *Eur Respir J* 1995;**8**: 1398–1420.

16 US Department of Labor. *Selected characteristics of occupations defined in the Dictionary of Occupational Titles*. Washington, DC: US Government Printing Office, 1981.

17 Cotes JE, Zejda J, King B. Lung function impairment as a guide to exercise limitation in work-related lung disorders. *Am Rev Respir Dis* 1988;**137**: 1089–1093.

18 Harber P. Respiratory disability: the uncoupling of oxygen consumption and disability. *Clin Chest Med* 1992;**13**: 367–376.

19 COPD Guidelines Group of the Standards Care Committee of the British Thoracic Society. BTS guidelines for the management of chronic obstructive pulmonary disease. *Thorax* 1997;**52**, suppl 5.

20 Health and Safety Executive. *Approved Code of Practice: The Control of Asbestos at Work Regulations 1987*, pp. 21–22. London: HMSO, 1988.

21 Wagner GR. *Screening and surveillance of workers exposed to mineral dusts.* Geneva: World Health Organization, 1996.
22 Health and Safety Executive. *Crystalline Silica*, p. 4. London: HMSO, 1992.
23 *Guidelines for the use of ILO international classification of radiographs of pneumoconioses.* Geneva: International Labour Office, 1980.
24 Research Committee of the British Thoracic Association. A study of a standardised contact procedure in tuberculosis. *Tubercle* 1978;**59**: 245–259.
25 Joint Tuberculosis Committee of the British Thoracic Society. Control and prevention of tuberculosis in the United Kingdom: Code of Practice 1994. *Thorax* 1994;**49**: 1193–1200.
26 *Diving Operations at Work Regulations.* London: HMSO, 1981.
27 Respiratory conditions. In: *Medical aspects of fitness for firefighting.* Association of Local authority Medical Advisers, 1983.

20

Renal and urological disease

R. Gokal and J. Hobson

The kidney has the vital function of excretion, and controls acid–base, fluid, and electrolyte balance. It also acts as an endocrine organ. Renal failure, with severe impairment of these functions, results from a number of different processes, most of which are acquired although some may be inherited. Glomerulonephritis, which presents with proteinuria, haematuria, or both, may be accompanied by hypertension and impaired renal function. Renal scarring is the end result of pyelonephritis. Additionally, systemic diseases such as diabetes, hypertension, and collagen disorders can affect the kidney. Polycystic kidney disease is the commonest inherited disorder leading to renal failure. Chronic renal failure implies permanent renal damage which is likely to be progressive and will eventually require renal replacement therapy.

Advances in the treatment of end-stage renal failure using haemo- and peritoneal dialysis, and the success of kidney transplantation, have improved the quality of life for patients and mean that many can expect to return to normal lives including work. Better management of urinary infections and calculi, prostatic obstruction, incontinence, and other complications of urinary tract disease enable the attending physician or surgeon to predict less time lost from work and less incapability.

The impact of renal and urinary tract disorders on work attendance and performance has been scantily reported in the literature, but national data indicate that disease of the genitourinary tract accounts for less than 2% of absence. Women have twice as many episodes of absence as men but account for only a quarter of total lost time. There are, however, few overall contra-indications to undertaking gainful employment for those with renal or urological disorders, and many opportunities for encouraging both an early return to work and continuing in the same job.

Reintegration of patients into the workforce following transplantation or dialysis offers an exciting and rewarding challenge to the wider health team.

Prevalence and morbidity

In general, major renal disease or malignancy is infrequent in those of working age and in the day to day work of occupational physicians or general practitioners. Currently, in the UK, between 80 and 100 new patients are accepted for **renal replacement therapy** per million of population each year (England: 8 – per million, Wales: 109 – per million).[1] The number of patients on therapy in the UK (1995) was 500 per million of the population, in contrast to over 600 per million in other European countries.[2]

In terms of claims for incapacity benefit, diseases of the genitourinary tract (ICD10 N00–N99) make up a small proportion of the total nationally. In 1995 and 1996 approximately 0.6% of claims were for diseases of the genitourinary tract in men (9000 claimants) and 1.3% in women (10 000 claimants).[3] Between 1985 and 1990 for each sex, certified incapacity due to sickness from genitourinary causes averaged about 3 million days annually where all causes of incapacity accounted for 290 million days in men and 100 million days in women.[4] In men, most time was lost in those aged 60–64 (800 000 days), whereas in women most days were lost in those aged 30–39 (900 000 days).

Although many **urinary tract infections** are symptomless, there is much morbidity from this condition. The size of the problem is difficult to ascertain. Up to 50% of women have symptoms at some stage in their lives. Occurrence is much less frequent in men but rises sharply after the age of 60 owing to lower urinary tract conditions, especially prostatic problems. It has been estimated that 12–60 per 1000 consultations in general practice are for symptoms suggestive of urinary tract infection[5] and an estimated 45 days per 100 people each year are lost from work from this cause.

Urolithiasis of the upper urinary tract is a fairly common condition in the UK, with a prevalence of 3.5–4%, but the incidence appears to be on the increase. The peak incidence in men occurs at the age of 35 years. Renal stones cause much morbidity, but with the widespread availability of lithotripsy, extensive renal surgery can be avoided in most cases and as a consequence time off work is considerably reduced.

Papilloma of the bladder is the only occupational cancer to reach double figures for annual disability benefit awards in England and Wales, apart from asbestos-related lung cancer.[6] In the 6 years between 1989 and 1995, 122 new cases were assessed for disablement as Prescribed Disease C23 (papilloma of the bladder). In 1994/5, 15 out of 19 cases received benefit for this condition. Under the Reporting of Injuries, Diseases and Dangerous Occurrences Regulations (RIDDOR) 1995, however, only 19 cases of papilloma of the bladder were reported in the ten years to 1996.

Benign prostatic hyperplasia (BPH), is the commonest prostatic problem after the fourth decade; 50% of men have BPH by the time they reach 51–60 years of age. Some 25% of 55 year olds notice some decrease in force of their urinary stream, and 29% of men who survive from the age of 40–80 will require prostatectomy.

Mortality

In 1995 there were 1563 male and 1720 female deaths (all ages) from glomerulonephritis, nephrotic syndrome, and chronic renal failure.[7] Even though 90% occurred over retirement age, much of the associated morbidity would have been incurred during the working years. These totals represent about half (46%) of all deaths from diseases of the genitourinary system.

In England and Wales during 1995, bladder cancer killed twice as many men (3261) as women (1548) in all age groups. Most of the deaths were in those over the age of 55 years. As a cause of death it was the fifth most common tumour for men (4% of male cancer deaths) and the eleventh for women (2% of female cancer deaths). However, only a minority of the male (14%) and female deaths (5%) occurred in the population of working age. Carcinoma of the body of the kidney caused fewer deaths—1554 men and 982 women during 1995.

During the 1980s there was a slight but steady increase in the number of registrations and deaths from bladder cancer. The rise was more marked in men than women and for incidence more than mortality. Undoubtedly improved final prognosis and extended survival times accounted for the discrepancy, but a change in nomenclature which previously excluded papilloma has also contributed. New cancer registrations in 1992 (latest figures available) were 8536 for men and 3476 for women in England and Wales. The relative 5-year survival rate rose from 38.7% in 1963 to 63.4% in 1984, and the ratio of new registrations to deaths in a given year is now more than two.

Complications and sequelae

The complications and sequelae of renal disease include hypertension, haematuria, and proteinuria. The discovery of asymptomatic haematuria, whether macroscopic or microscopic, and not related to urinary tract infections, requires further investigation. Initially microscopy and culture should be undertaken. If this is negative then nephro-urological investigations are necessary to identify any underlying pathology before making decisions about treatment and employment.

In one study, microscopic haematuria was detected by the strip technique in 3.5% of 2100 men over the age of 40 systematically examined at their place of work. Thirty-two agreed to undergo further investigations of whom a quarter were found to have urinary tract disease including two with kidney stones, two with prostatic adenoma, one with a vesical diverticulum, and two with bladder tumours. It was necessary to perform intravenous urography and cystoscopy to detect all these abnormalities. The conclusion was that even a single episode of microscopic haematuria in a man over 40 should be investigated with intravenous urography. If the results are normal and the subject is a smoker or has an occupational or familial risk of cancer, cytology and vesical echography should be performed and then cystoscopy if these are negative.[8] A nephrological referral is indicated if these investigations are negative or if there is associated proteinuria, hypertension or renal impairment.

Proteinuria needs to be quantified; if it is more than 0.3 g/24 hours, referral for further nephrological investigation is required.

Hypertension

Hypertension is a common sequel of renal parenchymatous disease, but is itself a cause of chronic renal failure in up to 20% of cases and this proportion has been increasing. Antihypertensive therapy, together with salt and water restriction, is usually necessary. The condition can sometimes be difficult to control and the drugs used may themselves cause side-effects, which may affect fitness for work in certain jobs. This is discussed more fully in Chapters 18 and 26.

End-stage renal failure

End-stage renal failure is reached when the glomerular filtration rate is irreversibly reduced to less than 5 ml/minute. Without renal replacement, death is inevitable. The main causes of renal failure are glomerulonephritis (25%), diabetes mellitus (25%),

Table 20.1   HD and CAPD and types of employment

Unsuitable (contra-indications)
Armed forces (active service)
Chemical exposure to renal toxins
Construction/building/scaffolding
Diving
Fire service
Furnace/smelting
Heavy labouring or heavy manual work
Mining
Police (on the beat)
Work in very hot environments

Possible (relative contra-indications)[a]
Catering trades[b]
Driving
Farm labouring[b]
Horticultural work
Motor repair (care with fistula in HD patients)
Nursing[b]
Painting and decorating[b]
Printing[b]
Refuse collection[b]
Shiftwork
Welding[b]

Suitable (no contra-indications)
Accountancy
Clerical/secretarial
Law
Light assembly
Light maintenance/ repair
Light manufacturing industry
Medicine
Middle and senior management
Packing
Receptionist
Retail trade
Sales
Supervising
Teaching

---

[a] Occupations in this category which entail much heavy lifting or manual work may be unsuitable.
[b] Not contra-indicated in HD.

hypertension and vascular disease (20%), polycystic kidney disease (10%), and pyelonephritis (10%). Renal replacement therapy can be achieved in one of three ways:

- **haemodialysis** performed at home, in hospital, or in specialized minimal care units
- **peritoneal dialysis,** the commonest form of which is continuous ambulatory peritoneal dialysis (CAPD), done at home or at work as a self-dialysis technique; an increasingly used modality within this category is automated peritoneal dialysis (APD) where a machine is used to cycle dialysis fluid at night with little or no dialysis during the day—an obvious advantage for working people
- **renal transplantation** (cadaveric, or from a living relative).

Renal dialysis

Dialysis improves many of the signs and symptoms of uraemia by removing solutes, water, and toxins which accumulate as a consequence of inadequate kidney function. Both peritoneal dialysis (PD) and haemodialysis (HD) are effective, each relying on a semipermeable membrane which separates blood from a dialysis solution (the dialysate). Removal of fluid (ultrafiltration) is achieved by osmosis in PD (glucose is the osmotic agent), or by applying transmembrane pressure in HD.

Impaired renal function leads to a progressive anaemia with haemoglobin values around 8–10 g/dl. Consequently, patients may be chronically tired and more quickly fatigued, which can impair work performance and make heavy manual and other physically demanding work unsuitable (see Table 20.1). However, the availability of recombinant human erythropoietin has made symptoms of anaemia a thing of the past, with substantial improvement in well-being and employment prospects.[9] In spite of regular dialysis, the biochemistry at no time returns to normal; at best, dialysis therapy imparts a renal function equivalent to a glomerular filtration rate of 5–7 ml/min. Dietary modifications of protein, fat, carbohydrate, sodium, potassium, phosphate, and vitamin intake, and restriction of fluid intake are therefore necessary. With control of dietary and fluid intake and adequate dialysis it is unusual to experience uraemic symptoms such as nausea, vomiting, itching, cramps and diarrhoea.

Several complications other than anaemia can affect dialysis patients. Vascular disease is a common problem, with angina, hypertension, peripheral vascular complications, and cardiovascular accidents. In a minority, disordered metabolism of vitamin D, parathyroid hormone, calcium, and phosphate can lead to osteodystrophy, which can present with bone pain, proximal myopathy, and, rarely, pathological fractures. These setbacks are more marked in the elderly and in those with other systemic disease such as diabetes mellitus.

Patients undergoing dialysis live a stressful life. Although most patients adjust to their dialysis regimes, some may have psychological problems related to dialysis itself. Other problems such as loss of libido and impotence may be superimposed. Such patients may thus be intolerant of small difficulties in their work situation.

A study of 100 haemodialysis patients found depression to be present in more than half at some stage and that psychiatric complications were worse in the 3-month period before, and the 12-month period following the start of HD. Absence from full-time work was found to predict psychiatric morbidity.[10]

Haemodialysis

Patients must undergo dialysis three times a week for 4–8 hours on each occasion. For those working full-time, home dialysis is done in the evenings and at weekends, while those dialysing in hospital during the day may only be able to manage part-time employment on non-dialysis days. It is not unusual for a haemodialysis patient to feel 'washed out' after a session of dialysis. This is related to the rapid removal of fluid and uraemic toxins (disequilibration). Although this usually passes off completely by the next day, it may linger and affect the patient's performance at work. Machine failure at home may also mean a return to hospital dialysis, requiring more time off work. After starting haemodialysis, patients may be unable to work for some 3–4 months while undergoing training for home therapy.

Continuous ambulatory peritoneal dialysis

CAPD entails 3–4 daily exchanges of about 2 litres of fluid drained in and out of the peritoneal cavity, each taking about 30 minutes to perform and being spaced out over the day. This usually means that at least one exchange must be done at work; this can often be conveniently fitted into the lunch break, but needs to be performed in a suitably clean and private area. APD is a modification of the routine, in which all the exchanges of fluid are done at night using a cycler machine, thus obviating the need for daytime exchanges. The apparatus is expensive, but can help those (e.g. salesmen and representatives) in occupations that involve much daytime travel. CAPD is flexible enough to allow an individual to do most types of work and is unlikely to cause problems in employment. The training period required for peritoneal dialysis is usually about 2 weeks, so work can resume quite soon.

Hospital admission

The main reasons for hospital admission in patients on peritoneal dialysis are peritonitis or catheter-related problems; for haemodialysis patients problems of vascular access predominate. Hospital admission is much commoner in patients with systemic disorders such as diabetes and cerebro- or cardiovascular disease. Patients receiving dialysis need frequent out-patient visits at first, but eventually stabilize to fewer visits (every 2–3 months). Although few figures are published, the hospitalization rate for dialysis patients is about 10–15 days per patient-year of treatment.[11] This would be the minimum time off work, as the figures do not include out-patient visits.

Table 20.2 Median survival time by age and diabetic status in patients on dialysis

Age	Non-diabetic	Diabetic
<55	14.2 years	7.4 years
55–65	7.4 years	3.5 years
>65	3.5 years	3.5 years

Table 20.3 Frequency of successful vocational rehabilitation in patients with end-stage renal failure undergoing dialysis or transplantation[14]

	Male	Female
Transplant	70%	33%
CAPD	35%	15%
Hospital haemodialysis	19%	11%

Survival in dialysis patients

In Europe, patients maintained on HD or CAPD have a similar survival of approximately 60% at 5 years and 30% at 10 years, measured from the start of dialysis. Survival, however, is related to age, disease, comorbidity and therapy. It is higher in younger age groups but lower in diabetics (Table 20.2).[12]

Both types of dialysis increase the chance of longevity and decrease the likelihood of serious morbidity; HD has now kept some patients alive for more than 20 years. Although the final goal is a successful renal transplant, which offers the opportunity of a full and normal working life, dialysis treatment itself is fully compatible with many types of employment.

Transplantation

In successfully transplanted patients renal function returns to normal, as does the haemoglobin level. These patients can thus lead a normal life to all intents and purposes, but need daily immunosuppressive therapy (prednisolone, azathioprine, cyclosporin A, tacrolimus, mycophenolate mofetil). Because of this, the transplant patient is more prone to common infections. Patients on prolonged immunosuppressive therapy have a slightly increased risk of developing malignancy (skin malignancies, non-Hodgkin's lymphoma, and possibly bladder cancer), cardiovascular disease, cataracts, and avascular necrosis of the hip.

After a transplant frequent out-patient visits are needed for the first 3–4 months to monitor renal function and to treat rejection episodes, which are more likely in that period. Most employers will understand this, and will be sympathetic and willing to accommodate the delay if the reasons are explained.

The 5-year survival of cadaveric transplant patients is 80%, but it is better in those who have received a transplant from a living relative. Kidney survival from cadaveric transplantation is about 65% at 5 years and 50% at 10 years after surgery.[2] Premature atherosclerosis, hypertension, and vascular disease are causes of excess morbidity and mortality.

Those with a successful transplant can lead a normal life at home and at work. The work situation should, however, carry no undue risk of blows or trauma to the lower abdomen, because the transplant site must be protected. The arteriovenous fistula at the wrist can be injured by sharp projections or tools, and cutting instruments need to be handled carefully using suitable protective clothing.

Renal failure and employment

The work record of those who have received a successful transplant is good. A transplant cannot now be accepted as a valid reason for denying employment, or of restricting work content, since transplant patients are capable of virtually any normal work. A useful simple guide for employers, patients, and their doctors has been published.[13]

In the US marked differences have also been found in successful vocational rehabilitation in end stage renal therapy patients,[14] with transplant patients faring better (Table 20.3). Thus the main problems surround those on dialysis. The special needs of these patients and their capabilities are less well understood and, thus far, little studied. A recent joint study from the Manchester and Oxford renal units[15] found that there was a sharp decline in the proportion of those working some 6–12 months after the start of CAPD (44% from 73%), or of HD (42% from 83%) compared to those in employment before therapy commenced. The figures seem to confirm the better employment prospects in successfully transplanted patients.[16] Predialysis intervention has been shown to be of benefit in assisting workers with end-stage renal failure; in a study from California, those who had social worker assessment, patient education and counselling, and renal unit orientation to the dialysis were almost three times more likely to continue work after starting HD.[17]

More recent data from the US Renal Data System (USRDS 1997) showed that 17.9% of dialysis patients under the age of 60 were in full-time employment, 5.1% in part-time employment, 3.5% looking for work, 8.3% retired, 47.2% disabled, and 9.5% keeping house.[18] Similar data from the UK are available in a study from Edinburgh where 113 patients on dialysis were assessed; 35% of patients considered themselves too ill for work and the bulk of them were of an age where this would be viewed as unusual.[19]

These statistics do not take into account the effect of patient selection, which favours fitter patients receiving a transplant, and higher risk patients receiving PD or hospital HD.

Other factors that impact on employment have been outlined in several studies. In a review from the US of post-transplant employment, 58% were working but 72% were considered capable of working—the difference was related to health insurance and disability allowances.[20] Another concern was raised by Friedman and Rogers who interviewed dialysis patients and employers about potential problems in the workplace; many employers expressed concerns about financial issues, reduced productivity and a high rate of absenteeism.[21] It appears that there are both variables and barriers (including education and the type of occupation) other than medical ones that impact on employment and vocational rehabilitation.[22]

Fitness for work and renal failure

For the younger patient with good family and hospital support, and without other serious medical problems, dialysis now offers the chance of increased longevity and a much better prospect of employment. With flexibility, adaptation, careful planning and support many more dialysis patients can work successfully. The aim should be to adapt both ways; the work to the patient's needs and the patient's treatment regime to the work, whichever direction best achieves a satisfactory outcome. Many employers, although sympathetic, underestimate what patients with chronic renal failure can achieve, and this in itself may preclude successful employment. There is thus a real need firstly to educate both doctors and employers about the work capabilities of such people, and secondly to encourage a positive attitude in the patients themselves. The close co-operation of all concerned (the patient, the renal unit, the general practitioner, occupational health staff, and the employer) is often needed to effect a successful placement. The occupational physician is usually best placed to catalyse the necessary adjustments and this is discussed further on p. 408.

The essential and relative employment contra-indications for dialysis patients are shown in Table 20.3.

Patients in irreversible renal failure are unsuited for work as firefighters, police on the beat, rescue personnel, or armed forces on active service, because of the high energy demands, extended hours, and the flexibility required for emergency duty imposed by these jobs. Similar restrictions may apply to particularly stressful jobs demanding a very high degree of vigilance (e.g. air traffic controllers). Jobs combining both a high radiant heat burden and high physical activity may also be contra-indicated. Patients in end-stage renal failure on dialysis are not fit to work underground, to dive, or to undertake other work in hyperbaric conditions such as tunnelling under pressure. They are also unlikely to meet the standards required for merchant shipping which may require lengthy periods at sea and in tropical and subtropical climates. Additionally, most seafarers nowadays will need to join and leave ships by air travel. Although air travel is not contra-indicated for those undertaking CAPD regimes, it imposes extra difficulties and the added inconvenience of carrying supplies of the dialysate solution. Also, in the context of travel abroad, the reduced dosage required for drug prophylaxis against malaria for those in renal failure should be recognized.

Drivers with chronic renal failure including CAPD and haemodialysis are subject to individual assessment by the DVLA for group 2 entitlement (large goods vehicles and passenger-carrying vehicles) and for group 1 entitlement (motor cars and motor cycles) the issue of a licence is dependent on medical enquiries.[23] Because of prolonged absences from home, fatigue, and the many hours spent at the driving wheel, LGV driving may be precluded in any case. The physical demands of loading and unloading wagons and constantly climbing in and out of cabs may also preclude similar work in transportation such as removals, warehouse storage, or dockyard labouring. Following renal transplant, drivers may hold group 1 and 2 licences subject to satisfactory medical enquiries.

The demands and restrictions on work are substantially similar for PD and HD, and depend on the dialysis schedules and the clinical state of the individual. CAPD requires the capacity to perform an exchange during the work day, which is not necessary for HD or APD. CAPD, because of the constant presence of fluid in the peritoneal cavity, is not appropriate for patients in jobs that may lead to increased intra-abdominal pressure (frequent bending or lifting). Tight or restrictive clothing should not be worn. Patients also need a clean area for performing their midday fluid exchange, as it is essential to prevent infection. The renal unit specialist nurse, in conjunction with the occupational health staff, should assess the suitability, both of the type of work and of the area for the exchange at the workplace.

HD patients can undertake full employment especially if they are dialysing at night or evenings but they need to be within easy reach of a dialysis facility, so work involving much distant travel and frequent periods away from home may not be suitable. If there are canteen facilities, it can be helpful to ensure that the necessary low-salt and high/low-protein foodstuffs are readily available.

There are no specific occupations that are contra-indicated in immunosuppressed transplant patients; however, in markedly dusty and potentially 'infected' environments (e.g. demolition jobs), there is a risk and caution is advised. Usually there are no restrictions to employment for people with only one kidney that functions well.

Renal disease and the DDA

The main renal condition which will cause disability within the definition of the DDA is chronic renal failure because of the extreme fatigue which it causes, and the disruption to daily activities, with or without renal dialysis. The types of work where application of the Act must be considered, and where appropriate adjustments may be required, are listed in Table 20.3. Even if a person has had a successful renal transplant and is to all intents and purposes normal, they are still protected by Schedule 1 para 6(1) which states, in effect, that even though a disability has been alleviated it is to be treated as having the effect it would have had if it had not been treated.

The types of adjustment that employers must consider making relate to physical work capacity, shiftwork, provision of suitable breaks, and facilities for dialysis. They may also need to make allowance for chronic fatigue and increased sickness absence. Employees receiving dialysis would need adjustment according to their work capacity, particularly, but not exclusively, if carrying out physical work, which should be alleviated by the maximum use of mechanical aids. This might also entail rotation of duties, reduced or part-time working, or job sharing. Shiftworkers requiring haemodialysis would need provision for their dialysis routines and may need to avoid night shifts. For those carrying out peritoneal dialysis the employer would need to look at providing suitable breaks if necessary during the working day and the provision of suitable clean areas for it to take place. Assessment of the facility would have to be carried out by a member of the renal team if there is no occupational health department. Finally, patients receiving dialysis will have higher absence levels for regular out-patient attendance and employers would be expected to make reasonable allowance for this.

Holidays

Most patients on PD can take a holiday without restrictions, but HD patients either need to make special arrangements for a dialysis facility at the holiday centre, or to arrange for the use of portable machines. Such provisions need to be planned well beforehand.

Shiftwork

Shiftworking is not generally contra-indicated for patients with renal or urinary tract disorders. Neither is shiftwork an absolute contra-indication to employment for PD patients, because their treatment can often be rescheduled to fit in with a regular shift rota. For patients on HD, shiftwork and extended hours may present problems requiring greater adaptation. Some patients have learnt to dialyse while asleep, using the built-in warning devices on the machine. Rapidly rotating shift systems can be more difficult to accommodate because of their constantly changing patterns, especially for patients on haemodialysis.

Drivers

Patients on peritoneal dialysis could seek an exemption under the Motor Vehicle (Wearing of Seat Belt) Regulations 1982, SI: 1982 Regulation 5, or under the Motor Vehicles (Wearing of Seat Belts in Rear Seats by Adults) Regulations 1991, SI: 1991 No 1255, by obtaining a valid medical certificate from a registered medical practitioner. However, the hazards of not wearing a seat belt must be weighed against any relatively minor inconvenience and restrictions. Adaptations to seat belt mountings can often solve any problems.

Urinary tract infections

Symptoms that relate to urinary infection are very common, but of serious importance only when there is an underlying anatomical abnormality. A small percentage of women suffer from repeated infections and remain symptomatic in spite of antibiotic therapy. Anatomical abnormalities (such as ureterovesical reflux, or obstruction) are associated with repeated infection, which can eventually lead to chronic renal failure later in life. Tuberculous infection of the urinary tract is now being seen again, but employment can continue because therapy is usually administered in the out-patient setting.

Urinary incontinence and retention

Better incontinence devices, more thorough investigation and improved therapy with anticholinergic drugs have greatly assisted sufferers to stay at work, although incontinence remains an unrecognized problem at work. The specialist continence nurse adviser can help to improve work attendance by giving advice, reassurance, practical help, and support. The value of intermittent self-catheterization for helping patients with poor bladder emptying, urinary retention and incontinence, or even voiding difficulties, often associated with a neuropathic or hypotonic bladder, is underestimated.[24] The technique is still much underused but, as awareness grows, it will be more frequently applied at the place of work. Those who learn the technique can become dry, gain more social acceptance, and, by establishing effective drainage, protect their kidneys from the effects of back pressure and urinary infection.

Urinary diversion procedures for incontinence are becoming more acceptable; the most acceptable one is the Mitrofanoff operation. The patient's bladder is left intact although the bladder neck may be closed off in some, but not all, situations. The right ureter is divided at its midpoint and joined to the left ureter, and the lower disconnected right ureter is brought out as a stoma in the right groin, above the inguinal ligament. Through this the patient can self-catheterize with a Lofric catheter. This is a form of continent diversion which is really quite acceptable for those who are unable to empty their bladder and get fed up with intermittent self-catheterization, or alternatively, those who are totally incontinent and whose bladder necks are closed off surgically.

Although disabled male patients in wheelchairs learn to catheterize themselves, and so improve their morale, quality of life, and ability to attend at their place of work, it is very difficult, perhaps impossible, for female disabled patients to self-catheterize. Clean and private provisions at the workplace will enable the technique to be properly and hygienically undertaken.

Those with incontinence, repeated urinary infections, ileal conduits, or catheterization need good toilet facilities and nearby access. Ileostomy bags may be compressed by low benches, or desks, or the sides of bins or boxes. Excess bending, crouching, or poor seating may inhibit the free flow of urine in the bag, or damage it, causing leakage. Mining, tunnelling, quarrying, or foundry work is contra-indicated for these patients, including those using intermittent self-catheterization, because a clean and private place is required to effect catheter changes and bag emptying. Many other jobs, however, can accommodate this requirement.

Urinary tract calculi

The main component of idiopathic renal calculi is calcium oxalate. The underlying causative factors are socio-economic (associated with affluence) and regional (associated with water hardness), but occupational factors such as a high ambient temperature, chronic dehydration, and physical inactivity because of sedentary work may also be implicated.

Urinary stone formation has been found to be increased in male marathon runners, lifeguards in Israel, hot-metal workers, and some British navy personnel. An Italian study of machinists at a glass plant found a prevalence of renal stones of 8.5% in those exposed to heat stress against 2.4% in controls working in normal temperatures.[25] In those exposed to heat stress, 39% of stones were uric acid and such workers were found to have significantly raised serum uric acid concentrations.

Those with a strong history of stone formation should be encouraged to increase their fluid intake liberally if they want to accept overseas postings in tropical climates and to maintain a high intake during their stay, especially when undertaking strenuous outdoor work. Fitness for furnace or other very hot work must be carefully assessed because of the relative dehydration and increased tendency for stone recurrence, but this should be easily preventable with increased fluid intake.[26] Patients need to be warned about becoming dehydrated on long-haul flights (>4 hours). Similarly, airline pilots should drink 600 ml/hour while they are in the cockpit.

The newer treatments of percutaneous nephrolithotomy, and especially extracorporeal shock-wave lithotripsy for urinary tract stones, now offer the prospect of dramatically improving on the historic picture of long periods off work and poor attendance. This is entirely an out-patient procedure, with minimal postoperative discomfort, and generally a resumption of normal activity is possible within a day or so.[27]

Tumours of the renal tract

Adenocarcinoma of the kidney is the commonest adult renal tumour. In the bladder more than 95% of tumours are urothelial in origin. Only about 4–5% are occupational in origin from former association with the chemical, dyestuffs, rubber, cable, and other industries, or from occupations where exposure to carcinogenic aromatic amines or polycyclic aromatic hydrocarbons has occurred.

In renal tract cancer the relative 5-year survival rate is now over two-thirds. Employees in certain industries with historic exposure to known bladder carcinogens, may be advised to provide regular samples for urine cytology. This is usually every 6 months and can be carried out by post if employees leave or retire. Routine urine cytology is also suggested for those exposed to 4,4-methylene bis(2)-chloro-aniline (MbOCA). In those who have had tumours an early warning of cytological change can herald recurrence and thus allow early treatment. Local treatment using bladder instillation therapy has proved helpful in some cases.

Advisory services

The staff of renal units, general practitioners, occupational health services, the Employment Services' Disability Employment Advisers, and the Employment Medical Advisory Service should collectively be able to provide advice on most aspects of employment and renal disease. The approach is usually spearheaded by members of the renal unit team: physician, specialist nurse, social worker, home dialysis administrator, and transplant co-ordinator. An occupational health physician or nurse is uniquely qualified to assess the suitability of a patient with renal or urinary tract disease for a particular job, as well as the ways and means to adapt it. The advice, guidance, and contacts of the social worker attached to renal units will be indispensable. Several associations offer useful advice and support, and their addresses and phone numbers are given in Appendix 7.

Social security provisions

There are particular social security provisions for patients undergoing haemodialysis or plasmapheresis to work through their illness (Regulations 3(3) and 15 of the Unemployment, Sickness and Invalidity Benefit Regulations 1983). Patients not capable of holding down a full-time job may do limited work, up to a maximum of 16 hours per week, with a doctor's encouragement. This is known as Therapeutic Earnings, for which a doctor's supporting letter and agreement from the Department of Social Security are required before entering the scheme. If incapacity benefit is also being claimed, there is an earnings limit—currently £58.00 in any week (1998).

Patients who can work more than 16 hours a week, but whose medical condition puts them at a disadvantage in getting a job may be able to get Disability Working Allowance (introduced in April 1992) to supplement their earnings. This provision is 'means tested' so advice is needed before making a claim, which, however, will not normally require any additional medical support on the first claim. Those on regular haemodialysis or plasma-pheresis which prevents them from working for 2 or more days in any 6 consecutive days (excluding Sundays) are allowed to claim Incapacity Benefit for those days.

Existing legislation: seafarers

Restrictions on the employment of people suffering from diseases of the genitourinary tract are imposed by the Merchant Shipping (Medical Examination Regulations) 1983, SI: 1983 808, which require a statutory examination for fitness to work (see Appendix 3). The Amendment Regulations 1990, SI: 1985 enable an approved medical practitioner to suspend or cancel a medical fitness certificate under certain circumstances—i.e. when the seafarer was not able to meet the appropriate standard, or if the certificate was incorrect. The medical standards for service in the tropics, or other conditions of high ambient temperature, would not be met by those with recurrent urinary tract infections, stone formation, urinary obstruction, renal transplant or intractable incontinence.

Conclusions and recommendations

Because of the great advances in dialysis and renal transplantation, most people with renal failure can now achieve significant rehabilitation, and often a degree of independence and quality of life sufficient to allow useful, gainful, and active employment.

Employers must be actively encouraged to accommodate those with renal tract disease who are generally fit for work, but who may otherwise experience minor inconveniences (like catheterization) or more frequent short absences from work. However, prejudice still abounds, and occasionally difficulty in arranging associated life insurance cover or joining pension schemes is cited as the reason for not employing someone in end-stage renal failure. It should be made clear to employers that none of the causes of renal failure are contagious, and so there is no risk to other workers. Thus, apart from the renal condition itself, those with renal failure should be regarded in the same way as anybody else. A successful transplant restores the recipient to full health with the same capability as their contemporaries.

There are now few absolute contra-indications to the successful employment of those with renal or urological disorders but the difference in employment rates between those with a transplant and those on dialysis suggests that problems in employment still exist for sufferers with renal disease.

Selected references

1	Roderick PJ, Ferris G, Feest TG. The provision of renal replacement therapy for adults in England and Wales: recent trends and future directions. *Q Journ Med* 1998;**91**: 581–587.
2	Valderabano F, Berthoux FC, Jones EPH, Mehls O. Report on management of renal failure in Europe, XXV, 1994: end-stage renal disease and dialysis report. *Nephrol Dial Transplant* 1996;**11**(suppl 1): 2–21.

3 Department of Social Security. *Social Security statistics 1997*, pp 171–172. London: Stationery Office, 1998.

4 Department of Social Security. *Social Security statistics 1991*, Tables D1. 11–16, pp 153–170. London: HMSO, 1992.

5 Cattell WR. Lower and upper urinary tract infections in the adult. In Cameron J.S *et al. Oxford textbook of clinical nephrology* Vol. 3, pp. 1676–1699. Oxford: Oxford University Press, 1992.

6 Health and Safety Commission/Government Statistical Service. *Health and Safety statistics 1995/96*, Tables 2.1, 2.2, 2.8. London: HMSO.

7 Office for National Statistics. *Mortality statistics for England and Wales: Cause, 1995*. Series DH2 No.22. London: Stationery Office.

8 Vallancien G, Cadranel J, Jardin A. Que faire en présence d'une hematurie microscopique isoleé chez l'homme en milieu de travail? [What should be done in the presence of isolated microscopic hematuria in man in the work environment?] *Presse Med* 1985;**14**(23): 1279–1281.

9 Canadian Erythropoietin Study Group. Association between recombinant human erythropoietin and quality of life and exercise capacity of patients receiving haemodialysis. *BMJ* 1990;**300**: 573–578.

10 Kaneko S, Sato T, Hirayama N *et al.* Psychiatric complications with chronic hemodialysis–importance of psychological and social care. *Jpn J Psychiatry Neurol* 1986 **40**(4): 559–570.

11 Gokal R, Jakubowski C, King J *et al.* Outcome in patients on continuous ambulatory peritoneal dialysis and haemodialysis: 4 year analysis of a prospective study. *Lancet* 1987;**ii**: 1105–1109.

12 Royal College of Physician of London and the Renal Association. *Treatment of adult patients with renal failure—recommended standards and audit measures*. London: Royal College of Physicians, 1997.

13 *MIMS: Pocket guide to chronic renal failure*. London: Haymarket Medical Publications, 1996.

14 Simmonds RG, Anderson CR, Abress LK. Quality of life and rehabilitation differences among four ESRD therapy groups. *Scand J Urol Nephrol (suppl)* 1990;**131**: 7–22.

15 Auer J, Gokal R, Stout JP *et al.* The Oxford–Manchester study of dialysis patients. *Scand J Urol Nephrol* 1990;**131** (suppl): 31–37.

16 Gokal R. Quality of life in patients undergoing renal replacement therapy. *Kidney Int* 1993;**38**(suppl 40): S23–S27.

17 Rasgon S, Schwankovsky L, James-Rogers A, Widrow L, Glick J, Butts E. An intervention for maintenance among blue-collar workers with end-stage renal disease. *Am J Kidney Dis* 1993;**22**: 403–412.

18 US Renal Data System. *Annual data report*. Bethesda, MD. National Institutes of Health, National Institute of Diabetes and Digestive and Kidney Diseases, 1997.

19 Final Report grant K/OPR/2/2/D86 to the Health Services and Public Health Research Committee of the Chief Scientist's Office, Scottish Home and Health Department.

20 Raiz L. The transplant trap: The impact of health policy on employment status following renal transplantation. *J Nephrol Social Work* 1997;**17**: 79–94.

21 Friedman N, Rogers TF. Dialysis and the world of work. *Contemp Dial Nephrol* 1988;**19**: 16–19.

22 King K Vocational rehabilitation in maintenance dialysis patients. *Adv Ren Replace Ther* 1994;**1**: 228–239.

23 *At a glance guide to the current standards of fitness to drive*. Swansea: DVLA Drivers Medical Unit, March 1998.

24 Intermittent self-catheterisation. *Drug Ther Bull* 1991;**29**(10): 37–39.

25 Borghi L, Meschi T, Amato F, Novarini A, Romanelli A, Cigala F. Hot occupation and nephrolithiasis. *J Urol* 1993;**150**(6): 1757–1760.

26 Pin NT, Ling NY, Siang LH. Dehydration from outdoor work and urinary stones in a tropical environment. *Occup Med* 1992;**42:** 30–32.

27 Wickham JEA. Minimally invasive surgery. Treatment of urinary tract stones. *BMJ* 1993;**307**: 1414–1417.

21

Obstetrics and gynaecology

L. H. Kapadia and P. Owen

In 1996 in the UK there were 11 million employed women, almost equal to the number of employed men. Half of these were part-time workers in clerical, sales, secretarial, and personnel positions. Women, whether working or not, still bear the greatest share of housework and childcare. Equal opportunities legislation in socially developed countries now allows women to enter almost any occupation and ensures job retention during and after pregnancy. Women in some countries, mainly developing ones, are the mainstay of the agricultural and engineering working populations and perform physically strenuous tasks traditionally performed by men elsewhere.

On average in the UK, women live longer than men (84 years as compared with 79 years), take a more active interest in their health, consult their general practitioners more often, take more time off work, and are more frequently admitted to hospital, although the reasons for these patterns of illness behaviour are not clear.

Obstetrics

Legislation

The Management of Health and Safety at Work Regulations 1992 (SI No. 2051) were amended with effect from 1 December 1994 to implement the European Directive on Pregnant Workers (SI No. 2865), Council Directive 92/85/EEC. The changes put a duty of care on employers to provide a safe system of work to all women of reproductive age, their unborn children, and all working mothers who are breast-feeding. It also introduces protection against loss of income, establishing a woman's right to return to her employment and to have time spent in antenatal care remunerated.

The statutory minimum maternity leave is currently 14 weeks (regardless of length of service and how much money is paid out), 6 weeks of which is paid at 90% of full-time salary.

Statutory Maternity Pay is given for 18 weeks which must be continuous, starting at the earliest 11 weeks before the expected week of confinement (EWC) and at the latest, in the week after the baby's birth. The woman is protected against dismissal for ill health during this time and has full contractual rights with regard to holiday, pensions, etc. Some employers improve on this for long-serving workers and create incentives for early return to work. If a redundancy situation arises the woman is entitled to be offered a suitable alternative where available.

The 1998 Employment Relations Bill (Bill 36) which is concerned with fairness at work, has reduced the service criteria from two years to one for the full 40 week maternity break entitlement, together with an extension of the minimum period of maternity leave from 14 to 18 weeks. The Bill also sets out the minimum requirements on parental leave and time off work on grounds of *force majeure,* as an important means of reconciling family life and promoting equal opportunities and equal treatment of men and women.

The Parental Leave Directive, which was also implemented in December 1999, provides for both parents to have unpaid leave for up to 13 weeks for the purpose of caring for a child or for the birth or adoption of a child. This Directive will apply to all parents with children under the age of 5, but for a child with a disability the 13 weeks leave can be taken until the child reaches the age of 18; it can be taken all at once or broken up into periods of weeks over 5 years. The minimum leave that can be taken is one week and only in exceptional circumstances can it be taken in odd days. It also gives both men and women the right to take a reasonable amount of unpaid leave for family emergencies affecting dependants.

A woman must give her employers written notice of the fact that she is pregnant, and of the expected week of birth, at least 21 days before she begins her maternity leave. The employer is entitled to ask for written medical certification. She should also inform them of the date she intends to commence her maternity leave at least 21 days in advance. This normally commences after week 29 of pregnancy unless there is a sickness absence issue which requires certification, or maternity leave commences from the first day of absence.

When delivery occurs before the expected date of confinement, maternity leave starts from the date of birth and the employer should be notified of this as well as the expected date of return to work after the confinement, at least 14–21 days before she returns.

Return to work after delivery should be no later than 29 weeks after the date of childbirth and notice should be submitted in writing. If the workforce consists of five or more employees she is entitled to return to work in an equivalent job after confinement. On return to work a risk assessment by the occupational health team is prudent, especially if the woman is still breast-feeding.

In Clause 9 and part 11 of Schedule 3 of the Employment Relations Bill, entitled *Time Off For Domestic Incidents*, all employees will be given the right to take a reasonable amount of time off work to deal with a domestic incident. The intention is to allow employees to take time off to deal with urgent problems where it is reasonable in all circumstances for them to do so. The type of incidents which are intended to be covered include under new section 57A:

- dealing with sudden illness or accident of a member of the employee's family or someone who relies on the employee
- domestic crises and issues needing the employee's immediate attendance, e.g. issues involving a child at school.

Laws on health and safety already cover most of these areas, as a safe workplace is one where both men's and women's health is taken into account. If a risk is identified in pregnancy it should be assessed in the spirit of the Control of Substances Hazardous to Health Regulations (COSHH) and the employer may need to adjust the woman's working conditions or hours, move her to an alternative job, or provide her with paid leave.

Night work, when contributing to a medical issue in pregnancy, may require a change to day work.

Pregnancy and incapacity for work

For state incapacity benefit purposes, pregnancy alone is not generally regarded as a cause of incapacity for work. A woman can be treated as incapable of work if, because of her pregnancy, there would be a serious risk to her health or the health of her unborn child if she did not refrain from work. Otherwise fitness decisions need to be based on the existence of pregnancy complications (e.g. hyperemesis, bleeding, hypertension) or pose a special risk to pregnant workers (e.g. diabetic complications, epilepsy).

Hazards in the workplace

A few specific workplace hazards pose a special risk to pregnant workers. Chemical hazards include lead, mercury, carbon monoxide, herbicides, and certain pesticides.

Lead is a classic example of a chemical hazard being a reproductive risk as it is associated with infertility, and it is a teratogen affecting fetal development in the early weeks of pregnancy, resulting specifically in abortion and stillbirth. There is also some evidence that excessive lead exposure in male workers may result in lowered sperm counts and other sperm abnormalities. Lead can also be passed on to the baby during breast-feeding and intellectual impairment in childhood has been associated with low-level lead exposure.

Special care to follow good working practices and a high standard of personal hygiene is important, along with regular, mandatory health surveillance. Lower action and suspension levels are required for women of reproductive age than for men, and it is against the UK Control of Lead at Work Regulations 1998 for women capable of having children, or young people under 18, to work in workplaces where potentially hazardous exposure to lead may occur, e.g. lead smelting and refining and most jobs in manufacturing lead–acid batteries. Lead-based solder fluxes used in the electronics industry cause serious health risks because of the high exposures that may occur even in a short period of time. The fumes can be extremely irritant both to the respiratory tract and to the eyes, allowing systemic absorption. The Approved Code of Practice associated with the Control of Lead at Work Regulations 1998, ensures that women who may become pregnant have low lead levels[*] and, once pregnancy is confirmed, women are suspended from work which exposes them to lead. COSHH assessments and control measures ensure minimal risk nowadays.

Physical hazards include ionizing radiation, lifting heavy loads, and repetitive and fatiguing muscular work. Women who have a long working week or whose work is physically tiring are thought to have a higher incidence of preterm births. Occupational stress, where there may be conflict or disparity between the demands of the job and a worker's ability to meet those demands is frequently cited as a cause of ill health. A recently completed European collaborative study (EUROPOP) investigating the relative effects of working practices and social conditions on preterm delivery risk demonstrated a small increased risk of delivery before 32 weeks' gestational age among women whose work

---

[*] The Control of Lead at Work Regulations specify an action level of 25 µg/100ml and a suspension level of 30 µg/100ml for women capable of having children.

was described as physically demanding or mentally stressful.[1] The magnitude of increased risk is small and is therefore unlikely to influence any advice on working practices given to women with no previous history of spontaneous preterm birth (SPB). The risk of SPB for a woman who has previously experienced a SPB is 15% (compared to an overall incidence of approximately 5%) and advice regarding limiting physical exertion during pregnancy in this group of women would appear justified.

Biological hazards

Exposure to infectious agents such as *chlamydia psittaci,* brucellosis, and *Toxoplasma gondii* may occur if work involves contact with animals (cats, parrots, lambs). Exposure to HIV and hepatitis B virus may occur from body fluids (mainly blood) and contact with listeria, *Salmonella, Campylobacter,* or scrombotoxins may occur in those in food preparation. Other high-risk groups include those who come into contact with school-children who may be carrying rubella, chickenpox, or human parvovirus B19.

Exposure to rubella or chickenpox is a common cause of concern and referral for medical advice. Rubella immunity is routinely ascertained at the booking antenatal visit; over 90% of women of childbearing age are immune. Seroconversion of the non-immune woman in the first trimester may be associated with teratogenic effects, whereas infection in later pregnancy may be associated with intrauterine growth retardation. Susceptibility to varicella zoster (chickenpox) is uncommon in pregnancy and immunity should be confirmed serologically if exposure occurs. If susceptible, zoster immune globulin should be administered. Expert advice should be sought if clinical infection occurs, since respiratory complications are more commonly encountered in pregnancy than at other times and may be particularly severe. Fetal infection in the first trimester may result in teratogenesis in approximately 2% of cases.

Vaccinations of killed or attenuated virus may be given in pregnancy. Live immunizations should be avoided, as should rubella, mumps and measles vaccines because of the risk of causing pyrexia, which can, theoretically at least, lead to spontaneous miscarriage.

Exposure to any potential organic or non-organic teratogen should be avoided in pregnancy, particularly in the first trimester (up to 12 weeks from the last menstrual period). Recent EC directives have laid responsibility on the employer to provide protection for pregnant women against specific harmful industrial agents and processes (see Box 21.1), and even wider prohibitions apply to breast-feeding mothers.

Box 21.1 Chemicals: reproductive risk[2]
Chemicals that may present a reproductive risk to women are labelled as follows:

R45   chemicals that may cause cancer
R61   chemicals that may cause harm to the unborn child
R63   chemicals that may possibly have a risk of harm to the unborn child
R64   chemicals that may cause harm to breast-fed babies.

Display screen equipment

Concern has been expressed in the past about the potential adverse effects of working with visual display units (VDUs). The energy of X-rays emitted from a VDU is about 25 keV and is not detectable beyond the glass screen of the tube. Other non-ionizing radiations are at background levels. Very low and extremely low-frequency electric and magnetic fields of the order of 1.8 kV/m and 10 millitesla are typically well below acceptable levels. For example, these figures equate 1 hour with a VDU to 1 minute with a food mixer. A large cohort study of the effect of VDUs on pregnant telephone operators revealed no significant difference in rates of adverse pregnancy outcome in the VDU-exposed group compared to the controls. Women can be confidently advised that there is no evidence that work with a VDU will jeopardize pregnancy.[3,4]

High-frequency non-ionizing radiation is used in healthcare (short-wave diathermy), some industry (thermal plastic sealing, glue hardening) and telecommunications.

The environment

Environmental working conditions and working systems must be as safe as reasonably practicable to comply with the provisions of the Health and Safety at Work Act 1974 and the Control of Substances Hazardous to Health Regulations (COSHH). When exclusionary policies are imposed they often ignore any effects on the male, which are just as important as the effects on females in respect of reproduction. For example work in environments which are hot enough to increase core body temperature in females or testicular temperature in males, such as laundry work, kitchen work and, sometimes hairdressing, may depress fertility. Tiredness in shiftworkers may diminish sexual activity and crossing time zones may disturb the menstrual cycle, both of which will contribute to conception failure.

General problems

There are several general, non-specific problems commonly associated with pregnancy. Women often tire more easily, and non-specific backache follows the alteration of the body's centre of gravity; the woman's size may make certain tasks difficult. Sickness in early pregnancy may lead to time off and occasionally needs hospital admission. It is important to consider all aspects of an employee's work as soon as she becomes pregnant to see if they require modification.

Most pregnant women can work their usual hours, but provision of a time for rest after lunch may be desirable in later pregnancy; in other instances shorter working hours or flexi-time are desirable to avoid tiring rush-hour travel. If work involves prolonged standing, alternative work or part-time sedentary work should be considered as pregnancy progresses. Any employer keen to maintain the best productivity from employees will suggest less physical work for a pregnant member of staff. Through modifications of such aspects of the pregnant employee's work most women should be able to continue working until the last weeks of pregnancy if desired and if the physical load is considered sufficiently light.

Diet

During pregnancy a woman should take a diet which is nutritious though not necessarily bulky or very calorific. In some workplaces, canteens provide enough variety for a pregnant woman to select appropriate food. However, in many instances employees buy their own lunches or snacks in nearby shops. Employers could help employees and improve their health by health promotion and good dietary advice. Specifically, the Department of Health has advised taking low doses of folate (0.4 mg folic acid daily) both when planning pregnancy and in the first 12 weeks of pregnancy, to reduce the risk of neural tube defects (NTDs). These women should be encouraged to eat more folate-rich foods, e.g. bread (soft grain), sprouts, cornflakes, branflakes and spinach.

Smoking

Smoking has harmful effects on pregnancy. There is an increased risk of preterm labour amongst smokers although it is difficult to separate the relative effects of adverse socio-economic status and smoking which often co-exist. A higher incidence of miscarriage, placental abruption, fetal growth retardation, and an increased perinatal mortality rate accompany cigarette consumption.[5] Smoking should be actively discouraged and employers can help by prohibiting smoking at work. The introduction of self-help programmes and leaflets has been demonstrated to increase the number of women who stop smoking during pregnancy.[6]

The effect of passive smoking in the workplace (if any) on pregnancy is not established.

Alcohol and drugs

Health promotion at work should also draw attention to the dangers of excess alcohol and the use of non-prescription drugs in pregnancy. Alcohol is a fetal teratogen in early gestation and has adverse effects on fetal growth throughout pregnancy. There is no absolute safe limit for the consumption of alcohol during pregnancy although Sulaiman *et al.*[7] were unable to show a detectable effect on the fetus or neonate of a consumption below 100 g per week. The fetal alcohol syndrome describes a group of neonatal features seen in association with higher alcohol consumption. Characteristic features are low birthweight for gestational age, microcephaly and microphthalmia, short nose, and narrow upper lip. Mental retardation and neuro-developmental delay may subsequently become evident. Identification of women at risk of excess alcohol consumption may be aided by the T-ACE questionnaire[8] (Box 21.2).

Box 21.2   The T-ACE questionnaire

T   How many drinks does it take to make you feel high? (score 2 if answer >2)
A   Have people annoyed you by criticising your drinking? (score 1 if yes)
C   Have you ever thought of cutting down your drinking? (score 1 if yes)
E   Have you ever had a drink first thing in the morning to steady your nerves or get rid of a hangover? (score 1 if yes)

70% of those scoring more than 2 will be 'heavy drinkers'.

Opiate abuse is associated with premature delivery, but it is difficult to dissociate this from the frequently co-existing poor socio-economic status of many abusers. A withdrawal syndrome is commonly seen amongst infants of mothers who continue to abuse opiates during pregnancy.

Travelling in pregnancy

Most airlines refuse women over 34 weeks of pregnancy on international routes and over 36 weeks on domestic flights; they may need certification from a doctor about the length of gestation. This is mainly because airline owners are worried that premature delivery might occur in flight. Air travellers should be advised to stretch their legs and to drink plenty of fluids. Gentle exercise of the lower limbs is recommended to avoid venous stasis and limit the subsequent risk of deep venous thrombosis.

Genetic counselling and prenatal diagnosis

Counselling may be requested for those who have a family history or a previously affected child with an inherited condition such as sickle cell anaemia, cystic fibrosis, or other inherited or non-recurrent disorders.

Chromosomal abnormality in the fetus increases with maternal age. The principal abnormality is Down's syndrome where the incidence at birth is 1/3000 at 25 years, 1/300 at 35 years, 1/100 at 40 years, and 1/40 at 45 years. Biochemical tests on maternal blood are used for screening all women at 15–18 weeks' gestation and their results combined with maternal age to give an individual prediction of risk for Down's syndrome. More recently, nuchal translucency screening employing ultrasound measurement at 10–14 weeks' gestation is being proposed as an effective method of screening for Down's syndrome. For the general obstetric population biochemical testing will identify 60–70% of Down's syndrome pregnancies by identifying the 5% of women who are at increased risk.[9] Although the test is an improvement on screening based on age alone, the vast majority of women found to be positive on screening do not carry babies with Down's syndrome. The prenatal diagnosis of Down's syndrome (and other chromosomal abnormalities) requires fetal or placental tissue for analysis. Chromosomal abnormalities can be detected by chorionic villus sampling (CVS) from 9–11 weeks of gestation or by amniocentesis from 14 weeks. Both are invasive tests with risks of miscarriage of 1–2 and 0.5–1% respectively. A day's rest is usually advised following these invasive procedures.

This screening is now offered routinely to women regardless of age, and it is an area that they are understandably reluctant to discuss with management at work but will usually confide in the occupational health nurse or physician. It may account for poor performance and anxiety or absence issues in early pregnancy, as results of tests are often delayed by up to 4 weeks, before the woman will know whether the karyotype is normal or not.

Pre-existing and co-existing illness

Diabetes

Preconceptual advice and improved periconceptual glycaemic control is important to reduce the risk of fetal abnormality, particularly cardiac defects and spina bifida. Good glycaemic control will improve pregnancy outcome. This will lower fetal loss from all causes, and so timing and dosage of insulin with meals is important. Regular meal breaks from work may be necessary at set times; this could interfere with some work timetables. Perinatal mortality used to be four times as high in diabetics as in the general population. The figure now approaches that of the non-diabetic population.

Heart disease

In cyanotic heart disease the miscarriage rate is minimal, but extra rest is mandatory. There may be problems in pregnancy for a woman with a heart of a fixed volume, high left atrial pressure, and pulmonary vascular obstruction. Despite this, the majority of women with stable cardiac problems do not experience additional difficulties during pregnancy. Preconceptual counselling from a cardiologist is frequently invaluable.

Tiredness, increased absence, breathlessness, and difficulties with work that requires physical effort or standing for prolonged periods may impact on work.

Asthma

Asthma is a common problem but seldom has any adverse influence on pregnancy. Equally, asthma is seldom exacerbated by pregnancy although a small number of women experience an exacerbation of symptoms during the puerperium. Inhaled bronchodilators and steroids should be used as required and courses of oral steroids should not be withheld when considered necessary for an exacerbation.

Hypertension

Women with hypertension are at increased risk of developing superimposed pre-eclampsia, although this is the exception rather than the rule. Antihypertensive medication should ideally be reviewed before pregnancy. There is often a physiological drop in blood pressure in the mid-trimester with a progressive rise towards prepregnancy levels at term, which may require modification of therapy. Labetalol, methyl-dopa, and calcium channel blockers are suitable antihypertensive agents in pregnancy

Breast-feeding

The benefits of breast-feeding to both mother and child are well established and fully justify the widespread promotion of breast-feeding by the World Health Organization. A reduction in infectious morbidity, particularly gastrointestinal, is seen amongst breast-fed infants together with a reduction in the incidence of atopic conditions in childhood. With appropriate encouragement and support, most mothers can successfully breast-feed although cultural and social pressures often result in either outright dismissal or early abandonment of breast-feeding. Breast-feeding mothers enjoy a reduced incidence of breast cancer in later life. Where possible, employers should encourage mothers to continue breast-feeding particularly if they have returned to work within a few weeks of the birth. The availability of flexible or part-time working together with the time and facilities for expression and storage of breast milk will encourage mothers both to initiate and to continue breast-feeding with subsequent benefit to both mother and her child. The provision of a suitable room where this can take place at the workplace is helpful.

Gynaecology

It is probable that women who are at work have a lower morbidity rate than those who are not employed (the healthy worker effect), but anyone employing many women is likely to encounter the consequences of several gynaecological conditions in their employees. Women undergoing treatment for subfertility and even malignancy often continue working. Day-case surgery and out-patient procedures provide for the rapid return of women to the workplace but may require temporary adjustment to working hours and practices.

Disability Discrimination Act 1995

Women with long-term urge or stress incontinence from prolapse, carcinoma or operative complications, terminal cancer, or psychological problems secondary to gynaecological pathology, may qualify as disabled under the Act, if such problems affect their ability to carry out normal day to day activities and have been present for more than a year. Suitable adjustment to working patterns, workstations and working hours may be needed.

Menstrual disorders

Menstrual bleeding usually occurs every 28–35 days and lasts for 4–7 days. On average, periods start at the age of 11 and menstruation does not usually cause clots or flooding or more than mild to moderate pain for more than the first 2 days. Many variations of menstruation may occur from absent or scanty periods to heavy, frequent, and irregular ones.

Scanty or absent periods often have an endocrine explanation: most commonly polycystic ovarian syndrome, hyperprolactinaemia, or premature menopause. Simple biochemical investigation will identify these cases. Psychological upsets and anorexia nervosa can also present in this way; here an occupational health physician or nurse may enable the woman to continue work and avoid lengthy absences. Counselling and advice for further referral help the employee to acknowledge the condition. A long period off work may be necessary if hospital admission is required for eating disorders; fortunately the majority are managed as out-patients nowadays.

The term **menorrhagia** describes excessively heavy or prolonged periods, which may cause problems at work especially if anaemia results. Menorrhagia is experienced by about 1 in 3 women at some stage of their lives and accounts for 15% of gynaecological referrals and half of the 90 000 hysterectomies performed in the UK each year. Menorrhagia can occur in 18–25 year old women, when it may be associated with anovulation.

More often (1 in 20 women) it is the 35–50 year-old who has these problems which may be linked with hormonal fluctuations and organic disease such as fibroids and endometriosis. Investigations are usually done as an out-patient procedure, including ultrasound, visualization of the uterine cavity (hysteroscopy), and endometrial biopsy. Often medication which may include hormones (combined contraceptive pill or progesterone in the form of tablets, injection, or coil), antiprostaglandins (mefenamic acid 500 mg taken three times a day on the days of heavy bleeding) or antifibrinolytic agents (tranexamic acid 1 g three times a day from day 1 during heavy flow), will help to control symptoms. The Mirena IUS is an intrauterine contraceptive device containing progestogen, which is increasingly being employed in the management of menorrhagia. If the woman is at the end of her reproductive life, a hysterectomy or endometrial ablation may be more appropriate.

In the UK 1 in 5 women will have a hysterectomy before the age of 60 years; over half of these operations are performed for menorrhagia. Hysterectomy is a major surgical procedure, which can be performed vaginally or abdominally. In uncomplicated cases the vaginal route is preferred by most experienced gynaecologists since it is associated with less morbidity and discomfort. Although there is no recommended duration of convalescence, a 6–8 week absence would be considered a minimum and considerably longer if the job involves heavy lifting. Return to work is sooner following endometrial ablation, which can be performed on a day-case basis. Satisfaction rates for both hysterectomy and endometrial ablation is high and many women can be offered endometrial ablation if they wish to avoid hysterectomy. The vast majority of women can expect to return to work within a week of this procedure, although a vaginal discharge may persist and cause discomfort for up to a month.

Laparoscopic or minimal-access surgery has revolutionized gynaecological investigations for unexplained abdominal pain, infertility, sterilization, and other problems such as ovarian cysts. Under general anaesthesia, a small incision is made below the umbilicus and a small telescopic instrument, the laparoscope, is introduced into the peritoneal cavity. One or more small incisions are usually made in the pelvic area as well. The woman is in hospital either as a day-case or occasionally overnight. Up to a week's convalescence may be necessary after laparoscopy.

Dysmenorrhoea

Dysmenorrhoea is painful menstruation. It presents as cramping low central abdominal pain in young women or teenagers just before the onset of a period. This is **primary dysmenorrhoea**, which, at its worst, is a debilitating pain associated with nausea, diarrhoea, and flushes. Painful periods starting after the age of 30 years are more commonly due to pelvic disease; there may be other symptoms such as heavy periods or pain on intercourse (dyspareunia). Primary dysmenorrhoea may cause regular monthly absence from work in some young women. Investigations to exclude other causes of pain in this area may be required, but often the diagnosis is obvious and treatment may be given in the form of the oral contraceptive pill or non-hormonal medication (antiprostaglandins). When the pain is **secondary** to fibroids, endometriosis, or pelvic infection, treatment is that of the primary cause. This may require laparoscopic or ultrasound examinations to confirm the diagnosis and any requirement for surgery. Dysmenorrhoea is a common reason for short-term absence and may be revealed by its monthly pattern. Management in the workplace is symptomatic with at least partial relief of symptoms achievable with oral non-steroidal anti-inflammatory agents (NSAIDs) such as mefenamic acid (500 mg three times a day) and time and place to rest quietly for an hour. Endometriosis is frequently treated medically with oral progestogens or danazol, although laparoscopic ablation is an alternative if medical treatment is unsuccessful or cannot be tolerated.

Premenstrual syndrome

Premenstrual syndrome (PMS) is a widely recognized but often misunderstood collection of somatic and psychological complaints. The quoted incidence of PMS varies widely, depending on the classification of symptom severity. Several aetiologies have been proposed but there is no firm basis to support any of the current theories. Cyclical ovarian activity appears to be necessary but PMS can occur in the absence of menstruation (e.g. after hysterectomy with ovarian conservation). A wide variety of symptoms may be reported, the commonest being anxiety, irritability, clumsiness, depression, fatigue, breast tenderness, abdominal bloating, and fluid retention. Differentiating between PMS and underlying psychological or psychiatric disorders is often difficult but the characteristic pattern of PMS symptoms is one of premenstrual exacerbation followed by relief with the onset of menstruation. Psychological illness may co-exist with PMS where the persistent symptoms of the latter are exacerbated premenstrually. Although some features of PMS are experienced by most premenopausal women, severe PMS can undoubtedly impair cognitive and physical performance on a regular, predictable basis; some adjustment to work schedules may then be necessary. Severe PMS can, on occasion, be defensible in law for unusual behaviour such as shoplifting.

Treatment varies according to the nature and severity of the woman's symptoms and her reproductive needs and treatment preferences. A placebo response is common in PMS and this has resulted in a large number of unsubstantiated claims for therapeutic success. Dietary and lifestyle adjustments may improve the woman's general well-being but rely on her self-motivation. Treatments with some objective basis for their effectiveness include non-hormonal treatments such as mefenamic acid, evening primrose oil and bromocriptine. Hormonal methods include oral contraceptives, danazol, oestrogen implants or patches and luteinizing hormone releasing hormone (LHRH) analogues with add-back hormone replacement. The severest cases may wish to undergo surgery to remove the ovaries. Psychological symptoms may improve with an antidepressant such as sertraline.[10]

Infections of the genital tract

Infections can affect the vulva, vagina, uterus, fallopian tubes, and ovaries or any combination of these sites. Usually the first two comprise lower genital tract infection and the last two pelvic inflammatory disease. Vaginal discharge is a common complaint amongst women of reproductive age.

- Vulva: **Pruritus vulva is a common presenting symptom. The causes may be:**
  - fungal (candida)

- viral (herpes genitalis)
- parasitic (scabies, pediculosis pubis, or threadworms)
- sexually transmitted diseases (e.g. trichomonas vaginalis or gonorrhoea.)
- premalignant and malignant lesions
- local skin atrophy (especially following the menopause)
- chronic skin conditions such as psoriasis, eczema, and lichen sclerosis.
- Vagina: **A discharge may be caused by:**
  - infection especially candida, trichomonas, and bacterial vaginosis
  - inflammation from rubber allergy (condom use)
  - foreign body (forgotten tampon)
  - 'physiological' effects, as in pregnancy and with a combined oral contraceptive.

True pathogens of the lower genital tract include *Chlamydia*, *Trichomonas*, *Herpes simplex* (Type 1 and II), gonorrhoea, and *Treponema pallidum*; these are sexually-transmitted diseases. Vulvovaginitis and vaginal discharge are common presenting complaints; they can be managed easily and corrected by the patient's general practitioner. Occasionally referral to a genitourinary clinic is advisable when the sexual history shows recent casual contact.

Discomfort and distress, along with fears that these infections generate, especially regarding future reproductive potential, can be allayed by simple explanations and consultation with the appropriate professional, although they may well be the cause of anxiety at work. Regular short-term absence may be its presentation at work.

Pelvic inflammatory disease

Pelvic inflammatory disease (PID) refers to infections of the uterus, tubes, ovaries and parametrium. It is non-reportable and regional incidences vary in parallel with the incidence of sexually-transmitted disease. It may be an acute febrile illness with pelvic pain and local signs of genital infection or a chronic condition typified by pelvic pain, dyspareunia and possibly infertility. The diagnostic accuracy of the clinical picture is poor.

Primary ascending infection from the lower genital tract tends to occur after delivery or miscarriage or following termination of pregnancy or insertion of an intrauterine device; 70% of cases are due to ascent of endogenous vaginal and perianal flora. The sequelae of PID include: **chronic pelvic pain** in 20% of affected women (of these, 60% will be infertile and suffer from deep dyspareunia); **heavy and painful periods** because of pelvic inflammation (although the mechanism is poorly understood); infertility which follows in 15–20% of cases, increasing to 60% after three attacks of PID, and **ectopic pregnancy** (rates increased 7–10-fold).

Accurate diagnosis and evaluation require laparoscopy. PID is treated with rest and elimination of active infection after identifying the causative organism. Microbiological cultures are frequently negative despite confirmed disease. Infection is usually with more than one organism, with *Chlamydia* being the most important in the UK. Doxycycline and metronidazole are frequently prescribed. Absence from work will be for variable duration depending on the severity of the infection. Definitive treatment of chronic disease is by hysterectomy and bilateral salpingectomy.

Infertility

Infertility affects 1 in 7 couples in the UK; in 40% of those investigated a female cause is found, in a further 30% there is a male cause, and among the rest no cause is discovered (unexplained infertility). The female factors include blocked fallopian tubes (14%) and non-ovulation (21%); in the male, there may be poor or absent sperm production.

Infertility does not produce physical symptoms but the emotional stress is considerable, particularly at the time of menstruation, when the woman is often depressed and disappointed that no pregnancy has occurred. Infertility does not intrude on a woman's work physically, but the mental stress and the repeated and often unpleasant investigations needed may affect work performance and come to the attention of the employer, because of time taken from work. Financial difficulties may result from treatment cost. General advice on weight loss, smoking cessation, and control of alcohol consumption is appropriate for men and women. The avoidance of occupational or social conditions causing testicular hyperthermia may improve semen quality and function.

Male reproductive factors

The contribution of the male gamete to successful pregnancy outcome is equally important. Well-established effects on male fertility are found with occupational exposure to the nematocide 1,2-dibromochloropropane (DBCP) and to lead. Employment in hot environments such as the steel industry may be associated with reduced sperm quality. Paternal occupation in the glass, clay, stone, textiles, and mining industries has been associated with an increased risk of premature delivery,[11] and the wives of workers exposed to vinyl chloride have increased miscarriage rates.

Contraception

Effective family planning is an essential part of any healthcare programme and uncontrolled fertility usually adds to the deprivation cycle. Although contraception is not relevant to fitness for work or placement, contraceptive enquiries are common problems for occupational health practitioners in companies with large female workforces. The occupational physician may need to advise about work situations where there may be a risk to a pregnant worker or her unborn baby.

Oral contraceptives

Steroidal contraception with synthetic oestrogens and progesterones is the commonest method among young women in the UK. There are three commonly used types of oral contraceptive—combined low-dose pills, progesterone-only pills, and triphasic pills. Low-dose pills have few side-effects and can be used by women well into their 40s unless there are specific contra-indications. Manipulation of the menstrual cycle will help occasionally during travel, in certain work situations (e.g. where there are poor hygiene facilities, situations such as diving, space expeditions, rescue/first aid workers/journalists in disaster or war situations), and in athletes. The combined oral contraceptive pill is best used for this. The intrauterine contraceptive device or hormone injection or implant will help in situations where supplies of the contraceptive pill are unavailable.

It is ideal advice to stop the pill at least 4–6 weeks before elective major surgery and up to about 4 weeks after an operation **provided alternative contraception is arranged**.

Injectable steroids such as Depo-Provera can be given 3 monthly; these are effective, although they can cause weight gain and irregularity of menstruation so that a third of users get episodes of amenorrhoea. Fertility usually returns to normal within 6 months of the last injection.

Postcoital contraception

Hormonal postcoital contraception (the 'morning after' pill) can be given within 72 hours of unprotected intercourse using two 12 hourly doses of 50 mg oestrogen (PC4) (which may cause nausea and vomiting) with 98% efficacy, or the antiprogesterone mifepristone. Alternatively the woman can be fitted with an IUCD which is almost 100% effective if inserted within 5 days of the earliest calculated date of ovulation after unprotected intercourse. Current data suggest that progesterone-only pills are more effective than the combined oestrogen/progesterone preparation (Microval 25 tablets taken right away and again at a 12 hour interval or Neogest 20 tablets). They are less likely to cause nausea, have fewer contra-indications, and are more effective, but are currently not licensed for general release in the UK although they can be prescribed on a named patient basis.[12]

Contraceptive advice and management of the complications and side-effects are issues that are commonly raised in a female workforce of reproductive age, especially now that emergency contraceptives are available.

Intrauterine devices

Intrauterine contraceptive devices (IUCD) are effective for 5 years with low failure rates of 2–4% per year. If pregnancy occurs with an IUCD in place, the risk of ectopic pregnancy is higher. Menstrual loss typically increases in IUCD users, which may limit its acceptability to some women. The Mirena IUS is an effective contraceptive and is associated with reduced menstrual loss. Other methods of contraception include chemical barriers to sperm, condoms, and diaphragms but these have higher failure rates than the oral contraceptive or IUCD.

Sterilization

Female sterilization is performed laparoscopically by occluding the fallopian tubes with a ring or clip; the operation means the woman is away from work for a few days only. A small number of women report heavier periods after the operation, which is usually a consequence of discontinuing the oral contraceptive.

Miscarriage and ectopic pregnancy

The exact incidence of spontaneous miscarriage is not known. Probably up to 50% of fertilized ova either do not implant or do not develop, and 10–20% of women who realize they are pregnant undergo a miscarriage characterized by vaginal bleeding and lower abdominal cramping pains. Treatment is often in hospital, with evacuation of the uterus, although conservative management with out-patient observation is often appropriate. A woman who has had a miscarriage will probably return to work 1 week after the evacuation unless physical or psychological complications occur. Recurrent miscarriage (three or more miscarriages) is experienced by 1% of women. Additional investigations are usually performed but are frequently negative with a good prognosis for subsequent pregnancies.

Ectopic pregnancy rates are rising, reflecting the increasing incidence of tubal disease following PID. Diagnosis is frequently made before tubal rupture, allowing more conservative medical or surgical procedures to be performed. Where surgery is necessary, the laparoscopic approach is preferred in order to minimize postoperative discomfort and shorten convalescence.

Shock, vibration, shiftwork, heavy physical work, long working hours, and work with display screen equipment have all been studied in relation to miscarriage, but no association has been proved to date. Chemicals such as lead and copper and ionizing radiation have a well-recognized association.

Legal abortion

In the UK, over 180 000 women have a therapeutic termination of pregnancy each year. If this is performed in the first trimester (before 12 weeks' gestation) it is usually an uncomplicated surgical procedure which involves the woman being off work for 3–4 days only. The psychological effects, however, may last longer. After 12 weeks' gestation, difficulties in performing a termination increase in parallel with the age of the pregnancy. Women may require up to 2–3 weeks' leave following a prostaglandin termination of pregnancy, which can exceptionally be legally performed up to 24 weeks' gestation. In the presence of a fetal abnormality likely to cause significant handicap if the child was born alive, there is no upper limit of gestational age for termination of pregnancy.

The antiprogesterone mifepristone is used as a non-surgical method of termination of pregnancy in women who are less than 9 weeks pregnant. It involves taking mifepristone orally and the insertion of vaginal prostaglandin pessaries 48 hours later. Vaginal bleeding and lower abdominal discomfort ensue; most women are managed as day cases and do not require anaesthesia or surgical intervention.

Menopause

The **menopause** is the time when menstruation ceases; the **climacteric** is the transitional period during which the woman's reproductive capacity ceases. The average age of the menopause has slowly increased since the mid 19th century, so that in the UK it is now 50 years; this is concomitant with women's life expectancy increasing from 45 to 84 years of age. There are approximately 10 million postmenopausal women in the UK, many of them still at work. Often those who were part-time workers while their family was growing up return to full-time paid work at this age.

Symptoms of the menopause frequently begin before the cessation of menses. Interlinked groups of symptoms are:

- **vasomotor:** hot flushes and night sweats lead to insomnia and tiredness so affecting work during the day
- **emotional**: lack of concentration, irritability, depression, and lability of mood can follow and these too may obviously affect work performance

- **sexual symptoms**: decreased libido and dyspareunia may cause anxiety but do not relate to work directly
- **urinary symptoms**: frequency and urgency of micturition may be a problem for women who have to do long shifts, and those who do not have easy access to lavatories
- **long-term effects**: these are principally an increasing incidence of ischaemic heart disease and osteoporotic fractures related to prolonged oestrogen deficiency.

The menopause can be premature (before 40 years of age) following oophorectomy or from early ovarian failure. Such women have a greater predisposition to osteoporosis and ischaemic heart disease, and hormone replacement treatment should be seriously considered.

Psychological symptoms in perimenopausal women may be related to sleep disturbance; difficulty in making decisions and loss of confidence may be features of the menopause itself. Equally, some psychological symptoms may be the result of co-existing socio-domestic changes, which frequently occur when a woman is in her late forties and are not necessarily attributable to declining hormone levels. For a significant number of women, the menopause is associated with few adverse symptoms and for those with heavy or painful menstruation the spontaneous cessation of menses often results in an increased sense of well-being.

Although 70–85% of women experience some climacteric symptoms, only a minority seek medical advice. Hormone replacement therapy (HRT) relieves 85–100% of a woman's symptoms although a significant placebo effect is encountered for those symptoms which are less easily attributable to hypo-oestrogenism. As well as treating the acute symptoms of hormonal decline, oestrogen replacement approximately halves the risk of osteoporotic fractures and possibly deaths from coronary heart disease.[13] Oestrogens are more beneficial than calcium or vitamin D in conserving bone and preventing fractures.

Oestrogen replacement can be given systemically as implants, oral therapy, or transdermal therapy. Local vulvo-vaginal therapy can be given as pessaries, rings, or creams for the relief of urogenital symptoms. In women who have not had a hysterectomy, it is important that a progestogen is given to prevent endometrial hyperplasia and carcinoma. This is often given cyclically, usually resulting in a monthly bleed, but this may prove unwelcome and result in impaired compliance. An alternative is to prescribe continuous combined therapy either orally or transdermally, which results in high rates of amenorrhoea after 6 months of treatment.

Contra-indications to HRT are oestrogen-dependent tumours such as breast and endometrial carcinomas and severe liver disease. A large number of other conditions commonly considered to be contra-indications have no objective basis for being considered as such. Even in women with a history of oestrogen-dependent tumours, HRT can be given in carefully selected cases following appropriate explanation and discussion if the benefits of therapy are believed to outweigh the possible risks.

Side-effects of HRT are usually of a minor nature and cannot always be explained by the recognized physiological effects of oestrogens and progestogens. The progestogenic component can cause symptoms similar to PMS such as irritability, mood swings, and possibly weight gain. There is a recognized increase in the incidence of deep venous thrombosis (DVT) among HRT users, but the overall risk to the individual woman with no other risk factors for DVT is very small. The incidence of breast cancer is increased with prolonged use of HRT (>5 years) and it is advisable to make these women aware of the risk and ensure they undergo screening with mammography.[14]

For some women menopausal symptoms may severely affect work performance; they may be inconvenienced to the extent of curtailing their career. Commonly this is because they have failed to seek help and advice, or are unhappy about taking medication, preferring the 'natural approach'. A short trial of HRT may demonstrate improvement in well-being and change their mind. Often women do not comply with treatment because of the inconvenience of menstruation returning. The newer 'no period' preparations on the market can then be helpful.

Prolapse and stress incontinence

Women who have had children may develop some weakness of the ligaments supporting the pelvic organs and develop a genital prolapse. Symptoms may be non-specific, such as backache or a low dragging pain in the lower pelvis; more specifically there can be an associated involuntary loss of urine on sneezing or coughing (stress incontinence). Examination and assessment of the degree of laxity make the diagnosis. A few women who are unfit, or those in the younger age group wishing for further pregnancies, may elect to try a vaginal pessary in an effort to compensate for the weakness. Such pessaries need changing at intervals; occupational health staff may help women to adjust to this, and are likely to recommend that employees with prolapses should avoid jobs that involve heavy lifting.

More commonly, corrective surgery is performed to reduce and support the prolapse. A vaginal hysterectomy is sometimes required, but alternatively an anterior and posterior wall buttress operation will support the organs. These operations will involve the woman being off work for 6–12 weeks depending on the extent of surgery performed. On return to work duties involving repetitive lifting, or standing in a fixed position without an opportunity to sit down periodically, should be avoided for about 3 months.

Gynaecological cancers

Gynaecological cancer usually affects women over 40 years old. Figures for registration and deaths in England and Wales are shown in Table 21.1.

Cancer of the ovary

Ovarian cancer is one of the commoner fatal cancers of women aged 50–70 and is the most common gynaecological malignancy in the UK. The disease is often asymptomatic

Table 21.1 New registrations (1992) and deaths (1995) for gynaecological cancers.

Cancer site	Registrations (1992)	Deaths (1995)
Ovary	5272	4350
Endometrium	3806	743
Cervix	3597	1339

Data taken from Cancer Research Campaign Fact Sheet 1997.

in the early stages, presenting with poorly defined ill health or swelling of the lower abdomen. It is often first diagnosed by feeling a mass on examination; the tumour is confirmed at laparotomy. Ultrasound screening can reveal pathology at an earlier stage and along with tumour markers in the blood, such as CA125, has been considered as a potential screening system in the general population. However, it is felt that the way forward is to concentrate screening on the relatives of women with ovarian cancer as they have a four-times greater risk of developing it than the population at large.

Following treatment with surgery and chemotherapy, women are likely to be off work for some weeks and will require time off for further follow-up. Survival rates vary greatly, depending on the spread of the tumour at the time of first treatment. Unfortunately, the tumour has often already spread widely when it is diagnosed and so it is associated with a poor prognosis. The overall survival rates are stage dependent and are shown in Table 21.2.[15]

Cancer of the endometrium

Endometrial cancer accounts for 25% of all gynaecological cancers, but only 4% of deaths. This is because 80% are diagnosed at an early stage. The median age is approximately 60 years. Of the one-quarter who are premenopausal, 5% are under 40 at the time of initial diagnosis.

In two-thirds of cases, endometrial cancer presents with postmenopausal bleeding, but if it starts before the menopause there may be prolonged or irregular menstrual bleeding. The diagnosis is confirmed at hysteroscopy and endometrial biopsy; surgical treatment is usually followed by radiotherapy. In a few cases, progestogens are given to reduce the symptoms of distant spread. This condition has a good prognosis and many women are back at work within 6–12 weeks of therapy. The range of survival rates is wide, but this tumour is commonly slow to metastasize and is detected early; thus the prognosis is generally better than other cancers of the genital tract.

Cancer of the cervix

Cervical cancer often presents in the younger woman, commonly aged 35–50 years, and is characterized by postcoital or intermenstrual vaginal bleeding. The diagnosis is made on vaginal examination or at colposcopy and confirmed by biopsy. Depending on the stage of the disease, treatment may be by radical pelvic surgery, by radiotherapy, or by a combination of the two.

Of all the gynaecological cancers, cervical cancer has the best chance of being prevented. Cervical smear screening programmes often detect the condition at a pre-invasive stage when treatment is simple and reproductive capacity conserved. The benefits to the working woman of providing this examination at the workplace are obvious

Table 21.2 Gynaecological cancer 5 year survival rates (%) 1996

Cancer site	Stage I	Stage II	Stage III	Stage IV
Cervix	90–100	65	35	15
Uterus	85	60	40	<10
Ovary	90	74	40	<5

because of the age and effectiveness of screening in the prevention of this condition. Good communication about normal as well as abnormal results between the screening doctor, the general practitioner, and the individual avoids misunderstanding. If screening is not available at the workplace, the working woman should be allowed time off to have this done at a clinic, or by her general practitioner. However, cervical screening at work remains a valuable adjunct to NHS facilities for those women who are unwilling to come forward for screening and usually have the highest risk of cancer and for whom the workplace is the ideal venue for the examination. Although the effectiveness of cervical cytology screening has never been established by randomized trials, epidemiological data strongly suggest a significant impact of a national screening programme in reducing the incidence and associated deaths from cervical cancer.[16]

Cancer of the vulva

Vulval cancer occurs in an older age group (usually over 60 years). The diagnosis is confirmed by biopsy and then usually treated with radical surgery. The woman may expect to be off work for several months. The prognosis is very variable, depending on the extent of the disease at presentation.

Selected references

1 Di Renzo GC, Moscioni P, Perazzi A *et al*. Risk factors for preterm delivery. *Prenat Neonat Med* 1998; **3** (suppl 2): 12 (abstract).

2 HSE. *Chemical hazard information and packaging,* 1995.

3 Schnoor TMI, Grajewski BA, Hornung RW *et al*. Video display terminals and risk of spontaneous abortion. *New Engl J Med* 1991; **324**: 727–733.

4 Roman E. Spontaneous abortion and working with VDUs. *Br J Indust Med* 1992; **49**: 507–517.

5 Cnattigus S, Haglund B, Meirik O. Cigarette smoking as a risk factor for late fetal and early neonatal death. *BMJ* 1988; **297**: 258–261.

6 Hjalmarson AIM, Hahn L, Svanberg B. Stopping smoking in pregnancy; effect of a self-help manual in controlled trial. *Br J Obstet Gynaecol* 1991; **98**; 260–264.

7 Sulaiman N, Florey C, Taylor D, Ogston S. Alcohol consumption in Dundee primigravidas *BMJ* 1988; **296**: 1500–1503.

8 Sokor RJ, Martier SS, Ager JW. The T-ACE questions: Practical prenatal detection of risk drinking. *Am J Obstet Gynecol* 1989; **160**: 863–870.

9 Whittle M, *Ultrasound screening for fetal abnormalities.* Report of the RCOG Working Party London: RCOG Press, 1997.

10 Yonkers KA, Halbreich U, Freeman E *et al*. Symptomatic improvement of premenstrual dysphoric disorder with sertraline treatment. *JAMA* 1997; **278**: 983–988.

11 Blond JP. Semen quality and sex hormones amongst steel and stainless steel welders. *Br J Indust Med* 1990; **47**: 508–514.

12 WHO Task Force on postovulatory methods of fertility regulation. Randomised controlled trial of levonorgestrel versus Yuzpe regime of combined oral contraceptives for emergency contraception *Lancet* 1998; **352**: 428–433.

13 Hemminiki E, McPherson K. Impact of postmenopausal hormone therapy on cardiovascular events and cancer; pooled data from clinical trials. *BMJ* 1997; **315**: 149–153.

14 Collaborative Group on Hormonal Factors in Breast Cancer. Breast cancer and hormone replacement therapy; collaborative re-analyses of data from 51 epidemiological studies of

52 705 women with breast cancer and 108 411 women without breast cancer. *Lancet* 1997; **350**: 1047–1059.

15 Piver MS (ed.) *Handbook of gynecologic oncology*, 2nd edn. Boston: Little, Brown, 1996.

16 Patrick J. Has screening for cervical cancer been successful ? *Br J Obstet Gynaecol* 1997; **104**: 876–878.

22

Surgery

M. Samuel and I. McColl

There is no general agreement among surgeons about the time interval between operation, ambulation, hospital discharge, and return to employment, but the trend towards early activity continues. During the Second World War an army order decreed that all patients had to be kept in bed for 21 days after inguinal herniorrhaphy, but by the 1950s early mobilization had become popular.[1] Advances in laparoscopic and electrocautery surgery, the removal of kidney stones by lithotripsy, and day-case surgery, are now contributing to earlier recovery and earlier return to work. Hernia repairs, appendicectomy, and cholecystectomy can all be performed through an endoscope thereby reducing the size of incisions and the amount of postoperative pain. The Royal College of Surgeons lists hernioplasty and laparoscopy amongst operations suitable for day-case surgery and states that up to 50% of elective surgery could be performed on a day-case basis.[2] In suitable patients laparoscopic cholecystectomy can also be done as a day case.

In England in 1994/95 there were 3.5 million ordinary hospital operations and 2.2 million day-case operations.[3] In the next decade the number of day-case procedures is likely to move steadily towards the 50% suggested by the Royal College of Surgeons. All these advances in treatment methods will gradually reduce the time taken to recover from surgery and facilitate earlier return to work.

Abdominal and hernia operations

Every year more than a quarter of a million patients require advice about the degrees of activity and exertion which may safely be undertaken during convalescence following surgery and many of them need guidance on the length of absence from work and on the type of work compatible with their surgical operations.

Factors which influence return to work after abdominal and hernia surgery are reviewed below.

Wound strength

Since 1945 the Shouldice Clinic in Toronto has advocated early postoperative activity, and in 1972 Iles described the procedure followed for 75 000 abdominal herniorrhaphies.[4] Repairs were carried out under local anaesthesia and patients were discharged from hospital 72 hours later and advised to resume immediately any activities they could carry out in reasonable comfort. By the fourth week, the most strenuous activity was permitted, including piano-moving. The Shouldice technique consists of a double-breasted repair of the fascia transversalis, followed by a Bassini-type procedure using a continuous suture.

Glassow[5] reported that survivors to 10 years whose hernias had been repaired by a consultant using this technique had a 99% expectation that the hernia would remain sound. Use of non-absorbable sutures is essential for early ambulation and also for early return to work.

A study of wound healing revealed that wound strength was 70% of normal immediately after operation, provided that non-absorbable sutures were used, whereas the strength of scar tissue alone improved slowly and after 8 weeks was only 41% of normal.[6] Three further studies in the literature confirm that return to any kind of employment 1 month after an operation for unilateral inguinal hernia does not increase the risk of a recurrence. Laparoscopic repair of inguinal hernias was introduced in 1990 and involves stapling mesh over the internal surface of the inguinal region. As this produces far less damage to tissue with no suturing or tension, postoperative pain is minimal and the patient can return to work within a week. The results of long-term follow up are awaited to see if laparoscopic repair will rival the recurrence rate of less than 1% of the Shouldice repair. Preliminary results suggest that laparoscopic repair for bilateral inguinal hernias may have advantages in terms of early return to work.

Size and location of scar

A small scar from a gridiron incision for appendicectomy can be expected to reach maximum strength quickly owing to the crossing layers of the abdominal wall. A **paramedian incision**, in which the rectus abdominis muscle is sandwiched between two layers of connective tissue, may also be expected to heal soundly with more strength than midline abdominal scars. **Transverse or oblique incisions** sever fewer nerve segments, even though muscle is divided, and are therefore less painful. A **midline incision** through the linea alba leaves a weak scar, but current surgical practice is to use a continuous nylon suture four times the length of the wound, with 2 cm bites, and this technique reduces the incidence of incisional hernia to the same order as that for paramedian incisions. Laparoscopy wounds do not significantly weaken the abdominal wall and rarely cause herniation except at the umbilicus where hernia may occur in 1–2% unless repaired with suture material which lasts for 3 months. Smaller incisions and trocar ports (<10 mm) reduce postoperative pain and expedite return to work.[7]

Wound dehiscence

Partial or complete disruption of the deeper layers of a wound can occur in the early postoperative period and may be symptomless. Unless the wound is immediately re-sutured an incisional hernia will develop and seriously prejudice the permanent strength of the abdominal wall (see p. 440).

Wound infection/haematoma

Superficial wound infection should not weaken the wound, but infection of the deep fascia and lower layers of the wound will delay healing and may lead to permanent weakness and recurrence. A haematoma of the deep layers of a wound also delays healing.

Persistent pain or paraesthesia

Pain and tenderness in the scar or paraesthesia or hypoaesthesia usually resolve rapidly following most surgical operations. Transverse abdominal incisions which divide few sensory nerves are the least painful in the postoperative period, whereas vertical incisions dividing numerous nerve branches are more painful. Operations for inguinal hernia sometimes divide or trap the scrotal branch of the ilioinguinal nerve and cause pain or hypoaesthesia which may delay a return to full activity. In occupations which involve leaning across benches or against machine guards, tenderness of abdominal scars may delay a return to work.

Occupation

In many occupations such as general clerical work (manual handling of files, shifting of small pieces of office equipment etc. packets of paper weighing less than 5 kg for men, 3 kg for women, etc.), the intra-abdominal pressure arising from exertion and the forces applied to the scar by muscular contraction are unlikely to exceed the forces generated by normal physiological functions such as defecation and coughing if not performed with bending or thrusting movements. In occupations which involve significant manual handling of loads, rapid build-up of trunk forces, jolting (e.g. when driving over uneven ground), sustained flexed postures, or work requiring manual handling while bending or twisting, the force applied to the scar is considerable.

Several studies have been conducted relating intra-abdominal pressure (IAP) and abdominal muscle activity to manual handling of loads and other forms of muscular effort. Cresswell[12] refers to the Valsalva manoeuvre as a deliberate intra-abdominal pressure building action (sometimes known as 'abdominal bracing') and a greater level of IAP can be achieved in the Valsalva manoeuvre than during a maximum isometric trunk task, e.g. pulling a loaded trolley or lifting from a confined space.

Generally the literature is unclear as to the mechanical physiological advantage of an elevated IAP[13]. However, it is stated that the IAP mechanism for stabilizing the lumbar spine appears preferable in tasks that demand trunk extension such as lifting or jumping[14].

Meuller[15] emphasizes that IAP is dependent on posture. A kyphotic back posture produces at least five times higher levels of pressure compared with an upright posture. Holding a 10 kilogram weight 25 centimetres in front of the body instead of close to the body doubles the IAP. Increasing the load from 10 to 20 kilograms significantly increases the IAP for all working postures.

Cresswell[16] suggests that in order to efficiently control the increase and decrease in IAP, the abdominal muscles need to be 'trained' for the necessary movements. It is clear from the literature that return to work programmes with specific work hardening for the tasks are advocated.[17,18]

Advice to patients

The most important factor determining the interval between surgical treatment and return to work is motivation. Some patients who have a keen interest in their work or career, or who cannot afford to lose money, will return to work very soon after an operation, sometimes on the next day. Others are more cautious and may appreciate professional advice; some will require persuasion. In practice, most patients will delay their return to work until it suits them, but preoperative advice is important in determining not only length of stay, but also time off work. For instance, a patient who is told that the operation will require 3 days in-patient treatment will be champing at the bit if kept any longer. Conversely, if told beforehand that the expected length of stay in hospital is 10 days, the patient will be perturbed if discharged after 3 days. The same principle applies to time off work, and much unnecessary absence from work could be avoided by counselling patients appropriately before their operation about expected time off work. Employers may also wish to know, from their occupational physician, how long an employee is likely to be off work after elective surgery.

Some guidelines are proposed below for patients who have made a normal recovery. Table 22.1 summarizes the average time off work which will be required following most surgical procedures. (Surgeons may sometimes deviate from these guidelines because of strong personal preferences or variations in surgical technique.)

Unilateral inguinal herniorrhaphy and epigastric hernia operations

More than 85 987 inguinal hernias were repaired in the year 1994/95.[3] Two long-term studies by Bourke *et al.*[8] and Taylor and Dewar[9] recommended a return to full activity and normal work within 28 and 21 days respectively. A leading article in the *Lancet* in 1985[10] stated that 'we should therefore recommend return to work within two weeks for sedentary workers and after four weeks for those in more strenuous occupations', but 'any physical activity that causes pain should be avoided'. Since most surgeons now use a nylon darn or a Bassini-type operation for repair of inguinal herniae, these recommendations are reasonable and evidence from the Shouldice Clinic[4] is most convincing that any occupation may be resumed safely after 4 weeks. Patients should be advised not to drive for 2 weeks following inguinal herniorrhaphy, as they may be slower to operate the brake due to wound discomfort. Most patients who have had a laparoscopic hernia repair return to work within a week.

Bilateral inguinal hernia operations

A prospective study of bilateral inguinal hernia repair concluded that repair of bilateral herniae can be carried out in a single operation with no greater morbidity than a unilateral repair and the return to normal activity is as rapid: hernias should be repaired in the same operation rather than in separate procedures.[11] After laparoscopic hernia repair most patients return to work within a week.

Reassurance

Some doctors recommend a period off work of up to 3 months, and of light work for 3–6 months, after operations for inguinal hernia. However, there is no evidence of clinical benefit from such a prolonged period of inactivity, and patients should be reassured that they do not increase the risk of recurrence, or of other complications by returning to normal work after a shorter interval. Patients who have residual discomfort in the scar due to peripheral nerve involvement should receive an explanation and reassurance that the discomfort can be ignored.

Table 22.1 Time off work following surgery

Condition	Procedure	Time off work (weeks) Return to light duties	Return to heavy duties
Achalasia of the cardia	Heller	2	4
Pneumonectomy		8	Probably not
Operations on salivary glands		2	
Open cholecystectomy		3	12
Laparoscopic cholecystectomy		2	4
Major abdominal conditions without surgery		6	12
Major abdominal surgery		6	12
Thyroidectomy		2	8
Haemorrhoidectomy		2	4
Manual dilatation of the anus or partial internal sphincterotomy		1	3
Fistula in ano	Laying open	2	2
Pilonidal sinus	Laying open	1	3
More radical operation for pilonidal sinus		3	6
Vasectomy		1	2
Prostatic enlargement	Transurethral resection	2	4
Testicular torsion		2	4
Excision of hydrocoele		2	
Orchidectomy		2	
Nephrectomy		6	12
Shockwave lithotripsy		2	
Open operation for removal of stone		8	12
Coronary artery disease	Coronary artery bypass grafting	Varies on consultation with cardiologist	Varies on consultation with cardiologist
Femoral popliteal bypass graft		4	12
Abdominal aneurysm		6	12
Any carotid surgery		4–5	8
Excision of lump in breast		1	2
Radical mastectomy		4–8	Depends on subsequent treatment
Simple mastectomy		<4	Depends on subsequent treatment
Inguinal hernia	Open repair	2	4
Inguinal hernia	Laparoscopic repair	1	2
Femoral hernia	Repair	2	3
Appendicitis	Appendicectomy	2	3
Appendicitis	Laparoscopic appendicectomy	1	2
Recurrent inguinal hernia	Open repair	3	12
Recurrent inguinal hernia	Laparoscopic repair	2	6
Small incisional hernia	Open repair	2	6
Large incisional hernia	Open repair	12	Never
Umbilical hernia	Open repair	2	6

Femoral hernia operations/uncomplicated appendicectomy with gridiron incision

More than 43 000 appendices were removed in the year 1994/95.[3] The majority of patients should be able to resume sedentary work after 2 weeks, and heavy occupations after 3 weeks. After laparoscopic appendicectomy most patients return to work within a week, but when the illness is complicated by peritonitis return to work may be delayed several weeks.

Umbilical hernia operations

The period of restriction tends to be longer and may be extended to 3 months for a large umbilical hernia.

Hernia scars weakened by infection or haematoma

The scar may be permanently weakened and healing will certainly be delayed if the procedure is complicated by wound infection or haematoma. Those employed in heavy occupations or indulging in strenuous leisure pursuits should be advised to avoid heavy exertion if they wish to reduce the risk of developing a further hernia, but for those who must return to heavy work there appears to be no advantage in reducing activity more than 3 months from the time of operation.

Operations for recurrent inguinal hernia

If an inguinal hernia has to be repaired for a second time, the scar is likely to be weaker than for a primary repair. Patients will also be more reluctant to risk a further recurrence due to heavy exertion. There is no reason why the patient should remain inactive during the postoperative period, but they should be advised against heavy exertion for a period of 3 months.

Recurrent hernias are best treated laparoscopically when return to work is usually possible after 2 weeks.

Operations for incisional hernia

Incisional hernias vary in size. Return to a sedentary occupation should be possible within 2 weeks following repair of the smallest hernias, and to more strenuous occupations after 6 weeks. Repair of a large incisional hernia is unlikely to achieve sufficient strength to withstand heavy manual exertion and there will remain a high probability of further breakdown of the scar. Ideally, heavy exertion should be avoided permanently, and return to any manual work delayed for 3 months. Use of a suitable corset can give some protection for those who must undertake heavy exertion. The results of laparoscopic repair of incisional herniae have been encouraging in reducing the length of stay. Some of the new meshes used are more expensive, but the savings are recouped in terms of a shorter stay. The results of long-term studies are awaited.

Cholecystectomy and cholecystitis

More than 35 772 gallbladders were removed in the year 1994/95.[3] Endoscopic cholecystectomy is rapidly replacing the traditional operation through a Kocher's incision, both for elective removal of gallstones and for acute cholecystitis.[19] Recovery is rapid and the patient is able to return to normal activity within a few days of surgery. The traditional transabdominal approach leaves a painful wound which restricts activity for about 6 weeks and most patients cannot work during this time; those in heavy manual occupations may not be able to resume work for 3 months from the time of operation.

Acute cholecystitis usually resolves in several weeks and a period of convalescence of 2 weeks may be required before the patient returns to work. Endoscopic cholecystectomy is now being performed in the acute phase in many centres and appears to shorten the period of recovery. In some cases patients have returned to work within 21 days of operation.

Operations on the stomach and duodenum

There were about 8000 open operations on the stomach and duodenum in the year 1994/95.[3] Operative wounds usually become pain-free within a month, enabling patients to resume general employment, with progression to heavy manual work within 3 months. Following partial gastrectomy small frequent meals are necessary and patients must take regular meal-breaks. Shiftworkers should be encouraged to work regular hours for a few weeks or longer if any digestive symptoms occur. This is not an absolute requirement for all patients as some seem to obtain more rest during daylight hours.

Postgastrectomy syndromes

Postoperative abdominal and vasomotor symptoms arise in the majority of patients following gastric surgery, but they usually diminish with time. Early symptoms occur shortly after a meal and these may persist in 5–12% of patients. To alleviate symptoms they need to eat small meals separate from drinks, and this may require concessions on the part of management when the patient returns to work. Patients should also avoid sugar. Late symptoms which occur about 2 hours after a meal are treated by taking food, and here too, when patients return to work they must be able to obtain food when required. Following gastric surgery it is common for patients to lose weight and to suffer from nutritional disturbances which may limit their capacity for physically strenuous work. Placement in alternative, less active work is sometimes desirable.

Resection of the colon and other major abdominal operations

At least 38 000 resections and other major abdominal operations are performed each year.[3] The recommendations are similar to those for conventional cholecystectomy, namely a return to sedentary occupations in 6 weeks, with a maximum of 3 months' avoidance of heavy exertion in manual occupations. Alteration of bowel function, causing more frequent bowel actions, sometimes requires immediate access to a toilet; this should be taken into consideration in job placement. This applies especially to low rectal anastomoses and operations in which the ileocaecal valve has been removed and to extensive intestinal resection for Crohn's disease and other pathology which also frequently results in malabsorption and loss of weight. Nevertheless, working capacity may be retained in half the patients. Permanent colostomy is discussed in Chapter 15, p. 310.

Pancreatitis

The course of this disease is so variable that no general rules can be given and each patient must be individually assessed.

Patients waiting for operations

Patients awaiting surgery may be unfit for work owing to the symptoms of their illness. Those who have some chronic illnesses such as ulcerative colitis or duodenal ulcer and are awaiting surgery, may fall within the protection of the Disability Discrimination Act (DDA) 1995 and every effort should be made by the employer to accommodate the employee during this period, e.g. homeworking, shortened hours, and in the case of industrial staff, minimizing offsite work, temporarily redeploying them to office-based work, etc. However, those awaiting hernia repair or cholecystectomy for example, do not usually fall within the definition of disability within the DDA and are capable of attending work normally. In the early stages during the development of an inguinal hernia patients may experience aching discomfort due to stretching of tissue as the hernia enlarges, and symptoms are increased by exertion. During this time the patient may be able to attend work if manual exertion and excessive walking can be avoided. As the hernia enlarges, symptoms may disappear and a return to any kind of work is possible, although it is usual to avoid heavy work while waiting for surgery. The patient should be warned, however, that if pain occurs in the hernia or abdomen, they should immediately lie down and reduce the hernia. If this is not possible or if the pain continues, medical advice must be obtained without delay. For this reason work in remote locations should be avoided. A truss is an acceptable aid to some patients waiting for repair of an inguinal hernia.

Anal region and pilonidal sinus

There are more than 86 000 operations per year for disorders of the anal region including 9500 for pilonidal sinus and 24 000 for haemorrhoids.

Haemorrhoids

Perianal haematoma has been described as the 5 day painful self-curing lesion of Milligan; most patients present after a week and need no treatment. Discomfort is increased by walking and sitting on hard surfaces. Absence from work is usually not justified, but in some cases alternative employment may be necessary for a few days.

Prolapsing internal haemorrhoids may cause disability. Usually symptoms can be relieved by immediate reduction, but if strangulation and/or thrombosis occur the patient will be unable to attend work. A diet with increased roughage will reduce the incidence of this condition.

Patients who suffer from recurrent prolapse of piles often assume that the condition will be aggravated by sitting on hard or warm surfaces. They should be reassured that their fears are groundless.

Operative treatment

Most prolapsing internal haemorrhoids are treated in the out-patient department using rubber band ligation, or injection. However, some patients require admission for day-case surgery including dilatation under general anaesthesia. These treatments cause little postoperative discomfort and the patient can return to any form of employment on the next day. Those requiring general anaesthesia may be unable to work for 2–3 days and should be advised not to drive for 48 hours. Following haemorrhoidectomy, the patient should be able to return to work without a restriction on activity or exertion after 2–3 weeks. A high roughage diet and administration of stool softeners will expedite recovery.

Ischiorectal abscess and perianal abscess

Following surgery for ischiorectal or perianal abscess, symptoms should rapidly disappear, and return to work will be determined by the availability of dressing facilities. If there is an occupational health unit at the place of work, the patient could be referred there by letter for wound dressing. Otherwise a return to work should be postponed until the patient can dress the wound without help. In occupations involving prolonged sitting, the patient should be advised to sit on a soft foam pad.

Fissure-in-ano and fistula-in-ano

Following anal dilatation or lateral partial internal sphincterotomy, the patient will normally be able to return to work within 2–3 days. Occasionally there may be temporary impaired control of faeces or flatus which would delay the return to work.

Most fistulae occur in the lower part of the anal canal, and following treatment of this kind of fistula patients can return to work in a week or two after operation. Earlier return may be possible if dressing facilities are available at work. Fistulae that are higher in the canal occasion a much longer period of absence from work.

Pilonidal sinus

There is no ideal treatment for pilonidal sinus. About half of all cases present with an abscess which is treated by incision, curettage, and drainage. Complete healing occurs within 1 month but 40% of patients will require further treatment. Sinuses treated by phenol injection or by laying-open will probably heal within 1–2 months. Excision with primary closure may be followed by healing within 2 weeks, whereas healing takes 2–3 months after excision and laying open.[20] It is possible for well-motivated patients to return to work quite soon after laying-open, and dressing facilities at work will assist. Patients treated by primary closure tend to return to work earlier, sometimes within 3 weeks of operation but 6–7 weeks is more usual. Pressure over the coccyx should be avoided by sitting on a soft foam pad.

Arterial system (See also Chapter 18)

Incidence of cardiovascular operations

At least 25 500 open heart operations are performed annually including 11 400 coronary artery bypass grafts (CABGs).[3]

Heart valve surgery

Between 65% and 80% of patients resume work after heart valve surgery. The avoidance of lengthy sick leave by operation at an early stage in the disease has been shown to improve the quality of life and the rate of return to work.

Coronary artery angioplasty and bypass surgery

The dilatation of narrowed coronary arteries by an inflatable balloon catheter (angioplasty) is now an established method of treatment for coronary artery disease. Compared to the bypass operation, angioplasty has the advantage of a shorter hospital stay, earlier return to work and lower psychological stress.

A randomized intervention trial compared coronary angioplasty (percutaneous transluminal coronary angioplasty or PTCA) with CABG[21] and found that 1 month after treatment the PTCA patients had higher mean exercise times, were more physically active and had less coronary-related unemployment than CABG patients. Recovery after CABG takes longer than after PTCA, but patients treated in the latter fashion required more supplementary revascularization procedures, and had more repeat diagnostic arteriography and more myocardial infarctions than CABG patients. After 1 year the mean exercise times of both groups had increased by 3 minutes. Mortality in the two groups was not significantly different. Patients need to be followed up for 3 years.

Following coronary artery bypass surgery for more extensive arterial disease, 47–79% resume work in 2–12 months after operation. In most studies more than 65% eventually resume work. In one series up to 97% returned to work in low-exertion jobs but only 47% in high-exertion jobs.[22]

Permanent unemployment after operation is a more likely outcome in patients who have lengthy sick leave prior to operation and for those with persistent angina. There is anecdotal evidence that vocational counselling by an occupational physician and rehabilitation including exercise between 2 and 6 months from the time of operation both benefit the patients and may improve the prospect of resuming work. Depending on the severity of the coronary artery disease, its chronicity and the impact which it has on daily activities, the provisions of the DDA may apply. Every effort should be made by the employer to accommodate the employee where possible by offering homeworking, shortened hours, and—particularly in the case of industrial staff—finding alternative sedentary duties with minimal manual effort.

Cardiac transplantation

The numbers of successful heart transplant operations is steadily increasing and many such patients are able to resume work. In one series of 250 patients, 45% were employed and most managed to return to their previous occupation.[23]

Patients may be anxious following heart surgery that physical activity and exertion could be harmful. Clear advice from the surgeon about suitable exercise and the type of employment that may safely be undertaken will help to reassure patients and encourage early return to full employment.

Aortic aneurysm

It is possible for patients in sedentary occupations to continue in employment while awaiting surgery, providing they are well, their blood pressure is controlled, and they avoid driving. Those employed on manual tasks that might raise blood pressure should not work.

Aortic grafts and aorto-iliac grafts

Patients should avoid all physical exertion for 4 weeks after aortic surgery. They are normally able to return to sedentary work after 6 weeks and any other work after 3 months.

The outcome after aorto-iliac grafting is excellent and should enable the patient to return to any form of employment. However, there may be a restriction on activity as a result of the underlying arterial disease. Cessation of smoking, control of weight and blood pressure, and a healthy low-fat diet are all thought to improve the prospects for a full recovery.

Femoropopliteal grafts

Patients with ischaemic limbs may be spared an amputation by femoropopliteal grafting. The results of surgery are less successful than for aorto-iliac grafts, but patients may be able to resume sedentary work in four weeks, and more active occupations in 12 weeks, depending on the symptoms and the degree of atherosclerosis affecting other organs. They should not return to occupations involving crouching and repetitive knee flexing.

Carotid stenosis

Ability to work in patients with carotid stenosis is liable to be determined by the underlying arterial disease and residual symptoms. Recovery from surgical operations on the internal carotid artery should be complete within 4–5 weeks.

Further care after cardiovascular surgery

Drug therapy is often required following cardiovascular surgery to prevent potential complications. This may include anticoagulant therapy to prevent emboli, antibiotics to prevent the infection of grafts, and immunosuppressive drugs following transplantation procedures. These therapies are compatible with most types of work, although the employee may need to take some time off work to attend special clinics for the monitoring and adjustment of dosage.

Driving is permissible in these patients as long as cardiovascular function is acceptable (see p. 365 *et seq*). Strenuous exertion may need to be avoided on immediate return to work, but moderate exercise is likely to be beneficial and activities should not be restricted unduly. Patients taking immunosuppressive drugs should not be employed in jobs where exposure to infectious agents is likely.

Breast

During 1994/95 there were over 12 500 total breast excisions and 63 000 other breast operations.[3]

Biopsy and surgery for innocent cysts and swellings

Lumpectomy, together with chemotherapy and radiotherapy, has drastically reduced the number of total breast excisions.

Aspiration of cysts need not lead to absence from work, but operations involving an incision may require an absence of a few days.

Simple mastectomy

Following simple mastectomy, the principal obstacle to resuming normal activity and work is motivation. It is usually in the patient's best interest to return to work as soon as the wound is healed. Breast reconstruction or fitting a prosthesis immediately after the operation will assist the patient to adjust to the disfigurement.

Evidence for the beneficial effect of psychological support is growing. Weekly group therapy with self-hypnosis for pain relief and psychological support by a well-trained nurse, has been shown to assist social recovery and return to work.[24]

Following simple mastectomy, it is common for a serous discharge to drain from the wound for up to 1 week or more. Patients should be warned about this, provided with suitable dressings, and reassured that it has no serious import.

Radical mastectomy

Radical mastectomy is not often undertaken now, but the operation sometimes leads to oedema of the arm and shoulder stiffness which may interfere with employment. Patients will usually require a period of absence of at least 2 months.

Radiotherapy

Radiotherapy and adjuvant therapy with either endocrine or cytotoxic drugs, are likely to delay a return to full activity owing to systemic disturbance.

After surgery for breast cancer, particularly in the case of radical mastectomy, the provisions of the DDA will apply and modifications may be necessary to the employee's workstation and tasks particularly if the work involves operating display screen equipment. In addition ergonomic assessment may need to be carried out to identify any functional mismatch as a result of shoulder and arm stiffness and appropriate corrective measures instituted.

Genitourinary tract

In the year 1994/95 more than 48 000 major open operations were performed altogether on the genitourinary tract, as well as 62 815 endoscopic operations on the prostate and 13 545 lithotripsy procedures.[3]

Shock wave lithotripsy

Major surgery to remove kidney stones is being superseded by ultrasonic shock wave destruction of stones. Patients are treated as day cases or may be admitted for 1–2 days. Fragments of stones are usually passed completely within 3 months but additional surgical procedures are required in about 8% of patients.[25] The majority return to normal work within 2 weeks. The traditional surgical operation usually leads to an absence of about 8 weeks.

Nephrectomy

Patients frequently complain of discomfort in the scar which is aggravated by bending and twisting movements. A return to clerical-type work should be possible within 6 weeks, but avoidance of repetitive stooping and heavy lifting for a further period of 6 weeks would be reasonable in some manual occupations.

Patients who have lost one kidney are anxious about possible injury to the remaining kidney. In practice the risk of injury to a kidney at work is remote. Patients can be reassured that loss of a kidney does not prevent manual work in any occupation (Chapter 20).

Laparoscopic nephrectomy is being carried out in some centres and results in much less morbidity than open surgery.

Prostatectomy

Following transurethral prostatectomy patients usually leave hospital within a week and will require at least a similar period of convalescence before resuming work. The chief considerations regarding return to work are adequate control of micturition and ready access to a toilet. The type of work is less important.

Testicular torsion

Following surgery to relieve testicular torsion the patient should be able to return to any kind of work when scar tenderness settles, usually within 2 weeks.

Hydrocoele

Simple aspiration of a hydrocoele should not lead to absence from work. Following an operation for excision, the scar will be tender and this will reduce activity for 1–2 weeks.

Orchidectomy

Orchidectomy only requires a reduction in activities such as walking until tenderness has diminished to an acceptable level—possibly a week or so. However, treatment of the underlying disease, for example by cytotoxic drugs or radiotherapy, may further delay return to work.

Vasectomy

One study showed that 46% of patients do not lose time from work following vasectomy, and the percentage could be much higher if the operation were performed on a Friday.[26] Those who were absent lost an average of about 5 days. It is possible that patients with more active manual occupations find it necessary to take time off work. The occurrence of a haematoma or of infection may cause an absence of up to 10 days.

Head and neck

During 1994/95 there were 9825 thyroid operations and more than 300 000 other operations excluding eye and dental operations, on the head and neck.[3]

Thyroidectomy

Patients usually make a rapid recovery from thyroidectomy, but convalescence may be prolonged if the patient previously had hyperthyroidism, especially if there have been symptoms of cardiac involvement. Most patients will be capable of normal work after 2 weeks, with a further restriction on heavy physical exertion for 2 months in all.

Operations on the salivary glands

Removal of stones from the ducts of salivary glands causes few operative problems, and patients should be capable of any type of work within 2 weeks.

Operations for malignant tumours

Depending on the site of the malignancy there is likely to be disfigurement and disability. Radical surgery for tumours of the sinuses and mandible is especially disfiguring, and early fitting of a prosthesis is highly beneficial. Reconstructive surgery by skin and muscle flap grafts is a major advance in cosmetic rehabilitation. Radical neck dissection, to remove tumour and lymphatic tissue, may cause persistent shoulder pain and many patients in manual occupations are forced to give up work, especially if the accessory nerve is divided. Patients in non-manual occupations should be able to return to work.

Excision of laryngeal tumours causes partial or complete loss of the voice which may damage promotion prospects in some occupations. Re-acquisition of speech has been shown to be an important factor for employment. Laryngectomy is usually performed on patients in their late fifties or older; nevertheless in one series 24 of 62 patients returned to employment.[27]

The surgical formation of a fistula between the oesophagus and the trachea together with the insertion of a stomal valve (speech button) enable the patient to force a greater volume of air into the oesophagus; up to 90% of patients achieve fluent speech. Dedicated and well-trained staff are required to provide a speech button maintenance service.[28]

Employees suffering from these conditions are subject to the provisions of the DDA and the employer would be expected to make reasonable adjustments to the employee's work activities to accommodate the disability (e.g. minimizing telephone work for laryngectomy cases, finding less manual duties for those who have undergone head and neck surgery, considering homeworking, etc.).

Craniotomy and operations on the circle of Willis

There are about 11 000 intracranial operations per annum including 1400 on brain aneurysms and arteries.[3]

Subarachnoid haemorrhage and operations to clip a berry aneurysm

Disability following surgical treatment for subarachnoid haemorrhage and aneurysm varies considerably. There may be residual neurological disability from the haemorrhage or from the surgery. This varies from minor symptoms, from which the patients may recover in a few weeks, to more serious disability, but most patients will require lengthy rehabilitation. A minimum absence of 2 months is to be expected.

Successful operations to clip the aneurysm will eliminate the need for any restriction on physical activity, but for a period of some 2 years thereafter the patient should be considered to be at increased risk of an epileptic seizure. Employers should be advised that the patient could fall without warning and should not, therefore, work at heights, work with unguarded moving machinery, or drive vehicles during this period (See also Chapter 8).

On returning to work, patients with a postoperative skull defect who are liable to bump their heads may require a padded cap or safety helmet.

Operations on the middle and inner ear

Operations to control infection of the middle ear or to close perforations of the tympanic membrane are normally followed by a resumption of work in about 2 weeks, but dressing facilities may be required and patients will not be able to wear ear protection in a noisy environment until healing is complete; avoidance of excessive noise is essential. Operations on the inner ear may be followed by disability lasting from weeks to several months. Patients have to avoid noise and hazardous situations in which loss of balance might lead to injury. For example, patients should not climb, drive, or work near moving parts of machines when they are unsteady. Hearing protection is necessary when resuming work in a noisy environment. Ear-muffs or plugs can be worn when there is no longer any risk of introducing or aggravating infection, but advice from the surgeon is essential.

The provisions of the DDA would apply in cases where there is interference with balance or communication is severely impaired through deafness. (See also Chapter 10.)

Ingrowing toenails

There are over 23 000 admissions per annum for nail operations.[3] Ingrowing toenails lead to a great deal of needless absence from work; absence for more than 24 hours is quite unnecessary for the majority of these patients. Symptoms are relieved almost immediately by excising a triangle of nail where it is irritating the nail fold; by contrast, avulsion of the nail causes tenderness of the nail bed and absence from work of at least 1 week. Recurrent ingrowing toenails often require additional treatment, such as cryotherapy or excision of a strip of nail and ablation of a small piece of the nail bed with phenol, and these procedures justify an absence of a few days until tenderness has cleared and the wound is healing. Complete removal of the nail bed requires an absence of at least 2 weeks and probably longer for patients whose work involves much walking.

Thorax

More than 30 000 surgical procedures per annum involve opening the chest. They include more than 11 000 coronary bypass grafts and 3000 excisions of lung.[3]

Thoracotomy scars

Incisions for pulmonary operations usually follow the dermatome, but injury to the sensory branches of intercostal nerves sometimes leaves residual tenderness and paraesthesia which may interfere with employment. An explanation of the cause of symptoms should help to convince the patient that there is no need to restrict activity or avoid heavy exertion.

Partial and total pneumonectomy

Following total pneumonectomy, in addition to symptoms from scar tissue, exercise tolerance may be limited. Pneumonectomy is commonly undertaken in middle life or in older people whose pulmonary reserve has already been compromised by smoking. Dyspnoea at rest or on very slight exertion will prevent travel to work or any physical activity. Nevertheless, a long-term study in the Netherlands revealed that of 37 male pneumonectomy patients 14 resumed full-time work and 9 part-time work.[29] Patients have better exercise tolerance and a better prospect of re-employment following partial pneumonectomy. The minimum period of absence is likely to be 2 months, extending to 6 months for those who are most disabled.

Hiatus hernia and reflux oesophagitis

As many as 1 in 14 of the population may have heartburn from reflux oesophagitis, but only 5% of patients referred to hospital need surgery.

Patients awaiting surgery for reflux should be able to attend work providing that there is no requirement to stoop to waist level or lower; symptoms are aggravated by reflux of acid while stooping. In those who fail to respond to medical treatment surgery will usually eliminate the symptoms from reflux. The surgery may involve an abdominal incision or a thoracotomy, and postoperative progress is mentioned on p. 435 and p. 450 respectively. A minimum absence of 6 weeks is to be anticipated for sedentary workers and up to 3 months for manual workers. Laparoscopic fundoplication has greatly reduced morbidity and patients can leave hospital after 2 days and return to work in a week or two.

Operations on the oesophagus

Operations on the oesophagus will usually require a transthoracic approach, and the factors described on p. 450 may apply. Postoperative disability depends on the extent of the operation and will be maximal following resection of a carcinoma. This usually entails a combined abdominal and thoracic approach, and may involve radiotherapy. Very few patients will return to work. After a laparoscopic Heller's operation for achalasia the patient can leave hospital in 2 days and return to work in a week or two.

Spontaneous pneumothorax

Following spontaneous pneumothorax the patient should be advised to avoid exertion for at least 2 weeks to allow full expansion of the lung. A further period of restriction is sensible to permit sound healing of the defect. An absence of 6 weeks would be reasonable for manual workers. Recurrent pneumothorax will require a longer period of protection from heavy physical activity, up to 12 months, and operative intervention may be indicated. Factors discussed on p. 450 may apply following operation. There are particular restrictions on divers and hyperbaric workers (see also chapter 19 and appendix 4).

Depending on their chronicity and their impact on everyday life, some of these conditions would be subject to the provisions of the DDA (e.g. permanent and substantially impaired mobility, due to poor exercise tolerance, in a patient who has had a pneumonectomy) and would require the employer to make reasonable provision to accommodate the employee's disability before and following surgery if some impairment remains (e.g. by finding more sedentary duties for such a worker).

Selected references

1 Farquharson EL. Early ambulation with special reference to herniorrhaphy as an outpatient procedure. *Lancet* 1955;**2**: 517–519.
2 *Report of the Working Party on Guidelines for Day Case Surgery* (revised edition), pp. 35–43. London: Royal College of Surgeons, March 1992.
3 *Hospital episode statistics. Volume 1: Finished consultant episodes by diagnosis and operative procedure. England: Financial year 1994/95.* London: Department of Health, 1993.
4 Iles JDH. Convalescence after herniorrhaphy. *JAMA* 1972;**219**(3): 385–358.
5 Glassow F. Inguinal hernia repair using local anaesthesia. *Ann R Coll Surg Eng* 1984;**66**: 382–387.

6 Lichtenstein IL, Herzikoff S, Shore JM, Jiron MW, Stuart S, Mizuno L. The dynamics of wound healing. *Surg Gynecol Obstet* 1970;**130**: 685–690.

7 Matsuda T, Ogura K, Uchida J, Fujita I, Terachi T, Yoshida O. Smaller ports result in shorter convalescence after laparoscopic varicoelectomy. *J Urol* 1995;**153**(4): 1175–1177.

8 Bourke JB, Lear PA, Taylor M. Effect of early return to work after elective repair of inguinal hernia: clinical and financial consequences at one year and three years. *Lancet* 1981;**2**: 623–625.

9 Taylor EW, Dewar EP. Early return to work after repair of a unilateral inguinal hernia. *Br J Surg* 1983;**70**: 599–600.

10 British hernias (editorial). *Lancet* 1985: **1**: 1080–1081.

11 Serpell JW, Johnson CD, Jarrett PE. A prospective study of bilateral inguinal hernia repair. *Ann R Coll Surg Eng* 1990;**72**(5): 299–303.

12 Cresswell AG, Grundstromöm H, Thorstensson A. Observations on intra-abdominal pressure and patterns of abdominal intra-muscular activity in man. *Act Physio Scand* 1992;**144**: 409–418.

13 Kumar S. The effect of sustained spinal load on the intra-abdominal pressure and EMG characteristics of trunk muscles. *Ergonomics* 1997;**40**(12): 1312–1334.

14 Cholewicki J, Juluru K, McGill SM. Intra-abdominal pressure mechanism for stabilising the lumbar spine. *J Biomech* 1999;**32**(1): 13–17.

15 Mueller G, Morlock MM, Vollmer M, Honl M, Hille E, Schneider E. Intramuscular pressure in the erector spinae and intra-abdominal pressure related to posture and load. *Spine* 1998;**23**(23): 2580–2590.

16 Cresswell AG, Blake PL, Thorestenson A. The effect of an abdominal muscle training programme on intra-abdominal pressure. *Scand J Rehabil. Med* 1994; **26**(2): 79–86.

17 Buckle P, Stubbs D. The contribution of ergonomics to the rehabilitation of back pain patients. *J Soc Occup Med* 1989;**39**(2): 56–60.

18 Clearly L, Thombs DL, Daniel EL, Zimmerli WH. Occupational low back disability: effective stratagies for reducing lost work time. *Am Ass Occup Health Nursing J* 1995;**43**(2): 87–94.

19 Wilson RG, Macintyre IMC, Nixon SJ, Saunders JH, Varma JS, King PM. Laparoscopic cholecystectomy as a safe and effective treatment for severe acute cholecystitis. *BMJ* 1992;**305**: 394–396.

20 Allen-Mersh TG. Pilonidal sinus: finding the right track for treatment. *Br J Surg* 1990;**77**(2): 123–130.

21 Coronary angioplasty versus coronary artery bypass surgery: The Randomised Intervention Treatment of Angina (RITA) Trial. *Lancet* 1993;**341**: 573–580.

22 Sim Munro W. Work before and after coronary artery bypass grafting. *J Soc Occup Med* 1990;**40**: 59–64.

23 Paris W, Woodbury A, Thompson S, Levick M, Nothegger S, Hutkin-Slade I, Arbuckle P, Cooper DK. Social rehabilitation and return to work after cardiac transplantation—a multi-centre survey. *Transplantation* 1992;**53**(2): 433–438.

24 Psychological factors in breast cancer (editorial). *BMJ* 1991;**302**: 1219–1220.

25 Rajagopal V, Bailey MJ. Mobile extracorporeal shockwave lithotripsy. *Br J Urol* 1991;**67**(1): 6–8.

26 Randall PE, Marcuson RW. Absence from work following vasectomy. *J Soc Occup Med* 1985;**35**: 77–78.

27 Goldberg RT. Vocational and social adjustment after laryngectomy. *Scand J Rehab Med* 1975;**7**: 1–8.

28 Voice after laryngectomy (editorial). *BMJ* 1992;**304**: 2–3.

29 Laros CD. The patient after total pneumonectomy. A long-term study. *Selected papers*, Vol 19. The Hague: Royal Netherlands Tuberculosis Association, 1979.

23

Dermatology

N. F. Davies and R. J. G. Rycroft

Less is known about the relationship between skin conditions (dermatoses) and employment than some dermatologists and occupational physicians care to admit. In the everyday practice of dermatology and occupational medicine there are many individual exceptions to the received dermatological wisdom. For example, Rystedt in Sweden found that, even in jobs known to entail a high risk of dermatitis, about a quarter of those who had moderate or severe atopic eczema in childhood did not develop a work-related dermatitis.[1] Hence there is often doubt as to whether a particular individual with a dermatosis will be able to tolerate a particular job. It is generally a wise course of action to give the individual the benefit of that doubt, in the interests both of the employee and the prospective employer. The recommendations that follow should not, therefore, be treated as prescriptive. A flexible approach allows individual circumstances to be considered properly and fosters good industrial relations.

Classification of skin conditions

Dermatoses can usefully be divided into two categories:

* **non-occupational**: not primarily caused by skin contact at work, though some (such as atopic eczema) may be aggravated by it.
* **occupational**: primarily caused by skin contact at work, though some (such as allergic contact dermatitis from chromate in cement) may continue even after this contact ceases.

The distinction between occupational and non-occupational dermatoses is often difficult to make, largely because the majority of occupational dermatoses and a sizeable proportion of non-occupational dermatoses have a similar clinical appearance. This clinical and histopathological entity is termed eczema or dermatitis; the two words are used synonymously by most dermatologists in this country. However, proper advice on fitness for work cannot be given until the distinction between occupational and non-occupational patterns of disease has been drawn as accurately as possible.

The interaction between individual constitution and the occupational environment is variable and unpredictable. **Exogenous** (contact) factors and **endogenous** (constitutional) factors appear to interact differently in different individuals. For example, of two individuals with the same occupational skin exposures, one might notice no adverse effects on a pre-existing psoriasis, whereas another might find that psoriasis developed on their palms for the first time (see p.457).

Skin conditions and employment

The relation between dermatoses and employment may be considered from two aspects:

- the effect of the common **non-occupational dermatoses** on fitness for work
- the effect of the common **occupational dermatoses** on fitness for work.

Skin conditions, especially those involving the hands and face, are obvious to prospective employers and fellow employees. They easily provoke aversion and prejudice, including groundless fears about contagion and poor personal hygiene. Thus, Cunliffe has demonstrated that unemployment levels are significantly higher among acne patients of both sexes than in controls.[2]

Severe disfigurement (whether facial or otherwise) is considered to be a substantial adverse effect within the definition of the Disability Discrimination Act 1995 (DDA). It is unlawful for employers to discriminate on these grounds for employment purposes, and this is therefore particularly relevant in the case of disfiguring skin disease. The severity of disfigurement may well be debatable, but employers may need to be reminded that, contrary to popular belief, the vast majority of dermatoses are not infectious or contagious. The emphasis should be shifted instead towards the accurate identification of the few dermatoses that can present real problems in specific occupations.

Similarly, fellow employees may need to be reassured, particularly about the sharing of washing and eating facilities. The occupational physician or general practitioner may accept the fitness for work of a prospective employee, but others, such as the personnel manager, supervisor, and fellow employees may be less receptive. In some cases, naive misconceptions will need to be dispelled—the level of accurate information about skin disease in the community is still low, particularly in relation to its visibility and prevalence.

Prevalence

General

Skin disease is common. Probably the best estimate of the prevalence of skin disease in the general population is that carried out on behalf of the National Center for Health Statistics in the US,[3] in which 20 000 adults from the general population were examined. Nearly one-third of the sample were found to have 'some skin pathology that should be evaluated by a physician at least once'. The commonest skin conditions were: acne vulgaris, tinea ('athlete's foot' or ringworm), benign and malignant tumours, seborrhoeic eczema, atopic eczema, contact dermatitis, and psoriasis.

The combined prevalence of seborrhoeic eczema, atopic eczema and contact dermatitis in the survey was 6%. The prevalence of psoriasis in the UK and other western European countries is around 2%. Skin conditions prompted 22.5% of all attendances at general practitioner surgeries in a London borough, and 20–30% of these consultations were for eczema.[4] Skin disease is thus very common but it is not always appropriately treated by non-specialists, sometimes resulting in unnecessarily prolonged absences from work.

Contact dermatitis

On direct examination of a sample of over 3000 adults from a mixture of urban and rural communities in the Netherlands,[5] 6.2% had eczema on the hands and/or arms, nearly two-thirds of whom were women. Contact irritants were considered to be a factor in more than half of all cases, but no patch testing was carried out. Reports on the prevalence of contact dermatitis based on patch testing of dermatological out-patients vary widely according to the views of individual dermatologists.

Contact urticaria

Contact urticaria from natural rubber latex (NRL) is a problem that affects up to 10% of occupations where glove wearing is widespread or mandatory: doctors, nurses, vets, pharmacists, cleaners, and many others.[6]

Occupational dermatoses

The prevalence of occupational dermatoses is not as well described as that of the common non-occupational dermatoses. This is due to the greater difficulty in diagnosing occupational dermatoses and to the lack of accurate reporting systems. Because more men are in paid employment than women more men have occupational dermatoses.

EPI-DERM is a surveillance and reporting system for dermatologists and occupational physicians, which provides useful data on patterns of occupational skin disease in the UK. Not surprisingly, contact dermatitis is the most commonly reported category, comprising more than 70% of reports. Trend analyses suggest that the causes of occupational dermatoses are remarkably uniform over time, although there is evidence of a decreasing proportion of cases arising from foods and flour, and an upward trend from rubber chemicals and NRL.[7]

In 1989, the Health and Safety Executive (HSE) commissioned a survey of occupational dermatitis presenting over a 6 month period to 73 general practitioners across the UK. This provided an annual estimate of 60 000[8] cases for the country as a whole. In high-risk groups such as construction workers 5–15% prevalence rates of occupational contact dermatitis have often been reported,[9] though similar rates of non-occupational dermatoses may occur by chance.

The rate of premature retirement due to skin disease is not known. Frequently, affected individuals can be found alternative employment, but some highly trained people such as toolmakers, laboratory technicians, and nurses with occupational contact dermatitis may be forced to give up their work. Some atopic eczema sufferers may eventually have to give up their work because exposure to irritants is unavoidable (shampoos in hairdressers, for example).

Clinical aspects affecting work capacity

The comments that follow apply mainly to prospective employees with a past history and current clinical evidence of the skin disease in question. If their conditions have cleared and remained clear without therapy for a long time (a year, for example) their dermatoses need not necessarily be considered a significant influence on their fitness for work. When a history of previous dermatosis is relevant and needs to be taken into consideration, it will be specifically indicated. Extreme climatic conditions may be contra-indicated for practically any of the skin conditions listed.

Effect of the common non-occupational dermatoses on fitness for work[10]

Eczema

Atopic eczema is considered to render the potential employee more susceptible to contact irritants, but only if the condition was severe in childhood and particularly if it involved the hands.[11] This increased susceptibility is not shared by other atopics—those with asthma or hayfever alone—and does not extend to contact allergens as well as contact irritants. Indeed, there is some evidence that it is harder for the atopic to become sensitized to contact allergens than the non-atopic. However, atopics are more susceptible to contact urticaria from NRL, and, in this situation, advice will be required not only about the prevention of urticaria but also about asthma and anaphylaxis.[12]

There are few jobs for which a history of severe childhood atopic eczema with hand involvement can be regarded as an absolute contra-indication, but three notable exceptions are hairdressing (shampoo), catering (wet work and detergent), and production engineering (soluble oil). In most other jobs the irritant exposure is insufficient to constitute a problem, even in employees with active atopic eczema, unless the hands are currently eczematous. Other occupations that entail significant exposure to contact skin irritants are domestic cleaning, nursing, construction work, motor vehicle maintenance, horticulture, and agriculture. The eczema of some atopic individuals worsens in response to hot occupational environments, whether dry or humid.

Involvement of the hands in atopic eczema can pose an entirely separate problem in certain occupations. Lesions of eczema are very frequently colonized or infected by *Staphylococcus aureus*, and sometimes by *Streptococcus pyogenes*. In certain eczematous lesions, carrier rates for *S. aureus* approach 100% and densities may exceed $10^6/cm^2$, leading to clinically apparent infection. In addition, such patients are colonized on clinically uninvolved skin at rates which may exceed 90%.[13]

Any organism which colonizes or contaminates the skin surface is dispersed into the environment on naturally shed skin scales.[14] This has implications in healthcare (patient infection), catering (food poisoning), and the pharmaceutical industry (product contamination). The risk to hospital patients is increased in the immunologically suppressed, though it is not confined to such patients. Hospitals with methicillin-resistant *S. aureus* (MRSA) strains need to be particularly vigilant as to staphylococcal carriage in staff.[15] The hazard posed by active eczema in these particular occupations is real and requires individual assessment of risk.

One further consideration may influence the advice given to atopic subjects. Rystedt[11] has pointed out that, even where the work provides no recognizable hazard to the skin, around half of atopics may develop hand eczema *de novo* or exacerbations of pre-existing hand eczema. When hand eczema develops in an atopic potentially exposed to any skin hazard at all, it is often difficult for the patient, their trades union representative, or the insurer to accept that the condition is not necessarily occupational. In such cases, industrial injury assessors and expert witnesses who give evidence in claims for compensation may allow the patient the benefit of the doubt. Many essentially endogenous dermatoses are then stated to be aggravated by work exposure, especially if there is known to be a high-risk substance, such as chromate, epoxy resin, or a powerful irritant, in the occupational environment.

Seborrhoeic eczema appears to be associated with an increased susceptibility to contact irritants, but to a lesser extent than for atopic eczema. Spread of seborrhoeic eczema from its localized chronic sites can occur in response to hot environments. Discharging otitis externa or profuse scalp scaling may raise problems of bacterial dispersal similar to those in atopic eczema.

Stasis (varicose) eczema can be aggravated by prolonged standing. Occupations that may pose a problem include work as a waiter, a shop assistant, or a machine operator in engineering. Such postural occupational factors can probably be countered effectively, however, with correct advice about the importance of appropriate exercise and adequately supportive legwear, and reasonable adjustments to the workplace.

Discoid (nummular) eczema has few, if any, implications for employment, unless associated with hand eczema, when similar considerations apply to those in atopic eczema.

Psoriasis

Mild psoriasis that does not affect the hands can probably be safely ignored from the point of view of fitness for work. Aggravation of psoriasis by physical or chemical trauma (Köbner phenomenon) can occur occupationally. Occupational factors may elicit it on the hands for the first time in psoriasis-prone individuals though patients with psoriasis vary widely in their liability to hand involvement. If it already involves the hands, work involving heavy manual labour, such as scaffolding, or contact with irritants (e.g. in production engineering) may aggravate it.

If psoriasis is (or has been) at all extensive, physically or emotionally demanding occupations can aggravate the disorder. When disease is extensive and associated with arthropathy, special consideration should be given to the requirements of the job.

Colonization of psoriatic lesions with potentially pathogenic bacteria is less of a problem than in atopic eczema and occurs chiefly in those with severe psoriasis who have been hospital in-patients. The density of *S. aureus* has been shown to be three times as heavy on psoriatic plaques as on clinically uninvolved skin, but still to be light in comparison with the density of colonization on eczematous skin.[16]

Psoriatics with well-controlled plaques do not generally present a risk from bacterial carriage. Psoriasis becomes a potential hazard in those working in hospitals, catering, or the pharmaceutical industry when lesions involve the hands, forearms or scalp (common), and face (rare). Nevertheless, the lesser degree of staphylococcal colonization in psoriasis compared to atopic eczema, as well as the wider spectrum of suppressive treatments that now exist for psoriasis, allow greater scope for employment of psoriatics even in such high-risk occupations. However, work in special areas such as operating theatres or caring for immunosuppressed patients increases the risk.

Other conditions

Chronic urticaria can be made worse by physical or emotional stresses at work. Its control with oral antihistamines, which tend to have the side-effect of drowsiness, may raise the question of fitness for work that requires a constant level of alertness, such as driving or machine operating. Some newer antihistamines are claimed to be non-sedative and many, though not all, patients can tolerate these safely (Chapter 26, p. 500).

Photosensitive dermatoses, and, to a lesser extent **vitiligo**, may make outdoor work in very sunny environments inadvisable, unless sufficient protection is provided by clothing or by high efficacy sunscreens. Dermatological advice can often assist subjects with light sensitivity. Those on drugs such as long-term tetracyclines for acne or amiodarone for arrhythmias may also exhibit photosensitivity.

Severe nodulocystic acne may be a contra-indication to work involving unavoidable exposure to hot climatic or microclimatic environments (e.g. diving in suits heated by hot water), which can severely exacerbate the disorder. Probably it also increases the susceptibility to oil acne, though this should be preventable by other means. Treatment with oral isotretinoin (Roaccutane) can now help to resolve even the worst cases of acne, including those formerly resistant to treatment. There is an increased prevalence of acne in the unemployed[2] and care should be taken to guard against unfair discrimination at the recruitment stage.

Multiple viral warts of the hands could be deemed to be a severe disfigurement and appropriate adjustments should be made for those in occupations involving food handling, patient care, or overt contact with the public. A specific group at risk are wholesale butchers, among whom viral warts can spread to become endemic. It would be unwise to allow anyone with viral warts on the hands to start working in a large butchery without prior treatment. Special arrangements may need to be considered for those in occupations involving shared showering or bathing facilities. Dermatological referral should eventually effect the removal of all but the most stubborn warts, allowing the patient to work in areas previously barred to them.

Tinea pedis is endemic in occupations involving shared showering or bathing facilities and in those that require occlusive footwear to be worn. The condition is common and it would not be justifiable to keep new employees away from work pending curative treatment. However, it should be recognized and treatment initiated, before employment starts.

Impetigo and other more serious **primary bacterial infections** of the skin, such as tuberculosis, may result in temporary debarment from employment. Adequate treatment of primary bacterial infections is needed before work is permitted which may render a risk to the health of others. Common skin infections such as impetigo can probably be regarded as non-infectious after two days of antibiotic treatment, but 2 weeks might be a safer interval in the case of rarer infections.

It is important to be clear that **zoonoses** such as cattle ringworm can be transferred between animals and humans, but not between humans. A zoonosis is not therefore a risk to fellow employees despite its appearance to the contrary.

Hyperhidrosis of the hands may be a liability in engineering, causing ferrous workpieces and materials to rust. It may also be a disadvantage in work such as sales or public relations, where frequent handshaking is required. Dermatological treatment can help, but often to a limited extent, and may fail to solve the occupational problem. As with acne, however, it is important to guard against unfair discrimination at job interviews.

Race and complexion

Experimental work has detected differences in the susceptibility of skins of different racial origin and complexion to contact irritants. However, these relatively small differences are not reliable enough to enable helpful decisions to be made on fitness for work.

Pre-employment skin testing

Patch testing

Patch testing prior to employment can detect previously acquired sensitization but cannot predict future sensitization. A recommendation for universal pre-employment patch testing is therefore based on a misunderstanding of these fundamental principles, as well as a lack of recognition of the expertise required to be proficient in the technique. Anyone who carries out any patch testing at all should be properly trained and continue to practise it as part of their regular professional routine. Patch testing may be indicated in individual cases prior to employment if a past or present dermatitis has not been adequately investigated.[17]

Prick testing

Prick testing prior to employment is not generally of value from the dermatological point of view. It may help to detect an atopic constitution, but it is the history or presence of atopic eczema which indicates an increased susceptibility to contact irritants, and not an atopic constitution *per se*. Prick testing should never be carried out without full resuscitation equipment being readily available.

Other skin testing

Although interesting research has been conducted applying various standard irritants to the skin, there is not as yet any simple practical skin test that can be used to predict susceptibility either to irritants or to allergens.

Effect of the common occupational dermatoses on fitness for work

An accurate assessment and determination of the causal factors of the dermatosis is essential. Once guided by a precise diagnosis, changes in working methods and other preventive measures (such as substitution, enclosure, mechanical handling, ventilation, rotation and personal protective equipment) can be helpful. The Control of Substances Hazardous to Health (COSHH) Regulations now provide the legislative mandate for such an assessment, and require that every employee should have adequate information, instruction and training on the substances they handle at work. For those at special risk, regular health surveillance may be required to identify any indication of disease at an early stage.

In most cases of occupational dermatoses continuation in the same employment is a realistic goal, sometimes with minor adjustments to work practices. This is particularly important in the many occupational dermatoses where prognosis is known to be little altered by change of job, such as allergic contact dermatitis caused by chromate in cement among construction workers. Carefully considered preventive skin care programmes make both the primary and the secondary prevention of occupational dermatoses more effective.

Occasionally a change of occupation may be in the best interests of the individual. It must be stressed that **this should always be preceded by accurate diagnosis**. There are certain groups in which a change of job is likely to be indicated. Those who have most of their working life ahead, such as first-year apprentices, may be well advised to give up a job that is already causing them persistent contact dermatitis. When the prognosis following avoidance of further contact with a highly specialized allergen is known to be good, as it is in epoxy, acrylic, or isocyanate resin dermatitis, a rapid change of job may be indicated once the allergy has been confirmed by patch testing. Equally, when the prognosis of continued exposure to contact irritants is almost certainly bad, as it is in workers with active or previously severe atopic eczema, the best advice may be to give up the unsuitable job as soon as possible. A change of occupation may also be forced on those who have an airborne contact dermatitis, from the Compositae (Asteraceae) group of plants such as chrysanthemums, because of the inherent difficulty of preventing such exposure.

When a decision has been made to advise a change of occupation, it is essential that the alternative occupation should genuinely be more suitable.[18] Clearly, the major requirement is avoidance of the original contact factor(s). This may need expert guidance, particularly when the contact factor is widely used, e.g. allergens such as formaldehyde or irritants such as detergents. A patient with atopic eczema may otherwise change occupation with little if any benefit, as might for example happen if a hairdresser became a chef.

Up-to-date tables of occupations with a high risk of contact dermatitis and of the irritants and allergens in various occupations are to be found in the textbook by Rycroft *et al.*[9]

Sometimes, in the case of common allergies, spurious work restrictions are suggested. For example, there is a misconception that nickel allergy, which has a prevalence of about 10% of north-western European women, implies a generally increased risk of dermatitis in the engineering industry. This is probably fallacious, given the very low amounts of biologically available nickel in most of the metals used in engineering. Only prolonged contact with nickel-plated objects or nickel plating itself is likely to constitute a risk. Few of those working in supermarket checkouts or banks seem to develop hand dermatitis from handling money continually, even though nickel is a constituent of most coinage.

Special work problems, restrictions, or needs caused by skin conditions

Certain types of work may be considered unsuitable from the point of view of the employer, the insurer, or the safety engineer, though skin conditions rarely pose a safety concern. Public health considerations in healthcare, catering, and pharmaceutical industries, as detailed above, may preclude or delay the employment of certain applicants, for example those with untreated hand eczema, otitis externa, or scalp psoriasis. People working with ionizing radiation may not be considered suitable for work in areas of potential contamination if they have widespread skin lesions since these may provide a portal of entry and can present difficulties if decontamination becomes necessary.

Rehabilitation

Rehabilitation of people with occupational dermatoses rarely requires special facilities. Patients need not necessarily achieve complete clearance of their dermatitis before returning to work, especially if they can temporarily be offered alternative work away from the offending irritant or allergen. Too often employees are advised to stay off work until all trace of abnormality is gone, causing unnecessary emotional and financial strain and endangering the patients' eventual chance of returning to their original jobs. Such action, although taken for what is thought to be the best of motives, can hinder rather than help recovery.

The aim of rehabilitation in occupational dermatology is to keep the patient in the same job if at all possible, but this can be irretrievably jeopardized by prolonged sickness absence. The foundations of successful rehabilitation are close working relationships between general practitioners, dermatologists, occupational physicians, occupational hygienists, and employers; maintenance of contact between the patient and the place of work during any periods of sickness absence; and monitoring the employees' progress on their return to work.

Conclusions and recommendations

Skin conditions require thorough dermatological investigation in order to achieve a diagnosis sufficiently accurate to give reliable medical advice about employment. Even after full investigation, there may remain sufficient doubt about the aetiology and prognosis to make medical advice on employment subject to error. Because of this, an individual should often be given the benefit of any doubt on fitness for work. Medico-legal considerations may prompt an overcautious approach that is not truly in the best interests of the employee or the employer. If possible, such prompting should be resisted in a rational manner which can be legally defended.

Dermatological treatment of many common dermatoses, such as acne and psoriasis, has advanced considerably in the last few years. A patient's fitness for work may in some cases be transformed by dermatological referral and treatment prior to final placement. Occasionally, however, it will be necessary for prospective employees to be refused for certain jobs on dermatological grounds; a patient with atopic hand eczema, for example, applying to be a production engineering machine operator working with soluble oil; or a patient with extensive psoriasis applying to be a marine commando. On these occasions it is sometimes invaluable for the physician to cite the published evidence. The emphasis should always be on the accurate identification of the few dermatoses that do have genuine implications for employment, rather than on a general bar on people with skin disease.

Any medical report on a patient, however informal, that is requested for the purposes of pre-employment assessment, should be supplied only with the patient's consent, after due consideration, and with great care not to mislead unwittingly. Uncertainty should not be disguised with general statements that cannot be supported either by published evidence or experience.

Selected references and further reading

1 Rystedt I. Work-related hand eczema in atopics. *Contact Dermatitis* 1985;**12**: 164–171.
2 Cunliffe WJ. Acne and unemployment. *Br J Dermatol* 1986;**115**: 386.
3 Johnson MLT. *Skin conditions and related needs for medical care among persons 1–74 years, United States, 1971–1974.* DHEW publications no. (PHS)79–1660 (series 11; no 212). Washington, DC: US Department of Health, Education and Welfare, 1977.
4 Champion RH, Burton JL, Burns DA, Breathnach SM (ed.) *Textbook of dermatology*, 6th edn, pp. 144–145. Oxford, Blackwell, 1998.
5 Coenraads PJ, Nater JP, van der Lende R. Prevalence of eczema and other dermatoses of the hands and arms in the Netherlands. Association with age and occupation. *Clin Exp Dermatol* 1983;**8**: 495–503.
6 Turjanmaa K, Alenius H, Mäkinen-Kiljunen S, Reunala T, Palosuo T. Natural rubber latex allergy. *Allergy* 1996;**51**: 593–602.
7 EPI-DERM quarterly reports, June-December 1997. Pub. Epi-derm, Ocup. & Environ. Health, Stopford Bldg., Oxford Rd., Manchester M13 9PT
8 Health and Safety Executive. Health and safety statistics 1989–90. *Employment Gazette, Occasional Supplement* No. 2, September 1991: 60.
9 Rycroft RJG. Occupational contact dermatitis. In: *Textbook of contact dermatitis*, ed. Rycroft RJG, Menné T, Frosch PJ, Benezra C, pp. 338–397. Berlin: Springer-Verlag, 1999.
10 Cotterill JA. Constitutional skin disease in industry. In: *Essentials of industrial dermatology*, ed. Griffiths WAD, Wilkinson DS, pp. 38–46. Oxford: Blackwell, 1985.
11 Rystedt I. Factors influencing the occurrence of hand eczema in adults with a history of atopic dermatitis in childhood. *Contact Dermatitis* 1985;**12**: 185–191.
12 Posch A, Chen Z, Raulf-Heimsoth M, Baur X. Latex allergens. *Clin Exp Allergy* 1998;**28**: 134–140.
13 Noble WC. *Microbiology of human skin*, p. 325. London: Lloyd Luke, 1981.
14 Noble WC. Dispersal of skin microorganisms. *Br J Dermatol* 1975;**93**: 477–485.
15 Are the epidemiology and microbiology of methicillin-resistant *Staphylococcus aureus* changing? (editorial). *JAMA* 1998;**279**: 623–624.
16 Noble WC, Savin JA. Carriage of *Staphylococcus aureus* in psoriasis. *BMJ* 1968;**1**: 417–419.
17 Rycroft RJG. Is patch testing necessary? In: *Recent advances in dermatology* **8**, ed. Champion RH, Pye RJ, pp. 101–111. Edinburgh: Churchill Livingstone, 1990.
18 Wall LM, Gebauer KA. A follow-up study of occupational skin disease in Western Australia. *Contact Dermatitis* 1991;**24**: 241–243.

24

Acquired immune deficiency syndrome (AIDS)

A. Cockroft and P. Griffiths

Fear, anxiety and ignorance still surround human immunodeficiency virus (HIV) and acquired immune deficiency syndrome (AIDS). In this chapter the spectrum of HIV disease is reviewed and the epidemic summarized. The main problem in the workplace is the concern of non-infected workers; this should be tackled by a clear policy and an effective education programme. The virus is only transmissible by certain limited means and occupational transmission is rare, even in the healthcare setting where the risk can be reduced by implementing guidelines for safe practice. In most workplaces employees with AIDS can continue at work as long as they are physically and mentally able, and the considerations for their work are the same as for any progressive debilitating illness. There are special considerations in the healthcare setting, where official guidelines advise that HIV-infected workers should not participate in certain invasive procedures. The management of HIV-infected healthcare workers requires a sensitive, informed approach. **Confidentiality is of particular importance in the occupational issues surrounding HIV infection.**

A major problem for workers infected with HIV is the general public's perception of AIDS. No other health problem has had such wide publicity or engendered so much fear and anxiety. There is still considerable ignorance about the risks of contracting infection with HIV. It is widely perceived as being contagious—transmissible by casual and accidental contact in everyday life—despite good evidence to the contrary. Additionally, in the western world HIV infection is most prevalent amongst male homosexuals and injecting drug users; the behaviour of these groups is seen by some as deviant or morally reprehensible. Prejudice and misconceptions often influence the way that people with HIV infection are treated by others.

In reality, HIV infection is concentrated in, but not confined to, certain high-risk groups. Although the prevalence of infection in 'low-risk groups' remains low, the rate of increase in the heterosexual population now exceeds that in the traditional risk groups. The virus is only transmissible by certain limited means and in the vast majority of jobs there is no risk of workers becoming infected or of transmitting the infection to others. In the healthcare and laboratory setting there is a risk of occupational transmission of the virus, but even here the risk is very low and can be further reduced by proper precautions.

Occupational health professionals must recognize and play a part in reducing the fear, ignorance and prejudice which still surround HIV disease. If employees discover or suspect that a colleague is HIV-infected, or even suspect that they are at greater risk of infection, considerable problems and disruption can occur. Stigmatization and ostracism of such individuals can increase the burden on their physical and mental well-being where infection does exist. Such problems can be prevented by pre-emptive

Fitness for work: the medical aspects

action in the workplace. This should include education about HIV infection for all employees and support for any that are infected with HIV. The employer must decide in principle how to tackle HIV infection in employees and review existing policies and procedures relating to ill health to ensure that they are robust enough to cope with HIV disease should it arise.

The HIV epidemic is a problem for everyone. Workplace initiatives can have an important influence. They can help the community to accept the need for the changes in attitude and behaviour that are necessary to control the spread of infection and to provide adequate care for those who are already infected or who may become so.

Spectrum of disease: clinical aspects affecting work capacity

Natural history of untreated HIV infection

HIV infection results in a spectrum of disease, over a variable but prolonged time[1] (see Fig. 24.1). Individuals with HIV infection often remain asymptomatic for many years and, even with symptoms, are often fit enough to continue at work. Most people with HIV infection can and should be in employment. During the asymptomatic phase many people are unaware that they are infected and work capacity is usually unaltered although anxiety and depression can lead to difficulties, especially soon after the diagnosis has been confirmed.

It seems reasonable to advise HIV-positive people to lead as healthy a lifestyle as possible, and to avoid unhealthy behaviour such as smoking and excessive drinking. Since

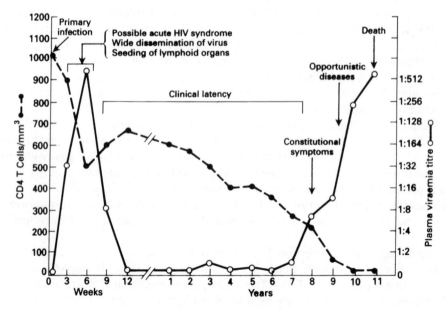

Fig. 24.1 Viraemia, CD4 lymphocyte count, and clinical disease in HIV infection (from the *New England Journal of Medicine*, 1993, pp. 328–329, reprinted by permission

stress can affect the immune system, it also seems wise to avoid stressful situations as far as possible, including those at work. Psychological symptoms may be prominent. Anxiety and depression are common, especially if individuals have not received adequate counselling before and after HIV testing. Psychological problems are often severe enough to affect work capacity, at least in the short term. Most HIV-infected individuals learn to cope with the diagnosis with the help of counselling, but problems in coping with work will be worsened if they receive a negative and unsympathetic response from employers and colleagues to whom they reveal their diagnosis.

In a proportion of those infected with HIV an initial acute retroviral illness occurs about 2–8 weeks after infection. It is self-limiting and may go unrecognized, often being attributed to influenza or glandular fever. Antibodies to HIV appear in the blood about 6 weeks after infection, while at the same time the viral load in the blood falls from the very high level that may occur soon after infection to a plateau (see Fig. 24.1). The higher the level at which the viral load plateaus, the more rapid is the subsequent progression to AIDS.[2] After a variable period of years, symptoms begin to appear and there is a further rise in the level of viraemia. Once the CD4 (T helper cell) lymphocyte count has declined to less than 200 x 10^6/litre, indicating extensive damage to the immune system, the risk of disease increases. The latest American definition of AIDS includes HIV infection with a CD4 count below 200 x 10^6/litre, even in the absence of other AIDS-defining features, but in the UK a low CD4 count alone is not considered sufficient to make the diagnosis.

Clinical syndromes related to AIDS[1] include persistent generalized lymphadenopathy (PGL), which can occur relatively early after infection and may be associated with fatigue which limits the capacity for full-time work, especially if it is physically taxing. Later symptoms include fever, night sweats, significant and rapid weight loss, malaise, and skin rashes. As AIDS progresses there may be repeated episodes of opportunistic infections, such as *Pneumocystis carinii* pneumonia, herpes zoster, cytomegalovirus (CMV) infections, systemic fungal infections, and infection with mycobacteria. Infection with *Mycobacterium tuberculosis* is an increasingly frequent feature of AIDS in the US and developing countries. Although tuberculosis is not yet a prominent feature in the UK AIDS epidemic, it may become so in the future. Malignancies such as Kaposi's sarcoma (caused by human herpes virus 8) and lymphoma (usually caused by Epstein–Barr virus) can affect almost any part of the body. Neurological involvement in AIDS includes dementia, specific neurological deficits, and psychotic syndromes. AIDS-related dementia can be caused by HIV itself or by CMV, and minor degrees of mental impairment are common in the late stages of HIV disease.

Once AIDS has developed, there is usually serious debility, even between acute episodes of infection, so that most people are unable to continue in full-time work. The prognosis of untreated AIDS is very poor, and more than half of AIDS cases die within 2 years of diagnosis.

Alteration of natural history by treating opportunistic infections

Better treatment and prophylaxis of opportunistic infections have improved the prognosis a little and led to an improved quality of remaining life. Improvements in survival can be attributed to:

- the 'learning curve' of physicians in recognizing new presentations of opportunistic disease and treating them promptly
- the strong beneficial effect of giving prophylaxis against *P. carinii* once the CD4 count declines to 200 x 10^6/litre
- the ability of acyclovir to inhibit herpes virus infections, which otherwise could act as cofactors, enhancing HIV and increasing its pathogenicity.

Alteration of natural history by potent antiretroviral drugs

Early studies with drugs such as zidovudine showed transient reductions in viral load with definite clinical benefits, but these were short-lived. Dual therapy with antiretroviral drugs proved some additional benefit but, again, only transiently. In contrast, the administration of three antiretroviral compounds has dramatically reduced HIV viral load, halted progressive damage to the immune system and allowed some immune recovery sufficient to prevent most opportunistic infections. At the time of writing, such **highly active antiretroviral therapy (HAART)** has had a profound effect on the prognosis of AIDS, allowing previously debilitated patients to return to work and leading to closure of in-patient facilities for AIDS patients in many cities.

Several antiretroviral drugs have produced these benefits. Some inhibit the reverse transcriptase enzyme because they resemble the natural substrates and so are termed nucleoside reverse transcriptase inhibitors (NRTIs). Others inhibit the same enzyme by binding to a different site; they are chemically diverse[3] and are termed non-nucleoside reverse transcriptase inhibitors (NNRTIs). The third group of drugs inhibit the protease enzyme of HIV and are termed protease inhibitors (PIs). Combination HAART usually involves one PI plus two NRTIs in current practice, but ongoing trials indicate that one NNRTI plus two NRTIs may also be effective. The objective of treatment is to bring the viral load down to the lowest possible level so that replication falls below the amount required to cause disease and below the amount necessary to generate resistant strains. Compliance with prescribed therapy will therefore be of major importance and the development of combination tablets (e.g. zidovudine plus lamivudine) should help this. In addition, there is no *a priori* reason to believe that three drugs will always be required; novel compounds with excellent potency such as abacavir (an NRTI) may form the basis of two-drug HAART regimes in the future.

The HIV / AIDS epidemic

HIV infection in the UK has been mainly spread by sexual intercourse, especially between men. However, increasing numbers of AIDS cases are being contracted through heterosexual intercourse and injecting drug use. The annual incidence of AIDS cases in the UK to the end of September 1998 is shown in Fig. 24.2. Coinciding with the availability of HAART at the end of 1995, the number of patients progressing to AIDS has decreased dramatically. Furthermore, the decreased death rate from AIDS due to HAART means that the overall prevalence of AIDS is now increasing rapidly. Figures for HIV-positive people are less reliable, based only on confidential reporting by physicians, but are clearly much higher than the number of AIDS cases. Table 24.1 shows the

Table 24.1 Frequency of HIV infection by exposure category and latest reported stage: UK data to end of December 1998

How HIV infection was probably acquired	Latest report stage number (%)				Total
	Infection only reported	AIDS reported	Death from reported AIDS	Death without reported AIDS	
Homosexual sex	11 109 (49)	2845 (13)	8181 (36)	584 (22)	22 719
Heterosexual sex	5019 (63)	1203 (15)	1535 (19)	199 (3)	7956
Injecting drug use	2072 (59)	293 (9)	731 (21)	393 (11)	3489
Blood products	480 (35)	60 (5)	585 (43)	229 (17)	1353
Blood/tissue transfusion	102 (38)	35 (13)	106 (39)	28 (10)	271
Mother to infant	232 (42)	169 (31)	137 (25)	8 (2)	546
Other/undetermined	805 (71)	34 (3)	121 (11)	171 (15)	1131
Total	19 819 (53)	4639 (12)	11 396 (30)	1612 (5)	37 465

Source: AIDS and HIV infection in the UK: monthly report. *Commun Dis Rep* 1999;**9**(5): 45, Table 1.

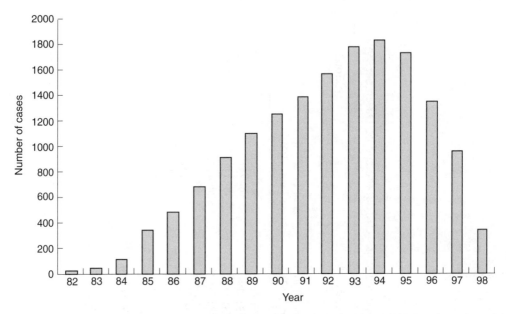

Fig. 24.2 AIDS cases in the UK by year of diagnosis (up to September 1998). Total number of cases 15 756. Source: PHLS AIDS and STD Centre—Communicable Disease Surveillance Centre, and Scottish Centre for Infection and Environmental Health. Unpublished Quarterly Surveillance Tables No. 41, 98/3, Table 2.

number of HIV infected people in the UK by exposure category and latest reported stage of disease to the end of December 1998.

Modes of transmission (general)

By far the commonest mode of transmission of HIV is by sexual contact, both between men and between men and women. Sexual contact between men has been particularly prominent as a means of transmitting HIV in the western world, but the majority of cases of HIV infection worldwide are acquired by heterosexual contact. Transmission can also occur via transfusion of infected blood or blood products (such as factor VIII). This is no longer a risk in the UK and in other developed countries where blood donations are screened and people who are at risk of HIV infection are discouraged from giving blood, but it continues to be a risk in some parts of the world. Transmission by blood or blood products occurs mainly when needles and other equipment are shared by injecting drug users; this has been an important mode of transmission in some UK cities and in continental Europe, especially Spain and Italy, where up to 60% of HIV infections occur in injecting drug users or their partners. Transmission can also occur from infected women to their children, occasionally *in utero* or more usually at delivery, or via infected breast milk after birth. None of these modes of transmission is likely to occur in the workplace, except in very specialized circumstances.

Workplace transmission

The risk of transmission of HIV in the workplace is very low. The risks are confined to accidental exposures to material containing live virus, namely

- inoculation injuries with contaminated sharp instruments or tissues (e.g. needlestick injuries)
- contamination of broken skin or mucous membranes.

It is clear that HIV is very much less transmissible than hepatitis B in these circumstances. Large prospective studies have found that the risk of transmission of HIV after a single infected needlestick is about 0.3%,[4] whereas the equivalent risk for hepatitis B (e antigen positive source) is up to 30%, and that for hepatitis C is around 3% (see p. 295–301).

Up to December 1997, 286 cases of occupational transmission of HIV from contact with infected blood had been reported worldwide, mostly related to needlestick or other percutaneous injuries (Table 24.2).[4] This is very likely an underestimate of the actual number of occupational infections that have occurred (especially in developing countries with poor reporting systems), but nevertheless the number is very small in relation to the many thousands of procedures carried out on patients with HIV infection, including circumstances where infection control provisions are inadequate.

Occupational transmission in the healthcare setting includes transfer of the infection in both directions—from patients to healthcare workers or from healthcare workers to patients. There are only two reported cases of the latter:

- a Florida dentist with AIDS who transmitted HIV to five of his patients in the course of his practice[5]
- an orthopaedic surgeon in France who transmitted HIV to an elderly woman during a surgical procedure.[6]

In the case of the dentist, the exact mode of transmission was unclear, although disinfection procedures were grossly inadequate. Clearly, the risk of occupational infection to healthcare workers is far greater than the risk of an HIV-infected healthcare worker infecting patients or colleagues. These two reported cases of HIV transmission to patients contrast with the steady stream of clusters of hepatitis B infection contracted from infected healthcare workers, mainly surgeons and dentists.[7]

Prevention of occupational HIV transmission in the healthcare setting relies on safe practice to avoid exposure to blood and body fluids.[8] Some people consider that a two-tier

Table 24.2 Occupational transmission of HIV up to December 1997[4]

	USA	UK	Rest of Europe	Rest of world	Total
Documented seroconversions (specific exposure incident)	52	4	28	11	95
Possible occupational infection (no lifestyle risks)	114	8	56	13	191
Totals	166	12	84	24	286

approach, with identification of infected patients and special precautions in their case, is both feasible and cost-effective. However, it is now increasingly accepted that a 'universal precautions' approach should be adopted.[9,10] This means that all blood is considered infectious and precautions to avoid needlesticks and skin or mucous membrane exposures to blood are taken with all patients and with all blood and tissue samples.[10] Local guidelines should be drawn up for safe practice in all situations where contact with blood or body fluids is possible; all employees who may have contact with blood or body fluids should be trained in these practices and the adherence to practice guidelines should be regularly reviewed. Protective equipment and clothing, such as gloves, gowns and eye protection, should be provided as necessary. Under the Control of Substances Hazardous to Health (COSHH) Regulations, employers are required to assess risks to the health of employees and others from hazardous substances and to take steps to reduce these risks. The regulations include biological hazards, such as blood that could contain infectious agents. The level of precautions required for a particular procedure will depend on the likelihood of blood exposure during that procedure. **In the healthcare setting the precautions taken to protect employees from infected patients will also serve to protect patients from any infected employees.**

Despite all precautions, accidental exposures to blood will continue to occur in healthcare work and related occupations. Such exposures cause great anxiety to employees, especially if the blood involved is known to be infected with HIV. Procedures for reporting and managing blood exposure incidents should be set up and publicized to employees.[11,12] There is evidence from a case-referent study, that a reduction in the rate of HIV seroconversion after HIV-positive needlestick injuries occurs when zidovudine is given.[13] Recent new guidance recommends the use of post-exposure prophylaxis after an exposure incident to HIV-infected blood.[14] The recommended regime is four weeks of zidovudine, lamivudine (both NRTIs), and indinavir (a PI). This regime has significant side-effects; a recent review of 15 healthcare workers taking post-exposure prophylaxis with the recommended three drugs found that three-quarters of them had to have time off work (often for most of the 4 weeks) due to disabling side-effects, especially nausea (Dr S. Williams, personal communication). Reports from the US suggest that many people there discontinue the regime before 4 weeks because of the side-effects.

There is no need to restrict temporarily the duties of healthcare workers who have had accidental exposure to HIV-infected blood, even if their duties involve invasive procedures where their blood could contact the patient's tissues ('exposure-prone invasive procedures').[14] The risk of seroconversion is so small (around 0.3% and lessened further by suitable post-exposure prophylaxis) and the risk of transmission to patients, if infected, is so small that the combined risk is virtually zero. Individuals who have had accidental exposure to HIV-infected blood may want to use condoms for a period to avoid any possible risk of transmission to their sexual partner. This issue should be raised with them while discussing the incident, leaving the final decision to them and their partners.

Healthcare workers who practice abroad in areas of high HIV endemicity and poor standards of infection control may be at a significant cumulative risk of contracting HIV from infected needlesticks and other accidental blood exposures. It has been suggested that this excess risk may be sufficient to justify their having a test for HIV antibodies on their return to the UK. A particular concern is with medical students on electives overseas, and it has been suggested that they should take with them a course of the recommended three-drug post-exposure prophylaxis in case of an infected needlestick. However, this raises several problems and many would argue that it is better for students to avoid going on electives to places with high rates of HIV infection and poor infection control and healthcare arrangements.

One special case of occupational transmission of HIV is in relation to sex workers. Studies have shown varying prevalences of HIV infection among prostitutes in different parts of the UK. Prostitutes are clearly at risk of HIV infection, as well as other sexually transmitted diseases, as are their clients. Preventive measures (i.e. safer sex practices such as the correct use of condoms and avoidance of activities likely to cause trauma or bleeding) are particularly important in this group.

Workplace education and dealing with prejudice

As indicated in the introduction to this chapter, the main problems in the workplace often arise from those employees who are not HIV infected rather than those who are.[15,16] Unreasonable and irrelevant demands may result from lack of accurate information, fear, or prejudice. The demands can relate not only to known infected individuals but also to individuals perceived to be at risk of being infected. Examples of such demands have included refusal to work with HIV-infected employees, with haemophiliacs, with gay men or those thought to be gay, and requests for separate work equipment, toilet facilities, or canteens.

Many of these difficulties can be successfully tackled by a combination of a clear policy in the organization, supported by senior management, and a programme of education for employees at all levels. Action is most effective if taken before problems arise. Many companies in the UK now have policies relating to HIV infection. These policies usually include statements about confidentiality, employment rights and the non-acceptability of workplace discrimination against colleagues with known or suspected HIV infection, and are often accompanied by a programme of employee education.[17] To be effective, policies need to be implemented should the need arise, to the extent of taking disciplinary action.

Box 24.1   Elements of a policy on HIV in the workplace

- Background information about modes of transmission, lack of risk in the workplace
- Employment policy regarding HIV in job applicants
- Statement on rights to confidentiality about all medical information, including HIV status
- Statement about rights of workers who become ill from any cause, e.g. right to redeployment, medical retirement
- Statement about non-acceptability of workplace discrimination on basis of known or suspected HIV status
- Statement on programme of education for staff about HIV issues
- Statement about arrangement for advising HIV-infected staff in confidence about any necessary work limitations (for healthcare setting only).

Workplace education programmes need involvement of all of the relevant parties, including occupational health professionals, human resources specialists, and others concerned with staff training. General public health campaigns in the UK have been designed to heighten awareness of the risks of transmission of HIV; in the workplace these messages need to be accompanied by more reassuring ones about the lack of risk from everyday activities at work. Programmes should be tailored to the level of the audience concerned and should include basic information about the nature of HIV and AIDS, the modes of transmission of HIV, the risks of transmission in different circumstances, and the need to treat colleagues with AIDS like anyone else with a serious illness. The opportunity can also be taken to inform employees about how to protect themselves from HIV infection in their own personal lives. This may be backed up for example, by provision of condom vending machines in the company toilets.

Education is needed particularly for employees who travel abroad as part of their work[16] (see Appendix 5). They need to be made aware of the risks of casual sexual encounters in countries where there is a high prevalence of HIV infection. They also need to know how to reduce the risk of having accidents which may result in the need for an emergency blood transfusion abroad; avoidance of excess alcohol before driving is important. Some companies have arrangements whereby employees stationed abroad act as a 'walking blood bank' for colleagues at nearby locations who may need transfusions. Employees travelling to areas with high endemic rates of HIV infection and poor healthcare facilities may wish to carry a travel kit containing sterile disposable syringes and needles, but should remember that these are of limited use should an accident occur that makes blood transfusion necessary.

Encouragingly, there is now evidence that programmes of education can improve knowledge and attitudes about HIV infection. In the authors' experience, there are now individuals with AIDS being given help and support by colleagues at all levels in an organization, whereas in the early years of the epidemic there were cases of physical intimidation of employees suspected of being HIVpositive.

Care of the HIV-infected employee

Modifications of working practices are not necessary to protect others from infection by HIV-infected workers, expect in very special circumstances (see below: HIV-infected healthcare workers). When these are necessary for their work, HIV-infected people can be given any of the licensed viral vaccines, although it is prudent that they be given the killed (rather than the usual live) polio vaccine, but they should not be given BCG. Modifications may be required by the Disability Discrimination Act 1995 (DDA) to allow HIV-infected individuals suffering physical and psychological problems to stay at work as long as possible. Individual workers with HIV infection should be able to discuss their diagnosis, in confidence, with an occupational physician and be given support and advice as necessary. The advice given will depend on the clinical stage of the disease and the individual's work circumstances. Liaison between the individual's general practitioner and specialist's team and the occupational physician will foster the best management. The individual's consent for such communication is, of course, necessary.

In the asymptomatic stage, support must be provided to deal with anxiety and depression. This can come from the clinical and counselling team concerned with the worker's care and from the occupational health service. Once symptoms of fatigue and malaise appear, it may be necessary to consider modified duties or reduced working hours. Work that involves heavy physical exertion or significant stress (such as time pressures or caring for ill patients) is usually best avoided if possible. It is helpful, with the individual's consent, to involve the immediate manager. When AIDS has developed, the individual will need to visit hospital frequently for treatment and monitoring and there will be episodes of acute illness. It is difficult to maintain work in this phase but some form of flexible work arrangement that utilizes the skills of the individual can be beneficial to both the worker and the organization. Neurological deficits are frequent in more advanced forms of HIV disease and these will affect the work an individual is able to undertake. Careful assessment and monitoring is necessary to ensure that the individual remains capable of the work and is not unsafe because of, for example, impaired memory or difficulties with concentration.

When work is no longer possible, retirement on ill health grounds should be arranged where this is available in the organization. In this respect AIDS is no different from any other progressive debilitating disease. In the authors' experience, it is useful to discuss with workers, while they are still relatively well, the work arrangement that can be made as they become ill. This should include the possibilities of part-time working and ill health retirement. Early discussion allows individuals to think about choices (for example about redeployment options) in advance and to feel more confident about what will happen as they become ill. This approach of dealing with 'dreaded issues' in advance is often used in general AIDS counselling.[18]

Pre-employment screening, HIV testing, and the DDA

The idea of HIV antibody testing as a condition of employment is controversial.[17,18] In support of such a policy, it is argued that this enables the employer to reject prospective employees who are infected, thus avoiding the eventual problems associated with future morbidity or mortality as well as trouble from other employees. A number of companies operate a policy of pre-employment HIV testing and this is legal so long as it is applied equally to men and women and to all races. Since HIV infection alone does not affect 'normal day to day activities' it does not fall within the DDA, so testing and refusing employment to people who are HIV positive remains lawful. Although HIV infection is specifically mentioned in the DDA *Definition of disability* booklet,[19] a person who is HIV positive would not be protected by the Act until they first develop symptoms that affect their ability to carry out normal day to day activities. Even the diagnosis of AIDS, by whatever criteria, would not bring a person within the meaning of the Act until the condition affected 'normal day to day activities'.

In addition, there are important ethical and other criticisms of pre-employment HIV screening.[20,21] The test may be negative for up to 3 months after infection and tested employees may become infected after employment. This may lead to calls for exclusion of so-called high-risk groups such as haemophiliacs or homosexual men, with or without HIV testing. It could even extend to excluding people with many sexual partners.

Being HIV infected does not affect work capacity, except in healthcare workers, unless disease develops, and there is no accurate way of determining prognosis regarding work capacity. If the occupational pension scheme is a concern, there is no longer a requirement for an employee to belong to the company scheme. To be consistent, employers enacting a policy of pre-employment HIV screening should also consider excluding other individuals with a high risk of future morbidity such as heavy smokers or those who consume large quantities of alcohol.

Occupational physicians and nurses have a duty of care towards candidates for employment.[21] Screening for HIV offers little advantage to the employer and may have disadvantages to the candidate, which are both psychological and social. Any testing must always be preceded by competent and informed consent. The candidate must be informed of the test result, strict confidentiality maintained and post-test counselling undertaken. **Routine pre-employment screening without adequate pre- and post-test counselling is not ethical, and occupational physicians should not lend themselves to such a policy.[21]**

Routine HIV screening of all donated blood is necessary to protect the safety of those requiring blood transfusion. However, it is important that those who have been at risk of acquiring infection do not donate blood; this reduces the risk of donations within the window period before antibodies appear. Blood donation sessions at work may lead to pressure on everyone to donate, including individuals who know themselves to have been at risk recently. Such undue pressure should be avoided. To help with this problem, the transfusion service will accept an individual's confidential instruction to discard donated blood if the donor is concerned about its safety.

Infected healthcare workers

There is considerable public concern about the risk of transmission of HIV from infected doctors and other healthcare workers to their patients. There is evidence from observational studies in operating theatres of a high rate of sharps injuries during surgical procedures (up to 10% in some specialties) with the sharp instrument re-contacting the patients' tissues in up to 30% of injuries, so giving a potential for transmission of infection from operator to patient.[22] In practice, there is only one reported case of transmission of HIV to a patient during a surgical procedure.[6] More than 19 000 patients of HIV-infected healthcare workers have been followed up, with no cases of transmission demonstrated.[23] In the few patients found to be HIV positive (as expected among 19 000), genetic sequencing indicated that they did not have the same strain of virus as the healthcare worker concerned.[23]

Official guidance about HIV-infected healthcare workers in both the US and the UK[24,25] is that those who are infected with HIV should not carry out invasive procedures where there is a risk that their blood may contact the patient's open tissues. Situations likely to be particularly risky are those where the operator's hands are incompletely visible in a restricted space within the body cavity. This may occur, for example, during gynaecological procedures in the pelvis or during dental procedures. Importantly, in neither the UK nor the US is screening of healthcare workers for HIV recommended. However, healthcare workers who suspect that they may be infected are expected to have themselves tested. If testing confirms infection, they have an ethical duty to seek professional advice about any limitation of their practice that may be necessary and to act on that advice.[26] Current UK guidance states that a doctor caring for a healthcare worker who is HIV infected and who does not take advice about ceasing to perform invasive procedures should inform the appropriate professional body and the employer.[25] There is an expert panel in the UK to provide advice about limitation of practice when this cannot be agreed locally.

Occupational physicians with responsibility for healthcare workers have an important role in the management of HIV-infected workers, as emphasized in the government guidance on the issue.[25] They must encourage workers who suspect or know themselves to be infected to come to them for sensitive and confidential advice. If limitation of practice is necessary, the occupational physician should advise management accordingly but without revealing any clinical information and with the agreement of the individual concerned. Each case should be dealt with individually after taking expert virological and other advice as necessary. A blanket view that all infected healthcare workers will automatically be banned from all surgical procedures, even modern minimally invasive procedures, is unhelpful and is likely to discourage concerned healthcare workers from coming forward for testing and seeking advice. There is already disquiet that the present official guidance in the UK and the US may be a disincentive to healthcare workers to have themselves tested for HIV, since it could be seen as penalizing the conscientious.

Where possible, infected healthcare workers who cannot continue with their normal duties should be re-deployed without loss of income. This will require a sympathetic approach by management, and the occupational physician has a role to protect workers. If it seems likely that the HIV infection was acquired occupationally, healthcare workers should be able to claim injuries benefit under the NHS Employees' Scheme even though HIV is not a disease prescribed for state benefit in the UK. Clearly however, this would not compensate the individual fully for loss of a career.

Confidentiality is of great importance when dealing with HIV infection, and healthcare workers have the same rights to confidentiality as anyone else.[20] Patients can be reassured that the routine precautions taken in their care protect them from the tiny risk of infection from their carers. Repeated routing screening of healthcare workers, which is sometimes demanded by pressure groups, cannot offer foolproof protection because infectivity precedes antibody development by several weeks; it is neither justifiable nor feasible. The decision concerning whether to notify and offer testing to patients who have been operated on by a surgeon found to be HIV-infected is a difficult one; incomplete follow-up testing is of limited value, but the anxiety caused to the patients may outweigh any possible benefits. Where healthcare workers known to be HIV-infected have been involved in invasive procedures, employers are officially advised that they must contact the patients concerned and offer them counselling and HIV testing if they wish it.[25] They must endeavour to preserve the confidentiality of the worker concerned, although in practice it is often difficult to prevent the individual's identity from becoming public knowledge.

The risk of transmission of HIV to patients is not the only consideration in the occupational management of an infected healthcare worker. Such workers should be under regular medical supervision. If they become immunosuppressed, they may be at risk of acquiring infections from patients and should not work in areas where such infections are frequently encountered; conversely, they may acquire infections, such as mycobacteria, that could be transmitted to patients and colleagues. Liaison is essential between the physician caring for the healthcare worker and the occupational physician.

Hepatitis B and healthcare workers (see also Chapter 15, p, 300)

Because of the similarities between HIV and hepatitis B and C viruses in mode of transmission and occupational risks, mention should be made of the situation in healthcare workers infected with hepatitis B and hepatitis C.

Official guidance in the UK is that healthcare workers who are 'high-infectivity' carriers of **hepatitis B**, indicated by the presence of the e antigen, should not participate in invasive procedures.[27] Recent reports show that healthcare workers who are HbsAg positive but HbeAg negative (so called 'low-infectivity' carriers) can sometimes transmit infection to patients during invasive procedures.[28] However, current guidance is that such low-infectivity carriers of hepatitis B can continue to undertake invasive procedures unless they are shown to transmit to patients.[27] This judgement has been made partly because the risk is apparently low and partly because there is no easy and reliable way at present of determining which of them is particularly likely to transmit infection. In the light of the accumulating evidence of transmission from some workers who are HbsAg positive, HbeAg negative, together with improvements in quantitative techniques for detecting DNA in the blood, revised guidelines are likely to be published soon. In addition, potent new antiviral drugs active against HBV are in clinical trial, so it is possible that some staff members may in the future be rendered non-infectious by new treatments.

In view of the availability of an effective vaccine and the substantial evidence of transmission of hepatitis B from healthcare workers to patients, the official guidance in the UK states that it should be a condition of employment in workers undertaking invasive procedures that they are immunized against hepatitis B and are not e antigen positive.[27] Experience in large programmes of hepatitis B immunization and antibody testing among healthcare workers suggests that e antigen positive individuals are rare. Since infection in early life is more often associated with the carrier state, many of the workers found to be carriers of hepatitis B (including the e antigen) come from countries with a high endemicity of hepatitis B. Occupational physicians should be involved in drawing up and implementing local policies about hepatitis B and employment in the healthcare setting and should provide confidential advice to healthcare workers who are found to be e antigen positive.[27]

In the case of **hepatitis C**, although there are two reported cases of transmission from infected healthcare workers to patients, the current UK guidance is that only hepatitis C infected healthcare workers who are shown to have transmitted to patients need be barred from undertaking invasive procedures. This guidance may change as more evidence accumulates and, perhaps, markers for particular infectivity of hepatitis C carriers are identified. Physicians advising healthcare workers who are 'low-infectivity' carriers of hepatitis B or who have antibodies to hepatitis C should make it clear to them that the guidelines may become more stringent in the future so that they would be unwise to embark on a career involving invasive procedures.

No vaccine is available for protection against hepatitis C infection, and there is evidence that healthcare workers in certain settings have an increased prevalence of antibodies to hepatitis C, related to occupational exposures. There is currently no recommendation in the UK to screen healthcare workers, even those undertaking invasive procedures, for antibodies to hepatitis C. There is also no sign yet of any potent antiviral drugs active against hepatitis C which could be used to treat healthcare workers.

Conclusions and recommendations

The background, natural history, and risks to life associated with HIV infection and related disease have predisposed to discrimination within the workplace and to stigmatization of perceived risk groups. Pre-emptive strategies to educate and inform people at work about HIV may prevent workplace problems and reduce stress for infected individuals and those at risk of infection. Occupational physicians have an important part to play in this process.

The continued employment of infected workers, with or without constitutional illness, is feasible. It is an important factor in the successful management of their condition and should be strongly encouraged. Indeed, a sympathetic and realistic approach to this problem may encourage at-risk workers to seek testing and advice about HIV, potentially leading to improved management of their condition. The modifications of work and environment which may be needed are not different in principle from those likely to be necessary for any employee with a progressive and debilitating condition. The possibility of neuropsychiatric manifestations may impose some restrictions on employment in certain occupations, particularly as these may appear relatively rapidly in a younger than usual age group.

Particular considerations apply in the healthcare setting, both to reduce the small risk of occupational infection and to ensure that HIV-infected workers do not pose any risk of infection to patients. Other blood-borne viral infections are also an issue in the healthcare setting, notably hepatitis B and hepatitis C.

Because of the fear and prejudice that are still associated with HIV infection, strict adherence to the normal professional duty of confidentiality is of particular importance for individuals with HIV infection, both in their clinical care and their occupational health management.

Selected references

1 Mindel A (ed). *AIDS: a pocketbook of diagnosis and management*. London: Edward Arnold, 1990.

2 Melors JW, Rinaldo CR Jr, Gupta P, White RM, Todd JA, Kingsley LA. Prognosis in HIV-1 infection predicted by the quality of virus in plasma. *Science* 1996;**272**: 1167–1170.

3 De Clercq E. What can be expected from non-nucleoside reverse transcriptase inhibitors (NNRTIs) in the treatment of human immunodeficiency virus type 1 (HIV-1) infections? *Rev Med Virol* 1996;**6**: 97–117.

4 PHLS AIDS and STC Centre at the Communicable Disease Surveillance Centre and Collaborators. *Occupational transmission of HIV: summary of published reports*. CDSC, London December 1997.

5 Ciesielski C, Marianos D, Ou C-Y *et al*. Transmission of human immunodeficiency virus in a dental practice. *Ann Intern Med* 1992;**116**: 798–805.
6 Anonymous. French patient contracts AIDS from surgeon. *BMJ* 1997;**314**: 250.
7 Heptonstall J. Outbreaks of hepatitis B virus infection associated with infected surgical staff. *Commun Dis Rep* 1991;1: R81–R85.
8 *A code of practice for the safe use and disposal of sharps*. London: British Medical Association, 1990.
9 Centers for Disease Control. Update: universal precautions for prevention of transmission of human immunodeficiency virus, hepatitis B virus and other blood borne pathogens in health care settings. *Morbidity Mortality Wkly Rep* 1988;**37**: 377–388.
10 UK Health Departments. *Guidance for clinical health care workers: protection against infection with blood-borne viruses. Recommendations of the Expert Advisory Group on AIDS and the Advisory Group on Hepatitis*. London: Department of Health, 1998.
11 Oakley K, Gooch C, Cockcroft A. A review of incidents involving exposure to blood in a London teaching hospital, 1989–91. *BMJ* 1992;**304**: 949–951.
12 Cockroft A, Williams S. Occupational transmission of HIV and management of accidental blood exposures. *Med Internat* 1993;**21**(1): 38–40.
13 Cardo DM, Culver DH, Ciesielski CA *et al*. A case-control study of HIV seroconversion in health care workers after percutaneous exposure. *New Engl J Med* 1997;**337**: 1485–1490.
14 UK Health Departments. *Guidance on post-exposure prophylaxis for health care workers occupationally exposed to HIV*. PL/CO (97). London: Department of Health, 1997.
15 Department of Employment and Health and Safety Executive. *AIDS and employment*. London: Central Office of Information, 1987.
16 *What employers should know about HIV and AIDS*. London: Society of Occupational Medicine, 1992.
17 Williams S, Cockcroft A. Policies for HIV and hepatitis B infected health care workers. *Occup Health Rev* 1992;**36**: 12–14.
18 Bor R, Miller R, Goldman G. *Theory and practice of HIV counselling: a systematic approach*. London: Cassell, 1992.
19 *The Disability Discrimination Act: definition of disability*. DL60. London: Minister for Disabled People, April 1996.
20 Sieghart P. *AIDS and human rights: a UK perspective*. London: British Medical Association Foundation for AIDS, 1989.
21 *HIV infection and AIDS: ethical considerations for the medical profession*, 2nd edn. London: British Medical Association Foundation for AIDS, 1992.
22 *HIV infection: hazards of transmission to patients and health care workers during invasive procedures. Report of a working group of the Royal College of Pathologists*. London: Royal College of Pathologists, 1992.
23 Centers for Disease Control. Update: investigations of persons treated by HIV-infected health care workers–United States. *Morbidity Mortality Wkly Rep* 1993;**42**: 329–337.
24 Centers for Disease Control. Recommendations for preventing transmission of human immunodeficiency virus and hepatitis B virus to patients during exposure-prone invasive procedures. *Morbidity Mortality Wkly Rep* 1991;**40**(RR-8).
25 UK Health Departments. *AIDS–HIV infected health care workers: guidance on the management of infected health care workers and patient notification*. London: Department of Health, December 1998.
26 *HIV infection and AIDS: the ethical considerations*. London: General Medical Council, October 1995.
27 UK Health Departments. *Protecting health care workers and patients from hepatitis B*. London: Department of Health, August 1993. Addendum under cover of EL(96)77, 1996.

28   The Incident Investigation Team and others. Transmission of hepatitis B to patients from four infected surgeons without hepatitis B e-antigen. *New Engl J Med* 1997;**336**: 178–184.

Further reading

Vitry-Henry C, Pénalba I, Béguinot S, Deschamps F. Relationships between work and HIV/AIDS status. *Occup Med* 1999 **49**(2): 115–116.

25

Alcohol and drug misuse

G. Smith and C. C. H. Cook

Misuse of alcohol and other drugs is of concern both to employers and to company medical officers and produces an adverse effect in the workplace, be it in terms of output and performance or other behaviour, such as interaction with colleagues. It also has an important impact on the health and well-being of employees, and carries significant legal implications for both employees and employers.

Alcohol and drug misuse is an important cost to industry in terms of lost production, reduced speed of work, mistakes in procedures, damaged equipment and compensation claims for accidents and injuries. Accident proneness, frequent sickness absence, poor work performance, and erratic behaviour should indicate to managers and occupational physicians the possibility that an employee may be drinking heavily, or misusing illicit or prescribed drugs. Alcohol has been implicated in a wide variety of industrial accidents especially drowning, falling from heights, burns, and road traffic accidents.

During any 12-month period about 12% of the population of the UK will suffer from a drinking problem. During a similar period, about 8% of men and 2% of women will experience alcohol dependence.[1] Occupational physicians should be concerned both with acute alcohol intoxication and with long-term misuse of alcohol. The former has an obvious and immediate effect on the handling of dangerous machinery and other activities requiring dexterity and judgement, whereas the latter leads to absenteeism and inefficiency, with colleagues often colluding with and covering up for the alcohol-dependent employee.

Features suggestive of a drinking problem include absenteeism, frequent accidents, obvious physical signs (such as tremulousness or the odour of alcohol), changes in personality, and erratic behaviour at work. Colleagues and supervisors might be aware of inappropriate talkativeness, and a tendency to be argumentative. Both alcohol and drug-using employees have a high absenteeism rate,[2,3] as well as having more accidents and injuries, causing breakages, demoralizing colleagues, and even stealing from them and their employers to support their addiction.

Certain occupations are associated with a substantially higher rate of problem drinking. Liver cirrhosis mortality is the best available indicator of the relative prevalence rates of alcoholism. Higher mortality from this condition is found in licensees, members of the catering and hotel trade, seamen, the armed services, sales representatives, brewers and distillers, journalists, and legal and medical practitioners. Factors contributing to this wide occupational spread include the availability of alcohol at work (sometimes even provided free or at a reduced price), social pressure to drink, and self-selection by people with established drink problems for entry into jobs where alcohol is easily or cheaply available. Freedom from supervision is a factor in independent professions such as medicine, the law, and journalism. Other groups, such as servicemen and seamen, who are separated from normal social relationships and have limited opportunities for recreation, may also resort to drinking excessively.

Alcohol and drugs in the occupational setting

Alcohol

The risk of causing a driving accident increases 3-, 10-, and 40-fold if the blood alcohol concentration (BAC) exceeds 80, 100, or 150 mg/100 ml respectively. In fact many skills and cognitive processes begin to decline at much lower BACs. In the US armed forces a blood alcohol level of 50 mg/100 ml or above indicates unfitness for duty and such a level merits disciplinary action. At this level memory transfer from immediate recall to permanent storage may be disturbed, causing impairment of long-term recall. Companies operating oil and gas rigs offshore ban alcohol completely and refuse access to the work site to anyone reporting for duty under the influence of alcohol. Studies of pilots in flight simulators indicate that performance is impaired at a BAC as low as 11 mg/100 ml, the equivalent of consuming only one standard drink.[4]

It has been shown that driving at levels below the prescribed blood alcohol level introduced in the Road Traffic Act 1967 (80 mg/100 ml) is not free from hazards. Even 'safe' levels of alcohol may be associated with significant impairment of driving ability. Drivers who have consumed moderate doses of alcohol and have BACs of 30–60 mg/100 ml have impaired ability to negotiate a test course with artificial hazards. Furthermore it has been shown that the combination of alcohol and cannabis (see below), even at low levels, has a hazardous effect on the driving task. The impairment created by the combination of these two drugs is much greater than that created by either drug alone.

A strong association has been demonstrated between a raised gamma-glutamyl transferase (GGT) and road traffic accidents in drivers aged over 30, indicating that many of these accidents may be caused by problem drinkers. Of even greater concern is that a high prevalence of raised liver enzyme activity has also been demonstrated in those over the age of 30 who apply for licences as drivers of large goods vehicles (LGVs) and passenger carrying vehicles (PCVs).

Cannabis

Cannabis use is now widespread in the UK. In 1995 drug seizures by police and HM Customs rose by 6% to a total of 115 000; 50% of these seizures involved cannabis.[5] Cannabis is attractive as a workplace drug of abuse because of its compact packaging and rapid onset of action.

In 1987 a series of 162 offshore oil and gas rig workers in the North Sea were subjected to urine analysis for cannabinoids immediately prior to deployment offshore. Positive results were found in over 9%.[6]

In another study, 10 experienced pilots each smoked a cigarette containing 19 mg of tetrahydrocannabinol (THC). Twenty-four hours later their performance on a simulated landing task showed trends towards impairment in all variables, of which they were unaware.[7]

Cannabis impairs the ability to drive, in a manner similar to alcohol. Cannabis-intoxicated drivers are over-represented in fatal accidents and it is potentially as dangerous as alcohol in this context, and more so when the two drugs are taken together. Cannabis users have been found to have twice the background frequency of road traffic accidents in the 6–12 months before conviction for cannabis use. In a study of 710 fatally-injured drivers in the US, over half had used alcohol, 8% were taking benzodiazepines, and 38% had also used cannabis.[8] On a driving simulator, cannabis has a much stronger effect than alcohol on the estimation of time and distance, and has correspondingly more potent effects on braking time. In controlled laboratory studies cannabis adversely affects perception, co-ordination, braking time, and other motor skills. **Cannabis is especially potent in its effects on these skills when combined with alcohol.**

There is an extensive literature on human performance under the influence of cannabis and effects on memory, attention span, and perception have been demonstrated. This has implications not only for operating complicated, heavy equipment but also for aircraft pilots, air traffic controllers, train drivers, and signalmen.

Two accidents in the US involving railroad crews performing complex tasks were associated with cannabis which was detected in the urine of a signalman on one occasion and of a driver on another. A pilot in a fatal commercial air crash was found to have smoked cannabis 24 hours before the crash, and there is concern that the use of this drug can lead to impaired piloting performance even after such a length of time.

Cannabis can have an adverse effect on any complex learnt psychomotor task involving memory, skill, concentration, sense of time, and orientation in three-dimensional space, and on the performance of multiple complex tasks. Cannabis impairs judgement, performance, and immediate recall whereas alcohol tends to affect the transfer process from short to long-term memory stores. There is no cerebellar dysfunction (slurred speech and ataxia) due to cannabis, but there is impairment of glare recovery, peripheral vision, and sense of time. Visual hallucinations and the intrusion of inappropriate memories can also occur.

Cannabis can cause temporal disorganization with disruption of the correct sequencing of events in time, and work requiring a high level of cognitive integration is adversely affected. A single 'joint' of cannabis can cause measurable impairment of skills for more than 10 hours. This cognitive impairment lasts for long after the euphoria has disappeared. Psychophysiological activities impaired by cannabis include tracking ability, complex reaction time, hand steadiness, complicated signal interpretation, and attention span. There are therefore deficiencies in perception, memory and cognition. Cannabis has a particularly deleterious effect on pilots who have to orientate themselves in three-dimensional space, which is particularly crucial for helicopter pilots.

In the intoxicated state cannabis, like alcohol, impairs short-term memory in proportion to the dose. However, unlike alcohol, moderate cannabis use is associated with selective short-term memory deficits that persist following a period of several weeks of abstinence.

Prescribed medication

Sedative psychoactive medication, like alcohol, reduces the overall level of alertness of the central nervous system. Certain antidepressants, anxiolytics, and hypnotics have side-effects which reduce skilled performance, concentration, memory, information processing ability, and motor activity as demonstrated in both volunteers and patient populations. All these effects increase the risk of driving accidents. It is for this reason that airline pilots are prohibited from flying while taking prescribed psychotropic medication. It is also known that the use of both prescribed and illicit drugs is associated with an increased liability to road traffic accidents[9] (see also Chapter 26, Medication).

The relative contributions of mental illness and psychotropic drug use as causes of accidents have not been analysed in many studies. It is possible that some mentally disturbed patients would pose a greater danger without treatment. On the other hand, after taking their drugs in normal therapeutic doses, these individuals may still present a risk to road safety. Laboratory studies on the effects of psychotropic drugs on driving-related skills of patients on long-term medication are rare. However, it has been demonstrated that patients receiving diazepam do perform more poorly, exhibiting impaired visual perception and impaired anticipation of dangerous events when driving.

In the official report of a railway accident in Scotland (March 1974, Glasgow Central Station) it was concluded that the use of diazepam by the train driver was a contributory cause; and Scandinavian researchers have found that serum concentrations of benzodiazepines are significantly greater in drivers involved in road traffic accidents than in control groups. Laboratory assessments of the effects of psychotropic drugs on sensory and motor skills, steering, brake reaction time, divided attention, and vigilance have shown specific impairment following the administration of minor tranquillizers and tricyclic antidepressants. Similar effects have been found to persist in the morning after taking benzodiazepine hypnotics. Data from Holland have shown that hypnotics, minor tranquillizers, and tricyclic antidepressants cause driving errors in real-life conditions on the open road, including a tendency to wander across the carriageway. Even fairly low doses of psychoactive drugs have a detrimental effect on the performance of car-driving tests and related measures of psychomotor ability.[10]

These detrimental effects have been demonstrated with the hypnotic nitrazepam in a dose as low as 5 mg, and with other psychotropic agents including flurazepam (30 mg), amitriptyline (50 mg), mianserin (10 mg), lorazepam (1 mg), diazepam (5 mg), and chlordiazepoxide (10 mg). The hypnotics were assessed for their residual activity the morning after night-time sedation, whereas the effects of the antidepressants and anxiolytics were measured during the day. The amnesic effect of some benzodiazepines is such that drivers fail to remember routines and cannot read maps competently.

The sleep disturbance caused by jet lag might lead pilots or other people whose work requires vigilance, motor skill, and a high level of decision-making to take a hypnotic. A benzodiazepine with a short half-life might appear to be an attractive option because of the reduction of daytime sedation, but amnesia may persist after the sedation has disappeared. For sedatives or hypnotics, the available data show that their use could more than double the road accident risk factor.

Whereas both amitriptyline and dothiepin impair performance on laboratory analogues of car-driving and related skills, the 5-hydroxytryptamine re-uptake inhibitor fluoxetine, in a dose of 40 mg, showed a lack of cognitive and psychomotor effects when administered in an acute dose to volunteers. However, since fluoxetine has a long half-life it is possible that if administered to patients over a therapeutic period, there might be some impairment of skill performance and car-handling ability.

Alcohol and drug policies in the workplace

The development and implementation of alcohol and drug policies in the workplace is essential, not only because of the legal implications, but also because of the benefits to any company and its employees. No employer can afford to overlook such concerns: however, some employers may wish to consider these issues within the context of their overall approach to health and safety, whereas others may wish to devise a completely separate policy. Some may wish to include smoking at work within the policy, but others may wish to treat that as a separate issue entirely. Nonetheless, it is recommended here that alcohol and drug misuse should be addressed in similar but separate policies, which may be combined or kept separate, and which should include both illicit drug use and legal drug misuse (including solvents, amyl nitrite, and ketamine). Misuse of prescribed medication should also be included. Problems related to appropriate and therapeutic use of medicinal drugs may be addressed within the drugs policy, and should certainly not be overlooked in any safety-sensitive industry.

Alcohol and drugs policies are introduced in order to:

- reduce the adverse effect of alcohol on the health and well-being of employees
- encourage safer and more sensible drinking
- minimize problems at work
- make employees aware of the problems
- identify employees with problems
- ensure fair and even-handed treatment
- offer early advice and access to help
- make staff aware of their responsibilities.

Comprehensive policies should:

- Provide some information about the nature of alcohol and drug use and misuse, and provide for education of the workforce.
- Consider preventive measures that may be introduced in a particular workplace.
- Explain how alcohol and drug problems may and will be identified in the workplace (including details of any screening programmes).
- Explain the reasons for the existence of the policies.
- Make clear how identified problems will be managed, clinically and administratively.
- Make clear what the responsibilities of the staff are in respect of implementing the policies.
- Clarify procedures of confidentiality and record keeping.

Implementation of a new policy

Implementation of a new alcohol and drug policy requires a careful prior assessment of the financial and other implications, and clear agreement on who will be responsible for drawing it up. The workforce should be educated and trained about the content and the implementation of the policy, which should thereafter be carefully monitored and reviewed. In setting up company alcohol and drug policies it is essential that wide consultation is held at the draft stages, particularly with staff associations or trade unions.

Their acceptance and co-operation is crucial to success and so they should be well-briefed.

The principle underlying the workplace management of alcohol and drug misuse is that both are considered as health-related problems and the onus is on the employee to co-operate with treatment and achieve abstinence. There is evidence that the costs of dismissing an employee who has a drink problem, including those relating to formal discipline, grievance procedures, and legal liability, are greater than the costs of rehabilitation, even allowing for impaired productivity, and any excess absenteeism and accidents.

Employers must also realize that it is a criminal offence for the occupier of any premises to allow the use, possession, or production of any controlled substance on those premises (Misuse of Drugs Act 1971). This includes cannabis, so an employer who condones or ignores the smoking of cannabis on their premises is committing a criminal offence.

It is also counter-productive to provide a bar with alcohol available at subsidized rates or to make it freely available for entertaining visitors.

If a manager suspects that an employee has a drug or alcohol problem, the employee should be referred to the occupational health service, either directly or through the personnel department. Quite often the problem only comes to light after a criminal offence has been committed or a serious breach of company rules has occurred. In such cases it is usually better to proceed with the disciplinary action, if appropriate, and then implement the rehabilitation process. Unfortunately in some organizations, particularly those with high safety sensitivity (e.g. the offshore gas and oil industry and the railways), the disciplinary process can mean summary dismissal. It is for this reason that staff are encouraged to self-declare problems in advance of dangerous incidents and managers are briefed on the early identification of problem drinkers or drug users so that help can be offered.

An employee who requests or is encouraged to seek professional help should be allowed time off work for treatment and follow-up appointments. If they have a relapse, further treatment should be offered providing the employee has co-operated up to that point. The management of dependency problems is best achieved as a 'partnership' or 'contract' between the employee, the manager, and the occupational health department. Failure of the employee to follow the treatment programme, maintain abstinence, and achieve regular attendance should lead to termination of the programme for that individual, followed by disciplinary measures or dismissal.

It may be advisable for some employers to include a term in the contract of employment that requires abstinence from alcohol for 12 hours before starting a shift. However, such alcohol-free intervals have their limitations. For example, the very heavy drinker who consumes 9–10 pints of beer 12 hours before attending for duty may still have a BAC above the legal drinking and driving limit on arrival at work. Similarly, the policy or contract may need to address the problems of prescribed medication with an extremely long half-life. In these cases, there is the additional need to obtain medical advice on the effects of the medication on the employee's performance, the risks of discontinuing it or altering the timing of the daily dosage, and the advisability of continuing at work whilst taking it.

Company drug screening programmes

There are many reasons why a company may wish to introduce a drug-screening programme. These include concern for public or staff safety, security, maintenance of work performance, public relations and corporate image, the requirements imposed by a third party (e.g. insurance or contractual obligation), observance of legal requirements, and general benefits of a 'drug-free workplace'. A screening programme should not be introduced without prior consideration of the action that will be required if an employee tests positive. **It is therefore necessary to introduce suitable alcohol and drug policies before implementing screening.**

A comprehensive company drug screening programme comprises a triad of measures, namely:

• pre-employment screening
• 'with-cause' screening when there are clinical or situational indications (e.g. following an accident)
• random or unannounced screening.

Only when all three components of the triad are in place can management consider it has maximized the opportunity to reduce drug misuse within its workforce to the lowest achievable level.

Pre-employment screening

Pre-employment screening is the easiest measure to introduce because, at the selection stage, there is no contractual relationship between the job applicant and the prospective employer. It also provides the opportunity for the organization to signal its position on drug misuse and make it clear to prospective new entrants that drug misuse will not be tolerated. It is therefore important that the screening policy is as open as possible, including the provision of information leaflets which clearly state the situation.

Drug users sometimes maintain abstinence long enough to pass the drug screening test and then resume their habit once they have been hired. National companies also need to be aware of the applicant who, having failed the screening test in one locality, re-applies in another part of the country. On the second occasion the applicant may pass the drug screening test if they have had a sufficient period of abstinence. The only effective way of avoiding this situation is to maintain good records of the pre-employment candidates who have been screened. Those who have failed the screening should be time-barred from a further application for some specified period (e.g. 3 years).

When screening for alcohol or drug misuse in a pre-employment medical examination, the informed consent of the job applicant has to be obtained. The physician should explain the nature of the blood and urine tests and should obtain the prospective employee's consent to disclosure of the test results to the prospective employer. Positive findings at a screening examination must be confirmed by a further laboratory analysis.

Screening when there are clinical or situational indications ('with-cause' screening)

In the workplace managers and supervisors often refer to 'post-incident' screening which is indeed, a major component of 'with-cause' screening. However, the latter term is more flexible, particularly as it avoids any argument as to whether a particular event constitutes an 'incident' or not.

'With-cause' screening is probably best described as the drug screening of staff at the behest of management when there is a situation in which the manager or supervisor feels that drug misuse might have occured or in which they wish to exclude drug misuse. It is sensible to screen for alcohol at the same time, as this is a more likely underlying cause of accidents than drug misuse.

No screening can be conducted without consent. However, the workplace policy must address the handling of cases where consent for a test is withheld whether 'with cause' or random. Where there are important safety considerations, policies often specify that refusal to undergo testing will be treated as if a positive result had been obtained.

Random (unannounced) screening

Random screening is possibly the most difficult element of the screening triad to introduce, in terms of both acceptability to staff and the scope of its application. The randomness of screening may be in terms both of the timing and the selection of employees who will be tested on any given occasion. However, plans should allow for all eligible employees to be screened at least once over a given period of time.

It is necessary to decide whether to screen the entire workforce or merely those in safety-sensitive jobs. The policy should also indicate whether or not contractors will be eligible for screening, a decision that has implications for the contracting process itself. The frequency of screening also needs to be considered. If screening is too infrequent then it loses its deterrent effect, as the factor of uncertainty will be blunted by a low expectation of being screened. On the other hand, if screening is too frequent it runs the risk of becoming irksome and intrusive and causes resentment rather than acceptance of a necessary part of a comprehensive drug misuse management programme. The most effective system for many companies may comprise an annual screen for everyone plus the possibility of second screening tests within the same year for, say, 10–20% of the same population. If the target population is relatively small then such a system is manageable, but size and the geographical dispersion of the workforce determine the feasibility and cost of such a programme.

Additional screening

In addition to the three basic components regarded as essential to a comprehensive screening programme, other opportunities to screen may also be taken—for example, when staff change jobs within the company and at a periodic medical assessment. It might be assumed that nothing will be detected because screening on such occasions is predictable and forewarned, but practical experience proves otherwise. The adoption of such a system also provides management with a further opportunity to demonstrate its refusal to tolerate drug misuse.

Role of the occupational physician

Drug screening is not an integral part of the occupational physician's role, or indeed a natural task for an occupational health department within a company, but such programmes do require medical involvement. In pre-employment screening, which can be done at the same time as the standard new entrant medical assessment, the drug screening process should be regarded as a management responsibility delegated to the occupational health department. Separation of function can be achieved by separately reporting results so that the drug-screening test is not perceived as part of the clinical procedure. It is then perfectly possible for a candidate to meet the medical fitness requirements of the post applied for in all respects, but fail to be offered the job by management because of a positive drug screening test.

In 'with cause' and random screening, the role of the occupational health department should, ideally, be rather more detached. Both are 'policing' activities which could compromise the rehabilitation role of the occupational health department in cases of alcohol and drug misuse. The best means of overcoming this objection is for the collection of samples to be undertaken by a separate organization, possibly external to the company. The occupational physician should help to select the contractor and set up the necessary procedures and protocols for sample collection. However, after this, it is often best that the only direct involvement of the occupational health department is to receive the screening results and report them to the employees and to line management which will ensure that the occupational health department is more securely placed to implement an appropriate rehabilitation programme in accordance with the company policy.

In addition to the need to maintain strict impartiality in the implementation of the alcohol and drugs policy, the occupational physician also has an active part to play in reporting results as the medical review officer (MRO). This role is crucially important as it provides confidential interpretation of both the analytical findings from the laboratory and the clinical information that the sample collection officer has obtained from the donor's completed pre-screening questionnaire. This information may include recent medically prescribed drugs as well as over-the-counter medication. The importance of this information cannot be overestimated, as it will become part of the structured dialogue that must take place between the MRO and the toxicologist responsible for the analysis of the donor's urine sample. The purpose of this discussion is to ensure that proper account is taken of any medication and dietary or other factors, so that false positive findings are recognized and correctly reported.

Employers who are considering the introduction of a drug screening policy require expert advice on the selection of the drugs to be screened for and their metabolites, as well as the collection of the biological specimens, their identification, storage, preservation, and transport, and the validity and reliability of the subsequent chemical analyses. They will also require advice on the reporting and interpretation of the laboratory-generated results. Although blood, breath, hair, saliva, and urine are all suitable biological specimens for drug testing, urine is most commonly used in both the military and civilian settings.

Commercial laboratories can screen for opiates, barbiturates, amphetamines, cannabis, and cocaine metabolites. Both heroin and codeine are metabolized to morphine and so both the heroin user and the cold sufferer can have a positive urine test for morphine. Any immunoassay test that produces a positive result must be confirmed by gas chromatography–mass spectrometry (GCMS) if the result is to be legally defensible. A urine test for cocaine metabolites can be positive for up to 72 hours; in a daily user of cannabis, urine can be positive for 2 weeks or more because the drug is deposited in fat stores. However, the results of urine tests alone cannot be used to determine whether or not the donor was actually impaired by drugs or their metabolites or was unfit to undertake any given task. Furthermore, a positive urine drugs test result cannot be used by itself to establish what dose of a drug was administered or when. On all these matters the judgement and advice of the company's occupational physician will be critical. The Faculty of Occupational Medicine has produced guidelines on this subject which cover the role of the occupational physician in the purpose and planning of drug screening programmes and the role of the occupational physician as well as the ethical issues and other matters.[11] Anyone considering preparing a drug misuse policy or programme is strongly recommended to consult this document.

Mechanics of alcohol and drug screening

The Road Traffic Acts and the Transport and Works Act 1992 (which applies to the railways), allow for samples of breath, blood, and urine to be screened for alcohol and blood and urine for drugs. In the workplace the most effective method for alcohol screening is an analysis of breath and for drugs an analysis of urine. Avoidance of venesection is recommended where possible, as it is time consuming and carries the risk of needlestick injury with all its attendant problems.

In collecting the urine samples for drug screening, it is essential to maintain 'chain of custody' security. This is an auditable process whereby the sample donated by each identified individual is uniquely identified and remains secure at all times, so that it cannot be adulterated, interfered with, or swapped. The chain of custody runs from the point of donation through the transit and despatch system, to the laboratory itself and finally the transmission of the findings back to the occupational health department. A common system uses barcode labels that are unique to the donor, and the code itself accompanies the sample throughout the entire process. Errors in the chain of custody procedure are the commonest reason for successful challenges of positive results.

The analytical procedure in the laboratory requires a one- or two-step process depending on the findings. The initial screening procedure, which is now largely automated to permit a high throughput of samples, is an immunoassay system, which detects a range of analytes. If no analytes are detected at the first pass nothing further needs be done and the laboratory will report the screen as negative. The sample is then usually retained for a period of up to 2 weeks before being destroyed.

Samples which test positive on immunoassay have to undergo a second entirely separate test using GCMS. This is the definitive method of identification and if the analytes initially discovered on immunoassay are confirmed to be present then the sample will be reported as positive. It is at this stage that discussion takes place between the MRO and the toxicologist at the laboratory. This ensures that the interaction of any previously disclosed medication, or other factors, can be taken into account. Consequently in some cases, laboratory 'positives' will be reported to management as negative because a satisfactory explanation has been found. The usual explanation for such 'positives' is the presence of a metabolite of either over-the-counter or prescribed medication, e.g. opioid analgesics. In those cases in which there is no obvious explanation mentioned by the donor on the pre-screening questionnaire, it would be advisable for the MRO to interview the donor to investigate the reason for the discrepancy. It is worth emphasizing that such results are not false positives: the laboratory findings are entirely correct, and the positive result is reported as negative to the line manager only because the MRO has obtained a satisfactory explanation for the presence of the drug in question.

In addition to the analytical process just described, laboratories can assist in the evaluation of samples which may have been tampered with to achieve a negative result. The commonest trick employed to conceal misuse is to dilute the urine with tap water. This method runs the risk of detection (as the sample's temperature will be outside the normal range), and an alternative approach is to dilute the urine by drinking copious amounts of water before voiding. However, this is also detectable because it alters the pH of the sample and also the level of creatinine both of which are routinely measured and reported by laboratories as part of the screening process.

Newer methods of screening

Although immunoassay and GCMS remain the mainstay of most drug screening programmes, using these methods it takes at least a day to establish a negative result. Confirmation by GCMS takes several days—sometimes 10 days or more. Inevitably tests with a faster response time have been sought. Such a capability is now available (referred to as unit test or rapid test screening, near-person screening or, more simply, as on-site screening).

Most of these screens involve dip-testing a slide in urine. A colour change denotes the interaction between the drug metabolite in the urine sample and the test substance impregnated into absorbent material on the device. One variation on this theme is a device that requires a moistened pad to be wiped on the skin in areas where there is natural perspiration such as the forehead or axilla. This method allows for screening of amphetamine, metamphetamine, benzodiazepines, cannabis, cocaine, and opiates. As with laboratory screening, immunoassay technology is involved, the particular technique being immunochromatographic.

Unfortunately, such tests do not approach the reliability and validity of laboratory-based methods, raising concerns about false positive and false negative findings. Of the two, it is the false negative test that is the most worrying, as it is only too easy to envisage a road, rail, or other accident in which a false negative result was misleading. False positives are much less dangerous, as such an error would almost certainly be corrected by later testing.

If, because of the very simplicity of these tests, there was a proliferation of screening, and if the false positive rate proved fairly high, then many employees might find themselves embarrassed and even stigmatized by the process and subsequent vindication by a negative confirmation test arriving several days later would probably do little to alleviate it. A job applicant who screens positive in one of these tests should be given the benefit of a confirmation test.

This new technology is already far more reliable than it was just a few years ago. Nevertheless, at present, it should not be seen as an automatic replacement for current laboratory-based screening programmes which are perfectly satisfactory in many situations and which enjoy the confidence and support of the workforce.

Early recognition and intervention in the problem drinker

Potentially the problem drinker may be identified in the workplace at an early stage of the development of their drinking problem. Identification may occur through the use of questionnaires, such as the AUDIT,[12] through the use of screening tests (breathalyser, GGT, etc.) or through the attentiveness of the manager or occupational physician who identifies characteristic signs of alcohol misuse.

The breathalyser may be employed in a similar fashion to the drug screening protocols described above, although it is not usually used as a part of the pre-employment screening programme. It is much easier to use than urine tests, and may be valuable for routine, random, or 'with-cause' screening in safety-sensitive contexts. It is the detection of acute intoxication in these circumstances, and thus the risk of performance impairment, which is important. The breathalyser enables recent consumption to be assessed but does not allow a diagnosis of long-term alcohol misuse to be made unless the context in which it was used is taken into account.

GGT testing (and other tests, such as carbohydrate-deficient transferrin), in contrast, identifies the individual who has been consuming large amounts of alcohol over a period of time. Elevated GGT does not necessarily demonstrate that work performance is impaired, but should be taken as grounds for further investigation of alcohol consumption and other possible alcohol-related problems. Furthermore, there is widespread individual variability in the sensitivity of GGT to alcohol consumption. An elevated GGT may reflect relatively modest alcohol consumption in some individuals, and a normal GGT may hide excessive consumption in other cases. 'False positive' GGT results also occur as a result of other factors, such as viral hepatitis or certain medications which lead to an elevated GGT level. Nonetheless, a health screening programme which identifies all individuals with a raised serum GGT as a means of identifying employees with drinking problems may reduce the absenteeism rate for all alcohol-related conditions by 50%, if it is combined with counselling about reduction of alcohol intake and serial GGT estimations at 3 monthly intervals to monitor progress.

When colleagues collude with the problem drinker to conceal the alcohol abuse, recognition of the problem is delayed. Markers of misuse include absenteeism, especially on Monday mornings, and also certain observable features including redness of eyes and tremulousness, irritability, indecisiveness, procrastination, errors, and poor productivity.

A crucial aspect of a company's alcohol policy is to get the employee to admit to and tackle their drinking. The link between the alcohol intake and presenting work problems, deterioration in general health, and social and domestic problems should be explored. It is valuable to teach the patient the concept of units (in the UK, 1 unit = 1 glass of wine or sherry, 1 measure of spirits, or 1/2 pint of beer) to maintain a drinking diary, and to identify emotional or social triggers for heavy drinking. To avoid futile debate about whether a particular employee is 'an alcoholic', it is more constructive to describe the presenting problem in terms of the damage, whether social (including occupational), psychological, or medical, which that particular individual's drinking is causing. Referral to a counselling agency and to organizations such as Alcoholics Anonymous can also be extremely helpful. Some physicians recommend a supervised programme of treatment with disulfiram. This chemical deterrent might have a place, provided its limitations are recognized.[13] It should, however, be regarded as a short-term measure to provide a respite from drinking while counselling with both the individual and their partner begins to take effect. It is certainly not a substitute for counselling and education.

Drug and alcohol rehabilitation programmes

When setting up a programme of alcohol or drug screening for employees it is essential also to set up a formal rehabilitation programme to provide help for those who self-declare a problem, and for those found to be positive on screening. The nature and scope of the rehabilitation programme will depend on the management style of the company and also the nature of its activities. However, irrespective of whether rehabilitation is offered as an in-house service or through outside agencies, responsibility for managing the programme must be retained within the company and not devolved to an external provider. This is needed to ensure proper follow-up and compliance with the terms of the programme. Management must be kept informed of progress as serious default may lead to termination of employment.

The corporate occupational health service is the most appropriate vehicle through which to manage company alcohol and drug rehabilitation programmes and to facilitate communication between the employee concerned, the management, any external agency that might be involved, and the occupational health department itself.

In principle, there should be little difference between a rehabilitation programme for staff with alcohol misuse and one for staff with drug misuse. However, employers and trade unions seem to be much more accepting of the reformed problem drinker than the reformed drug user. It seems that drug dependency is commonly perceived as a lifelong, irretrievable addiction whereas alcohol dependency is not. However, the occupational health service should endeavour to convince managers that dependency problems need to be treated in a uniform way, with the outcome of each judged on its merits, particularly when the employee has scrupulously complied with the rehabilitation programme.

It is not possible here to describe the full range of alcohol/drug rehabilitation programmes. However, the occupational physician should become acquainted both with the particular programme(s) used by their company, and also the broad spectrum of approaches to rehabilitation which are available.[14-16]

Conclusions

Alcohol and drug misuse is a serious concern in the workplace, because of its financial and commercial costs, and also because of the human suffering and its impact on the social milieu. However, there are greater opportunities for prevention, early identification and effective treatment than exist in many other areas of medical practice. It is important for all occupational physicians to be well informed about these matters. Similarly, no company can afford to be without properly considered and carefully implemented alcohol and drug policies.

Selected references

1 Meltzer H, Gill B, Pettigrew M, Hinds K. *The prevalence of psychiatric morbidity among adults living in private households*. OPCS surveys of psychiatric morbidity among adults living in private households, 1. London: HMSO, 1995.

2 Banta WF, Tennant F. *Complete handbook for combating substance abuse in the workplace*. Lexington: Lexington Books, 1989.

3 Hore BD, Plant MA. (ed.) *Alcohol problems in employment*. London: Croom Helm, 1981.

4 Davenport M, Harris D. The effect of low blood alcohol levels on pilot performance in a series of simulated approach and landing trials. *Int J Aviat Psychol* 1992; **2**: 271–280.

5 *Home Office Bulletin–Issue 25/91. Statistics of drugs seizures and offenders dealt with. United Kingdom 1995*. London: Home Office, 1995.

6 Calder IM, Ramsey J. A survey of cannabis use in offshore rig workers. *Br J Addict* 1987; **82**: 159–161.

7 Yesavage JA, Leirer VO, Denari M, Hollister LE. Carry-over effects of marijuana intoxication on aircraft pilot performance: A preliminary report. *Am J Psychiatry* 1985; **142**: 1325–9.

8 Glauz WD, Blackburn RR. *Drug use among drivers*. Technical contract report to the National Highway Traffic Safety Administration. Washington DC: Department of Transportation, 1975.

9 Skegg DCG, Richards SM, Doll R. Minor tranquillisers and road accidents. *BMJ* 1979; **1**: 917–919.

10 Hindmarch I. The effects of psychoactive drugs on car handling and related psychomotor ability. In: *Drugs and driving*, ed. O'Hanlon JF, de Gier JJ, pp. 71–79. London: Taylor and Francis, 1986.

11 *Guidelines on testing for drugs of abuse in the workplace*. London: Faculty of Occupational Medicine, Royal College of Physicians, 1994.

12 Babor TF, de la Fuente JR, Saunders J, Grant M. *AUDIT The Alcohol Use Disorders Identification Test: Guidelines for use in primary health care*. Geneva: World Health Organisation, 1989.

13 Hughes J, Cook CCH. Disulfiram in the management of alcohol misuse—a review. *Addiction* 1997; **92**: 381–395.

14 Cook CCH. The Minnesota model in the management of drug and alcohol dependency: miracle method or myth? Part I. The philosophy and the programme. *Br J Addict* 1988; **83**: 625–634.

15 Cook CCH. The Minnesota model in the management of drug and alcohol dependency: miracle method or myth? Part II. Evidence and conclusions. *Br J Addict* 1988; **83**: 735–748.

16 Edwards G, Marshall EJ, Cook CCH. *The treatment of drinking problems*, 3rd edn. Cambridge: Cambridge University Press, 1997.

26

Medication

I. G. Rennie and G. T. McInnes

Most people at work do not take regular medication. However, many people work while taking medication and many can only work because of their medication. Additionally, many people have to take medication because of their work, e.g. those who travel regularly to areas of the world where malaria is endemic.

The benefits of being at work must be balanced against the risks of side-effects and other consequences of taking medication, or the health consequences of omitting the medication altogether. There are very few studies which help in making such an assessment. Moreover, most treatments are ordered by general practitioners and hospital doctors who rarely have sufficient knowledge of the patients' work and working environment to assess the consequences of any incompatibility between medication and work.

The risks associated with alcohol and other medication, particularly psychotropic drugs, impairing performance, skills, and memory have led to particular concerns for those taking such drugs[1] (see Chapter 25). As a consequence the World Health Organization (1983) gave advice and guidance in a booklet (*Drugs, driving and traffic safety*). This publication is concerned with drugs and driving; such advice is relevant to those who fly aircraft, operate machinery or perform skilled tasks, and those who must remain vigilant at a workstation.

Prevalence of medication in society

Use of medicines continues to rise in all developed countries. In 1963, the average number of prescriptions per head for UK National Health Service patients was 4.6; in 1996 it was estimated to be 9.5.[2] This estimate covers the entire population, however, and the extent of drug consumption among those at work has rarely been investigated. A study in the 1970s[3] indicated that 55% of a sample population had taken or used some medication during the 24 hours before the interview, whereas a study by Rennie in 1984[4] indicated that 20% of a factory population were taking medication.

The frequency of drug taking within a working population is dependent on a number of factors, in particular age and sex. Lader[5] found that psychotropics were the most commonly taken drugs in a female working population. In a mainly male population cardiovascular drugs, especially beta-blockers, are commoner.[4] Both groups of drugs can affect performance adversely.

Clinical aspects affecting work capacity

Unwanted effects of medication fall into two main categories: those which are predictable and usually dose-related, and those which are unpredictable and not usually dose-related.[6] In addition, unwanted effects may result from interactions with other drugs, with alcohol, and with other chemical substances which may be encountered at work. Of particular concern to the patient at work are effects on performance, especially for those who operate machinery, drive vehicles, or fly aircraft, or whose sound judgement or vigilance is imperative. Some drugs may produce particular problems for patients in specific jobs. Any doctor prescribing medication, or any occupational physician reviewing an individual returning to work, should consider whether there might be hazards to the patient from drug effects, e.g. slowing of reaction time, drowsiness, or altered thermoregulatory systems. In addition, because people differ in their response to drugs, particularly in reactions to psychoactive drugs, any potentially dangerous occupation should be avoided for at least a week after starting such therapy. Thereafter, treatment can be reviewed.

The Disability Discrimination Act 1995 and medication

To qualify within the scope of the Disability Discrimination Act 1995 (DDA), an employee must have, or have had, a physical or mental impairment causing a substantial and long-term adverse effect on their ability to carry out normal day to day activities. Long-term means that the impairment must have lasted for, or be likely to last for, 12 months or more.

The use of medication and the successful control of a disability by medication does not invalidate the protection afforded to such people by the DDA. Examples such as diabetes and epilepsy were considered during the committee stage of the Act. In addition, whereas drug addiction is normally excluded from the Act, any addiction which was originally the result of administration of medically prescribed drugs or other medical treatment is covered by the Act.

The DDA requires employers to make reasonable adjustments to enable qualifying employees to remain at work. Such adjustments may require alterations in working hours or type of work if the effects of the medication lead to problems at work. The employer, however, does need to consider the requirements of the Health and Safety at Work Act etc. (HSAWA) in reviewing whether it is possible to make 'reasonable adjustments' to the job and not place the individuals taking the medication at risk to themselves or others.

General effects of medication on performance

Circadian rhythm

Changes in performance occur naturally as part of the circadian rhythm. Scores for most simple tasks rise during the day to a peak between 12.00 and 21.00 hours and fall to a trough between 03.00 and 06.00 hours,[7] correlating with body temperature. During the day increased arousal partly compensates for the effect of prolonged work, whereas at night the normal circadian decrease in alertness may aggravate the effect. Problems may occur in shiftwork, submarines, aircraft, and space flight; the actions of drugs which affect performance may be additive in such circumstances.

There is also evidence that the absorption and elimination, as well as the pharmacological effect, of some drugs are influenced by circadian rhythms. For example, blood levels of amitriptyline are higher after a morning dose than after an evening dose and this difference is associated with greater sedative and anticholinergic effects.[8] The mechanism is unknown, as is the relevance to shiftworkers.

In patients on long-term corticosteroid treatment, suppression of the hypothalamic–pituitary–adrenal axis can be minimized by giving the steroid as a single daily dose in the early morning, after the diurnal peak of ACTH secretion which occurs just prior to waking. In long-term night workers the diurnal rhythm is reversed, and the steroid should then be given in the evening, immediately on waking.

Testing drugs to assess their effect on performance

Drug testing is complex and time consuming. Tests fall into two main categories: those that measure the effects of drugs on individual components of psychomotor function, and those which measure their effects on activities of everyday life, such as car driving. Assessing the effects of drugs on real-life activities has many problems, but there is now much evidence that some laboratory tests of psychomotor function correlate well with, for example, driving ability. The components of psychomotor function measured by laboratory tests include cognitive information processing, short-term memory and learning, motor function, and activities involving sensory, central, and motor abilities. Such well-controlled psychopharmacological tests can now indicate with reasonable reliability those drugs which may affect regular activities such as driving and operating machinery.[9,10]

Laboratory testing in carefully placebo-controlled conditions has been used to assess the effects of various benzodiazepine hypnotics and antihypertensive drugs in air-force pilots. This has led to recommendations which are discussed in later sections (see p. 507). In theory, similar approaches could be used to screen workers taking essential long-term medication such as anticonvulsants in professions where safety is critical e.g. train drivers, air traffic controllers, or even doctors, or where impaired cognitive function may have major commercial consequences e.g. company executives or accountants. However, marked variability in responses between individuals greatly reduces the precision of such tests and only gross abnormalities are likely to be detected with confidence. Laboratory assessments therefore have a limited role in determining suitability for a particular employment.

Effects of environmental chemicals on drug response

Most drugs are inactivated by detoxication in the liver. Drug metabolism can be affected by factors which increase or reduce the activity of the responsible hepatic enzyme systems. Many environmental chemicals have been shown to be enzyme inducers which increase the rate of metabolism of many drugs in animals. These include polycyclic aromatic hydrocarbons and organochlorine and other pesticides. Studies of workers engaged in pesticide manufacture have demonstrated enzyme induction,[11] but its practical importance is unknown.

In theory, any drug metabolized by the liver might be involved in such interactions but examples most likely to be relevant in the work environment include warfarin, sulfonylureas, and cyclosporin. The main danger arises when exposure to the enzyme-inducing agent is discontinued with the result that plasma concentrations increase and toxicity can occur.

Effects on work capacity

Drugs which primarily affect the central nervous system (CNS) causing lethargy and drowsiness are likely to reduce work capacity. However, other commonly prescribed drugs, such as beta-blockers, can also affect the capacity to work.

Effects on adaptation to extremes of temperature

The human body temperature is maintained within limits of $\pm0.5°C$, despite wide ambient changes superimposed on the circadian rhythm which is individually consistent.[12] Drugs which affect the control of body temperature may place patients at risk if they are working in an inhospitable environment. Drugs can influence body temperature either by interfering directly with effector pathways or through the central control of temperature.

Effector pathways

- **Sweating** provides coarse control of heat loss; it is under cholinergic control and hence may be diminished by drugs with anticholinergic (antimuscarinic or atropine-like) properties. Thus antiparkinsonism agents, antihistamines, tricyclic antidepressants, and neuroleptics such as chlorpromazine can cause heat intolerance. However, as most of these drugs cross the blood–brain barrier their effects on body temperature may also involve central effects.
- **Cutaneous blood flow** is responsible for fine control of heat loss, and drugs which act on the peripheral sympathetic nervous system, e.g. the adrenergic neurone-blocking drugs such as bethanidine, α-adrenoreceptor antagonists such as prazosin; and those which act on the vasculature e.g. direct vasodilators such as hydralazine and calcium antagonists such as nifedipine, may impair the vasomotor response to cold exposure. Normally, however, reflex mechanisms compensate for these effects.
- The cutaneous vasoconstriction which occurs following administration of β-adrenoreceptor antagonists does not affect body temperature but may cause local signs and symptoms such as cold extremities, chilblains, and Raynaud's phenomenon. Those working in cold environments should be warned of potential side-effects, and the suitability of such work for individuals requiring β-blockers must be assessed.

Central mechanisms

Virtually all drugs with cerebral depressant properties may alter thermoregulation when given in sufficient doses. Body temperature is influenced by the surroundings. The mechanisms involved are complex. In therapeutic doses barbiturates, benzodiazepines, and neuroleptics may all impair central temperature regulation. Tricyclic antidepressants and monoamine oxidase inhibitors may precipitate hyperthermia both singly, and more commonly, in combination.

Effects due to occupational exposure to CNS depressants

Employees who work with solvents, (e.g. in degreasing plants, printing, paint spraying, or with adhesives) and those who work in atmospheres where there may be a potential build-up of gases or fumes that can depress the CNS may be at risk; this risk may be potentiated if they also take medications which depress the CNS. Safe exposure levels at work are based on occupational exposure limits: these have been derived from animal experiments and experiments on humans who are not on medication. An interaction with the CNS depressant action of medication may place the treated worker at increased risk (see also Chapter 6, p. 108).

Hypnotics and sedatives

Hypnotic and sedative drugs are all CNS depressants and most have been shown to inhibit psychomotor function, retard responsiveness, and impair motor skills, co-ordination, and responses concerned with self-preservation. As a result, such drugs may affect the ability to drive or operate machinery. Moreover, the hangover effects of a night dose may impair driving and other skilled tasks the following day. The duration of effect after a single dose depends on the plasma half-life of the drug and on the dose, but most hypnotics produce residual effects the following morning. Effects on psychomotor function persist during long-term administration although some tolerance or habituation occurs. These are more marked in elderly patients and are potentiated by alcohol.

Barbiturates have a greater effect on performance than benzodiazepines do and should not be used in patients who drive or operate machinery. Long-term barbiturates have a very limited role in modern therapeutics. These drugs are not recommended as hypnotics or anxiolytics.

The individual benzodiazepines differ in effects on psychomotor performance. When used as hypnotics, short-acting drugs such as temazepam and lormetazepam are less likely than nitrazepam, flunitrazepam, and flurazepam to produce effects the following morning. When used during the day as an anxiolytic, clobazam appears to have less effect on performance than other benzodiazepines. However, all these drugs can affect performance in susceptible patients and differences are of degree only. Benzodiazepines and newer hypnotics and anxiolytics such as zolpidem, zopiclone, and buspirone may cause dizziness, light-headedness, and vertigo, confusion, visual disturbances, and amnesic effects which are to a certain extent independent of sedative actions. Lorazepam and diazepam severely affect performance in memory-based tests. Less is known about other benzodiazepines but some, e.g. clobazam, appear to have less effect on memory. Effects on memory are unlikely to produce problems when benzodiazepines are used as nocturnal hypnotics but the effects of daytime use on immediate memory could affect performance in a wide range of activities. Temazepam, because of its short activity time, is the only hypnotic approved by the Royal Air Force for use in pilots.

The study from Dundee[13] on the association of road traffic accidents with benzodiazepine use has provided useful guidance as to the risk of using such medication not only for drivers but also, potentially, for those working in other hazardous situations. This study found a significant increase in the risk of having a road traffic accident amongst those in the study population taking anxiolytic benzodiazepines; users of hypnotic benzodiazepines were not at increased risk (probably because they had little residual pharmacological effect the next day). However, the short-acting hypnotic zopiclone, included in the study even though it is a cyclopyrrolone rather than a benzodiazepine, because it acts on the same receptors as benzodiazepines, did have residual effects that impair car-driving. There was no increase in road traffic accident rate amongst users of tricyclic antidepressant medication or selective serotonin re-uptake inhibitors. It is likely that anxiolytic benzodiazepine exposure is causally related to road traffic accidents and that those using long half-life anxiolytic benzodiazepines and zopiclone should be advised not to drive.

Particular problems can arise when these drugs are stopped. Benzodiazepine withdrawal can produce a characteristic syndrome of anxiety, sleeplessness, perceptual disturbances, depersonalization, and general malaise. When severe, these effects can markedly impair work performance.

Barbiturates can interfere with central thermoregulation, and this may occasionally be a problem with benzodiazepines.

Antipsychotics

The antipsychotics include the phenothiazines, such as chlorpromazine; the butyrophenones, such as haloperidol; and similar drugs, such as pimozide and fluspirilene, which are used mainly to treat schizophrenia and other psychotic illnesses.

Many of these drugs impair psychomotor performance and the degree to which they do so probably depends on the degree of sedation produced. Thus, flupenthixol and low doses of sulpiride, which have a predominantly alerting effect, may have less effect on performance than the more sedative phenothiazines such as chlorpromazine. Psychotic patients show impairment of psychomotor function even without drugs and in some this will be improved by treatment. This needs to be considered when advising such patients about the possible risks of working or driving while taking antipsychotic medication. Lithium probably has little effect on performance, though impairment of some laboratory tests of psychomotor function has been described.

The extrapyramidal side-effects of antipsychotic drugs, particularly tremor, may interfere with precision work and affect driving. Lithium rarely produces extrapyramidal effects but commonly produces tremor. Postural hypotension may cause problems, particularly in hot environments. Patients taking lithium should maintain an adequate fluid consumption and avoid dietary changes which might alter sodium intake.

Interference with temperature regulation is more profound than with the hypnotic/sedative drugs. Neuroleptics interfere both with hypothalamic temperature regulation and with cholinergic control of sweating. Either hyperthermia or hypothermia can occur when environmental temperatures are extreme.

Chlorpromazine and thioridazine can cause visual disturbances through various mechanisms. The antimuscarinic effects of chlorpromazine may result in blurred vision; corneal and lens opacities may occur during chronic high dose therapy. Pigmentary retinopathy with thioridazine is associated with reduced visual acuity.

Antidepressants

Many antidepressants produce sedation, especially when treatment is started, and this is markedly potentiated by alcohol. Psychomotor impairment has been demonstrated and seems to be related to the sedative effect. Of the tricyclic antidepressants, amitriptyline, doxepin, mianserin, trazodone, and trimipramine are the most sedative and imipramine, nortriptyline, protriptyline, and viloxazine the least. Monoamine oxidase inhibitors usually have a stimulant effect although phenelzine can sometimes be sedative. The newer serotonin re-uptake inhibitors such as fluoxetine and paroxetine do not usually produce sedation and appear to have little effect on performance. As tolerance to the sedative effects develops, it seems sensible to advise patients not to drive or to undertake work which could be affected by sedation during the first few days of treatment with the more sedative agents.

Tremor due to antidepressants may be a problem in some types of work. Many antidepressants produce blurring of near vision which may affect driving and the performance of other tasks. Those with anticholinergic (antimuscarinic) effects interfere with sweating and can also affect central temperature regulation. All can produce postural hypotension, but this is more likely to occur with the monoamine oxidase inhibitors and with imipramine and amitriptyline than with nortriptyline or some of the newer antidepressants, such as mianserin or maprotiline.

Antihistamines and anticholinergic (antimuscarinic) anti-emetics

The tendency of these drugs to cause blurred vision, the sedative effects, and the potentiating effect of alcohol are well recognized. The effects vary, depending on individual susceptibility and the properties of the individual drugs. Antihistamines that produce less blurred vision and sedation, such as astemizole and terfenadine, should be used where driving cannot be avoided. Otherwise, patients should be warned that their ability to drive or operate machinery is likely to be impaired. Although it produces some sedation, hyoscine is thought to have less effect on driving skills than most antihistamines and is the anti-emetic of choice for drivers with travel sickness.

Stimulants and appetite suppressants

Amphetamines and other stimulants increase risk-taking behaviour and can be expected to diminish work performance and driving safety, especially if combined with alcohol. Fenfluramine produces sedation but its effects on psychomotor function are unknown.

It should be remembered that theophylline and related substances have stimulant properties. Tremor, dizziness, anxiety, agitation, insomnia, visual disturbances, and even seizures are common.

Analgesics and anti-inflammatory drugs

The more powerful opioid analgesics, such as morphine, produce marked sedation, and patients requiring these drugs should not drive or undertake work likely to be affected adversely. Of the milder opioid analgesics codeine is known to affect driving-related skills and others, such as dextropropoxyphene, may also do so. Alcohol potentiates the effects of all these analgesics, even dextropropoxyphene.

Phenylbutazone and indomethacin have been reported to impair laboratory tests of driving-related skills. The effects of other anti-inflammatory analgesics are unknown. All non-steroidal anti-inflammatory drugs (NSAIDs) have caused nervous system effects and can cause dizziness and vertigo. Even over-the-counter preparations such as ibuprofen can provoke symptoms of drowsiness, fatigue, and blurred vision. These reactions can be hazardous in workers where safety is critical, e.g. train drivers, or lead to commercial loss in other occupations, e.g. management. Recognition of such risks in advance is important because NSAIDs are widely self-prescribed for minor musculoskeletal injuries.

Anticonvulsants

Studies of cognitive function, both in normal volunteers and in patients on chronic anticonvulsant therapy, have shown impairment of concentration and sustained attention, and other aspects of psychomotor performance. Impairment is greater in patients on polytherapy than in those treated with a single drug, and there is some evidence that it is greater with phenytoin than with carbamazepine. The importance of these effects in patients well controlled on long-term monotherapy is unknown. Driving must be temporarily suspended if treatment is changed until there has been a fit-free interval of 1 year (see pp. 163 and 530).

Excessive doses of phenytoin, carbamazepine, and newer drugs such as lamotrigine or gabapentin produce drowsiness, tremor, ataxia, and double vision. Patients affected by drowsiness should not drive or operate machinery. It may be necessary to ensure that blood levels are within the therapeutic range in patients at work.

Anaesthetics

As a general rule patients should not drive or operate machinery for 24–48 hours after general anaesthesia for minor out-patient surgery, but this depends to some extent on the drug used, the duration of anaesthesia, and the response of the individual patient. Clear, written instructions should be provided for the patient at the time of discharge from the day surgery centre.

Antihypertensive drugs

Modern antihypertensive drugs (low dose thiazides, calcium channel blockers, α-blockers, ACE inhibitors, and angiotensin receptor blockers) do not have important central effects and do not appear to affect performance. Older drugs such as methyldopa, clonidine, guanethidine, bethanidine, debrisoquine, and indoramin produce sedation, and methyldopa has been shown to impair driving performance. The newly introduced imidazoline (I_1) receptor antagonist moxonidine has sedative properties but these are less than those seen with clonidine.

β-blockers, especially the more lipophilic agents such as propranolol, can affect psychomotor function but this returns to normal after 3 weeks' administration. Aircrew are permitted by the Civil Aviation Authority to take specified β-blockers, but only after careful specialist evaluation and simulation testing. A period of ground duties should be undertaken first to allow for stabilization and habituation[14] (see also Appendix 2.)

In a small proportion of patients β-blockers have other side-effects which could impair work capacity. These include general fatigue, malaise, tiredness, and muscle fatigue. Reduced exercise tolerance has been reported with all β-blockers and there is no good evidence that the cardioselective drugs such as metoprolol have lesser effects than those of non-selective drugs such as propranolol. Both types of β-blocker significantly increase the sense of fatigue during exercise compared with placebo, and a given workload appears subjectively more difficult to achieve. Fatigue has been reported in about 5% of patients on β-blockers but minor unreported symptoms are probably more common, and it is important to be aware of the potential effect of these drugs on work capacity.

β-blockers can produce bronchospasm in susceptible people, and this should be considered when they are prescribed for patients working in irritant atmospheres. α-blockers and β-blockers with α-blocking properties, such as carvedilol and labetalol, can cause postural hypotension which may affect work performance.

All antihypertensive drugs may cause unexpected hypotension but the risks with modern drugs at current recommended doses have probably been exaggerated. Patients should not drive or operate machinery in the first few hours after beginning treatment or after a dose increment. Particular care should be taken if the patient works in a hot environment. Most antihypertensive drugs affect cutaneous blood flow and can impair the vasomotor response to cold exposure. Diuretics increase the risk of dehydration at high temperatures and are not the antihypertensive of choice for patients working in a hot environment (see p.357) .

Antidiabetic drugs

Loss of warning of hypoglycaemia is a common problem among insulin-treated patients and can be a serious hazard, especially for drivers. The cause is not known but very tight control of blood sugar appears to lower the threshold needed to trigger hypoglycaemic symptoms. Some patients have reported loss of warning of hypoglycaemia after transfer to human insulin. β-blockers can blunt hypoglycaemic awareness and delay recovery.

Car drivers and operators of machinery need to take particular care to avoid hypoglycaemia. Drivers should check blood sugar before starting and at intervals of approximately 2 hours on long journeys and they should ensure that a supply of sugar is always available. If hypoglycaemia occurs, the driver or operator should stop immediately and wait until recovery is complete. Driving is not allowed when hypoglycaemia awareness has been lost. (See also Appendix 1.)

Anticoagulants

Consideration must be given to the suitability for employment of people taking anticoagulants. Usually the underlying condition is the limiting factor. Should bleeding occur, the guidelines given in the *British National Formulary* should be followed. It is advisable for employees taking such medication to carry anticoagulant treatment cards, or other means to indicate that they are receiving this treatment (see Chapter 17, p. 347).

Any occupation which involves potential hazards that significantly increase the risk of injury and bleeding should be reviewed for suitability while the individual is taking the anticoagulant. Such jobs might include, for example, fishing, mining, foundry working, and labouring activities. If such hazards are present it would be appropriate, where possible, for adjustments to be made to the job to reduce the risk; if that is not possible, alternative work should be recommended whilst the individual is taking the medication. Those individuals whose work involves foreign travel should not undertake such travel until their anticoagulant medication is stabilized; in addition they should remember to take sufficient medication with them on the trip. Once stabilized on the medication it is more likely to be the underlying medical condition or the available medical facilities in the countries to be visited that may be the deciding factors as to whether travel is advised.

Specific jobs, because of safety or isolation issues, require particular consideration e.g. flight crew prescribed anticoagulants must discuss with an Authorized Medical Examiner (AME) both the reason for taking the medication and the risks associated with taking it, because flight safety implications will require removal from operational activity until the AME believes it is safe to resume flight crew duties. Similarly, those prescribed anticoagulants who work offshore are considered unsuitable for such work; in addition, because of the risks associated both with the underlying medical condition and the unsupervised taking of anticoagulants for long periods, it is considered inappropriate for serving seafarers on long sea journeys to undertake such work—those working on shorter ferry crossings should seek the advice of a Department of Transport Medical Referee.

Anticancer medication

A significant number of employees remain at work while undergoing chemotherapy. Sometimes the patient needs admission to hospital for intravenous therapy but most frequently the medication is taken orally. Employees taking such medication require support and understanding from their employer in view of potential side-effects. For instance, the widely used oestrogen receptor antagonist tamoxifen is associated with light-headedness and visual disturbances (corneal opacities, cataracts, and retinopathy). Frequently work patterns have to be adjusted, as the employee often feels temporarily unwell as a result of therapy, and will require support when such worrying side-effects as hair loss occur. Continuity of therapy is essential and must not be interrupted in those whose work takes them overseas, for example.

Continuous ambulatory infusion therapy

Some employees wish to return to work while receiving medication via continuous ambulatory infusion. In such circumstances a discussion between the employee's general practitioner or consultant and the occupational health adviser or the employer should identify the potential needs of the employee receiving the therapy to allow a risk assessment of the working environment and arrangements for changing of infusion bags in a safe environment.

Antimigraine drugs

The $5HT_1$ agonists naratriptan, sumatriptan, and zolmitriptan can cause drowsiness which may affect performance of skilled tasks such as driving. Other drugs such as ergotamine, isometheptene (Midrid), pizotifen, clonidine, and methysergide are associated with dizziness, vertigo, and postural hypotension.

Drugs for Parkinsonism

Hypotensive reactions with cabergoline, lysuride, pergolide, and ropinirole may be disturbing in some patients during the first few days of treatment and particular care should be exercised when driving or operating machinery. Troublesome hypotension may also be encountered with levodopa (and combinations with DOPA decarboxylase inhibitors) and selegiline. Blurred vision may complicate the use of most antiparkinsonism drugs including amantadine and antimuscarinics such as benhexol, benzatropine, and orphenadrine.

Cardiovascular drugs

Most patients treated with amiodarone develop corneal microcrystals. Drivers may be dazzled by headlights at night. Visual disturbances also occur with disopyramide, flecainide, propafenone, and gemifibrozil. Fibrates, statins, and dipryidamole cause myalgia or myositis which can affect ability to perform physical work. Many cardiovascular drugs can cause dizziness and hypotension, e.g. disopyramide, flecainide, propafenone, nicorandil, dipyridamole, and nitrates.

Respiratory drugs

The anti-asthmatic drug ketotifen causes drowsiness which can affect performance of skilled tasks such as driving. The fine tremor caused by β_2-agonists and ephedrine can cause difficulty with precise tasks.

Anti-infective agents

The antituberculosis drug ethambutol is associated with visual disturbances in the form of loss of acuity, colour blindness, and restriction of visual fields. Patients should be advised to discontinue therapy immediately if vision deteriorates.

The 4-quinolone antibiotics, such as ciprofloxacin, may affect performance of skilled tasks such as driving. The effect of alcohol is enhanced. The risk of convulsions is increased particularly if used with NSAIDs.

Many diverse antimicrobials can cause dizziness which may affect performance. Examples include the penicillins, cephalosporins, metronidazole, 4-quinolones, griseofulvin, and itraconazole.

Endocrine drugs

The dopamine receptor stimulants bromocriptine, cabergoline, and quinagolide can cause dizziness and postural hypotension. Hypotensive reactions with quinagolide may be disturbing during the first few days of treatment and after dose increments; particular care is needed with driving and operating machinery; tolerance is reduced by alcohol. High-dose steroids cause cataracts which can affect performance of skilled tasks.

Other drugs

The muscle relaxants baclofen, dantrolene, and methocarbamol produce sedation and muscle weakness and make driving and operating machinery dangerous. Mydriatic eye-drops such as homatropine, atropine, and cyclopentolate paralyse accommodation and produce blurred vision. Blurred vision due to antimuscarinic actions is also seen with oxybutynin and flavoxate for urinary incontinence and pilocarpine tablets used for dry mouth. With pilocarpine, blurred vision may affect the ability to drive, particularly at night, and to perform hazardous activities in reduced light. It should also be remembered that the effects of ototoxic drugs, such as gentamicin or salicylates, will summate with any effects of noise on the middle ear.

Malaria prophylaxis

Drugs used for prophylaxis of malaria can cause symptoms which may affect ability to work. Chloroquine is often associated with visual disturbances. Dizziness or disturbed sense of balance after mefloquine may affect performance of skilled tasks such as driving. Dizziness is to some extent dose-related but neuropsychiatric reactions can occur even during prophylactic use. The incidence of minor symptoms is 20–90%. Severe transient neuropsychiatric reactions are less common with an estimated frequency of 1 in 13 000 during prophylactic use but 1 in 215 with therapeutic use. Symptoms include non-cognition, disorientation, mental confusion, hallucinations, agitation, and decreased consciousness. A single dose can be all that is needed to evoke a mental reaction. Unpredictable reactions can be provoked by concomitant use of CNS-active drugs and alcohol. Because of these potential side-effects caution is required prior to prescription with a risk assessment comparing benefits to risk based on past medical history. In addition, it is good practice for individuals to commence taking this medication 2 weeks prior to travel rather than the usual 1 week so that any potential side-effects can be detected and alternative medication prescribed before leaving the UK.

Prospective travellers should consult their general practitioner or a specialist in tropical diseases who will determine the appropriate prophylactic drug and its dosage according to the area to be visited and the time to be spent away, also taking into consideration any drug contra-indications. It is advisable to start medication a week before departure if the patient has not taken antimalarials before. The recommended prophylactic drug for malaria protection varies according to the type of malaria present in the area to be visited and the sensitivity of the parasites. The traveller's age and previous exposure to antimalarial drugs, the duration of stay, and other conditions will need to be taken into account.

Drug prophylaxis should begin, at the latest, on the day of travel to the endemic area and continue for at least 4 weeks after returning. Whether drugs are taken daily or weekly, it is advisable to take them at the same time each day, or the same day each week. The correct dosage should be strictly observed. Whatever drug is taken it must be taken with unfailing regularity to be fully effective. Drugs should be taken with liquids after a meal in order to reduce the occurrence of nausea and vomiting or mild gastrointestinal upsets, particularly if chloroquine is used.

See Appendix 5 for advice regarding medical care of overseas employees, and Appendix 7 for agencies from whom further information can be obtained.

Patient pack prescribing and provision of patient information leaflets

Since December 1998 patients must be provided with detailed written information about drugs that are dispensed to them,[15–17] bringing the UK into line with EU legislation. All drugs in the *British National Formulary* dispensed by general practitioners are now covered. The full scheme does not apply to medication dispensed through hospitals. Patients now receive packs of medicines containing an information sheet describing side-effects, interactions, etc. in simple terms. The wording on the pack and the leaflet must be approved by the Medicines Control Agency. These leaflets should provide patients with a better understanding of the risks of working with machines or driving. Patients who cannot read English or with poor sight will require risks to be explained.

Special problems in specific occupations

Flying (see also Appendix 2)

All medication that affects performance is likely to be a hazard to aircrew. In addition, environmental factors such as pressure, gravity, and temperature may all affect the performance of those flying, together with the potential additive effects of the medication. The Civil Aviation Authority (CAA) gives guidance to aircrew and states that accidents and incidents have occurred as a result of pilots flying while medically unfit, and that the majority have been associated with minor ailments rather than overwhelming medical catastrophes. In addition the Civil Aviation Authority Aeronautical Information Circular 20/1997, *Modern Medical Practice and Flight Safety,* states that 'any regular use of medication' requires the advice of a CAA Authorized Medical Examiner (AME) before duty resumes—this applies to both flight crew and air traffic control officers. The following advice is taken from the Civil Aviation Authority Aeronautical Information Circular—AIC 114/1996, which gives guidance on medication, alcohol, and flying:

- **Antibiotics**: Apart from any potential effects of the antibiotics, the effects from the infection will almost always mean that the pilot is not fit to fly.
- **Tranquillizers, antidepressants, and sedatives**: Because of their effects on performance those who are required to fly must not take them.
- **Stimulants** (e.g. caffeine and amphetamine): the use of such 'pep' pills while flying cannot be permitted.
- **Antihistamines**: many cause drowsiness. In many cases the condition requiring treatment precludes flying and if treatment is necessary, expert advice should be sought.
- **Drugs for the control of high blood pressure**: If the blood pressure is such that drugs are needed, the pilot must be temporarily grounded. Any treatment instituted should be discussed with an expert in aviation medicine before return to flying.
- **Analgesics**: The more potent analgesics may have marked effects on performance. In any case, the pain for which they are being taken is likely to indicate a condition which is a bar to flying.
- **Anaesthetics**: Following dental and other anaesthesia, at least 24 hours should elapse before return to flying after a local anaesthetic, and 48 hours after a general anaesthetic.
- **Antimalarials**: *AIC 2/1995 Malaria* provides advice on this subject with reference to flying. In particular it states that mefloquine (Larium) is not recommended for aircrew because of the potential neuropsychiatric side-effects. All aircrew need to take precautions and seek up-to-date advice if travelling to malarious areas.
- **Other medication**: if there is any change in medication or dosage or if any other medication is taken, those flying are exhorted not to take such medication unless they are completely familiar with the effect on their own body. Those taking such medication should ask three questions:
  - Do I feel fit to fly?
  - Do I really need to take medicine at all?
  - Have I given this particular medication a personal trial on the ground for at least 24 hours before flying, to ensure it will not have any adverse effects whatsoever on my ability to fly?

In certain selected cases, aircrew who are under the care of cardiologists and consultants in aviation medicine may be allowed β-blockers. Additionally, the use of temazepam as a hypnotic by aircrew in the Royal Air Force has been shown by Nicholson to have no residual effects on performance.[18] It is, however, most important that, before issuing hypnotics to aircrew, the cause for the requirement should be sought as this may be work-related and amenable to change, e.g. unusual work rosters. Similar advice is given by the CAA regarding medication and air traffic controllers.[19]

The position regarding cabin crew is different, as these staff are unlicensed and each company sets its own health standards. However, Air Navigation (No 2) Order 1995: Article 57(2) states:

A person shall not, when acting as a member of the crew of any aircraft or being carried in any aircraft for the purpose of so acting, be under the influence of drink or a drug to such an extent as to impair his capacity so to act.

The question of risks from medication to cabin crew is less relevant than their health status. The same applies to those travelling as passengers as part of their job.

Merchant navy (see also Appendix 3)

The fitness of merchant seafarers to serve at sea is determined more by the underlying condition than any medication, but it is doubtful if it is ever wise to commence seafaring if the loss of an essential drug could cause a rapid deterioration of health. Where medication is acceptable for serving seafarers, arrangements should be made for a reserve stock of the prescribed drugs to be held in a safe place, with the agreement of the ship's master.

Diving (see also Appendix 4)

Any medication that may affect performance is a potential hazard to those who dive. Additionally, environmental temperature and pressure and the use of gas combinations, e.g. oxygen/helium, may cause further problems. Guidance is given on Form MAI from the Employment Medical Advisory Service (EMAS) on the medical examination of divers where it is stated in Note 3: 'The diver should be asked specifically for details of any current medication'. In general, it is the medical condition rather than the medication that is the bar to diving.

The question of the effect and use of drugs in hyperbaric conditions is an interesting but practical problem for those who have to treat sick divers under pressure. Cox[20] lists drugs that have been used by divers; the depths to which they have been used; and whether there were any untoward effects.

Offshore workers (see also Appendix 4)

Guidance is given by the UK Offshore Operators Association in its *Guidelines for medical aspects of fitness for offshore work*. Referring to medicines, it states the following:

- Individuals on anticoagulants, cytotoxic agents, insulin, anticonvulsants, immuno-suppressants, and oral steroids are unacceptable for offshore work.
- Individuals on psychotropic medication e.g. tranquillizers, antidepressants, narcotics, and hypnotics are also unacceptable. A previous history of such treatment will require further consideration.
- Individuals taking medication must ensure they have an adequate supply and must report any adverse drug reaction to the offshore medic.

Those who work in the Norwegian and Dutch sectors of the North Sea come within the similar legislation of those countries.

Driving

Ordinary driving licences

- Section 5 of the Road Traffic Act 1972: refers to 'Driving or being in charge under the influence of a drug'.
- The Poisons Rules (1972) require a number of substances containing antihistamines to be labelled with the words 'Caution, may cause drowsiness, if affected do not drive or operate machinery'.

Advice from the Drivers Medical Unit of the Driver and Vehicle Licencing Agency (DVLA) for medical practitioners on medication[21] states:

- Driving while unfit through drugs provided or illicit is an offence and may lead to prosecution.
- All CNS-active drugs can impair alertness, concentration and driving performance. This is particularly so within the first month of starting or increasing the dose. It is important to cease driving during this time if adversely affected.
- Benzodiazepines are most dangerous and are overrepresented in drivers involved in road traffic accidents.
- Drugs having anticholinergic side-effects should be avoided in drivers. These include tricyclic antidepressants and phenothiazines. Antihistamine effects of some antidepressants may cause drowsiness and care must be taken.
- SSRIs, MAOIs, and nonadrenaline re-uptake inhibitors have fewer side-effects and are safer. However, some patients have idiosyncratic responses, and should be advised accordingly.
- Long-acting depot neuroleptics and the new antipsychotic drugs can impair driving, but sedation usually diminishes after approximately 3 months. Parkinsonian side-effects can be dangerous. Drivers on these drugs should be carefully assessed clinically. A formal driving assessment may be required.
- The interaction of all CNS-active drugs with alcohol will increase impairment and affect driving ability.
- Drivers with psychiatric illnesses are usually safer when well and on regular psychotropic medication than when they are ill. Inadequate treatment or lack of compliance may render the driver impaired by both illness and medication.
- Doctors who fail to advise their patients of the dangers of side-effects of psychotropic medication may have serious medico-legal difficulties should an accident occur.

Drivers of LGVs, PCVs, and taxis

Much stricter criteria have to be applied to professional than to private drivers. As a class they have to drive for longer hours, so the risks of adverse drug reactions or interactions coinciding with a situation in which other road users could be injured by loss of control is far greater. Furthermore, it is not so easy for a professional driver to stop driving when feeling unwell as a result of adverse effects of drugs.

Where there is a need for long-term medication, the issue of whether it is safe for vocational driving to continue may not arise as the driver will often be excluded from holding an LGV or PCV licence as a result of the medical condition requiring treatment. *Medical aspects of fitness to drive*[22] deals with the desirability or otherwise of LGV or PCV drivers being allowed to drive under treatment, and should be consulted where appropriate.

In the case of short-term medication, the safest course is to certify the driver as unfit to drive for an initial period if it seems at all likely that the treatment might impair driving ability. If treatment has to continue, a decision about returning to work can then be taken in the light of any adverse reactions which may have occurred in the initial stage of treatment.

Someone who has to take insulin, hypotensive drugs (except diuretics and β-blockers) or drugs that affect the CNS is not likely to be fit to drive vocationally.

Conclusions and recommendations

Suggestions for advice to patients taking drugs which affect the CNS

- Do not exceed the stated dose.
- Do not drive, fly, or operate machinery until the nature and extent of any side-effects are known.
- Do not take any other medication or drugs unless prescribed for you.

General principles of prescribing for people at work

- Always enquire into the patient's occupation, and be aware of drug effects which can be hazardous in the work environment.
- Make sure the patient understands what to expect and what action to take.
- Be particularly careful with all drugs which act on the CNS and avoid polypharmacy as this may have unintended additive effects.
- Keep treatment regimens simple and, where possible, avoid more than two daily doses to increase compliance.
- If a hypnotic is required, use one with a short duration of effect.
- Avoid unsupervised use of drugs; give a minimum of repeat prescriptions and supervise regularly.
- Avoid the use of antihistamines in those who have to operate machinery, drive, or fly. Where they are essential, favour less-sedating agents.
- Reserves of medication must be carried by those whose occupation takes them abroad for long periods of time, e.g. those on board ship. Reserves should also be

available for emergency use for those working in isolated or dangerous situations where evacuation may be delayed.

Selected references

1   Edwards F. Risks at work from medication. *J R Coll Physicians Lond* 1978; **12**: 219–229.
2   Kirkness B (ed.) *Pharma facts and figures.* London: Association of the British Pharmaceutical Industry, 1997.
3   Dunnell K, Cartwright A. *Medicine takers, prescribers and hoarders.* London: Routledge and Kegan Paul, 1972.
4   Rennie IG. Accidents at work—risks from medication. Royal College of Physicians, Faculty of Occupational Medicine, MFOM Dissertation, 1985.
5   Lader M. Benzodiazepines—long-term use and problems of withdrawal. *MIMS Magazine* 1985, March.
6   Rawlins MD, Thompson JW. In: *Textbook of adverse drug reactions*, 4th edn, ed. Davies DM. Oxford: Oxford University Press, 1991.
7   Nicholson AM, Stone BM. Disturbance of circadian rhythms and sleep. *Proc R Soc Edinburgh* 1985; **82BL**: 135–139.
8   Nakano S. Time of day effect on psychotherapeutic drug response and kinetics in man. In: *Towards chronopharmacology*, ed. Takahashi R, Holberg F, Walker CA. *Adv Biosci* 1982; **41**: 51–59.
9   Hindmarch I. Psychomotor function and psychoactive drugs. *Br J Clin Pharmacol* 1980; **10**: 189–209.
10 Broadbent DE. Performance and its measurement. *Br J Clin Pharmacol* 1984; **18**: 5S–9S.
11 Hunter J, Maxwell JD, Stewart DA. Increased hepatic microsomal enzyme activity from occupational exposure to certain organochlorine pesticides. *Nature* 1972; **237**: 399–401.
12 Blain PG, Rawlins MD. Drug-induced body temperature changes. Prescribers Journal 1981; **21**: 204.
13 Barbone F, McMahon AD, Davey PG et al.. Association of road-traffic accidents with benzodiazepine use. *Lancet* 1998; **352**: 1331–1336.
14 Second European Workshop in Aviation Cardiology. *Eur Heart J Vol 1.SuppD.* 1999.
15 *The patient pack initiative.* London, Medicines Control Agency, 1995.
16 Council Directive 92/27 EEC. *Official J Eur Community* 1992 L113/8-/12.
17 *Medicines. The Medicines for Human Use (marketing authorisations, etc.) Regulations 1994.* Statutory Instrument No.30144. London: HMSO, 1994.
18 Nicholson AN. Long periods of work and disturbed sleep. *Ergonomics* 1984; **27**: 629–630.
19 *Medication and air traffic control.* Aeronautical Information Circular, United Kingdom Civil Aviation Authority 12/1991.
20 Cox RAF (ed.) *Offshore medicine; medical care of employees in the offshore oil industry*, 2nd edn. Berlin: Springer-Verlag, 1987.
21 *At a glance guide to the current medical standards of fitness to drive.* DVLA, Swansea, 1998.
22 Taylor JF. *Medical aspects of fitness to drive*, 5th edn. Medical Commission on Accident Prevention, London, 1995.

27

Work and the older employee

W. J. A. Goedhard

Although average life expectancy has increased considerably in the twentieth century, especially in developed countries, fewer years are spent at work. People start to work later because of longer periods of education and training, but in most countries they do not retire later. On the contrary, during the last few decades early retirement (at the age of 55–65) has become a popular, well-accepted policy in most western countries. Little thought has therefore been given to the needs of older employees.

This situation is changing rapidly, however, and early retirement is less likely in the future[1]. Lower birth rates since the 1960s and prolonged life expectation have led to an unprecedented ageing of populations, and consequently the average age of employees is increasing. For example, the age profile of employees in a Dutch chemical company, DSM, with 8 500 employees will change as shown in Table 27.1 (derived from De Vroom and Walker[2,3]). Such changes in age profiles warrant the timely development of appropriate policies.

The trend is towards an increasing age of employees in most countries, although economic aspects may cause differences between countries.

- Levels of economic activity among people aged 50 and over in France, Germany, and the Netherlands are lower than in the UK.[4] This may be partly due to differences in national government policies.
- In Finland the workforce shows a much bigger increase in average age than in most other countries; between 1980 and 2000 the percentage of workers aged 45–60 years in Finland will increase from 32% to 41%.[5]
- In Japan between 1996 and 2025 the median age of the workforce will probably increase from 39 to 45 years.[6]
- In the OECD countries the percentage of workers between 45 and 64 years will increase from 32% to 35.5% between 1980 and 2000. A further rise towards 41% is expected by 2025.[7]

Furthermore, in many countries economic growth in the 1990s has increased the demand for labour. This situation may also vary from country to country: in the

Table 27.1 Age profile of employees in a Dutch chemical company

Age category	1995	2000
20–34 years	36%	21%
35–49 years	48%	55%
50–64 years	16%	24%

Netherlands, for example, many workers between 55 and 65 were made redundant between 1978 and 1993 and many others left the labour market with attractive early retirement schemes. Unemployment figures for younger employees were too high. However, between 1994 and 1998 half a million new jobs were created (i.e. about 8% of the total workforce) and unemployment has now dropped below 5%. Early retirement schemes will soon disappear and people will remain employed until the age of mandatory retirement. In the future many workers may still be actively employed beyond the traditional age of retirement. Table 27.2 shows some data on the forecast of labour participation in the Netherlands, and there are similar data for other countries.

These trends raise two important issues:

- Can these changes be accomplished without the help of occupational health services?
- Can older employees cope with the work demands?

These questions pose important challenges to policy makers, companies (management and personnel officers), and occupational health services.

Ageing and work

What is an 'older employee'? Trying to define an age limit is probably not very useful. It can be assumed that employees beyond the age of 45–50 years are in the final third of their professional career. Between 45 and 65–70 years many age-associated changes occur in the human body, some of which affect the ability to work. The effects vary in different types of work. Very heavy physical work cannot usually be performed by workers over 60, because the functional performance of many body systems declines with age. However, there is much inter-individual variation, and this seems to increase with chronological age. It is essential that occupational health physicians who are dealing with older employees have a sound knowledge of age-associated changes in the body.

Gerontological information is the basis for the proper management of older employees. Both physiological and psychological changes occur with advancing age. For example, psychomotor performance related to the central integration of perceptual and motor functions tends to decrease with age.[9] Examples of age-associated changes are increased reaction time, and declines in short-term memory and visual search speed. Fine motor speed was found to decrease by 2–7% in a 4-year follow-up study on workers

Table 27.2 Projected age profile of the workforce in the Netherlands, based on a balanced growth model[8]

Year	1990	2005	2020
Median age	35 years	39 years	39–40 years
% of total workforce	66	71	75
Workers			
aged 15–29 years (%)	36	26	26
aged 50–64 years (%)	14	19	27

between 51 and 55 years.[10] Other physiological functions also tend to change with age. Pulmonary function, maximum oxygen uptake capacity, and cardiac output decrease, though the rate of decrease is slowed by regular physical exercise.[11]

Ageing in specific physiological functions has effects on work ability.

Vision

Visual function tends to decrease with age. Changes are observed in light adaptation, dark adaptation, accommodation of the lens, and visual acuity.[12] Dark adaptation, and to a lesser extent light adaptation, show a linear decrease with age from the beginning of adulthood (over 20 years of age). Loss of lens accommodation starts early in life, beginning at the age of 10, resulting in a virtually complete loss of accommodation for near vision at the age of 55 years. The near vision point, which is at 8 cm on the average at 16 years, shifts to over 25 cm for people over 45 years.[13] The comfortable working distance from a computer screen is usually 40–70 cm, so older employees may experience difficulties in the use of visual display units (VDUs) and computers. Reading glasses often do not provide appropriate correction, but this can be overcome by using separate glasses for computer tasks (see Chapter 9, p. 175).

The decline in visual acuity usually begins around 25 years and becomes even more pronounced beyond the age of 60 years. The loss of visual acuity may be partly compensated by an increase of light intensity; this will also increase contrast sensitivity.

Changes in visual abilities may have consequences in different occupations. For professional drivers and airline pilots changes may lead to loss of work ability; workers in the electronics industry, where components are increasingly miniaturized, may experience difficulties in performance, especially if the work demands also include good colour perception. However, in most professions age-associated changes in visual functions will probably not lead to a diminished work ability.

Hearing acuity

Loss of hearing associated with ageing is called **presbycusis**. The prevalence of hearing problems increases, from 1/10 000 at 35 years to 10/10 000 at 65 years,[12] and becomes increasingly prominent in people over 65. This may result in speech comprehension problems, but probably has little effect on work ability. Disability figures indicate that only a small percentage of workers become disabled because of hearing problems, although there may be some underestimation (see Chapter 10, p, 185).

It is debatable whether all age-associated hearing losses can be attributed to the ageing process. Our modern, noisy industrial society might be partly responsible for some loss in hearing function.

Intellectual performance and learning ability

Basic cognitive abilities show an average decline with age.[14] However, it is also reported by Salthouse that in some occupations the most capable workers are older adults. There appears to be little relation between age and measures of work performance. Although a positive relation can be assumed between basic cognitive processes and work performance, experience probably also has a considerable influence. Since experience usually increases with age, this may partly compensate for the decline in cognitive abilities.

Learning new technologies, for example in computer-aided secretarial work, may be a problem for older workers,. It is not quite clear whether age is a causative factor in any decline in learning ability. In the past, the lower educational levels of older workers may have induced learning anxiety during training of new skills.[15] Preparatory training of older employees is particularly advocated before technological changes are implemented,[16] though there is not yet much knowledge available about the right procedures to be followed when dealing with an ageing workforce in relation to new technological developments. A fundamental problem in studies on age in relation to work performance seems to be the difference in educational level of different age-cohorts. Studies on intelligence and aptitudes are often based on cross-sectional studies. This may influence test results more than the actual ageing process.[17] What is lacking is a systematic body of knowledge that ties age-related changes in skills and abilities to the skill requirements of jobs.[18]

Locomotor performance and diminishing mobility

Locomotor performance is a complex process which involves the functioning of the nervous system, muscles, joints, and bones. The various tissues and organs are known to change with age. For example, muscle strength declines with increasing age. Peak of muscle strength occurs at the age of 20–30 years.[19]

Musculoskeletal capacity was found to decrease by 16–22% in 4 years in a Finnish group of workers between 51 and 55 years, i.e. 4–5% per year.[20] This may strongly affect work ability.[21] Without training, muscle power deteriorates at a rapid rate, but regular physical exercise opposes these age-associated effects.[11] Training has beneficial effects on strength, power, and speed of movement ('use it or lose it'). Work itself is not enough to maintain locomotor performance. Physical exercise should therefore be promoted and undertaken apart from work; for example, by participating in fitness programmes, especially for workers aged 50 years and above.

Since musculoskeletal complaints in the elderly often result in diminished working capacity and are responsible for many cases of disability, special attention should be focused on workers at high risk. In the Netherlands 32% of all disability cases are caused by locomotor disorders, the biggest group of disabled workers. Over the age of 50 years women are even more at risk than men.[22] De Zwart recommends four measures to reduce disability figures:

- ergonomic interventions aimed at reducing the workload
- career planning aimed at changing the workload
- shortening of exposure time
- physical exercise during leisure time.

Diminishing cardiopulmonary performance and physical fitness

Cardiopulmonary performance is dependent on age-associated changes as well as lifestyle. For a long time it was assumed that cardiac output decreased linearly with age.

However, later studies confirmed that, in healthy individuals, cardiac output with exercise is maintained with advancing age.[23]

Nevertheless, cardiopulmonary performance shows a decrease with age in most people, because of independent pathological changes, but there is much individual variation which depends on both genetic factors and environmental factors. Longitudinal studies on endurance capacity have shown that there is an average decrease with age,[24] but regular physical exercise can increase cardiopulmonary performance by as much as 20%. Environmental factors, such as lifestyle and work exposures, may affect cardiopulmonary functioning as much as age does.[24] Good performance starts with a healthy lifestyle, refraining from smoking and avoiding an adverse work environment. Various chemical and physical exposures at work, and also psychosocial work stress, may affect cardiopulmonary function and a healthy work environment will prevent deterioration in cardiopulmonary function[25].

A positive relation between physical fitness and work ability is likely. In a study of 49 overtly healthy workers a positive relationship was found between the work ability index (WAI) score and VO_2 max (i.e. maximum oxygen uptake capacity). In the group with low VO_2 max values and low WAI score a sickness percentage of nearly 10% per year was observed,[26] which suggests that companies should ensure optimum physical fitness of their employees.

Psychological changes

Cognitive abilities, when tested under laboratory circumstances, also show age-related declines in performance. Thus, older individuals have more difficulty in memorizing a series of unrelated words or numbers. Even the IQs of older individuals have been found to be lower than those in a young reference group.[14] These changes are reflected in work performance. However, as Salthouse has pointed out, there is apparently little relation between age alone and measures of work performance. In some occupations, older employees are more capable than their younger colleagues. Thus, although ageing in general has a negative influence on basic cognitive processes, this is often compensated by the greater experience of older employees. This may result in a strong positive influence of age on work performance, which is a complex, multifactorial concept. A simplified model is shown in Fig. 27.1.

Effects of disease

In similar models, disease and its effects are examined.[27] It can be argued that age-associated diseases may have an adverse impact on work performance (e.g. osteoarthritis or diabetes mellitus). However, the relationships are often more complicated than they at first appear. Diseases are not merely induced by age, but usually depend on many other risk factors such as adverse ergonomics, chemical exposures, psychological work stress, obesity, and adverse lifestyle. It may help to define and consider several different aspects of ageing:

- healthy ageing
- productive ageing
- successful ageing

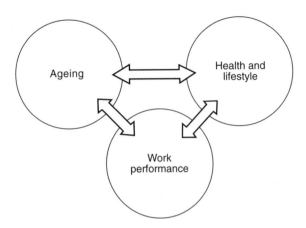

Fig. 27.1 Model of the relations between ageing, health, and work performance. Ageing has effects on biological, social, and psychological functions.

Healthy ageing

The way people age differs considerably, and this variation increases with age. Why? What is ageing? Gerontology, the science dealing with the study of the ageing process, cannot yet provide us with a clear answer about what causes the ageing process. There are many ageing theories but none of them can explain satisfactorily why biological organisms age. The best we can say is that the ageing process depends on both genetic and environmental factors.[28,29]

Genetic factors primarily define the maximum lifespan of a species; humans may very occasionally live for 120 years, mice only 4 years. Furthermore, genetic factors are responsible for important morphological and physiological changes of the ageing process.

Environmental factors are also very important in relation to the ageing process. These factors can probably increase or decrease the process of ageing and determine its rate. This has become quite clear in the twentieth century, during which life expectancy at birth has increased considerably, especially in developed countries. This increase has mainly been achieved by the reduction of infant mortality. However, other measures in later life, including improvements to working conditions, have contributed favourably to improved life expectancy. A major problem, however, remains the lack of good health in old age. On the average we live longer, but many of the extra years are subject to chronic diseases. These include osteoarthritis, diabetes mellitus, cardiovascular diseases, hypertension, chronic obstructive pulmonary disease, and malignancy. We should distinguish, therefore, between average life expectancy and healthy life expectancy. It is estimated that the latter at present is only 60 years.[30] This means that many older workers will be affected by one or more chronic disorders during their professional life. Often this will end in disablement and involuntary early retirement. It is a challenge to occupational health professionals both to prevent the development of such chronic disorders and to minimize their effects.

What can be done to promote healthy ageing? The various environmental factors that may affect health are described below.

Smoking

Smoking is the most important factor. The prevalence of smoking differs according to socio-economic status (SES) and level of educational attainment. Data reported from the Netherlands are shown in Table 27.3.[31] Smoking is still very common, despite intensive promotional campaigns to give it up, and it is commoner in blue-collar workers than in white-collar workers. Other adverse working conditions may also be more prevalent in the less educated group.

Diet and obesity

It is beyond the scope of this chapter to review in great detail the possible effects of diet on health and disease. Control of body weight is important for work performance. Obesity is an increasing problem, mostly in the lowest SES groups.[31] Typically, in western Europe, about 13% of men and 16% of women are obese, where obesity is defined as having a body mass index (BMI) > 30 kg/m^2. Obesity increases the risk of cardiovascular diseases, arthritis, and diabetes mellitus. For elderly workers the BMI should be below 27 kg/m^2. From animal experiments it is known that reduction of energy intake (food restriction) is inversely related to longevity.[28] It is not known whether these findings can be applied to humans as well.

Physical exercise

Physical inactivity, or a sedentary lifestyle, is a phenomenon of developed societies. In the US the majority of men (56%) and women (62%) are not engaged in regular physical exercise (defined as at least three times a week for 20 minutes)[32]. Regular physical exercise will increase fitness, aerobic power, and muscular strength and will thus have beneficial effects on workers' health. With advancing age, the tendency towards a sedentary lifestyle increases, and it is therefore essential that special attention is paid to this problem in elderly employees. Some workers, especially in physically demanding jobs, believe that their work already requires enough physical exercise. However, this view cannot usually be supported: in many jobs the heavy physical demands necessary to maintain an optimal physical condition arise only occasionally.[33] Special physical exercise training programmes are therefore warranted. Such company-encouraged programmes have beneficial effects on health, productivity, absenteeism, and work ability.

Table 27.3 Frequency of smoking in relation to sex and level of education

Educational status	Men (%)	Women (%)
Low (only basic education)	50	47
High (university degree)	29	31

Productive ageing

Productive ageing can be defined in a wide or narrower sense. The wide definition is 'engagement over a lifetime in paid or unpaid activities that produce valued goods or services'.[34] A narrower definition, referring to professional activities and elderly employees only, could then be 'engagement in paid activities that produce valued goods or services after the age of 45 years'.

Maintenance of work ability

For many workers it is obviously difficult to satisfy the above definition until retirement. Many older workers are compelled to retire prematurely through disability. Maintenance of work ability is thus a particularly important issue in relation to older employees.

Work capacity and work demands

Theoretically the ability to perform professional tasks should decrease with advancing age. If, for reasons of simplicity, working capacity is considered as the total sum of all physiological functions, the ratio of work demands to work capacity would become more and more unfavourable during the course of life. Figure 27.2a presents the theoretical ratio of job demands and work capacity. On the basis of this model, the solution would be to adapt the job demands continuously to the age-associated work capacity (Fig. 27.2b). However, the situation is more complex, as work ability is determined not only by physiological functions and their changes with age.

Older employees can be likened to precious cars. They have many good qualities, which are valued, preserved, and used, but at the same time they are at risk of breakdown if they do not receive proper care. They should be serviced with more than average dedication and at shorter intervals.

Work ability is a complex entity. This is shown in a schematic model (see Fig. 27.3). As can be seen, maintenance of work ability depends on the work in question and the work environment; the organization's culture, and the individual worker. Action plans can be devised for each of these areas, and specifically targeted at ageing workers.

Work and environment

The working environment includes physical workload, chemical and biological exposures, and ergonomics. The specific needs of older employees and these various aspects of the work environment should be evaluated. Interventions can then be undertaken. An example of such an evaluation is a study on refuse collectors.[35] It was found that few refuse collectors were able to continue working after the age of 45 years because of health problems. Different systems of collecting were studied in various age groups. Based on the study's findings, recommendations were made such as:

* reducing the workload of older workers during their career, taking into account the age-dependent loss of work capacity
* introducing a rotation schedule of heavy and light tasks (job rotation).

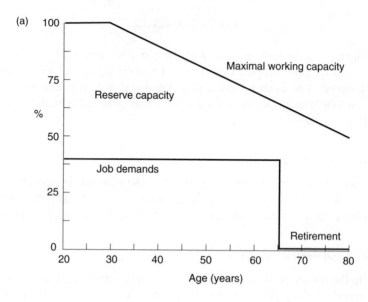

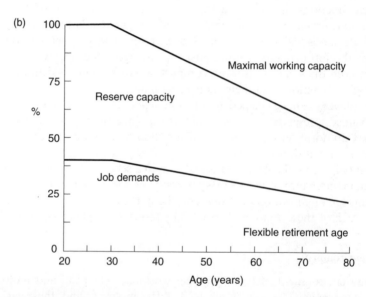

Fig. 27.2 (a) Physiological functions decrease with age at a rate of about 1% per year after the age of 30, and this affects working capacity. If work demands remain at the same level, the ratio of demands to capacity deteriorates with age. (b) The solution to the dilemma is to adapt work demands by reducing them with age, and introducing a flexible retirement age.

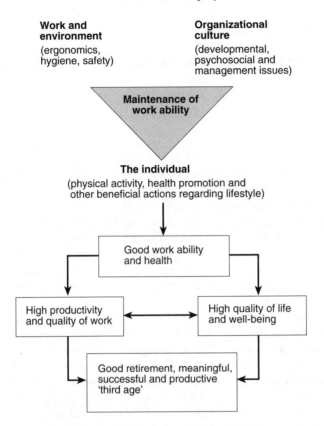

Fig. 27.3   Factors contributing to the maintenance of work ability. See text for details.

Implementation of such recommendations enabled the older employees to continue at work.

Organizational culture

The culture of the workplace encompasses management issues, leadership and psychosocial factors such as work stress. Maintaining work ability is not only a matter of occupational healthcare but also includes other aspects of personnel care. An important facet is the way older workers are treated within an organization. In the 1970s and 1980s older workers were readily made redundant, which had consequences on matters such as training and development.

Training and development of older workers

In a study on middle and higher level functions in employees over 40 years old it was found that the amount of training and development offered decreased considerably with age.[36] This subsequently greatly reduced their flexibility and, in the event of reorganization, made their positions vulnerable. According to the authors, senior managers neglect action that could lead to timely development of the elderly worker's potential. A possible reason for this is the stereotyped belief that the ability or motivation to learn new skills deteriorates with age. The principal results of this study are presented in Table 27.4.

Work stress

Work stress is also an important aspect of work ability. In the present economic circumstances psychological stresses on most workers have increased. In many countries, as in the Netherlands, excessive levels of work stress have become a major cause of disablement. Work stress affects both young and older workers. Older workers are probably better able to cope with stress owing to greater experience on the job; younger workers tend to develop depressive disorders when exposed to high work stress. However, stress may be more dangerous for elderly workers by affecting physiological systems such as the cardiovascular system. Work stress can be assessed by questionnaires. In a study on Dutch employees of a national research organization, a questionnaire developed by Frommer et al.[37] was used to measure the following stress factors on a five-point scale (1 = no stress; 5 = high stress) (Box 27.1).

Stress scores above 2.0 were found to indicate a significantly increased level of perceived stress, and more than one stress factor has to be increased to qualify for a diagnosis of increased work stress.[38] This is analogous to the model of Karasek[39] (see Table 27.5). In that particular model two stress factors were examined, namely workload (work demands) and decision latitude (work control). If workers are exposed to high workloads but can make their own work arrangements (i.e. are in control of their work), they do not usually experience excessive work stress. This group was said to be 'active'.

Social support has beneficial effects on the perception of stress. In the study mentioned above the relationship between work stress and absenteeism was also quantitatively examined (see Table 27. 6). In the active group a very low figure was observed; in the high strain group the figure was much higher. It is clear that work stress tends to increase absenteeism.

Table 27.4 Utility value, learning value, training and development of 308 workers with middle-level positions in ten large scale industries in The Netherlands (derived from Boerlijst and van der Heijden[36])

Age range (years)	40–46	47–52	53+
Numbers ($n = 308$)	100	91	117
Utility value[a] (%)	75%	70%	55%
Learning value[b] (%)	35%	45%	30%
Mobility[c]	Medium	Low	Very low
Training and development provided			
(>5 days per year) (%)	45%	50%	35%

[a] Utility value: the value of a function within the framework of the organization or the department in which the function is positioned.
[b] Learning value: the value of a function as a basis for the employee's further development.
[c] (Functional) mobility: the transition to another position or function (job mobility).

> **Box 27.1 Stress factors**
> - Boredom
> - Lack of support
> - Quantitative overload
> - Qualitative overload
> - Unsatisfactory prospects or remuneration
> - Unsatisfactory physical working conditions

Shiftwork and ageing

It is well known that shiftworkers usually run into problems when they have to continue in shiftwork schedules after the age of 40–50 years. This is probably due to the changes in sleep pattern with advancing age. The number of arousals during sleep increases with age, and this must reduce the ability to cope with a shift superimposed on the biological circadian rhythm.[40,41] There are several reports in the literature about physiological changes induced by shiftwork. However, there is virtually no information on how to overcome the negative consequences, such as the deterioration of health. Health problems associated with shiftwork include gastrointestinal disturbances, cardiovascular disorders, and neurological disorders, which may result in disablement and ceasing work. One aim of good occupational health practice is to prevent disability. This may be achieved by pre-employment examination of the worker, which will reveal disorders not compatible with shiftwork, such as diabetes mellitus, peptic ulcers, and epilepsy. The main problem arises if a worker, after many years on the job, can no longer cope with the sleep disturbances of shiftwork. The best solution is secondary prevention following early detection by periodic occupational health examination of the ageing employee. A useful instrument is the work ability index.

Table 27.5 Model of stress factors according to Karasek[39]

Control	Work demands	
	Low	High
High	Low strain (relaxed)	Active[a]
Low	Passive	High strain

[a]Active: in control of their work.

Table 27.6 Average number of sickness claims per year in relation to work stress[39]

Lack of support	Quantitative overload	
	No	Yes
No	1.5 (relaxed)	0.7 (active)
Yes	1.2 (passive)	2.4 (high strain)

Work ability index[42-44]

The WAI is an instrument developed by researchers of the Finnish Institute of Occupational Health.[42] The WAI has been developed with the particular aim of promoting and maintaining the ability of older employees to work. Like many other western countries, Finland faces a rise in the average age of the workforce. A comprehensive longitudinal study was conducted on more than 6000 workers aged 45–58 years and led to the development of the WAI which consists of a questionnaire comprising seven items. The questionnaire is administered by an occupational health professional and each item is scored and the overall WAI score, which varies between 7 and 49, is obtained by adding the seven scores (Table 27.7).

The compilers of the WAI are very positive about its usefulness, and the instrument has been used a great deal in Finland. Reports on longitudinal studies indicate an inverse relationship between the WAI score and the risk of premature retirement because of disability. Based on these findings, workers could be classified into four categories and suitable management goals planned to keep the worker gainfully employed (see Table 27.8).

The WAI has also been translated into several other languages. The Dutch version became available in 1995 and experience with the instrument so far is promising. Table 27.9 presents some data from a Dutch study. There are two preliminary conclusions based on this study:

- nearly 1 out of 8 (12%) workers have a poor to moderate work ability
- blue-collar workers are at higher risk of unfavourable work ability than white-collar workers (the differences may be even more marked if the healthy worker effect is taken into account).

Age and work ability

An important question concerns the rate of change in work ability in relation to age. Physiological functions (such as pulmonary function, maximal endurance capacity, and maximal heart rate) usually decrease by about 1% per year after the age of 30. In the Finnish study, as well as in the Dutch study, a much smaller decrease in work ability was observed. The average decrease was about 0.3% per year. Work ability seems to be deter-

Table 27.7 The WAI items[42]

Item	Description	Scale
1	Present work ability compared with life time best	0–10
2	Work ability in relation to physical and mental work demands	2–10
3	Number of diagnosed diseases	1–7
4	Work impairment due to disease	1–6
5	Sickness absence during last 12 months	1–5
6	Prognosis of work ability after 2 years	1–7
7	Psychological resources (spirit, optimism about the future)	1–4
Total	WAI score	7–49

Table 27.8 Relation between WAI score, work ability, and the ageing worker's future needs[42]

WAI score measures	Work ability	Objective of
7–27	Poor	Restore work ability
28–36	Moderate	Improve work ability
37–43	Good	Support work ability
44–49	Excellent	Maintain work ability

Table 27.9 Study in 207 older[a] Dutch workers of the frequency of WAI score by employment status[42]

WAI score	Work ability	Number (%)	Number Blue collar	White collar
7–27	Poor	3 (1.4)	3	0
28–36	Moderate	22 (10.6)	18	4
37–43	Good	65 (31.4)	41	24
44–49	Excellent	117 (56.5)	50	67

[a]Mean age 42 years.

mined mainly by muscular strength or physical endurance capacity (VO_2 max), but psychological influences such as work stress or motivation may also play an important role.

These findings give us hope for the future. The ability to continue working beyond the age that has traditionally been set as the start of retirement (65 years) is clearly possible, but much will depend on the proper care of older employees.

This includes not only the regular assessment of the WAI score, but also on-going advice and follow-up. From Table 27.8 it is apparent that workers with poor to moderate WAI scores should receive appropriate advice, which will depend on the individual's needs and will be in one or more of the action groups indicated (work environment, organization, and individual worker). Sometimes workers will be advised to improve their health by changing their lifestyle, or the work environment may have to be improved, e.g. by ergonomic measures. A third, more complex, group of actions may comprise change of job contents and training. An overview of possible measures for older workers is summarized in Box 27.2.

Conclusion: successful ageing

In the nineteeth century Benjamin Franklin said, 'All would like to live long, but none would like to be old'; but this a matter of opinion depending on a person's perception of successful ageing. An objective definition might describe the concept as reaching one's potential and arriving at a level of physical, social and psychological well-being in old age.[34]

Box 27.2   Some instruments for developing good policies for older workers in
companies (derived from De Vroom[2] and Walker[3])
- Recruitment and selection:
  - raise the age limit on vacancies
  - remove age limits
  - offer temporary employment to older workers
- Training and career development:
  - develop specific training courses for older workers
  - encourage age-conscious personnel policies
- Flexibility:
  - improve the work environment and workload
  - make adaptations to jobs
- Control of negative image-building:
  - conduct or report research on the good productivity of older workers
  - conduct campaigns aimed at changing negative attitudes to ageing
- Changes in retirement policy:
  - raise the age of early retirement
  - raise the mandatory retirement age

According to the model depicted in Fig. 27.3, reaching a good retirement is already an expression of successful ageing. From the active working period the perspective is directed primarily at the phase immediately following retirement. Modern occupational health services should promote health in such a way that the expected life after retirement will be full, healthy, and independent. Ideally, occupational healthcare should be extended beyond the age of retirement. This would also facilitate study of the possible long-term effects of work exposures. Employees, employers, and occupational health services together are jointly responsible for ensuring that the worker arrives at the age of retirement in good shape. An important question is when retirement should be. There are many reasons why a worker will retire. In the case of mandatory retirement it is just a formal matter. However, the trend will probably be towards workers choosing their own age of retirement. Legislation can be expected that will prevent age discrimination and enable workers voluntarily to continue working beyond the traditional age limits. On the other hand, for workers who wish to consider early retirement, the possibilities of flexible retirement between 55 and 65 are emerging. Such policies are in accordance with the different aspirations and capabilities of older workers.[45] The period between 55 and 75 ('young old age') is an important phase of life. This phase has long been neglected in society. Now, with a growing interest in employees belonging to this phase it will be essential to provide many options for workers in this age group.

Selected references

1   Thomas A, Pearson M, Meegan R. *Older workers: Conditions of work and transition to retirement. Country Report. United Kingdom.* Geneva: International Labour Office, 1992.

2   Vroom B de. *Work and age in the Netherlands* [in Dutch]. Enschede: University of Twente, 1997.

3   Walker A. Work after 45—a sociological perspective. In: *Work after 45?*, ed. Kilbom A *et al.*, Vol. 1. pp. 29–48. Stockholm; Arbetslivinstitutet, 1997.

4   Grattan P. United Kingdom. In: *Projects assisting older workers in the European Community*, ed. Taylor P, pp. 84–87. Luxembourg: . Official Publisher for the European Community, 1998.

5   Rantanen J. Opening address. In: *Ageing and Work*, ed. Ilmarinen J, pp. 1–4. Helsinki: FIOH, 1992.

6   Kumashiro M. A practical ergonomic approach to developing supporting equipment for older workers. In: *Work after 45?*, ed. Kilbom A *et al.*, pp. 200–206. Stockholm: Arbetslivinstitutet, 1997.

7   Ilmarinen J. Background and objectives of the Finnish research project on ageing workers in municipal occupation. *Scand J Work Environ Health* 1991;Suppl. 1: 7–11.

8   Wetenschappelijke Raad voor het Regeringsbeleid [Scientific Council for Governmental Policy]. *The elderly for the elderly. Demographic developments and policy* (in Dutch). The Hague: Sdu, 1993.

9   Ilmarinen J. Productivity in late adulthood—physical and mental potentials after the age of 55 years. In *Ageing and Work* 3, ed. Goedhard WJA, pp. 3–18. The Hague: Pasmans, 1996.

10 Suvanto S, Huuhtanen P, Nygard C-H, Ilmarinen J. Performance efficiency and its changes among ageing municipal employees. *Scand J Work Environ Health* 1991;**17**: 118–121.

11 Skinner JS, Tipton CM, Vailas AC. Exercise, physical training and the ageing process. In *Lectures on Gerontology*, ed. Viidik A, vol. 1, pp. 407–440. London: Academic Press, 1982.

12 Meisami E. Ageing of the nervous system: sensory changes. In: *Physiological basis of ageing and geriatrics*, ed. Timiras PS, pp. 156–178. New York: Macmillan, 1988.

13 Kroemer KHE, Grandjean E. Fitting the task to the human. In: *A Textbook of Occupational Ergonomics*, 5th edn. London, Taylor & Francis, 1997.

14 Salthouse TA. Implications of adult age differences in cognition for work performance. In: *Work after 45?*, ed. Kilbom A *et al.*, Vol. 1. pp. 15–28. Stockholm; Arbetslivinstitutet, 1997.

15 Delgoulet C, Marquie JC, Escribe C. Training older workers. Relationships between age, other trainee characteristics, and learning anxiety. In *Work after 45?*, ed. Kilbom A *et al.*, Vol. 1. pp. 70–78. Stockholm; Arbetslivinstitutet, 1997.

16 Itoh KH. Adaptation to change in the work environment for senior white collar employees. In *Work after 45?*, ed. Kilbom A *et al.*, Vol. 1. pp. 186–192. Stockholm: Arbetslivinstitutet, 1997.

17 Huuhtanen P. Psychological issues of ageing and work. In: *Preparation for ageing*, ed. Heikkinen E *et al.*, pp. 205–214. New York: Plenum Press, 1995.

18 Czaja SJ (ed.). *Human factors research needs for an ageing population*. Washington, DC: National Academy Press, 1990.

19 Timiras PS Ageing of the skeleton, joints and muscles. In: *Physiological basis of ageing and geriatrics*, ed Timiras PS, pp. 349–370. New York: Macmillan, 1988.

20 Nygard CH, Luoparjarvi T, Ilmarinen J. Musculoskeletal capacity and its changes among ageing municipal employees in different work categories. *Scand J Work Environ Health* 1991;**17(suppl 1)**: 110–117.

21 Ilmarinen J. A new concept for productive ageing at work. In: *Preparation for ageing*, ed. Heikkinen E *et al.*, pp. 215–222. New York: Plenum Press, 1995.

22 De Zwart BCH. Ageing in physically demanding work. Thesis, University of Amsterdam, 1997.

23 Rodeheffer RJ, Gerstenblith G, Becker LC, Fleg JL, Lakatta EG. Exercise cardiac output is maintained with advancing age in healthy human subjects. *Circulation* 1985;**69**: 203–213.

24 Astrand PO, Rodahl K. *Textbook of work physiology*. New York; McGraw-Hill, 1970.

25 Goedhard WJA, Rijpstra TSHW, Puttiger PHJ. Work ability and its relationship with age and maximal oxygen uptake. In: *Work after 45?*, ed. Kilbom A *et al.*, Vol. 1. pp. 106–111. Stockholm Arbetslivinstitutet, 1997.

26 Lakatta EG. An integrated approach toward understanding myocardial ageing. In: *Dimensions in ageing*, ed. Bergener M *et al.*, pp. 105–132. London: Academic Press, 1986.

27 *Ageing and working capacity*. Report No. 835. Geneva: World Health Organization, 1993.

28 Hall DA. *The biomedical basis of gerontology*. Bristol: Wright PSG, 1984.

29 Bergeman CS. *Ageing, genetic and environmental influences*. London: Sage, 1997.

30 Water HPA, van de Boshuizen HC, Perenboom RJM. Health and life expectancy [in Dutch]. In: *Volksgezondheid toekomst verkenning*, ed. Ruwaard D, Kramers PGN, pp. 203–211. The Hague. Sdu, 1993.

31 Ruwaard D, Kramer PGN (ed.) *Volksgezondheid toekomst verkenning* [Public health future reconnaissance]. The Hague: Sdu, 1993.

32 Berg RL, Cassells JS (ed.) *The second fifty years*. Washington DC: National Academic Press, 1992.

33 Shephard RJ. Ageing and productivity. In: *Ageing and Work*, ed. Ilmarinen J, pp. 11–24. Helsinki: FIOH, 1992.

34 Gibson RC. Promoting successful ageing in minority populations. In: *Promoting successful and productive ageing*, ed. Bond LA *et al.*, pp. 279–288. London: Sage, 1995.

35 Kemper HCG. Physical work and the consequences for the ageing worker. In: *Work and ageing*, ed. Snel J, Cremer R, pp. 31–46. London: Taylor & Francis, 1994.

36 Boerlijst G, Heijden V van der (1997). Impediments of growth and development of over-forties in organisations. In: *Work after 45?*, ed. Kilbom A *et al.*, Vol. 1. pp. 55–62. Stockholm; Arbetslivinstitutet, 1997.

37 Frommer S, Edye B, Mandryk JA, Berry G, Ferguson DA. Systolic blood pressure in relation to occupation and perceived work stress. *Scand J Work Environ Health* 1986;**12**: 476–485.

38 Goedhard WJA. The relation between psychosocial stress and ageing in a working population. In *Ageing and work*, ed. Ilmarinen J, pp. 25–32. Helsinki: FIOH, 1992.

39 Karasek RA. Job demands, job decision latitude and mental strain implication for job redesign. *Adm Sci Quart* 1979;**24**: 185–308.

40 Zwart BCH de, Meijman TF. The ageing shiftworker: adjustment or selection? In: *Work and ageing*, ed Snel J, Cremer R, pp. 107–120. London: Taylor & Francis, 1994.

41 Harma M, Hakola T. Ageing decreases sleep length and alertness after consecutive night shifts. In *Ageing and work*, ed. Ilmarinen J, pp. 226–231. Helsinki: FIOH, 1992.

42 Tuomi K *et al.* (ed.). *Work ability index*, 2nd edn. Helsinki: FIOH, 1997.

43 Ilmarinen J, Tuomi K. Work Ability Index for ageing workers. In: *Ageing and work*, ed. Ilmarinen J, pp. 142–151. Helsinki: FIOH, 1992.

44 Goedhard WJA, Puttiger PHJ, Rijpstra TSHW. Application of the Finnish Work Ability Index in the Netherlands. In: *Advances in Occupational Ergonomics and Safety*, ed. Mital A *et al.*, pp. 27–32. Cincinnati, OH: Int Soc Occ Erg and Safety, 1996.

45 Walker A, Taylor PH. *Combating age barriers in employment. A European portfolio of good practice*. Dublin: European Foundation for the Improvement of Living and Working Conditions, 1998.

Appendix 1

Driving: standards of fitness required for British driving licence holders and applicants

P. A. M. Diamond

The licensing authority for driving licences is the Secretary of State for Transport, who delegates this function to the Driver and Vehicle Licensing Agency (DVLA). The medical assessment of drivers is done by the Agency's Drivers Medical Unit (address in Appendix 7), comprising a team of doctors. The Road Traffic (Driver Licensing and Information System) Act 1989 amended the Road Traffic Act 1988 so that the DVLA now issues all driving entitlements, and these are shown in an EC Model Licence in terms of categories. Previously, heavy goods and public service vehicle drivers had to have separate licences issued by the Traffic Commissioners.

The duty of applicants for licences

The application for a licence is made on Form D1 obtainable from a Post Office. An application for a licence to drive large goods vehicles (LGVs) or passenger-carrying vehicles (PCVs) has to include a medical report form (D4), also available from Post Offices. The address and telephone number for medical enquiries are given in Appendix 7. A leaflet explaining the medical and other aspects of driver licensing (D100) is also available from Post Offices.

Duration of driving licences

The motorcar and motorcycle driving licence normally runs until the age of 70, but people with medical conditions likely to be progressive or intermittent may, at the discretion of the licensing authority, have their licences restricted to 1, 2, or 3 years. After the age of 70 these licences are renewable, normally on a 3 yearly basis on payment of a fee. A fee is not charged for medically restricted short period licences.

Categories of licence

The EEC Directive on Driving Licensing has two categories of licence:

* group 1 covers motorcars and motorcycles
* group 2 covers LGVs and PCVs.

Each category has its own medical standard, and these are further enshrined in each member state's standards. In most member states, group 2 vehicles have always included those LGVs with a laden weight of 3.5 metric tonnes and above, and those PCVs with 9 or more passenger seats. In the UK, however, LGVs are those with laden weight of 7.5 metric tonnes or above, and PCVs those with 15 or more passenger seats; additionally there are separate categories, C1 (vehicles with laden weight 3.5–7.5 metric tonnes) and D1 (vehicles with 9–15 passenger seats). Formerly any holder of a group 1 licence was entitled to drive a C1 or D1 vehicle. Following implementation of the Directive on 1 January 1997, those who apply for a Group 1 licence must make a separate application to drive C1 and D1 vehicles, and meet certain additional requirements, which include group 2 medical standards. Those who already held a licence on 31 December 1996 retain their right to drive C1 and D1 vehicles. However, this entitlement ceases if a driver for any reason has to reapply for a licence after this date, when they must apply separately for C1 and D1. This includes renewal at 70 years, and renewal of short period licences granted for medical reasons, when group 2 medical standards will apply. Those with medically restricted licences were granted an extra year, until 1 January 1998, before they lost this entitlement, to give them time to rearrange their commitments.

Qualifying criteria

Generally the minimum age for holding an LGV or PCV licence is 21, although in certain circumstances it can be 18. It will normally expire after the 45th birthday and is renewable every 5 years up to the age of 65, and annually thereafter. Each application has to include a medical report on form D4, completed by a registered medical practitioner, usually the applicant's general practitioner. If a company doctor is not familiar with an applicant's medical history it is advisable to consult the patient's general practitioner.

Ambulances, taxis, and police cars are not specifically singled out in driver licensing legislation, but taxi drivers are licensed by local authorities under local government legislation; and for drivers of all these vehicles the Medical Commission on Accident Prevention recommends that the higher LGV/PCV public standards should apply.

Duties of the applicant and licence holder

The licensing authority is bound to refuse or revoke the application or licence when a person is unfit to drive because of a relevant disability. Relevant disabilities are prescribed in law or, alternatively, comprise **any other medical disease or disability likely to cause the driving of a motor vehicle by the applicant or licence holder to be a source of danger to the public.**

The following prescribed disabilities bar drivers of motorcars and motorcycles (group 1 as defined in the EC Directive):

- a person who is suffering from epilepsy, and
  - is not free from any attack for at least one year or

- has not established a pattern of attacks asleep and not awake for more than 3 years or
- is likely to be a danger to the public when driving
- severe mental disorder, including arrested or incomplete development of the mind, such that a person is incapable of leading an independent life or of guarding against serious exploitation
- liability to sudden attacks of disabling giddiness or fainting caused by any disorder (but if they are caused by a heart disorder which can be controlled by an implanted pacemaker, the bar is lifted subject to the person undertaking to have regular medical assessments at a pacemaker clinic and having a 3 year licence)
- inability to read in good daylight (with the aid of glasses or contact lenses if worn) a registration mark fixed to a vehicle containing figures and letters 79.4 millimetres high at a distance of 20.5 metres generally, except that for those applying to drive pedestrian controlled vehicles, such as milk floats or motor-propelled mowing machines, the distance is 12.3 metres
- in addition, as mentioned above, the person must not suffer from any other disease or disability likely to cause them to be a source of danger to the public when driving or in pursuance of a driver's licence.

LGV/PCV prescribed disabilities (group 2 requirements in the EEC Directive) include all those above for group 1, and, in addition, the following:

- any liability to epileptic seizures, which will usually be interpreted as positive if the applicant has:
  - had any epileptic attack in the last 10 years or
  - has taken any medication to prevent epilepsy in the last 10 years or
  - if a consultant has confirmed there is a continuing liability to epileptic seizur
- abnormal sight in one or both eyes where:
  - the visual acuity is worse than 6/9 in the better eye and worse than 6/12 in the worse eye and, if corrective lenses are worn, the uncorrected acuity in either eye tested separately is worse than 3/60.

If a driver held a group 2 licence before 31 December 1996 then a lower standard may apply, because there exist several 'grandfather' rights relating to the different dates of previous legislation. To retain entitlement, a driver must have held the licence continuously from the qualifying date, the visual status must have remained the same, and there must be no intercurrent pathology. The full standards of 'grandfather' rights are included in *Medical aspects of fitness to drive*[1] and further advice may be obtained from the Drivers' Medical Unit, DVLA.

In all driving licence legislation measurements of visual acuity refer to visual acuity measured on the Snellen scale.

- people with diabetes requiring insulin treatment, unless the person in question held, on 1 April 1991, an existing licence and the Traffic Commissioner in whose area he resided or the Traffic Commissioner who granted the licence knew of the disability before 1 January 1991 (subject to regular review by DVLA).

In very exceptional cases, drivers of C1 vehicles who can show that they were in full-time occupation in this capacity at the time of renewal may be permitted to continue to drive, subject to regular review by the DVLA. The EC definition of 'very exceptional case' is that it refers only to the clinical condition, and not to the circumstances of driving.

Notification of disabilities to the Licensing Centre

The Road Traffic Act 1988 places a statutory obligation on driving licence holders and applicants to notify any disability likely to affect safe driving, either now or at some future date, to the DVLA as soon as the person becomes aware of the condition. Awareness normally involves being told it is relevant or prospectively relevant by a medical practitioner. Only temporary disabilities not expected to last more than 3 months, such as fractured bones, are exceptions to this rule. However, conditions such as strokes with underlying cerebrovascular disease, or conditions such as sleep apnoea, unless permanently cured by surgery, are not exempt from this 3-month rule. Licence holders are also required to notify the licensing centre if any disability previously notified becomes worse.

Procedure for medical assessment

When the DVLA receives information about a disability from an applicant/licence holder or third party, it may require the applicant or licence holder to authorize their doctor to provide information about the disability to the Medical Advisory Branch at the centre. If the applicant or licence holder fails to do so, or if the information available from the doctor does not conclusively confirm their fitness to drive, the DVLA may require them to have a medical examination by a nominated doctor or doctors. If necessary, to establish the effect of the disability on ability to drive, the DVLA may require them to take another driving test. If the licence holder or applicant refuses to give consent to the release of a medical report to the DVLA, or fails to attend a medical examination without reasonable excuse, this will usually result in a driving licence being withheld or withdrawn.

Loss of a limb due to trauma

Applicants for licences who have a static limb disability enjoy an automatic right in Great Britain to hold a provisional driving licence for the purpose of taking a driving test to prove their ability to drive (if they do not already hold a full licence). Normally provisional licences run until the applicant's 70th birthday, but the motorcycle entitlement only runs for 2 years and cannot be renewed until a further year has elapsed unless the applicant has passed a test.

Doctor notification without the patient's consent

Sometimes a doctor tells a patient not to drive and to report a relevant disability to the DVLA, only to find that the patient has disregarded the advice and is continuing to drive to the danger of the public. In such cases it is advisable for the doctor to repeat the advice, to place it in writing, and to seek the medical opinion of their professional indemnity association. The defence bodies normally advise direct notification, without the consent of the patient, but that the patient be informed of the action taken. The authoritative document for reference is the General Medical Council (GMC) pamphlet *Professional conduct and discipline; fitness to practice*. The Guidance Notes produced by the GMC in October 1995, *Duties of a doctor*, specifically advise on notifying the DVLA in Appendix 1 (page 11) of the section on Confidentiality. The address of the GMC is provided in Appendix 7.

Medical appeal provisions

Where a driving licence is refused or revoked on medical grounds or restricted in period of duration, there is a right of appeal to a Magistrates Court in England and Wales or to a Sheriff Court in Scotland.

Medical aspects of fitness to drive

More details on medical fitness to drive and UK driver licensing standards are contained in *Medical aspects of fitness to drive*,[1] a guide for medical practitioners published by the Medical Commission on Accident Prevention. (Copies of the booklet can be obtained from the DVLA.) Details of the assessment of cardiac fitness for vocational driving are contained in the Appendix to Chapter 18 (p. 365).

Reference

1 Taylor JF. *Medical aspects of fitness to drive*, 5th edn. London: Medical Commission on Accident Prevention, 1995.

Appendix 2

Civil aviation

K. Edgington

The civil aviation industry has a well-developed and tested system of medical standards that undergoes close and regular scrutiny. The main reason for this is to preserve the safety of the travelling public. In the first instance, this is addressed by the national authorities responsible for air safety—in the UK, the Civil Aviation Authority (CAA)—which is concerned to ensure that a licence holder can function effectively and is not likely to suffer sudden incapacitation during the short period (6–12 months) for which their medical certificate is valid. An employer has a different viewpoint, seeking not only to satisfy the safety requirement but to recruit an employee who will remain fit through a long-term career. This is particularly important when the very high cost of training a public transport jet aircraft pilot is considered. An individual with a progressive disability might be given a pilot's licence subject to regular reviews, but would not be employed by a major airline. Guidance is often needed on this subject and would be given by the CAA.

Risk

Risk management is the main principle of aviation licensing. It is not possible, nor is it policy, to seek a zero defect system (complete absence of risk). The best airlines operating the best aircraft now achieve a fatal accident rate close to or even better than the CAA safety target of 1 fatal accident in 10 million flights[1]. Many factors contribute to accident causation. The flight crew can be considered to be one of the 10 major systems of an aircraft, so the safety target for accidents arising from medical conditions is 1 in 100 million flights or less.[2] This risk can be managed by larger aircraft carrying two or more pilots, by solutions to incapacitation scenarios being rehearsed during routine simulator training, and by licensing only pilots with medical conditions that carry a sudden incapacitation risk of 1% per year or less. This has become known as the 1% 'rule' and, by the use of this rule, the medical certification assessment process can match the safety traget.[3]

Risk mismatch

One issue of regular concern for occupational physicians undertaking licensing assessments is that applicants are often falsely advised by other doctors that the complications of a particular condition do not affect their fitness to hold a licence. This does not stem from a wish to mislead, but rather a wish to reassure and to prevent minimal risks interfering with the enjoyment of everyday life and work. A mismatch occurs when an individual with a very small risk of developing some medical complications discovers that they fall outside the aviation risk criteria currently in place and is, therefore, denied a licence. Handling this situation demands a considerable amount of experience, tact, and skill. An individual's career may be interrupted, albeit temporarily, for a reason that is apparent to the physician but puzzling to the patient. Similar problems arise when individuals present for licensing assessments and part of the assessment reveals an abnormality that has not caused any symptoms. Individuals in this position often find it difficult to accept that there is a latent risk of future incapacitation. Again, the experienced occupational physician will be familiar with this situation, and will explain and discuss the situation with tact and care.

Pilots

The medical standards for pilots (and for flight engineers and air traffic control officers) are internationally agreed and are contained in Annex 1 to the Convention on International Civil Aviation.[4] A few, such as the visual requirements, are specific but many are couched in general terms such as 'cases of metabolic nutritional or endocrine disorders likely to interfere with the safe exercise of the applicant's licence privileges shall be assessed as unfit'. There is also a waiver clause which allows a national authority to issue a licence, even if the standards are not met, if it believes it is safe to do so. The International Civil Aviation Organization, a United Nations organization, issues a manual of guidance material[5] on the interpretation of the standards.

Possible exposure to a harsh environment, notably hypoxia, high G-forces, and sudden changes of pressure and temperature, requires very good cardiovascular function and freedom from conditions likely to be aggravated by sudden changes such as middle ear and sinus disorders, lung bullae, bowel herniation, etc.

The special senses, especially vision, are clearly important. Uncorrected distant visual acuity must in some countries be 6/60 (20/200) or better. Correction to 6/9 (20/30) or better is required, and there are near and intermediate requirements. A correction of refractive error by the use of spectacles or contact lenses is allowed within certain limits. Normal colour vision is not always necessary provided the candidate can reliably distinguish signals that are red, white, and green. Experienced pilots who lose an eye can often continue to fly satisfactorily by day but may have difficulty landing at night.

Pilots with disabilities resulting from orthopaedic or neurological conditions are given a practical test in each aircraft type they wish to fly.

The lifestyle of a professional pilot is necessarily irregular and this excludes applicants with some gastrointestinal and metabolic disorders. Insulin-dependent diabetes is absolutely disqualifying and diabetes controlled by oral therapy is usually so.

Because the continual exercise of judgement and self-discipline is so vital to the pilot's task, significant mental and personality disorders are unacceptable. A history of psychosis is permanently disqualifying. Neurotic illness is assessed on the probability of recurrence, as is alcohol and drug abuse. HIV infection may first manifest itself with neuropsychiatric symptoms and is considered disqualifying in many countries.

A pilot's licence is temporarily suspended on presumption of pregnancy but flying in a two-pilot aircraft is usually possible in the middle trimester.

Commonly used therapeutic agents are often unacceptable because of their side-effects. Performance testing in a flight simulator may be carried out, if necessary, to assess this. In many cases the disorder requiring the therapy will be disqualifying, at least temporarily. As examples, antihypertensive therapy may well be acceptable depending on the severity of the condition and its response to treatment, the side-effects of the therapy, and the proof of satisfactory task performance while the pilot is taking the therapy. Conversely, antidepressant therapy is unacceptable in that the underlying condition is not compatible with the safe operation of an aircraft regardless of the efficacy of any therapeutic agents. Short-acting hypnotics such as temazepam may well be acceptable, depending on the reason for their being prescribed. The underlying condition and the dosage of such a hypnotic should be assessed by a physician experienced in aviation medicine.

Conditions likely to cause incapacitation, either sudden or subtle, are usually disqualifying. Passenger aircraft smaller than 5700 kg (air-taxi size) sometimes carry only one pilot, whose incapacitation would inevitably result in an accident. Larger aircraft must carry two pilots. As mentioned earlier, simulated incapacitation training in the aircraft simulator is now a routine practice and research has indicated that on only fewer than 1 occasion in 100 of sudden pilot incapacitation may an accident result.[6]

Experience indicates that the risk of accidents increases directly as the total number of medical disabilities rises. It also falls dramatically with increasing age and experience up to age 60, when most professional pilots retire. Hence the ill-considered removal of middle-aged pilots on medical grounds and their replacement by younger, less experienced pilots may be positively detrimental to air safety.

The medical standards for pilots engaged in flying instruction and non-passenger-carrying activities, such as banner-towing, were more relaxed prior to 1 July 1999, but from that date the harmonized European medical requirements of the Joint Aviation Authorities (JAA) xame into force in the UK and the current standards are now more in line with those described above.

The initial medical examination for a professional pilot's licence (and those of flight engineers and air traffic control officers) is carried out in the UK by the CAA. Airline transport pilots and commercial pilots are examined annually below the age of 40 and 6-monthly above the age of 40, the renewal examinations being undertaken by medical examiners who have had postgraduate training in aviation medicine and who are authorized by the CAA.

Flight engineers

Flight engineers play an important role in monitoring the actions of the pilots as well as controlling the aircraft's systems. The required medical standards for these crew members are therefore essentially similar to those of pilots, but because they do not physically handle the flying controls at critical stages of flight, their sudden incapacitation does not present the same threat to safety as it would for pilots. They may, therefore, continue to fly with conditions which present a somewhat greater risk of incapacitation.

Air traffic control officers

The increasing congestion of air traffic means that air traffic control officers have responsibility for maintaining safety that are almost as great as those of pilots. Medical fitness standards are therefore similar. Some controllers work in teams and in these circumstances a risk of incapacitation comparable to that for pilots of larger aircraft may be acceptable.

Cabin crew

Aircraft cabin staff do not hold licences and formal medical standards are not laid down. The CAA merely requires airlines to ensure by medical examination that they are fit to carry out their assigned duties. Good cardiorespiratory function and freedom from conditions aggravated by pressure changes and the effects of irregular working and worldwide travel are important. Uncorrected distance vision of 6/60 (20/200) or better is necessary, as spectacles and contact lenses may be lost in an accident where the cabin crew's effectiveness is vital to passenger survival.

European dimension

For several years there has been a process of harmonization that covers all aspects of civil aviation in Europe. Licensing and medical certification are covered by this process and, as from 1 July 1999, the 30 European states that form the Joint Aviation Authorities (JAA) - the European Community 15 states plus 15 other European nations - have been required to implement identical licensing and medical standards (known as Joint Aviation Requirements - Flight Crew Licensing Par 3 (Medical). The UK and Denmark were able to conform to these new standards on time; the other states are expected to conform, as the necesssary processes are established and inspected, during 2000 and 2001. This harmonization will allow the 30 states to accept each others' licenses without further test or expense. A new code has assured primacy and states are not allowed to vary the standard unilaterally. However, this will not limit national authorities' discretion under the waiver clause. An age limit of 65 has been established for two-pilot and multi-crew operations.

It appears likely that an EC proposal will be adopted, leading to the establishment of a single European Aviation Safety Authority (EASA) with greater executive and enforcement powers than the current JAA. At present, under the JAA arrangements, each state will run the licensing and medical certification processes according to the harmonized requirements, the standards and policy being determined by committees made up of members of each state's authorities. If EASA becomes established, there is likely to be a much stronger central policy unit with responsibility for setting, maintaining and enforcing the standards. The European states with major aviation industries will continue to have a major influence and involvement in this process.

Legislation

The Disability Discrimination Act 1995 does not apply to employment on board a ship, aircraft, or hovercraft (Section 68(2) of the Act). Civil aviation legislation (Civil Aviation Act 1982 and Air Navigation (No 2) Order 1995) specify the requirements for licensed jobs. The Joint Aviation Requirements - Flight Crew Licensing Part 3 (Medical) are now effective in the UK and have been incorporated into the Air Navigation (No2) Order 1995. Denmark has also implemented them and the other 28 JAA states will be implementing them during 2000 and 2001, leading to a fully harmonized European scene.

Selected references

1 Bennett G. Medical-cause accidents in commercial aviation. In: *First European workshop in aviation cardiology*, ed. Joy M. *Eur Heart J* 1992; **13**(suppl H): 13–15.
2 Chaplin JC. In perspective—the safety of aircraft pilots and their hearts. *Eur Heart J* 1988; **9**(suppl G): 17–20.
3 Tunstall Pedoe H. Acceptable cardiovascular risk in aircrew. In: *Second United Kingdom workshop in aviation cardiology*, ed. Joy M, Bennett G. *Eur Heart J*, 1988; **9**(suppl G): 9–11.
4 *Annex 1 to the Treaty on International Civil Aviation*, 8th edn. Montreal: International Civil Aviation Organisation, 1988.
5 *Manual of civil aviation medicine*, 2nd edn. Montreal: International Civil Aviation Organisation, 1985.
6 Bennett G. Pilot incapacitation and aircraft accidents. *Eur Heart J* 1988; **9**(suppl G): 21–24.

Appendix 3

Medical standards for entry into the Merchant Navy and for serving seafarers

P. A. M. Diamond

The Department of the Environment, Transport and the Regions (DETR) is responsible for the statutory medical standards for seafarers which were introduced under the Merchant Shipping (Medical Examination) Regulations 1983, SI 1983, No 808. Revised standards were published in April 1998 in a new Merchant Shipping Notice (MSN 1712(M)) which is available from the address in Appendix 7. These standards apply throughout to serving seafarers and provide the legal basis for the issue of medical certificates in accordance with Article 3 of the International Maritime Organization (IMO) Convention 73.

Previously the standards had been agreed by a panel of doctors working within the industry. Member companies of the then General Council of British Shipping (GBS) examined seafarers to these standards in their employment by agreement with the trade unions. When examination became a statutory requirement the standards were revised by a Joint Working Party comprising representatives of the GBS and the Faculty of Occupational Medicine. Subsequent revision has been undertaken by the panel of Medical Referees (see below) in discussion with clinical specialists and those involved with working conditions and treatment at sea, radio medical advice, and rescue. There is full consultation with the shipping industry, trade unions, and other interested parties. Very few changes have been made, but the entire standard has been reviewed. Many employers of seafarers have their own agreed medical standards and continue to undertake company medical examinations at pre-employment, after sickness, and on other occasions, but the statutory certificate is still, of course, necessary.

DETR recognizes that the medical assessment of those in a potentially hazardous occupation requires special experience and a panel of about 300 doctors is appointed by the Secretary of State for the Environment, Transport and the Regions to undertake this. Each appointment is personal and the work cannot be delegated. There is a recommended fee for the medical examination for which the seafarer is responsible. The doctors are known as approved doctors and are required to meet certain criteria which may be audited. Each doctor is responsible for the issue of certificates, and must keep full records for 6 years. Returns of all examination results are made on the appropriate form and sent to the Maritime and Coastguard Agency (MCA) for record. A serving seafarer has the right of appeal if declared permanently unfit or fit for restricted service only. The appeal is heard by one of a panel of Medical Referees, again personally appointed by the Secretary of State. The function of a referee is to ensure a diagnosis is established beyond reasonable doubt in accordance with the available medical evidence and to determine whether the standards have been properly interpreted. Thus, there is a limited margin for judgement, but no scope for changing the standard in an individual case.

Occupational physicians, general practitioners, and specialists may encounter established seafarers and new applicants. (The revised standards place responsibility on a serving seafarer who suffers from a medical condition covered by the Regulations which precludes seafaring to arrange for further approved examination as soon as possible.) The information that follows may assist in career advice, although the statutory examination which will determine the applicant's eligibility for seafaring must be undertaken by an approved doctor. (The list of doctors is available from Marine Offices.)

Procedures

Frequency of examination

- <18 years: yearly medical examination
- 18–40 years: intervals not exceeding 5 years
- >40 years: intervals not exceeding 2 years.

In addition, seafarers serving on bulk chemical carriers are required to have medical examinations, which may include blood tests, at yearly intervals or more often, depending on the nature of the cargo.

If seafarers develop a condition during the term of their licence covered by the Merchant Shipping Notice ('M' Notice) and which precludes service at sea, they must arrange a further examination as soon as possible so that a revised certificate can be issued.

A seafarer who holds an ENG3 (failure) or an ENG 7 (final failure on appeal) certificate, is responsible for declaring it to the examining doctor. (ENG stands for Engineering and Nautical Group, now obsolete, but the classification still remains.) Otherwise, any subsequent certificate is not valid.

Categories of medical fitness

The approved doctor will issue one of the following certificates:

A   unrestricted service

A(T)   unrestricted service subject to medical surveillance

E   restricted service only (with definition of restriction)

B   permanently unfit

C   indefinitely unfit, subject to review in .... months

D   temporarily unfit, subject to review in .... weeks.

The employer must observe the conditions imposed by the category of the certificate. Periodic surveillance, medical investigation, and length of treatment which precludes service at sea, will have a considerable impact on the individual seafarer, who may regard the ship, rather than land, as their natural home. Liaison between treating physicians, the examining approved doctor and the employer is essential to achieve an early and effective return to work.

Medical fitness of seafarers

The standard covers safety aspects, occupational requirements, the secondary safety concern of reduction in crew size, and constraints of medical treatment at sea. There is considerable inherent risk in the general occupation of seafaring. A ship can be a hazardous environment in normal circumstances, but in an emergency each crew member has a specific and often extremely hazardous duty to perform, and must be in good health to undertake this without imposing additional demands on others and putting themselves in unnecessary danger. Article 4 of IMO Convention 73 states that 'due regard shall be had to the age of the person to be examined and the nature of the duties to be performed.' Careful occupational assessment is very important, particularly as there are no 'light duties' on board ship, and no substitute crew. (Restrictions applied to certificates normally relate to the type of vessel or the location but not to the specific employment.)

Due regard must also be given to medical conditions which could be aggravated by work at sea. Most ships run the minimum complement of crew. When one member is sick, this places extra demands on the rest. If the sick person requires constant attention, for example because of acute mental illness, the demand is even greater. Very few merchant ships carry doctors. Acute illness or injury is dealt with by designated ships' officers whose training is limited to first aid or medical aid treatment. Any medical condition with risk of serious exacerbation which requires expert treatment should be excluded. Too much reliance can be placed on helicopter evacuation and removal to the nearest port as a form of solution. The distance and weather conditions determine whether evacuation is a viable option but, even so, the patient suffers a very uncomfortable and frightening experience, sometimes with total immersion for a short period. Many serious medical conditions, such as acute asthma, cannot be transported. Medical treatment on shore in some parts of the world also falls short of the desired standard.

General living conditions on board ship must be considered. The crew is a closed community, seldom quiet or still. Individual eating habits, dietary needs, and tastes cannot easily be met. Facilities for leisure physical activities are limited, forced ventilation systems are used, and the tedium of routine can often become oppressive in the absence of normal diversion enjoyed by those ashore. An inability to fit in, take responsibility, or accept a reasonable degree of discipline may impair the safe and efficient working of the ship. However, many people adapt wholeheartedly and are happiest when at sea; for them it is enforced time on shore that can have a deleterious effect.

The medical standards cover the main conditions likely to cause serious or sudden incapacity, alteration or loss of consciousness, physical constraint (including diminished sight or hearing and persistent or recurrent pain), and disturbance of judgement. Eyesight standards have recently been slightly relaxed and now permit resumption of work, but not entrance into employment, after loss of sight in one eye, providing the vision in the remaining eye reaches a certain standard and good stabilization is achieved. Requirements for colour vision have been reviewed, but remain strict for those on deck. The standards for engineers and radio officers are slightly more relaxed.

If a seafarer is dependent on medication, or where lack of it might precipitate rapid deterioration of their condition, then service is not normally permitted. Those who do take medication to sea should always inform the ship's master, so that arrangements can be made for a reserve stock of prescribed drugs to be held in a safe place in case the voyage is unexpectedly extended. Some trades require lengthy periods in tropical climates and most seafarers will need to join and leave their ships by air travel, and should not suffer from any condition which precludes work in hot climates or flying. Infectious and contagious diseases must be excluded where possible in such closed communities. Many employers have strict alcohol and drug policies, but in all cases persistent alcohol abuse and/or a history of drug dependence in the past 5 years is a permanent bar.

The DDA does not apply to employment on board a ship (Section 68(2)).

Although the Medical Standards Regulations are applied by a specially selected panel of doctors, other doctors may encounter patients seeking medical advice about seafaring. The foregoing information may serve as a guide, but the complete standards and procedures are available to all intending and serving seafarers on request without charge, and from the address in Appendix 7. A summary note for seafarers is also included in the notice which is to be read before arranging an appointment for statutory examination; in some cases, this may prevent the applicant from incurring unnecessary expense.

Appendix 4

Fitness for work offshore and in commercial diving

N. K. I. McIver and D. Bracher

Offshore workers

The offshore environment is remote and medical conditions which are easily managed onshore may be life-threatening on an offshore installation owing to the limited medical facilities and the hazards of emergency evacuation in adverse weather conditions.

All offshore installations in the UK sector of the North Sea that have more than 25 workers on them must have a trained offshore paramedic (known as a medic). All medics are specially trained for working offshore and many have exceptional skills; most companies equip the sick-bays to complement these very high standards. Nevertheless, it is difficult for a single medic to deal with very serious or multiple emergencies even with the help of advanced first aiders and advice from an experienced physician based onshore. The Search and Rescue Service will attempt to evacuate patients in the most hazardous weather conditions though this can put the lives of the helicopter crew and the medical attendants at risk. Medical evacuations (medevacs) for illness outweigh those for injury and the RGIT Ltd (previously Robert Gordon Institute of Technology) statistics for the 12 months to August 1998 showed that out of 245 medevacs 70% were for illness. This is in contrast to an RGIT study from 1987–1992 when illness accounted for only 55% of 3979 medevacs. Injury offshore is becoming less common and the number of medevacs could be reduced further by ensuring proper assessment of fitness to work offshore.

The required standard of fitness is higher than that required for similar work onshore. There is a need to take fitness for survival in emergency situations into account and offshore workers have to complete a practical survival training course.

In determining fitness to work offshore it is necessary to consider the effect of any medical condition on the safety of individuals and their colleagues as well as the effect of the work and the environment on the medical condition, including transportation, usually by helicopter, to the workplace.

Other factors to be considered include physical demands of the work and the requirement to cope with awkward walkways, steep outside stairways, work at heights, and shiftwork. Psychological or mental problems may arise from absence from family support and, in some cases the experience of external control by the operator, of all aspects of living for 24 hours every day. Other aspects include weather, climatic exposure, and methods of travel. Claustrophobia, agoraphobia, limitation of privacy through sharing cabins, and peer pressure are also important. Hence, the fitness requirements for working offshore truly present a special situation.

The Health Advisory Committee of the UK Offshore Operators Association (UKOOA) has drawn up guidelines on medical standards for offshore work.[1] Divers and hyperbaric chamber operating staff connected with a diving operation are covered by the requirements of the Diving at Work Regulations 1997. Other countries bordering the North Sea, such as Norway and the Netherlands, have similar regulations and guidelines.

Offshore operators often adopt standards which exceed those recommended by the UKOOA Health Advisory Committee and the final decision on fitness of an individual to work offshore is that of the operator, who has ultimate responsibility for the safety of the installation and of all people on it. The operator usually delegates the responsibility for health-related matters to its company occupational physician. UKOOA has also introduced an appeals procedure.

UKOOA has recently adopted a system of approved doctors with special knowledge of working conditions offshore to examine offshore workers. A list of those who are suitably qualified can be obtained from its London office (see Appendix 7).

Norwegian and Dutch authorities also approve doctors in the UK. The examination of commercial divers must be performed by doctors known as Medical Examiners of Divers.

In addition to assessing general fitness to work offshore it is necessary to consider the specific medical fitness requirements of the particular job being undertaken. In many cases this will already have been assessed by the company doctor. This is particularly true of itinerant workers who have similar duties onshore, for example equipment maintenance staff who service the same machinery wherever it is located. Some companies do not have their own occupational health staff and may rely on the physician performing the offshore medical examination to determine fitness to follow a specific occupation offshore, e.g. catering or crane driving. The examining physician needs to understand the requirement clearly and to ensure that they are appropriately qualified to provide an opinion. It is important in the case of work involving lead, asbestos, or radiation that they also comply with the respective regulations for certifying fitness, and, if necessary, apply to become a Health and Safety Executive (HSE) appointed doctor for the purpose.

Medical assessment of offshore workers

A detailed past medical history should be obtained, as well as an accurate occupational and social history. Completion of a questionnaire with explanation of any positive answers, together with a declaration signed by the examinee, should form a part of the assessment.

Proof of identity should be obtained at the time of the examination. UKOOA states a minimum age of 18 is required for working offshore. All offshore employees should be in possession of an in-date medical certificate of fitness.

The frequency of examination recommended by UKOOA is: before offshore placement; then 3 yearly up to 39 years, 2 yearly between 40 and 50, and annually thereafter.

The examining physician can recommend more frequent assessments and a re-assessment should always be made following significant absence due to injury or illness.

Clinical medical examination

The examination includes measurement of height, weight, and body mass index (BMI), visual acuity, colour vision, and systematic physical examination. Investigations should include urinalysis, pulmonary function, and audiometric testing.

Certification of dental fitness is required by some operators, and some require proof of ongoing routine dental surveillance.

Specific occupations may require additional examination and investigations, for example UKOOA recommends catering staff to have at least one stool sample cultured for pathogens and subsequently if there is clinical suspicion of gastrointestinal infection or possible carrier status.

General considerations

An assessment should be made of body fat in addition to fitness, because of its effect on exercise tolerance and mobility. Body mass index (BMI), calculated as weight in kilograms divided by the square of the height in metres (see Box A4.1), is often used. A BMI greater than 30 is described as 'obese with increased health risk'. Some companies use bio-impedance as a measure of body fat. Excessive weight is of significance in emergency evacuation from either the installation or a helicopter..

For offshore workers a BMI greater than 35 should be regarded as unacceptable. A number of companies have more stringent standards and encourage their workforce to have a BMI of less than 30.

Box A4.1 Body mass index (BMI)
The BMI is measured as $[\text{weight (kg)}]/[\text{height (m)}]^2$, where:

A BMI of	Means
$<18 \text{ kg/m}^2$	Underweight
$19{-}25 \text{ kg/m}^2$	A desirable BMI figure indicating a healthy weight
$26{-}30 \text{ kg/m}^2$	Overweight, health could suffer. Some weight loss should now be considered
$31{-}40 \text{ kg/m}^2$	Obese; health is at risk. Losing weight now should be seriously considered
$>41 \text{ kg/m}^2$	Losing weight immediately is essential

Adapted from health implications of obesity in: Garrow J. S. *Obesity and related diseases* Churchill Livingstone, Edinburgh, 1988.

Infectious diseases

Any intercurrent infection should be assessed and treated before allowing the person to work offshore.

HIV

A diagnosis of HIV positivity does not necessarily debar from employment offshore. However, the development of symptoms or signs of AIDS related complex debars and the usual care is necessary offshore in dealing with blood spillages and contamination from body fluids.

Malignancy

Patients with malignant conditions are not ordinarily considered fit for work offshore but each case needs to be assessed individually, taking into account the nature of the tumour, disability, progress, and treatment.

Alcoholism and substance abuse

Alcohol and substance abuse pose a major risk to health and safety offshore and many companies have introduced screening programmes for substance abuse as part of their routine medical assessment. Some companies have a system of testing following accident or injury and randomly at other times. These tests must be carried out under carefully controlled conditions observing a complete chain of custody. Samples must be available to the examinee for independent analysis and for confirmatory tests if required.

The introduction of pre-employment screening procedures has reduced the proportion of tests later found to be positive for recreational drug abuse. Breath testing at heliports has reduced the incidence of acute alcohol intoxication and acute symptoms of withdrawal. Most companies have alcohol and drug policies which include assistance for employees who come forward and admit that they have a problem.

Alcohol is not permitted offshore and companies have different policies for dealing with employees with alcohol-related problems. These may include referring the employee to the occupational health department for advice and supervision during rehabilitation or requiring the employee to report to the department before going offshore to determine whether they are under the influence of alcohol. Such policies operate in addition to the routine checks at heliports.

Medications

Certain medications may pose unacceptable risks in offshore workers as may the underlying condition. The possible consequences of running out of the medication also need to be considered.

Approved medication should be declared to the heliport security staff prior to departure and to the offshore medic on arrival on the installation. More medication should be taken offshore than needed for the expected length of stay.

Workers who require anticoagulants, cytotoxic agents, immunosuppressants, insulin, anticonvulsants, or oral steroids are unfit to work offshore. Those who routinely use psychotropic agents, tranquillizers, narcotics, and hypnotics are similarly unfit. A history of previous use of any of these must be investigated.

Systematic assessment

Ear, nose, and throat

Acute infections require treatment before acceptance, and any symptomatic chronic ear disease or vertigo is unacceptable. Dry perforation of the tympanic membrane may be acceptable. Significant symptomatic nasal airway obstruction or recurrent or chronic sinus infection is unacceptable until corrected. Hayfever which responds to therapy (without side-effects) is usually acceptable.

Hearing must be adequate to interpret speech and to detect an audible alarm. Audiometric testing is advised at pre-employment and at subsequent periodic medical examinations as part of a hearing conservation programme. Audiometric assessment should be made in accordance with the HSE guidelines.[2] Where the measured loss in the better ear is greater than 35 dBA for lower frequencies or 60 dBA for higher frequencies then the individual is unlikely to be fit for work offshore.

The use of an intrinsically safe hearing aid, that is one which will not cause an explosion in a volatile atmosphere, may be permissible, but safety warnings must be audible without the use of a hearing aid.

Chronic or recurrent ear, nose and throat (ENT) problems (including tonsillar infection) should be treated adequately before working offshore.

Dental fitness

Dental caries represents a significant cause of morbidity in offshore workers. In the first 6 months of 1992 there were 114 medical evacuations from the UK sector of the North Sea because of disorders of the digestive system, of which 43% were due to dental problems.[3] Dental problems should be treated before proceeding offshore.

Digestive system

Active peptic ulceration, or the need for clinical maintenance treatment, is not acceptable. Other conditions which would normally disbar from employment offshore include active inflammatory bowel disease, symptomatic hiatus hernia, haemorrhoids, fistulae or anal fissures, cholelithiasis, and pancreatitis.

Abdominal herniae require repair; patients with stomas need to be individually assessed, as they may cause problems offshore.

Cardiovascular system

Cardiac problems generally debar employment offshore. Congenital heart disease, if associated with symptoms or haemodynamic effects, is not acceptable. Corrected valvular disease may be acceptable for work offshore, but not usually individuals who have a cardiac myopathy or who have had a heart transplant.

Coronary artery events are not uncommon offshore and a history of myocardial ischaemia, including angina, myocardial infarction, coronary artery bypass, and coronary artery angioplasty, will usually preclude employment in such a remote, hostile environment.

However, a person with a history of coronary heart disease may be fit to work offshore if several conditions are satisfied. These include:

- absence of symptoms for at least 6 months
- a normal resting ECG
- a satisfactory exercise ECG (stage III on the Bruce Protocol)
- in some circumstances a coronary angiogram will be required to demonstrate non-threatening coronary vascular anatomy.

All will require cardiological assessment before returning to work offshore and annual reassessment by a cardiologist thereafter. The annual reassessment should include successful completion of Stage III of the Bruce Protocol. If symptoms are controlled only by medication, a ban will usually apply. All offshore workers must complete survival training; this includes those with a medical history of coronary heart disease.

Cardiac arrhythmias require specialist assessment and individual consideration, as does the use of a cardiac pacemaker. Not only does the underlying pathology need to be considered, but also the effect of the working environment on the pacemaker.

A single pulmonary embolic event needs careful assessment. Permission to work offshore would depend on the underlying cause but any recurrence would be a bar, as would any cerebrovascular event.

Cardiovascular examination for offshore work does not usually include an ECG (except for the Dutch authorities) unless clinically indicated, but if there are symptoms suggestive of ischaemic heart disease an exercise ECG is required and possibly a coronary aniogram.

Exercise testing

Exercise testing is not usually performed for offshore workers unless required for special tasks such as fire and emergency response work. However some companies have included sub-maximal exercise testing as part of the assessment of general fitness and to encourage individuals to improve physical fitness.

Peripheral vascular disease

Varicose veins with ulceration, varicose eczema or active deep vein thrombosis are, bars to working offshore as is arterial claudication.

Hypertension

As a guideline blood pressure should not be greater than 140/90 mmHg (fifth phase diastolic). Persons with treated hypertension and who have no target organ damage with sustained blood pressure levels below 150/90 should be acceptable for offshore work.

Respiratory system

The upper respiratory tract, lung structure, and anatomy should essentially be normal and with unimpaired respiratory function and gas exchange. Conditions that may give rise to a medical emergency will be a bar to offshore employment. Chronic sinus problems, snoring, and sleep apnoea may also be problematic.

Assessment should include a history, clinical examination and standard spirometry. Measurements of forced expiratory volume in 1 second (FEV_1) below 65% of predicted and forced vital capacity (FVC) below 70% of predicted are unacceptable for offshore work. Symptomatic obstructive or restrictive airways disease, even if reversible and only in response to exertion, are unacceptable. Similarly, symptomatic fibrotic lung disease is unacceptable. Conditions in these categories include chronic obstructive pulmonary disease, emphysema, bronchiectasis, pulmonary tuberculosis and active pulmonary sarcoidosis.

Asthma

Asthma requires individual assessment if it occurs beyond childhood, involves atopy or is occupationally related. Reversible airways obstruction may occur in response to cold, exertion, stress, and inhalation of emissions; it may also be provoked by inhaling dry gas through breathing apparatus.

For offshore workers in general the prophylactic use of an inhaled steroid may be acceptable. Those who require intermittent medical intervention such as oral steroids, hospital admission, or use β-agonists require individual assessment. There should be normal exercise capacity without inducing symptoms.

Spontaneous pneumothorax

A history of spontaneous pneumothorax is a bar except for a single episode without recurrence for a year or after a successful surgical procedure.

Central nervous system and organs of special sense

Any employee with an acute or chronic neurological disease, significant motor or sensory deficit, impairment of neuromuscular co-ordination, or intellectual impairment is likely to be unfit for work offshore.

Migraine

A history of migraine which does not affect efficiency and safety at work may be acceptable.

Epilepsy

Any disturbance of conscious level, or a confirmed diagnosis of epilepsy, apart from a febrile convulsion under the age of 5, will exclude a person from work offshore. This would include any stroboscopically induced seizure and epilepsy or fits occurring after alcohol withdrawal. However, after more than 3 years without recurrence or treatment an employee may be fit for 'low risk' duties. For those workers on 'high risk' duties, such as working at heights or crane operators, who have been more than 10 years without recurrence, offshore work may be permitted after specialist assessment. Also cases of childhood *petit mal* which did not extend into adult life might be acceptable after specialist assessment.

Mental disorders

As a general rule any acute or chronic psychosis or neurosis is not acceptable offshore unless the patient is fully recovered, off all therapy, and free of all symptoms for at least a year. A current history of alcohol or drug abuse is not acceptable.

Work offshore is sometimes stressful and may be exacerbated by the remote location and its inherent hazards and risks. Domestic difficulties at home and long separations may also be contributory factors. Those with a tendency to anxiety or depression may be more vulnerable. An established history or clinical evidence of personality disorder, psychosis, phobia, chronic anxiety state, or recurrent depression cannot be accepted in the offshore worker.

Cerebrovascular disease

Any cerebrovascular disease would be a bar to work offshore.

Vision

Vision must be adequate for task. Correction is allowable but the offshore worker must be capable of wearing safety spectacles, and must have adequate uncorrected vision to be able to escape safely without spectacles in an emergency. Binocular vision is preferable, but monocular vision is acceptable for some tasks, but only after specialist occupational health advice.

Corneal surgery

Where myopia has been corrected by a procedure such as photoreactive keratotomy (PRK) using an excimer laser, fitness for work offshore may be certified once the corneal structure has adequate strength and there is no risk of infection.

Cataract surgery

Following lens implant procedures, once the wounds are healed and visual acuity is stable, work offshore is permitted but corrected visual acuity must be at least 6/12 (20/40) in the better eye.

Genitourinary system

A history or investigation of renal disease requires detailed assessment. Dipstick urinalysis for glucose, protein, and blood should be undertaken routinely.

Any renal disease which could lead to renal failure (e.g. progressive or recurrent nephritis, nephrosis, polycystic disease, or hydronephrosis) is unacceptable for working offshore. The following conditions are relative contra-indications until treated or corrected:

- renal, ureteric or vesical calculi
- renal colic
- recurring urinary tract infection
- hydrocele or testicular abnormality
- transmissible genitourinary infection

The following are absolute contra-indications to working offshore:

- renal transplantation
- enuresis or incontinence
- gynaecological disorders such as disabling dysmenorrhoea or pelvic inflammatory disease
- confirmed pregnancy (because of risk factors to mother and fetus)
- urethral or prostatic pathology–inflammation, hypertrophic or malignant conditions, urethral stricture with incomplete bladder voiding.

A single kidney is acceptable if shown to be functioning normally. Any case of haematuria or haemospermia must be fully investigated.

Musculoskeletal system, fitness, and training

Offshore tasks are specialized and require training, skill, self-reliance, and aptitude, with adequate reserves to cope in an emergency.

There must be no deformity or amputation of a limb or digit which might affect performance or safety, including emergency evacuation procedures offshore. Hence prostheses are usually unacceptable. Similarly any acute, chronic, or recurring pain or restriction of movement (e.g. low back pain) will be unacceptable. The incidence of recurrent back pain is predicted by the Troup criteria.[4] Recurrence of back pain is greater if there is:

- a history of two or more previous attacks
- pain is caused by a fall on the buttocks or back
- sickness absence in excess of 5 weeks with previous low back pain
- residual pain in the leg

The following features on examination also indicate an active problem:

- restriction of pain-free straight-leg raising to less than 45°
- pain or weakness on resisted hip flexion
- inability to sit up from lying flat
- back pain on lumbar extension

Macdonald[5] suggests that in assessing fitness after a back pain episode the following criteria should be considered:

- recurrent back pain
- the Troup criteria
- arthralgia on spinal compression.

Endocrine and metabolic disorders

Adequate control and absence of target organ damage or environmental risk are the considerations here, as are the possible effects of temporary absence of replacement therapy. Any abnormality must be carefully assessed, but, for example, well-controlled thyroid disease may be acceptable offshore if carefully monitored. Other endocrine abnormalities such as Addison's disease, Cushing's disease, acromegaly, diabetes insipidus, pancreatitis, or adrenal pathology leading to hypoglycaemia preclude offshore employment.

People with diabetes controlled by diet alone, are fit for general employment offshore, provided there is no target organ damage. If oral therapy is required, individual assessment is recommended, but workers who require insulin would normally be barred.

Haematology

A routine full blood count is a useful screening measure and may identify some remediable conditions.

Anaemia
Anaemia is the most commonly discovered haematological condition and requires

investigation. Iron deficiency may be due to occult gastrointestinal blood loss. Pernicious anaemia is rare in the age group working offshore.

Polycythaemia

Primary and secondary polycythaemia may be associated with transient ischaemic attacks, visual disturbances, and peripheral vascular disease which would be hazardous offshore.

The mean corpuscular volume (MCV) may be raised in vitamin B_{12} deficiency, folic acid deficiency, and excessive alcohol intake. This requires investigation; successful treatment would enable general work offshore, except in alcohol abusers.

Blood dyscrasias

Leukaemia, lymphoma, multiple myeloma, and disorders of the reticuloendothelial system are normally incompatible with any work offshore, but individual consideration should be given to those in long-term remission and under regular review. Patients are not fit to work offshore while taking cytotoxic or immunosuppressive agents.

Splenectomy

There is an increased risk of overwhelming infection and such employees should have antibiotic prophylaxis and should be fully vaccinated (haemophilus influenzae b, meningococcus A and C, pneumococcus, and influenza) (see also Chapter 17, p. 338).

Thalassaemia and haemoglobinopathies

Carriers of the sickle-cell or thalassaemia trait are not thought to be at significantly increased risk when working offshore.

Coagulation disorders (haemophilia A and B, Christmas disease)

Accidental trauma may cause profound haemorrhage in haemophiliacs and facilities do not exist offshore to manage such an emergency. Coagulation defects that pose an increased risk of clotting are another contra-indication to work offshore.

Skin

The skin must be healthy, intact and not show signs of contact dermatitis to oil-based muds or detergents.

Acute or chronic infections may lead to rejection, as will severe exfoliative disorders such as psoriasis and active eczema.

Preventive aspects

An appreciation of patterns of illness is of value in healthcare planning for isolated populations. For example, Cooper[3] found that preventive measures resulted in fewer hospitalizations for mental illness than expected in the South Atlantic during the Falklands campaign. Alcohol abuse was also shown to be a major factor associated with *grand mal* epilepsy and fatal injuries; ischaemic heart disease was found to be an important cause of morbidity in the North Sea; and dental conditions caused 43% of North Sea medevacs for digestive system disorders, as compared with 6% for the South

Atlantic where routine dental surveillance was combined with rapid local access to dental treatment.

It is further recommended that:

- An intensive health education programme for all offshore personnel be implemented to counter, in particular, tobacco consumption, alcohol abuse, obesity, sexually transmitted disease, and stressful life patterns.
- Offshore rig medics should be trained in counselling skills, particularly to deal with psychological stress.
- There should be a general improvement in dental hygiene in offshore workers.

Conclusion

Despite the tendency towards de-manning of established production installations, offshore exploration continues both in shallow and in deep waters, in remote locations. Medical surveillance, health screening, and lifestyle health risk assessments aim to identify those lifestyles which can contribute to ill health and which can be modified to prevent illness and to promote good health.[6] Although hazardous incidents continue to occur, offshore injury rates are falling.[7]

The final decision regarding offshore employment or visits will be taken by the operator, taking into account medical advice from the examining physician, and any relevant contractual implications.

Extra stresses may arise in an ageing workforce required to 'multiskill' and learn new tasks. Medical assessment for offshore workers must reflect the national desire for workers in general to be healthy, and to perform effectively in an increasingly safety-conscious environment. Fitness for work offshore is summarized in Table A4.1.

Divers

All employed divers are covered by the Diving Operations at Work Regulations 1997 (SI 1997, No. 2776). These regulations stipulate that no person shall take part in any diving operation as a diver unless they have a valid certificate of medical fitness to dive (Regulation 12(1)(b)). This certificate can be issued only after a medical examination in accordance with the HSE Guidelines, performed by a Medical Examiner of Divers (which is the HSE's new name for the Approved Diving Doctor of previous regulations).

The Regulations also impose a duty on people who have responsibility for, or control over, diving operations to ensure that diving is safe so far as is reasonably practicable, and the diver has a responsibility to declare if they are unfit to dive on any diving operation.

Examination and certification mechanism

The medical examination of divers should be carried out in accordance with the recommendations in the HSE document MA1.[8]

A network of doctors approved to carry out diving medical examinations and issue certificates of fitness where appropriate extends throughout the UK and some other countries. Such certificates are entered in the diver's personal log-book and their validity must not exceed 12 months. Before approval as a Medical Examiner of Divers by the HSE, a doctor must demonstrate knowledge and experience of diving medicine, have attended a recognized course in the subject, and show that they meet the continuing clinical requirements of the HSE and have access to the necessary equipment for special examinations including electrocardiography and audiometry.

Medical considerations

Before the first diving medical examination the examining physician should obtain documentary evidence of the candidate's medical history from their general practitioner. At subsequent annual examinations the doctor must have a copy of the previous examination results.

Diving requires superior levels of physical fitness, self-reliance, and aptitude with reserves to cope in an emergency. The effects of immersion, increased breathing resistance, and exercise at depth produce physiological changes which require training for optimal performance. Once divers descend to their worksites the work they must perform may require strength, agility, judgement, observation, and accuracy without distraction. These requirements are reflected in the demanding standards of fitness required for pre-employment selection to a career in diving. In general, this standard is applicable to all divers. However, there may be divers who, although not meeting these standards fully, are fit for restricted diving, e.g. short dives at shallow depths. An examining doctor who is in doubt about a diver's fitness is recommended to obtain a further opinion from a second approved medical examiner or advice from a relevant specialist. Great importance is attached to the baseline medical examination. Updated guidance is issued to approved medical examiners of divers from time to time.

The HSE does not specify any minimum age limit for diving work, although approved medical examiners are advised that it is unlikely that anyone under 18 would be suitable. Nor is any upper age limit specified, provided that all the medical standards can be met.

The same general fitness criteria apply to both male and female divers, apart from relating size and strength to the type of professional diving involved. Available evidence, however, supports the view that no pregnant woman should dive.

Medical examination

There should be a standard enquiry into past and current health, occupational history, social history (including smoking and alcohol), and any details of past decompression illness.

Investigations which are required at the initial examination are: full blood count, HbS assessment, urinalysis, audiometry, chest radiograph, resting ECG, pulmonary function testing (FEV_1, FVC) and, for saturation diving, long bone radiographs.

At subsequent examinations: urinalysis, pulmonary function testing, audiometry, (but only after an episode of aural barotrauma), and resting ECG (if over the age of 40 and otherwise every 5 years unless there is a clinical indication). Haematology and radiology of the long bones and chest are required only if clinically indicated.

HIV positivity would not necessarily debar from diving, although the development of symptoms or signs of AIDS related complex would[9].

Examination by system

Physical fitness

Physical fitness is particularly important in divers where the effects of immersion, increased breathing resistance, and exercise produce physiological changes which require training for optimal performance. The diver's work may require strength, agility, mobility, and judgement. These standards are reflected in the physical requirements for unrestricted diving and limits on depth and duration, or type of exposure which may be imposed by the examining doctor if they perceive a risk to in-water safety[10].

A commercial diver must not be obese and where a lack of fitness, stamina, or athletic physique is observed, further assessment will be required. Estimation of fat content by skinfold thickness, ultrasound or impedance should be performed on those with a BMI in excess of 30. The diver must be physically fit and trained for hard work. The effects of immersion, cold, and increased work of breathing make aerobic fitness even more important.

Exercise testing

Exercise testing of commercial divers is routine. A commercial diver must be able to meet the physical requirements of the task and those arising in an emergency situation. An assessment of exercise capacity must be carried out at the preliminary examination and at each subsequent annual assessment. Where possible an assessment of maximum oxygen uptake (either direct or indirect) should be carried out. A diver should be able to achieve an exercise level equivalent to 13 Mets or 45 ml $kg^{-1}min^{-1}$ (lean body mass) oxygen consumption. These results should be considered in conjunction with other aspects of general fitness such as blood pressure, obesity (BMI), and lung function.

Where any respiratory symptoms result from exercise, peak expiratory flow rate (PEFR) before, and 5 and 10 minutes after the exercise test, provides a useful screen for exercise-induced wheeze. Acceptable exercise testing protocols include the army physical fitness test, Master two-step test, cycle ergometer test—direct or indirect assessment of oxygen uptake, treadmill test, and timed swimming test.

The chosen exercise test should be repeated at subsequent assessments to aid comparison. Medical examiners must satisfy themselves beyond reasonable doubt that the candidate is fit enough for the task.

Ear, nose, and throat

Divers should be able to clear their ears in order to equalize the pressure across the tympanic membrane and to cope with the changing barometric pressures in the water or in a chamber. Complications of otitis media such as glue ear, deafness, perforation, and persistent discharge debar diving under UK Regulatory Standards. Disease of the mastoid cavities is also a reason for restriction. The following points should be covered during an assessment of otological fitness:

• The external auditory meati should appear normal. If wax is present, it is not necessary to disturb it unless it is excessive or obstructing the canal. Acute or chronic otitis externa is a bar to diving until resolved. Exostoses are not harmful unless the canal is occluded, when the diver should be referred for their removal.

- The ear-drum should be inspected: well-healed scars are acceptable. New entrants must demonstrate the ability to clear their ears. A similar requirement exists after infection or barotrauma.
- The diver should be able to hear and understand normal conversation, and communication systems. Vestibular function should be normal.
- Audiometry should be carried out at each annual examination, using equipment covering the frequencies 500–6000 Hz[2] (and ideally 250–8000 Hz), and according to the recognized procedure. Particular attention should be given to divers who have unilateral hearing loss; the risks of further hearing damage should be discussed with the diver.

Vision

Visual acuity of 6/9 (20/30), or better, in both eyes is required for diving. A prescription faceplate may be used in a dive mask. Any history of glaucoma, uveitis, optic neuritis, or other retinal pathology requires individual assessment.

For divers, underwater vision is limited and binocular vision is ordinarily required. Divers must be able to read gauges and colour perception should be adequate for the task (trade testing can be used). Patients with visual field defects due to neurological disease may be inherently unfit to dive.

- **Contact lenses** are not encouraged in divers because of the risk of slippage and of infection especially in saturation diving. Hard impermeable lenses are not suitable, but disposable lenses may reduce the risk of infection and soft, gas-permeable types of lens may be acceptable subject to precautions. Surgical or laser corrections must be individually assessed.[11]
- **Corneal surgery** for correction of myopia has been practised since 1953. One common procedure is RK. However, concerns have been expressed that this may weaken the corneal structure and encourage infection which would be exacerbated by diving. Myopic correction using PRK is now more common, and less likely to cause infection, so thus should replace RK. PRK is not thought to be a contra-indication to diving.
- **Cataract surgery** is the commonest operation in the world today. A lens implant procedure is frequently performed in these cases. Although the majority of patients are over 60 there are younger patients also. The corneal wounds heal well and have considerable strength. Since the eye is fluid filled there are no special problems with compression effects after a lens implant procedure, but avoidance of mask squeeze is advised.

Alimentary and dental

- **Dental care** is important in commercial divers, and dental caries and periodontal disease need to be treated. Changes in pressure can cause pain in teeth which have been filled leaving small pockets of air trapped within the tooth. This can lead to dental barotrauma and collapse of the tooth.

- **Peptic ulceration** is not acceptable, but the relapse rate after a course of triple therapy is sufficiently low to allow return to air diving.
- Active inflammatory bowel diseases, symptomatic hiatus hernia, haemorrhoids, fistulae or anal fissures, cholelithiasis, and pancreatitis are **contra-indications** to diving.
- **Stomas** need to be individually assessed particularly in saturation diving.

Skin

The skin must be healthy and free of dermatoses which may be exacerbated by immersion or high humidity.

Respiratory system

There must be general fitness for vigorous swimming on the surface, and no conditions likely to lead to localized air trapping and barotrauma on ascent. Fibrotic lung disease, chronic obstructive airways disease, and reversible airways obstruction are absolute contra-indications.

A history of childhood asthma needs full assessment and perhaps lung provocation tests, as does exertion-induced bronchospasm. Any history suggestive of asthma in adulthood should be investigated by flow volume loops and gas transfer factor measurements. In certain circumstances only, and with specialist approval using precise criteria,[12] diving may be permitted.

There should be no significant past history of respiratory disease and no evidence of disorder causing obstruction, restriction or reduction of compliance or gas transfer capacity. A previous history of spontaneous pneumothorax presents a contra-indication, as does the existence of bullous lung disease. A penetrating chest injury which results in pleural adhesions or pulmonary scarring is similarly unacceptable. A history of previous chest surgery should be assessed by a chest physician with experience of diving medicine.

Lung function testing for diving

A full-size posterior–anterior chest radiograph in both inspiration and expiration should be performed at the preliminary examination. Spirometry should be performed at the preliminary examination and at each subsequent examination. As a routine FEV_1 and FVC should both be at least 80% of the predicted normal and the FEV_1/FVC ratio should be at least 70%. Anyone not achieving these standards should be referred to a diving respiratory specialist.

Cardiovascular system

A history, or discovery at examination, of ischaemic valvular or myocardial heart disease would be a bar even if successfully treated by medication or surgery. However, some percutaneous procedures may be acceptable. The assessment should include a resting ECG. Any variation from normal on examination, or investigation including disorders of rhythm, should be referred for specialist cardiological review and if risk factors such as poor family history, smoking, and obesity are present a supervised monitored exercise tolerance test should be performed with measurement of oxygen uptake if possible.

Such a test may, occasionally, demonstrate unsuspected evidence of myocardial ischaemia. Any subject with risk factors for coronary artery disease should be tested to an equivalent of stage IV on the Bruce Protocol (13 Mets).

Conditions which permit intracardiac shunting from right to left, such as an atrial septal defect, may be a cause for rejection and may account for previously unexplained acute decompression illness, but are not sought routinely in the medical screening of diving candidates.

Peripheral vascular disease

Intermittent claudication or other evidence of ischaemia of the lower extremities is a bar to diving. Minimal varicose veins may be acceptable but any history of deep vein thrombosis or any skin changes would be unacceptable.

Hypertension

The resting blood pressure (BP) should not be greater than 140 mmHg systolic or 80 mmHg diastolic (fifth phase). Patients on medication for hypertension which could cause side-effects incompatible with diving (e.g. β-blockers) are not acceptable.

Neurological system

Assessment of the CNS is one of the most important aspects of fitness assessment; a careful history and examination are essential as the more subtle and serious forms of decompression illness may involve the CNS. All modalities should be tested: cranial nerves, motor and sensory systems, balance, co-ordination, gait, and proprioception.

Sensation should be tested for light touch, pain, temperature, vibration, position and two-point discrimination. Reflex testing should include pupillary, tendon reflexes, abdominals, cremasters, and perianal reflexes.

Neuropsychometric assessment is important following a dysbaric event, and so a baseline observation is valuable and should be attempted. The diver's manner, attitude, and verbal and intellectual response form part of the examination. Any pertinent observation should be recorded. Where doubt exists, a specialist neuropsychometric assessment should be made.

Causes for rejection would include:

- Claustrophobia or severe motion sickness.
- Epilepsy (other than febrile convulsion occurring up to the age of 5 years). If off treatment and symptom free for 10 years then in certain circumstances diving may be permitted, subject to specialist investigation and advice. Single seizures are assessed in a different manner from established epilepsy. A single seizure has a recurrence risk of between 23% and 80%,[13] most second seizures occurring within 1 year of the first. Enquiry must be made into predisposing factors (family history, EEG abnormality, or past history of febrile convulsion) and a specialist assessment made. This is to exclude genetic or constitutional predisposition to subsequent seizures. Without recurrence after 3 years, diving may be permitted.
- Migraine with neurological symptoms or signs.
- Any intracranial surgical procedure or depressed skull fracture.
- A head injury where there has been brain damage or a risk of post-traumatic epilepsy:

- depressed skull fracture
- intracranial haematoma
- loss of consciousness or PTA of $>$ 30 minutes
- focal neurological signs.
- After less severe head injury than above (loss of consciousness or post-traumatic amnesia [PTA] of $<$30 minutes) the diver should be declared temporarily unfit for a minimum of 4 weeks subject to medical review, and evidence then sought of any cognitive dysfunction.
- Any evidence of cerebrovascular accident, significant spinal cord trauma, spondyloses with myelopathy, demyelination (multiple sclerosis), or neurodegenerative disease (Parkinson's disease).

Psychiatric illness

Any psychiatric risk to the individual's or buddy's safety should be assessed, together with the risk of recurrence of psychiatric or psychological disorder. Divers should be free from psychiatric illness and cognitive impairment, and should not be suffering from psychological or personality problems that would interfere with their own in-water safety or that of others.[14]

The following conditions are absolute contra-indications to diving even while quiescent:

- schizophrenia
- bipolar affective disorder
- unipolar affective disorder
- disorders that still require treatment.

A past history of certain disorders may be compatible with diving, subject to specialist assessment and provided there has been resolution:

- adjustment reactions
- parasuicide
- premenstrual dysphoric disorder
- phobias
- isolated psychotic episode.

No diver using any psychotropic medication should be passed as fit to dive.

Cerebrovascular disease

Any cerebrovascular disease is a bar to diving.

Endocrine

In diving there are numerous neurological and hormonal responses to the effects of immersion and thermoregulation which must be considered. Uncomplicated thyroid disease if adequately controlled may be acceptable if carefully monitored.

Commercial diving candidates who are diabetic, whether controlled by insulin, oral hypoglycaemic agents or diet alone, are not considered fit to dive. If a professional diver develops hyperglycaemia which can be controlled by diet alone, diving may be permitted subject to continous monitoring and as long as there is no evidence of target organ damage.

Haematology

Baseline haematological investigations are required for commercial divers at initial examination.

Blood dyscrasias, even in remission, will be cause for rejection and people with frank haemoglobinopathies should also be excluded. **Polycythaemia** will increase the risk of acute decompression illness. **Coagulation disorders**, whether they increase or decrease the bleeding tendency are incompatible with diving.

Divers who have had a **splenectomy** are at an increased risk of overwhelming infection from pseudomonas and should carry appropriate antibiotics (4-quinolones, ciprofloxacin, for example). This is not compatible with saturation diving.

Any disorder which impairs oxygen transport in the blood would bar from diving. **Thalassaemia major** and **sickle-cell anaemia sufferers** would not be fit for diving. Carriers of the sickle-cell and thalassaemia traits are not thought to be at significantly increased risk in diving.

Genitourinary system

A history of renal disease or of urinary tract investigation is a reason for more detailed questioning and examination. Dipstick urine analysis for glucose, protein, and blood should be undertaken routinely. Venereal disease will debar until adequately treated. The presence of renal, ureteric, or vesicular calculi and other genitourinary diseases is usually a cause for rejection. The presence of a single kidney which is normally functioning is acceptable for diving work, but any case of haematuria or haemospermia must be fully investigated.

Malignancy

Cases of malignancy should be individually assessed for factors affecting in-water safety (surface orientated diving) or extended stay in an isolated environment and especially saturation diving.

Infection control

The examining doctor must be satisfied that the diver is not suffering from a communicable disease. All cases should be excluded from diving until treated.

Hyperbaric chamber workers

The use of hyperbaric chambers within diving projects is covered by the Diving Regulations and people who may be routinely subjected to hyperbaric conditions need to have the same level of medical fitness.

Hyperbaric chambers in hospitals are not covered by the Diving Regulations but the British Hyperbaric Association (BHA) recommends that medical attendants working in such chambers undergo medical examinations and that the standards are similar to those for commercial divers.[15]

Conclusion

The statutory diving medical examination is designed to exclude factors which might affect the diver's safety in the water. To this is added the need to avoid jeopardy to others

Table A4.1 Fitness for diving and work offshore

	Absolute contra-indication		Relative contra-indication	
	Diving	Offshore	Diving	Offshore
Cardiovascular system				
Ischaemic heart disease	*	*		
Congenital heart disease			*	*
Uncontrolled hypertension	*	*		
Respiratory system				
Asthma	*			*
COAD	*	*		
History of pneumothorax	*			*
Alimentary system				
Dental decay			*	*
Active upper GI disease	*	*		
Active inflammatory bowel disease	*	*		
Stoma			*	*
ENT				
Deafness			*	*
Inflammation/perforation	*			*
Balance	*	*		
Vision				
Monocular vision			*	*
Visual field defects	*	*		
Colour blindness			*	*
Refractive errors			*	*
Central nervous system				
Epilepsy	*	*		
Cerebrovascular disease	*	*		
Other neurological diseases	*			*
Musculoskeletal				
Chronic back pain	*	*		
Amputation of limb	*	*		
Amputation of digit			*	*
Genitourinary system				
Calculi			*	*
Haematuria	*	*		
Infections	*	*		
Endocrine system				
Insulin-dependent diabetes	*	*		
Diabetics on oral hypoglycaemics	*			*
Diabetics on diet alone			*	*
Addison's disease	*	*		
Other			*	*
Skin				
Eczema/psoriasis			*	*
Malignancy				
Active/chemotherapy	*	*		
Remission/cured			*	*

Table A4.1 *Continued*

	Absolute contra-indication		Relative contra-indication	
	Diving	Offshore	Diving	Offshore
Other				
Pregnancy	*	*		
Clotting disorders	*	*		
Psychosis	*	*		
Alcoholism/substance abuse	*	*		
bmi > 30			*	*

Fitness for work offshore does not confer fitness for occupation. See text for details.

who might become involved in possible rescue. Finally, the long-term health effects should be monitored by comparing results of each year's examination.

Divers have an obligation to declare any factor of which they are aware that might affect their own personal safety, and the employer has the responsibility for ensuring that a diving operation is carried out in as safe a manner as is reasonably practicable.

The HSE has placed much emphasis on the promotion of safe diving practices and on the medical assessment of divers.

Fitness for diving is summarized in Table A4.1.

Selected references and further reading

References

1   *Guidelines for medical aspects of fitness for offshore work, issue 4*. London: UK Offshore Operators Association Limited, Health Advisory Committee, 2000.
2   *A guide to audiometric testing programmes*. Guidance Note MS26. Sheffield: Health and Safety Executive, 1995.
3   Cooper NK. Secondary medical referrals from the British service population of the South Atlantic 1986–1990. A comparison with medevacs from oil and gas rigs of the British sector of the North Sea 1992. MFOM dissertation, Faculty of Occupational Medicine, Royal College of Physicians, 1993.
4   Troup JDG, Edwards FC. *Manual handling and lifting*. London: Health and Safety Executive, 1985.
5   Macdonald E. Musculoskeletal back pain. In *Medical assessment of fitness to dive*, ed. Elliot DH, pp. 171–183. Guildford: Biomedical Seminars, 1995.
6   Bell JG *et al*. A systematic approach to health surveillance in the workplace. *Occup Med* 1995; **45**(6): 305–310.
7   *Offshore accident and incident statistics report*. Publication No. OTO 97951. Sheffield: Health and Safety Executive, 1997.
8   *The medical examination and assessment of divers*. MA1 (03.98). Sheffield: Health and Safety Executive, 1998.
9   HIV infection and diving. Ind(G). 101L C150 3.91 Bootle: Health and Safety Executive Medical Division, 1991.

10   Elliott DH. Medical evaluation for commercial diving. In: *Diving medicine*, ed. Bove AA, 3rd edn, pp. 361–371. Philadelphia, Saunders, 1997.

11   Le May M. Ophthalmological aspects of fitness to dive. *South Pacific Underwater Medicine Society Incorporated Journal* 1996; **26**(4): 253–259.

12   Harries M. Why asthmatics should be allowed to dive. In: *Are asthmatics fit to dive*, ed. Elliott DH. Proceedings of the Underseas and Hyperbaric Medicine Society, 1996, pp. 7–15.

13   Hauser WA, Rich SS, Annegers JF, Anderson VE. Seizure recurrence after a 1st unprovoked seizure: an extended follow-up. *Neurology* 1990; **40**: 1163–1170.

14   Lunn B. Mental fitness to dive. In: *Medical assessment of fitness to dive*, ed. Elliott DH, pp. 215–242. Guildford: Biomedical Seminars, 1995.

15   Colvin AP. Pre-employment assessment of hyperbaric healthcare workers. *British Hyperbaric Association Newsletter*, June 1996, 10–18.

Further reading

Cox Report. A report of the Faculty of Occupational Medicine: a code of good working practice for the operation and staffing of hyperbaric chambers for therapeutic purposes: a report to the Faculty of Occupational Medicine of the Royal College of Physicians, pp. 11–13. London: Faculty of Occupational Medicine of the Royal College of Physicians, 1994.

Medical assessment of fitness to dive. In *The Proceedings of Conference, Edinburgh*, eds. Elliott DH. Biomedical Seminars, Guildford: 1995.

Appendix 5

General aspects of fitness for work overseas

R. A. F. Cox

Although most of the comments in this appendix apply to companies and their employees overseas, it must be remembered that many people are working overseas, often in hostile areas, without any support from well-organized parent organizations. Such people may include the self-employed, academics, missionaries, students, and professional adventurers. An excellent and fascinating account of the hazards facing anthropologists is given by Howell (see Further reading). Any person planning to work overseas should make careful preparation for the preservation of their health and the provision of medical care in the event of illness, before departure.

A list of centres from which essential medical advice can be obtained and useful books which may be consulted during the planning of an overseas assignment can be found at the end of this appendix.

Companies who send employees overseas, however long or short the assignment may be, retain a responsibility for them while they are abroad, as some companies have recently discovered to their cost. It is therefore essential that they ensure, as far as possible, that potential expatriates are fit for their overseas duties and that proper arrangements are in place to take care of them, if they are ill or injured.

Disability *per se* should not be a bar to travelling or working overseas though some medical conditions may not be compatible with some overseas locations. Those disabled by multiple sclerosis, for example, are likely to be worse in hot climates, though the progress of the disease is not affected. Each case must clearly be considered individually but employers would be expected to make 'reasonable adjustments' to enable disabled employees to travel or transfer overseas, especially where this is an integral part of their job or an important step in their career. 'Reasonable adjustment' might include, for example, providing transport to and from airports, making special arrangements with airlines, and, if necessary, buying seats with more leg room or closer to the aircraft toilets, even if this means upgrading. Similarly, obtaining accommodation for a disabled employee close to the place of work, even if this were more expensive, would be regarded as a 'reasonable adjustment'. On the other hand, putting disabled employees' health at risk by posting them to a place where they are unable to obtain essential medical care would be regarded as unreasonable. Like any other employees, those with disabilities should be carefully assessed by an occupational physician before a decision is made to allow them to travel or to transfer overseas. They should not be rejected, simply because they have a disability, without being given the opportunity of a skilled assessment by an occupational physician.

There are a great number of factors to be considered when a company is planning an overseas operation, and the medical requirements tend to be relegated to the end of the list even though concerns for general health will be a major anxiety of any potential expatriates and their families.

The company must, therefore, not only find out about diseases and medical conditions which may be prevalent in the areas of their operations but it must also review the local medical and hospital facilities and services and appoint a local doctor to act on its behalf. In many areas of the world this will require a visit by a doctor from the home country on behalf of the company.

Any company which embarks on overseas operations should appoint a doctor at its home base, if it does not already have its own occupational physician. This is necessary not only so that they can determine whether employees are fit to transfer overseas but to liaise with the local overseas doctor and to advise on the numerous health queries which will inevitably arise in the course of a foreign operation.

No matter how thorough the pre-departure medical screening and examinations may have been, some illness will still occur, requiring decisions regarding treatment, possible repatriation, and liaison with doctors and relatives in the home country. Even if illness does not occur, injury, especially from road traffic accidents, is a constant risk and the commonest reason for emergency repatriations. Policies and procedures for dealing with such contingencies must be in place before the operation begins. It may be fatal to wait until such an emergency arises. Such policies must include the mechanism by which the costs of local medical care are to be met. It is essential that all overseas assignees and regular travellers have adequate medical insurance cover, which is available from any of the major health insurers. In most countries this has to be purchased and, in many places payment, or a guarantee of payment, is required before admission to hospital can be arranged or treatment commenced.

There are a number of air ambulance services available, but two of the largest established ones, Swiss Air Rescue Organization and SOS Assistance are based in Switzerland (addresses in Appendix 7).

Before departure, or the establishment of an overseas operation, arrangements should be made with one of these, or a similar organization, for the emergency evacuation of sick and injured personnel.

People's behaviour changes as soon as they are overseas. The different culture, climate, food, and social activities include psychological and physiological changes which often result in health effects. Even the most demure people seem to relax their usual standards of conventional sexual behaviour when abroad, particularly if they are not accompanied by their usual sexual partners.

Some people will seek overseas employment to escape from domestic or financial crises or because they have drinking problems or established psychiatric conditions. Such people are likely to be disastrous choices for overseas assignments and should be rigorously excluded. The enquiries of the pre-departure medical examiner should be particularly oriented towards revealing these factors.

Staying well is taken for granted in western countries, because of their excellent public health and medical care systems, but staying well in many undeveloped and tropical countries requires strict self-discipline and personal vigilance. Standards of personal and domestic hygiene must be greater, and risks which may be quite acceptable in Europe or North America may lead to dire consequences in tropical Africa. People who may have difficulty in adjusting to this very different environment should be counselled before departure. A trivial and easily managed illness in the UK can be a major problem for the patient, their family and their employers when it occurs overseas. In no other circumstance is the hackneyed cliché 'prevention is better than cure' more true. The emergency evacuation of a sick employee is often a hazardous experience for the patient and always an expensive, worrying, and very time-consuming exercise for those responsible for the organization of the repatriation.

The essential medical examination should be arranged well in advance of departure and should be conducted by a doctor experienced in travel medicine who is instructed to perform the examination on behalf of the company, to which they should make their report. This should preferably be in confidence to the company's own medical adviser but, if not, it should be in the form of a non-confidential report to the personnel manager or other appropriate senior person. As long as the report is made by a person who has not had clinical care of the employee it will not fall within the Access to Medical Reports Act.

The examining doctor must be aware of the local conditions at the overseas place of residence, preferably through first-hand experience. It may be quite acceptable to transfer someone with quite significant health problems to a location where medical care of an equivalent standard to that at the home base is available, although the same health problem would be an absolute bar to transfer to other places. A totally different standard of medical fitness must be expected in a geologist who may be moving to an office job in Chicago, if they were instead to lead a survey party in Niger.

The medical examination should be designed and performed to reveal actual or potential health problems which may occur during the course of the overseas assignment. In this respect the examination for transfer overseas differs from an employment examination which is designed to determine only a person's fitness for work. Because of the different environmental and physiological demands, many employees who are perfectly fit to work in the UK would not be fit to do the same work overseas. The examination must also be performed sufficiently ahead of departure that remediable conditions can be treated.

Any person who is suffering from a medical condition which requires regular medical supervision should not be permitted to transfer overseas unless the examining doctor is quite certain that such supervision, and of an acceptable standard, is available.

If companies with international operations keep their employees under regular health surveillance they can be very rapidly processed for overseas service and may not even need an examination. However, unless the doctor who has to decide on the potential expatriate's fitness for overseas work is very familiar with their current medical state or has access to notes of a recent examination, the employee must have a comprehensive medical review including a physical examination. Screening by questionnaire is not in the experience of this author adequate.

Even more important is the examination of family members, if the employee is to be accompanied, though there is an increasing tendency for employees to transfer overseas on 'bachelor status' with 2 weeks home leave every 3 months. Children normally adapt to living overseas very well but may have medical conditions which could be a liability, and in many undeveloped countries the facilities for the medical care of children are even less adequate than those for adults, so that children who are ill must either be nursed at home or repatriated. Expatriate mothers must, therefore, be not only capable, confident, resourceful, and very adaptable but they must also be very fit. Thorough and detailed review and examination of spouses is just as important as for employees.

When the family have been deemed 'fit to travel', appropriate prophylactic immunizations must be administered and essential emergency medical equipment in the way of drugs, dressings, and other items provided. Medicines and other medical items, readily available and taken for granted in the UK, are often unavailable or of very inferior quality in developing countries and every expatriate and family should carry essential supplies from their home base. The exact list should be recommended by the company medical officer and will depend on the location and the anticipated requirements of the family. The course of immunizations should also be completed in good time so that any untoward reactions are over before departure.

Although this is not the place for detailed advice about recommended immunizations, which changes regularly anyway, and which can be obtained from any of the centres listed in Appendix 7, some comments on some of the latest vaccines is not out of place.

- **Hepatitis A** vaccine should be given to all long-term assignees (i.e. more than 6 months stay) and travellers to areas where the food and water hygiene may be less than ideal. Immune globulin (γ globulin) should now only be used to protect unprotected travellers departing at short notice.
- **Hepatitis B** vaccine should be given to all regular travellers and long-term assignees (i.e. more than 6 months) to all areas of the world except North America, Australia, New Zealand, and Northern Europe; also to travellers who may put themselves at risk because of their behaviour, or who may need medical or dental treatment abroad.
- The modern **rabies** vaccine is safe and effective and it should be given to all longer-term travellers to developing areas of the world. Administering this vaccine prophylactically obviates the need for giving a blood product (rabies immunoglobulin) in the event of a bite, which is particularly reassuring in the current AIDS climate. However, the traveller must be warned that further doses of vaccine are always advised post-exposure.
- Although group B **meningitis**, for which there is no available vaccine, is the commonest strain in the UK, the other strains, A and C, for which there is an effective vaccine, are commoner in some areas of the world. Meningitis vaccine should be given to overseas assignees or regular travellers to east, west and central Africa, the Delhi area of India, Nepal, and pilgrims to Mecca.
- Vaccination against **Japanese encephalitis** should be considered for people embarking on rural travel in Asia from India to Japan, but individual advice should be sought from one of the centres already mentioned.
- **Yellow fever** vaccine is mandatory for many countries within the endemic zones of tropical Africa or South America. A single injection lasts for 10 years and it is so often neglected until immediately before urgent travel that it is mentioned here to emphasize the importance of taking the vaccine in advance, if there is any likelihood of travelling to a yellow fever area. Even where the vaccine is not mandatory, it is advised for personal protection for travel within the zones. The only exceptions are short trips to capital cities at high altitude.
- **AIDS** is covered elsewhere in this book, but it is spreading rapidly in both sexes in some areas of Africa, Asia, the Caribbean and eastern Europe and the importance

of not taking risks cannot be overemphasized for the regular traveller or overseas assignee. (As a side issue, some international operators, in areas of the world where the prevalence of HIV positivity is reported to be a high as 40% of the population, may have to consider whether it would be any advantage to screen local employees for HIV prior to employment. For more detail on pre-employment screening see Chapter 24.)

The medical processing of potential overseas expatriates is an essential prerequisite which should be completed well in advance of departure and must include every member of the family who is travelling. The cost of such a procedure is small compared with the cost of medical repatriation which such screening could have prevented.

Summary

- Local medical facilities must be reviewed.
- Appoint a local doctor.
- Establish liaison between the local overseas doctor and the company's occupational physician.
- Arrange adequate medical insurance cover.
- Prepare contingency plans for medical evacuation/repatriation.
- Arrange thorough medical examinations, well in advance of departure, for all members of the family who are going.

Further reading

Generally for travellers

Dawood R (ed.) *Travellers' health*. Oxford: Oxford University Press, 1992.
Health advice for travellers. London: Department of Health (updated regularly).
Werner D. *Where there is no doctor*. London: Macmillan, 1993.
Wilson-Howarth J, Ellis M. *Your child's health abroad*. Chalfont St. Peter: Bradt UK, 1998.

Generally for health professionals

Guidelines for the prevention of malaria in travellers from the United Kingdom PHLS (Communicable Disease Report 19.9.1997).
Health information for overseas travel. London: HMSO, 1995 (the UK Yellow Book).
Howell N. *Surviving fieldwork, a report on health and safety in fieldwork*. Washington, DC: American Anthropological Association, 1990.
Immunisation against infectious disease. London: Stationery Office, 1996.
The yellow book. Health information for international travel. Washington, DC: US Department of Health and Human Services, Public Health Service. Regularly updated. (Beware of significant differences in recommended practice between the US and Europe).
Walker E, Williams G and Raeside F *The ABC of Healthy Travel*. London: BMJ Publishing, 1993.

Appendix 6

Ill health retirement guidance

K. J. Pilling and P. A. Wynn

From time to time all doctors are called on to offer an opinion on fitness to work and on retirement on medical grounds, but advising managers and employees on these issues is a regular responsibility of occupational physicians. For an employee, ill health retirement is a major life event which hinges on the doctor's opinion and clinical judgement, and on a manager's interpretation of this advice after taking account of company policy. Some cases will be straightforward but others will require careful consideration of all the circumstances. Most companies do not have a clear and detailed set of rules available to help those involved in the ill health retirement process to reach a fair, consistent, and auditable decision.

Despite the profound impact of early retirement on the individual, the employing organization, and the pension scheme, an essentially subjective approach is usually taken. This introduces bias which can significantly influence company ill health retirement rates. This inconsistency has been attributed to, amongst other causes, the difficulty in defining such terms as 'permanent incapacity' and allowing individual doctors to adopt either 'dove' or 'hawk' stances. In addition, a lack of formal guidance has been identified for occupational health physicians in this significant area of their work.

The following guidance is intended to help all parties involved in decision-making and to promote equity and confidence in the process.

Ten key questions and guidance notes

1 What guidance, if any, does the pension scheme provide in relation to criteria for eligibility and the interpretation of its rules?

Pension scheme medical advisers should always know what the criteria and rules are for eligibility for a pension, and should use them in order to guide them in making their ill health retirement decisions. Where pension scheme guidance is unclear or requires only a yes/no answer the physician, in discussion with the pension fund trustees, may wish to alter the criteria for qualification or develop consensus guidelines to allow consistency of approach. However, in the short term, if guidance is open to individual interpretation, the following nine additional questions will help the examining physician to provide fair and considered advice to management and trustees, who ultimately have to decide whether or not to retire an employee on ill health grounds.

2 Is the employee currently able to perform the duties for which they were most recently employed?

It is important to have an accurate knowledge of the current work content of the post, especially the physical and psychological demands and skills required to enable the employee to work effectively. It is important to discuss these matters with the employee and management. Managers will often be in the best position to assess performance. It is important for physicians to be familiar with an employee's work, but it is impossible to know how individuals are coping when they are not being observed.

3 Is this situation likely to be permanent or to continue for the foreseeable future?

Some physicians are expected to work to extremely strict criteria that only qualify an employee who will never be fit to work again. If this is taken literally, then an ill health retirement pension can only be awarded to those with extreme ill health or disability. Even in these cases it is sometimes impossible, as a result of improved treatments, to state that a return to work is impossible. For example, advanced heart disease, liver disease, and kidney disease treated by transplantation can result in individuals making a successful return to their original jobs. A more pragmatic approach is to consider whether a return to any type of available work is likely in the foreseeable future. Clearly, employers are unable to keep posts open indefinitely and sick, pensionable employees should not remain on sick leave for prolonged periods if improvement is not observed or likely. The particular difficulties in prognosis of psychiatric disorders, chronic fatigue syndrome, back pain etc. have recently been fully discussed. Poole *et al.* 1997[1] is a useful source of advice and should be consulted.

4 Is the employee's medical condition likely to be aggravated by remaining in the present post?

When occupational factors may have contributed to the poor health of an employee considered for ill health retirement it is obviously unsound practice to allow the employee to remain exposed to those factors in the same post. If the risk factors cannot be controlled, relocation is advisable. Similarly, those workers with non-occupational conditions that could be aggravated by the workplace should be transferred to alternative work if process control measures do not resolve the problem. If no suitable alternative work is available and no reasonable accommodation can be made, termination of contract on ill health grounds may be a fair reason for dismissal under employment protection legislation and under the Disability Discrimination Act 1995 (DDA).

5 Does the medical condition make it unsafe, either for themselves or for others, for the employee to continue as before?

When the health of an employee impairs performance in such a way that the individual is unable to work safely and risks injuring themself or colleagues, it is inappropriate and possibly unlawful for that person to continue as before. A credible attempt at finding alternative work should be made. Employers should be mindful of their common law duty not to be negligent by placing the employee or others at risk.

6 Can the content, working hours, or location of the employee's job be changed or is the employee fit for any other post the company may reasonably offer having regard to the individual's skills, experience, and terms of contract?

The majority of companies have some provision for alternative employment or in-house rehabilitation for employees returning to work after illness.

In general:

- Occupational physicians, managers, and the employee should communicate as openly as possible and share the responsibilities, difficulties, and successes of the rehabilitation process.
- Short-term redeployment is much easier for most companies to support than long-term, and employers should be given the best possible medical advice on the likely duration of an employee's reduced capacity.
- Arrangements can frequently be offered for employees to return to work on shorter hours and lighter duties can frequently be offered. Careful observation, support, and modification of duties are essential so that targets can be set, monitored and reviewed. Where progress is unsatisfactory ill health retirement can be considered.
- In practice, an employee's personal qualities, qualifications, past attendance record, and performance will have an impact on how much effort and support is provided for rehabilitation. In times of economic hardship, recession, contracting labour force, and use of contractors in non-critical jobs, rehabilitation is becoming more difficult. These days it is rare for companies to operate redeployment panels or have in-house convalescent facilities.

7 Has the employee been accurately informed about the financial consequences of ill health retirement?

It is important for sick employees to be aware not only of the financial benefits that will accrue on accepting ill health retirement but also the implications of remaining at work if this is a viable alternative.

For employees attempting to remain at work or on rehabilitation programmes, temporary reduction of hours or modification of duties when recommended by a medical adviser and supported by management should not normally incur financial penalty. If an employee is ultimately downgraded, employers should not reduce salary but freeze income until the job value increases to equal the frozen salary. A decision should be made on whether company benefits, such as a company car, would be retained. Shift-workers who move on to day work would expect to lose the shift allowance. Although understandable, this may have serious consequences from loss of earnings. The financial consequences must be explained if there are valid medical and performance reasons for retiring an employee.

8 Is the employee in favour of ill health retirement?

Whenever possible it is best that all parties involved in the ill health retirement decision are in agreement. The majority of sick employees initiate the ill health retirement option. Some employees are retired on grounds of ill health without their consent, but employers must behave responsibly and reasonably if this course of action is pursued, as it is likely that in these circumstances the employee will seek legal advice on the matter. Employers should be mindful of the provisions of the DDA.

In practice, this legal concern is of practical importance only if the medical grounds for ill health retirement are in doubt. If an individual cannot perform such duties as are available there may be no other option but to terminate service. However, permanent health insurance (PHI) schemes may offer alternative financial compensation.

9 Is the employee's general practitioner in favour of ill health retirement, and has the general practitioner or specialist sent written comments to the occupational physician on the employee's current medical condition and prognosis?

In cases of ill health retirement occupational physicians should be aware of all relevant medical details before advising management. Once the employee's written consent has been given this may involve the occupational physician discussing the case with the employee's general practitioner and/or consultant. A consensus view on the appropriateness or otherwise of ill health retirement from all medical practitioners involved is to be recommended, and this is even more important if the employee is to be ill health retired against their wishes. Advice should be based on objective medical evidence and not on feelings of benevolence toward the applicant, on their illness behaviour, or on financial consideration. Where there are two conflicting medical opinions, pension schemes tend to take the advice of their own medical adviser. However, in cases of dispute there are three situations where a reasonable employer ought to take a third medical opinion from another specialist:

- Where the occupational physician's report is vague or unhelpful.
- Where the occupational physician or the general practitioner has looked only at the medical files and has not personally interviewed or conducted a medical examination on the employee.
- Where the employee is undergoing specialist treatment and that specialist has not been asked to give an opinion. Even in cases where the employee's general practitioner and the company medical adviser agree, an employee may wish to present a specialist's report when this may make a significant difference to views of the prognosis.

10 After considering the physical, social and mental aspects of the application for ill health retirement, has any underlying problem with work practices or the working environment been a contributory factor?

Differential rates of ill health early retirement are well recognized between different occupations. The audit of such retirement by the occupational health department will allow the identification of the largest sources of morbidity—be they workplace related or otherwise—and the appropriate allocation of resources for primary prevention and/or early identification.

The consideration of the physical, social, and mental aspects in each case may allow the identification of systematic problems within an organization in the treatment of older workers. This could include failure of the enterprise to consider the change in the physical capability of their older workers and inappropriate or ill-considered job progression. Other factors may include poor skills development and lack of recognition and support. Identification of such problems and feedback to central and line management may avoid retirement in specific cases and improve the quality of employee care in general. The value of retaining trained and experienced staff, and the savings to the pension scheme, should not be underestimated by management or occupational heath care professionals.

Reference

1   Poole CJM, Baron CE *et al*. Ill health retirement—guidelines for occupational physicians. *Occup Med* 1996;**46**: 402–406.

Further reading

Elder AG, Symington IS, Symington EH. Do occupational physicians agree about ill-health retiral? A study of simulated retirement assessments. *Occup Med* 1994; **44**: 231–235.
Hudson D. Long term absence and ill health retirement—an employer's nightmare? *Occup Health Rev* 1994; September/October: 21–24.
The Disability Discrimination Act 1995. London: HMSO.

Appendix 7

Addresses and contact details

Chapter 1   **Introduction**
Chapter 2   **Legal aspects of fitness for work**
Chapter 3   **The Disability Discrimination Act 1995**
Chapter 4   **Vocational rehabilitation services**

Office of the Chief Medical Adviser
Department of Social Security
1–11 John Adam Street
London WC2N 6HT
Tel: 020 7834 9144

SEMA Group
Medical Director
SEMA Medical Services
Government Buildings
1 Cop Lane
Penwortham
Preston PR1 0SP
Tel: 01772 237 963
Fax: 01772 237839

CancerBACUP
3 Bath Place
Rivington Street
London EC2A 3DR
Cancer Support Service: 020 7613 2121
Freephone: 0808 800 1234
Employee Support Scheme: 020 7920 7213
Publications: 020 7696 9003
CancerBACUP Scotland (counselling service) 0141 553 1553
Web: www.cancerbacup.org.uk

Employment Medical Advisory Service
Offices located in each of HSE Regions. Details of local office in telephone directory.

National Council for Voluntary Organisations (NCVO)
Regents Wharf
8 All Saints Street
London N1 9RL

Tel: 020 7713 6161
Voluntary Sector Helpdesk 0845 600 4500
Fax: 020 7278 0211

RADAR (The Royal Association for Disability and Rehabilitation)
12 City Forum
250 City Road
London ECIV 8AF
Tel: 020 7250 3222
Fax: 020 7250 0212
Minicom: 020 7250 4119
e-mail: RADAR@radar.org.uk
Web: www.radar.org.uk

SKILL: National Bureau for Students with Disabilities
Chapter House
18–20 Crucifix Lane
London SE1 3JW
Info: 0800 328 5050 (voice)
Info: 0800 068 2422 (text)
Office voice/text: 020 7450 0620
Fax: 020 7450 0650

Employment Opportunities for People with Disabilities
1 Bank Buildings
Princes Street
London EC2R 8EU
Tel: 020 7726 4961
Fax: 020 7726 4961
Minicom: 020 7726 4963

Health and Safety Executive (HSE)
Information Centre
Broad Lane
Sheffield S3 7HQ
Tel: 0541 545500—Infoline
Fax: 0114 289 2333
Web: www.open.gov.uk/hse/hsehome.htm

Disability Information Trust
Mary Marlborough Centre
Nuffield Orthopaedic Centre
Headington
Oxford OX3 7LD
Tel: 01865 227 592
Fax: 01865 227 596
e-mail: ditrust@btconnect.com

Employers' Forum on Disability
60 Gainsford Street
London SE7 2NY
Tel: 020 7403 3020
Fax: 0120 7403 0404
e-mail: efd@employers-forum.co.uk

Disabled Living Foundation
380–384 Harrow Road
London W9 2HU
Tel: 020 7289 6111
Fax: 020 7266 2922
Minicom: 020 7432 8009
e-mail: dlfinfo@dlf.org.uk

Finchale Training College
Durham DH1 5RX
Tel: 0191 386 2634
Fax: 0191 386 4962

Queen Elizabeth's Training College (training disabled adults 18–64 for work)
Leatherhead Court
Leatherhead
Surrey KT22 0BN
Tel: 01372 841 100
Fax: 01372 841 156
Minicom: 01372 843 483

St Loye's College (training disabled people for employment)
Topsham Road
Exeter
Devon EX2 6EP
Tel: 01392 255428
Fax: 01392 420889

Vocational assessment centres
(NB: very few of the following organizations have specific Functional Capacity Assessment equipment, but they may be able to offer standardized physical assessments or know someone in their area who could help).

Crawford TGH
Healthcare Division
Lloyds Court
1 Goodmans Yard
London E1 8AT

Dept of OT
Glasgow Caledonian University
Southblane Campus
Jordan Hill
Glasgow G13 1PP

Enham Resource Centre
Enham Alamein
Andover
Hants SP11 6JS

Lambeth Accord
336 Brixton Road
London SW9 7AA

Langman HRD Ltd
Robert House
Acorn Business Park
Woodseats Close
Sheffield S8 0TB

Oakleaf Enterprises
101 Walnut Tree Close
Guildford
Surrey GU1 4HQ

Physical Evaluation Systems
Clipper House
66 London Street
Reading RG1 4SQ

Queen Elizabeth's Foundation for Disabled People
Leatherhead Court
Leatherhead
Surrey KT22 0BN

Rehab UK
Tabard House
116 Southwark Street
London SE1 0TA

Rehab Scotland
Melrose House
Cadogan Street
Glasgow G2 6QQ

UNUM
Milton Court
Dorking
Surrey RH4 3LZ

Chapter 5 Ethics for occupational physicians

Faculty of Occupational Medicine
6 St Andrews Place
Regent's Park
London NW1 4LB
Tel : 020 7317 5890
Fax: 020 7317 5899
e-mail: FOM@compuserve.com

Society of Occupational Medicine
6 St Andrews Place
Regent's Park
London NWI 4LB
Tel: 020 7486 2641
Fax: 020 7486 0028

Chapter 6 Neurological disorders

Parkinson's Disease Society of the United Kingdom
215 Vauxhall Bridge Road
London SWIV 1EJ
Tel: 020 7931 8080
Fax: 020 7233 9908
e-mail: mailbox@pdsuk.demon.uk

Motor Neurone Disease Association
PO Box 246
Northampton NN1 2PR
Tel: 01604 250 505
Fax: 01604 624 726

Multiple Sclerosis Society of Great Britain and Northern Ireland
25 Effie Road
Fulham
London SW6 1EE
Tel: 020 7610 7171
Fax: 020 7736 9861
e-mail: info@mssociety.org.uk

ME Association
4 Corringham Road
Stanford-le-Hope
Essex SS17 0AH
Tel: 01375 642466
Fax: 01375 360256

The Stroke Association
Stroke House
Whitecross Street
London ECIY 8JJ
Tel: 020 7566 0300
Fax: 020 7490 2686
e-mail: stroke@stroke.org.uk

British Guillain–Barré Syndrome Support Group
Churchgate House
Old Harlow
Essex CM17 0JT
Tel: 01279 427148

Chapter 7   Psychiatric disorders

Mind (National Association for Mental Health)
15–19 Broadway
London E15 4BQ
Tel: 020 8519 2122
Fax: 020 8522 1725
Mind Info Line: 0345 660 163 (Monday–Friday 0915–1645)

The Samaritans
24 hour confidential National Helpline: 0345 909090 (calls charged at local rate).
Volunteers are also available for face to face befriending. Local telephone numbers and
    details can be found in your local telephone directory.
e-mail: jo@samaritans.org
Web: www.samaritans.org.uk

The British Stammering Association
15 Old Ford Road
London E2 9PJ
Tel: 020 8983 1003
Fax: 020 8983 3591
Helpline no: 0845 603 2001 (local rate)
e-mail: mail@stammer.demon.co.uk

Chapter 8   Epilepsy

British Epilepsy Association
New Anstey House
Gateway Drive
Yeadon
Leeds LS19 7XY
Tel: 0113 2108800
Fax: 0113 3910300

The David Lewis Centre for Epilepsy
Mill Lane
Warford
Nr. Alderley Edge
Cheshire SK9 7UD
Tel: 01565 640000
Fax: 01565 640100
e-mail: enquiries@davidlewis.org.uk

St Piers
St Piers Lane
Lingfield
Surrey RH7 6PW
Tel: 01342 832243
Fax: 01342 834639
Website: www.stpiers.org.uk

The National Institute for Epilepsy
Chalfont St Peter
Gerrards Cross
Bucks SL9 0RJ
Tel: 01494 601 300
Fax: 01494 871 927

Park Road Hospital for Children
Old Road
Headington
Oxfordshire OX3 7LQ

Bootham Park Hospital
Bootham
York YO30 7BY

Chapter 9   Vision and eye disorders

Royal National Institute for the Blind
224 Great Portland Street
London WIN 6AA
Tel: 020 7388 8316
Fax: 020 7388 8316
Helpline: 0345 66 99 99

Royal National College for the Blind (RNC)
College Road
Hereford HR1 1EB
Tel: 01432 265 725
Fax: 01432 353 478
minicom: 01432 276 532
e-mail: md@rncb.ac.uk

Queen Alexandra College
Court Oak Road
Harborne
Birmingham B17 9TG
Tel: 0121 428 5050
Fax: 0121 428 5048
e-mail: enquiries@qac.ac.uk
Web: www.qac.ac.uk

Keeler Ltd
Chewer Hill Road
Windsor
Berks SL4 4AA
Tel: 01753 857177
Fax: 01753 857817

International Glaucoma Association
King's College Hospital
Denmark Hill
London SE5 9RS
Tel: 020 7737 3265
Fax: 020 7346 5929
Web: www.iga.org.uk/iga/

Chapter 10   Hearing and vestibular disorders

The Royal National Institute for Deaf People
19–23 Featherstone Street
London ECIY 8SL
Tel: 020 7296 8000
Fax: 020 7296 8199
Textphone: 020 7296 8001

RNID Court Grange College
Abbotskerswell
Newton Abbot
Devon TQ12 5NH
Tel: 01626 353401
Fax: 01626 360895
Minicom: 01626 367677
e-mail: lizyardley@rnid.freeserve.co.uk

British Deaf Association
1–3 Worship Street
London EC2A 2AB
Tel: 020 7588 3520
Fax: 020 7588 3527
Minicom: 020 7588 3529

Medical Devices Agency
Hannibal House
Elephant and Castle
London SE1 6QT
Tel: 020 7972 8100

Chapter 11   Spinal disorders

National Ankylosing Spondylitis Society (NASS)
PO Box 179
Mayfield
East Sussex TN20 6ZL
Tel: 01435 873527
Fax: 01435 873027
e-mail: nasslon@aol.com
Web: web.ukonline.co.uk/nass

National Back Pain Association
16 Elmtree Road
Teddington
Middlesex TW11 8ST
Tel: 020 8977 5474
Fax: 020 8943 5318

Arthritis Care
18 Stephenson Way
London NW1 2HD
Tel: 020 7916 1500
Fax: 020 7916 1505

Arthritis Research Campaign
Copeman House
St Marys Court
St Marys Gate
Chesterfield
Derbyshire S41 7TD
Tel: 01246 558033
Fax: 01246 558007
e-mail: info@arc.org.uk
Web: www.arc.org.uk

Banstead Mobility Centre
Damson Way
Fountain Drive
Carshalton
Surrey SM5 4NR
Tel: 020 8770 1151
Fax: 020 8770 1211

Spinal Injuries Association
76 St James's Lane
London N10 3DF
Tel: 020 8444 2121
Fax: 020 8444 3761
e-mail: sia@spinali.demon.co.uk
Web: jgrweb.com/sia

MEDesign Ltd
Clock Tower Works
Railway Street
Southport
Merseyside PR8 5BB
Tel: 01704 542 373
Fax: 01704 545 214
e-mail: postbox@medesign.co.uk

Chapter 13   Trauma

The Royal Society for the Prevention of Accidents (RoSPA)
RoSPA House
353 Bristol Road
Edgbaston
Birmingham B5 7ST
Tel: 0121 248 2000
Fax: 0121 248 2001
e-mail: help@rospa.com

Headway National Head Injuries Association
4 King Edward Court
King Edward Street
Nottingham N51 1EW
Tel: 0115 924 0800
Fax: 0115 9584446
e-mail: www.headway.org.uk

Chapter 15   Gastrointestinal and liver disorders

National Association for Colitis and Crohn's Disease
4 Beaumont House
Sutton Road
St Albans Herts AL1 5HH
Tel: 01727 844 296 (Information and answerphone)
Tel: 01727 830 038 (Administration and Press)
Fax: 01727 862 550
e-mail: nacc@nacc.org.uk
Web: www.nacc.org.uk

The Ileostomy and Internal Pouch Support Group
P O Box 132
Scunthorpe DN15 9YW
Tel: 0800 018 4724
Fax: 01724 721 601

Digestive Disorders Foundation (previously the British Digestive Foundation)
3 St Andrews Place
Regent's Park
London NW1 4LB
Tel: 020 7486 0341
Fax: 020 7224 2012

Chapter 16   Diabetes mellitus and other endocrine disorders

British Diabetic Association
10 Queen Anne Street
London WIM OBD
Tel: 020 7323 1531
Fax: 020 7637 3644
Careline: 020 7636 6112 (for information about diabetes and diabetes care)

Chapter 17   Haematological disorders
Haemophilia Society
Chesterfield House
385 Euston Road
London NW1 3AU
Tel: 020 7380 0600
Fax: 020 7387 8220
e-mail: info@haemophilia.org.uk

Sickle Cell Society
54 Station Road
London NW10 4UA
Tel: 020 8961 7795
Fax: 020 8961 8346
e-mail: sicklecellsoc@btinternet.org
Web: www.sicklecellsociety.org

Leukaemia Research Fund
43 Great Ormond Street
London WIN 3JJ
Tel: 020 7405 0101
Fax: 020 7405 3139

Chapter 18   Cardiovascular disorders

British Heart Foundation
14 Fitzhardinge Street
London WIH 4DH

Tel: 020 7935 0185
Web: www.bhf.org.uk

The British Pacing and Electrophysiology Group (BPEG)
9 Fitzroy Square
London WIP 5AH
Tel: 020 8980 0654
Fax: 020 8980 0725
e-mail: 101712.3304@compuserve.com

Chapter 19   Respiratory disorders

National Asthma Campaign
Providence House
Providence Place
London N1 0NT
Tel: 020 7226 2260
Fax: 020 7704 0740
Web: www.asthma.org.uk

Cystic Fibrosis Trust
11 London Road
Bromley
Kent BR1 1BY
Tel: 020 8464 7211
Fax: 020 8313 0472
e-mail: enquiries@cftrust.org.uk
Web: www.cftrust.org.uk

Action on Smoking and Health (ASH)
102 Clifton Street
London EC2A 4HW
Tel: 020 7739 5902
Fax: 020 7613 0531
Web: www.ash.org.uk

Quit
Victory House
170 Tottenham Court Road
London WIP 0HA
Tel: 020 7388 5775
Fax: 020 7388 5995
Quit – Smokers' quit-line 0800 00 22 00

Chapter 20   Renal and urological disease

British Renal Association
Guy's, King's and St Thomas' Department of Nephrology and Transplantation
Floor 5
Thomas Guy House
Guy's Hospital
London SE1 9RT
Tel: 020 7955 4305
Fax: 020 7955 4303

National Kidney Federation
6 Stanley Street
Worksop
Notts S81 7HX
Tel: 01909 487795
Fax: 01909 481723

British Kidney Patient Association
Bordon
Hampshire GU35 6JZ
Tel: 01420 472 021/2
Fax: 01420 475 831

The Continence Foundation
307 Hatton Square
16 Baldwins Gardens
London ECIN 7RJ
Tel: 020 7404 6875
Fax: 020 7404 6876
e-mail: continence.foundation@dial.pipex.com
Helpline: 020 7831 9831 (Monday–Friday 0930–1630)

Association for Continence Advice (an organization for those professionally involved in
    continence services)
Winchester House
Kennington Park
Cranmer Road
London SW9 6EJ
Tel: 020 7820 8113
Fax: 020 7820 0442

Enuresis Resource and Information Centre (ERIC) (advice on bedwetting, soiling, and
    other bladder and bowel problems in children)
34 Old School House
Britannia Road
Kingswood
Bristol BS15 2DB
Tel: 0117 960 3060
Fax: 0117 960 0401

Incontact (an organization for consumers of continence services, quarterly magazine, and other schemes)
St Pancras Hospital
London NW1 OPE
Tel: 020 7530 3401
Fax: 020 7530 3980

Chapter 21   Obstetrics and gynaecology

Wellbeing
The Health Research Charity for Women and Babies
27 Sussex Place
Regent's Park
London NWI 4SP
Tel: 020 7262 5337
Fax: 020 7724 7725

Women's Nationwide Cancer Control Campaign
128–130 Curtain Road
London EC2A 3AR
Tel: 020 7729 4688
Fax: 020 7613 0771
Helpline: 020 7729 2229

Chapter 22   Surgery

CancerBACUP
3 Bath Place
Rivington Street
London EC2A 3DR
Cancer Support Service: 020 7613 2121
Freephone: 0808 800 1234
Employee Support Scheme: 020 7920 7213
Publications: 020 7696 9003
CancerBACUP Scotland (counselling service) 0141 553 1553
Web: www.cancerbacup.org.uk

Macmillan Cancer Relief
Anchor House
15–19 Britten Street
London SW3 3TZ
Tel: 020 7351 7811
Fax: 020 7376 8098
Information line: 0845 601 6161

British Colostomy Association
15 Station Road
Reading
Berks RG1 1LG
Tel: 0118 939 1537
Fax: 0118 956 9095

Chapter 23   Dermatology

National Eczema Society
163 Eversholt Street
London NW1 1BU
Tel: 020 7388 4097
Fax: 020 7388 5882
Web: www.eczema.org

The Psoriasis Association
Milton House
7 Milton Street
Northampton NN2 7JG
Tel: 01604 711 129
Fax: 01604 792 894

The Vitiligo Society
125 Kennington Road
London SE11 6SF
Tel: 020 7840 0855
Fax: 020 7840 0866
e-mail: all@vitiligosociety.org.uk
Web: www.vitiligosociety.org.uk

Acne Support Group
16 Dufour's Place
Broadwick Street
London W1V 1FE
Tel: 020 8743 2030

Chapter 24   Acquired immune deficiency syndrome (AIDS)

Terrence Higgins Trust
52–54 Grays Inn Road
London WCIX 8JU
Tel: 020 7831 0330 (administration)
Helpline: 020 7242 1010 (1200–2200)
Web: www.tht.org.uk

The Stationery Office
Publication Centre
PO Box 276
London SW8 5DT
Tel: 020 7873 9090
Fax: 020 7873 8200
Web: www.national-publishing.co.uk

Chapter 25   Alcohol and drug misuse

Accept Services
724 Fulham Road
London
SW6 5SE
Tel: 020 7371 7477

Al-Anon Family Groups UK and Eire
61 Great Dover Street
London SE1 4YF
Tel: 020 7403 0888 (24 hour helpline)
Fax: 020 7387 9910
e-mail: alanonuk@aol.com
Website: www.hexnet.co.uk/alanon

Chapter 26   Medication

British Airways Travel Clinics
156 Regent Street
London WIR 6LB
Tel: 020 7434 4719
Fax: 020 7439 9584

**Appendix 1   Driving: standards of fitness required for British driving licence holders
and applicants**

The Medical Adviser (for medical enquiries)
Drivers' Medical Unit
DVLA
Longview Road
Swansea SA99 1TU
Tel: 01792 783686 (answerphone after hours).

General Medical Council
178 Great Portland Street
London W1N 6JE
Tel: 020 7580 7642
Fax: 020 7915 3641

Appendix 2   Civil aviation

Civil Aviation Authority
CAA House
45–59 Kingsway
London WC2B 6TE
Tel: 020 7379 7311

Appendix 3   Medical standards for entry into the Merchant Navy and for serving seafarers

Eros Marketing Support Services
Unit B
Imber Court Trading Estate
Orchard Lane
East Molesey
Surrey KT8 0BN
Tel: 020 8957 5008 / 5028
Fax: 020 8957 5012

Appendix 4   Fitness for work offshore and in commercial diving

UK Offshore Operators Association (UKOOA)
30 Buckingham Gate
London SWIE 6NN
Tel: 020 7802 2400

Diving Medical Advisory Committee
177a High Street
Beckenham
Kent BR3 1AH
Tel: 020 8663 3859

Appendix 5   General aspects of fitness for work overseas

Centres from which health professionals can obtain essential medical advice
PHLS Communicable Diseases Surveillance Travel Medicine Section
61 Colindale Avenue
London NW9 5EQ
Tel: 020 8200 6868

PHLS Malaria Reference Laboratory
London School of Hygiene and Tropical Medicine
Keppel Street
London WC1E 7HT
Tel: 020 7636 3924

Communicable Diseases (Scotland) Unit and Department of Tropical Medicine
Clifton House
Clifton Place
Glasgow G3 7LN
Tel: 0141 300 1100

Department of Tropical Diseases
Birmingham Heartlands Hospital
Bordesley Green Road
Birmingham B9 5ST
Tel: 0121 766 6611

Department of Infectious Diseases and Tropical Medicine
North Manchester General Hospital
Delaunays Road
Crumpsall
Manchester M8 5RB
Tel: 0161 795 4567

Liverpool School of Tropical Medicine
Pembroke Place
Liverpool L3 5QA
Tel: 0151 708 9393

Hospital for Tropical Diseases
Mortimer Market
Capper Street
London WCIE 6AV
Tel: 020 7387 4411 (for clinical advice regarding ill or returning travellers)

Advice lines for travellers
Hospital for Tropical Diseases
Tel: 0839 337733

Medical Advisory Service for Travellers Abroad (MASTA)
Tel: 09068 224100

Department of Health (for copies of *Health advice for travellers*)
Tel: 0800 555 777

Air ambulance services
Swiss Air Rescue Organization
Mainaustrasse 21
CH-8008 Zurich
Tel: 00 41 1 385 8585

SOS Assistance
12 Chemin Riantbosson
1217 Meyrin 1
Geneva
Tel: 00 41 22 736 3333 or 00 41 22 347 6161

Appendix 8

ABI	Association of British Insurers
ABR	auditory brainstem responses
ACC	Accident Compensation Corporation (New Zealand)
ACE	angiotensin converting enzyme
ACOP	Approved Code of Practice
ADA	Americans with Disabilities Act
AIDS	acquired immune deficiency syndrome
ALAMA	Association of Local Authority Medical Advisers
ALL	acute lymphoblastic leukaemia
AMAS	activity matching ability system
AME	authorized medical examiner
AML	acute myeloid leukaemia
ANHOPS	Association of National Health Occupational Physicians
APD	automated peritoneal dialysis
AVC	additional voluntary contribution
AWT	all work test
BAC	blood alcohol concentration
BEA	British Epilepsy Association
BMI	body mass index
BPT	bronchial provocation challenge test
BHA	British Hyperbaric Association
CAA	Civil Aviation Authority
CABG	coronary artery bypass grafting
CAPD	continuous ambulatory peritoneal dialysis
CBI	Confederation of British Industry
CCDC	Consultant in Communicable Disease Control
CEDP	committee for the employment of disabled people
CFC	chlorofluorocarbons
CFS	chronic fatigue syndrome
CHD	coronary heart disease
CI	confidence interval
CLL	chronic lymphatic leukaemia
CML	chronic myeloid leukaemia
CMV	cytomegalovirus
CNS	central nervous system
COPD	chronic obstructive pulmonary disease
CORAD	Committee on Restrictions against Disabled People
COSHH	Control of Substances Hazardous to Health
CPAP	continuous positive airways pressure
CRE	Commission for Racial Equality
CSF	cerebrospinal fluid
CT	computed tomography

CTEV	congenital talipes equinovarus (clubfoot)
CVS	chorionic villus sampling
DAS	Disability Advisory Service
DBCP	1,2-dibromochloropropane
DDA	Disability Discrimination Act 1995
DDH	developmental dysplasia of the hip
DEA	Disability Employment Adviser
DETR	Department of the Environment, Transport and the Regions
DfEE	Department for Education and Employment
DIP	distal interphalangeal joint
DIT	Disability Information Trust
DLA	Disability Living Allowance
DLF	Disabled Living Foundation
DOTS	directly observed short-course treatment
DRG	dorsal root ganglion
DRO	Disablement Resettlement Officer
DSA	Disablement Services Authority
DSE	display screen equipment
DSM	*Diagnostic and statistical manual* (American Psychological Association)
DSS	Department of Social Security
DST	Disability Service Team
DVLA	Driving and Vehicle Licensing Agency
DVT	deep venous thrombosis
EAA	extrinsic allergic alveolitis
EASA	European Aviation Safety Authority
EAT	Employment Appeal Tribunal
ECJ	European Court of Justice
ECSC	European Coal and Steel Commumity
EEG	electroencephalography
EFA	Epilepsy Foundation of America
ELISA	enzyme-linked immunosorbent assay
EMAS	Employment Medical Advisory Service
EMG	electromyogram
ENT	ear, nose, and throat
EOC	Equal Opportunities Commission
ERC	Employment Rehabilitation Centres
ESR	erythrocyte sedimentation rate
ETS	environmental tobacco smoke
EU	European Union
EWC	expected week of confinement
FCA	functional capacity assessment
FEFC	Further Education Funding Council
FEV_1	volume of gas expired in the first second
FRC	functional residual capacity
FVC	forced vital capacity

GBS	General Council of British Shipping
GCMS	gas chromatography–mass spectrometry
GCS	Glasgow Coma Scale
GGT	gamma-glutamyl transferase
GMC	General Medical Council
HAART	highly active anti-retroviral therapy
HD	haemodialysis; Hodgkin's' disease
HIV	human immunodeficiency virus
HRT	hormone replacement therapy
HSAWA	Health and Safety at Work Act 1974
HSC	Health and Safety Commission
HSE	Health and Safety Executive
HTL	hearing threshold level
IAP	intra-abdominal pressure
IB	Incapacity Benefit
IBE	International Bureau for Epilepsy
IBS	irritable bowel syndrome
ICD	implantable cardioverter defibrillator
ICD-10	*International classification of diseases* (WHO)
ICOH	International Commission on Occupational Health
IDDM	insulin-dependent diabetes mellitus
IIDB	Industrial Injury Disablement Benefit
ILO	International Labour Office; International Labour Organization
IMO	International Maritime Organization
IT	information technology
ITP	idiopathic thrombocytopenic purpura
IUCD	intrauterine contraceptive device
JAA	Joint Aviation Authorities
JCA	juvenile chronic arthritis
JRA	juvenile rheumatoid arthritis
K_{CO}	carbon monoxide transfer coefficient
LASIK	laser *in situ* keratomileusis
LGV	large goods vehicle
LLI	leg length inequality
LTD	long-term disability
MAOI	monoamine oxidase inhibitor
MCA	Maritime and Coastguard Agency
MCH	mean corpuscular haemoglobin
MCV	mean corpuscular volume
ME	myeloencephalitis
MIT	multiple injection treatment
MND	motor neurone disease
MRC	Medical Research Council
MRI	magnetic resonance imaging
MRO	Medical Review Officer
MS	multiple sclerosis

MTP	metatarsophalangeal joint
NGO	non-governmental organization
NGPSE	National General Practice Study of Epilepsy
NHS	National Health Service
NIDDM	non-insulin dependent diabetes mellitus
NIOSH	National Institute of Occupational Safety and Health (US)
NMR	nuclear magnetic resonance
NNRTI	non-nucleoside reverse transcriptase inhibitor
NRL	natural rubber latex
NRR	noise reduction ratio
NRTI	nucleoside reverse transcriptase inhibitor
NSAID	non-steroidal anti-inflammatory drugs
NSE	National Society for Epilepsy
NSH	National Study of Hearing
NTD	neural tube defects
OA	osteoarthritis
OHA	oral hypoglycaemic agent
OHS	occupational health services
OPCS	Office of Population Censuses and Surveys
PACT	Placing, Assessment and Counselling Team
PCV	passenger carrying vehicle
PD	peritoneal dialysis
PE	pulmonary embolism
PEF	peak expiratory flow
PEFR	peak expiratory flow rate
PGL	persistent generalized lymphadenopathy
PHI	permanent health insurance
PI	protease inhibitor
PID	pelvic inflammatory disease
PIP	proximal interphalangeal joint
PMS	premenstrual syndrome
POBA	plain old balloon angioplasty
PRK	photorefractive keratectomy
PRV	polycythaemia rubra vera
PTA	post-traumatic amnesia
PTCA	percutaneous transluminal coronary angioplasty
RA	rheumatoid arthritis
RADAR	Royal Association for Disability and Rehabilitation
RADS	reactive airways dysfunction syndrome
RAST	radioallergosorbent tests
RIDDOR	Reporting of Injuries, Diseases and Dangerous Occurrences Regulations 1995
RK	radial keratotomy
RNIB	Royal National Institute for the Blind
RPE	respiratory protective equipment
RSD	reflex sympathetic dystrophy

RSI	repetitive strain injury
RTI	reverse transcriptase inhibitor
RV	residual volume
S/N	signal-to-noise (ratio)
SCBA	self-contained breathing apparatus
SDA	Severe Disablement Allowance
SES	socio-economic status
SIG	Sheltered Industrial Group
SLE	systemic lupus erythematosus
SPB	spontaneous preterm birth
SPL	sound pressure level
SSP	Statutory Sick Pay
SSRI	serotonin selective re-uptake inhibitor
TEC	Training and Enterprise Council
TENS	transcutaneous electrical nerve stimulation
TfW	Training for Work programme
THC	tetrahydrocannabinol
TIA	transient ischaemic attacks
TLC	total lung capacity
T_{LCO}	carbon monoxide transfer factor
TUC	Trades Union Congress
UKOOA	UK Offshore Operators Association
V_{CO_2}	carbon dioxide production
VDU	visual display unit
V_{O_2}	oxygen consumption
WAI	work ability index
WHO	World Health Organization
WRULD	work-related upper limb disorder
YOI	Young Offenders Institution

Index

Brief contents

KU-078-571

Contents

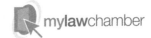

Visit the *Criminal Law*, ninth edition mylawchamber site at **www.mylawchamber.co.uk/jefferson** to access valuable learning material.

FOR STUDENTS

Do you want to give yourself a head start come exam time?

Companion website support
- Use the exam-style questions with answer guidance to prepare for exam success.
- Test yourself with practice multiple-choice quizzes on the main topics in criminal law.
- Check updates to major changes in the law to make sure you are ahead of the game by knowing the latest developments.
- Live weblinks direct you to online resources where you can read more widely around the subject.
- Use the online glossary for quick reference to key terms in criminal law.
- Use the flashcards to improve your recall and comprehension of key terms in criminal law.

Worried about getting to grips with cases?

Case Navigator*
This unique online support helps you to improve your case reading and analysis skills.
- **Direct deep links** to the core cases in criminal law.
- **Short introductions** provide guidance on what you should look out for while reading the case.
- **Questions** help you to test your understanding of the case, and provide feedback on what you should have grasped.
- **Summaries** contextualise the case and point you to further reading so that you are fully prepared for seminars and discussions.

Also: The regularly maintained Companion Website provides the following features:
- Search tool to help locate specific items of content.
- Online help and support to assist with website usage and troubleshooting.

For more information please contact your local Pearson Education sales representative or visit **www.mylawchamber.co.uk/jefferson**.

*Please note that access to Case Navigator is free with the purchase of this book, but you must register with us for access. Full registration instructions are available on the website. The LexisNexis element of Case Navigator is only available to those who currently subscribe to LexisNexis Butterworths online.

Preface

This book is written for LLB, CPE, Diploma and BA students sitting examinations on English criminal law in their first or second year whether in England and Wales or abroad. It is hoped that persons with little or no access to law libraries will find the text helpful. The text is also useful for those studying for other qualifications by private study including distance learning. Extracts of law reform reports may be of especial use to such students. The book, which is analytical in nature, covers those areas of substantive criminal law which are traditionally covered on a criminal law course, and those topics are presented in the way in which English law subjects are normally taught. Criminal law is fast-moving and fast-growing and there has to be some selection among topics. The focus is on the rules of criminal law and criticism of them. English criminal law is replete with inconsistencies, and this book reflects those issues. Students must grapple with such difficulties, for a superficial treatment will lead to wrong law and low marks. Attention is focused on what is sometimes called the 'internal critique of the law', in order that such inconsistencies are brought out, and on those areas which present difficulties. There are many areas of controversy such as the definition of recklessness and the width of defences. The arrangement of topics may differ from the order in which the subjects are taught on your course. However, because of the House of Lords decision in *G* (2004) some rearrangement of topics was made in the previous edition. In particular, the consideration of intention and recklessness in the context of murder and criminal damage respectively has been abolished. This 'unique selling point' of the text was intended to encourage readers to focus their minds on the results that the accused had to intend or on to which he had to be reckless. For example, as an examiner I saw too many students writing: 'the *mens rea* for murder is intent'. Besides being incorrect (if it were true, an intent say to touch would be malice aforethought), the statement reveals an ignorance as to how precisely the elements of a crime are defined. Whether this experiment was successful is for others to judge. As things are now, namely the law has returned to the pre-*Caldwell* position, opportunity was taken to reorder the book. This reordering is maintained in the current edition.

Among differences from other textbooks are the following:

(a) There is a concentration on one or two topics which have been unjustifiably neglected in recent years in comparison with some other matters. Offences of strict liability are instanced. Some issues which this book considers have over the past 20 years come to the fore: corporate criminal liability is one obvious instance.

(b) Emphasis is laid on suggestions for reform and on criticism both of individual decisions and the ambit of offences. Criminal law needs to be evaluated and criticised. Proposals contained in Law Commission Consultation Papers and Reports are analysed. It is in the context particularly of reform that the European Convention on Human Rights is looked at. Some attempt is made to uncover the underlying purposes behind offences: if that purpose is not served by current law, reform is due.

(c) There is some reference to Commonwealth and US cases and commentators.

(d) The student is introduced to some of the concepts of theoretical criminal law, such as the distinction between excuses and justifications. There is a growing body of academic criticism and this book introduces the reader to some of the major issues. There is discussion of gender issues, particularly in the law concerned with battered women. This is not, however, a book on criminal law theory. Readers are referred to the further reading at the end of each chapter.

(e) I hope that values and policies underlying the rules of criminal law are brought out.

This book deals with, as stated earlier, substantive criminal law; that is, it is concerned with the question of whether an accused is guilty of a particular offence. It does not deal with the following, all of which are important topics in their own right.

(a) *Bringing the accused to trial* and *procedure at trial*. Such topics are generally covered in courses of varying names such as English Legal System, Criminal Justice and Criminal Process. Arrest may be dealt with in constitutional or public law. Similarly excluded are the choice of charges, the workings of the police, the Crown Prosecution Service, the Director of Public Prosecutions, and the investigation of crime, including forensic jurisprudence.

(b) *Sentence*. The methods of disposal after trial are usually dealt with, if at all, in criminology or perhaps jurisprudence courses. Why people commit offences is also part of criminology. Victimology is also not part of substantive criminal law.

(c) *Evidence*. The opening chapter of this book looks at the evidential and legal burdens of proof so that readers can understand the terms when they meet them in, e.g., Chapter 9, which deals with the defences of insanity, diminished responsibility and automatism. The remainder of the law of evidence is for a course on evidence.

(d) *Public order*. Criminal law can be seen as a way in which the state controls citizens and how officials control state officers. Offences against public order are usually covered by courses on public law.

All these excluded topics are interesting in their own right. For example, why was the Commissioner of Police for the Metropolis charged with endangering the public contrary to s 3 of the Health and Safety at Work Act 1971 rather than murder when his officers put seven bullets into the head of the Brazilian Jean Charles de Menezes at Stockwell underground station in south London in 2005? The remainder of a possibly very wide course forms substantive criminal law. It is that area of law which has to be applied by the triers of fact, the jury in the Crown Court and the justices of the peace in the magistrates' courts, in order to determine whether the accused is guilty. A jury may have to determine whether the accused is to be convicted of murder or whether he has the defence of provocation. Substantive criminal law is concerned with *what* has to be shown in order to find the accused guilty or not. *How* a matter of substantive criminal law is to be proved is part of the law of evidence. A person may confess to murder, have the crime proved against him in court, and so on. Those matters are ones of evidence. What has to be proved is part of substantive law. If when reading substantive criminal law you find difficulty accepting what it is said the accused thought or did, don't worry: assume that the prosecution has proved to the satisfaction of the triers of fact what the accused did or thought.

This book is part of the *Foundation Studies in Law Series* which has a Companion Website at: www.mylawchamber.co.uk/jefferson.

Errors and omissions are my own.

When originally submitted to the publishers, this book was written in what I considered to be a non-sexist style. However, to conform to series style, the traditional use of 'he' to refer to both sexes was reverted to at editing stage.

I would like to thank Christine Statham and Anita Atkinson at Pearson for their professionalism and patience, and the anonymous students who read the book with 'student eyes' on the text.

Michael Jefferson
4 January 2009

Guided tour

Case summaries highlight the facts and key legal principles of essential cases that you need to be aware of in your study of criminal law.

> ### Nedrick
>
> Lord Scarman in *Hancock and Shankland* thought that guidelines had little place in criminal law, yet the Court of Appeal laid down such principles in *Nedrick*, above, which was followed in *Barr* (1989) 88 Cr App R 362 (CA), a decision from 1986.
>
> *Nedrick* [1986] 1 WLR 1075
>
> The accused poured paraffin through the letter box of a house and on to the front door. He set it alight. The house blazed up and a child was killed. He was convicted of murder after a direction by the trial judge which followed the pre-*Moloney* law laid down in *Hyam v DPP*, above, a case with similar facts, that foresight of grievous bodily harm was to be treated as an intention to cause it. (The case was heard before *Moloney*.) The Appeal Court allowed the appeal on the grounds that, following *Moloney*, foresight was not to be equated with intention. Foresight was merely a step on the way towards proving intent.
>
> The court gave advice to trial judges as to how they should direct juries when the defendant does a dangerous act, as a result of which someone dies. As ever, it should be

Clear headings and subheadings keep you firmly focused and constantly aware of the context and structure of each chapter.

> In general a prosecution is no bar to civil proceedings and vice versa. There are exceptionally provisions found in ss 44–45 of the Offences Against the Person Act 1861 which stipulate that a civil action for assault or battery may not be brought when the accused has been tried in a magistrates' court and has either obtained a certificate of dismissal of the complaint or been punished.
>
> ### Hierarchy of the criminal courts: the appeal system
>
> After the decision is taken in which court the case is to be heard, the accused is tried. The process of appeal depends on whether the case was tried in the magistrates' court or at the Crown Court. The final Anglo-Welsh court on criminal matters is the House of Lords, which during the currency of this book may become the Supreme Court.
>
> #### Magistrates' courts
>
> There are two possible routes of appeal. The usual one is to the Crown Court, which for this purpose is composed of a judge and (usually) two magistrates. Only the accused can appeal, and the grounds are (a) on the points of fact or law against conviction, or (b) against sentence. The first ground may be used only if the accused pleaded not guilty. The format is a rehearing, i.e. a new, full trial (a trial *de novo*). The alternative appeal is to the Divisional Court of the Queen's Bench Division of the High Court. The appeal is called 'by way of case stated'. Either side may appeal, but the grounds are solely (a) on a point of law, or (b) that the magistrates exceeded their jurisdiction. If the prosecution succeeds, the magistrates are directed to convict and give the appropriate sentence. There is also an appeal by way of case stated from the Crown Court to the Divisional Court. There were 188 such appeals in 1998. Appeal from the Divisional Court is to the House of Lords. Either side may appeal, but only on points of law. There are two other prerequisites: the Divisional Court must certify that the point is of general public importance and either that Court or the Lords must grant leave to appeal. There are about ten such appeals a year.
>
> #### Crown Court
>
> Appeals from this Court lie to the Court of Appeal (Criminal Division). Appeal against conviction lies on the ground that the conviction was 'unsafe'. It does not matter that the accused might nevertheless have been found guilty by the jury. Only the accused may appeal. The appeal may be against conviction on a point of law, or against conviction on a point of fact or mixed law and fact; or against sentence. Retrials are possible but rare. They are, however, a growing phenomenon. Under the Criminal Justice Act 1972, s 36, the Attorney-General may refer a point of law to have the matter clarified. If the court decides that the Crown Court should have convicted, the accused's acquittal is not affected. Under the Criminal Justice Act 1988, ss 35–36, the Attorney-General can refer

Marginal cross-references direct you to other places in the text where the same subject is discussed, helping you to make connections and understand how the material fits together.

> See Figure 12.3 in Chapter 12 for a diagram illustrating constructive (unlawful act) manslaughter.
>
>
>
> a father was found not guilty in *Lowe* [
> for the purposes of the crime of unlaw
> even a deliberate one, such as failing to
> clear. Finally, the defendants would no
> to let the victim stay in their house. To
> (inadequate) best seems almost cruel. T
> selves, never mind the male defendant
>
> A more recent case than *Stone and*
> The victim had injected a mixture of c

Figures and diagrams are used to strengthen your understanding of complex legal processes and areas in criminal law.

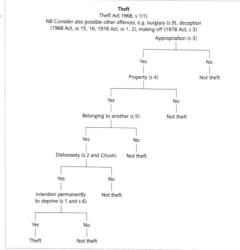

CHAPTER 15 THEFT AND ROBBERY

Theft
Theft Act 1968, s 1(1)
NB Consider also possible other offences, e.g. burglary (s 9), deception
(1968 Act, ss 15, 16; 1978 Act, ss 1, 2), making off (1978 Act, s 3)

Appropriation (s 3)

Yes — No
Property (s 4) — Not theft

Yes — No
Belonging to another (s 5) — Not theft

Yes — No
Dishonesty (s 2 and *Ghosh*) — Not theft

Yes — No
Intention permanently — Not theft
to deprive (s 1 and s 6)

Yes — No
Theft — Not theft

Figure 15.1 Theft

Chapter summaries located at the end of each chapter draw together the key points that you should be aware of following your reading, and act as a useful checklist for revision.

Summary

This is the second chapter concerned with the 'building blocks' of criminal law. This time the concentration is not on the physical side but on the mental side. What state of mind did the accused have when he or she was committing the *actus reus*? Each crime is composed of an *actus reus* and usually of a *mens rea* but not just does the *actus reus* differ from offence to offence, but so does the *mens rea*. For example, the *mens rea* of murder is either the intent to kill or the intent to cause grievous bodily harm, but the *mens rea* of theft is dishonesty and the intent permanently to deprive. The student has to know both the *actus reus* and the *mens rea* for the crimes taught on his or her course. The discussion then concentrates on the major *mens rea* words in criminal law: intent, recklessness, knowledge, wilfulness and negligence, though with regard to the last there is debate whether or not a lack of a state of mind ('I didn't think') may be regarded as a state of mind, a *mens rea*. The chapter concludes with an explanation of various issues surrounding *mens rea*, including the need for contemporaneity of *actus reus* and *mens rea* and the doctrine usually known as transferred malice.

- Definition of *mens rea*: *Mens rea* may be defined as 'the mental state which is required by the definition of the offence to accompany the act which produces or threatens harm' (S. H. Kadish).

- Examples of *mens rea*: The *mens rea* of murder, also known as malice aforethought, is in part composed of an intent to kill or commit grievous bodily harm. In theft, the mental element is 'dishonesty' and 'intention permanently to deprive'. The *mens rea*, like the *actus reus*, differs from crime to crime.

- Motive: In general the motive of the accused is irrelevant in criminal law. For instance, it does not matter if I kill you to get your money or your lover or if I do so in order to save you from a life filled with pain. Some offences do, however, make motive relevant in the sense that they are defined in such a way that the triers of fact have to consider the reason why the defendant behaved as she did. An illustration is blackmail. If the accused believed she was warranted in acting as she did, there is no offence and 'warranted' covers the accused's motive.
  Modern statutes sometimes make crimes more serious when the accused acted out of a certain motive, e.g. racially motivated crimes.

- Intent: The definition of intention is one basic to English criminal law, partly because

Suggestions for **Further reading** at the end of each chapter encourage you to delve deeper into the topic and read articles that will help you to gain higher marks in both exams and assessments.

Further reading

Arlidge, A. 'The trial of Dr David Moor' [2000] Crim LR 31. (See also response by Sir John Smith, 'A comment on Dr Moor's case' [2000] Crim LR 41.)
Ashworth, A. 'Reform of the law of murder' [1990] Crim LR 75
Ashworth, A. and Mitchell, B. *Rethinking English Homicide Law* (Clarendon Press, 2000)
Bingham, Lord http://www.open.gov.uk/lcd/judicial/speeches/mansent.htm
Brudner, A. 'Subjective fault for crime: a reinterpretation' [2008] 14 *Legal theory* 1
Buxton, R. 'Some simple thoughts on intention' [1988] Crim LR 484
Chiu E. M. 'The challenge of motive in criminal law' (2005) 8 Buff Crim LR 653
Ferzan, K. K. 'Beyond intention' (2008) 29 Cardozo L Rev 1147
Gledhill, K. 'Criminal carelessness' [2007] 157 NLJ 41
Horder, J. 'Intention in criminal law: a rejoinder' (1995) 58 MLR 678
Horder, J. 'Transferred malice and the remoteness of unexpected outcomes' [2006] Crim LR 383
Kaveny, M. C. 'Inferring intention from foresight' (2004) 120 LQR 81

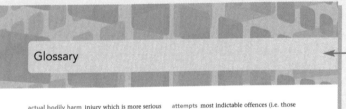

Reference sections have a stepped coloured tab to allow you to navigate quickly to key information within the text.

Glossary

A full **Glossary** located at the back of the book can be used throughout your reading to clarify unfamiliar terms.

actual bodily harm injury which is more serious than a touching but less serious than grievous bodily harm (q.v.). 'Bodily' is read widely to cover not just the flesh and bones but also psychiatric matters. The crime of assault occasioning actual bodily harm is contrary to s 47 of the Offences Against the Person Act 1861.

actus reus this Latin term means the act, omission or state of affairs required by the offence. It is distinguished from the *mens rea* or mental element of the crime. The *actus reus* differs from crime to crime. For example, in theft it comprises three elements: appropriation, property and belonging to another.

age the age of criminal responsibility is 10. The Crime and Disorder Act 1998, s 34, abolished

attempts most indictable offences (i.e. those triable in the Crown Court) are committable as attempted crimes when the accused intends to commit the offence and performs a 'more than merely preparatory' step on the way towards committing the offence. For example, I, having made my mind up to kill you, am stopped from shooting you dead just before I pull the trigger. I intend to kill you and I have performed a more than merely preparatory step on the way towards killing you. Similarly, if I shoot to kill but miss, I can be found guilty of attempted murder. It should be noted that the crime of attempted murder's *mens rea* is intent to kill even though murder itself may be committed by either an intent to kill or an intent to cause grievous bodily harm. All attempts

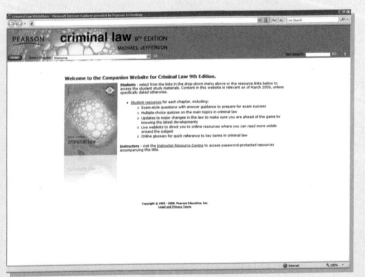

Companion website
Use the **Companion Website** at **www.mylawchamber.co.uk/jefferson** to find extensive resources designed to assist you with your study, including exam style questions with answer guidance, multiple choice quizzes, web links to useful resources, and regular legal updates on developments in criminal law.

Case Navigator provides access and guidance to key cases in the subject to improve your case reading and analysis skills. Cases which can be found in Case Navigator are highlighted in the text and marked with the Case Navigator icon.

Table of cases

Case Navigator cases are highlighted in bold.

For ease of reference this table of cases includes authorities from different jurisdictions. Reference is to readily accessible series.

Table of legislation

Table of Statutory Instruments

Table of European Legislation

Table of International Legislation

Part 1

Preliminary matters

1   Introduction to criminal law

Introduction to criminal law

The fundamental principles of criminal liability

There are some 5 million crimes notified to the police each year. The figure for the year ending July 2008 was almost 5 million. (The British Crime Survey, which includes unreported and unrecorded crimes, estimated that there were 10.1 million offences in 2007–08 and the 2001 Survey estimated that only half of crimes are reported to the police and the proportion may be less than that. Perhaps one in thirty crimes lead to a conviction, though many people are cautioned.) Most of these crimes are committed by men and boys. Offences against property comprise some 75 per cent, of which half involve theft. Violent crimes make up 5 per cent. Violent crimes rose by 2 per cent, 2004–05 to 2005–06 but decreased by 8 per cent in 2007–08, according to the British Crime Survey. In recent years violent crimes have been increasing and there is a public fear in some cities such as London, Manchester and Nottingham of gun and knife crime by young males (but are still well below the level of 1995, the peak year), and non-violent offences decreasing. Contrary to the popular view the number of crimes committed is not rising year on year, but what is increasing is the number of offences created by Parliament.

Criminal law can be seen as a series, perhaps not a system, of rules aimed at controlling misconduct. From the other end of the telescope criminal law also controls the behaviour of those involved in the criminal justice system such as the police and judges. It ensures that the stigma of a conviction is attached only to those to whom it should be attached.

Crime is big. Criminal law was for many years regarded as undeveloped in terms of theory. The jury's verdict – guilty or not guilty – cannot be explored. Jury instructions are not strong precedents. It was not until 1907 that there was a Court of Criminal Appeal and until 1960 appeals to the House of Lords were few. Until the mid-1960s textbooks for both students and practitioners were largely lists of rules with authorities. Since then there has been an exponential growth in academic interest and analysis. Despite this development and perhaps because of it, a substantial amount of criminal law is unclear. Should the person who attempts to kill but fails be treated in the same manner as one who succeeds? Why is murder more serious than manslaughter? Is sexual intercourse a part of life or part of a crime? Accordingly rules, principles and policies have to be investigated. Attention in this book is focused on those offences normally discussed in a criminal law course, but there are thousands of others and no one book can deal with all of them.

Which principles are to be considered when looking at criminal law? Some argue that there are no principles, and certainly Parliament is subject to few international or other constraints when making law, others that such principles as exist are subject to large exceptions. In his book *Philosophy of Criminal Law* (Rowman & Littlefield, 1987), the American D.N. Husak, largely in reliance on Jerome Hall's *Foundations of Jurisprudence* (Bobbs-Merrill, 1973) postulates eight principles of liberal philosophy underlying US criminal law. They are generally based on the autonomy of the individual. They can be taken to represent aspirations of some of those involved in creating, applying and teaching criminal law in the UK and elsewhere. These principles are not constrained by country, time or politics. It should however, be stressed that these principles are not always applied. Parliament is rarely concerned with these general principles of criminal law. It may, for example, try to prohibit an activity which many people indulge in on an almost daily basis such as speeding on motorways. It presumably saw criminal law as being the most efficient means of bearing down on speeding, despite the fact that many do not see conviction for this crime as containing stigma. Why criminalisation takes place is an important area of study for all concerned in the criminal law. Criminal law cannot be divorced from its political, sociological and economic context. Some control of the creation of new offences and the increase in width of old ones is provided by the European Convention on Human Rights; its influence as yet has been minimal but may increase in the next few years.

Legality

This principle is that persons must not be held to be criminally liable and punished without there first being a law so holding (see also below). It prevents arbitrary state power. Husak derives four subsidiary conditions: (a) laws must not be vague; (b) the legislature must not create offences to cover wrongdoing retrospectively; (c) the judiciary must not create new offences; and perhaps (d) criminal statutes should be strictly construed. (Others derive different sub-rules: for example, laws must be published and laws must not be impossible to obey.) English law does not adopt the first subsidiary principle, and the others are doubtful. For example, it could be said that in **Preddy** [1996] AC 815 the House of Lords strictly construed the Theft Act 1968 (with the effect that mortgage fraudsters were not convicted of an offence of deception), whereas the House has at times extended the criminal law by defining statutory offences broadly, as occurred in **Hinks** [2001] AC 241 where 'appropriation' in the same Act was read broadly to cover a gift. Many of the offences have uncertain boundaries. For example, murder is a very serious crime, but the state of mind needed for it has been the subject of change over the past 30 years. As a matter of parliamentary sovereignty, the government acting through Parliament can create laws which apply retroactively. Judges are not consistent in their interpretation of statutes, but have more or less given up the privilege of law-making (see further below). Judges in the House of Lords have recently extended criminal liability in several cases, yet in **Clegg** [1995] 1 AC 482 the House of Lords refused to change the law in favour of the accused. In **Ireland; Burstow** [1998] AC 147 the House of Lords, disregarding the learning of centuries, extended assault to cover frightening by words including words spoken over the phone. In **R** [1992] 1 AC 599 the House of Lords in effect retrospectively abolished the long-standing immunity of the husband on a charge of rape of his wife, a breach of the principle of strict construction of penal statutes and of the principle against retroactivity, though its reasoning was that the exemption did not exist at the time of the accused's act; in **Gotts** [1992] 2 AC 412 the House of Lords held that duress was no defence to attempted murder, thereby altering the common law; in **Woollin** [1999] AC 82 the House of Lords on one view extended the boundaries of murder. The cases in this paragraph are further explained in the relevant chapters.

However, decisions of the House of Lords are not uniformly in favour of widening criminal liability and when in **C v DPP** the Divisional Court abrogated the principle that children aged over 10 but under 14 were not guilty unless they had mischievous discretion, the House of Lords restored the previous law ([1996] 1 AC 1). Both offences and defences are subject to change, with the result that a person would be guilty one day, but not guilty on the next because of a change in the law made by the judiciary. If the accused in **R v R** (above), the case involving the marital immunity in rape, had asked a lawyer for advice whether he would be guilty, the reply before the case would have been in the negative, despite the House of Lords ruling that the immunity did not exist at the time when the husband committed an act which would otherwise have been rape. These rulings were not predictable. If one had asked a lawyer before the speeches of the Lords in **R** whether the husband in the circumstances which existed on the facts would be guilty of rape, the answer would have been in the negative. The contrary argument is that expressed by Lord Keith in **R** (above): 'The common law is capable of evolving in the light of changing social, economic and cultural developments.' Changing the common law keeps it up to date.

As can be seen from this brief discussion, criminal law does not always consist of hard and fast rules, and the extension of the law to previously exempt categories is inconsistent with Article 7(1) of the European Convention on Human Rights, to which the UK is a signatory. Article 7 of the European Convention on Human Rights is an embodiment of the principle of legality. It provides that no one can be convicted of an offence which was not an offence at the time when the act or omission allegedly constituting the crime was committed. The Human Rights Act 1998, which came into force in October 2000, obliges the courts to give effect to the European Convention on Human Rights. At present it remains uncertain what effect the statute will have. It is suggested that it will affect strict liability, the age of consent to sexual activities as well as the laws of insanity and self-defence, but as yet English criminal courts have been tentative in their approach to construing the definitional elements of offences in conformity with the Convention. The general judicial view seems to be that as a rule the *substantive* law is largely unaffected. See the discussion of the Human Rights Act 1998 later in this chapter. The courts must construe statutes and interpret the common law consistently with the Convention and can issue declarations of incompatibility if a statute is inconsistent with the provisions of the Convention. The Convention must be read in accordance with modern conditions. Therefore, what was once Convention law need not be so now, and authorities are not to be used as precedents. An example is **Sutherland v UK** [1998] EHRLR 117. The European Court of Human Rights ruled that a ban on homosexual behaviour among males until the age of 18 when heterosexuals were legally permitted to have sexual intercourse from the age of 16 was a breach of Article 8(1), the right to respect for private life, despite the fact that other Convention decisions supported the ban.

Article 7 can be used to prevent a court from making a statutory offence have retrospective effect. It would also seem to ban, for example, the penalisation of marital rape as occurred in **R**. However, the European Court of Human Rights ruled in **SW v United Kingdom** [1996] 1 FLR 434 that 'however clearly drafted a legal provision may be, in any system of law, including criminal law, there is an inevitable element of judicial interpretation' and Article 7 did not prohibit the clarification of the law over time and the final abolition of the marital immunity in rape constituted a gradual clarification. What the Lords had done in *R* was to declare that the marital exemption had disappeared over time and Article 7 permitted them to do so because there was no retroactivity. As the Court put it:

> The essentially debasing character of rape is so manifest that the result of the decisions of the Court of Appeal and the House of Lords [which abrogated the marital immunity] cannot be said to be at variance with the object and purpose of Article 7 of the Convention, namely to ensure that no one should be subjected to arbitrary prosecution, conviction or punishment. What is more, the abandonment of the unacceptable idea of a husband being immune against prosecution . . . was in conformity not only with a civilised concept of marriage but also, and above all, with the fundamental objectives of the Convention, the very essence of which is respect for human dignity . . .

In *Misra* [2005] 1 WLR 1 the court said:

> Vague laws which purport to create criminal liability are undesirable, and in extreme cases . . . their very vagueness may make it impossible to identify the conduct which is prohibited by a criminal sanction. . . . That said, however, the requirement is for sufficiency rather than absolute certainty.

It was held that the crime of gross negligence manslaughter, which is discussed in Chapter 12, did not contravene Article 7.

Another aspect of Article 7 is that it appears to prohibit the restriction of defences. If so, cases such as *Gotts* [1992] 2 AC 412, the authority on whether duress is a defence to attempted murder, are incorrect. It should be noted that there is an exception to non-retrospectivity. This occurs where the act 'was criminal according to the general principles of law recognised by civilised nations'. This exception was held in *C* [2004] 1 WLR 2098 (CA) to cover the judicial abolition of the marital immunity from conviction for rape. Judge LJ said:

> Article 7(2) provides ample justification for a husband's trial and punishment for the rape of his wife, according to the general principles recognised by civilised nations. Indeed, . . . it would be surprising to discover that the law in any civilised country protected a woman from rape, with the solitary and glaring exception of rape by a man who had promised to love and comfort her.

UK jurisprudence on Article 7 so far is disappointing to those who expected the Human Rights Act 1998 to restrain judicial legislation. *C* so demonstrates. In this case a man was found guilty in 2003 of raping his wife in 1970 when, had he been charged in 1970, he would not have been convicted. In *Rimmington* [2006] 1 AC 459 the House of Lords did, however, amend the common law crime of public nuisance to bring it into line with Article 7. The Law Lords found that they had no common law powers to abolish offences, but they could overrule cases to bring the common law into line with Article 7. *C* is inconsistent with *Rimmington* where Lord Bingham stressed that: 'There are two guiding principles: no one should be punished under a law unless it is sufficiently clear and certain to enable him to know what conduct is forbidden before he does it; and no one should be punished for any act which was not clearly and ascertainably punishable when the act was done.' The second principle is contrary to the ratio of *C. C*, however, may be upheld on the basis provided by the European Court of Human Rights in *SW v UK*, namely, that what the accused did was 'criminal according to the general principles of law recognised by civilised nations', as Article 7(2) ECHR states. *Rimmington* is also authority for the proposition that the crime of causing a public nuisance was not too vague to satisfy Article 6. As the ECHR said in **Kokkinakis v Greece** (1993) 17 EHRR 397, 'where the individual can know from the wording of the relevant provision and, if need be, with the assistance of the courts' interpretation of it, what acts and omissions will make him liable', then Article 7 is satisfied but Article 7 is breached if 'the criminal law [is] extensively construed to the accused's detriment, for instance by analogy'.

Actus reus

The accused is guilty only if he has acted or has brought about a state of affairs, (*actus reus*). He is not liable for just being as he is (e.g. poor, religious, black). People are not punished for mere thoughts. The nearest English law has come to penalising people for thinking is one form of treason, encompassing the Queen's death, and conspiracy. Partly on account of this principle there have arisen problems about the scope of criminal liability for omissions (see Chapter 2), attempts (see Chapter 10), and involuntary acts (see automatism in Chapter 9). The US Supreme Court has held that a crime without an *actus reus* is unconstitutional. In English law, where the *actus reus* is an act or an omission, the accused is guilty only if he had at least some control over his behaviour. There must be a willed act, a voluntary act.

Mens rea

A wrongful mental state, **mens rea**, is required in almost all serious crimes. People should not be punished unless they are at fault. Only people who act intentionally or who know that they run a risk are at fault. Justice is not done if persons are punished by the state when they have not acted in a blameworthy way. Criminal responsibility is largely founded on moral culpability. There are, however, many exceptions: strict liability offences minor or serious do not require *mens rea* as to one or more parts of the *actus reus* (see Chapter 4). It has been questioned whether negligence is properly to be classified as a state of mind. It is also thought that if the law requires that an accused has a defence only if he acted reasonably as in duress (see Chapter 7), the *mens rea* condition is excluded in relation to this matter. It is sometimes argued that an accused should not be guilty when he is not blameworthy and offences which do so convict him should be abrogated.

Concurrence

In English law the basic rule is that the *actus reus* and *mens rea* must be simultaneous. There are, however, several exceptions discussed in Chapter 3.

Harm

In many offences a person or thing is harmed. In murder someone is killed; in criminal damage property is destroyed or damaged. One purpose of the law is to allow people to act free from harm. Aggressors are to be deterred. As the European Court of Human Rights stated in **Laskey v United Kingdom** (1997) 24 EHRR 39: 'one of the roles which the state is unquestionably entitled to undertake is to seek to regulate, through the operation of the criminal law, activities which involve the infliction of physical harm'. There are several offences which are not predicated on harm to others. The Terrorism Act 2006 creates the offence of glorifying terrorism, a vague term, but one which does not require any victim to be injured or killed. No one need be harmed in the inchoate offences (Chapter 10) and dangerous driving, and there is argument about so-called 'victimless offences' such as possessing marijuana. Some 'victimless' offences are treated as ones where the harm is to others. If one does not wear a seatbelt and, as a result, one is more seriously injured than otherwise, one becomes a burden to others. An alternative view is to contend that the state has an interest in the well-being of its citizens (see N. Lacey, *State Punishment* (Routledge, 1988), in which Lacey argues in favour of a concept of 'welfare': the state is entitled to intervene to provide for the physical welfare of its citizens by such means as ordering the wearing of seatbelts and penalising violations). Moreover, health costs and absences from work are prevented by such means. Some harms may be trivial on the facts. Others may be serious, e.g. pollution. One aim of the criminal law is to prevent certain harms such as interferences with the person or property by penalising infractions.

Some academics also derive a principle of proportionality. In other words, some crimes are more serious than others. For example, murder is more serious than assault occasioning actual bodily harm. Therefore, murder should be punished more severely than actual bodily harm. Perhaps linked closely with this principle is that of fair labelling; namely, that the name given to the crime should correspond to the wrong encapsulated by the offence.

Jurisprudential discussion of the 'harm' principle over the past 50 years is extensive. Some jurists have sought to justify offences based on morality or offensiveness. Readers are referred to the Further reading at the end of this chapter for discussion.

Causation

In result crimes it must be proved that the accused committed the *actus reus* (see Chapter 2). It is not always clear who caused an event. Causation in pollution cases seems to be wider than the doctrine found elsewhere in criminal law. Transferred malice can be seen as exceptional: the accused intends to harm one person but harms another. There are also difficulties with omissions (Chapter 2).

Defences

These are examined in Chapters 7–9.

Jurisprudential discussion of the 'harm principle' over the past 50 years is extensive. Some jurists have sought to justify offences based on morality or offensiveness. Readers are referred to the further reading at the end of this chapter for discussion.

Proof (beyond reasonable doubt)

This is dealt with in this chapter. All the elements of the offence charged must be proved beyond reasonable doubt. What has to be proved varies from crime to crime, and that may change from time to time. For example, since 1994 men can be the victims of rape; before then only women could be.

The principles of criminal law and criminalisation

Alan Norrie summarised these norms in *Crime, Reason and History* (2nd edn, Butterworths, 2001) 10: 'Criminal law is, at heart, a practical application of liberal political philosophy.' These principles restrain the power of the state expressed through its agencies, such as the police and the judiciary. Without them criminal law would have no bounds and the powers of the agents of the state would be limitless. The democratic enactment of offences justifies the use of state power to punish lawbreakers. Punishment after conviction for an offence is a substantial power in the hands of the state and may take the form of imprisonment, which deprives the offender of his freedom. There is attached to all serious and some less serious crimes the stigma of being convicted. Most people shun murderers and rapists. The principles also allow citizens, to some degree, to be able to foresee whether their conduct will be criminal or not. In *Jackson* (1994) *The Independent*, 25 May, the Court of Appeal said that legal certainty was a fundamental principle of criminal law. One may criticise criminal law textbooks for being positivistic, that is, describing the law as it exists (in all its detail), but one would surely not wish to be convicted because some people say that what one has done is not in line with their moral stance. Liability should not depend on 'speculation or inquiry' or the politics of the moment. Even the 'bad man' ought to know whether he is breaking the criminal law. (See below for judicial interpretation of Acts of Parliament.) The principles are not, however, uniformly applied. The American jurist, Oliver Wendell Holmes, formulated the aphorism that the life of the law has been experience, not logic. Criminal law is an exemplar of this proposition. It is not consistent or logical, as this book amply demonstrates. Much of the law is complex, sometimes needlessly, as the chapter on non-fatal offences demonstrates. In reading this book you may consider that there is little which can be said of the general principles said by Husak to underlie criminal law. Students who start on criminal law courses are often of the belief that they know a good deal about the subject, but find difficulty with the course because they are not prepared for a mass of difficult law, such as that on intent. There is a trend towards consistency, encouraged by the Law Commission, but the government has not felt the need to reform the law, even when such reform would save money. Criminal law is therefore concerned with the setting of standards, and punishment is for those who break such norms.

While these principles inform the substance of the law, they do not delimit its width. That width is sometimes a matter of history. For example, the law on dangerous dogs is a response to a small number of horrific attacks by certain breeds of dogs on children. Whether behaviour is criminal should be a matter of policy. Most would agree that murder and rape are not good things. The Law Commission's draft Criminal Code (see later in this chapter) did not focus on what the criminal law *ought* to do. Some attempt to consider when criminal liability should be imposed must be made because otherwise the power of the criminal law to punish wrongdoers is diminished and its condemnatory function is undermined. Moreover, in a democracy there must be some control over the agents of the state who could otherwise use the strongest of state sanctions against trivial offenders. The most authoritative exposition of the aims of criminal law from a liberal viewpoint is the *Report of the (Wolfenden) Committee on Homosexual Offences and Prostitution*, Cmnd 247, 1957, which led to the decriminalisation of adult male homosexual practices in private. Criminal law existed:

> ... to preserve public order and decency, to protect the citizen from what is injurious and to provide sufficient safeguards against exploitation or corruption of others ... It is not ... the function of the law to intervene in the private lives of citizens ... further than is necessary to carry out [these] purposes ... (paras 13–14).

 It can be argued that the majority of the House of Lords in **Brown** [1994] AC 212, discussed in Chapter 13, broke these principles when they penalised homosexual sado-masochism. The reduction of the age of consent for male homosexuals from 21 to 18 came into force when the Criminal Justice and Public Order Act 1994 received Royal Assent (3 November 1994). The then difference in the age of consent for heterosexual (16) and homosexual intercourse (18) was condemned by the European Court of Human Rights as being contrary to Article 8 of the Convention, respect for private life, and contrary to the parasitic Article 14, non-discrimination: *Sutherland* v *United Kingdom*

[1998] EHRLR 117. The Sexual Offences (Amendment) Act 2000 reduced the age to 16. The Wolfenden Committee's main contention was that the criminal law should not be used to enforce the morality even of a majority of the members of society. Lord Hobhouse (dissenting) in **Hinks** [2001] 2 AC 241 stated: 'To treat otherwise lawful conduct as criminal merely because it is open to . . . disapprobation [by ordinary right-thinking citizens] would be contrary to principle and open to the objection that it fails to achieve the objective and transparent certainty required of the criminal law by the principles basic to human rights.'

The US Model Penal Code, which seeks to encapsulate best practice in state jurisdictions, famously states that the criminal law has five aims (spelling anglicised):

(a) to forbid and prevent conduct which unjustifiably and inexcusably inflicts or threatens to inflict harm to public interests;

(b) to subject to public control persons whose conduct indicates that they are disposed to commit crimes;

(c) to safeguard conduct that is without fault from condemnation as criminal;

(d) to give fair warning of the nature of the conduct declared to be an offence;

(e) to differentiate on reasonable grounds between serious and minor offences.

As the Commentaries explain, this part of the Code 'undertakes to state the most pervasive general objectives of the Code'. It is also meant to control official discretion and to aid interpretation of the Code. Some of these principles are broken by current English law, which does not have any written aims. For example, maliciously inflicting grievous bodily harm is a more serious offence than occasioning actual bodily harm, yet both have the same maximum punishment. Sometimes the principles conflict, and there may be disagreement about the scope of each principle. Some people argue that smoking marijuana does not harm the public interest. The Court of Appeal in **Kingston** [1994] QB 81, in a passage which was not criticised by the House of Lords, said that 'the purpose of the criminal law is to inhibit, by proscription and by penal sanction, antisocial acts which individuals may otherwise commit'. Unfortunately the common law has not developed principles such as those found in the Model Penal Code. The same is true of Parliament. Therefore, one cannot draw in advance the line between criminalising conduct and not doing so. Criminal law sets norms, standards of behaviour, to which natural and juristic persons must conform. Largely it tells people what not to do, not what they should do.

It is highly important that criminal law is kept within bounds. Police resources would be even more stretched than at present if the law were widened unnecessarily, and the powers of arrest and prosecution could become more arbitrary than they are at present. Criminal law is a strong form of state control. After all people can be deprived of their liberty for life and there is still the possibility of the sentence of death for treason. There is stigma attached to a criminal conviction. One's name may be in the local paper even for trivial offences. Society condemns a person for offending. For these reasons citizens must know which conduct is criminally unlawful. Areas of law such as dishonesty, conspiracy to corrupt public morals and intent where the definition is not clear are scrutinised in this book, as are occasions when judges are seen to 'stretch' the law to cover 'manifestly guilty' persons who are charged with the wrong offence. A case on insider-trading provides useful material for discussion. Until Parliament penalised the use of confidential information to buy shares at a low price there was no offence directed specifically at this form of behaviour. This way of making money was acceptable to those who did it. Does the insider-trader's conduct fall within the scope of criminal law adumbrated by the Wolfenden Committee? Within Husak's fifth principle, harm, who is harmed? The reader is invited to consider what would happen if there was no criminal law. Indeed, as a general rule misappropriating confidential information is not a crime. Nevertheless, it must be said that whatever the answer to the insider-trading conundrum not all offences are serious socially or economically, and sometimes it might be better to use training and administrative measures rather than criminal sanctions. Governments of all persuasions seem to have a tendency to criminalise behaviour which they cannot control otherwise, even when there is no consensus in society that certain forms of conduct should be visited by penal sanctions. Criminal law has developed in a piecemeal fashion without regard to theory. Some criminal laws epitomise kneejerk reaction to perceived crises such as dangerous dogs, stalking, raves, anti-roads protesters and 'hippie' convoys. In the jargon such offences are 'historically contingent': their arrival on the scene marks some kind of campaign, not rational and principled inquiry. As can be seen, modern criminal law is vast in scope. It covers both serious and non-serious offences by individuals, and is also used as a means of regulating business.

Furthermore, Parliament, while rarely abolishing offences, also creates new offences, with the consequence that the boundaries of criminal law are ever widening. There were some 7,000 offences in 1980; it is estimated that there were about 8,000 in 2000. The current figure seems to be about 11,000: see *The Independent*, p. 1, 16 August 2006. It was estimated that the government has created 3,023 crimes since 1997. Senior members of the police have called for the decriminalisation of the possession and inhalation of so-called soft drugs such as cannabis. In a rational system of law, if one wanted to penalise the possession of drugs, one might start with criminalising alcohol (look at any volume of the Criminal Appeal Reports or issues of *Criminal Law Review* for what people do when drunk), or if one wanted to stop violence, one might easily conclude that boxing should be illegal. After all, politicians, and to some extent judges, make law (we no longer believe the fairy tale that judges do not make law) and they have their own predilections and are subject to moral panics. In a Written Answer the then Minister of State at the Home Office, Lord Williams of Mostyn, stated that new offences 'should be created only when absolutely necessary' (*Hansard*, HL Deb, 18 June 1999, WA 57). It remains to be seen whether the pledge is honoured. In summary, the creation of new law by Parliament may depend on politics, not principle. It is interesting to see how much parliamentary time can be given to a subject in the news such as, say, dangerous dogs, whereas no time can be found to enact well-considered proposals for law reform, such as those put forward by the Law Commission, discussed in the last part of this chapter.

Human Rights Act 1998

This statute does not entrench the European Convention on Human Rights into UK law: it is not a constitution or a higher law. What the Act does is to oblige courts to interpret legislation in accordance with the Convention 'so far as . . . possible' (s 3(1)). If the impugned statute cannot be so construed, the High Court (and the Court of Appeal and the House of Lords) is to make a declaration of incompatibility. That declaration does not, however, affect the validity of the statute (s 4(1)). Parliament then has the option of deciding whether to amend the law or not. This power has not so far been used in a substantive criminal case. Public bodies, a term which includes courts, must act consistently with the Convention (s 6). The Human Rights Act 1998 does not only permit the accused to argue that certain offences are contrary to the Act but it also allows a victim to argue that the state has not protected his rights. An example of the latter method is the law relating to a parent's chastisement of his child. The state's protection of the child leads to a narrowing of the circumstances in which a child could be punished by his parent (or other person *in loco parentis*).

It should be noted that the 1998 Act does not directly apply to the common law. A way to avoid this non-application is as follows. Take insanity as an example. Current law may be incompatible with the Convention. Article 5 stipulates that everyone has a right to liberty and to security of the person. If a verdict of insanity would be inconsistent with the Convention, then since the courts are public bodies, they must act in conformity with it. In *H* [2002] 2 Cr App R (S) 59 the Court of Appeal accepted that using s 6 was a legitimate way of proceeding.

It is suggested that in the next few years the following areas of criminal law which form part of this book may be affected by the European Convention on Human Rights: the defence of self-defence/prevention of crime (by Article 2, right to life), strict liability (by Article 3, right not to be subjected to inhuman and degrading punishment: Arden J writing extrajudicially in [1999] Crim LR 439 thought that the courts could create a defence of due diligence but UK courts have not gone so far as yet in criminal law), insanity (by Article 5, above), strict liability and burden of proof (by Article 7, right to a fair hearing and presumption of innocence), conspiracy to defraud, corrupt public morals and outrage public decency and offences of dishonesty (by Article 7, non-retroactivity), and consent to non-fatal and sexual offences and offences of dishonesty (by Article 8, respect for private life). As an illustration the defence of prevention of crime will fall foul of Article 2 because (a) killing in defence of property is not justifiable under the Convention and (b) case law, including *McCann v United Kingdom* (1995) 21 EHRR 97, demands a belief based on reasonable grounds whereas in present law an honest belief suffices. Much of the case law at present deals with Article 6, the right to a fair trial, which to a large extent is outside the scope of this book, but it is mentioned where relevant, such as in the discussion of the burden of proof. It should be noted that the Convention is interpreted in the light of current social conditions. Therefore old precedents may no longer be of value.

The 1998 Act does not affect the right to petition the European Court of Human Rights in Strasbourg but Article 34 of the Convention provides that domestic remedies must be exhausted first. Therefore, an applicant must use the English courts first.

If a court considers that an English precedent is inconsistent with the Convention, it should follow the precedent and give leave to appeal: *Lambeth London Borough Council v Kay* [2006] 4 All ER 128 (HL).

Attempted definitions of a crime

Definitions are said to be unfashionable, but without them the reader may be misled into thinking that a violation of one of the Ten Commandments is *per se* a crime or that a breach of contract is a crime. There have been several attempts at defining crimes, most of which are to the effect that a crime may give rise to criminal proceedings which may lead to (criminal) punishment. Blackstone wrote that a crime was 'a violation of the public rights and duties due to the whole community considered as a community'. This definition came from the mid-eighteenth century from one of the leading commentators on English law. More up to date are the definitions which include 'a breach of duty imposed by law for the benefit of the community at large' and a wrong 'whose sanction is punitive and is no way remissible by any private person, but is remissible by the Crown alone if remissible at all'. Punishment by the state makes criminal law important in society. 'Remissible' means that the sanction granted by the court can be reduced. The House of Lords, the highest English tribunal for most criminal law purposes, essayed a definition in **Board of Trade v Owen** [1957] AC 602: 'an unlawful act or default which is an offence against the public and renders the person guilty of the act liable to legal punishment'. Such a definition tells us nothing about why conduct is made criminal. A crime may cause less harm than a tort or breach of contract. If employers dismiss their employees in breach of their service agreements, loss is caused to them, their families, local shops and so on, but punches in a pub car park at closing time may not even cause bruises except to self-esteem.

One of the leading writers on criminal law, Glanville Williams in 'The definition of a crime' [1955] CLP 107, stated that a crime was 'a legal wrong that can be followed by criminal proceedings which may result in punishment', while a leading American, H. M. Hart 'The Aims of the Criminal Law' (1958) 23 L & CP 401 at 405, considered that a crime is 'conduct which . . . will incur a formal and solemn pronouncement of the moral condemnation of the community'. Therefore, criminal law is imbued with symbolism: a convicted accused is condemned by the state and that condemnation has a public aspect. Such a definition may be rejected on the basis that strict offences (see Chapter 4) may not be morally wrong, yet they are crimes. It should be noted that these definitions do not say that a penalty, punishment, must follow after conviction and that there is no necessity that crimes are always prosecuted and even if the accused is prosecuted, he may escape conviction. For example, breaches of safety legislation are often dealt with administratively without recourse to enforcing criminal law. Compliance with the law and not punishment for it is the driving force. A work which summarises the whole of English law is *Halsbury's Laws of England*, vol. 11(1), para. 1 (Butterworths, 1990 re-issue). The fourth edition contains the following:

> Ordinarily a crime is a wrong which affects the security or well-being of the public generally so that the public has an interest in its suppression . . . However, . . . an act may be made criminal by Parliament simply because it is criminal process, rather than civil, which offers the more effective means of controlling the conduct in question.

Effectiveness can be seen in crimes such as those controlling road traffic and insider-dealing. By enacting a law, Parliament is seen to be doing something about a social problem. Parliament may convert a tort into a crime or what was previously lawful into one, or it may make lawful that which was previously illegal. What was previously redressable only civilly may be converted into a crime, and the public becomes involved in suppressing what Parliament has deemed to be unlawful behaviour. Moreover, it is not always clear why an offence has been created. Sometimes it seems simpler to institute an offence than to do anything else.

The more modern definitions are admittedly circular and do not lay down rules on what types of behaviour should be criminalised. An offence is a breach of a legal duty which may be followed by criminal proceedings and sentence. Criminal procedure defines what is criminal law. Unfortunately, we do not know whether criminal proceedings are needed until we know that the criminal law has been broken. The definitions do not resolve the doubt whether a matter is civil or criminal. Further, knowing that there are procedural differences between criminal and civil law does not justify distinguishing the two types of law in terms of substance. Williams noted that he could give only a list of factors indicating on which side of the line an issue fell but sometimes features indicating criminal law had to be balanced against factors indicating civil law. Nevertheless, in most instances the criminal law is like an elephant: we know it when we see it. Accepting that it is difficult to define a crime for all purposes, the following suffices for our purposes: 'a legal wrong the remedy for which is the punishment of the offender at the instance of the state' (Professor Cross). Professor Cross's words are echoed in the seventeenth edition of Card, Cross and Jones: *Criminal Law* (OUP, 2006), pp 1–2: '. . . a crime is a legal wrong . . . the principal legal consequence of a crime is that the offender . . . is prosecuted by or in the name of the State.' Accordingly there must be (a) some wrongdoing, or indeed a wrongful situation; (b) 'a legal wrong'; (c) a wrong where the state in whichever guise intervenes to punish the wrongdoer; and (d) a remedy for the wrong in terms of punishment. Compensation is, therefore, a mark of civil, not criminal, law. Punishment marks out or stigmatises the defendant as a criminal. Criminal law is that part of the law which cannot be left to private individuals to enforce.

See p584 in Chapter 15 for a definition of theft.

Take, for example, the offence of theft. The accused has stolen something. The state has decreed that this wrongdoing is punishable, the prosecution proves that the accused committed the offence beyond reasonable doubt and the accused receives a sentence such as a fine or imprisonment. The victim of the offence normally gets nothing out of the criminal justice system either from the state or from the accused, though there are exceptions, such as a restitution order of the thing stolen under s 28 of the Theft Act 1968 or in some cases money from the Criminal Injuries Compensation Board. The accused may be prosecuted either at the instance of the state (normally the Crown Prosecution Service or the Director of Public Prosecutions, the DPP) or by private individuals or companies, such as when a high-street shop prosecutes for shoplifting. On the definition given earlier, theft is a crime because it may be followed by criminal proceedings.

One term in Cross's definition needs more explanation. The wrong must be a legal wrong. This phrase points to one of the differences between criminal law and morals (or what the majority of society think). A crime is a breach of the criminal law, whether that law was laid down by Parliament or the courts. It need not be a moral wrong, a breach of a duty imposed by an ethical system. Criminal law covers a vast range of situations not all of which are condemned as breaches of morals. Some crimes are not seen by all people as moral wrongs. For example, euthanasia as when a daughter kills her terminally ill mother who is suffering great pain is not seen by everyone as morally wrong, but it is a breach of one of the criminal laws: it is murder. Taking food to feed a starving baby is theft. Morality can, however, be taken into account at the sentencing stage. No doubt a person who stole to feed a starving child would receive less punishment than one who stole to satisfy greed. Indeed, many crimes have no moral content whatsoever. Drivers in the UK drive on a side of the road different from that in the USA and continental Europe but there is no morality behind the difference. While not all crimes are breaches of all forms of morality, similarly not all moral wrongs are crimes. Selfishness, lying, breaking promises and adultery may be morally wrong, but they are not crimes. Yet, the same event may be both a crime and a moral wrong. Rape is a crime, and presumably most people would also say that rape is morally wrong. Therefore, although crime and morality are not the same, there are some areas of overlap.

It is sometimes said that a crime affects the public and civil law affects one person, but this proposition is easily disproved. For example, a fight between two people in a pub car park may lead to injuries such as cuts, bruises and perhaps concussion. These injuries constitute one or more non-fatal offences. It cannot be said that the whole public is affected. However, an oil spillage will affect many more people than a punch-up in a car park despite its being a tort.

Just as some aspects of morality change, so does the criminal law. The usual example is homosexuality. Until quite recently it was an offence among consenting males, of whatever age, to perform homosexual acts wherever in England and Wales. In 1967 Parliament changed the law to make homosexual activities in private between two men over 21 lawful. The age was reduced to 18 in 1994 and later to 16. It should be noted that these changes in the law can be consistent with the European Convention. The Convention is a living document which has to be interpreted as society now exists and not as how matters were at the time of its drafting. Generally speaking, homosexuality was illegal in the states which signed the Convention in the 1950s and the European Commission on Human Rights permitted such laws. However, just as national laws have changed, so has the interpretation of the Convention with the result that states can, for instance, no longer lay down separate ages of consent for heterosexual and homosexual intercourse. Similarly, heterosexual buggery was illegal until 3 November 1994, since when it has been lawful, subject to conditions: both partners must be over 18 and the activity must take place in private and be consensual. (Lesbianism has never been a crime though sometimes indecent assault charges were brought. The crime of indecent assault is now that of sexual assault, and it is unlikely that charges will be brought.) In a different area of criminal law, dishonesty under the Theft Acts, the courts have said that juries can take into account current standards of behaviour. It could be that a jury in 1972 would not convict on the same facts on which a jury would convict now. An example might be the practice of asking for more shares than one had money to pay for at the time when the shares would be allotted in the expectation that the full amount of shares requested would not be allocated to the accused so that he would have sufficient money to pay for the shares which he did obtain. In this way he would get the shares he really wanted. If he had just put in for that number, he would not have got all of them in the event of oversubscription. Which forms of behaviour are criminal is a matter for Parliament and the courts. Sometimes coverage is non-existent. If I misappropriate trade secrets, I am not guilty of theft. Sometimes coverage is only partial. If I tell lies to have sexual intercourse, I am not guilty of rape, unless I lie about the nature or purpose of the act or my identity. If I tell lies to gain an item of property, I may be guilty of fraud. One aspect of the problem is that Parliament and the courts create offences of enormous width with the result that acts of vastly different depravity are included within the same offence. Two illustrations suffice. In manslaughter the crime covers misconduct on the border of murder (and even acts which not much more than 20 years ago would have been murder) as well as the scenario where there is a brief fist fight, the victim is punched, falls on the ground, hits his head on a brick by mischance, and dies. The best-known example is, however, murder which covers the worst terrorist outrage and the most compassionate mercy-killing.

There is also the fact that the criminal law is changed only slowly and partially by Parliament to reflect social developments. There was no Computer Misuse Act until 1990. The language both in judge-made and Parliament-made criminal law may be out of date. 'Malice aforethought', the state of mind required for murder, is not based on spite or premeditated killing. Similarly the term 'maliciously' in the Offences Against the Person Act 1861 was with hindsight badly chosen, for there is no need for malice. Some areas of the law have been updated and the language modernised in recent years, e.g. theft, criminal damage, but some parts use old-fashioned vocabulary. Even if the present draft Criminal Code should be enacted, that new body of law would not cover all areas of criminal law (see later in this chapter). Since the development of the law has been piecemeal over centuries it is not surprising that there is no single definition which encapsulates why this conduct is a crime and that conduct is not.

Parliament has not defined a crime. There is, however, a provision now found in s 18(1)(a) of the Supreme Court Act 1981 by which subject to exceptions there is no appeal from the High Court to the Court of Appeal (Civil Division) in any 'criminal cause or matter'. Cases, the principal one being *Amand v Home Secretary and Minister of Defence of the Royal Netherlands Government* [1943] AC 147 (HL), decide that if the proceedings may lead to punishment, they constitute a criminal cause or matter. Even if Parliament did define a crime, that definition would now be subject to the European Convention on Human Rights.

Article 6(2) of the European Convention on Human Rights applies only to persons 'charged with a criminal offence'. It gives greater protection to those accused of crimes than to defendants in civil cases. For example, the accused is subject to the presumption of innocence and must be provided with a lawyer free of charge if he cannot afford one. The definition of 'criminal offence' is an autonomous one, not tied to that found in national law. The nature of the proceedings, the severity of the penalty and the classification by national law are all taken into account, but the first consideration is the most vital. An example is *Benham v UK* (1996) 22 EHRR 293 (ECHR). The accused was put into prison when bailiffs could not find goods of sufficient value to pay his community charge ('poll tax'). English law says that such proceedings, although they take place in the magistrates' court, are civil in nature: as the ECHR put it, 'The purpose of the detention was to coerce the appellant into paying the tax owed, rather than to punish him for not having paid it.' Nevertheless, the Court held that the proceedings were criminal ones and, therefore, Article 6 of the Convention applied. The nature of the proceedings was very important. The proceedings were brought by a public authority and had a punitive element in that the magistrates could commit to prison and the defendant could be imprisoned for a maximum of three months. (The European Court called this maximum 'relatively severe'.) The classification according to English domestic law was not decisive. *Benham* was distinguished by the House of Lords in *Clingham v Royal Borough of Kensington and Chelsea* [2003] 1 AC 787. The making of an anti-social behaviour order was a civil law matter, though a breach of it led to proceedings of a criminal nature: there was no penalty until that later stage. As yet, the European Court of Human Rights and the English courts have not been divided as to whether there is or is not a 'criminal offence'. There will be more jurisprudence on this issue over time.

Differences between criminal and civil law

Modern legal systems throughout the world distinguish between civil and criminal law and England and Wales is no different. One might assume that a breach of criminal law would necessarily be more serious than a breach of civil law but that does not necessarily follow. Criminal and civil law do not necessarily differ in the sorts of behaviour they are intended to control. The same act can be both a crime and a tort, what is sometimes called a civil wrong. If I assault you, I am guilty of a crime and of a tort. If the bus driver who drove you home this evening carelessly crashed and you were injured, there may be several crimes relating to the driving and the harm as well as tort and a breach of contract by the bus company to transport you safely.

However, there are important differences in some respects which may be listed as follows:

(a) *The courts are not the same.* In civil law the two courts which are the first to hear cases are the High Court and the county court. The distinction between the two changed greatly in 1991, but the basic division remains that the High Court hears cases involving high monetary amounts, the county court hears the rest. Under the wing of the county court exists the small claims court, the jurisdiction of which is limited. Appeals are to the Court of Appeal (Civil Division) and thence to the House of Lords. When the Constitutional Reform Act 2005, Part 3, is in force, the House of Lords as a judicial body will be replaced by the Supreme Court. There is also a possibility of a reference from any of these courts to the European Court of Justice at Luxembourg on a matter of European Community law. The basic rule is that a court below the House of Lords *may* refer the matter, whereas the House *must* refer unless in general the issue has been clearly resolved previously (*acte clair*).

The hierarchy and relationship of criminal law courts are outlined later in this chapter. In brief the courts which hear matters first (courts of first instance) are the Crown Court and the magistrates' courts. In both these courts the majority of defendants plead guilty. There is appeal to the Divisional Court or Court of Appeal (Criminal Division), with most appeals from magistrates going to the Crown Court. The court of last resort, the final appeal court, is the House of Lords. There was no true Court of Appeal in criminal matters until 1907 when the Court of Criminal Appeal was established. That court was replaced in 1966 by the present intermediate Court of Appeal. It was not until 1960 that the House of Lords gained its present full appellate jurisdiction in criminal matters. Criminal law has hardly been touched by European Community law, but that law does now, for example, affect the law on fishing.

(b) *The terminology is different.* In criminal law the prosecution prosecutes the accused (or defendant). In civil law the claimant sues the defendant.

(c) *The outcome is different.* In civil law if the claimant wins, he usually receives damages or an injunction. Damages at civil law may well exceed criminal law fines. In criminal law the accused, if guilty, is (usually though not always) sentenced. The aim of civil law is normally to compensate the victim, whereas in criminal law punishment is the objective. There are several exceptions. The accused may be ordered to restore the stolen item (Theft Act 1968, s 28) or any item taken (Police (Property) Act 1897, s 1), or to compensate the victim (Powers of Criminal Courts (Sentencing) Act 2000, s 130), but although compensation orders are often made in magistrates' courts, in most criminal cases the victim receives nothing from the offender. Moreover, convictions usually bear a greater stigma than do unsuccessful civil law claims or defences. Because punishment is not a necessary consequence of conviction, it is suggested that criminal law and punishment are not as inextricably linked as some believe.

(d) *Procedural matters differ.* As we have seen, it is normally the state which prosecutes, whereas it is private individuals or companies which sue, and the Crown can commute a sentence in criminal law but not in civil law. Another distinction is that once started criminal proceedings cannot be stopped except by the Attorney-General issuing what is called a *nolle prosequi* ('do not prosecute'), whereas civil proceedings can be settled at any time by the parties. The defendant can be compelled to give evidence in a civil but not a criminal matter. It may be said that the state has an interest in criminal proceedings which the wishes of the non-state parties cannot override.

PART 1 PRELIMINARY MATTERS

(e) Breach of the criminal law is a symbol of state power. Conviction communicates the state's displeasure at certain forms of conduct. Being found civilly liable does not serve this purpose.

(f) The victim has little role to play in criminal law, whereas the claimant has the leading role in civil law.

In general a prosecution is no bar to civil proceedings and vice versa. There are exceptionally provisions found in ss 44–45 of the Offences Against the Person Act 1861 which stipulate that a civil action for assault or battery may not be brought when the accused has been tried in a magistrates' court and has either obtained a certificate of dismissal of the complaint or been punished.

Hierarchy of the criminal courts: the appeal system

After the decision is taken in which court the case is to be heard, the accused is tried. The process of appeal depends on whether the case was tried in the magistrates' court or at the Crown Court. The final Anglo-Welsh court on criminal matters is the House of Lords, which during the currency of this book may become the Supreme Court.

Magistrates' courts

There are two possible routes of appeal. The usual one is to the Crown Court, which for this purpose is composed of a judge and (usually) two magistrates. Only the accused can appeal, and the grounds are (a) on the points of fact or law against conviction, or (b) against sentence. The first ground may be used only if the accused pleaded not guilty. The format is a rehearing, i.e. a new, full trial (a trial *de novo*). The alternative appeal is to the Divisional Court of the Queen's Bench Division of the High Court. The appeal is called 'by way of case stated'. Either side may appeal, but the grounds are solely (a) on a point of law, or (b) that the magistrates exceeded their jurisdiction. If the prosecution succeeds, the magistrates are directed to convict and give the appropriate sentence. There is also an appeal by way of case stated from the Crown Court to the Divisional Court. There were 188 such appeals in 1998. Appeal from the Divisional Court is to the House of Lords. Either side may appeal, but only on points of law. There are two other prerequisites: the Divisional Court must certify that the point is of general public importance and either that Court or the Lords must grant leave to appeal. There are about ten such appeals a year.

Crown Court

Appeals from this Court lie to the Court of Appeal (Criminal Division). Appeal against conviction lies on the ground that the conviction was 'unsafe'. It does not matter that the accused might nevertheless have been found guilty by the jury. Only the accused may appeal. The appeal may be against conviction on a point of law, or against conviction on a point of fact or mixed law and fact; or against sentence. Retrials are possible but rare. They are, however, a growing phenomenon. Under the Criminal Justice Act 1972, s 36, the Attorney-General may refer a point of law to have the matter clarified. If the court decides that the Crown Court should have convicted, the accused's acquittal is not affected. Under the Criminal Justice Act 1988, ss 35–36, the Attorney-General can refer sentences to the Court of Appeal if he believes them to be unduly lenient. This power exists only in relation to certain serious offences. The Court of Appeal may impose any sentence which the Crown Court could have imposed.

Appeal from the Court of Appeal is to the House of Lords. The point must be one of law, and either side may appeal. Again there are two requirements: the Court of Appeal must certify that there is a point of law of general public importance, and either that court or the House of Lords must grant leave. There were three such appeals in 1998. Attorney-General's References on law or sentence may go to the House of Lords. An example of a reference is *Attorney-General's Reference (No. 1 of 1988)* [1989] AC 971 (HL), which is discussed below.

Precedent in criminal law

Decisions of magistrates' courts are not binding on any court. Decisions of the Crown Court are not binding, though judges may well follow them if they know of them. Such decisions are rarely reported, but see Chapter 14 on rape for modern exceptions. Decisions of the Divisional Court and Court of Appeal (Criminal Division) bind courts below them in the hierarchy (see previous section). It is said, but not always adopted, that the Court of Appeal (Criminal Division) will not adhere as closely to its previous decisions as the civil side does because of its supposed bias in favour of the accused, in favour of liberty: *Gould* [1968] 2 QB 65. It seems that a five-person court can overrule a three-person court. The House of Lords binds courts below it. Since 1966 it has not been bound by its own decisions: *Practice Statement* [1966] 1 WLR 1234. However, that Practice Statement declares that the House of Lords will take into account the especial need for certainty in the criminal law. That is, in criminal law matters more than civil law ones it will strive not to depart from its previous judgments. The effect of the Practice Statement is that their Lordships seek to uphold previous decisions under which people have been convicted, even though the result is unjust. However, the House of Lords has on one

See pp 432–33 in Chapter 10 for a detailed explanation of impossible attempts.

occasion very rapidly done just that, overruling its decision on impossible attempts in *Anderton v Ryan* [1985] AC 560 in *Shivpuri* [1987] AC 1. The House of Lords has, like the Court of Appeal, often convicted persons by not adhering to a strict interpretation of a statute (e.g. *Ayres* [1984] AC 447 and *MPC v Charles* [1977] AC 177), or indeed a strict reliance on previous (non-binding) cases: see *MPC v Caldwell* [1982] AC 341. It is uncertain whether a lower court is bound by the court immediately above it or by the court above that one. On the civil side the former rule applies.

In criminal cases the Court of Appeal has stated that it is bound by earlier Court of Appeal decisions and not by the advice of the Privy Council: *Campbell* [1997] 1 Cr App R 199. The rule is otherwise in the civil law, and there is no apparent reason for the difference. However, very recently the Court of Appeal has, amazingly to some, followed the advice of the Privy Council and not the decision of the House of Lords: see *James* [2006] EWCA Crim 14 on provocation. The court stressed the following: there were nine Law Lords in the Privy Council; the majority explicitly said that their advice was the law of England and Wales, and the majority constituted more than half the Law Lords.

In terms of orthodox theory of precedent there are doubts about the precedential value of Attorney-General's References, but they have been treated as being equivalent to authorities from the courts in which they were heard.

English 'courts should, in the absence of some special circumstances, follow any clear and constant jurisprudence of the Strasbourg Court' (per Lord Nicholls in *Kay v London*

Borough of Lambeth [2006] UKHL 10), unless there is a domestic precedent, in which case the court should apply the precedent, give its view and give leave of appeal: see Lord Bingham in the same case at [43].

The interpretation of criminal statutes

Most parts of the criminal law are based on statutes, and the enactment of the draft Criminal Code would accelerate the trend towards having criminal law based on Acts of Parliament. If enacted (and neither Conservative nor Labour governments have shown any readiness), it would not change the basic role of the judge in interpreting statutes as there is no special rule attached to the draft which the judge must follow. The Code would not apply to 'pre-Code' offences, of which there are, as of 2009, some 11,000, which would continue to be interpreted in the usual fashion. Under either system words are open-textured: 'what is reasonable self-defence?', 'is this person dishonest?'

Since statutes do not apply automatically, someone has to explain their width to the triers of fact, whether Justices of the Peace (or District Judges (Magistrates' Court)) in the Magistrates' Courts, or juries in the Crown Court, in order that they can apply the law to the facts. Moreover, Parliament often misses out fundamental matters such as which party bears the burden of proof and what the *mens rea*, if any, is. Sometimes too statutes become outdated by technology. The judge is in a difficult position. He has to apply the law impartially but he forms part of the state order, part of the mechanism for repressing crime. There is still room for judicial creativity for Parliament cannot legislate for every eventuality. It used to be said that in England criminal law should be construed strictly, or at least in favour of the accused (sometimes put as 'in favour of liberty'). That is, that criminal statutes had to be read narrowly so as to cover only those areas where it was clear that Parliament wanted the law to apply. There seem to be several reasons why such a view was taken. In the era of capital punishment it did not appear just to hang a person when Parliament had not expressly laid down a rule which covered the situation. In the time when parliamentary intervention was rare, and even today murder is a common law offence, judges said that the law they made was the epitome of reason, and any changes made by Parliament should be narrowly read. Lord Reid said in *Sweet v Parsley* [1970] AC 132 (HL): 'It is a universal principle that if a penal provision is reasonably capable of two interpretations, that interpretation which is most favourable to the accused must be adopted.' Modern-day judges seem at times to have gone to the other extreme: 'Here is a naughty or nasty person; he ought to be guilty of something; therefore let's make him guilty of something.' Examples can be taken especially from Chapter 15 on theft, where the judges have sought to sustain charges which look as if they should have been brought under different sections. The effect is to make the law both unclear and, at times, inconsistent. The House of Lords' decision in *Kassim* [1992] 1 AC 9 may do something to halt this development. The accused was charged with procuring the execution of valuable securities, cheques, by deception contrary to s 20(2) of the Theft Act 1968 (see now the Fraud Act 2006). Lord Ackner allowed the accused's appeal on the ground that 'execution' bore a specific meaning which did not cover paying out under a cheque. The correct charge was under s 15 of the same Act, obtaining property (money) by deception (see now the crime of fraud contrary to s 1 of the Fraud Act 2006).

The lawyers had by the middle of the twentieth century adopted what is called the literal approach to the construction of statutes. *Fisher v Bell* [1961] 1 QB 394 exemplifies this literal rule. A shopkeeper was charged with the offence of offering a flick-knife for sale when he had displayed it in his window. Parliament had decided that flick-knives were dangerous and it wanted them not to be sold. One might have thought that the Divisional Court would reason like this: 'A flick-knife is dangerous; a person who puts one into his shop window wishes to sell a dangerous item; therefore he is guilty of offering that knife for sale.' However, Lord Parker C. J. ruled that what the shopkeeper had done was not to offer the knife for sale, but to invite passers-by to come into the shop and offer to buy it, therefore the accused was not guilty. His method of analysis is sometimes known as 'conceptual'. He worked from one category to the next with the result that the accused was set free (to the evident chagrin of Parliament which changed the law the following year: the accused would now be guilty). Besides issues of sovereignty of Parliament, there was no compulsion on Lord Parker C. J. to adopt the categories of contract law in criminal law, but his use of such categories demonstrates how statutes can be interpreted to convict or acquit the accused. For a recent House of Lords decision applying the literal rule, see **Bentham** [2005] 1 WLR 1057. It was held that the accused did not have 'in his possession, an imitation firearm' when he pointed his fingers under his jacket at the time of a robbery. He did not possess his own fingers within the meaning of the statute.

The House of Lords took a different approach with regard to criminal statutes. In *Attorney-General's Reference (No. 1 of 1988)* cited above, it adopted what is called the 'purposive' approach. Lord Lowry said that judges should use the context of the offence in the statute in order to effect Parliament's purpose.

The case involved insider-dealing. The accused had received confidential information about prices of shares. A company was on the point of being taken over. He was charged with obtaining such information. The trial judge ruled that he had not obtained the information 'by purpose and effort'. He had simply received it while talking to a person from a merchant bank. The Attorney-General referred the matter to the Court of Appeal and it went to the House of Lords, the principal speech being delivered by Lord Lowry. He said:

(a) The dictionary definition of 'obtained' covered both getting possession by effort and acquiring (with or without effort). In other words, there were two meanings of 'obtained' in ordinary language. The former was the primary meaning, the latter the secondary or general one.

(b) The principle about the strict construction of penal statutes applied only in cases of real doubt. It was not sufficient that there was an ambiguity.

(c) The question therefore was whether Parliament intended to use the word in its primary or secondary meaning. Only if it was the latter was the accused guilty. The undesirability of the information being used did not depend on whether the accused had acquired it effortfully or effortlessly. The White Paper on which the relevant statute was based contemplated the mischief as being the possession of the information, not the mode of acquisition. The act of procuring is not the actus reus ('guilty act'): why should the accused be prohibited from using only some of the confidential information? 'The object of the legislation must be partially defeated if the narrow meaning of "obtained" is adopted.' The narrow meaning would also lead to fine distinctions.

The contrary arguments were rebutted. 'Obtain' can mean 'obtain by endeavour' in some statutes, e.g. Theft Act 1968, s 15 (now repealed), but that meaning does not apply in all contexts. The case was not one of a proper meaning and a loose (or inaccurate) one:

it was of a primary and secondary meaning, both of which were correct. Accordingly, the wider meaning was adopted, with the effect that those who received snippets of confidential information from insider-traders were liable, and the matter should not have been withdrawn from the jury.

In *Attorney-General's Reference (No. 1 of 1991)* [1993] QB 94 (CA) the accused entered keystrokes in a computer to give himself a 70 per cent discount at his former firm. The trial judge said that the offence charged was directed at computer hacking. Hacking required access to one computer by means of another. The accused had, however, accessed only one computer. The Court of Appeal would have convicted. 'The plain and natural meaning' of the statutory words was clear. Access to one computer was sufficient. Since there was no ambiguity, there was no need to discuss the mischief against which the trial court thought Parliament had acted. Indeed the mischief goes wider than hacking: it includes industrial espionage through the use of a computer, whether that computer is accessed by another or otherwise.

There is a tension between the freedom of the individual and not letting the 'obviously guilty' go. Part of this tension was noted by Professor Ashworth 'Interpreting criminal statutes: a crisis of legality?' (1991) 107 LQR 419 at 443–444:

> If one of the aims of the criminal law is to convict those who culpably cause harm, this con-stitutes a policy goal which should form part of the doctrine of criminal law and which may properly enter into decisions on interpretation. The claim here is not that criminal laws should be extended retrospectively to citizens' conduct, but rather that people who knowingly 'sail close to the wind' should not be surprised if the law is interpreted so as to include their conduct.

Furthermore:

> There are several points on which modern systems typically depart from the principle of maximum certainty (e.g. the requirement for causation, the distinction between prepara-tion and attempt, the definition of recklessness [see Chapters 2, 10 and 3 respectively]). To aim for maximum certainty in all these cases might minimise judicial discretion (and with it discriminatory practices and casual inconsistency), but it might equally lead to inflexible provisions which fail to draw distinctions in fair places and which result in the acquittal of some persons who should be convicted.

The strict construction of criminal statutes imposing liability never extended to defences, few of which are statutory. The Law Commission, always ready to reduce the width of fault terms, especially recklessness, continues to propose that some defences should not be defined in statute in order to allow for judicial development. One must not be misled by such protestations. It is as easy to find examples of courts narrowing defences (e.g. duress) as it is to see their widening them (e.g. provocation: see *Camplin* [1978] AC 705 (HL)).

As on the civil side, criminal courts may look at *Hansard* and law reform reports to find the mischief that an Act of Parliament was designed to fill but cannot use them to determine the width of the statutory words where there is no ambiguity, obscurity or absurdity: *Pepper* v *Hart* [1993] AC 593 (HL). There is recent authority that this rule should not be used to extend criminal liability when the words of the statute on their own are not such that the accused is guilty: *Thet* v *DPP* [2007] 2 All ER 425 (DC). However, *Thet* v *DPP* was distinguished in **Tabnack** [2007] 2 Cr App R 34. It was said that *Thet* applied when the prosecution sought to rely on parliamentary debates, not where the defence did.

Classification of offences by origin: can judges make new criminal laws?

Common law crimes are those created by judges such as murder laws (see Chapter 11). There are other ways in which 'common law' is used, but it is this sense which is used in this book. Statutory offences are those created by Parliament such as criminal damage (see Chapter 18). By far the vast majority of offences nowadays are statutory ones. Parliament often creates offences; it rarely unmakes them.

Judges have renounced the power to make new criminal offences: *Knuller (Publishing, Printing and Promotions) Ltd* v *DPP* [1973] AC 435 and *DPP* v *Withers* [1975] AC 842, both decisions of the House of Lords. A more recent House of Lords authority is *Jones* [2006] UKHL 16. This abnegation contrasts sharply with the strongly expressed view of the same court in *Shaw* v *DPP* [1962] AC 220, a case involving the publication of the names, addresses and sexual services of female prostitutes, that 'there remains in the courts of law a residual power to enforce the supreme and fundamental purpose of the law to conserve not only the safety and order but also the moral welfare of the state'. The case involved a controversial social problem, and a matter on which Parliament had had its say only a short while previously. On both counts the House of Lords should not have intervened. *Shaw* v *DPP* was a breach of the principle of legality discussed on the first page of this book. There is nowadays little doubt that there exists a crime of outraging public decency, but that determination took 30 years after *Shaw* to occur. The Court of Appeal, while saying that it was not doing so, reasserted the power to create new crimes when it held in *R* [1991] 2 All ER 257 that husbands were liable when they had sexual intercourse with their wives without their consent. The judgment was upheld by the House of Lords ([1992] 1 AC 599), despite the fact that since the early eighteenth century at the latest the general rule had been that a husband was exempt from conviction for rape of his wife. The removal of exceptions is equivalent to creating new offences, and both lead to uncertainty in the law. Compare the stance of Lord Reid in *Shaw*: '[w]here Parliament fears to tread it is not for the Courts to rush in'. *Shaw* and *Knuller* are presumably wrong now that the courts in England and Wales have been given the duty to apply the European Convention on Human Rights by the Human Rights Act 1998.

In *C* v *DPP* [1996] 1 AC 1, a decision before the Human Rights Act 1998 came into force, Lord Lowry, with whom the other Law Lords concurred, laid down five principles:

(1) If the solution is doubtful, the judges should beware of imposing their own remedy; (2) caution should prevail if Parliament has rejected opportunities of clearing up a known difficulty or has legislated while leaving the difficulty untouched; (3) disputed matters of social policy are less suitable areas for judicial intervention than purely legal problems; (4) fundamental legal doctrines should not be lightly set aside; (5) judges should not make a change unless they can achieve finality and certainty.

For all these reasons Lord Lowry rejected a lower court's attempt to abolish the rebuttable presumption that children aged over 10 but under 14 are legally incapable of committing crimes. (It was for similar reasons that the House of Lords in *Kingston* [1995] 2 AC 355 refused to create a broad involuntary intoxication defence and in *Clegg* [1995] 1 AC 482 denied a defence of excessive self-defence because the decision to reduce the offence from murder to manslaughter in such circumstances was one for Parliament, though Lord Lloyd was willing to change the law, even where questions of social policy are involved.) Cases such as *Shaw* would not survive the application of Lord Lowry's five principles: at least principle (3) was broken. It is interesting to compare these guidelines with recent judge-made changes in the law. For example, the reader is invited to consider how many of them were breached when the House of Lords abolished the husband's immunity in rape (*R* [1992] 1 AC 599). This decision was not foreseeable in, say, 1970. It has to be said that the major judicial changes to the law in the last 40 years would probably not all fall foul of these guidelines. The various attempts to define intention and recklessness, discussed in Chapter 3, would be permissible under them.

The House of Lords in *Jones* [2006] UKHL 16 said that the courts could no longer create offences. That task was for Parliament. That was so even when what was proposed to be introduced in Anglo-Welsh law was already a crime in customary international law, that of aggression against a state. It is 'an important democratic principle in this country', said Lord Bingham, 'that it is for those representing the people of the country in Parliament, not the executive and not the judges, to decide what conduct should be treated as lying so far outside the bounds of what is acceptable in our society as to attract criminal penalties.'

Power in the judges to create new offences is not needed in a democracy, and the judiciary realises that it should not in theory invent new criminal laws. That is the reason why in *R* the court maintained that it was not doing so. Courts do not have the socioeconomic information which Parliament has when deciding to enact Bills, e.g. England has no 'Brandeis' brief which the USA has to decide the effect of decisions either way, though the growing practice in some areas of law to have a barrister briefed as *amicus curiae* (literally 'friend of the court') may go some way to remedy this lack, and they do not have the power to supervise the implementation of their judgments which Parliament has in order to implement statutes. Parliament does not always pass statutes on controversial matters and some statutes are not drafted well or integrated into existing law, but the constitutional theory is plain: Parliament enacts laws and the courts apply them. This doctrine of parliamentary legislative sovereignty is under attack in European Union matters, but in criminal law the thesis stands. Parliament, moreover, can legislate whenever it wishes and in such manner as the government of the day thinks fit. It does not have to wait for the point to be brought before it by the prosecution as the courts do. And the judges are restricted to dealing with the very point before them: any point which is not relevant to the decision is called an *obiter dictum*, which need not be applied in later cases (see also the next section). Parliament can therefore enact statutes directed at evils, often called mischiefs, if the government so wishes. In the not too distant past, it fairly quickly passed, e.g., the Prohibition of Female Circumcision Act 1985, the Computer Misuse Act 1990 and the Theft (Amendment) Act 1996. To allow the judiciary, which is not democratically accountable, to invent new offences gives it too much power.

Sometimes, however, Parliament does not act and the courts may, with some reluctance, decide as a result to change the law. Lord Millett in *K* [2002] 1 AC 462 made a heartfelt plea:

> ... The age of consent has long since ceased to reflect ordinary life, and in this respect Parliament has signally failed to discharge its responsibility for keeping the criminal law in touch with the needs of society. I am persuaded that the piecemeal introduction of the various elements of s 14 [of the Sexual Offences Act 1956, the crime of indecent assault, since repealed], coupled with the persistent failure of Parliament to rationalise this branch of the law even to the extent of removing absurdities which the courts have identified, means that we ought not to strain after internal coherence even in a single offence. Injustice is too high a price to pay for consistency.

The general acceptance by the judges that they are constitutionally unable to create new crimes does not extend to two matters. The first is that they can apply present law to new circumstances though the line between not creating new crimes and extending old ones may be narrow. There are offences under ss 23–24 of the Offences Against the Person Act 1861 of administering a noxious thing to a person. If the accused made up a bag containing glue and invited his best friend to sniff it, the court would have to decide whether the glue was a noxious thing and whether, if so, it was administered within the meaning of the statute. The law is already in existence but the problem is new. A similar decision was reached by the House of Lords in *Ireland*; *Burstow* [1998] 1 AC 147, where it was held that although the drafter of the 1861 statute did not have psychiatric harm in mind, nevertheless the statute was to be interpreted according to late twentieth-century definitions and therefore 'harm' included 'psychiatric harm.' In the jargon of the law the 1861 Act is 'ever-speaking'. (For a statute dealing with selling glue-sniffing kits, see the Intoxicating Substances (Supply) Act 1985: English courts could not have phrased the crime in the way Parliament did.) Secondly, the judges have not eschewed the creation of new defences. The development of the defence of duress of circumstances (see Chapter 7) has largely undercut the previous general non-recognition of necessity as a defence. The Law Commission proposed in its Report No. 218, *Legislating the Criminal Code – Offences against the Person and General Principles*, 1993, to endorse the judicial creation and development of defences 'either to recognise changing circumstances or to piece out unjustified gaps in the existing defences' (para 27.8). The three principles of non-creation of new offences, the application of old offences to new facts, and the possible development of new defences, will be maintained under the draft Criminal Code, if enacted (see later in this chapter). Perhaps the ability to create new defences should be restricted to excuses (see Chapter 7), where one is looking at the mental state of the accused, not at whether his behaviour was justified. The law should lay down what is justified.

The enactment of the draft Criminal Code (see later in this chapter) would not abolish common law offences. Wide offences such as public nuisance and conspiracy to defraud would remain.

Evidential and legal burdens of proof

English criminal law to a large extent gives the accused the benefit of the doubt (the work of Ashworth and Blake cited in the Further Reading section does, however, demonstrate that 40 per cent of the offences triable on indictment reverse the presumption of innocence; the authors write of the casual manner in which Parliament has placed the burden of persuasion on the accused). Triers of fact, whether juries, magistrates or District Judges (Magistrates' Court), are to convict only if they are sure of the accused's guilt. Punishment should be applied only when it is certain that the accused committed the offence. The principle and exceptions to it are detailed in this section.

There is a distinction between the evidential and legal burden of proof. The difference may be illustrated by reference to automatism (see Chapter 9). Before the accused can rely on this defence, he must put forward some evidence that he was acting automatically when he, say, hit his lover over the head with a heavy ashtray. The evidence might consist of a witness's saying that he saw what happened or a psychiatrist's drafting a report. In legal terms he has to adduce or lead evidence. If he does not adduce such evidence, his plea will fail at that stage and the prosecution does not have to lead evidence

For more on automatism as a defence, see Chapter 9. This is illustrated in Figure 9.3 on p 380.

that his plea ought not to succeed. If he does, the prosecution has to disprove that he was acting automatically. His burden is called the evidential burden or onus of proof. The prosecution's burden is the legal one.

Evidential burden

The evidential burden means that the accused has to adduce evidence that may raise a doubt in the minds of reasonable jurors. As can be seen from the above, in most offences the Crown does not need to negative any defence the accused might have. It has to show the *actus reus* and *mens rea*, if any. If the defendant wishes to rely on a defence, he must raise it and show evidence in support, as Lord Diplock said with regard to mistake in **Sweet v Parsley** [1970] AC 132. The same can be said about self-defence, automatism and duress.

Legal burden

In most areas of the criminal law the prosecution must prove both the *actus reus* and the *mens rea* 'beyond reasonable doubt'. That means that the triers of fact (jury or magistrates) must be sure that the accused was guilty. If authority is needed for this proposition, it may be found in the famous speech of Viscount Simon in **Mancini v DPP** [1942] AC 1, which changed previous law:

> No matter what the charge or where the trial the principle that the prosecution must prove the guilt of the prisoner [the old-fashioned word for the accused] is part of the common law of England and no attempt to whittle it down can be entertained.

The 'Golden Thread' of English criminal law is the duty of the prosecution to prove guilt beyond a reasonable doubt. As regards the decision of **Mancini v DPP**, J. C. Smith wrote ('The presumption of innocence' (1987) 38 NILQ 223 at 224): 'Never, in my opinion, has the House of Lords done more noble a deed in the field of criminal law than on that day.' A more modern statement is that of Hodgson LJ in **More** [1987] 1 WLR 1578: 'The prosecution's first task is to satisfy each juror . . . that every ingredient of the offence has been made out.' This principle also applies to inchoate offences (see Chapter 10) even when Parliament has placed the burden on the accused in respect of the full crime.

The same principle applies to most defences. The prosecution has, e.g., to disprove duress and self-defence. Older cases to the contrary are no longer authoritative. To this principle there are three, perhaps four, exceptions. These exceptions have come in for criticism. Article 6(2) of the European Convention on Human Rights states that anyone 'charged with a criminal offence shall be presumed innocent until proved guilty according to the law'. The jurisprudence of the European Court of Human Rights is unhelpful to the accused: no challenge to placing the burden on defendants has so far been successful. However, the House of Lords by a majority of four to one ruled in **Lambert** [2002] 2 AC 545, in reliance on Article 6(2), that the phrase 'it shall be a defence for the accused to prove . . .' in s 28(2) of the Misuse of Drugs Act 1971 was to be interpreted contrary to previous authorities as imposing only an evidential burden on the accused. This is a remarkable interpretation, despite the presumption of innocence found in Article 6(2). See also the discussion below. It was unclear at the time whether or not this decision changed all other reverse onus decisions. It is thought not. Lord Steyn expressly spoke to that effect and no one disagreed. It was an extremely important decision. In **C** [2002] Crim LR 316 it was held that placing the onus on the accused to prove the lack of an intent to defraud once the prosecution had proved the concealment of a debt breached Article 6(2). However, the same Court in *L v DPP* [2002] Crim LR 320 decided that placing the burden on the accused to prove that he had a good reason or lawful authority to carry a lock-knife in a public place once the prosecution had proved that he did possess that type of knife in a public place did not contravene Article 6(2). The court said that it was not disproportionate to place the onus on the accused. Similar is *Sliney v Havering London Borough Council* (2002) 20 November, unreported (CA). The court took into account the provision's social context, the effectiveness of the law and the maximum sentence.

There has been something of a retreat from *Lambert* and the current position is that reverse burdens of proof can be justified under Article 6(2). In *Johnstone* [2003] 1 WLR 1736 (HL) Lord Nicholls said: 'The court will reach a different conclusion from the legislature [as to the reverse burden] only when it is apparent the legislature has attached insufficient importance to the fundamental right of an individual to be presumed innocent until proven guilty.' The Court of Appeal followed *Johnstone* in preference to *Lambert* in *Attorney-General's Reference (No. 4 of 2004)* [2005] 1 WLR 2819 as being the later authority. The case provides a list of factors. On appeal, where the case is also known as *Sheldrake*, [2005] 1 AC 264 the Lords said that the true question for each offence was whether a reverse burden was consistent with a fair trial. They resurrected *Lambert*, holding that due deference should be paid to the fact that Parliament has imposed onus on the accused. Previous cases mentioned in the last paragraph were approved. The law was summarised by Lord Bingham: 'relevant to any judgment on reasonableness or proportionality will be the opportunity given to the defendant to rebut the presumption, maintenance of the rights of the defendant, flexibility in the application of the presumption, retention by the court of a power to assess the evidence, the importance of what is at stake and the difficulty which a prosecution may face in the absence of a presumption'. The latest case is *Keogh* [2007] EWCA Crim 528. The court held that ss 2–3 of the Official Secrets Act 1989, which placed the legal burden of proof on the accused, were to be read as imposing only an evidential burden on him because to place the legal burden on him would be 'disproportionate and unjustifiable' particularly because the accused would have to disprove a major element of the offence.

Insanity

For more on insanity as a defence, see Chapter 9. This is illustrated in Figure 9.1 on p 356.

For the accused to have this defence he must show that he was insane at the time of the offence. The standard of proof is on the 'balance of probabilities'. That phrase means in effect that if it is more likely than not that the accused was insane, he has the defence. This standard was stated in cases such as *Sodeman v R* [1936] 2 All ER 1138, a decision of the Privy Council (PC) which has been accepted as stating English law. The legal reason assigned for this exception is that every person is presumed to be sane; therefore, the accused must prove insanity: *M'Naghten* (1843) [1843–60] All ER Rep 229. The effect is that if the jurors are not certain either way, the accused does not have this defence. The principal justification for reversing the burden of proof is that the accused has some particular knowledge. For instance, in the crime of possessing articles for suspected terrorist purposes, the defendant has to prove that the articles were not for a terrorist purpose; that information is within his knowledge. In *DPP, ex parte Kebilene* [2000] 2 AC 326 (HL) Lord Hope referred to the nature of the threat (e.g. terrorism) which the statutory provision is designed to combat. Lord Steyn, with whom Lords Slynn and Cooke agreed, said that the reverse burden of proof found in the Prevention of Terrorism Act 1989 could be read as merely placing the evidential burden on the accused.

Parliament's expressly placing the burden on the accused

As stated in Viscount Simon's speech in **Mancini v DPP**, quoted above, the general rule about onus of proof is a matter of the common law. Parliament can alter the burden by statute and has done so on several occasions. The following are examples. Section 4(1) of the Explosive Substances Act 1883 affords a defence if the accused is able to prove that he made the material for a lawful purpose. By s 2 of the Homicide Act 1957 the accused must prove that he has the defence of diminished responsibility. This reverse burden of proof does not violate Article 6(1) of the European Convention on Human Rights. One problem with s 2 occurs when the defence of diminished responsibility and provocation are pleaded together. The prosecution has to disprove provocation and the defence has to prove diminished responsibility. Yet both may arise out of the same facts. By s 1 of the Prevention of Crime Act 1953, the accused has a defence if he can show that he had lawful authority or reasonable excuse to carry an offensive weapon. By s 6 of the Public Order Act 1986 which defines riot:

For more on the defence of diminished responsibility, see Chapter 9. This is illustrated in Figure 9.2 on p 368.

> . . . a person whose awareness is impaired by intoxication shall be taken to be aware of that which he would be aware if not intoxicated, unless he shows either that his intoxication was not self-induced or that it was caused solely by the taking or administering of a substance in the course of medical treatment.

'Shows' was meant to place the legal burden on the accused, but it could be read as placing only the evidential burden on him. The Law Commission proposed in its Report No. 229, *Legislating the Criminal Code: Intoxication and Criminal Liability*, 1995, that the burden should be placed on the prosecution.

Following **Lambert** presumably many legal burdens placed on the defence when an element of the offence is under discussion should now be read as imposing only evidential burdens. While these provisions are seen as exceptional, that perception is not necessarily true. Andrew Ashworth ('Is criminal law a lost cause?' (2000) 116 LQR 225 at 228) reported the outcome of a survey he carried out of crimes created in 1997. He found that 'the bulk of new offences is characterised by . . . reverse onus provisions for exculpation. [Such a feature lies] a considerable distance from the conception of criminal law held by many university teachers and criminal practitioners. Indeed [it is] inconsistent with prominent elements of English criminal law – . . . that . . . the prosecution bears the burden of proving guilt.' Where Parliament places the burden of proof on the accused, the standard of proof is on the balance of probabilities, unless Parliament states otherwise.

'Exception, exemption, proviso, excuse or qualification' in a statutory offence

In **Hunt** [1987] AC 352 the accused was charged with the unlawful possession of morphine contrary to s 5(2) of the Misuse of Drugs Act 1971. The Misuse of Drugs Regulations 1973, Sch 1, para 3 provided:

> [a]ny preparation of medicinal . . . morphine containing not more than 0.2 per cent of morphine . . . being a preparation compounded with one or more . . . ingredients in such a way that . . . the morphine cannot be recovered by readily applicable means or in a yield which would constitute a risk to health . . .

was not within s 5. The prosecution did not lead evidence to show the percentage of morphine in the powder in possession of which the accused had been found. The other ingredients in the powder were caffeine and atropine. The House of Lords allowed his appeal.

The simplest speech was delivered by Lord Templeman. The prosecution had put forward facts which might or might not show that the accused was guilty. It was not proved that the accused possessed more than 0.2 per cent of morphine. Lord Ackner held that Parliament could place the burden of proof on the accused either expressly or 'by necessary implication'. When deciding whether the burden was by implication on the accused, the court had to look not just at the language of the enactment but also at its substance and effect. The practical consequences could also be investigated.

> If the result of holding that the burden of proof . . . would make the prosecution . . . particularly difficult or burdensome with the consequence that the purpose of the legislation would be significantly frustrated, then this would be a relevant consideration to weigh against the grammatical form of legislation.

On the facts the prosecution had merely to obtain an analyst's report. Therefore, the burden remained on the Crown.

The principal speech was delivered by Lord Griffiths, with whom Lords Keith and Mackay agreed.

(a) Statute could place the burden of proof impliedly on the accused. Previous authorities have so held and if the rule were otherwise the laws in the Crown Court and magistrates' courts would be out of line (see (c) below). In criticism, it may be said that this implied exception represents a serious unravelling of the 'golden thread' that the burden of proof is on the prosecution.

(b) Lord Wilberforce was correct to say in **Nimmo v Alexander Cowan & Sons Ltd** [1968] AC 107 (HL on appeal from Scotland) that 'exceptions etc., are to be set up by those who rely on them'.

(c) The Court of Appeal in **Edwards** [1975] QB 27, which was to be upheld on its own facts, had said that the burden lay on the accused when Parliament had enacted offences 'which prohibit the doing of an act save in specified circumstances or by persons of specified classes or with specified qualifications or with the licence or permission of specified authorities'. This rule, which the Court of Appeal had treated as being one of law, was in truth a guide to construction for 'each case must turn upon the construction of the particular legislation'.

The rule in **Edwards** in any case suffered from the defect that it did not rest on a solid distinction between the definition of the offence and the exception to that definition. For instance, suppose that there is a law providing that 'no one shall enter the County of North Yorkshire without a passport'. This law could be rephrased as 'no one shall enter the County of North Yorkshire, except when that person has obtained a passport'. The two versions mean the same thing, but if the rule in **Edwards** were correct, the accused would have to prove that he had a passport in the second version, whereas in the first version the prosecution would have to disprove that he did have a passport. The illustration shows how absurd **Edwards** was. One can reformulate offence and defence into a narrow offence.

The same rule applies whether trial is on indictment or summary: that is, whether in the Crown Court or in the Magistrates' Courts. If the former, **Hunt** applies. If the latter, s 101 of the Magistrates' Courts Act 1980 stipulates that:

> Where the defendant . . . relies for his defence on any exception, exemption, proviso, excuse or qualification . . . , the burden of proving the exception [etc] shall be on him.

J. C. Smith, in his 1987 article above, noted the failure to apply s 101, especially to lawful excuse and lawful authority defences. An example is belief in the consent of the victim, had he known of the circumstances, in the offence of criminal damage. However, in general the main effect of **Hunt** is to place the burden on the accused when a statutory defence is provided.

After **Hunt**, therefore, the rule about exceptions is one of construction, not of law: it is one of statutory interpretation. Either way offences (ones which may be tried either in the Crown Court or the Magistrates' Courts) are therefore treated the same in the Crown Court and magistrates' courts.

(d) Where Parliament places the burden of proof on the accused, he bears the legal burden and not just the evidential one.

(e) On the facts the burden of proof remained on the prosecution. As it is an offence to have morphine in one form but not in another, the prosecution must prove that the morphine was in the prohibited form. If it could not do so, the accused was acquitted. It was easy for the accused, for the substance may have been seized by the police or may be in too small a quantity for further analysis or might have been destroyed by analysis. Moreover, since possession of drugs was a strict offence (see Chapter 4), ambiguity should be resolved in the accused's favour. Paragraph 3 of Sch 1 to the Misuse of Drugs Regulations 1973, therefore, did not state the exception but what the prosecution had to prove.

The types of argument utilised in **Hunt** will be used in later cases to decide whether an exception in a statute (the rule is inapplicable to common law offences, since it is one of statutory construction) places the burden of proof on the accused. Doing so has to be justified and could not be justified simply on the basis of the grammar of the section containing the offence. In deciding whether Parliament intended to place the burden on the accused, one should look at the practicalities. If one side would have serious difficulty in proving something, there was an inference that that party did not bear the burden. It was also a factor whether the crime was serious or not. If it was serious, it was more likely than not that the prosecution bore the onus. The burden was not likely to be placed on the accused, for it ought not easily to be held that Parliament did not intend to protect the innocent. However, it has to be said that the House of Lords in **Hunt** could have put the burden of proof on the prosecution, subject to Parliament expressly stating otherwise. It would have then been for Parliament and not the courts to decide. It should be for the elected government to make such choices. **Hunt** will no doubt come in for more and more criticism as the thrust of **Lambert** is accepted by the English courts.

The first case to apply **Hunt** was **Alath Construction Ltd** [1990] 1 WLR 1255. Developers were charged with felling a tree which was subject to a preservation order, contrary to the Town and Country Planning Act 1971. The accused company contended that it was not guilty because it had a defence within that statute that the tree was dangerous. The Court of Appeal ruled that this defence was an exception for the purposes of **Hunt** and accordingly the burden was on the accused. The court considered that its decision was justified by the structure of the Act (the crime was in one section, the defence in another), the language of the defence (the terms of the subsection which created the defence began 'without prejudice to any other exceptions . . .', implying that the defence granted was also an exception), and the practicalities of knowing whether the tree was dangerous (developers were more likely to know of the danger than the local authority, which has the duty to safeguard protected trees). The court distinguished **Hunt** on the ground that it concerned dangerous drugs, which had nothing to do with tree preservation orders.

From the viewpoint of **Hunt**, **Alath** is open to criticism.

(a) In **Hunt** it did not matter that the offence and defence were in separate sections, while in **Alath** the separation was used to justify holding the defence to be an exception.

(b) **Hunt** frowned on the use of the statute's language to determine whether the defence was an exception for the purposes of allocating the burden of proof, yet the Court of Appeal in **Alath** did just that. Moreover, the wording of the exception reads like a narrowing of the definition of the offence rather than an exemption to the offence: the accused is not guilty because the tree was dangerous, not the accused is exempt from conviction because the tree was dangerous.

It might also be argued that since Parliament did not determine which party should bear the burden of proof, Parliament impliedly left the onus on the prosecution as a matter of the law of evidence.

Lord Steyn in **Lambert** expressly stated that the revision of the law found in that case did not affect the law laid down in **Edwards**.

Autrefois acquit and autrefois convict

It may be that the burden of proof lies on the accused to prove that he has been previously acquitted or convicted in a criminal trial.

Two matters concerning the burden of proof

(a) Before 1935 it was said that where the accused had caused the victim's death, he had to show that he did not have the *mens rea* for murder. This burden was placed on the prosecution in **Woolmington v DPP** [1935] AC 462.

> Throughout the web of the English criminal law one golden thread is always to be seen, that is the duty of the prosecution to prove the prisoner's guilt.

Those words of Lord Sankey have often been repeated, but they do not explain why the golden thread does not run through insanity and the statutory exceptions. The contrary argument, which is not tied to murder, is that the accused is best placed to explain his conduct. If, e.g., the victim is shot dead by a bullet from a smoking gun held by the accused, who coveted his wife, one might say that to put the burden of proof onto the prosecution is absurd. No doubt the triers of fact take a robust view on such facts.

(b) Under the influence of **DPP v Smith** [1961] AC 290 (HL) it was thought that a person intended to do what the natural consequences of his behaviour were. In legal terms a man was presumed to intend the natural consequences of his behaviour. If this presumption was ever irrebuttable, s 8 of the Criminal Justice Act 1967 abolished it.

> A court or jury in determining whether a person has committed an offence (a) shall not be bound in law to infer that he intended or foresaw a result of his actions by reason only of its being a natural and probable consequence of those actions, but (b) shall decide whether he did intend or foresee that result by reference to all the evidence, drawing such inferences from the evidence as appear properly in the circumstances.

Section 8 deals with *how* to prove intention or foresight. It deals with the law of evidence or procedure. It is not concerned with the substantive criminal law, which is the subject of this book. Therefore, it does not affect the substantive law of murder. One might have expected that since s 8 does not affect the substantive law of murder, the ruling in *DPP v Smith* that the *mens rea* for murder includes what a reasonable person in the position of the accused would have foreseen would continue to apply after the 1957 Act, but in fact courts quickly held that this part of *DPP v Smith* was overruled by s 8. This surprising stance continues to be taken, as can be seen in the decision of the House of Lords in *Woollin* [1999] AC 82.

The section applies only to the accused's intention or foresight. Beyond those states of mind the common law governs. Section 8 is stated to apply to intention and foresight of results, but the same rule applies at common law to circumstances: *DPP v Morgan* [1976] AC 182 (HL). It does not apply where the accused does not have to intend or foresee a consequence. In manslaughter by gross negligence the accused is guilty whether or not he realised that death might result. The same is true of crimes of negligence. As a result of judicial construction s 8 does not apply where the accused was intoxicated. The section refers to the jury's taking into account 'all the evidence'. The House of Lords in *DPP v Majewski* [1977] AC 433 determined that 'all the evidence' meant 'all the legally relevant evidence'. Since intoxication is no defence to so-called basic intent offences it is not part of the evidence with regard to the offences.

Reform

The Law Commission's draft Criminal Code, cl 13, provides:

(1) Unless otherwise provided –
  (a) the burden of proving every element of an offence and any other fact alleged or relied on by the prosecution is on the prosecution;
  (b) where evidence is given (whether by the defendant or the prosecution) of a defence or any other fact alleged or relied on by the defendant the burden is on the prosecution to prove that an element of the defence or such other fact did not exist.

(2) Evidence is given of a defence or any other fact alleged or relied on by the defendant when there is such evidence as might lead a court or jury to conclude that there is a reasonable possibility that the element of the defence or such other fact existed.

There is a saving for pre-Code offences in which case s 101 of the Magistrates' Courts Act 1980 or 'any corresponding rule or interpretation applying on trial on indictment' (i.e. *Hunt*) continues to apply (cl 13(6)). The standard of proof is, unless otherwise provided, beyond reasonable doubt if the prosecution bears the legal burden or on the balance of probabilities if the accused bears it (cl 13(4)), except if a defence is wholly or partly based on showing that someone else was guilty, in which event the burden of proof is beyond reasonable doubt (cl 13(5)).

Section 8 of the Criminal Justice Act 1967 is preserved and reformulated in cl 14.

A court or jury, in determining whether a person had, or may have had, a particular state of mind, shall have regard to all the evidence including, where appropriate, the presence or absence of reasonable grounds for having that state of mind.

The draft Code therefore reaffirms the presumption of innocence laid down in *Woolmington v DPP*, above, and widens s 8 of the 1967 Act to cover all 'Code' states of mind. Section 1(2) of the Sexual Offences (Amendment) Act 1976, which stated that a jury may take into account the reasonableness of the mistake in deciding whether the accused (honestly) made a mistake, fell within cl 14; however, the Sexual Offences Act 2003 gives a defence to rape only when the accused formed his belief as to the victim's consent on reasonable grounds. The draft Code also retains the present standards of proof – beyond reasonable doubt when the burden is on the prosecution; on the balance of probabilities when it is on the accused (cl 13(4)).

Article 6(2) of the European Convention on Human Rights states: 'Everyone charged with a criminal offence shall be presumed innocent until proven guilty according to law.' The Convention was incorporated into UK law by the Human Rights Act 1998, which came into force in England on 2 October 2000. Placing the burden of proof on the accused is inconsistent with Article 6(2). The Lords held in *Lambert*, above, that burdens of proof on the accused were evidential and not legal ones. *Lambert* has come in for criticism. Simply substituting 'introduce sufficient evidence' (which is what the evidential burden means) for 'prove' (the legal burden) does not do what their Lordships apparently think it does. They wanted the accused to have a defence only if the jurors were in reasonable doubt; they did not intend the accused to have a defence but to adduce evidence that *may* raise a reasonable doubt.

Criminal law reform, the Law Commission and the draft Criminal Code

The Criminal Law Revision Committee was the first body to take on reform, doing sterling work on the first Theft Act (1968) but it now is moribund. The Law Commission, which was established in 1965, has taken over its role in criminal law and has promoted several major reforms over the last 30 and more years, such as the Criminal Damage Act 1971. Its approach was summarised in Report No. 228, *Conspiracy to Defraud*, 1994, para 1.18:

> The Commission has seen codification of the criminal law as a central feature of [its] work ... The criminal law controls the exercise of state power against citizens, and the protection of citizens against unlawful behaviour, and it is important that its rules should be determined by Parliament and not by the sometimes haphazard methods of common law. This can be achieved only if the law is put into statutory form in a comprehensive manner. It is also important from the standpoints of efficiency, economy and the proper administration of justice that the law should be stated in clear and easily accessible terms.

A comment was made by Buxton J who said extrajudicially ('The Human Rights Act and the substantive criminal law' [2000] Crim LR 331): '. . . the present jumble of ancient statutes, more modern accretions to them, and the acres of judicial pronouncements should be replaced by a criminal code that would set out the criminal law in rational, accessible and modern language'. Arden J wrote to similar effect in 'Criminal law at the crossroads: the impact of human rights from the Law Commission's perspective and the need for a Code' [1999] Crim LR 489: the criminal law should be 'well considered, consistent, coherent and modern', not as it is, 'seriously defective and out of date'. She correctly added that political will is needed.

The Report, *A Criminal Code for England and Wales* (Law Com. No. 177), was published in 1989. A team of three academics had drawn up the preliminary version in *Codification of the Criminal Law: A Report to the Law Commission* Law Com. No. 143, 1985. To emphasise that it is not part of English law but is a body of rules which may in the future be enacted, it is called the draft Criminal Code in this book. The Report consists of a draft Bill, examples of the application of the Bill, and a commentary. General principles are found in Part I of the draft Code. Part II deals with particular offences. The general principles apply to all offences treated in the Code and those created afterwards, including those crimes such as road traffic offences not contained in Part II. It is expected that some crimes not in Part II at present will in time be embodied in it, but that some areas of law, e.g. road traffic offences, will continue to be treated separately because of convenience to the users of legislation. If enacted, the Code will apply to 90 per cent of all indictable offences. It is fairly comprehensive of earlier work of the Commission in areas such as criminal damage, attempts and forgery. The law is not simply restated. There are amendments aimed at clarifying and reforming some parts of the law. For example, the proposals of law reform institutions such as the Criminal Law Revision Committee are incorporated. However, the Law Commission on this occasion did not incorporate all the amendments it thought were called for in criminal law, e.g. in relation to the liability of accomplices. The Law Commission took the view that such changes were for Parliament. It hoped that the draft Code's enactment would reduce the length of trials and appeals and improve access to and understanding of the criminal law. The themes of the draft Code are stated to be accessibility, comprehensibility, consistency and certainty. The need for certainty is of especial importance in the criminal law, which regulates, in part, the relationship between the citizen and the state.

The draft Code came under criticism on several grounds. Under whatever type of Code people in England and Wales live, there will be difficulties of access and coverage. Even with computer monitors it is unlikely that everyone all the time will have access to all the law on a certain topic, and because of the flexibility of the language it may be impossible to tell whether a person is guilty of an offence until he has been tried. If a law bans vehicles from parks, is a child's bicycle, a unicycle, a horse, a horse and cart, a vehicle? The malleability of English language will be reflected in any penal code. The draft Code may, however, be criticised on other grounds. Not all offences are included. Road traffic offences constitute the main omission. (It must be questioned why a serious offence such as causing death by dangerous driving is not to be included, especially when many minor offences are.) Also excluded are *inter alia* drugs offences, many highly specific crimes such as offences in sports stadia and crimes concerned with companies. The Law Commission considered that it would inconvenience users to have such crimes dealt with in the Code, for users would wish to see the excluded parts of the law contained in separate statutes. However, it may be argued that it would be best to have all crimes in one place. The draft Code is not a reforming instrument. Some parts are revised in accordance with recommendations (above), but others which have not been subject to proposals are left unreformed. The draft Code remains open to judicial interpretation on key terms such as intention, and the possibility of inconsistent verdicts on dishonesty in theft remains. The choices of the Law Commission between different views of the law are not always justified by the members. If one form of recklessness is preferred to another in the interests of consistency, it would be just as consistent to choose the second form over the first. The choice should be justified on policy grounds. Those values need to be articulated and applied.

At present the development of criminal law is ill-disciplined. Nevertheless, the attempt to cut out anomalies, put the law into the form it would have been in had the recommendations of reform bodies been enacted, and restate the law in authoritative form is worthwhile. What the draft Code should not do is to lead to preferring the formal virtues of a code to principles of justice. It is no use having an accessible code, a comprehensive code, a consistent code, a certain code, if the values it contains do not strike a balance between social protection and the liberty of the individual. The formal virtues show where the line between the two is: they do not draw it for us. Moreover, the great argument against codification, that it puts the law into a straitjacket, misses the point when it is understood that constitutionally the role of judges in criminal law is not to make law for that is Parliament's task. If Parliament fears to tread, even more strongly the courts should fear to tread. It is suggested that since the coming into force of the Human Rights Act 1998 the need for codification is even stronger than before. The Law Commission has sought to make its recommendations consonant with the European Convention on Human Rights. However, Parliament and the Home Secretaries have rarely listened to the Law Commission's criminal law reports.

Changes from present law

The changes which are proposed in the draft Code, if it were ever to become law, are dealt with in the appropriate place. The following details the changes which affect liability.

(a) *Burden of proof.* The evidential burden in relation to the defence of involuntary intoxication is placed on the accused.

(b) *Minimum fault element.* Unless Parliament ordains differently, the accused will not be guilty unless he adverted to the risk ('subjective recklessness'). The Law Commission used to be strong upholders of the doctrine of 'subjectivism'. An accused was not guilty when he intended to commit the crime or if he knew that he ran the risk of a certain result occurring. In fact the Commission has never fully debated the merits or otherwise of subjectivism as the base line for criminal liability. Since 1989, the Law Commission has sometimes resiled from this proposition. It proposed a new offence of killing by gross carelessness (and a similar offence for companies), recommended that only reasonable mistakes as to consent should give the accused a defence to rape and indecent assault (which indeed became the law as a result of the Sexual Offences Act 2003 but it is doubtful if those who voted in favour of the Bill had the Commission's arguments in mind), and in its Report No. 229 on intoxication has gone back on its proposal in Consultation Paper No. 127 to afford a defence of drunkenness whenever the defendant did not have the state of mind required in the definition of the crime (both the Consultation Paper and the Report were called *Intoxication and the Criminal Law*).

> Subjective recklessness is explained in Chapter 3.

(c) *Defences.* Mistake is to be a defence to all crimes where the accused honestly erred. Reasonableness is not demanded. The law on insanity is completely redrafted. There are changes in the law of duress and intoxication.

(d) *Vicarious and corporate liability.* The doctrine of delegation is abolished. The law on corporations is modified.

(e) *Participation.* Recklessness as to circumstances will be sufficient if sufficient for the principal crime. A person will be exempt if he acts 'with the purpose of avoiding or limiting any harmful consequences of the offence and without the purpose of furthering its commission'.

(f) *Inchoate offences.* The law on so-called 'double inchoate' law is rationalised. Recklessness as to circumstances will be part of the fault element if it is sufficient for the full offence. There will be liability for conspiracy with one's spouse, the victim, and a child under 10. The rule in *Curr* [1968] 2 QB 944 is reversed: the person incited will no longer have to have the fault element of the crime incited. *Fitzmaurice* [1983] QB 1083 will be reversed: impossibility will no longer be a defence to incitement.

(g) *Offences against the person.* The law is substantially revised. The Home Office unusually published a consultation paper in 1998 called *Violence: Reforming the Offences against the Person Act 1861*, with a view to reforming non-fatal offences but at the time of writing there has been no progress. It should be said that this area of law is the most in need of modernisation.

(h) *Sexual offences.* There are some changes but the Sexual Offences Act 2003 and various statutory and judicial changes in the period 1989–2003 have rendered the recommendations somewhat superfluous.

(i) *Theft and other property offences.* Very minor alterations.

The flow of papers and reports from the Law Commission, many of which were handled by the former Commissioner who is now Buxton LJ, has continued unabated. Reports enacted are those which led to the abolition of the year-and-a-day rule in homicide and to the penalisation of mortgage fraudsters. Because of the perceived lack of parliamentary time the Law Commission proposes not to have the Code enacted in one statute but to put forward Bills dealing with various areas which will in the end be consolidated into a code. The approach has been criticised as selective. The first tranche is the Criminal Law Bill found in Report No. 218, *Legislating the Criminal Code – Offences against the Person and General Principles*, 1993. The Home Office consultation paper mentioned above contains the non-fatal offences part of this Report, together with a draft Bill, but the part on general matters is omitted. Later Reports also contain Bills ready for enactment. The government has not enacted any part of the draft Criminal Code, though at the time of writing there is a Bill on corporate killing extant, which is based in part on a Law Commission Report.

As the former chair of the Law Commission, Brooke J, said in (1994) 158 JP 345, much criminal law 'is a disgrace, when judged in terms of simplicity, clarity and accessibility'. Money is being wasted and justice denied because of uncertainties in the law. As Henry LJ said in *Lynsey* [1995] 2 Cr App R 667 in the context of non-fatal offences, courts have better things to do than to administer bad laws. These words were echoed by Brooke LJ in *Baker* [1997] Crim LR 497 (CA). Brooke J was still in charge of the Law Commission when it put forward the second instalment of its attempt to have enacted parts of the 1989 draft Code when it stated that its aim especially in the criminal law was 'to make the law simpler, fairer and cheaper to use': *Legislating the Criminal Code: Intoxication and Criminal Liability*, Report No. 229, 1995, para 1.3. The text of this book demonstrates the truth of his statement. A previous chair of the Law Commission said that unless the government acted quickly, it demonstrated that it was content 'to leave the courts fighting twenty-first century crime with nineteenth-century weapons' ((2000) *The Times*, 15 June, quoted in J. Rowbotham and K. Stevenson 'Social dystopias and legal utopias?' (2000) 9 Nottingham LJ 25 at 37 n 63).

The Law Commission is still working on a code, and since 2002 it has been working on seven parts which would revise the 1989 Draft Criminal Code: external elements especially causation, fault, parties to crime, incapacity and mental disorder, defences, preliminary offences and proof. Work has proceeded slowly because of other projects: partial defences to murder, assisting and encouraging crime, and non-accidental death or serious injury to children. Consultation papers and reports have been published but the government, despite saying in *Criminal Justice: The Way Ahead*, Home Office, 2001, that it favoured a criminal code, is not giving a lead. It prefers to legislate on matters of media concern rather than law reform in the round: that is why the archaic Offences Against the Person Act 1861 remains unrevised.

The next part of this book, General Principles, outlines that area of criminal law which is often called 'the general part'. It is sometimes contended that there is no such concept as 'the general part', merely a wilderness of single instances. Whether there is or is not one is for debate, but the distinction between the general principles and specific offences helps to organise material. One does not need, for example, to repeat the law on duress or accessorial liability each time an offence is mentioned.

Summary

This chapter is concerned with introducing the reader to possible definitions of substantive criminal law and the distinctions between civil and criminal law and to the basic principles or building blocks of the law, in particular the concepts of *actus reus*, *mens rea* and defence, concepts which underlie most of the remainder of the book (see especially Chapters 2–4 and 7–9). Other introductory matters include the appeal system in criminal matters, judicial interpretation of criminal law statutes, the scope for judge-made law in the criminal field, and the effect of the Human Rights Act 1998 on criminal law. It concludes with discussions of the evidential and legal burdens of proof (focusing on the effect of the Human Rights Act on judicial interpretation of statutes) and of codification, especially the role of the Law Commission in constructing the draft Criminal Code 1989 and later attempts at partial codification.

- Fundamental principles of criminal law: Using the approach of Husak in his *Philosophy of Criminal Law* the author guides the reader through the principal constraints on the law of crime: legality, *actus reus*, *mens rea*, concurrence (usually known in England and Wales as 'contemporaneity'), harm, causation, defences, and proof beyond reasonable doubt). Many of these elements such as *actus reus*, *mens rea* and defences are discussed at length in later chapters but here the focus is on legality, particularly in the context of Article 7(1) of the European Convention on Human Rights (ECHR), the right not to be convicted of an offence which did not previously exist, the right against retrospectivity of the criminal law.

- Human Rights Act 1998: This statute 'brings home' particularly those human rights found in the European Convention. The Act has not had a major effect so far (for example, it is not contrary to the Convention to have offences of strict liability: see Chapter 4 for the meaning of such crimes) but it could greatly affect current definitions of offences and defences, e.g. the law on consent may be contrary to Article 8, respect for private life, and insanity looks certain to be contrary to Article 5, the right to liberty.

- Attempted definitions of a crime: Over the years various definitions of a 'crime' have been made but the standard definition is the circular one of 'a legal wrong that can be followed by criminal proceedings which may result in punishment'. (Glanville Williams).

- Differences between criminal and civil law: Among differences are terminology, courts, procedure and outcome of trials.

- Hierachy of courts: The vast majority of criminal law cases start in the magistrates' courts where cases are heard by magistrates or by District Judges (Magistrates' Court), who were previously called 'stipendiaries'; only the very serious offences are heard in the Crown Court, where the decision is taken by the jury after hearing the judge's instruction. Appeals from the Crown Court lie to the Court of Appeal and thence to the House of Lords.

- Precedent in criminal law: The normal rules of precedent exist in criminal law except that the Court of Appeal (Criminal Division) does not consider itself as bound by its predecessors' decisions as does the Civil Division. In very recent times the Court of Appeal decided to follow a Privy Council case in preference to a House of Lords one.

- The interpretation of criminal law statutes: It is sometimes said that statutes creating offences are read in favour of liberty; that is, in favour of the accused. However, many cases may be found which go the other way, i.e. convict the 'manifestly guilty' even when the statute could be construed in favour of the accused.

- Classification of offences: There are several methods of classifying crimes, including by their source (statutory or common law).

- May judges create crimes? The short answer in the last quarter of a century is 'no, but they may apply the law to new scenarios.' The virtual ban on creating offences, however, does not apply to new defences and the development of duress of circumstances exemplifies how new defences can be created.

- Proof: In criminal law the burden of proof normally rests on the prosecution and the standard of proof is that the Crown must prove each element of the offence beyond reasonable doubt. Indeed, this principle applies even to defences: for most defences the prosecution must disprove each element beyond reasonable doubt. Therefore, in respect even of defences the accused does not need to prove anything: he or she is afforded the defence if the prosecution cannot disprove beyond reasonable doubt that he or she has the defence. However, since Parliament can do anything, it can put the burden of proof on to the defendant, both with regard to offences and defences. For example, Parliament has placed the burden on the accused to prove that he or she falls within the defence of diminished responsibility. Whenever the burden is on the accused, the standard of proof is the civil law one of 'on the balance of probabilities'. There is one exceptional defence, insanity, where the burden lies on the accused as a matter of common law and the reason behind this rule seems to be that everyone is presumed to be sane: therefore, the accused must prove that he or she was insane. Wherever the burden in criminal law is on the accused, there is the possibility of conflict with Article 6(2) of the ECHR, the presumption of innocence, and English courts including the House of Lords have struggled to fit situations where the burden is on the accused with the ECHR.

- The draft Criminal Code: The Law Commission published the *draft* Criminal Code in 1989. It has not been enacted. The Law Commission currently sees no prospect of Parliament's enacting the whole of it in one go but has published several consultation papers and reports on various aspects of criminal law since 1989 and it hopes that these smaller tranches will be enacted and will over time form a code.

References

Reports

Home Office *Criminal Justice: The Way Ahead* (2001)

Law Commission Consultation Paper no. 127, *Intoxication and Criminal Liability* (1993)

Law Commission Report no. 143, *Criminal Law: Codification of the Criminal Law – A Report to the Law Commission* (1985)

Law Commission Report no. 177, *A Criminal Code for England & Wales* (1989)

Law Commission Report no. 218, *Legislating the Criminal Code – Offences against the Person* (1993)

Law Commission Report no. 228, *Conspiracy to Defraud* (1994)

Law Commission Report no. 229, *Intoxication and Criminal Responsibility* (1995)

Report of the Committee on Homosexual Offences and Prostitution (Wolfenden) Cmnd 247 (1957)

Books

Card, R., Cross, R. and Jones, P. A. *Criminal Law* 18th edn (Oxford University Press, 2008)

Hall, J. *Foundations of Jurisprudence* (Bobbs-Merrill, 1973)

Husak, D. N. *Philosophy of Criminal Law* (Rowman & Littlefield, 1987)

Lacey, N. *State Punishment* (Routledge, 1988)

Norrie, A. *Crime, Reason and History* 2nd edn (Butterworths, 2001)

Journals

Arden, J. 'Criminal Law at the Crossroads' [1999] Crim LR 489

Ashworth, A. 'Is Criminal Law a lost Cause?' (2000) 116 LQR 225

Buxton, J. 'The Human Rights Act and the substantive Criminal Law' [2000] Crim LR 331

Hart, H. M. 'The Aims of the Criminal Law' (1958) 23 L & CP 401

Rowbotham, J. and Stevenson, K. 'Social Dystopias and Legal Utopias?' (2000) 9 *Nottingham Law Journal* 25

Smith, J. C. 'The Presumption of Innocence' (1987) 38 NILQ 223

Williams, G. 'The Definition of a Crime' [1955] CLP 107

Further reading

Alldridge, P. 'What's wrong with the traditional criminal law course?' (1990) 10 LS 38

Alldridge, P. *Relocating Criminal Law* (Ashgate, 2000)

Arden, Mrs Justice 'Criminal law at the crossroads: the impact of human rights from the Law Commission's perspective and the need for a code' [1999] Crim LR 439

Ashworth, A. 'Interpreting criminal statutes' (1991) 107 LQR 419

Ashworth, A. 'Is the criminal law a lost cause?' (2000) 116 LQR 228

Ashworth, A. 'The Human Rights Act and the substantive criminal law: a non-minimalist view' [2000] Crim LR 564

Ashworth, A. Case comment on *Attorney-General's Reference (No. 4 of 2002)* [2005] Crim LR 215

Ashworth, A. and Blake, M. 'The presumption of innocence in criminal law' [1996] Crim LR 306

Bingham, Lord 'A criminal code: must we wait forever?' [1998] Crim LR 694

Brownsword, R. 'Who says penal statutes are construed restrictively?' (1977) 28 NILQ 73

Burca, G. de and Gardner, S. 'The codification of the criminal law' (1990) 10 OJLS 559

Buxton, R. 'The Human Rights Act and the substantive criminal law' [2000] Crim LR 331

Chalmers, J. and Leverick, F. 'Fair labelling in criminal law' (2008) 71 MLR 217

Dennis, I. 'The critical condition of criminal law' [1997] CLP 213

Dennis, I. 'Reverse onuses and the presumption of innocence: in search of principle' [2005] Crim LR 901

Doran, S. 'Alternative defences' [1991] Crim LR 878

Duff, A. 'Theorising criminal law' (2005) 25 OJLS 353

Duff, R. A. 'Theories of criminal law' Stanford Encyclopaedia of Philosophy (available online to UK higher and further education institutions)

Duff, R. A. 'Crime, prohibition, and punishment', (2002) 19 J Applied Phil 97

Etherton, J. 'Law reform in England and Wales: a shattered dream or triumph of political vision?' (2008) 73 *Amicus Curiae* 3

Farmer, L. 'The obsession with definition' (1996) 5 *Social and Legal Studies* 57–73

Gandhi, P. R. and James, J. A. 'Marital rape and responsibility' (1997) 9 *Child and Family Law Quarterly* 17

Husak, D. 'The criminal law as a last resort' (2004) 24 OJLS 207

Husak, D. 'Crimes outside the core' (2004) 39 Tulsa L Rev 755

Husak, D. 'Why criminal law: a question of content?' (2008) 2 Crim Law and Philos 99

Lamond, G. 'What is a crime?' (2007) 27 OJLS 609

Law Commission of Canada *What is a Crime?* Discussion paper (2003)

Roberts, P. 'Taking the burden of proof seriously' [1995] Crim LR 783

Robinson, P. H. *Structure and Function in Criminal Law* (Clarendon, 1997)

Schünemann, B. 'Alternative project for a European criminal law and procedure' (2007) 18 Crim LF 227

Smith, A. T. H. 'The case for a Code' [1986] Crim LR 285

Smith, A. T. H. 'Criminal law: the future' [2004] Crim LR 971

Tierney, S. and Tadros, V. 'The presumption of innocence and the Human Rights Act' (2004) 67 MLR 402

Toulson, R. 'Forty years on: what progress in delivering accessible and principled criminal law?' [2006] Stat LR 61

Uglow, S *Criminal Justice* 2nd edn (Sweet & Maxwell, 2002)

Williams, G. 'The definition of crime' (1955) 8 CLP 107. (For a criticism of his definition of a crime, see J. Dine [1994] JBL 325.)

Williams, G. 'The logic of exceptions' [1988] CLJ 261

For a critique of criminal law as a rational and principled enterprise see A. Norrie, *Crime, Reason and History* (Butterworths, 2nd edn, 2001). He argues that in criminal law 'the "extraordinary" is as much the norm as the ordinary' (p. 7) and that English criminal law is a product of the epoch in which we live (p. 8). There is also a good discussion of what he calls 'orthodox subjectivism' and its rivals such as practical indifference. See also the collection edited by S. Shute and A. P. Simester, *Criminal Law Theory: Doctrines of the General Part* (Oxford University Press, 2002).

For more discussion of harm and morality in criminal law see P. Devlin, *The Enforcement of Morals* (Oxford University Press, 1965). H. L. A. Hart, *Law, Liberty and Morality* (Oxford University Press, 1963), and the sequence of books by J. Feinberg, *Harm to Others* (Oxford University Press, 1984), *Harm to Self* (Oxford University Press, 1986), *Harmless Wrongdoing* (Oxford University Press, 1988), and *Offense to Others* (Oxford University Press, 1985).

Visit **www.mylawchamber.co.uk/jefferson** to access
exam-style questions with answer guidance, multiple
choice quizzes, live weblinks, an online glossary,
and regular updates to the law.

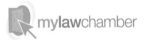

Use **Case Navigator** to read in full some of the key cases referenced in
this chapter:

DPP v *Majewski* [1976] 2 All ER 142
DPP v *Morgan* [1975] 2 All ER 347
R v *Brown* [1993] 2 All ER 75
R v *Woollin* [1998] 4 All ER 103

Part 2

General principles

2

Actus reus

Introduction

The general aim of the criminal law is to forbid certain types of conduct, but in most serious crimes the accused must also have been legally at fault. Offences therefore have two sides: conduct and fault. The 'conduct' requirement means that an accused is not criminally liable for merely thinking about committing a crime. Sometimes defences such as lack of consent are seen as failures to prove one or other of these ingredients. However, some defences cannot easily be seen as negating either conduct or fault. For the purpose of examining and explaining criminal law, it has become orthodox in the twenty-first century to divide the constituent elements of a crime into these two parts, which are called *actus reus* (the conduct element in the definition of the crime) and *mens rea* (the mental element in the definition of the crime). Both ingredients must be present. If one crashes into one's neighbour's car, one is not necessarily guilty of criminal damage. If one does so intentionally or recklessly, one is. In criminal damage one is guilty only if one has the requisite state of mind, the *mens rea* or 'fault element', as the Law Commission draft Criminal Code (Law Com. No. 177, 1989), cl 6, calls it. The *actus reus* is called the 'external element', which is the heading to cl 15. It is not defined in the definition clause, cl 6. The *mens rea* is the state of mind, or in the case of negligence the failure to attain a certain standard of behaviour, which the definition requires before the accused can be convicted. The *actus reus* is sometimes defined negatively as the remainder of the offence once the *mens rea* has been subtracted.

- Since there may be a defence which is not defined in terms of vitiating the *mens rea* or *actus reus* or both, it may be better to regard the *actus reus* as the act (such as causing death in murder), the omission (as in not displaying a valid tax disc), or the state of affairs (as in possessing a controlled drug) rather than negatively.

- In most offences both must exist. Crimes where there is no *mens rea* as to one or more parts of the *actus reus* are called strict offences (see Chapter 4).

- Usually the *actus reus* and *mens rea* must be contemporaneous (see Chapter 3).

- The two parts do not exist separately. The *mens rea* qualifies the *actus reus*. For example, in the offence of rape, the accused among other matters must intend sexual intercourse, and know that the victim does not consent. The 'sexual intercourse', 'woman' or 'man' and 'consent' points constitute the *actus reus*. The intention, recklessness and other

45

relevant states of mind are designated the *mens rea* of the offences. To find out which mental element is required in relation to each element of the *actus reus* is a task for the law student, for each external element may have a different *mens rea* attached to it.

● There are difficulties in dividing all elements of a crime into *mens rea* and *actus reus*. The element of possessing a proscribed drug looks like *actus reus*, but it hides an aspect of *mens rea*: one does not possess something unless one knows one possesses it, and knowledge is part of *mens rea*. This difficulty is explored in the next section (Some Problems) of this book.

The terms '*actus reus*' and '*mens rea*' are purely shorthand, useful for exposition. They are convenient for lawyers. This point was well put a long time ago by Rollin Perkins, ('A rationale of *mens rea*' (1939) 52 Harv LR 905):

> Some years ago the *mens rea* doctrine was criticized on the ground that the Latin phrase is 'misleading'. If the words '*mens rea*' were to be regarded as self-explanatory they would be open to this objection, but they are to be considered merely as a convenient label attached to any psychical fact sufficient for criminal guilt . . . This includes a field too complex for any brief self-explanatory phrase, and since it is important to have some sort of dialectic shorthand to express the idea, this time-honored label will do as well as any. (American spelling retained)

As has been seen, however, to what extent these elements must be shown to exist, if at all, depends on an analysis of the particular offence with which the accused is charged. Moreover, whether an element of an offence is classified as *actus reus* or *mens rea* does not normally matter for in either case the accused is not guilty. One exception is the developing doctrine of procuring the *actus reus* of a crime discussed in Chapter 5, but that doctrine may not survive challenge in the House of Lords.

There are also problems with the effect of mistake as to *actus reus* and *mens rea*. Normally even an unreasonable mistake exculpates, but if the crime is one of negligence, the accused has a defence only if the mistake was made on reasonable grounds.

Since the terms are legal ones, there is no need to use them before laypeople. Lord Diplock deprecated their use in court in **Miller** [1983] 2 AC 161.

> It would . . . be conducive to clarity of analysis of the ingredients of a crime that is created by statute, as are the great majority of criminal offences today, if we were to avoid bad Latin and instead to think and speak . . . about the conduct of the accused and his state of mind at the time of that conduct, instead of speaking about actus reus and mens rea.

His wish has been granted in the draft Criminal Code, but there is more usage of the term in the courts today than there was over a decade ago when Lord Diplock made his remarks, no doubt because practitioners were once students who were taught these terms. Certainly the terms could be dropped. The use can be illustrated thus:

Murder: *actus reus* (in part) = causing death
        mens rea (in part) = intentionally causing death or serious bodily harm

The terms *actus reus* and *mens rea* need not be used, and indeed the draft Criminal Code does not use them. One could just say that murder was defined in part as causing death with the intention to cause death or to cause grievous bodily harm. Since the terms are used in courts and the academic world of law, they are utilised in this book as a handy way of distinguishing the accused's behaviour and the circumstances of the offence from his state of mind.

Some problems

(a) There are difficulties in defining the *actus reus* as the offence minus the *mens rea*. The *actus reus* of an offence may go beyond what the accused did. The *actus reus* can cover the mental state of the victim. In rape the victim must not be consenting. The victim's consent is a state of mind, but not the accused's state of mind. It is also arguable that in some crimes it is unclear whether something constitutes the *actus reus* or *mens rea*. In the offence of driving without due care and attention, is the element 'without due care and attention' a state of mind? It could be said that it means 'carelessly'. If negligence ('without due care and attention') is a state of mind (see Chapter 3), the element is *mens rea*. It might be said, however, that the phrase qualifies 'driving'. One is driving in such a manner that the driving falls short of the standard of due care and attention. One can only possess something such as a controlled drug if one knows one possesses it: the accused's state of mind is part of the *actus reus*. It does not matter whether knowledge is part of the *mens rea* or *actus reus*. The prosecution has to prove it no matter how commentators define it. In conspiracy the element of 'agreement' is normally treated as part of the *actus reus*, but it also refers to a mental state. One form of aggravated burglary occurs when the accused has with him a weapon of offence. Whether an article is one of offence depends on the accused's intention. The *actus reus* includes the accused's state of mind. The division into *actus reus* and *mens rea* may not always be clearcut.

In some offences it is only the *mens rea* which is wrongful – the *actus reus* is perfectly innocent. A good illustration is theft. If the accused picks a tin of beans from a supermarket shelf, there is nothing wrong in what he has done: most people act similarly indeed every day. However, the addition of (part of) the *mens rea*, dishonesty, converts the *actus reus* into a crime. If only for this reason, readers should not translate *actus reus* as 'guilty act'. There may be nothing 'guilty' about it.

Some defences also create difficulties. In duress the accused seems to have the intention to commit the crime and to have caused it, but he has a defence. This defence goes beyond *mens rea* and *actus reus*. Some defences are not failures to show *actus reus* and *mens rea*. Where does automatism fit? It could be a denial of the *actus reus*: the accused was not in truth 'driving' because he was being attacked by a swarm of bees, an example given a new lease of life in **Bell** [1984] 3 All ER 842. It could be a denial of *mens rea*: when attacked by bees he has no state of mind (there could be a problem with strict offences in this regard). It could even be what might be called a true defence: he was driving and he knew he was driving badly, but he has the defence of automatism. Another view is to say that the correct analysis is that before the stages of *actus reus* and *mens rea* are reached, it must be shown that the accused loses control of his bodily movements. As Lord Denning put it in **Bratty v A-G for Northern Ireland** [1963] AC 386: '. . . the category of involuntary acts is very limited'. In most cases control is not at issue, and unless the accused raises doubt about his control, the prosecution need not prove affirmatively that he was in control. If, however, he was being attacked by a swarm of bees with the result that he was not in charge of his vehicle, he will be acquitted unless the prosecution can disprove his evidence. This ingredient is sometimes phrased as: was the accused acting voluntarily? He is not acting voluntarily if he is being attacked by bees. It should be noted that this type of involuntariness is different from that in duress, where the accused's behaviour is determined by threat which obliges the accused to act in a certain way.

In automatism the accused's voluntary conduct is negated by loss of conscious control. In duress the accused may have conscious control over his movements but his acts are directed by coercion.

Because the relationship between automatism and the definition of an offence is not yet solved, automatism cannot be neatly fitted into the distinction between justifications and excuses noted in Chapter 7. For further discussion of automatism see Chapter 9.

(b) The *actus reus* differs from crime to crime. In burglary the accused must enter a building or part of a building without the consent of the owner. In theft the defendant must appropriate property belonging to another. To say that all crimes have an *actus reus* does not inform us what that *actus reus* is in each offence. One has to look at each offence to determine what the *actus reus* is. One *actus reus* may suffice for several offences. In murder, manslaughter and other homicide offences the accused must cause the victim's death. The *actus reus* may also cover how a situation arose. Criminal damage caused by fire constitutes the offence of arson (Criminal Damage Act 1971, s 1(3)).

(c) As stated above, *actus reus* is not just a 'guilty act', as students sometimes say. It can cover a state of affairs, such as having with one articles for use in burglaries, being in possession of a controlled drug, membership of a proscribed terrorist organisation, and an omission (see below). The difference between these forms of behaviour may not be clearcut, and one may have difficulty distinguishing between acts and omissions, when one is guilty if one acts but not guilty if one fails to act (see **Fagan v MPC** [1969] 1 QB 439, discussed later in this chapter). Is drink-driving an act or is it a state of affairs? Also included in the *actus reus* are the legally relevant circumstances. In bigamy the accused must already be married. In rape the sexual intercourse must be without the consent of the victim.

(d) The *actus reus* must be proved. **Deller** is the authority normally given to illustrate this proposition.

Deller (1952) 36 Cr App R 184

The accused was charged with what was then false pretences and is now obtaining by deception contrary to s 15 of the Theft Act 1968. When he took his car in for a trade-in, he represented that there was no money owing on it. He believed that there were payments outstanding. It looked as if he had made a false pretence. In fact the loan on the car was void and in law did not exist. Therefore, he did not owe any money. His representation turned out to be true, though he mistakenly believed it to be false. The Court of Criminal Appeal quashed his conviction. The prosecution had failed to prove that the pretence was false.

One is not guilty of an offence simply because one believes oneself to be guilty. The prosecution must prove the whole of the *actus reus* and, on the facts, one element was missing. **Deller** can stand for the proposition that one is not guilty for having guilty thoughts. *Mens rea* alone is insufficient. The charge nowadays would be one of attempt under the Criminal Attempts Act 1981.

A more modern instance of the law stated in **Deller** is **McKoy** (2002), *The Times*, 17 June. The accused apparently thought he was being lawfully arrested when a police officer held his arm. In fact he was being unlawfully restrained. He used force to escape. The Court of Appeal held that he was entitled to use reasonable force to escape the unlawful restraint. The accused's mistake was irrelevant, because on the facts which actually existed he was entitled to use reasonable force. This belief did not make a lawful act unlawful. Unfortunately, as the court did not refer to *Dadson*, which is dealt with next, its authority is diminished.

The case always contrasted with *Deller* is *Dadson*. The distinction between the two authorities is often stated to be that in *Deller* there was an absence of an element of the offence whereas in *Dadson* there was an absence of an element of a defence. This distinction is crucial for the accused was not guilty in *Deller* but was guilty in *Dadson*.

Dadson (1850) 4 Cox CC 358

A constable was guarding a copse from which wood had been stolen on several occasions in the past. The constable saw the victim come out of the copse carrying wood. The wood had been stolen by the victim. He shot at the victim, who was injured. He was charged with shooting with intent to cause grievous bodily harm. At that time it was thought lawful for a constable to shoot an escaping felon. Stealing wood became a felony only if a person had two previous convictions, which the victim had. The constable did not know that the victim had the prior convictions. The constable was found guilty. In the Court for Crown Cases Reserved, where judges gathered to discuss points of criminal law, it was held that an accused did not have a defence unless he was aware of the facts justifying the defence at the time of the offence. (The conviction seems to be in line with policy, for persons should ask questions first and shoot later.)

The actual result in *Dadson* is now governed by s 24(4) of the Police and Criminal Evidence Act 1984 (PACE) (though cf. J. C. Smith's commentary on *Chapman v DPP* [1988] Crim LR 843), which deals with arrestable offences. The accused no longer needs reasonable grounds for suspecting that the victim has committed an arrestable offence when he uses force to effect the arrest if the victim in fact was committing one when arrested (though the arrest might still be unlawful because it cannot be stated what the grounds of arrest were at the time under s 28). Nevertheless the principle stands elsewhere: the accused must know the circumstances which justify his conduct.

Dadson is authority for the proposition that circumstances of justification are treated as part of the mental element, not as part of the *actus reus*. The accused must know of the circumstances of justification to obtain a defence. Accordingly, the accused is guilty of battery if he trips up the thief of a book from the library but does not know of the theft. It has often been suggested that *Dadson* is wrong. The victim was a felon and therefore it was lawful to use deadly force to arrest him. He was not doing anything forbidden by law. There was no *actus reus* and the case is on all fours with *Deller*. The court, however, held that the accused was guilty unless he knew that the victim was a felon: there was no need for the court so to rule; it could have held that the accused had a defence if the victim was in fact a felon. If *Dadson* is wrong, there would be no gap in the law, for nowadays the accused would be guilty of the attempt to commit the offence.

The Law Commission's draft Criminal Code (Law Com. No. 177, 1989), if enacted would reverse the general principle in *Dadson*, thereby giving the accused a defence when he did not know of the circumstances which justified his conduct. The Law

Commission believed (incorrectly) that PACE (see above) had overruled **Dadson** as to the lawfulness of the arrest. In order to bring the law into line with self-defence, however, the Law Commission later changed its mind and **Dadson** is preserved by the Criminal Law Bill attached to Report No. 218, 1993. The policy behind **Dadson** was aptly and succinctly stated in para 39.11 of the Report: 'citizens who react unreasonably to circumstances should not be exculpated by accidents of facts of which they were unaware.'

(e)   There are times when a person other than the accused committed the *actus reus* but the accused is nevertheless guilty of the offence of which the other party committed the *actus reus*. The obvious example is vicarious liability, discussed in Chapter 6.

(f)   The *actus reus* may help to prove the *mens rea*. If the accused stabs his victim through the heart at close range, there is some evidence that the accused had the *mens rea* of murder.

'Conduct' and 'result' crimes

It is becoming usual to divide offences into 'conduct' and 'result' offences. 'Conduct' crimes are those where only the forbidden conduct need be proved: no harm need be caused. An example is dangerous driving, contrary to s 2 of the Road Traffic Act 1988 (as amended), which provides in relation to the *actus reus* that a person is guilty when he is 'driving a mechanically propelled vehicle on a road'. One does not have to show that anything else occurred. The accused is guilty if he drove a motor vehicle dangerously on a road. There need be no harmful consequences, such as the accused drove a car on a public road so dangerously that someone was knocked down. In perjury the accused is guilty if he makes a statement on oath, knowing or believing it to be false. The outcome of the case need not be affected. Perjury is therefore a conduct crime. In 'result' crimes, because a forbidden consequence is part of the *actus reus*, the specified harm must be shown. In murder someone must be killed. The forbidden result must be caused.

With regard to conduct crimes, there is no problem normally with causation, since no result need be proved. In result crimes the accused must be proved to have caused the prohibited consequence. In s 1 of the Road Traffic Act 1988 (as amended), the prosecution must show that the accused drove dangerously and thereby occasioned the death of a person. (For causation generally, see below.)

One issue which has arisen in result crimes occurs where the definition of those offences contains the concept of unlawfulness. As late as **Albert v Lavin** [1981] 1 All ER 628 the Divisional Court thought that this word emphasised that the outcome of what would otherwise be crimes could be lawful. In murder, for instance, one is not guilty if one killed by performing service as public executioner or in self-defence. Such a defence would arise whether or not the word 'unlawfully' appeared in the definition of the offence. However, both **Kimber** [1983] 1 WLR 1118 (CA), where the issue of consent in the then existing crime of indecent assault was under discussion, and **Williams** [1987] 3 All ER 411 (CA) decided that 'unlawfully' is part of the *actus reus* (see Chapter 8 for the effect). This means that matters such as self-defence form part of the *actus reus*. If the accused falls within the boundaries of self-defence, the prosecution has failed to prove the whole of the *actus reus*. To call self-defence a 'defence' is a misnomer if by the term is meant a third concept beyond *actus reus* and *mens rea*. Nevertheless, the accused bears the evidential burden.

See p 70 later in this chapter for a more detailed explanation of omission.

Some offences can be committed by a failure to act, and others such as possessing cannabis are status or state of affairs ones. It is difficult to describe these offences as 'conduct' ones. Omission involves the opposite, a lack of conduct.

The draft Criminal Code and *actus reus*

By cl 15, 'act' in the draft Criminal Code means 'act' and 'also, where the context permits . . . any result of the act, and any circumstance in which the act is done or the result occurs, that is an element of the offence'. By cl 16 'act' is to be read as covering an omission (see later), state of affairs, or occurrence if the crime is so defined.

Causation

There is no more intractable problem in the law than causation (Criminal Law and Penal Methods Reform Committee, South Australia, Fourth Report, *The Substantive Criminal Law*, 1977, 50, quoted in E. Colvin 'Causation in criminal law' (1989) 1 Bond LR 253).

Questions of causation arise in many different legal contexts and no single theory of causation will provide a ready-made answer to the question whether [the accused's] action is to be treated as the cause or a cause of some ensuing event. The approach must necessarily be pragmatic . . . (Lord Bridge in ***Attorney-General of Hong Kong* v *Tse Hung-lit*** [1986] 1 AC 876 (PC)).

The law in deciding questions of causation selects one or more causes out of the total sum of conditions according to the purpose in hand . . . (McGarvie and O'Bryan JJ in ***Demirian*** [1989] VR 97, 110).

Introduction

Causation is in some sense a difficult area of the law (Fig. 2.1), yet according to the Court of Appeal in ***Cato*** [1976] 1 WLR 110, ***Pagett*** (1983) 76 Cr App R 279 and ***Cheshire*** [1991] 1 WLR 844 the issue of factual cause is largely one for the jury once the court has determined that there is sufficient evidence to be left to them, and since 'cause' is an ordinary English word, in most cases no direction need be given. As Lord Salmon put it in ***Alphacell Ltd* v *Woodward*** [1972] AC 824 (HL) in a passage approved by the House of Lords in ***Environment Agency* v *Empress Car Co (Abertillery) Ltd*** [1999] 2 AC 22, 'What or who has caused a certain event to occur is essentially a practical question of fact which can best be answered by ordinary common sense rather than by abstract meta-physical theory.' Nevertheless, as Lord Hoffmann in the ***Empress*** case recognised, there are principles of law involved too, and some of these may be complicated. The answer may depend on the question asked. Whether a person caused pollution and whether he caused a death may require different rules of attribution. A third party's intervention may prevent the latter being guilty but not the former. Doctors may give evidence of what they consider to be the cause, but the decision is for the jury. Similarly, whether an organisation had caused effluent to enter a river is a question of fact. In the ***Empress*** case the Lords held that the magistrates were entitled to find that the defendants had caused pollution to a river. Only if the act of the third party was 'extraordinary' and not 'a matter of ordinary occurrence' were the defendants not liable. They had built a tank for diesel oil in a place where the oil would flow into a river if someone turned a tap. Someone did. The failure to install a lock on the tank caused the pollution. This case has come in for

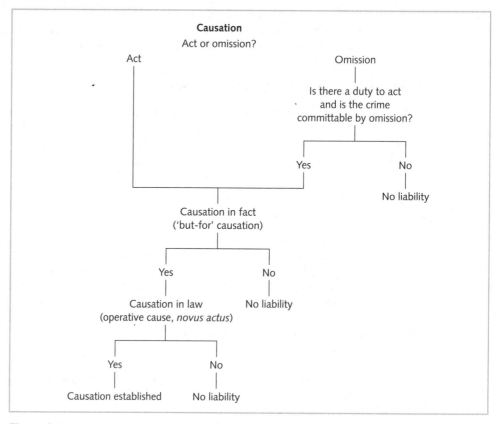

Figure 2.1 Causation

strong criticism because the 'free, deliberate and informed' act of a third party had released the oil: this act would seem to be a *novus actus interveniens,* a concept which is discussed below, but the phrase basically means that the accused is held not to have caused the prohibited result. It seems very strange to have an accused's criminal liability depend on the act of an unknown third party. ***Empress*** is confined to instances of pollution: ***Kennedy (No. 2)*** [2008] 1 AC 269, discussed below. An alternative view is to say that their Lordships were wrong because they hardly dealt with the standard authorities on causation: the installation of the tank was merely the setting for the pollution, not the cause of it.

The issue of legal causation can be withdrawn from the jury when the judge decides that the accused's act or omission was not the legal cause. The courts have readily stated what is and what is not a cause. There are principles of law operating. These principles may not cohere into doctrine, for the courts may increase or review their scope in order to catch or exculpate the accused. If a lorry driver falls asleep at the wheel and kills a motorist, is he liable or the employer who insures him to drive, or even the capitalist system which obliges him to work? (For the law on causation for secondary offences see Chapter 5.)

Cases on causation tend to arise in homicide, but the principles are applicable generally to result crimes, including strict offences, though pollution may be an exception. (The same can be said of the concept of intention. Knowing the law of murder is a great step towards the whole of criminal law.) It is not true to say that causation is always required. Some crimes ('conduct crimes', see above) do not require a consequence to be caused, and some crimes which are result crimes do not require causation. A person is vicariously liable, that is, criminally responsible for another's act, even though he did not occasion the wrongful act: the courts look for both 'but-for' causation (e.g. the victim would not have died but for the accused's shooting him – this aspect is sometimes called 'causation-in-fact') and legal causation (i.e. does the law attribute this cause to this defendant?). If the 'but-for' test were used alone, it would pick up too many accuseds. For example, if I am shot by a bankrobber, I would not have been shot if I had stayed in bed. One would not say that my failure to stay in bed caused the shooting. Common sense comes into play in the jury's decision. In most scenarios it is evident as a matter of common-sense that the accused caused the crime, for instance, by pulling the trigger. When there is no difficulty in determining causation, no direction is given. In some instances it is not simple to determine who caused death. If a person refuses a life-saving blood transfusion, one could contend that he caused his own death. The judges look further and give a direction on causation which potentially inculpates the accused who so injured the victim that he had to choose between a transfusion and death. It must be noted that there can be more than one cause of a consequence. In criminal law the inquiry is whether this accused contributed more than negligibly to the result, not whether or not there was any other significant contribution.

If the accused did not in fact cause the result, he is not guilty of the principal offence. In **White** [1910] 2 KB 124, the accused put potassium cyanide into lemonade, intending to kill his victim. She died, not through drinking the poison, but from natural causes. Therefore the accused had not caused her death, despite what he intended and did. The charge should be one of attempted murder. Similar is **Shoukatellie v R** [1962] AC 81 (PC), where the intended victim had died before the accused struck what would otherwise have been a fatal blow. A case which demonstrates 'but-for' causation is the Australian one of **Hallett** [1969] SASR 141. The victim had allegedly made a homosexual advance to the accused while they were drinking on a beach at night. The accused beat him up, leaving him unconscious. The tide came in and drowned him. The accused had caused his death: but for what the accused had done the victim would not have drowned. He would not have been guilty, had there been a tsunami. In **Dyson** [1908] 2 KB 959 the Court of Criminal Appeal held that the accused had caused the victim's death even though the latter would shortly afterwards have died of meningitis. The former had accelerated his death. As part of the 'but-for' test one should always remember **Dalloway** (1847) 3 Cox CC 273: the accused must have been able to prevent the crime. On the facts the accused did not cause the death of a child, whom he ran over. He was careless but his negligent driving did not cause death. The victim would have died anyway under the wheels of the cart for even had the defendant been driving properly, there was nothing he could have done to prevent the accident. Despite the accused's negligence, the child still would have died. In modern terms an accused is not guilty of causing death by dangerous driving if, though he is driving dangerously, a child unexpectedly dashes out and is killed under the car's wheels. Causation is lacking. A modern application of **Dalloway** is **Marchant** [2004] 1 WLR 442 (CA). The accused, the driver of an agricultural vehicle with a grab unit at the front, was not guilty of causing death by dangerous driving when a motor cyclist impaled himself on a metre-long spike on the grab unit. The spike was not covered by a guard. The court held that, even if it had been, the collision would still have occurred; and the driver's appeal was allowed. One phrase sometimes used is that the accused's act must be the *sine qua non* (a precondition) of the death. As we shall see, even if it can be said that the accused did in fact cause the death, he may not be responsible in criminal law for it because, e.g., there was in the court's words in *Jordan* (1956) 40 Cr App R 152 'palpably wrong' medical treatment, breaking the chain of causation and rendering the accused not liable. Accordingly, there are two stages: factual causation and legal causation. Proving factual or 'but-for' causation does not prove legal causation. Legal causation is concerned with whether criminal responsibility can fairly be ascribed to the accused.

The same rules apply in both murder and manslaughter as well as causing death by dangerous driving. In these crimes part of the *actus reus* is 'causing death'. Since it is certain that we are all going to die one day, the *actus reus* is better expressed as the accused accelerating death. Since the acceleration of death is the kingpin, it does not matter that the victim was suffering from a terminal illness, such as cancer: *Adams* [1957] Crim LR 365. In the words of Lord Widgery CJ in *Cato* (above), 'It was sufficient if the prosecution could establish that it was a cause, provided it was a cause outside the *de minimis* range and effectively bearing on the acceleration of the moment of the victim's death.' (*De minimis* means so trivial that no account should be taken of it.) Another result flowing from the definition, though not one totally accepted by Devlin J in *Adams*, is that a doctor who gives pain-killing drugs to a dying patient performs this part of the *actus reus* of murder if those drugs incidentally shorten life by a more than trifling period. If a doctor prescribes pain-killers in order to accelerate death, there is no problem. He has caused the patient's death. This is so despite any request from the patient and the severity of the pain. One might argue that the doctor should have a defence of necessity, or perhaps his motive should exculpate him. The law remains uncertain. There seems to be a move towards giving a doctor a defence when even though he knows that the treatment will accelerate death, he believes that he is undertaking the correct treatment to reduce pain. See the trial of *Moor* (unreported) before Hooper J discussed by Arlidge 'The trial of Dr David Moor' [2000] Crim LR 31. It is also uncertain whether, if this rule restricted to doctors exists, the civil case of *Re A* [2001] Fam 167 (CA) has affected it. The surgeons realised that separating conjoined twins would kill one of them. Two of the Lords Justices stated that once a jury found that the doctors knew that it was (virtually) certain that one twin would die, they intended to kill. (Of course, normally a doctor will not have the *mens rea* for murder.) It may be that a trifling acceleration is insufficient. Devlin J. said in *Adams* that an acceleration of death by 'minutes, hours or even, perhaps, days' by pain-killing drugs is not a cause of death. It is certainly arguable that Devlin J confused motive (the desire to stop the patient suffering unbelievable pain) with causation. Surely he would not have said the same about an accused who was not a doctor who fed her mother death-accelerating, pain-killing tablets to receive her inheritance 'perhaps days' earlier than she would otherwise have done? Devlin J emphasised that cause was a matter of common sense to be determined by the jury. It 'means nothing philosophical or technical or scientific'.

Again, because the accused must be shown only to have caused death, it does not matter which of his acts caused death as long as one did. In *Attorney-General's Reference (No. 4 of 1980)* [1981] 2 All ER 617 the accused pushed the victim backwards, strangled her and cut her throat, but was guilty whichever act caused death. (In light of the requirement of contemporaneity of *mens rea* and *actus reus*, we must assume that the accused had *mens rea* throughout the series of acts unless all the acts can be regarded as the same transaction. The concept of an indivisible transaction is discussed below. The case was not decided on that basis which would convict him if he had the *mens rea* at the time of the first attack and thereafter thought he was disposing of a corpse which in fact was a live body.) If the accused did not have *mens rea* at the start of the series of acts or through-out them, he is acquitted. If, however, the prosecution cannot prove beyond reasonable doubt that the accused's blow caused the victim's death when there were two blows from different persons, either of which might have occasioned death, the accused is not guilty: *Dyos* [1979] Crim LR 660 (Old Bailey). The prosecution could not prove that it was the accused's blow which caused the victim's death.

It is not essential that the accused's act is the sole, major or even a substantial cause of death: *Pagett*, above. In *Benge* (1865) 176 ER 665 the accused, a foreman of a plate-laying gang, was guilty of manslaughter through his carelessness even though others had contributed to the victims' death. It was irrelevant that no one would have been killed if others had acted differently. (The others such as the train-driver and a signalman could also have been liable for manslaughter because they too had significantly contributed to the victims' death.) The term 'substantial' means only that the cause must be more than *de minimis*: *Notman* [1994] Crim LR 518 (CA). Therefore, it is not a misdirection to use 'substantial' in this sense. In *Malcherek* [1981] 2 All ER 422 the Court of Appeal expressly held that the cause need not be a substantial one. The same court held in *Kimsey* [1996] Crim LR 35 that while the term 'substantial' could be used, it was a dangerous expression in that it might lead the jury to think that the cause really had to be substantial. What it really means is that the accused's conduct had to be more than *de minimis*, which the trial judge correctly translated as 'slight or trifling'. Similarly in *Cheshire*, above, the same court emphasised that the act of the accused need not be the sole or main cause of death. It is sufficient if his act contributed significantly to the victim's demise. 'Significantly' simply meant 'more than negligibly'. Therefore, there was no requirement to show that the defendant's act was the dominant or even substantial cause of death. The victim was shot in the thigh and stomach by the accused. A tracheotomy was per-formed in order to allow him to breathe. He died from the narrowing of the windpipe at the operation scar. Despite the hospital's failure to diagnose what was wrong with the victim, the accused's acts still contributed significantly to the victim's death. It can be argued that the facts of *Cheshire* resemble those of *Jordan*. The injuries continued to exist but they did not threaten the victim's life, and the hospital had been negligent. The distinction resides in the grossness of the doctors' negligence in *Jordan*, which broke the chain of causation.

In *Armstrong* [1989] Crim LR 149, a Crown Court decision, the accused supplied the victim with heroin and the means of injecting it. The case proceeded on the basis that the victim injected himself. Evidence showed that the death was caused primarily by the victim's drinking alcohol. The heroin was not a significant enough cause of death. (Experts were unsure whether heroin accelerated death appreciably: the case may therefore be authority for the proposition that in causation *de minimis non curat lex*: 'the law is not concerned with trifles'.) It is possible that *Armstrong* is out of line with *Blaue* [1975] 3 All ER 446 discussed below. In *Armstrong* the victim was under the influence of drugs. Why did not the accused take his victim as he found him? Compare also *Cato* above (which was distinguished in *Armstrong*) where the Court of Appeal looked for 'a cause' in a heroin-related death, not for 'but-for' causation in order to convict the accused of manslaughter. Again the court stressed that the issue was not one of substantial causation. In *Armstrong* the accused supplied the victim with the heroin and the means of injecting it but was found not guilty. In *Cato* the victim supplied the drug and mixed it, yet the accused was found guilty. On this analysis the cases look the wrong way round! In fact the distinction according to the courts resides in the iden-tity of the person who injected the drug.

Normally, if the accused was the factual cause of death, he is also the legal cause. There are, however, some circumstances where this conclusion cannot always be drawn, and these form the subject of the next section of this chapter.

Finally, it should be noted that when the courts are dealing with causation, particularly legal causation, they are not really asking: Did this accused cause the death? They are asking: Is it fair to attribute the death to this accused? Questions of attribution are ones of morality, not of fact.

Some special problems in causation

(a) *Novus actus interveniens*

This Latin phrase has become a legal term. What it means is that the intervening 'act was so independent of the act of the accused that it should be regarded in law as the cause of the victim's death to the exclusion of the act of the accused' (*per* Robert Goff L. J. in *Pagett* (1983) 76 Cr App R 279). When some event breaks the chain of causation, that is called a *novus actus interveniens*. The accused's conduct was no longer the operating cause of death, but merely part of the history. The judge noted that academic commentators spoke of the chain of causation being broken where the intervention was 'free, deliberate and informed'. Such intervention must be abnormal. In water cases the damage done by vandals has rendered factory owners not liable for polluting rivers. An example taken from the South Australian Full Court case of *Hallett* [1969] SASR 141 is of a victim left unconscious above the highwater mark who was drowned by a tidal wave. If, however, the victim had been left unconscious below that mark and had drowned, the accused who had left him unconscious would be liable when the incoming tide overwhelmed him.

The problem is illustrated by *Pagett*. The police shot and killed a girl being used as a shield by the accused. The court held that their action in shooting her was instinctive, was a reasonable act of self-defence or indeed self-preservation and was reasonably foreseeable. Alternatively, the shooting was an act done to prevent crime. Therefore, her death was attributable to the accused, who had shot at the police. It was as if the accused had pushed the victim under a tube train. In legal jargon the chain of causation was not broken by the police's shooting of the victim. What the police did was instinctive therefore, it was not 'free, deliberate and informed'. (Cf. *Empress*, where, despite the oil's release being caused by an unknown third party, the company was still liable. *Pagett* reiterates orthodox law; *Empress* is out of line.) Whether the police had a hand in the victim's death was therefore irrelevant. Had the police shot the victim dead in a grossly negligent fashion, then the chain of causation may have been broken. Similarly, a reasonable act of self-preservation, such as trying to escape from the accused's violence, will not break the chain of causation: see (b) 'The escape cases', below. It is interesting to note that in the civil action relating to *Pagett* reported in *The Guardian*, 4 December 1990, the police marksmen were held liable for negligence. They did not know that the victim was the defendant's former girlfriend; they ignored her mother's advice; there was no supervision of armed officers; the officer in charge had no experience of sieges; the officers could not see where the victim was standing because there was no light on the floors of the flats where the deceased was killed. Of course the police were not on trial in *Pagett* itself, just as the doctors were not in *Malcherek*, in which the position of the negligent doctors was not discussed. In *Malcherek* it could also be said that the doctors' intervention, the turning off of the life-support system, was free, deliberate and informed. Both cases demonstrate how in criminal law there can be more than one cause.

The fact that the police were negligent for the purposes of civil law did not of itself affect the accused's guilt in criminal law. (See also (f) 'Contributory negligence', below.) In **Pagett**, the human shield case, the marksmen acted instinctively to preserve their own lives. Though they were the immediate cause of death, the defendant was held to have been the legal cause of death. Even if the shooting of the victim was unlawful, it appears that he would still be criminally liable because he also unlawfully caused the death.

The basic rule is that the accused escapes liability only if the supervening event was highly abnormal or, put differently, unforeseeable or if there has occurred what has become known as 'free, deliberate and informed' intervention. The phrase is that of Hart and Honoré in the second edition of their treatise *Causation in the Law* (OUP 1985). Where the concept of foreseeability is used, the test is an objective one. The accused's characteristics, such as youth, stupidity or gender, are not taken into account: **Marjoram** [2000] Crim LR 372 (CA). Lord Parker CJ in **Smith** [1959] 2 QB 35 in the Courts-Martial Appeal Court said that:

> Only if the second cause is so overwhelming as to make the original wound merely part of the history can it be said that the death does not flow from the wound.

Otherwise, the accused's act will remain the effective or operative cause. On the facts of **Smith** the accused was guilty despite the 'thoroughly bad' treatment and despite the victim's good chance of recovery before that treatment. There were two concurrent causes of death, but because the wound made by the accused's stabbing the victim was still operative, the accused had caused his death. The jury does not choose which is the dominant cause. It answers the question whether the accused's acts contributed significantly to the death.

Smith was applied in **Gowans** [2003] EWCA Crim 3935. The defendants robbed a pizza delivery man, the victim. They put him into a coma. While in hospital he contracted septicaemia and died. The source of the infection was unknown. Evidence was led that the victim's condition required treatment which carried a risk of life-threatening infections. Kay LJ held that the jury had been directed properly. The attack made the victim vulnerable to infections; therefore, the death was attributable to the defendants. It would have been different if the attack was in the words of **Smith** 'merely the setting in which another cause operates'.

Another illustration is **Dear** [1996] Crim LR 595 (CA). The accused heard that the victim had sexually interfered with his young daughter. He slashed him repeatedly with a knife. The victim died from his wounds two days later. The accused argued that the chain of causation had been broken either by the victim's reopening his wounds (i.e., he committed suicide) or by failure to stop the blood from flowing. The court held that the injuries caused by the accused remained the operating and significant cause of death, whether or not the victim had reopened the wound. As long as the accused's acts had contributed significantly to the victim's death, the questions of whether the victim had acted in a negligent or grossly negligent manner or whether the intervening behaviour of the victim was foreseeable were irrelevant. It may be argued that if it were true that the victim did reopen his wounds, his behaviour was, in the words of **Roberts** (1971) 56 Cr App R 95 (CA), 'daft' and the accused should not have been convicted: suicide was not reasonably foreseeable. **Roberts** is discussed at (b) below. If the argument is accepted that as long as the accused's acts contributed significantly to the victim's death, the accused is liable, the law has moved on, for the previous law was that the chain of causation was broken when the victim's behaviour was not reasonably foreseeable. The contrary contention is that the accused must take his victim as he finds him, as noted at (e) 'The accused must take his victim as he finds him', below. If taking one's victim as one finds him means 'taking the whole of the victim including his mental state as one finds him', there is no scope for *Roberts*, for unreasonable behaviour (e.g. to escape) is part of the whole man. The rules can lead to different results. For example, if the accused sexually assaults the victim and the latter runs across a busy road and is killed, the facts look like a *Roberts* scenario: the accused is guilty if the victim's actions were reasonably foreseeable. If, however, the victim was suffering mental anguish at the time of the assault, the case resembles *Blaue* and the accused is guilty whether or not the death was reasonably foreseeable. Which rule applied was not discussed in *Dear*. In fact *Dear* is an unsatisfactory decision. The court said that 'the concepts of *novus actus interveniens* and foreseeability' should not 'invade the criminal law', yet these concepts have been used for many years.

For a case where it was suggested that suicide could be triggered by the accused's wounding the victim, see *Dhaliwal* [2006] EWCA Crim 1139. The discussion was *obiter*.

The chain of causation is also broken by a completely voluntary act of the victim. This principle was, however, not applied by the Court of Appeal in *Kennedy* [1999] Crim LR 65, a much criticised decision. The accused prepared for the victim a syringe containing heroin and water. The victim knew the contents of the syringe and injected herself. She died. The court held that the accused had caused the victim's death and that he was guilty of manslaughter. The court stressed that the accused supplied the drug to the victim for immediate use. These facts constituted encouragement to the victim to inject herself. (The position, the court thought, would have been different if the supply was for later use and therefore there was no encouragement.) What it should have said was that the voluntary act of the victim was a *novus actus*; therefore, the accused did not cause the victim's death. What he did was to bring about the facts which were the setting for the death but, leaving aside cases on pollution, that is not sufficient to constitute a cause of death. This case looks like one where the judges considered the accused to be morally at fault and so they made him legally guilty.

 Kennedy was referred by the Criminal Cases Review Commission to the Court of Appeal where it is reported as *Kennedy (No. 2)* [2005] 1 WLR 2159. The judgment of Lord Woolf CJ was very strange. He said that the parties were 'jointly engaged in administering the heroin' and therefore the accused caused the victim's death. This was novel law. In the words of M. J. Allen and S. Cooper, *Elliott & Wood's Cases and Materials on Criminal Law* (Thomson, 9th edn, 2006), p. v, 'The Court of Appeal surprised itself by creating confusion in three areas of law – causation, unlawful act manslaughter, and accessorial liability – with the coining of a new concept of "acting in concert".' Fortunately, the House of Lords strongly reasserted the primacy of the principle of 'free, deliberate and informed' intervention of the victim.

The House restored orthodoxy in *Kennedy (No. 2)* [2008] 1 AC 269. The facts are those of the *Kennedy* case mentioned above. The Court of Appeal asked the following question of general public importance: 'When is it appropriate to find someone guilty of manslaughter where that person has been involved in the supply of a . . . controlled drug, which is then freely and voluntarily self-administered by the person to whom it was supplied, and the administration then causes his death?' The Lords strongly and unanimously replied in a speech delivered by Lord Bingham: 'In the case of a fully informed and responsible adult, never'! The heroin was prepared by the accused and he passed the syringe to the victim, who then voluntarily self-administered the drug. The chain of causation was broken. Although scenarios existed where the accused could be said to have been jointly engaged in administering heroin, on the facts the accused had supplied the drug to the victim, who had a free choice whether to inject or not. There was no joint administration: 'the deceased . . . had a choice, knowing the facts, whether to inject himself or not. The heroin was, as the certified question correctly recognises, self-administered, not jointly administered.' Indeed, the Law Lords restricted liability in joint administration cases to rare facts: they overruled *Rogers* [2003] 1 WLR 1374, where the accused had tied the tourniquet on the victim's arm and the victim had then injected self-administered. If such a case cannot be seen as one on joint administration, it will be seldom that there can be liability of the accused when he jointly administered the drug.

The House, while not wishing 'to throw any doubt' on the authority, also took the opportunity to restrict the *Empress* case, above, to facts involving environmental offences. In Lord Bingham's words, the case does not 'lay down any general rules governing causation in criminal law'. Again, orthodoxy has been restored, but with a policy-based exception: 'causation is not a single, unvarying concept to be mechanically applied without regard to the context in which the question arises.' There is therefore some room for argument as to whether the general *Kennedy (No. 2)* principle or the *Empress* exception applies. Indeed, there is some possibility of further debate because the Lords did not define why drugs manslaughter cases fall within the orthodox rule.

An example of 'free, deliberate and informed' intervention occurred in *Latif* [1996] 1 WLR 104. The accused was charged with importing heroin into the UK. The drugs were given to a British customs officer in Pakistan and he brought them into the jurisdiction. The House of Lords held that the accused who had arranged for the heroin to be passed to a US Drugs Enforcement Administration officer who then passed them to the British officer was not guilty of the full offence, though he might have been guilty of the attempt to commit the full offence. Lord Steyn stated: 'The general principle is that the free, deliberate and informed intervention of a second person, who intends to exploit the situation created by the first, but is not acting in concert with him, is held to relieve the first actor of criminal responsibility.' The words from 'the free . . .' onwards are those of Hart and Honoré in *Causation in the Law*, though Lord Steyn omitted 'normally' before 'relieves'. This decision is inconsistent with the House of Lords ruling in the *Empress* case. In the latter case the act of a vandal should have broken the chain of causation. Instead the Lords held the defendants were liable for the vandal's act because such behaviour was not unforeseeable. Lord Nicholls in *Empress* may have confused the law on natural occurrences (where the test is one of reasonable foreseeability) and the law on third parties (where the test is one that 'free deliberate and informed intervention' breaks the chain of causation). As stated above, the Lords in *Kennedy (No. 2)* restricted *Empress* to environmental offences.

An illustration of this area of law is medical malpractice. Beldam LJ in *Cheshire*, above, said that only 'in the most extraordinary and unusual case' would negligent treatment, even if the immediate cause of death, be so independent of the acts of the accused that it could be regarded in law as the cause of the victim's death to the exclusion of the accused's acts. The maltreatment must be 'so potent in causing death that [the jury] regard the contribution made by his acts as insignificant'. Medical negligence by itself will not break the chain of causation. It does so only if it is so 'extraordinary' that the maltreatment made the accused's acts insignificant in causing death. (This rule would seem to be one which protects medical staff from the consequences of their carelessness.) The jury should look at the consequences of the treatment, and not at its degree of fault. In *Cheshire* the trial judge had directed the jury in terms of the recklessness of the treatment. He should have instructed them to consider whether it was the cause of death to the exclusion of the accused's acts. The Court of Appeal's test may be difficult to apply. The jurors have to use their judgment to determine whether or not the carelessness was 'so potent', and on the same facts different juries may disagree, with the result that one defendant is guilty of murder or manslaughter, whereas another is acquitted. Similar criticism may be made of 'so independent' and 'extraordinary'. The issue becomes one of normative attributions, not 'but-for' causation. A further criticism of **Cheshire** is that at the time of the victim's death, the acts of the accused no longer were 'potent' enough to cause death. As the court said, it was the negligent treatment which was the 'immediate' cause of death. Nevertheless, the accused was guilty. Furthermore, the accused shot the victim in the chest and leg; death was caused by a reaction to the insertion of a tube in his windpipe to aid breathing. The immediate cause of death, therefore, was not the accused's act, yet the accused was guilty because he had made a 'significant contribution' to the death.

One of the rare instances where medical mistreatment did break the chain of causation was in the following case, **Jordan**.

Jordan (1956) 40 Cr App R 152

The accused stabbed the victim, but the wound had largely healed. However, while undergoing treatment, the victim was injected with a drug and a large quantity of liquid, and died. The accused was not guilty of murder, because the treatment was so abnormal and so negligent ('palpably wrong') that the wound was merely the scene of the cause of death, not the cause itself.

Jordan has been called 'a very particular case depending upon its exact facts': **Blaue**, above. This was an attempt to distinguish **Jordan** out of existence. In **Malcherek**, above, the court said that if it were obliged to choose between **Jordan** and **Smith**, it would choose the latter; it did, however, recognise that both cases remained good law. **Jordan** is therefore the exceptional case. Only if, as occurred in **Jordan**, the treatment was 'palpably wrong' will it be a *novus actus interveniens*. (It should be noted that the medical treatment in **Smith** was said to be 'thoroughly bad', which seems the same as 'palpably wrong', yet in **Smith** the accused was convicted.) **Jordan** has been criticised for placing emphasis on the actions of the medical staff when it is the accused, and not the staff, who is on trial. **Jordan** is not too dissimilar from **Cheshire**, yet in the latter case the accused was convicted but not in the former. Presumably the question to be asked after **Cheshire** should be phrased as not 'Was the treatment palpably wrong?' but 'Was it so independent of the acts of the accused and so potent in causing death that the contribution of those acts was insignificant?'

The basic rule in **Smith**, that medical mistreatment does not break the chain of causation, was applied in **Cheshire**, above. Similarly, in **Mellor** [1996] 2 Cr App R 245 (CA) the accused was guilty when the victim of his beating up died of aspiration pneumonia, even though there had been a 90 per cent chance of his survival if he had been given oxygen, the correct treatment. The court held that the prosecution did not have to prove that the medical maltreatment was not a significant cause of death; it had to prove that what the accused did was a significant contribution to the death. In the New Zealand case of **Kirikiri** [1982] 2 NZLR 648 the accused *inter alia* battered his wife's face with a rifle. To help her breathe a plastic pipe was inserted by the hospital through her neck into her windpipe. Somehow the pipe became dislodged and the victim died. Jeffries J in the High Court applied **Smith**. The original wound was still the operating cause: 'death can properly be said to be the result of the wound, albeit that some other cause of death is also operating', as Lord Parker CJ put it.

An interesting application is **Malcherek**, where the doctors turned off the life-support system of patients who were already brain-dead. (Presumably the same applies to patients in a persistent vegetative state.) This act was held not to be the operative cause of death. The assault which put the victim into hospital was. Lord Lane CJ thought it bizarre to say that a doctor who was doing his or her best to save life was the cause of the victim's death. The courts seem to be pulling the law on causation to exculpate doctors and the police in order to catch the attacker.

If a pre-existing medical condition of the victim cannot be treated because of the accused's injuring him, the accused remains liable for his death unless, it seems, the refusal to operate was 'extraordinary and unusual': **McKechnie** (1992) 94 Cr App R 51 (CA). The victim's ulcer would have been treated, had he not been put into hospital by the accused beating him over the head with a TV set. It was immaterial whether the lack of treatment was correct provided that it was reasonable as it was on the facts: the doctors thought the victim might die under anaesthesia. The case illustrates the principle that a person's death may have more than one cause. Alternatively, one might say that the immediate cause of death was the refusal to operate, but the operative cause of that immediate cause was what the accused did.

An interesting comparison is with the law relating to refusal of medical treatment. The accused takes the risk that the victim will not undergo treatment, but not of independent and potent maltreatment. A case like **McKechnie** is also important for demonstrating that an accused can be held to be the cause of a consequence even though he did not cause the death in medical terms. The medical cause was a duodenal ulcer which burst. The accused has no control over the doctor, yet liability can turn on the doctor's competence.

Finally on medical treatment, attention should be drawn to the issue of the competence of the doctors. If the victim dies through their gross negligence, is it just to say that the accused contributed significantly to the death and therefore he or she is guilty of murder or manslaughter? In any case, even if not guilty of a fatal offence, he will be guilty of a non-fatal offence.

One fact-situation which has not yet troubled the English courts is whether an omission by a third party may constitute a *novus actus*. It is thought that such an omission does not break the chain of causation because the accused's act remains a significant contribution to the death or injury. The third party may also be guilty of an offence, depending on the facts.

Students should not get too worked up about this area of law. The Latin term *novus actus interveniens* is merely shorthand for a full statement of the law. As the Court of Appeal said in **Kennedy** [1999] Crim LR 65: 'Whether one talks of *novus actus interveniens* or simply in terms of causation . . . the critical question to which the jury must direct its mind, where (as in the instant case) there is an act causative of death performed by in this case the deceased himself, is whether the defendant can be said to be jointly responsible for the carrying out of that act.' The same applies where a third party jointly performs an act leading to death.

(b) The 'escape' cases

These are illustrative of the problem of *novus actus interveniens*. The accused is guilty when the victim is killed trying to escape, unless the escape was not foreseeable by a reasonable person. There are several cases, the principal English one being **Mackie** (1973) 57 Cr App R 453. A three-year-old boy fell downstairs and died in an attempt to escape a thrashing. The accused was found guilty of manslaughter. See also the discussion of **Roberts** (1971) 56 Cr App R 95 in the context of assault occasioning actual bodily harm, below. In **Roberts** the escape by a girl from a moving car (she suffered concussion and abrasions and had to stay in hospital for three days) as a result of sexual advances made by the accused was said to break the chain of causation only when it was voluntary and 'daft'. If 'the victim does something so "daft" . . . that no reasonable person could be expected to foresee it . . . then, it is really occasioned by a voluntary act on the part of the victim'. If the act is reasonably foreseeable the chain of causation is not broken. However, in some of the cases on drugs where the accused supplies the victim with heroin and paraphernalia, he has been held liable despite the victim's injection being voluntary, as we have seen. The accused was guilty if the escape was the 'natural result of what the alleged assailant said and did in the sense that it was something that could reasonably have been foreseen as the consequence of what he was doing or saying'. Roch LJ in **Marjoram**, above, approved the *ratio* of **Roberts**. The chain of causation is broken only if the victim does something so unexpected that it is 'daft'. The Court of Appeal in **Evans** [1992] Crim LR 659 seems to have been asking for the escape to be a 'natural consequence' of the accused's behaviour. In **Corbett** [1996] Crim LR 594 (CA), the victim was a mentally handicapped man with an alcohol problem. He argued with the accused with whom he had been drinking all day. The accused head-butted him without of course intending to kill him and as he fled he fell into the gutter. He was struck and killed by a passing car. The accused argued that the jury should have been instructed to inquire whether the death of the victim was the natural consequence of his conduct and that he should have been acquitted if that death was not the natural consequence. The court followed **Roberts**. As long as what the victim did was within the range of foreseeable actions, the chain of causation remained unbroken. Only if the victim's act was 'daft' was the chain broken. His disability and intoxication did not make his reaction daft. The prosecution did not have to prove that the death of the victim was *the* natural consequence of the accused's conduct. Accordingly, the accused's appeal was dismissed.

The principal Commonwealth authority involving an escape is the decision of the High Court of Australia in **Royall**, in which English cases were discussed.

Royall v *R* (1991) 65 ALJR 451

The victim was found on the ground below the bathroom window of the flat in which she and the accused had lived for the previous four months. There were many signs of a struggle. The accused, while not denying that he was present, said that the victim had voluntarily jumped out of the window and that he did not intend to kill or harm her.

Mason CJ clearly and succinctly opined (at 455):

[g]enerally speaking an act done by a person in the interests of self-protection, in the face of violence or threats of violence on the part of another, which results in the death of the first person, does not negative causal connection between the violence or threats of violence and the death. The intervening act of the deceased does not break the chain of causation.

English cases state that a reasonable act performed to escape does not break the chain (**Pagett** (1983) 76 Cr App R 279); similarly if the act of escape was reasonably foreseeable (**Roberts**, above, endorsed in **DPP v Daley** [1980] AC 237). If the test is one of reasonable foreseeability, **Pagett** can also be explained on this ground. It is reasonably foreseeable that if one shoots at armed police they will return fire.

Mason CJ continued (**Royall** at 456):

[i]n the context of causation the principle is best formulated as follows: where the conduct of the accused induces in the victim a well-founded apprehension of physical harm such as to make it a natural consequence (or reasonable) that the victim would seek to escape and the victim is injured in the course of escaping, the injury is caused by the accused's conduct. Whether it is necessary for the prosecution to establish also that the mode of escape adopted is a natural consequence of the victim's apprehension for his or her safety does not arise here for the deceased had no means of escape other than jumping out of the window in the situation posited. The question could arise only in circumstances where the victim does something irrational or unexpected, in which event it might be more difficult to establish that the injury sustained was a consequence of the accused's act and not the product of the victim's voluntary act. In such a situation much may turn on the nature and extent of the well-founded apprehension of the victim; and it is to be expected that persons fearful for their own safety forced to react on the spur of the moment will not always make a sound or sensible judgment and may act irrationally.

In the English cases the natural consequence test has been linked to the concept of foreseeability. Because the natural consequence test inevitably invites conjecture about the likelihood of an occurrence, it is impossible to divorce completely the application of the test from the concept of foreseeability. However, in my view, to invite the jury to consider foreseeability would be more likely, at least in the majority of cases, to confuse than to clarify the issue of causation. In many cases, for much the same reason, I see no point in linking that issue to the accused's state of mind. On the other hand, in some situations, the accused's state of mind will be relevant to that issue as, for example, where there is evidence that the accused intended that injury should result in the way in which it did and where, in the absence of evidence of intention, the facts would raise a doubt about causation.

Brennan J used the foreseeability test (at 460).

The question whether an accused whose conduct has led to a death is criminally responsible for the death when the death has been caused by a final fatal step taken by the victim thus depends on the reasonableness (or proportionality) of the victim's attempt at self-preservation and the accused's foresight, or the reasonable foreseeability, of the possibility that a final fatal step might be taken by the victim in response to the accused's conduct.

Deane and Dawson JJ wished foreseeability to be excised from the test. The question was whether the fear was well grounded, well founded or reasonable (at 464–465). Toohey and Gaudron JJ (at 471) said that: '. . . the jury may be told that if the victim's reaction to the act of the accused said to have caused the death was quite disproportionate to the act or was unreasonable, the chain of causation was broken'. The most thorough analysis was by McHugh J. He noted four tests:

(a) operating and substantial test (i.e. more than *de minimis*);

(b) natural consequence test, as in **Beech** (1912) 7 Cr App R 197;

(c) reasonable foresight test, as in **Roberts**, above, **Mackie** (1973) 57 Cr App R 453, and **DPP v Daley**, above;

(d) *novus actus interveniens* test – see **Dalby** [1982] 1 WLR 425 (CA), where the court held that the taking of a drug by the victim broke the chain. As Waller LJ put it, '. . . the supply of drugs would itself have caused no harm unless the deceased had subsequently used the drugs in a form and quality which was dangerous.' **Dalby** is still correct on this point: **Khan** [1998] Crim LR 830 and both of these authorities cannot be reconciled with **Kennedy**, in the Court of Appeal, which is wrong. In **Dalby** the accused supplied drugs to the victim, who injected himself. He died. The court held that the supply of the drug did not cause the victim's death; it was the victim's injecting himself which did. That act broke the chain of causation. In **Kennedy**, above, the Court of Appeal again agreed that **Dalby** remained good law. However, it distinguished it on the ground that in **Kennedy** it was the accused who prepared the syringe and handed it to the victim, who then injected himself. The distinction between supplying drugs (**Dalby**) and both supplying and preparing them is not a strong one. Both cases involve the accused encouraging the victim to take illegal drugs.

Because of the number of different tests the way was open for the High Court of Australia to rule what the law was in escape or fright cases. McHugh J preferred the reasonable foreseeability test, which had the weight of authority in its favour, over the natural consequence test, because of the latter's ambiguity (very likely to occur or might occur?). Despite observations to the contrary in **Dalby** it was not a *novus actus interveniens* that the victim acted unreasonably. Suicide and the refusal of medical treatment need not break the chain of causation. 'In determining whether a reasonable person could have foreseen the harm suffered by the victim, any irrational or unreasonable conduct of the victim will be a variable factor to be weighed according to all the circumstances of the case' (at 482).

The High Court of Australia was therefore split on the issue. The same court did, however, state in **McAuliffe v R** (1995) 69 ALJR 621 that **Royall** was authority for the proposition that 'in fright, escape or self-preservation cases, it is ordinarily undesirable to focus attention upon foreseeability'. Until challenged English law adopts the reasonable foreseeability test in escape cases.

It is suggested that there are strong *dicta* in **Environment Agency v Empress Car Co (Abertillery) Ltd** [1999] 2 AC 22, discussed above, which should lead to the demise of the 'foreseeability' test. Lord Clyde stated (and Lord Hoffmann spoke to similar effect):

> In deciding whether some particular factor has played so important a part that any activity by the defendant should be seen as entirely superseded as a causative element, it is not a consideration of the foreseeability, or reasonable foreseeability, of the extraneous factor which seems to me to be appropriate, but rather its unnatural, extraordinary or unusual character.

It may be that the House of Lords was restricting its remarks to pollution cases (indeed, the Lords seem to be striving to prevent pollution), though that was not the view taken by the Court of Appeal in **Finlay**, above. Lord Hoffmann said that when determining causation, the purpose of the law has to be ascertained. The purpose in this case was to stop pollution entering controlled waters. Therefore, a company which played a part in the pollution caused that event (as did the third party who opened the tap, thereby allowing diesel to run into a river). Normally one would expect the intervention of a third party to break the chain of causation. On the facts it was not extraordinary that an unknown third party would turn the tap on a tank containing diesel, allowing the fuel to pollute a river. Looking at the issue from a different angle, a third party could make the accused guilty of a crime by choosing to cause pollution. (Does a householder cause burglary by owning a home? It is foreseeable that burglary may take place in houses including this one.) And it may be hard to distinguish unforeseeable and extraordinary occurrences contrary to the view of the House of Lords. If **Empress** and **Finlay** are correct, the intervention of a third party, including the victim, would not break the chain of causation except in extraordinary circumstances even when that third party acted in a 'free, deliberate and informed' manner. Such extensions to the law should not be made *ad hoc*, as they certainly were in **Finlay** (see, however, **Kennedy (No. 2)** above), and require justifying.

There is no need to give an instruction on the test in **Roberts** where the facts do not call for it. For example, in **Notman** [1994] Crim LR 518, the accused, who had been banned from a shop, created a disturbance with others in it. A constable put out his foot to stop the accused charging at him and sustained an injury to his ankle. The accused was guilty of assault occasioning actual bodily harm. The case was an easy one, not requiring an elaborate direction on causation: the injury was caused by the defendant or it was not.

Whichever test English law adopts, the law will be flexible. Judges will be able to use concepts such as 'daft' and 'foreseeable' to convict those whom they wish to find guilty and to exonerate those whom they do not. In the **Roberts** case the victim jumped out of a car which was travelling fairly slowly when the accused tried to take off her coat as part of a sexual attack. If the vehicle had been travelling fast, it is thought that in the words of the court her jumping out would have been 'daft'. The result is that victims ought not to try to escape from sexual assault when the vehicle is being driven quickly, but are at liberty to escape from a slow-moving car. Yet in both situations the factual cause of the attempted escape is the accused's act, and the question whether the accused is guilty becomes one of legal policy. In terms of policy, the accused, it might be argued, should be guilty, no matter how fast the vehicle is going, for women should have the right to escape from sexual assaults in all situations and it is neither unforeseeable nor daft that they should do so. It should also be stated that the reasonably foreseeable test in **Roberts** is out of line with the operative cause test in **Smith**, above, and that the court made no reference to **Smith**. Certainly English judges, who may not have seen that they were faced in the cases with different tests, have not chosen which one should govern. Indeed, in **Williams** [1992] 1 WLR 380 (CA), Stuart-Smith LJ said that the accused was guilty if the deceased victim's attempted escape from a moving car travelling at some 30 mph was 'proportionate to the threat, that is to say, that it was within the ambit of reasonableness and not so daft as to make it his own voluntary act which amounted to a *novus actus interveniens*'. In judging whether the victim acted reasonably in trying to flee from an attempted robbery, the jury were to take into account 'any particular characteristic of the victim and the fact that in the agony of the moment he may act without thought and deliberation'. (Similar is **Marjoram**, above.) While the jury is to bear in mind the victim's characteristics, they must not take into consideration the accused's characteristics. The test is a reasonable person one, not one which as in provocation involves a reasonable or ordinary person imbued with most of the characteristics of the accused. Readers who have studied the law of negligence in tort will be able to draw parallels. There may be a difference between a range-of-reasonable-responses test as in this case and a no-reasonable-man-could-be-expected-to-foresee-the-victim's-act test in **Roberts**. On the facts of **Williams**, though the conviction for manslaughter was quashed, it is not easy to see whether the victim acted reasonably. He was dead, and the three defendants' statements were not uniform as to the threat which they made to him. Without knowing the nature of the threat, the jury could not say whether the reaction was daft or proportionate. The contrast with cases concerned with the rule that one takes one's victim as one finds him is obvious. In the latter type of case one does not inquire whether the victim's behaviour, such as refusing a blood transfusion, was 'daft', whereas in the escape cases an over-reaction caused by the accused's overtimidity breaks the chain of causation.

(c) Indivisible transactions

The general rule is that 'the intent and the act must both concur to constitute the crime': *Fowler* v *Padget* (1798) 101 ER 1103, 1106. There is no defence where a series of actions culminate in death and are classified by the court as being inseparable. (See also the section on contemporaneity.) The authority establishing this point was *Thabo Meli* v *R* [1954] 1 All ER 373. The acts of rendering the victim unconscious and pushing him over a cliff at the bottom of which he died of exposure were classified by the Privy Council as being indivisible. The accused were guilty of murder even though the actual cause of death was not their act. That case was followed in *Church* [1966] 1 QB 59 by the Court of Criminal Appeal. Unlike in *Thabo Meli* there was no antecedent plan – to throw the female victim into the river – but *Thabo Meli* was extended from murder to manslaughter. *Thabo Meli* was also followed in *Moore* [1975] Crim LR 229 (CA), where the defendants apparently intended only to assault, not to kill. The first accused had a grudge against the victim and arranged a meeting with him. The second defendant accompanied the first. They took with them breeze-blocks, a plastic bag and a length of rope. The victim got into a van and the first accused knocked him unconscious with a truncheon. The first defendant thought he had killed him. He weighted him with the breeze-blocks and threw him into a harbour, where he died of drowning. Both defendants were found guilty of murder.

A case which applied the *Thabo Meli* principle was *Le Brun* [1992] QB 61 (CA). During an argument the accused struck his wife on the jaw, causing her to sink to her knees. He dropped her while trying to drag her into the house. She died of a fractured skull. The accused had battered her but did not intend seriously to hurt her. He had not dropped her intentionally. The court held that he had caused her death and took the view that the blow, dropping the victim, and the death were all part of the same transaction. Accordingly, the principle of indivisible transactions applies outside of the area of disposal of a supposed corpse. Under *Thabo Meli* it was sufficient that the accused had the *mens rea* of the crime, in this case manslaughter, at the start of the sequence of events. Alternatively the court adopted the first principle stated above, that when the accused dropped his wife there was no break in the chain of causation which prevented the blow being the cause of death. Death was reasonably foreseeable. The court thought that if the accused had been trying to help his wife into the house to make her better, the dropping might have been a *novus actus interveniens*. As things were, his action was an attempt to conceal his attack on her, or the completion of his argument with her. On this point the court confused motive and causation. It said that if the accused had a good motive, seeking medical help, he was not liable because he did not cause her death; if, however, he picked her up with a bad motive, such as concealing his attack on her, he was guilty, for then he would have caused her death. The reasoning makes the accused's state of mind relevant to causation but the rule is that causation forms part of the *actus reus*. (Presumably he was also guilty of gross negligence manslaughter. His dropping of her was grossly negligent, if the jury so held. If this supposition is correct, there was no need to argue about the intention to batter and the cause of death being separate in time, for under this type of manslaughter they were contemporaneous.)

Current authorities are concerned with homicide, but the principles apply to other offences.

(d) Refusal of medical treatment

An old case is **Holland** (1841) 2 Mood & R 351. The victim refused treatment for a wound to the finger and died of tetanus. The accused was convicted of murder at Liverpool Assizes on the grounds that the wound was the ultimate cause of death. The same applies where the victim will not undergo treatment for religious or psychological reasons. The most authoritative case is **Blaue**, above, where a Jehovah's Witness refused a blood transfusion. The Court of Appeal held that the accused must take his victim as he finds him (see (e) below), a proposition similar to the eggshell skull rule in tort. Therefore, it was the stab wound which caused the victim's death. Lawton LJ said: 'The fact that the victim refused to stop this end coming about did not break the causal connection between the act and death.' The court rejected the argument that since medical treatment had improved in the years since **Holland**, the law in that case had also changed. It might be said that **Blaue** exemplifies English law's policy of religious freedom. It is not to the point that the victim's refusal was unreasonable. This rule distinguishes this area of law from the 'escape cases' discussed above. To make the attacker guilty of murder, could the victim refuse to have a tourniquet applied, an unlikely but possible scenario? Why should an accused be guilty of murder when the victim unreasonably refuses to seek medical attention? Why is the refusal not a *novus actus interveniens* when very poor treatment may be? Should the accused be guilty even though he did not foresee and a reasonable person would not have foreseen the refusal? Why should liability for homicide depend on whether the victim refuses to look after himself?

(e) The accused must take his victim as he finds him

This rule of causation is sometimes called the 'eggshell skull' rule and is the same as in tort. If, for example, the victim had a thin skull and no one including the accused knew of this fact, if the victim dies as a result of the accused's hitting her over the head with a baseball bat but she would not have died, had she not had a thin skull, then the accused is deemed to be responsible for the death, even though he did not know of the thinness of the skull (and even though a reasonable person would not have known). As we can see from **Blaue**, the rule is not restricted to physical condition (such as haemophilia) but most situations will in practice involve the physical well-being of the victim where she is in a poor state of health. Presumably the rule may be extended to a situation where a woman, on being raped, kills herself: see also **Dear** [1996] Crim LR 595, discussed above. Certainly the accused must act at his peril where the victim has a pre-existing mental condition such as depression. It is questionable whether or not the principle applies where it is a third party who is the immediate cause of death, such as would happen where an infant's parent or guardian who was a Jehovah's Witness refused a blood transfusion for him. If the principle in **Blaue** is not applied because it leads to unfair outcomes, the accused is still guilty of attempted murder and wounding with intent to cause grievous bodily harm.

A justification for the rule was put forward by McLachlin J in the Supreme Court of Canada in **Creighton** (1993) 105 DLR (4th) 632. She said that the eggshell skull rule 'requires aggressors, once embarked on their dangerous course of conduct which may foreseeably injure others, to take responsibility for all the consequences that ensue, even to death'. Current law stops the court, rightly many think, from investigating the merits of religious beliefs. Although the scenario is unlikely, if the victim refused a transfusion out of spite towards the accused, the latter would still on these principles have caused the death of the former. It is arguable that, though the accused has factually caused death (because the transfusion issue would not otherwise have arisen), death ought not to be legally ascribed to him. Hart and Honoré, *Causation in the Law*, 2nd edn (OUP, 1985) 332, consider that a person who refuses a transfusion on religious grounds is not acting voluntarily because of the pressure of his religion. Therefore, they argue that the spiteful victim is acting voluntarily. They contend, as already indicated, that the chain of causation is broken by 'a free, deliberate and informed act of a human being' (at 136). The epithets are, it may be said, to some extent normative and not purely descriptive. 'Voluntary' and 'involuntary' are, however, chameleon words, and if the accused is deemed to take his victim as he finds him, why cannot he find him spiteful and so be guilty? Is a person of a certain religious persuasion acting freely if she refuses a blood transfusion? Applying **Cheshire** the eggshell skull is 'independent' of the act of the accused. Moreover, if the accused in **Blaue** had to take his victim as he found her, why does not the same rule apply to the speeding motorist who is sexually assaulting a passenger (see **Roberts**, above)? These rules, both of which turn on the victim's response, are inconsistent. An eggshell skull is not reasonably foreseeable. It may not be reasonably foreseeable for a woman to kill herself after being raped but, following **Blaue**, the rapist would be guilty of manslaughter. **Blaue** has the potential to swallow the rule in **Roberts**. One possibility is that the accused does not take a 'daft' victim as he finds him. An example would occur if the victim thought that cancer could be caught by breathing her cancerous attacker's exhalations. Another attempt to reconcile **Blaue** and **Roberts** is to say that in **Blaue** the victim refused to act whereas in **Roberts** the victim did act, and therefore the distinction turns on whether there is an act or an omission. Alternatively if the victim must react reasonably in escape cases, why not in cases of refusing treatment? A linked argument is that if a daft escape breaks the chain of causation, why does not a voluntary decision not to have a transfusion break it? Surely it would have been broken if the victim had refused treatment because she did not like the colour of the hospital walls? Another way of reconciling **Blaue** and **Roberts** is to argue that **Blaue** is a special case concerned with freedom of religion. See D. Klimchuk 'Causation: thin skulls and equality' (1998) 11 Canadian Journal of Law and Jurisprudence 115. It is suggested that the 'take your victim' test should not apply where the outcome would offend common sense; therefore, if the victim has acted in a 'daft' manner the accused should not be guilty of the offence charged, though he may still be guilty of a lesser offence or of the attempt. It is also suggested that whether the victim has a weak heart, refuses blood transfusions and the like does not affect the accused's moral culpability.

This area of law can be usefully compared with that of negligent medical treatment. The accused takes the doctor as he finds him; that is, the competence of the doctor is (normally) irrelevant to criminal liability, just as the victim's personality is immaterial.

(f) Contributory negligence

The fact that the victim was contributorily negligent in causing her own death does not absolve the accused from criminal liability. In **Swindall and Osborne** (1846) 2 Cox CC 141 the victim was run over and killed by one of the two defendants. The jury was instructed that it did not matter whether the deceased was deaf, drunk or careless and whether his being so contributed to his death. If, however, the contributory negligence is gross, the chain of causation may be broken, gross negligence being seen as a *novus actus* (see above).

Difficulties of proof in causation

One can see the difficulty in proving causation and the effect of such a failure in *Fisher*.

Fisher [1987] Crim LR 334

The defendant, a nightclub bouncer, intervened in a fight involving the victim. The bouncer banged the victim's head several times on the stairs while dragging him down them. By the time they got to the bottom of the stairs, the victim was dead. If death was partly caused by dragging the victim downstairs the accused was guilty of manslaughter. If, however, the victim was killed by a blow landed by the accused in self-defence, he was not guilty. Since the prosecution could not prove the former, the Court of Appeal ruled that the accused was not guilty.

Similar is *Bunn* (1989) *The Times*, 11 May. The defendant hit the victim over the head with a snooker cue. Perhaps as a result, the victim developed a mental disease and committed suicide over three months later. The prosecution abandoned its case because it was not sure that a reasonable jury would convict because it was uncertain whether the blow caused the death. In *Evans* [1992] Crim LR 659 (CA), the Crown could not prove that the accused's behaviour caused the victim to jump out of the window to his death. Where the victim has committed suicide, it may be particularly problematic to attribute the victim's death to the accused.

Proposals for the reform of causation

In the Law Commission's draft Criminal Code, Law Com. No. 177, 1989, cl 17 reads in part:

(1) . . . a person causes a result which is an element of an offence when . . .
   (a) he does an act which makes a more than negligible contribution to its occurrence; or
   (b) he omits to do an act which might prevent its occurrence and which he is under a duty to do according to the law relating to the offence.
(2) A person does not cause a result where, after he does such an act or makes such an omission, an act or event occurs . . .
   (a) which is the immediate and sufficient cause of the result;
   (b) which he did not foresee, and
   (c) which could not in the circumstances reasonably have been foreseen.

In its commentary the Law Commission (p 188) showed that it wished to restate present law in relation to causation-in-fact, taking one's victim as one finds him, intervening acts including the escape cases, medical mistreatment including the principle in *Jordan*, above, and the refusal of treatment. The restatement does not readily demonstrate that the choice of the act is an essentially normative exercise, not a factual one. A cause is selected and attributed to the accused or it is not. Current law is sometimes criticised for not being a straightforward application of scientific principles, but it is doubtful that one could reach the stage where science alone solves causation problems. Causation-in-fact is not sufficient by itself, and to say that the accused caused something is not necessarily a statement of fact. One might say that the accused was guilty in *Smith* only because the brawl was in Germany, a fortuitous circumstance, where treatment was at that time poor, another fortuitous circumstance, and of course neither the UK nor the (then) West German government was put on trial for not providing a good standard of medical care. For criticism of the scope of cl 17(2) see Glanville Williams *'Finis* for *novus actus'*, [1989] CLJ 391. Certainly phrases such as 'negligible' and 'immediate and sufficient' are open to interpretation.

Omission

One must be careful when translating *actus reus* into English. It looks like 'guilty act'. However, the accused may also be guilty when he fails or omits to do something (omission). If in orthodox theory the criminal law imposes a duty to act and the accused does not perform that act he is guilty. There has to be a duty to act; otherwise all who did nothing would cause the *actus reus* to happen. English law traditionally does not always hold a person guilty for failing to act. There are exceptional cases where the accused is liable provided that he has the requisite *mens rea*. These exceptions have grown in recent years, but the general principle remains that generally a person is not guilty for omitting to do something.

> Generations of law students have been thrilled by the spine-chilling tale of individuals watching a small child drown in an inch of water . . .

is how C. Ryan, *Criminal Law*, 4th edn (Blackstone Press, 1995) 45, puts it. Yet a parent is guilty if he lets his child drown in such circumstances. (Whether a child would have the *actus reus* of murder if he let his parent drown in similar circumstances is more debatable.) It should not be thought that omissions are always less serious than commissions. Starving a person to death may be more morally unacceptable than mercy-killing. Nevertheless, Anglo-Welsh criminal law draws a distinction between an act (such as stabbing) and an omission (such as not feeding a baby). This distinction is based on the view that a hard-and-fast line can be drawn between an act and an omission, which was the prevalent view until recently among the judiciary: see Phillimore LJ in *Lowe* [1973] QB 702 (CA).

The general rule is exemplified by *Wychavon DC v National Rivers Authority* [1993] 1 WLR 125. The council was charged with causing polluted matter to enter any controlled water contrary to the Water Act 1989, s 107(1)(c). Watkins LJ in the Divisional Court held that failing to prevent or to take steps to clear a blockage in a system for which it was responsible did not constitute the offence. There was no positive or deliberate act which caused the sewage to enter the river. This decision turns on the construction of the statute, 'causes or knowingly permits': normally 'causes' does include both acts and omissions. (Possibly the case itself would nowadays be decided differently: see *inter alia*, *National Rivers Authority v Yorkshire Water Services Ltd* [1995] 1 AC 444 (HL); however, the principle stands.) The position would have been different had the council been charged with knowingly permitting polluted matter to enter controlled waters: *Environment Agency v Empress Car Co (Abertillery) Ltd* [1999] 2 AC 22 (HL) (this case is also known as *Empress Car Co (Abertillery) Ltd v National Rivers Authority*). 'Mere tacit standing by and looking on' is not 'causing': *Price v Cromack* [1975] 1 WLR 988 (DC). One can permit something to happen by failing to prevent it. This aspect of the case falls within (b) below.

The established exceptions are now detailed.

Points (a)–(d) detail offences which may be committed by an omission. Points (e)–(i) state when a person is under a duty to act in relation to those offences, which are normally committed by an act, but which are capable of being committed by an omission, failing to intervene. The list of situations where a legal duty to act is imposed is not closed: *Khan* [1998] Crim LR 830 (CA). It is normally said that it is for the judge to rule whether such a duty exists but in *Khan* it was held that whether a duty of care was owed by a drug dealer to his client was a matter of fact which depended on the circumstances. It is suggested that *Khan* is wrong. Juries cannot expand and contract the various duties to act. For example, juries cannot alter the outcome in Ryan's example, quoted above, by changing the law.

(a) Because of legislative supremacy Parliament can change the general law that a person is not guilty for omitting to do something. Statute has created offences which can be committed only by omissions such as dishonestly retaining a wrongful credit contrary to s 24A of the Theft Act 1968 as inserted by the Theft (Amendment) Act 1996 or failing to produce a breath specimen. Usually liability is imposed on a certain type of person, such as an occupier or a driver. Under the Merchant Shipping Act 1995, s 58(2)(b), a master or seaman who omits to do anything required to save a ship from loss or serious damage is guilty of an offence. A person may be guilty of the offence of failing to report a traffic accident in which he was involved and which caused injury or damage: Road Traffic Act 1988, s 170. A failure to look after one's child is an offence under the Children and Young Persons Act 1933, s 1(1). This is the crime of wilful neglect which is discussed in the next chapter. In each of these offences it should be noted on whom the duty is imposed: masters or seamen, drivers and parents. Passers-by are not liable. The duty is restricted to a certain class of persons. A failure to disclose information relating to terrorism is a crime contrary to the Terrorism Act 2000, s 20, if the information comes to the accused in the course of his trade, profession, business or employment and he does not disclose it to the police as soon as reasonably practicable. The width of the duty depends on construction and may include the whole world, as this statute demonstrates.

(b) In some offences the language of the statute can be read as imposing liability for not doing something. One permits one's drivers to break the law if one does not take reasonable steps to prevent breaches: *Vehicle Inspectorate* v *Nuttall* [1999] 1 WLR 629 (HL). One is guilty of handling by 'assisting in the retention' of stolen goods when one leaves money in one's Post Office account: *Pitchley* (1972) 57 Cr App R 30 (CA). Similarly one can obstruct the highway by not removing a collapsed wall after being given notice to remove it: *Gully* v *Smith* (1883) 12 QBD 121. There is a crime of dishonestly retaining a wrongful credit: see Chapter 17. In *Firth* (1990) 91 Cr App R 217 (CA) a doctor deceived by non-disclosure of the true facts. Another case is *Shama* [1990] 1 WLR 661 (CA). The accused was guilty of the crime of falsifying a document required for an accounting purpose contrary to s 17(1)(a) of the Theft Act 1968 when he failed to fill in a form, it being his duty to do so. On the wording of the crime it is, however, difficult to say that he falsified a document when he did nothing. In *Greener* v *DPP* (1996) 160 JP 265 the Divisional Court held that the crime of allowing a dangerous dog to enter a place which is not a public place, but where it is not permitted to be, covered a failure by the accused to take adequate precautions to secure the dog to a chain with the effect that it broke out of his back garden and bit the face of a child who was in a garden nearby. Some verbs can be read as including failures to act. See 'causing' in (c) below.

There are a couple of problematical cases. In **Speck** [1977] 2 All ER 859, the Court of Appeal held that the accused was guilty of gross indecency when he failed to prevent a child doing such an act with him. A young girl had placed her hand on his penis. He had an erection. He was found guilty under s 1 of the Indecency with Children Act 1960. That statute required an 'act of gross indecency'. The court decided that his failure to remove the girl's hand, an omission, was an invitation to her to undertake the act. Therefore, there was an act. This interpretation in view of the facts looks like stretching words to catch the accused. In **Yuthiwattana** (1984) 80 Cr App R 55, the Court of Appeal held that a failure to replace a key amounted to an act calculated to interfere with a tenant's peace and comfort. It may be that the court did not see the point at issue, and in **Ahmad** (1986) 84 Cr App R 64, the same court determined that failure to provide a bathroom was not an act calculated to interfere with peace and comfort. Failing to complete repairs was not an 'act'. The words in the statute creating the offence were clear, and statutes creating crimes should be strictly construed. **Ahmad** would seem to lay down a general rule of criminal law that where a statute states 'act', that term cannot be construed as including an omission. For further discussion in the context of attempts see Chapter 10. The court in **Ahmad** distinguished **Miller** [1983] 2 AC 161, see below, on the grounds that **Miller** did not apply where a statute expressly required an act. The accused in **Ahmad** was under no duty to act as the accused was in **Miller** because by its words the statute did not impose such an obligation. However, if one uses the so-called 'continuing (or continuous) act' theory one can find support for convicting the accused in **Ahmad**. He is guilty if he intentionally does an act and fails to take reasonable measures to prevent the *actus reus*. The situation is deemed to be an intentional act. Accordingly it may depend on which theory of omissions one uses to see whether the accused is guilty. Lord Diplock in **Miller** chose the duty theory on the ground that it was simpler than the other to explain to juries. A different court might be persuaded to adopt the continuous act theory if it wished to convict the accused. However that may be, **Yuthiwattana** seems incorrect. Parliament stipulated 'act'. If what the accused did cannot sensibly be described as an 'act', he should not be guilty.

It is thought that some offences cannot be construed as imposing criminal liability for omissions. It is impossible to conceive of a person's committing robbery (s 8 of the Theft Act 1968) or burglary (s 9) by omission. There is a crime of throwing missiles at a football match. This offence cannot be committed by an omission. One might have expected that it would be impossible to rape by omission because rape involves penetration, but the Privy Council held on appeal from New Zealand in **Kaitamaki v R** [1985] AC 147 that a man could rape when he did not withdraw on request. This advice related to the pre-2003 definition of rape but the law does apply under the Sexual Offences Act 2003, for the accused is guilty only if he 'penetrates the vagina, anus or mouth of another person with his penis'. For further discussion see Chapter 14.

(c) Sometimes the courts construe common law or statutory offences as imposing liability for omissions. If one part of the *actus reus* of murder and manslaughter is 'causing death' (rather than 'killing' which seems more to require a positive act, though one can 'kill' by an omission), one can cause death by failing to prevent death occurring. For more on this see gross negligence manslaughter (Chapter 12), but unlawful act manslaughter cannot be committed by an omission: **Lowe** [1973] QB 702 (CA). 'Causing' is therefore sometimes read as requiring an act (see **Wychavon**, above) but sometimes as covering an omission. It is suggested that it is construed in the latter sense when the *actus reus* is defined solely in terms of 'causing' something to happen, but in the former sense when the offence consists of 'causing or permitting'; 'permitting' covers a failure to act but here 'causing' does not. This was the view of the House of Lords in *Environment Agency* v *Empress Car Co (Abertillery) Ltd* [1999] 2 AC 22.

Since death may be caused by omission, so also may the lesser statutory offence of causing grievous bodily harm with intent contrary to s 18 of the Offences Against the Person Act 1861. 'Inflict' and 'wound' are debatable. It used to be said that 'inflict' requires an assault, which apparently can be committed only by an act, but the House of Lords in *Wilson* [1984] AC 242 held that an assault was not an essential element in inflicting grievous bodily harm. It is not certain whether other non-fatal offences, be they common law or statutory, may be committed by omission. The Court of Appeal in *Fagan* v *MPC* [1969] 1 QB 439 held that a battery (and therefore too assault occasioning actual bodily harm which requires an assault or a battery) could not be committed by an omission (the case is now regarded as one which falls within (h) below, though the *ratio* of the court was that what the accused did when he unwittingly parked his car on a police officer's booted foot was an act, a continuing act, and not a failure to move the car) but in *DPP* v *K* [1990] 1 WLR 1067 the Divisional Court did not doubt that assault (a term which includes battery) occasioning actual bodily harm could be committed by failing to clean a hand drier into which the accused had poured acid. The situation was analogous to setting a trap into which the victim fell. If liability for a battery needs an act, it is strange that the much more serious offence of murder can be committed by an act or omission. If one took this principle too far, one would undermine the general principle that one is not liable for omission. For that reason the courts' restriction that there has to be a duty impedes the development of liability for homicide where one has omitted to save the victim. There are also problems with the width of causation in such cases in that potentially a lot of people could be guilty of homicide. A simpler example of a common law offence is cheating the Revenue by failing to provide a tax return: *Mavji* [1987] 2 All ER 758 (CA).

(d) A rare common law offence committable by omission is misprision of treason. If a person fails to report treason to the authorities, he is guilty of this crime. It is also an offence to fail to assist a constable when he calls for assistance. It is suggested that the accused would not be guilty if he had a lawful excuse or if helping was physically impossible. There are very few common law offences of omission, and in practice neither of the two mentioned has been used for many years.

(e) Liability is imposed for failing to perform a duty one has undertaken voluntarily. The more one does, the more likely it is that one will be liable for an omission. In other words, no duty will arise if the accused refused to accept the obligation to take care of another but it will arise if he does so and performs it poorly. The old authority is *Instan* [1893] 1 QB 450, where a niece had failed in her duty to look after an aunt. Lord Coleridge in the Court for Crown Cases Reserved said that the accused:

> ... was under a moral obligation to the deceased from which arose a legal duty towards her; that legal duty the prisoner has wilfully and deliberately left unperformed with the consequence that there has been an acceleration of the death of the deceased owing to the non-performance of that legal duty.

A more modern case with the same result is one which Lord Mustill in *Airedale NHS Trust* v *Bland* [1993] AC 789 called troubling, *Stone and Dobinson* [1977] QB

354, which has grisly facts and an uncertain *ratio*. The Court of Appeal held a man and his mistress guilty of manslaughter when the victim died after they had failed to summon medical attention. The man was deaf, blind, and had learning difficulties; the woman was described as inadequate and ineffective. The man was the brother of the victim (liability, however, was not based by the court on the blood relationship). The victim gave the male accused £1.50 a week towards her rent, but liability was not based on contract, as to which, see (f) below. They lived in the same house. The female accused had tried to look after the victim by leaving food for her to eat, calling for a doctor and washing her. She had thereby undertaken an obligation to care for the victim. (However, only if she had embarked on looking after the sister would she have been found quilty.) The victim had paid money towards the rent, but the case was not decided on the contractual approach noted below – and one cannot really see the court imposing liability on absent landlords to look after their tenants. Since the accused persons were, at the least, lacking in intelligence and could not use a telephone, presumably the law is that one must act as a reasonable person would have acted, not as a person of limited intelligence and so on would have acted. This point presumably applies to the remaining exceptions. It is unclear law as to how the defendants could have terminated their duty to look after the deceased. Perhaps it would have been sufficient for one of them to inform the social worker who came to see the male accused's son. Moreover, the victim refused to eat properly and could not use a phone. Did this fact release the accused from their obligation? However, a father was found not guilty in **Lowe** [1973] QB 702 (CA): Phillimore LJ drew a line for the purposes of the crime of unlawful act manslaughter between an omission, even a deliberate one, such as failing to call a doctor, and commission. The law is not clear. Finally, the defendants would not have been found guilty if they had refused to let the victim stay in their house. To make them guilty when they were doing their (inadequate) best seems almost cruel. The defendants could hardly look after themselves, never mind the male defendant's sister (or his mentally ill son).

See Figure 12.3 in Chapter 12 for a diagram illustrating constructive (unlawful act) manslaughter.

A more recent case than **Stone and Dobinson** is **Ruffell** [2003] EWCA Crim 122. The victim had injected a mixture of cocaine and heroin at the accused's house. He had become ill during the night, lapsed into unconsciousness, and the accused had tried to revive him. The next morning the accused put the victim outside of his house where he died from opiate intoxication and hypothermia. It was held that the jury could on the facts find that the accused had assumed a duty of care. The victim was a guest in his house and the accused had tried to revive him by splashing water on his face, putting him next to a radiator for warmth, putting him by an open window for air, and covering him in towels.

This head of liability might be extended in the future to cover, e.g., joint participation in dangerous sports such as pot-holing. The Court of Appeal in **Khan** [1998] Crim LR 830 left open the possibility of a drug dealer's owing a duty to summon medical assistance to a person who had fallen into a coma as a result of taking heroin he had supplied. One difficulty, which was not discussed, was whether a duty can arise out of an illegal situation. The defendants were guilty of supplying drugs, the victim of possessing them. It is suggested, however, that this obstacle is not insuperable. In other areas of law such as illegal contracts the courts do take account of unlawful behaviour. (**Khan** can also be seen as an application of the **Miller** principle discussed at (h) below.) The Court of Appeal held in **Sinclair** [1998] NLJ 1353 that an attempt to assist the victim does not *per se* give rise to liability. On the facts, however, the accused did owe a duty of care to the victim. Rose LJ said:

'... [the accused] was a close friend of the deceased for many years and the two had lived together almost as brothers. It was Sinclair who paid for and supplied the deceased with the first dose of methadone and helped him to obtain the second dose. He knew that the deceased was not an addict. He remained with the deceased through-out the period of his unconsciousness and, for a substantial period, was the only person with him.... [T]here was ... material on which the jury ... could have found that Sinclair owed the deceased a legal duty of care.'

One problematical question concerns whether, and if so how, a person can give up a duty once he has undertaken it. Must one tell, e.g., the Department of Social Security that one is going to stop looking after an elderly relative several weeks in advance? Another question concerns how far, once one has voluntarily embarked on a duty, one must perform it. If the rescue of a fellow pot-holer is dangerous, must a person nevertheless attempt it? Is one obliged to spend all one's money looking after the relative? Is it sufficient merely to call for the doctor or must one provide the best expertise? If the answer is to do what is reasonable for the accused in all the circum-stances including any risk of danger, **Stone and Dobinson** looks out of line, for they may have done the best they could. It is uncertain if the law is that the accused has to do what a reasonable person would have done or that the reasonable person possesses the characteristics such as the lack of intelligence which afflicted the defendants in that case. Whichever rule it is, the court held that they fell short of the required standard.

(f) If one fails to perform a duty imposed by contract, one is guilty. The case always cited for this proposition is **Pittwood** (1902) 19 TLR 37 at Assizes. Wright J rejected the argument that the accused did not owe a duty to the victim, and spoke of 'gross and criminal negligence' when an employee of a railway company failed to open a level-crossing gate. He seemed to be implying that the case was not one for pure non-feasance (not doing) but one of misfeasance (doing something wrongly). The accused opened the gate for road traffic. The victim's haywain came through and he was then killed because the accused had not closed the gate to trains. The accused therefore caused the accident through doing his job badly in not closing the gate having pre-viously opened it. The contract need not be and was not in **Pittwood** owed to the victim. Presumably a lifeguard employed by a local authority at a pool or a seaside resort or a doctor whether employed by the NHS or privately would be guilty of manslaughter under this exception. This exception developed out of the one in (e) and **Instan** was cited as authority for liability arising *ex contractu*. It should be noted that **Pittwood** can nowadays be justified as a case falling within (h), below, creating a dangerous situation.

(g) Liability will be imposed if one fails to perform a duty imposed by law. Responsibility may arise out of a blood or marital relationship or be generated by common law in other ways. There is, e.g., an offence called misconduct in a public office. A police officer off duty was found guilty of this offence when he did not go to the rescue of a man being kicked to death by a bouncer at a club: **Dytham** [1979] QB 722 (CA). The ambit of this duty is unclear. Does it apply to prison officers, doctors, nurses, St John Ambulance persons? Does it apply when the accused is not contractually bound to be on duty? **Dytham** suggests that the defendant will not be liable 'if the circumstances contain a greater danger than a man of ordinary firmness ... may be expected to encounter'. Yet surely one would expect a police officer to go beyond what an ordinary person would do to save someone's life? In this era of AIDS would it be expected of anyone that he gives mouth to mouth resuscitation? There is as yet no solution to the problem of how much risk the accused has to run before he is absolved of the duty. *Dytham* also does not answer the question of whether a person is to be convicted when he starts out to help, finds the task too arduous, and stops. Does it matter that the intervention led others not to join in? A further criticism of *Dytham* is the difficulty in correctly labelling the accused's conduct. The facts do not in themselves suggest that he misconducted himself in a public office. An offence which looks closer to the facts is manslaughter but there is a problem with causation. Not attempting to save the victim did not 'cause' the death of the victim: he would have died even if the constable were on holiday in Ibiza.

A more recent authority is *Singh* [1999] Crim LR 582 (CA). The appellant's father ran a boarding house. The appellant collected the rent and did the maintenance. While his father was away a complaint was made about a gas fire in one of the rooms. The appellant found nothing wrong. Ten days later another lodger in another room was killed by carbon monoxide poisoning. The court held that all of his roles had to be conglomerated and out of that conglomeration arose a duty of care. That duty could have been fulfilled by calling in expert help. But he had not done so. Therefore, by his omission he was guilty of gross negligence manslaughter. There was an obvious and serious risk of death, and the accused had caused the death.

The main illustration of a duty imposed by law is the obligation of a parent to feed his young child. In *Gibbins and Proctor* (1918) 13 Cr App R 134, the Court of Criminal Appeal held the father guilty of murder when he starved his child to death. (The father's mistress was guilty under the principle in (e) above because she had accepted money to buy food.) This case demonstrates that an accused can be liable for an omission when he deliberately refused to act. Not all omissions signify a poor imagination or lack of sympathy. It is uncertain whether children owe reciprocal obligations to their parents. It is also unclear whether the father would have been guilty if the child had been a normal 16-year-old able to fend for himself. An old case is *Shepherd* (1862) 9 Cox CC 123 where it was held that a mother did not owe a duty to act to her 18-year-old daughter. There is old law that a brother does not owe a duty of care to his sister: *Smith* (1826) 172 ER 203. It is uncertain whether students sharing a flat would be liable for failing to look after one of the flatmates. Liability may depend upon how close the relationship was. It is questionable whether the courts would find such a duty between cohabitees or even married couples living apart, but the exceptions for voluntary undertakings or contract could apply.

It is unclear how far 'special relationships' extend. In *Curtis* (1885) 15 Cox CC 746, a child died after a relieving officer failed to perform his duty under Victorian poor law to summon medical assistance to a child of destitute parents. He would have been convicted of manslaughter, had the judge not directed the jury that the accused did not cause the death of the victim (causation in omission offences is difficult: see below). Parents have been tried for manslaughter on the grounds that they wilfully refused to give their daughter insulin. Presumably the duty of parents covers guardians, though there is as yet no precedent.

A case to compare with *Curtis* is *Smith* [1979] Crim LR 251. The wife refused to see a doctor after childbirth. She then gave permission for her husband to call a doctor, but she died. The husband was charged with manslaughter. The judge directed the jury that, if the wife was not too ill, she could direct her husband not to call the doctor. Thereby he would be released from his duty, which was not automatically imposed by virtue of their spousal relationship but which could be easily inferred from the facts, to take care of her. Exactly how persons can be released from their duty is debatable. *Smith* is not well reasoned. If the husband owed his wife no duty while she was mentally capable, it could be said that as she drew near death, she was no longer mentally capable and therefore the duty again arose. Moreover, if his duty only arose when she was no longer mentally capable, there was no proof that he had *caused* her death, and causation is part of the *actus reus* of any form of manslaughter.

Support for this principle of termination of duty comes *obiter* from *Airedale NHS Trust* v *Bland* [1993] AC 789 (HL). The House of Lords, in an attempt to protect doctors from being convicted of murder when they turned off lifesupport systems, treated the withdrawal of food and drink and ventilation as omissions, likening them to their non-provision in the first place (the argument is that not feeding the patient simply restored him to the position he was in when he was brought into the hospital), though this is moot. Apparently this is also the view of the medical profession. Lord Goff, who drew a line between ending treatment (an act) and not continuing it (an omission), a distinction difficult to accept (see the speech of Lord Mustill, who considered that an act and an omission were 'indistinguishable' from an ethical viewpoint), said: 'the doctor is simply allowing his patient to die . . . and as a matter of general principle an omission such as this will not be unlawful unless it constitutes a breach of duty to the patient'. The cause of death was not the turning off of lifesupport but was the reason why the victim had to be placed on life-support in the first place. On the facts there was no breach because it was not in the patient's best interests to continue life-support treatment when there was no chance that he might recover. (It can hardly be said that not feeding him was in the patient's best interests.) Certainly the House of Lords condemned active steps to kill a patient (such as giving a lethal injection), but it may be argued that the removing of a feeding tube or a ventilator is an active step, but *Bland* treats such a step as an omission: the doctors are omitting to supply food or an instrument for breathing. Yet, the House of Lords said that if the doctors' act had been performed by a stranger, that would have been an act! (It is thought that *Bland* does not breach Article 2 of the European Convention on Human Rights because while there is a right to life, there is no positive duty on the state to prolong life; there is no breach of Article 3, the prohibition of inhuman and degrading punishment, because the victim must be aware of the mistreatment. These points have been made in a civil case, *NHS Trust A* v *M* [2001] Fam 348 (High Court).)

While this authority is not a criminal case, there was some support in the speeches for the duty of care to be terminated by the patient himself and indeed by close relatives when the patient was incapable of appreciating the situation. It was suggested in *Bland* that continued treatment by the doctor contrary to the patient's wishes would be (at least) a battery, but that proposition has not yet been tested. It is uncertain whether this case can be applied generally. What if a person of sound mind tells his partner to let him die if at some time in the future he suffers from senile dementia? It is uncertain how far this case may be generalised so as to provide an endpoint to all duties to act however arising. If a lifeguard has gone off duty and has been replaced but is still at the edge of the pool, is he divested of the duty of care? Is there a duty to act until the moment of the termination of his contract of employment? The cases are not helpful. There is no doubt that a parent has a duty to intervene if his or her child is drowning but what if the parent is heavily pregnant? Is she released from her duty if she shouts for help? Alternatively, should we say that no duty arose on the facts? Again the authorities do not provide guidance. Does the duty end when the accused divorces his wife and the child goes to live with her? If he is on business in Paris, is he still responsible? It is thought that the duty terminates when the situation which gave rise to it terminates. Therefore, in answer to the last two questions the duty is expunged on divorce but not by a business trip.

The generally accepted basis for liability in (e)–(g) is that the accused is guilty because he and the victim were living together, or were connected in some way, which gave rise to the duty to take care of the victim. Contracts and blood relation ships, e.g., are in themselves merely matters going towards proving the assumption of a duty. This basis explains how duties can end. A parent no longer owes a duty to a child who is, say, married and living away from home, even though the blood relationship continues to exist. This principle applies even though the child is a minor.

(h) If one unwittingly (i.e. without *mens rea*) creates a dangerous situation, one is under a duty to put it right: *Miller*, above (see also Chapter 3). A squatter who set fire to a mattress and walked away was held guilty of arson when he did nothing to put the fire out. It was his physical act which caused the fire originally. It was held that he was under a duty to act. The issue of withdrawal in the event of the task becoming too onerous was not discussed in *Miller*. The recent cases on the *Miller* principle are *DPP v Santana-Bermudez* [2004] Crim LR 471 (DC) and *Matthews* [2003] 2 Cr App R 461 (CA). In the former case the victim, a police officer, asked the accused to turn out his pockets, which he did. She then asked: 'Are you sure that you do not have any needles or sharps on you?' He said that he did not. She started searching him but pricked her finger on a syringe. The court found him guilty of assault occasioning actual bodily harm. His failure to inform her of the hypodermic was the *actus reus* of the offences. The accused owed a duty of care as laid down by *Miller* to his victim. In *Matthews* the accused pushed the victim into a river, not knowing that he could not swim. When they did realise, they were under a duty to act as in *Miller* and, because they intended to kill or cause grievous bodily harm, they were guilty of murder.

It is uncertain whether an accused is guilty if it was his omission to act which led to the dangerous situation. If he fails to shore up a dangerous building, hears a cracking sound, sees children whom he hates playing where the building is going to fall, then decides not to warn them, arguably he is guilty of murder if a child is killed and he had malice aforethought, on the *Miller* principle, despite the fact that it was not his physical act which started the train of events which led to the child's death. He could have been found guilty under what might be called the reverse of *Thabo Meli v R* [1954] 1 WLR 228 (see Chapter 3). In the latter case an earlier *mens rea* was added to a later *actus reus*. In *Miller* an earlier *actus reus* could have been added to a later *mens rea*. *Speck*, above, is different. There the girl had initiated the touching, not the accused. *Gully v Smith*, above, could also be taken to illustrate this principle: the accused had adopted the nuisance by not removing it. *DPP v K* above is an illustration of the *Miller* principle. The accused had created a dangerous situation by putting acid into a hand dryer. He had then failed to remove it (or to warn that it was there).

If enacted, the draft Offences against the Person Bill attached to the Home Office Consultation Document, *Violence: Reforming the Offences against the Person Act 1861*, 1998, will put *Miller* into statutory form. The government has, however, shown little interest in reforming this part of the law, which really does cry out for change.

(i) The general rule is that one is not liable for failing to intervene to prevent a crime. Mere presence at the scene of the offence does not entail liability. There is, however, an exception. Where a person has a right of control over the action of another he is liable for failing to exercise that control when the other commits an offence. *Tuck v Robson* [1970] 1 All ER 1171 exemplifies this situation. A landlord did not require his customers to leave after closing time. Perhaps surprisingly, failing to do so is not an offence. It is the customers who are guilty of the substantive offence of consuming alcohol after hours, but the Divisional Court held that the landlord was guilty of aiding and abetting the offence. Cases falling within this category often involve driving. The owner who is a passenger in a car may have a right of control over the driver. In *Halmo* [1941] 3 DLR 6 the Ontario Court of Appeal held that the accused was guilty of being a secondary party to manslaughter when he was in the car at the time when his drunken chauffeur killed the victim. In England the law extends to the right of an instructor to control a learner driver: *Rubie v Faulkner* [1940] 1 KB 571.

The Court of Appeal held in *Khan*, above, that whether a duty of care arises out of a certain set of facts is a question for the jury. However, a later Court of Appeal ruled in *Singh*, above, that the crime was one for the judge. It is suggested that *Singh* represents the better view, because *Khan* might lead to a jury saying that because the victim is dead, there must have arisen a duty to prevent that death.

The American theorist G. Fletcher, in *Rethinking Criminal Law* (Little, Brown & Co, 1978) 421, has provided a taxonomy of liability for omissions. Some are breaches of a duty to act. For example, the non-reporting of an accident is a breach of a statutory duty to act. There need be no harm. The accused is punished for the breach. The second form is 'commission by omission'. The accused has a duty to act to prevent the occurrence of harm, such as death. This classification may be useful for the exposition of the law to categorise when the law intervenes. It may be useful for the courts in determining whether harm is necessary for liability.

The draft Criminal Code, 1989, did not attempt to state when an accused was liable for omissions. The Law Commission preferred to leave this area of law for judicial development rather than for a statutory formulation. Therefore, both the list provided above and the recommendations of the Law Commission do not restrict the development of the law: the list is not closed. One might expect that not restricting situations in which criminal liability for omissions can be found would breach Article 7 of the European Convention on Human Rights, the principle of non-retroactivity, but the European Court of Human Rights has ruled that common law extensions to liability do not breach that Article: *SW v United Kingdom* [1996] 1 FLR 434.

Causation in omissions

Even where there is potentially liability for an omission, it must be proved in result crimes that the accused 'caused' the omission which led to the harm. Proving causation may be difficult. For example, if a police constable stands by while a victim is kicked to death, does he cause her death? 'But for' his non-intervention would the victim still be alive?

Morby (1882) 15 Cox CC 35

A child was dying of smallpox. The father refused to summon medical aid. He was a member of a sect called the 'Peculiar People' who believed that prayer and anointment were sufficient to cure illness. The doctor gave evidence that the chances of the boy's survival would have been increased had a doctor been summoned. The father was tried for manslaughter. The

Court for Crown Cases Reserved agreed with the direction of Hawkins J. The question was whether the child's death was accelerated by the accused's neglect. Lord Coleridge said:

> [I]t is not enough to sustain the charge of manslaughter to know that the parent has neglected to use all reasonable means of saving the life of his child; it was necessary to show that what the parent neglected had the effect of shortening the child's life.

The prosecution had failed to prove beyond reasonable doubt that the child died because of neglect.

Therefore, the normal rules of factual and legal causation apply. The principal English theorists on this topic see no difference between acts and omissions: Hart and Honoré, *Causation in the Law*, 2nd edn (Clarendon Press, 1985) 5. As an example one can use the facts of *Pittwood*, above: the victim, the driver of the haycart, would not have been killed by the train, had the accused, the level-crossing gatekeeper, closed the gate. It is, however, sometimes argued that one cannot cause something by omission. If I watch my child drown, how have I occasioned its death? I did not push the child in; I did not even create the pond. My child would still have drowned, had I been in Italy rather than walking by the pond. One response is to say that what occurred is an exceptional deviation from the behaviour expected of a parent. This view is advanced by Hart and Honoré (at 37). English courts have not tackled this potential source of difficulty. One argument which might succeed is that with regard to acts the accused has more control over the effects than he has in relation to omissions. The accused, for instance, could have exerted control over his movements to stop him pushing his victim into a pond but may not be in a position to exert control when someone else has pushed a child into the water. Several people may be responsible for causing an omission.

The Law Commission in the draft Criminal Code proposed to replace the 'but-for' test in *Morby* with the rule that the accused would be guilty if he might have prevented the *actus reus*. The result would be to have liability for omissions in this respect to be wider than that for acts, which seems strange. Clause 17(1) states:

> . . . a person causes a result . . . when . . .
> (b) he omits to do an act which might prevent its occurrence and which he is under a duty to do according to the law relating to the offence.

The provision will ease the position of a court faced with a plea that the accused did not cause something by omitting to prevent it.

The policy behind general non-liability for omissions

There is a debate between those who wish to extend the law to cover criminal omissions and those who do not. This debate may be summed up by using the views of two protagonists. Professor Ashworth 'The scope of criminal liability for omissions' (1989) 105 LQR 424 argued in favour of mutual assistance that:

> [T]he general principle in criminal law should be that omissions liability should be possible if a duty is established, because in those circumstances there is no fundamental moral distinction between failing to perform an act with foreseen bad consequences and performing an act with identical foreseen bad consequences.

In his view life is of such a basic value that it must be preserved. The saving of life is a public good which outweighs the public good of liberty not to act. The behaviour of the non-rescuer is so reprehensible that criminal sanctions should be available. It has also been argued that since one of the aims of the criminal law is to improve standards of behaviour, liability for failing to attain those standards should be imposed. A person should rescue if there is no danger to him. It is the socially responsible thing to do. Other countries have laws in respect of failure to rescue. Those chasing the Princess of Wales through Paris when she was killed were charged with failing to assist a person in danger. William Wilson, *Criminal Law: Doctrine and Theory*, 3rd edn (Pearson, 2008) 80, also pointed out that omissions may be morally worse than acts. 'What is morally worse/causally more significant: shooting a child to prevent the agony of her burning to death in a flaming inferno one is powerless to prevent, or failing to save a similar child from a similar fate by the simple mechanism of unlocking the door behind which she is trapped?'

It is not always easy to see the difference between an act and an omission. Does one fail to stop at a red light or does one drive through a red light? Glanville Williams responded 'Criminal omissions – the conventional view' (1991) 107 LQR 86 in defence of individualism.

(a) There is a difference even on Ashworth's approach. Omissions give rise to liability only where there is a duty. No duty is needed for acts. (One could in the view of the author of this book invent one, but certainly the problem does not arise in positive acts: there is a duty not to commit murder. There is no need to refer to the duty.)

(b) There is a moral distinction between killing and letting die (except perhaps between parent and child). My shooting you with a gun is more blameworthy than my permitting you to starve to death. My pushing you overboard in the middle of the ocean is more reprehensible than my not rescuing you when a third party has pushed you in.

(c) It may be difficult to distinguish acts from omissions (e.g. is disconnecting a drip-feed an act or omission?), but the problem is inherent in all moral principles.

(d) The criminal law should be directed at active wrongdoing. It is not well suited to getting people to do things. Moreover, obliging people to perform acts is secondary to the primary purpose of suppressing bad behaviour.

(e) Everyone could be liable for omissions. By not selling one's house and giving the proceeds to aid agencies, one has failed to prevent a famine in Sudan.

(f) It is unfair to label non-doers as wrongdoers where statutory language is couched in active terms.

(g) The police, Crown Prosecution Service, courts and prisons would be overwhelmed if criminal liability for omissions were the norm. The clash of values is between inter-personal duties and personal autonomy.

Moreover, people should not be obliged to act when they do not so wish, especially if acting involves the expenditure of time and effort, as it does in this area of law. They would have to change their lives to accommodate what others were doing. Making people liable for omissions would encourage others to interfere in matters which do not concern them. Should it really be the law that if one hears a baby crying in a locked house, one should break down the door to check that it is not being ill-treated? People should be allowed to put their own interests and the interests of those they hold dear above strangers. In terms of the principles discussed at the start of Chapter 1, judicial extension of legal duties to act is a breach of the principle of legality.

The orthodox statement that English criminal law does not oblige people to do good but only prevents them from behaving badly is under attack but the principle survives.

Reform of liability for omissions
(See also under 'Causation in omissions', above)

The law of omissions has developed over time without much regard for principle. The Criminal Law Revision Committee in its Fourteenth Report, *Offences Against the Person*, Cmnd 7844, 1980, paras 252–255, recommended that in such crimes liability for omissions should be imposed only for murder, manslaughter, causing serious injury with intent (which was to replace grievous bodily harm and wounding with intent), kidnapping and abduction and unlawful detention. (The common law was to be left free to develop *when* an accused was under a duty to act. As has been seen, the draft Criminal Code adopted the latter proposition.) Since an accused was not to be liable for more minor offences against the person, he was also not to be liable for criminal damage.

The Law Commission in the draft Criminal Code, 1989, proposed a general provision on omissions which would not be restricted to those recommended by the Criminal Law Revision Committee. 'Causing' criminal damage and 'causing' death are to be used as the redrafted *actus reus* of criminal damage and murder and manslaughter to avoid any problem that those offences could not be committed by omission (for example, it may be difficult as a matter of language to say that a father *killed* his daughter when he starved her to death). This proposal is very much on the lines of the present law. The policy of imposing liability for omissions only in major crimes was reiterated by the Law Commission in *Legislating the Criminal Code – Offences against the Person and General Principles*, Report No. 218, 1993. The Non-Fatal Offences against the Person Bill would if enacted not impose liability for omissions in respect of the proposed crimes of recklessly causing serious injury, intentionally or recklessly causing injury and assault. No list of duties to act was recommended. It would be left to the common law to determine when a duty arose. The 1993 Report also confirmed the **Miller** principle about supervening fault.

One would hope in a true reform of the law that the position would be clarified by express words imposing liability for omissions. It should, however, be emphasised that simply making explicit what is implicit will not resolve some of the concerns about liability for omissions. Whether a person watching a small child drown in an inch of water is criminally liable should be based on principle and policy. It is the values the criminal law ought to incorporate which should be discussed. This is the reason why liability for omissions remains a controversial topic. Although changing the law from 'damaging' to 'causing criminal damage' resolves one issue, it does not alter the fact that the question of causation is dealt with in the draft Code in what looks like an over-inclusive way. ('Might prevent': see above.) Whether present law is retained or the draft Code enacted, to revert to the start of this chapter, a definition of the *actus reus* in terms of physical or bodily movement is incorrect for it fails to deal with criminal liability for omissions. If one cannot define 'act', one cannot define 'omission to act'. Lord Mustill in **Bland** said that 'the current state of the law is unsatisfactory both morally and intellectually', and that the distinction between act and omission was dubious: do you agree?

Summary

The reader is guided through the definition of *actus reus* (conduct, circumstances, state of affairs) with examples. The academic distinction between 'conduct' and 'result' crimes is rehearsed. The two major problems in considering *actus reus*, causation and omissions, are dealt with at length. Causation is explained using the standard factual and legal causation vocabulary and the case law is discussed. The emphasis is on drawing out the different definitions of causative factors, principles which can lead to different outcomes. The general rules on omissions liability are set out: for example, how some statutes can be read as imposing liability for omissions whereas some cannot. The legal duties are explicated, e.g. the liability for failure to act where the accused is a parent of the victim. The link between causation and omissions is explored: how can one be culpable when one is merely in a crowd which watches a child drown? There is discussion of the policies behind the Anglo-Welsh law on omissions, concentrating on the arguments advanced by Glanville Williams and Andrew Ashworth.

- Introduction: Criminal law is concerned with forbidding various forms of behaviour, whether that consists of acts, omissions or states of affairs. These are called *actus reus* or the external element(s) of offences. When added to the *mens rea*, there is an offence (though note Chapter 4 on strict liability); there may also be a defence.

- Some problems: The *actus reus* must not be read as meaning solely the conduct of the accused: it can, for example, cover the behaviour of the victim. An illustration is rape, which includes lack of consent by the alleged victim. Similarly, when considering defences, it is difficult to match some defences with the analysis of *actus reus*; *mens rea*; and defence. Some defences, e.g. mistake, seem not to be separate at all from the offence: they are not a third ingredient. Rather they negate either the *actus reus* or *mens rea* or both. For example, mistake seems to exist as a failure to prove the offence. Duress can be seen, however, as a defence available as a third ingredient: the accused did the prohibited conduct and had the relevant state of mind but she had a defence because she was forced to do what she did.

  Other problems include these. 'Actus' must not be translated as 'act' because it is wider than that; it covers 'non-acts', omissions. The *actus reus* varies from crime to crime: knowing that part of the *actus reus* for theft is 'property' does not help with the *actus reus* of murder. The *actus reus*, obviously, must be proved: for students, this proposition is to be taken as meaning that all elements of the *actus reus* (and *mens rea*) must be considered.

- Conduct and result crimes: A modern division of offences is into those where the prosecution must prove that the accused caused something to happen ('result' crimes) and ones where it does not ('conduct' crimes). The obvious example of the former is murder; it must be shown that the defendant caused the death of the victim. An example of the latter is dangerous driving: no one need be harmed, no damage to property need be occasioned.

  Compare the crime of causing death by dangerous driving. This is a result crime because a certain consequence, death, forms part of the *actus reus* of the offence.

- Causation: Causation is not a problem in conduct crimes, only in result crimes. English law divides causation into two parts: causation in fact and causation in law. The former, often known as 'but for' causation, asks: but for the act of the accused, would the victim be dead (etc.); if so, the triers of fact consider the second issue, that of legal causation. Usually but not always the question at this stage is: did the accused contribute significantly to the death (etc.)? There are exceptional principles, particularly the one which states that 'the accused must take his victim as he finds him', a principle often called the thin-skull rule. An example from the cases is the refusal of a Jehovah's Witness to receive a blood transfusion. Not all the cases are straightforwardly reconcilable, but in general a *novus actus interveniens* will break the chain of causation. For example, if the victim makes a free, deliberate and informed act, the so-called chain of causation is broken. This long-accepted statement of the law has come under increasing strain in recent years, especially in relation to suppliers of drugs present at the death of the drug-taker, but authorities which are to the effect that the accused remains guilty even when the victim refuses medical treatment may be seen as similar. Escape cases form a well-established principle that if the victim injures or kills herself while escaping from the accused, the latter is liable unless the former has done something 'daft'. Some causation cases exemplify the desire of the courts to convict those who have created dangerous situations even when the *actus reus* and *mens rea* are not contemporaneous. Once the prosecution has proved causation, all the other elements of the *actus reus* must be proved.

- Omissions: The general rule of English law is that no defendant is criminally liable for failing to act. To this rule there are exceptions. The starting point is that since Parliament can do anything, it can make persons guilty for not doing something. An example is the crime of failing to report a road traffic accident. Sometimes verbs in the definition of crimes can be interpreted as including failures to act. For example, one can obstruct a highway by not removing a blockage which has occurred naturally. Common law crimes of omission are very rare: the most common one, though rarely prosecuted, is that of not assisting a constable on request. However, the main difficulty surrounds liability for omissions when there may or may not be a duty to act. The law has been developed rapidly over the last quarter of a century or so by the courts and current situations where there is a duty to act comprise blood relationships, contractual relationships (not necessarily just encompassing the two parties), voluntary assumption of a duty of care, statutory duties, and dangerous situations which the accused has created. Outside these situations the law remains obscure, e.g. does a supplier of drugs have a duty to take care of his or her customer? Similarly obscure are the issues: how far must one go to fulfil the duty? And may the victim release the accused from the duty? The law remains open-ended, a scenario which may be in breach of Art. 7 of the ECHR, the principle of non-retroactivity.

  Causation in omissions is potentially a difficult issue. It might be said that I have caused your death if I fail to rescue you from drowning, and English law, insofar as the point has been considered, has held that the normal rules of factual and legal causation apply.

  Whether people ought to be liable for not doing something has exercised the mind of legal theorists. The issue tends to crystallise as: is there a moral difference between killing and allowing to die? Arguments in favour of current law that liability arises when there is a duty to act but not otherwise include: why should anyone be obliged to act, particularly when to do so may be dangerous as may occur when attempting to rescue a drowning child?

References

Books

Allen, M. J. and Cooper, S. *Elliott & Wood's Cases and Materials on Criminal Law* 9th edn (Thomson, 2006)

Fletcher, G. *Rethinking Criminal Law* (Little, Brown & Co., 1978)

Hart, H. L. A. and Honore, T. *Causation in the Law* 2nd edn (Oxford University Press, 1985)

Ryan, C. *Criminal Law* 4th edn (Blackstone Press, 1995)

Wilson, W. *Criminal Law: Doctrine and Theory* 3rd edn (Pearson, 2008)

Journals

Arlidge, A. 'The trial of Dr David Moor' [2000] Crim LR 31

Ashworth, A. 'The scope of criminal liability for omissions' (1989) 105 LQR 424

Colvin, E. 'Causation in criminal law' (1989) 1 Bond LR 253

Klimchuk, D. 'Causation: Thin skulls and equality' (1998) 11 Can JL&J 115

Perkins, R. 'A rationale of *mens rea*' (1939) 52 Harv LR 905

Smith, J. C. 'Comment' [1988] Crim LR 843

Williams, G. 'Criminal omissions – the conventional view' (1991) 107 LQR 86

Williams, G. *'Finis* for *novus actus*' [1989] CLJ 391

Further reading

Ashworth, A. 'The scope of criminal liability for omissions' (1989) 105 LQR 424

Busuttil, A. and McCall Smith, A. 'Flight, stress and homicide' (1990) 54 JCL 374

Finn, J. 'Culpable non-intervention: reconsidering the basis for party liability by omission' (1994) 18 Crim LJ 90

Hogan, B. 'The *Dadson* principle' (1989) Crim LR 679

Horder, J. and McGowan, L. 'Manslaughter by causing another's suicide' [2006] Crim LR 235

Hughes, G. 'Criminal omissions' (1958) 67 Yale LJ 590

Jones, T. H. 'Causation, homicide and the supply of drugs' (2006) 26 LS 139

Leavens, A. 'A causation approach to criminal omissions' (1988) 76 Cal LR 547

McCutcheon, J. P. 'Omissions and criminal liability' (1993–5) xxviii–xxx IJ 54

Moore, M. *Act and Crime* (Oxford University Press, 1993)

Norrie, A. 'A critique of criminal causation' (1991) 54 MLR 685

Ormerod, D. 'Manslaughter: suicide resulting from prolonged abuse' [2006] Crim LR 923

Smith, J. C. 'Liability for omissions in the criminal law' (1984) 4 LS 88

Spellman, S. and Kincannon, A. 'The relation between counterfactual "but for" and causal reasoning: experimental findings and implications for jurors' decisions' (2001) 64 *Law and Contemporary Problems* 241

Williams, G. 'Criminal omissions: the conventional view' (1991) 107 LQR 86

Williams, R. 'Policy and principle in drugs manslaughter cases' [2005] CLJ 66

The standard work, if long in the tooth, in causation is H. L. A. Hart and A. M. Honoré, *Causation in the Law* (Oxford University Press, 2nd edn, 1985). For a theoretical explanation of omissions, voluntariness and causation see W. Wilson, *Central Issues in Criminal Theory* (Hart, 2002), chs 3, 4, 6 respectively. For a brief and more up-to-date version of Tony Honoré's views, see 'Causation in the law', *Stanford Encyclopedia of Philosophy*, 2001.

Visit **www.mylawchamber.co.uk/jefferson** to access exam-style questions with answer guidance, multiple choice quizzes, live weblinks, an online glossary, and regular updates to the law.

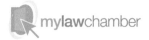

Use **Case Navigator** to read in full some of the key cases referenced in this chapter:

Fagan v *Metropolitan Police Commissioner* [1968] 3 All ER 442
R v *Blaue* [1975] 3 All ER 446
R v *Dear* [1996] Crim LR 595
R v *Kennedy (No. 2)* [2005] 1 WLR 2159
R v *Pagett* (1983) 76 Cr App Rep 279
R v *Ruffell* [2003] All ER (D) 139 (Jan)
R v *White* [1910] 2 KB 124

3

Mens rea

Introduction

> There is no term fraught with greater ambiguity than that venerable Latin phrase that haunts Anglo-American criminal law: *mens rea*. (George Fletcher, *Rethinking Criminal Law* (Little, Brown & Co, 1978) 398)

Mens rea or the mental element in crime is one of the most important concepts of substantive criminal law. In general terms, an accused is liable only if he has *mens rea*. This principle ensures that the accused is guilty only when he is at fault, and the lack of it in respect of one or more elements of the *actus reus* provides one of the planks of subjectivists' critique of strict liability (see the next chapter). The actual form of *mens rea* varies from crime to crime. Two types, intention and recklessness, are discussed below. Doctrinal discussion of these two fault elements has led to an overconcentration on those terms. Expressing mental elements in those terms in law reform projects has obscured the fact that present law is distinguished by a multitude of words indicating culpability. Strict liability, where there is no *mens rea* as to one or more elements of the *actus reus*, forms the subject of the next chapter. The specific mental element for each offence is tackled in the relevant chapter. It should be noted that different parts of the *actus reus* may have different states of mind attached to them. Even strict offences have some mental element in their definition. The *mens rea* doctrine ensures that those who cause the *actus reus* are legally responsible for doing so. This chapter, besides dealing with other general forms of *mens rea* including negligence, considers several problems relating to *mens rea* such as the so-called doctrine of transferred malice and the issue of contemporaneity or concurrence, whereby it is stated that in English law the *mens rea* and *actus reus* have to coincide in time.

The state of mind of the accused is relevant in several areas of criminal law.

(a) The mental capacity of the accused may be investigated. For example, a child under 10 is never criminally liable; one aged 10 to 14 used to be so liable only if he had 'mischievous discretion' though the latter changed in 1998 (see Chapter 7).

(b) The mentally disordered state of mind may be looked at, e.g. in the defences of insanity and diminished responsibility (see Chapter 9).

(c) At times the state of mind is relevant to the question of voluntariness. Is the accused acting of his own free will? This issue is discussed in Chapters 2 and 9.

(d) The fourth meaning concerns the particular state of mind required in relation to the other ingredients of the offence. This is a definition of *mens rea*. Sometimes the *mens rea* is expressly stated; sometimes it is implicit in the definition of the offence.

The philosophical foundation for *mens rea* is that the accused can control his conduct. He can decide whether to engage in conduct which breaks the criminal law. On one approach the law is to prevent harmful behaviour. A person acting when he is in control of his movements and adverts to the possible harmful consequences of his behaviour is more culpable than someone who acts objectively recklessly or carelessly, and he is deserving of more punishment than a person who has so acted. He as an autonomous human being has chosen certain forms of behaviour and should be penalised and deterred. It is usually said that penalising conduct without *mens rea* is inefficacious and unjust, e.g. H. Packer 'Mens rea and the Supreme Court' [1962] Sup Ct Rev 107 at 109. The accused will not be deterred from behaving in like fashion again; others will not be deterred; the defendant is not necessarily a dangerous person who needs to be reformed; and two other bases of punishment, prevention and retribution, do not work. It is thought to be unjust because it is wrong to impose the stigma of criminal conviction on someone who was not morally blameworthy.

As was seen in the previous chapter, the division between *actus reus* and *mens rea*, though convenient for exposition, is artificial and has been frowned on at the House of Lords level. Both terms continue to be used. They should be used in conjunction, for often the '*actus*' is not '*reus*' without a *mens rea*. For instance, in theft, the appropriation of property belonging to another, the *actus reus*, is neutral without the addition of the mental element. If you take your spouse's car, you are not guilty of theft. It is the addition of the *mens rea*, dishonesty and the intention permanently to deprive, which converts the legally neutral activity into a crime. Some *actus reus* words, such as 'possessing' and 'permitting', have within them a *mens rea* element, e.g. one cannot 'permit' something without knowing of its existence.

Definitions of *mens rea*

A literal translation of *mens rea* is 'guilty mind'. There is, however, no need for the accused to feel morally guilty or to know that what he is doing is morally blameworthy. As the Courts-Martial Appeal Court said in **Dodman** [1998] 2 Cr App R 338: '*mens rea* does not . . . involve blameworthiness'. The same applies *vice versa*: a person may be morally innocent but have *mens rea*. An example is an undercover police officer who joins a criminal gang. He is liable, for example, for conspiring to import drugs: **Yip Chiu-Cheung v R** [1995] 1 AC 111 (PC). Smith and Hogan, *Criminal Law*, 10th edn (Butterworths, 2002) 88 (not in the 12th edn (OUP, 2008) by David Ormerod) provided a working definition:

Intention, knowledge or recklessness with respect to all the elements of the offence *together with any ulterior intent which the definition of the crime requires.* [Italics in original.]

The phrase 'elements of the offence' is a reference to what those writers used to call 'all the consequences and circumstances of the accused's acts (or state of affairs) which constitute the *actus reus*'. As previously noted there are, however, many *mens rea* words in English law which are not 'intention, knowledge or recklessness'. The term 'ulterior

For a basic definition of rape, see p 573 in Chapter 14.

intent' will be discussed shortly. An example of the ap[...] from rape, which can be rephrased something along th[...] if he has sexual intercourse whether vaginal or anal (ac[...] knowing that it is unlawful sexual intercourse (*mens rea*) *reus*) knowing her to be a woman or knowing him to be a[...] consent (*actus reus*), knowing that the victim does not con[...] may not consent, or not caring less whether they consent [...] noted that using the term 'mind' as a translation of *mens* is [...] to denote not just states of mind but also negligence, whic[...] certain standard. The modern phrase of 'fault element' is m[...] this aspect of *mens rea* than is 'guilty mind'.

There are other definitions. Lord Simon in **DPP v Majewsk**[...] [...]C 443 said that '*mens rea* is . . . the state of mind stigmatised as wrongful by the criminal law which, when compounded with the relevant prohibited conduct, constitutes a particular offence'. S. H. Kadish 'The decline of innocence' [1968] CLJ 273 at 274, stated: '*Mens rea* refers only to the mental state which is required by the definition of the offence to accompany the act which produces or threatens the harm.' These definitions stress that *mens rea* is concerned with the criminality of the act, not its morality, as was confirmed by the House of Lords in **Kingston** [1995] 2 AC 355. All definitions may be criticised. If *mens rea* is defined in terms of 'intentionally, recklessly, and knowingly', automatically negligence is not *mens rea*. There are also other words in statutes which may not fit easily into a *mens rea* definition, e.g. if the crime is defined in terms of 'permitting', does one permit something to happen only if one knows one is permitting it? 'Maliciously' has been defined as meaning both intentionally and recklessly. 'Wilfully' is dealt with below. If one excludes certain frames of mind which are needed for conviction from the definition of *mens rea*, one necessarily inquires why they form part of criminal law when one would not ask that question if *mens rea* were defined in such terms as to include them.

Whichever definition is used, it does not get us far towards knowing what the *mens rea* required for each crime is, for it varies from crime to crime just as the *actus reus* varies from crime to crime. Its meaning in each crime must be determined by looking at statutes and cases. *Mens rea* is at heart an analytical tool, not a prescriptive norm.

To repeat a point mentioned already, *mens rea* does not mean morally wrongful mind, just as 'maliciously' in criminal law does not mean 'spitefully'. One can have *mens rea* even if one believes one's act to be morally right such as euthanasia: 'The criminal law represents an objective ethic which must sometimes oppose individual convictions of right' (J. Hall, *General Principles of Criminal Law*, 2nd edn (Bobbs-Merrill, 1960) 385). No *mens rea* term, not even the most currently used ones such as intention and recklessness, has been statutorily defined. One must, therefore, investigate the cases to see how judges have defined each mental state required by the offence's definition. Unfortunately, as Lord Simon put it in **DPP for Northern Ireland v Lynch** [1975] AC 653: 'A principal difficulty in this branch of the law is the chaotic terminology, whether in judgments [or] academic writings . . .'.

Examples of *mens rea*

Murder is a common law offence. Its *mens rea*, called malice aforethought, is the intention to kill or commit grievous bodily harm (see Chapters 3 and 11). In theft *mens rea* comprises two elements, dishonesty and intention permanently to deprive. Section 20 of the Offences Against the Person Act 1861 penalises the malicious infliction of grievous harm. 'Maliciously' means intentionally or recklessly in the **Cunningham** sense (*Cunningham* [1957] 2 QB 396 (CCA)). Section 18 of the same Act concerns among other things malicious wounding with intent to cause grievous bodily harm. Intention is the part of the *mens rea* in s 18. The phrase 'with intent' means that the *mens rea* is called 'ulterior intent' or 'further intent' as within Smith and Hogan's definition of *mens rea* above. In s 20 the accused need foresee only some harm, whereas in s 18 he must intend grievous bodily harm. The difference between ss 18 and 20 is reflected in the maximum sentence of imprisonment, life and five years respectively.

Sometimes the mental element is not laid down by Parliament. Problems arise as to which *mens rea*, if any, is called for. Illustrations include bigamy contrary to s 57 of the Offences Against the Person Act 1861 and assault occasioning actual bodily harm contrary to s 47 of the same Act. Even modern statutes do not always expressly state the mental element required. Section 9(1)(a) of the Theft Act 1968 creates one form of burglary, entering a building as a trespasser with intent to do one or more of several offences such as theft. No *mens rea* is attached to 'entering a building as a trespasser'. Must the accused intend to enter a building as a trespasser or is it enough that he is aware that he may be entering as a trespasser?

One must be careful not to think that the *actus reus* and *mens rea* are coextensive. In murder the intent to cause serious harm is sufficient, whereas part of the *actus reus* is killing. In s 20 of the Offences Against the Person Act 1861 the *actus reus* is in part causing grievous bodily harm but the *mens rea* is intentionally or recklessly causing any physical harm, grievous or less. Where the mental element is not as extensive as the *actus reus*, the crime is sometimes called a 'half strict' or 'half *mens rea*' one. Such offences are instances of constructive liability. The accused is guilty whether or not he intended to cause or was reckless as to causing grievous bodily harm. The name of the crime is something of a misnomer.

As examples of the difficulty of knowing how the courts will react to *mens rea* when Parliament has failed to express it, two famous contrasting cases may be instanced. In **Sherras v de Rutzen** [1895] 1 QB 918, a police officer went into a pub and ordered beer. It was an offence contrary to s 16(2) of the Licensing Act 1872 to sell alcohol to constables on duty. Normally police officers off duty who went into pubs did not wear their armbands. The present constable was on duty but did not wear his armband. The publican was charged with the offence. The Divisional Court read *mens rea* into the offence. The landlord had to know that the police officer was on duty before he could be convicted, according to Wright J. In **Cundy v Le Cocq** (1884) 13 QBD 207, which concerned the same Act but s 13, the court dealt with the offence of serving alcohol to drunks. As in s 16(2), there was no *mens rea* stated in the section. The landlord was held guilty even though he did not know that the man was drunk. Not only is the intentional, reckless and careless landlord caught, but so is the landlord who considered the question whether the customer was drunk or not and deemed that he was not. The type of crime at issue in **Cundy v Le Cocq** is called an offence of strict liability (see Chapter 4). Even if one does know what the *mens rea* is, there are difficulties in knowing the width of those expressions. Intention and recklessness are dealt with below. Two other *mens rea* words are 'knowingly' and 'wilfully', which are also discussed below.

Summary

The notion that a court should not find a person guilty of an offence against the criminal law unless he has a blameworthy state of mind is common to all civilised penal systems. It is founded upon respect for the person and for the freedom of the human will . . . [T]o be criminal, the wrongdoing must have been consciously committed. To subject the offender to punishment, a mental element as well as a physical element is an essential concomitant of the crime.

So said Dickson J in the Supreme Court of Canada in *Leary* v *R* (1977) 74 DLR (3rd) 103, 116. The next topic, motive, deals with a matter which looks like *mens rea* but is treated as not being relevant. Negligence is sometimes treated as *mens rea* and sometimes not, while the next chapter is the exception to Dickson J's rule.

Motive

While the criminal law takes into account *mens rea*, as a general rule it disregards motive. The problem is therefore to distinguish motive from *mens rea*. An accused can have *mens rea* despite having a good motive. Therefore, *mens rea* does not mean a morally 'guilty mind'. It is often easy to state that the accused's ultimate purpose was the motive. Why did this woman steal a loaf of bread? She stole because she wanted to feed her starving children, or she was greedy, and so on. Why did this accused put a bomb on a plane? He did so in order to kill his wife or to claim the insurance, wishing to set up home with his mistress. In *Mohan* [1976] QB 1, the Court of Appeal said that intention connoted 'a decision to bring about . . . the commission of the offence . . . , no matter whether the accused desired that consequence of his act or not'. What the accused desired is the motive for the crime. Generally speaking, motive is defined in such a way that it is excluded from *mens rea*. By definition it is irrelevant. A recent illustration is *A-G* v *Scotcher* [2005] 1 WLR 1867 (HL), where a juror was guilty of contempt of court even though she had disclosed jury deliberations in an effort to prevent a miscarriage of justice. An example of a motive being irrelevant is the Privy Council case *Wai Yu-Tsang* v *R* [1992] 1 AC 269. The accused was convicted of conspiring to defraud when his motive was to stop a run on the bank at which he was the chief accountant. Lord Goff drew a line between 'underlying purpose' (motive) and 'immediate purpose' (intention). If his immediate purpose involved a crime, he was guilty despite his honourable underlying purpose. A more recent and English authority is *Hales* [2005] EWCA Crim 1118. The accused ran over and killed a policeman attempting to arrest him. Since he was 'prepared to kill to escape' (Keene LJ), he intended to kill. His motive, trying to escape, was immaterial to the offence charged. In *Sood* [1998] 2 Cr App R 355 the accused, a doctor, certified that he had seen the deceased on the day of her death. In fact he had not. What he did was in accordance with standard practice. The Court of Appeal held that he was guilty of wilfully and knowingly making a false declaration. His belief that the practice was acceptable was his motive. As the Court said, 'concepts of motive, blame and moral culpability' go to punishment, not to guilt. In *Yip Chiu-Cheung* v *R* [1995] 1 AC 111 the Privy Council advised that a person who was an undercover drugs enforcement officer would be guilty of conspiracy to traffic in drugs despite his good motive. This case is further discussed in Chapter 10, where it is noted that the Law Commission proposes to reverse it by legislation.

Sometimes, however, the courts have, it seems, interpreted offences as including motive. In *Steane* [1947] KB 997, a British national was forced by the Nazis to broadcast in favour of them under the threat of the concentration camp for his family and himself. He was charged under a wartime regulation which created the offence of 'doing acts likely to assist the enemy with intent to assist the enemy'. Did he intend to assist the enemy? Under the definition in **Mohan** he did make up his mind to assist the enemy. He did not desire to do so. Indeed he was under pressure. The Court of Criminal Appeal quashed his conviction. Lord Goddard CJ held that the accused did not intend to aid the enemy. The outcome may be reconciled with general principles by holding that the accused was acting under duress. The Lord Chief Justice did not think that defence was available, but in the light of the present state of the law it seems that the accused would have this defence to the charge. **Steane** is out of line with the general definition of intention (see below), though it well illustrates how courts sympathetic to the accused's plight can alter the meaning of intent by calling the accused's motive his 'intent'. Moreover, if the accused's good motive led to his conviction being quashed, any motive good or bad would give the accused a defence. In Glanville Williams's example, if the accused broadcast for the Nazis for a packet of cigarettes, the court ought consistently to hold that the accused did not intend to broadcast for the Nazis. A defence of **Steane** can, however, be put up based on the drafting of the crime. The regulation penalised 'doing acts likely to assist the enemy with intent to assist the enemy'. If motive was to be excluded, the law would have been drafted as 'intentionally doing acts likely to assist the enemy'. The actual phrasing left the way open for Lord Goddard CJ's judgment. It is certainly to be expected that the drafting of wartime regulations will not be perfect. The result is still that there are two possible interpretations of intention in the criminal law, just as there are two if not three definitions of recklessness. Until the enactment of the draft Criminal Code or something similar, the problem of competing definitions will remain.

While **Steane** can be seen as a decision that motive was relevant, **Chandler v DPP** [1963] AC 763 exemplifies the opposite. A statute was phrased in such a way that motive appeared relevant but was construed as not requiring an investigation of motive. The defendants were charged with conspiring to enter a prohibited place 'for a purpose prejudicial to the safety of the state', contrary to s 1 of the Official Secrets Act 1911. They had held a protest at an airforce base and stopped planes landing or taking off for six hours in order to demonstrate against nuclear weapons. Lord Devlin said that if 'purpose' meant motive, a spy who gathered information for money would not be guilty; that interpretation could not be right. Lord Radcliffe, with the other Law Lords agreeing, held that the accused's immediate purpose was to block the airfield, which was prejudicial to the safety of the state. One did not have to inquire whether the defendants' long-term purpose was prejudicial or not. Both speeches led to the same conclusion that the appellants were guilty. However, there is a problem in the speeches which demonstrates the difficulty of differentiating *mens rea* (in this case 'purpose') from motive. What if a person entered the airfield to stop a plane with a bomb on board taking off? Lord Radcliffe said that preventing the plane's leaving was not the purpose of that person. The purpose was to save life, the prevention of take-off was the means to that end. Lord Devlin differed. The purpose was to prevent the take-off, but that purpose was not prejudicial to the safety of the state.

A cynic might argue, in conclusion, that the courts in these cases were simply giving vent to their prejudices. In one case the accused had a motive the judges approved, in the other they did not. A less cynical view would be to note how the courts can manipulate the law to exculpate defendants, should they so wish. Certainly by refusing to look at the defendants' purpose in **Chandler** the Lords did not have to get involved in political discussion of nuclear arms.

There are exceptions to the rule that motive is irrelevant. In blackmail, the accused has a defence if the demand was warranted. His belief that he has reasonable grounds for making the demand may be based on his motive. In the former crime of indecent assault, where the events were equivocal as to their indecency, the accused was guilty only if he had an indecent motive, such as buttock fetish. The 'racially motivated offence' created by the Crime and Disorder Act 1998 is a crime listed in that Act which was committed with a racial motive. For example, criminal damage is made a more serious offence than usual when the accused demonstrated hostility based on membership of a religious group or if the offence was motivated wholly or in part by hostility towards members of a certain racial group. Here motive is expressly made part of the definition of the offence. Elsewhere motive can be 'smuggled' into the law through concepts such as dishonesty in theft and the defence of necessity. Therefore, Parliament can make the law expressly or implicitly take motive into account. The motive of preventing the victim from hitting one may ground a defence of self-defence.

The exclusion of motive from consideration can be seen as part of the 'objectivisation' of criminal conduct. The accused's behaviour is extracted from its context such as hunger and avarice in the examples given at the start of this section.

Intent

Intention is an often used word in the English language. Its meaning in law despite its importance as a fundamental concept is problematic, though arguably less problematic than it used to be. The basic definition, its 'natural and ordinary' one, according to Robert Walker LJ in the civil case of *Re A* [2001] Fam 147 is 'purpose'. *Moloney* [1985] AC 905, besides confirming that malice aforethought has two forms and stating that the term malice aforethought is 'anachronistic and now wholly inappropriate', also determined that intention alone suffices. Foresight of consequences as probable was not sufficient. Foresight of even a virtually or highly probable consequence was neither intention nor the equivalent of intention after *Moloney*. However, 'intention' was not defined. Lord Bridge told judges that in most cases they could leave the definition to 'the jury's good sense'. For example, if the accused had a motive for killing the victim, cut her throat, and did know what the consequence of doing so would be, it is legitimate for the jury to say that he did intend to kill. In *Dudley and Stephens* (1884) 14 QBD 273 the defendants did intend to kill the cabin boy, but the motive was to eat him in order to survive. They argued that their intention was to preserve their lives, but the court rejected that contention. They would have been happy not to kill if they could have survived otherwise, but they did make up their minds to kill the boy in order to feast off his body. More up to date is *Wright* [2000] Crim LR 928 (CA). The victim was found unconscious on the floor of his prison cell. The accused said that he had nothing to do with what had happened. Accordingly, either he had made up his mind to kill or he had not. There was no room for a direction on oblique intent (see below). Intention covers the state of mind where the accused aims or decides to kill ('direct intent'). Accordingly, if the accused decides or sets out to achieve a result or if that consequence is his aim or purpose, he intends that outcome to occur. There was no attempt in *Moloney* or subsequent cases to overturn the concept of direct intent. As Lloyd LJ stated in *Walker and Hayles* (1990) 90 Cr App R 226, 'It has never been suggested that a man does not intend what he is trying to achieve.' Brennan J in *He Kaw Teh* (1985) 157 CLR 523 (at 569) HCA gave this definition of this form of intent: 'Intent . . . connotes a decision to bring about a situation, so far as it is possible to do so, to bring about an act of a particular kind or a particular result. Such a decision implies a desire or wish to do such an act or bring about such a result.'

It is still intention even though he thought that the chance of the harm occurring was slight. Presumably, it is not intention if the accused knows that the result is impossible, but it will be if he has a direct intent but considers that the chance of his achieving his objective is low, as when he, being a poor shot, fires at a person many yards away.

Since trial judges ought not to give any definition of intention, juries may reach different conclusions on the same facts, and the Court of Appeal is powerless to intervene. As Lord Bridge emphasised, 'intention' bears its ordinary meaning, whatever that is. Lord Scarman in **Hancock and Shankland** [1986] AC 455 said that jurors have to use their common sense to reach their decision. General guidelines could not replace the jury's use of common sense on the facts of each case. Accordingly, it can be said at this point in the analysis that intention as part of the law of murder does not bear and must not be given a technical meaning. Judges must not use synonyms such as purpose or aim. No doubt juries will use such synonyms. Unless told differently they will apply ordinary language definitions.

It was sometimes said that intention in criminal law (though perhaps not in ordinary language) also covers the state of mind of a person who thinks it virtually certain that the victim will die, the usual example being a person who plants a bomb on a plane to recoup insurance money on the cargo. He does not want the passengers to die and will be very happy if they survive but he demonstrates that he does not put any value on life. This state of mind in relation to the passengers, which goes often by the term 'oblique intent', was called by Glanville Williams (who was the first to use it in criminal law) the 'side-effect' of the accused's intent ('Oblique intention' [1987] CLJ 417). The same writer in *Criminal Law: The General Part*, 2nd edn (Stevens, 1961) 40, stressed that 'mere philosophical doubt, or the intervention of extraordinary chance, is to be ignored'. A case law example is **Mohan** [1976] QB 1 (CA). The case facts resemble those in **Hales**, above. In order to escape, the accused drove his car at a police officer. His purpose was to escape. The side-effect of his direct intent was an attempt to cause grievous bodily harm with intent to do some bodily harm. The constable might step aside but if he did not, he would be knocked down. In different words, the accused acted *in order to* escape. The italicised words show what his intent was and that the running down of the constable was not his intent. He did not drive as he did in order to run over the police officer. This mental element, foresight of a virtual certainty, is sometimes called 'oblique intent', though not all writers agree on its width. Moreover, not all commentators agree whether oblique intent is intent. If this form of intent is part of the *mens rea* of murder there may be difficult cases on the borderline between foresight of a virtual certainty and foresight of a consequence as highly probable, the latter not amounting to evidence of intent. (Students should be careful in their reading because the latter type of foresight is also sometimes called 'oblique intent'. 'Oblique intent' is also the term used for the state of mind which occurs when there is no possible way of achieving one's end, a breach of the law, without violating another law. For example, to shoot dead a rival the accused may have to shoot through a fixed window. The direct intent is to kill, the oblique to cause criminal damage.) 'Virtual' or moral certainty means 'certainty excepting the unforeseeable results of action', e.g. all passengers survive the blast and the plane lands safely. It is unsatisfactory that depending on the author different frames of mind are called by the same name. Moreover, intention and foresight, even of a certainty, can be completely different concepts. By imbibing alcohol you may foresee a hangover as a certain result, but one would not say that you intend to have a hangover. C. Finkelstein wrote in 'No Harm No Foul? Objectivism and the Law of Attempts' (1999) 18 Law and Philosophy 69, 75: 'Oblique intention is not really any kind of intention at all. It is a label for a different sort of mental state altogether, namely foresight. . . . Calling it a species of intention is pure obfuscation'. Nevertheless, some commentators consider that direct intent and foresight of a virtual certainty cannot be distinguished; both are morally wrong in that both represent a complete disregard for human life.

To gain an appreciation of what intention does mean one must consider five important cases: *Moloney*, the facts of which are stated in Chapter 11, *Hancock and Shankland*, *Nedrick* [1986] 1 WLR 1025, *Walker and Hayles* (1990) 90 Cr App R 226 (a case which is less important now than it was originally) and *Woollin* [1999] AC 82. A lot more could be said but the exegesis below omits the history of the topic except in so far as a knowledge of earlier authorities is necessary to understand present law.

Moloney

Despite criticism of *Moloney* in *Hancock and Shankland*, it remains an important case for several reasons.

(a) It abolished the previous law whereby foresight of death or grievous bodily harm was sufficient malice aforethought. It affirmed the view of Wien J in *Belfon* [1976] 3 All ER 46 on non-fatal offences that foresight was not part of intention. Foresight of the likelihood of injury is part of the evidence going towards proving intent, not a variety of intent itself. As Lord Hailsham put it: 'Foresight and foreseeability are not the same thing as intention.' Lord Bridge stressed that: 'No one has yet suggested that recklessness can furnish the necessary element in the crime of murder.' The contrary view, that in ordinary language foresight of a probability was intention, a view which had received support from at least one Law Lord, was rejected.

(b) The accused's foresight was, however, one part, but only one part, of the evidence which may be taken into account by the jury in determining whether the accused did intend to kill or cause grievous bodily harm. Accordingly, intent *may* be inferred from foresight, but proof of foresight, even of a virtual certainty, was not proof of intent. Juries did find difficulty with this notion and asked the trial judge for guidance in *Moloney*, *Hancock and Shankland* and *Nedrick*. It remains to be seen whether juries will require such help after *Woollin*.

(c) In order to avoid confusion in the minds of the jury there was no need, except in exceptional cases, for the judge to give a direction on the meaning of 'intent'. In this respect the House of Lords confirmed what had been the previous law: *Beer* (1976) 63 Cr App R 222 (CA), which the Privy Council had approved in *Leung Kam Kwok v R* (1984) 81 Cr App R 83. *Nedrick*, above, *O'Connor* [1991] Crim LR 135, *Bowden* [1993] Crim LR 380 (CA), *Hawkins* [1993] Crim LR 888 and *Fallon* [1994] Crim LR 519 have more recently upheld this proposition. Lord Bridge put it this way in *Moloney*:

> The golden rule should be that . . . the judge should avoid any elaboration or paraphrase of what is meant by intent and leave it to the jury's good sense to decide whether the accused acted with the necessary intent.

The exception was meant to deal with an instruction on natural consequences, but refer to *Hancock and Shankland*, below, for further elaboration of this point. On this point *Moloney* is as correct today as it was then. The 'golden rule' is: the jury should not be directed in *Moloney* and *Hancock and Shankland* terms unless there is evidence that the accused intended to do something other than the crime alleged. If the prosecution alleges that he intended to kill or commit grievous bodily harm but the defendant denies that allegation, there is no need for elaboration. If, however, he says that he did not so intend but wanted to put a bomb onto a plane to claim insurance money, there is a need for a ***Moloney/Hancock and Shankland*** direction.

(d) In murder there was no requirement that the accused should 'aim' at the victim. There were *dicta* of Viscount Kilmuir in ***DPP v Smith*** [1961] AC 290 and of Lord Hailsham in ***Hyam v DPP*** [1975] AC 55 to the effect that the victim must be the target of the accused, but Lord Hailsham withdrew his remarks and the rest of the House of Lords agreed unanimously with his withdrawal. This concession left the way open for the conviction of the terrorist who planted a bomb, even though he did not direct the bomb at the actual victim.

(e) The House of Lords disapproved of Lord Hailsham's view in ***Hyam*** that an intention to expose a potential victim to a serious risk of grievous bodily harm was part of the *mens rea* of murder. The House of Lords thought that if this type of malice aforethought were accepted, reckless drivers who killed could be convicted of murder, a result which they abhorred.

(f) Their Lordships continued to distinguish intention from motive and desire. In Lord Bridge's 'homely example':

> A man who, at London airport, boards a plane which he knows to be bound for Manchester clearly intends to travel to Manchester even though Manchester is the last place he wants to be and his motive for boarding the plane is simply to escape pursuit.

(Lord Bridge said that getting on the Manchester plane 'conclusively demonstrates his intention to go there, because it is a moral certainty that that is where he will arrive'. This statement seems to mix up the concept of intention and that of deriving intent from foresight of a moral certainty. This point is discussed below, particularly in reference to ***Woollin***.)

An even homelier example is: you may intend to go to the dentist without having the least desire to go to the dentist's. Indeed, it may terrify you to sit in the dentist's chair! The emotional reason – greed, jealousy, ambition and the like – behind the killing is disregarded. Only the intent to kill or to commit grievous bodily harm is considered.

A quick summary of ***Moloney*** would be that foresight and motive are not intention and except in rare cases 'intention' should be left to the jury. The principal difficulty was to understand and apply some of Lord Bridge's phraseology. At one point of his speech – unfortunately an important point, for he was stating what judges ought to tell juries in exceptional cases – he used the term 'natural consequence'. Did the defendant foresee death or really serious harm as a natural consequence of his act and was it in fact a natural consequence? What he seemed to have meant is that a result will occur 'unless something unexpected supervenes to prevent it', as he put it elsewhere (in this sense 'natural' means the same as 'virtually certain'), but it could mean that the accused was guilty where the death was indeed a natural, i.e. direct, consequence, without that consequence being morally certain (or even highly likely) to occur. To use a commentator's illustration, 'Conception is a natural consequence of sexual intercourse but it is not necessarily probable' (Glanville Williams 'Oblique intention' [1987] CLJ 417). In this second sense 'natural' does not include a virtual certainty. The term 'morally certain' means unless something unexpected supervenes. In another place in his speech he stated that the accused is guilty only if he foresaw the probability of an outcome as little short of overwhelming. Lord Hailsham said the same in **Hyam v DPP**, above.

Another difficulty with the speech of Lord Bridge was that he referred when defining intent not only to foresight of natural consequences but also to the fact that the harm was a natural consequence. It is uncertain why that fact should be relevant to the accused's *mens rea*. Another problem with **Moloney** is that the accused did not foresee the risk of death or grievous bodily harm at all; therefore, anything said about foresight of consequences, natural or otherwise, was *obiter*. Lord Bridge used the example of a terrorist bomber who leaves a bomb which has not yet exploded. He intends to scare people and phones a warning to the police. The bomb squad is summoned. While attempting to defuse the bomb, a soldier is killed. Lord Bridge assumed that the crime was murder. However, it is suggested that the offence is manslaughter: the terrorist did not foresee death or GBH of the soldier as a virtually certain consequence.

Despite the confusion which **Moloney** occasioned, it remains a highly important decision for the clarification of the points noted above and after all it was on its facts a simple case. The question for the jury was one of fact: what was in the accused's mind when he pulled the trigger? If he knew that the gun was pointing at the stepfather's head, the jury in the words of Lord Bridge 'were bound to convict him of murder. If, on the other hand, they thought it might be true that, in the appellant's drunken condition and in the context of [the] ridiculous challenge, it never entered the appellant's head when he pulled the trigger that the gun was pointing at his [stepfather], he should have been acquitted of murder and convicted of manslaughter.' A **Moloney** direction was not relevant on the facts of **Moloney**!

Hancock and Shankland

The House of Lords picked up on this point in the next case in this sequence. This case involved two striking Welsh miners, who during the 1984–85 miners' strike pushed a concrete block over a parapet onto a motorway with the purpose of encouraging a working miner to stop work. The driver of the taxi in which the miner was being carried was killed. They were held to be guilty of murder by the jury, but the House of Lords disagreed. The leading speech was delivered by Lord Scarman. Like the House of Lords in **Moloney**, he distinguished the *mens rea* of intention from the evidence needed to prove it. In **Moloney** their Lordships had stated that the jurors had to ask themselves in the exceptional case where they had to consider such matters (in the normal run of cases it is obvious that, say, the defendant stabbed the victim, intending to kill or cause grievous bodily harm) whether the result was a natural outcome of the accused's act. Lord Scarman added to this question that the death or injury had also to be a probable consequence of the act. Otherwise, the defendant would be liable for mere direct consequences, whereas the true import of Lord Bridge's speech in **Moloney** was that the accused was liable only where the jury inferred intent from his foresight of a virtually certain consequence.

While not laying down the minimum amount of foresight a jury could take into account, Lord Scarman emphasised that it was for the jury to determine on the facts, including the accused's degree of foresight, whether he intended to kill or cause grievous bodily harm. The greater the degree of foresight the more likely it was that the jury would reach the conclusion that the accused did have that intent. Lord Scarman said: 'If the likelihood that death or serious injury will result is high, the probability of that result may . . . be seen as overwhelmingly evidence of the existence of the intent to kill or injure.' However, the question remained one of evidence, not of substantive law. The issue for the jury in **Hancock and Shankland**, as in **Moloney**, was not a complex one: did they believe the prosecution's case or the defendants'? If the former was believed, the crime was murder; if the latter, the crime was manslaughter. The possibility of inconsistent verdicts remained: one jury might infer intent, another might not, from the same facts, yet the courts were powerless to intervene. Judgments on which side of the line something falls are difficult in law, but the problem is exacerbated in intention where the judge cannot instruct the jury as to the meaning of intent. Furthermore, Lord Scarman said that a jury could infer intention from a high probability, a lower test than Lord Bridge's one of virtual certainty.

Nedrick

Lord Scarman in **Hancock and Shankland** thought that guidelines had little place in criminal law, yet the Court of Appeal laid down such principles in **Nedrick**, above, which was followed in **Barr** (1989) 88 Cr App R 362 (CA), a decision from 1986.

Nedrick [1986] 1 WLR 1075

The accused poured paraffin through the letter box of a house and on to the front door. He set it alight. The house blazed up and a child was killed. He was convicted of murder after a direction by the trial judge which followed the pre-**Moloney** law laid down in **Hyam v DPP**, above, a case with similar facts, that foresight of grievous bodily harm was to be treated as an intention to cause it. (The case was heard before **Moloney**.) The Appeal Court allowed the appeal on the grounds that, following **Moloney**, foresight was not to be equated with intention. Foresight was merely a step on the way towards proving intent.

The court gave advice to trial judges as to how they should direct juries when the defendant does a dangerous act, as a result of which someone dies. As ever, it should be noted that if the accused had a direct intent to kill or commit grievous bodily harm, the judge should not refer to these guidelines. They are used only when the consequences which occurred were not the accused's purpose.

(a) A person could intend to kill or cause grievous bodily harm even though he did not desire that result.

(b) The more probable that consequence was, the more likely it was that the accused foresaw it; and if the consequence was foreseen, the greater the probability was that the accused intended it. (This statement follows **Hancock and Shankland** if it means that a jury may infer intent from foresight of a virtual certainty. If, however, it means that an accused intends something when he foresees the consequence as virtually certain, it is inconsistent with **Moloney**.)

(c) If the accused did not foresee death or grievous bodily harm he did not intend it.

(d) If the accused did foresee it, but thought that the risk of it occurring was slight, the jury could easily conclude that he did not intend it.

(e) If the accused realised that death or serious injury was a virtual certainty ('barring some unforeseen intervention'), the jury might find it easy to say, to infer, that he intended that consequence. In this regard the court approved Lord Bridge's phrases in **Moloney** that the result has to be a 'moral certainty' or 'little short of overwhelming'. This proposition may be paraphrased in this way. In life few things are certain. Unforeseen circumstances may arise which prevent something happening.

Passengers may live when a bomb explodes on a plane at 30,000 feet but barring unforeseen circumstances they will die. The planter of the bomb can still intend to kill even though he realises that there is a very slight possibility of the passengers surviving. This type of foresight is thus different from foresight of something occurring as a (very) high probability. On the facts of *Nedrick*, the outcome is that the accused did not have the requisite intent for murder because he did not foresee death or grievous bodily harm as a virtual certainty; therefore, intent could not be inferred.

(If the jury is entitled to infer intention from foresight of a virtual certainty, logically intention cannot include foresight of a virtual certainty.)

The Court of Appeal concluded, in a couple of sentences in which it came near to proclaiming that foresight of a virtual certainty is a form of intent, that:

> Where a man realises that it is for all practical purposes inevitable that his actions will result in death or serious harm, the inference may be irresistible that he intended that result, however little he may have desired or wished it to happen. The decision is one for the jury to be reached upon a consideration of all the evidence.

This quote may not be consistent with *Hancock and Shankland*, which is not necessarily restricted to deriving intent from foresight of virtual certainty, but may include deriving intent from a lesser degree of foresight than foresight of a virtual certainty. The Court of Appeal did, however, purport to apply that authority. *Nedrick* emphasised that not even foresight of a virtually certain consequence constitutes intention. In other words, foresight of a virtual certainty is not in itself intent but only part of the evidence as to whether the accused did intend the prohibited outcome. This ruling was not absolutely clear in *Moloney* where the question for the House of Lords was whether the *mens rea* for murder was established by proof of foresight 'that death or serious harm would probably occur'. The House of Lords rejected such foresight as malice aforethought. The guidelines are inconsistent with the speech of Lord Scarman in *Hancock and Shankland*, where he deprecated the use of guidelines. Lord Lane CJ, the leading member of the court in *Nedrick*, later said extrajudicially that he could not have been as clear as he would have liked because he was faced with two House of Lords decisions.

The Court of Appeal in *Purcell* (1986) 83 Cr App R 45 did not lay down detailed guidelines, while the same court in *Ward* (1987) 85 Cr App R 71 reiterated the view taken in all authorities that except in difficult cases only a simple direction of an intent was necessary: there was no need for an instruction on the difference between wanting and intending, unless such a distinction was called for by the facts. A more recent example is *Fallon* [1994] Crim LR 519. The prosecution alleged that the accused intended to kill a constable who was searching him by firing a pistol. The accused contended that the shooting was accidental. The Court of Appeal held that on these facts either the shooting was deliberate or it was not. In neither case did the defendant's foresight enter into the matter. Therefore, the trial judge was wrong to direct the jury as to foresight.

Walker and Hayles

The fourth case involved defendants who threw their victim from a third-floor balcony. They were tried for attempted murder. The sole mental element for that offence is the intention to kill. The Court of Appeal said:

(a) echoing *Belfon* [1976] 3 All ER 46, see above, that ordinary people find no difficulty in knowing what intent means; the core meaning of intent is 'purpose'. In the words of the court: 'It has never been suggested that a man does not intend what he is try-ing to achieve.' It was only in rare cases that an elaborate direction on intent was needed. The exceptional case is one where the accused achieves a result which he did not try to obtain. A request from the jury for such an instruction does not make the case into an exceptional one;

(b) it was not a misdirection for a judge to direct that a very high degree of probability of a result happening was required, provided that intention remained a matter for the jury and that the line between intent and recklessness was drawn. Foresight was not to be equated with intent. However, it was better to use the phrase 'virtual certainty', as *Nedrick* had done. Again the court stressed that foresight of a virtually certain consequence was not intent.

In effect the court equated 'virtual certainty' and 'a very high degree of probability'. Yet there is a substantial difference between a virtual certainty and a high probability. If something is virtually certain, it is almost inevitable that it will occur. If an event will highly probably occur, it is only highly likely that it will. The two concepts are not the same. As the bomb-on-the-plane hypothetical illustration shows, because of, e.g., chance occurrences few results are certain. An assassin can intend to kill an emperor, even though at the last second the empress leans across and takes the full force of the bullet. Foresight of a very high degree of probability looks like the *mens rea* of one form of manslaughter. As a result juries might have been uncertain as to what is the minimum degree of fore-sight needed before they may infer intent from foresight. Can one infer intent when the accused foresaw a result as probable, likely, on the cards, and so on? Perhaps judges should use the formulation of Lord Lane CJ in *Nedrick*: did the accused think that the consequence – death or grievous bodily harm – was 'inevitable'? Indeed Lord Lane CJ, the judge in *Nedrick*, said in the House of Lords debate on the Nathan Report (*Report of the Select Committee of the House of Lords on Murder and Life Imprisonment*, 1989) that he did not consider virtual certainty and high probability as covering the same ground. Otherwise, jurors in some cases might think that a virtual certainty is required, while in others they may believe that it is sufficient that the result was very likely. *Walker and Hayles* was not a helpful decision in elucidating intention and (b) above is wrong after *Woollin*. The defendants would nowadays be guilty of manslaughter and not of murder.

A case to compare with *Walker and Hayles* is *Donnelly* [1989] Crim LR 739. The accused and another committed armed robbery. The other hit a security guard several times over the head with a gun. The gun went off, killing the guard. The Court of Appeal held that it was wrong to say that if he was using the gun as a club, not intending to commit serious harm, the jury could find that he intended to shoot. There was no evidence that the probability of the gun going off was a 'virtual certainty'. Therefore, he was not guilty of murder but of manslaughter. If, however, he had used the gun as a club intending to cause grievous bodily harm and it had gone off accidentally, he would have been guilty of murder. The cause was irrelevant. The prosecution would have proved causation, death, and one form of malice aforethought. On this approach it was irrelev-ant whether it was possible or otherwise that the gun would go off.

Woollin

Woollin [1999] 1 AC 82

The accused's baby began to choke on some food. The accused became angry and threw the baby towards his pram, which was against a wall. The baby's head hit the wall or possibly the floor. The baby died. At the trial for murder the accused alleged that he did not intend to cause death or grievous bodily harm. The prosecution did not seek to prove that he did. The judge ruled that the jury could infer intent if the defendant foresaw serious harm as a 'substantial risk' of his actions. The jury convicted. The Court of Appeal dismissed the appeal, but the House of Lords allowed it because the conviction was unsafe.

The principal speech was delivered by Lord Steyn.

(a) The judge's reference to 'substantial risk' was wrong. He had blurred the distinction between intent and recklessness. The accused was guilty of manslaughter, not of murder.

(b) *Nedrick* was correct in holding that the prosecution had to prove foresight of a virtual certainty before the jury might find that the accused intended a consequence. In different words, references to 'high probability' and other degrees of likelihood are incorrect. While *Woollin* did not expressly overrule *Walker and Hayles*, that authority must be taken to have been overruled.

(c) A judge should not direct a jury as to foresight where the accused did desire a result. In that situation no definition of intent should be given to the jury, who in accordance with *Moloney* have to use their good sense to determine whether or not the accused did intend to kill or cause grievous bodily harm. A post-*Woollin* illustration is *Hales* [2005] EWCA Crim 1118. The accused drove his Volvo car at a policeman in order to escape. He either intended to kill or he did not. There was no space for a direction about foresight. A *Nedrick* direction was needed only when the accused 'may not have had the desire to achieve that result'.

(d) Lord Lane CJ was, however, wrong in *Nedrick* to refer to how probable the consequences were (which is a matter of *actus reus*) and to whether the accused foresaw that consequence. These issues were unhelpful to the jury.

(e) Lord Lane's direction in *Nedrick*, which Lord Steyn thought was of 'valuable assistance to trial judges', was modified. He had said: 'the jury should be directed that they are not entitled to infer the necessary intention unless they feel sure that death or serious injury was a virtual certainty'. The House of Lords stated that 'infer' should be replaced by 'find'. ('Infer', as used in *Nedrick*, is also the language of the Criminal Justice Act 1967, s 8, that 'A . . . jury . . . shall not be bound in law to infer that [the accused] intended . . . a result of his actions by reason only of its being a natural and probable consequence of those actions . . .'.) A terrorist who does not foresee the death of a bomb disposal expert as a virtually certain consequence of planting a bomb is not guilty of murder, contrary to the opinion of Lord Bridge in *Moloney*.

(f) There has been debate about whether Lord Scarman in *Hancock and Shankland* meant that a jury could find intent when the evidence disclosed something less than foresight of a virtual certainty. The House of Lords in *Woollin* stated that since Lord Scarman had approved everything which Lord Bridge said in *Moloney* except the reference to 'natural consequences', he had approved the minimum threshold of foresight of a virtual certainty (or otherwise put, where the probability of a consequence's occurring is little short of overwhelming) for finding intent.

(g) *Hancock and Shankland* did not rule out the framing of model directions.

(h) *Nedrick* is consistent with s 8 of the Criminal Justice Act 1967 because the jury has to take all the evidence into account.

(i) The Court of Appeal has been wrong to distinguish between cases where the only evidence is that of the accused and of the consequence (where **Nedrick** was necessary) and cases in which there was other evidence (where a **Nedrick** instruction was not necessary).

(j) Lord Steyn said that the definition of intent may vary throughout the criminal law. This aspect is dealt with below.

The major clarification lies in (e), above. Lord Steyn thought that he was merely clarifying the law, but on the most common interpretation of **Woollin** he was changing it. No longer is foresight just evidence of intent. The jury may now find intent from foresight of a virtual certainty. One interpretation of this phrase is that there are again two forms of intent for murder and most other crimes of intent. First, there is direct intent, where 'intent' means 'aim', 'purpose' or 'desire'; secondly, there is oblique intent, where the accused foresaw a consequence as virtually certain. This approach is that there is a change in substantive law. It is not that the second state of mind is a way of showing that the accused had the intent, but that there is a separate form of intent. The law would be clear and there would be no problem of inferring one state of mind from another state of mind. This interpretation comes from the substitution of 'find' for 'infer' in (e), the approval of Lord Bridge's speech in **Moloney** that if a person foresees the probability of a consequence as little short of overwhelming, this 'will suffice to *establish* the necessary intent', and the statement by Lord Steyn that the effect of **Nedrick** was that 'a result foreseen as virtually certain is an intended result'. The alternative view is that the second state of mind is still only evidence of the first frame of mind. Foresight of a virtual certainty is not a definition of intent, only evidence from which a jury may, but need not, find intent. This interpretation is supported by the approval of the rest of Lord Lane's sentence, quoted above, that the inference of intent '*may* be irresistible'. There is nothing here about 'must be irresistible', even if one substitutes 'finding' for 'inference'. The jury may hold, therefore, that a consequence foreseen by the accused as virtually certain is not intended by him though presumably in most cases it will be so. Had Lord Steyn wished to change the law he would have said that a jury *must* find intent, not that they were entitled to find intent. The problem is that Lord Steyn and the rest of the Law Lords do not seem to understand that there is a difference between foresight being intent and foresight being evidence of intent. Authorities such as **Moloney** and **Hancock and Shankland** were not overruled as being inconsistent with **Woollin**.

In the year or two following **Woollin** it was suggested that **Woollin** took the former approach: the accused does have intent if he foresees a result as a virtually certain consequence. This would have brought the law into line with that proposed by the Law Commission in cl 18(b) of the draft Criminal Code 1989, quoted below. This outcome would certainly clarify the law, as Lord Steyn desired. It was also the approach taken in the first Court of Appeal decision after **Woollin**: *Re A (Children) (Conjoined Twins: Medical Treatment)* [2001] Fam 147 (CA), a civil case. Surgeons separating conjoined twins intended to kill when they foresaw the death of one as a virtually certain consequence. There was no discussion of whether on the facts a jury would be 'entitled to find' intent. Ward LJ said: 'The test . . . is . . . whether . . . the doctors recognise that death or serious harm will be virtually certain (barring some unforeseen intervention) to result from carrying out this operation. If so, the doctors intend to kill or to do that serious harm . . .' Brooke LJ spoke to similar effect and therefore there was a majority in favour of equating the two states of mind. Robert Walker LJ, however, said that despite the death of one twin being certain, the doctors did not intend for death because that was not their purpose. There is, however, strong recent contrary authority in the form of *Matthews* [2003] 2 Cr App R 461 (CA), in which *Re A* was not mentioned: foresight of virtual certainty remains evidence of intent and is not, *per se*, intent. The defendants had thrown the victim into a river despite his telling them he could not swim. He drowned. They did not desire his death; they did not make up their minds to kill him. They were convicted at first instance. While the trial judge had equated foresight of a virtual certainty with intent, the Court of Appeal held that the jury would have been sure that the defendants knew of the virtual certainty on the facts that the victim would die and that the jury would have found that the defendants intended to kill. However, the model direction given in *Nedrick* and amended in *Woollin* ('infer' becoming 'find') was not a rule of substantive law but one of evidence. As pointed out by the court on the facts of certain cases such as *Matthews*, the line between a rule of substantive law and one of evidence is not wide: it was very easy, perhaps irresistible, for the jury to find intent when the accused threw the victim, who they knew could not swim, into a river. On the facts it was just about impossible for the jury not to find that the defendant foresaw the victim's death as a virtual certainty. It would be more difficult for a jury to find intent when the accused acted for a good purpose.

Brief summary

The House of Lords in *Moloney* and *Hancock and Shankland* quashed the idea that as a matter of law oblique intention was sufficient for malice aforethought. The jury may, but need not, infer intent from all the facts, including what the defendant foresaw. As we have seen, *Woollin* may have resurrected the notion that foresight of a virtual certainty is intent, and not merely evidence of intent. In *Moloney* it seems, however, that the jury could infer intent from a virtual certainty, but this requirement has been diluted in later cases. The principal criticism is that without more it is impossible to infer one juristic concept from another if the two concepts are distinct. If foresight was not intent, proving foresight even of a virtual certainty did not prove intent. The extra which the prosecution had to prove remained undefined. However, it remains that only in exceptional cases need the judge direct the jury in respect of foresight, for normally there is no doubt that the accused's purpose was to kill or commit grievous bodily harm. If the accused stuck a knife into the victim's stomach, the question is: did he have the requisite intent? Either he did or he did not. The issue is one of fact. It is only where the accused's aim was not to kill or cause grievous bodily harm that a *Woollin* direction is called for. Yet the judge cannot even tell the jury that if the accused's purpose was so-and-so he intended that consequence. In exceptional cases the jurors are to be instructed that foresight is not intent but they are informed that the second state of mind *may* be the first when they are sure that the accused foresaw the result as a virtually certain outcome.

It must be remembered that if the accused *did* intend to kill or commit GBH, that is the end of the question: *Woollin* is irrelevant. The trial judge in such cases should steer the jury away from 'the chameleon-like concepts of . . . foresight of consequences and awareness of risk' (*Wright* [2000] EWCA Crim 28).

Since intent is a question for the jury, medical evidence may not be led as to whether an ordinary person intended a result. However, said the Court of Appeal in *Toner* (1991) 93 Cr App R 382, it may be adduced to discover the effect of a mild hypoglycaemic episode on intent because such a state of mind was outside the experience of ordinary jurors.

One may encapsulate the law by saying, as did **Matthews**, that jurors 'are not entitled to find the necessary intention unless they [feel] sure that death or serious bodily harm was a virtual certainty as a result of [the accused's] actions and that [he] appreciated that this was the case'. Even then the jurors may reject the evidence and hold that he did not intend the consequence.

Criticism

Moloney and its progeny do not reflect creditably on English law. Lord Bingham CJ in 'Lord Chief Justice calls for a criminal code' (1998) 148 NLJ 1134 stated: 'even the most breathless admirer of the common law must regard it as a reproach that after seven hundred years of judicial decision-making our highest tribunal should have been called upon time and time again in recent years to consider the mental ingredients of murder, the oldest and most serious of crimes.' Why cannot the judiciary define the core concept in this extremely serious case? Juries may acquit or convict on the same facts. Because there is no set definition, unmeritorious defendants may win appeals against judges' directions when they might not have been able to even bring an appeal had the law been clear. C. M. V. Clarkson's criticism of **Moloney et al.** remains apposite:

> A concept such as 'dishonesty' involves value judgments . . . and the jury, as the mouthpiece of community values, is probably the most appropriate body to express such judgments. But the same is not true of intention . . . In the interests of certainty and predictability it is surely for *the law* to determine what intention means . . . The House of Lords, by leaving intention undefined, is trying to retain maximum flexibility so that juries do not have to resort to perverse verdicts to convict those felt deserving of conviction. Many . . . terrorist bombers who do not necessarily mean to kill . . . could escape liability for murder if a clear and narrow definition of intention were laid down . . . This is an intolerable position inviting prejudice, discrimination and abuse. It involves the abandoning of all standards in an area of law where it is crucial that standards be clearly laid down. (*Understanding Criminal Law* (Fontana, 1987) 62)

Slightly different words appear in the fourth edition (2005), Thomson, 61–3. There is nothing to stop a jury from, as it were, taking the law into its own hands and convicting defendants of murder even though they did not purposely seek to kill or cause grievous bodily harm.

The next criticism has often been made. If one is dealing with oblique intent, by definition there is no direct intent. Therefore, 'purpose', 'aim', 'decision' and the like are not oblique intent. Moreover, as a general rule motive or desire is irrelevant to guilt; therefore, they too cannot constitute oblique intent. Since aim, purpose, decision, motive and desire are ruled out, what is the ingredient which juries use to determine whether what the accused foresaw as a virtually certain consequence which converts such a state of mind into intent? In other words, one state of mind, intent, cannot be inferred from another, foresight of a virtual certainty.

What about where the accused knew that a result was virtually certain to occur but intended the opposite? For example, assume that I am a novice at archery and I expect to miss the target on most occasions; nevertheless, I do intend to hit the target, even though I know that it is virtually certain that I will miss it. Accordingly, I intend to hit but I know at the same time that it is virtually certain that I will miss. Yet after **Woollin** the courts could say that I intend to hit (desire or purpose) and at the same time I intend to miss (my foresight of a virtual certainty). The outcome is illogical!

Criticism may also be directed at the width of oblique intent. This point is very well put by S. Uniacke 'Was Mary's death murder?' (2001) 9 Medical LR 208, 217: '... to regard all killing that is foreseen by the actor as a virtual certainty as intended killing seems to include too much. For instance, if my car brakes fail I might deliberately swerve onto the footpath, foreseeing that I will kill one person who would not be able to get out of the way in time, rather than steer a straight course and run into a group of school children on a pedestrian crossing.'

Another criticism is that in present law the accused may be guilty if he foresees a consequence as a virtual certainty. In addition, there is the statement that the result must actually be a virtually certain consequence before the accused can be guilty. This objective test is inconsistent with the subjective nature of intent. If the terrorist plants a bomb, knowing that it is virtually certain that a person will be killed, why should it affect liability that a bomb-proof barrier has been erected that day between the bomb and the intended victim? His state of mind has not changed. All that has changed is something external to him.

As J. Stannard wrote in *Recent Developments in Criminal Law* (SLS, 1988) 38, malice aforethought is a confusing area because the courts are shifting the boundaries to catch persons whom they wish to be convicted of murder, while exculpating others. There is tension in the law. Some people wish the law to be flexible, to have in the words of Jeremy Horder ('Intention in criminal law: a rejoinder' (1995) 58 MLR 678) 'moral elbowroom' within which the jury can work. The contrary approach is that since murder is a particularly serious crime, it must be defined exactly: in other words, whether a person is convicted of murder should not depend on the jury's likes and dislikes. What a jury does is to consider the accused's moral sense; it should, however, according to **Woollin** consider which particular degree of foresight the accused had when he acted. The main problem involves terrorists. Lord Bridge in **Moloney**, as we have seen, gave the illustration of a bomber who gave a warning. Is he guilty of murdering the bomb disposal expert whom he expected to be called in? Lord Bridge seems to think he is, as did Lord Hope in **Woollin**, but on his definition the bomber did not have malice aforethought. There is neither the desire or aim to cause death or serious injury nor foresight of death or serious harm as virtually certain. The position remains the same after **Woollin**: death or grievous bodily harm is not foreseen as a virtually certain consequence. The courts wish to make terrorists guilty of murder, but exculpate persons like Moloney from that charge. However, terrorists could be found guilty of manslaughter and sentenced to life imprisonment, thereby maintaining a 'pure' concept of intention. Moreover, if the concept of intent is being expanded and contracted to reach a desirable outcome, why was Mrs Hyam found guilty of murder? Perhaps as suggested by C. Fennell 'Intention in murder: chaos, confusion and complexity' (1990) 41 NILQ 325 at 337–338 there should be an offence of second degree murder if the accused was aware of the risk of death or intended to cause fear. This proposal would catch terrorists who took a risk that someone may be killed or seriously injured.

It is unfortunate that the modern definition of intent has largely been laid down in murder cases. The result may have been 'pulled' by the facts, yet the law in these cases applies throughout the criminal law. If one looks at Lord Bridge's example in **Moloney** of a terrorist who plants a bomb and gives a warning, he foresees that someone may seek to defuse it but he does not foresee death or serious harm as being virtually certain. Bomb disposal experts do not become bomb disposal experts by getting killed or injured! Yet Lord Bridge would convict the terrorist of murder if the expert died. The difficulty lies in reconciling the core meaning of murder as deliberate killing and the need to satisfy public opinion that those who take a risk and kill (such as terrorists) are guilty of murder. The desire to convict terrorists of murder 'pulls' the law one way; the desire not to convict doctors of murder pulls it another way. In **Moor**, noted above, the trial judge in a case of a doctor's prescribing pain-killing drugs to a patient he believed to be terminally ill directed the jury in terms of direct intent but failed to mention foresight of a virtually certain consequence, oblique intent. Yet had he done so, a jury should have found that the doctor knew that acceleration of death was virtually certain.

To quote Lord Mustill in **Attorney-General's Reference (No. 3 of 1994)** [1998] AC 245:

> Murder is widely thought to be the gravest of crimes. One could expect a developed system to embody a law of murder clear enough to yield an unequivocal result on a given set of facts, a result which conforms with apparent justice and has a sound intellectual base. This is not so in England where the law of homicide is permeated by anomaly, fiction, misnomer and obsolete reasoning.

This is a real problem for judges and juries. Judges have to use ordinary English words so that juries understand the instruction, but 'intention' continues to elude clear judicial definition.

Does the definition of 'intent' in murder extend throughout the criminal law?

The House of Lords in **Moloney** and **Hancock and Shankland** did not restrict its remarks to murder. Its definition has been applied generally. In **AMK (Property Management) Ltd** [1985] Crim LR 600, the Court of Appeal applied this law to the offence under s 1(3) of the Protection from Eviction Act 1977: doing acts calculated to interfere with the peace or comfort of a residential occupier with intent to cause him to give up occupation. (See, however, below.) In **Bryson** [1985] Crim LR 669, the same court applied the law to wounding with intent to do grievous bodily harm, contrary to the Offences Against the Person Act 1861, s 18, when the accused drove at and knocked down four men celebrating the forthcoming wedding of one of their group. As we have seen, **Walker and Hayles**, above, involved attempted murder, where the sole *mens rea* is the intent to kill. The Court of Appeal of Northern Ireland held in **Murphy** [1993] NI 57 that 'common sense, reality and experience' led to the conclusion that when the IRA launched rockets and fired rifles at police stations they did intend to kill. No warning was given, and the weapons used were not ones for destroying buildings. Presumably the definition applies also where the term 'intent' does not stand alone in the definition of the offence but the crime is stated in terms of 'intentionally or recklessly' such as criminal damage. In these situations, however, the definition of intent is less important than in the three crimes just mentioned where the accused is not guilty if he acts recklessly. In **Woollin** the House of Lords confined its remarks to murder. If **Woollin** does not apply, the problem is to discover which test does apply. Perhaps in relation to the crime of attempt only direct intent suffices with regard to consequences. That is, the accused's aim must be to cause the forbidden result; it is not sufficient that he foresaw it as a virtually certain consequence.

Refer back to p 91 earlier in this chapter for a discussion of the *Steane* case. Note how a definition may vary from offence to offence.   In **Moloney** the Lords approved **Steane** [1947] KB 997, where the Court of Criminal Appeal laid down a narrower definition of intent. As a result, there is no one definition which applies across the criminal law. The accused was convicted of doing acts likely to assist the enemy when he did a broadcast for the Nazis in order to save his family from the concentration camp. The Court of Criminal Appeal quashed the conviction. It held that his intention was to save his family, that intent was not part of the *mens rea* of the crime; therefore, he did not intend to assist the enemy. However, his intention was not simply to save his family; he also intended to assist the enemy by broadcasting for them. The accused did not desire to help the Nazis, but current law is to the effect that the desire or motive of the defendant is immaterial to 'intent'. One can intend something without desiring it: *Mohan*, above, and *Nedrick*, the relevant part of which is quoted above. The accused's good motive, protecting his family, is irrelevant. Similarly, a bad motive, say, a wish to get rid of a wife in favour of a younger person, is immaterial. For more on 'desire' see the section on motive in Chapter 3. Under the *Moloney* approach surely he did foresee that it was (at least) virtually certain that he would be helping the enemy, and a jury could infer that he did intend to aid. Moreover, Lord Bridge in *Moloney* said that the accused intended to go to Manchester if the sole way he could escape the police was to go there, 'even though Manchester is the last place he wants to be'. Did not the accused in *Steane* intend to broadcast for the Nazis even though it was the last thing he wanted to do? *Steane* looks like a case of narrowing the law to exculpate the accused. The court wished to ensure that the accused's conviction could not be upheld, and to do so it manipulated the meaning of intention. It was able to do that because there is no one definition of intent which is accepted for all offences. *Steane* confuses an already confused area and should be overruled. *Steane* is also inconsistent with modern cases on duress which hold that that defence does not operate to negate intent. The accused did intend, but he has a defence.

More recently in the civil case of *Airedale NHS Trust* v *Bland* [1993] AC 789 (HL) Lord Goff said that it was an 'established rule' that a doctor could prescribe painkilling drugs knowing that they would shorten life, yet not be guilty of murder. *Re A*, above, the case of the conjoined twins, is similar: the surgeons knew that on separation one of the twins would die, but the Court of Appeal struggled to find a rule or rules which would exculpate doctors if they were put on trial. *Moor*, cited above, is a criminal case of a doctor's accelerating death but being found not guilty. The trial judge Hooper J, said: 'a person intends to kill another person if he does an act . . . for the purpose of killing that person. If [the accused] thought . . . that it was only highly probable that death would follow . . ., then the prosecution would not have proved that he intended to kill . . .'. This looks like the judge saying that proper treatment, including providing pain-killing drugs which incidentally shorten life, does not constitute an intent to murder. If so this defence needs public discussion.

The type of intention in *Steane*, sometimes called 'direct intent', may apply elsewhere. In the well-known case of *Ahlers* [1915] 1 KB 616 (CCA) the court held that a German consul was not guilty of treason when he assisted fellow nationals to return to their native land. He did not intend to aid the UK's enemies, merely to perform his consular duties. Applying modern law, the accused should have been found guilty. Alternatively, a different definition of intent, namely 'purpose', applies to this offence. Some statutes seem to require a certain purpose. In burglary, one form of the crime is trespassory entry with intent to commit one of a list of offences. It must be that intent in this context means 'purpose'. In blackmail the accused must act with 'intent' to gain or to cause loss. 'Intent' means direct intent. Similarly in the Protection from Eviction Act 1977, mentioned above, 'intent' means 'purpose' and the accused is not liable if he did not act with the purpose of getting the tenant out, even if he foresaw it as virtually certain that that result would occur. In the crime of using or threatening violence for the purpose of securing entry into premises only direct intent suffices. In such cases oblique intent will not suffice. The point is that *Steane* is not an isolated decision and *Moloney et al.* do not apply to all 'intent' crimes. There is debate among academics as to whether and if so which crimes are satisfied only when the accused acted with direct intent.

Proposals for defining intention

The *Report of the House of Lords Select Committee on Murder and Life Imprisonment* (HL Paper 78–1, 1989) and the Law Commission's Report, *A Criminal Code for England and Wales* (Law Com. No. 177, 1989) both recommended that foresight of a virtual certainty should amount to intention. The enactment of this recommendation would mean that foresight would again be part of substantive law, not merely part of evidence. The Law Commission stated that 'intention' should be defined in the interests of clarity and consistency. The Select Committee also wished to abolish the head of malice aforethought which is the intent to cause grievous bodily harm, and replace it by the intent to cause serious personal harm, being aware that death may be caused. The Select Committee approved, therefore, cl 54(1) of the draft Criminal Code, which states:

[a] person is guilty of murder if he causes the death of another –
   (a) intending to cause death; or
   (b) intending to cause serious personal harm and being aware that he may cause death.

The definition was approved by Lord Steyn in ***Powell***; ***English*** [1998] AC 147. In his view, 'the present definition of the mental element of murder results in defendants being classified as murderers who are in truth not murderers'. 'Being aware' connotes subjective knowledge. It would not be sufficient that a reasonable person would have known but the accused did not. It may be that the test will be hard to apply. Furthermore, there seems to be little, if any, moral difference between intending to cause serious harm being aware that one may cause death and simply being aware that one may cause death. Both states of mind are ones of taking a risk, recklessness.

Intention is defined by cl 18(b) as covering both direct intent and oblique intent:

[a] person acts 'intentionally' with respect to . . .
   (ii) a result when he acts either in order to bring it about or being aware that it will occur in the ordinary course of events.

Intention is therefore to be defined as to go beyond direct intent, something which it does not do in ordinary language. The accused in ***Steane*** would be guilty. The Law Commission thought that this change was demanded by justice. It would exclude foresight of anything less than a virtual certainty. This definition received the approval of Lord Lane CJ in the debate on the Select Committee's Report. Clause 18(b) would not cover the terrorist who plants a bomb intending to damage property and cause fear but not to kill or injure. Professor Smith criticised the width of the formulation. He wanted it to cover the terrorist who knows that half of his bombs will not explode. 'In the ordinary course of events' he is not virtually certain that a victim will die. He proposed to redraft (ii) as including the situation where 'his purpose is to cause some other result and he knows that, if he succeeds, his act will, in the ordinary course of events, cause that result' ([1990] Crim LR 85). The Law Commission accepted this revision in *Legislating the Criminal Code – Offences against the Person and General Principles*, Law Com. No. 218, 1993. Clause 1(a) of the Criminal Law Bill attached to the Report states:

A person acts 'intentionally' with respect to a result when –
   (i) it is his purpose to cause it, or
   (ii) although it is not his purpose to cause that result, he knows that it would occur in the ordinary course of events if he were to succeed in his purpose of causing some other result.

The replacement of 'in order to' with 'purpose' was thought to aid clarity; 'knows' replaced 'is aware' because the Law Commission thought that the awareness connoted a less clear appreciation than knowledge; and knowledge is linked to purpose, unlike in the draft Criminal Code, in order to disabuse people that intention might cover recklessness. The Law Commission rejected extending intention to awareness of any degree of probability less than virtual certainty. Such forethought would constitute recklessness. Therefore, the word used is 'would'. The accused has to know that an event would definitely occur unless something extraordinary occurred. The boundary between the concepts of intent and recklessness would be clearly drawn. Had the draft been 'he knows that it *might* occur', that state of mind is recklessness.

The Law Commission published its Report no. 306 *Murder, Manslaughter and Infanticide* in November 2006. It is based on its Consultation Paper of December 2005, *A New Homicide Act for England and Wales?* The Commission's view was that the mental element for first degree murder should be intent to kill and intent to cause serious injury, being aware that one's conduct involves a serious risk of causing death. Second degree murder would also comprise states of mind defined in terms of intent: intent to cause serious injury, and intent to cause injury, fear of injury or a risk of injury, being aware that one's conduct involves a serious risk of death. Therefore, intent would remain the *mens rea* of murder but there would be gradations in murder dependent on the state of mind of the accused.

The Commission was then faced with defining 'intent'. It had postulated two definitions in the Consultation Paper but having determined that current law could not to be left to common law, it decided to codify current law (though no supporting argument was given in the Report as to why the common law had to be codified) and it decided not to provide an extended meaning, which had been one of the options canvassed in the Paper. The revised definition is set out in para. 3.27:

(1) A person should be taken to intend a result if he or she acts in order to bring it about.

(2) In cases where the judge believes that justice may not be done unless an expanded understanding of intention is given, the jury should be directed as follows: an intention to bring about a result may be found if it is shown that the defendant thought that the result was a virtually certain consequence of his or her action.

This definition therefore covers an accused in this situation (para. 3.13):

> D is in the process of stealing V's car. V leaps onto the car bonnet to deter D from driving off. D accelerates to 100 miles per hour and V falls off the car. The fall kills V. D claims he did not intend to kill V or cause V serious injury but was simply determined to escape come what may.

Common law leaves this issue to the jury, and if enacted, the recommendations in the Report would do similarly. It should also be remembered that as is the case with current law, it will be rare for a 'virtually certain' instruction: normally, only the first direction ('in order to bring it about') will be needed, which again is the same as current law. Incidentally, the Law Commission opines that the jury would find intent in the example given (see para. 3.14) but it remains the case that the issue is one for the jury. The Commission also clarified that a person thinks a consequence is virtually certain to occur 'so long as he or she thinks that it will be virtually certain *if they do as they mean to do*. E.g., if someone plants a bomb on a plane intending to detonate it when the plane is in mid-air, given that they mean to detonate it, they can be taken to foresee the deaths of the passengers if they realise that the home-made bomb is unreliable and might fail to detonate as planned.' (footnote 9 on p. 56) The Commission recognises that their proposed approach leaves discretion in the juries' hands but says (at para. 3.21): '. . . it is sometimes necessary and desirable that juries should have the element of discretion if the alternative is a more complex set of legal rules that they must apply. It is the price of avoiding complexity.'

There have been calls for other definitions from academics. For example, in *Criminal Law: Text and Materials*, 6th edn (Thomson, 2007) pp. 142–44, C. M. V. Clarkson, H. Keating and S. R. Cunningham propose a definition which does not stray too far from ordinary language: aim. They would also include foreseeing a consequence as certain, but not foresight as virtually certain. Would this proposal prevent the aircraft bomber who kills in order to collect the insurance money being convicted of murder? One may wonder whether there is a conceptual difference between foresight as certain and foresight as virtually certain. There has also been a lengthy campaign to reduce the forms of malice aforethought to one: the intent to kill, the reason being that the term 'murder' should be reserved for the gravest killers. So restricting the definition would also mean that there would be no need to draw lines between different frames of mind, foresight of a consequence as virtually certain and foresight of a consequence as less than virtually certain. Whatever happens, 'it is in the interests of clarity and the consistent application of criminal law to define intention', as the Law Commission put it (at 193). Present law lacks that clarity. As Stanley Yeo wrote in *Fault in Homicide* (Federation Press, 1997) 50: 'The law lacks a clear definition of intention which is a gross failure on the part of the English courts given the pivotal role that this concept plays in determining culpability for murder and, indeed, for many other offences.'

Brief summary

Under present law a person who kills foreseeing death or grievous bodily harm as virtually certain may be a murderer. Under the reformed scheme he would be a murderer.

Recklessness

 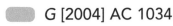

G [2004] AC 1034

Seriously avid readers of this textbook will have noted the downgrading of **Caldwell** [1982] AC 341 (HL) from 'the most important case' in Anglo-Welsh criminal law to 'for a decade thought to be the most important case'. The House of Lords has now overruled **Caldwell**, making it in practice one of the least important cases in Anglo-Welsh criminal law. Nevertheless, the 20 or so years of **Caldwell** remain significant theoretically and even after its demise the law of objective **recklessness** remains of importance, as will shortly be explained.

Facts and decision

See p 671 in Chapter 18 for more information on the relationship between arson and the Criminal Damage Act 1971.

Like **Caldwell** the facts of **G** are simple. Two boys, aged 11 and 12, set fire to some newspapers in the back yard of a shop. They threw the lit papers under a rubbish bin. The fire spread to the shop and some £1 million worth of damage was caused. The boys were charged with arson contrary to s 1(1) and (3) of the Criminal Damage Act 1971. They were found guilty at first instance, the trial judge directing the jury in accordance with

Caldwell. The House of Lords overruled *Caldwell* and held that the boys were not guilty of arson. They did not foresee criminal damage. The House adopted the Law Commission's draft Criminal Code (Report No. 177, 1989) definition: 'A person acts recklessly . . . with respect to

(i)   a circumstance when he is aware of a risk that it exists or will exist;
(ii) a result when he is aware of a risk that it will occur,
and it is, in the circumstance known to him, unreasonable to take the risk.'

Actually there is one way in which the boys could have been convicted of arson. If they adverted to the risk that by throwing lit newspapers they would set fire to rubbish underneath the bin, then this would set fire to the bin itself, and then they would be reckless as to criminal damage (to the bin), and as this fire caused damage to the shop, then they should have been convicted of arson to the shop.

What did *Caldwell* decide?

Caldwell held that for the purposes of s 1 of the Criminal Damage Act 1971 a person acted recklessly if (1) there was an obvious (and serious) risk of damage and either (2a) he gave no thought to the possibility of such a risk or (2b) he recognised that there was a risk but nevertheless went ahead. This is a short form of the definition given by Lord Diplock and for a full exegesis of this definition the reader is advised to read pp. 118–26 of the sixth edition of *Criminal Law*. (2b) is sometimes known as 'subjective recklessness' – did this accused foresee the relevant risk? This type of recklessness has existed for more than a century and the principal authority remains *Cunningham* [1957] 2 QB 396 (CCA). The words used were: 'The accused has foreseen that the particular kind of harm might be done and yet has gone on to take the risk of it.' (2a) is objective recklessness: might a reasonable person foresee a risk of some harm occurring? *G* overruled (2a), often known as *Caldwell*-recklessness. Subjective recklessness (2b) remains. Since the boys did not foresee the risk of damage, they were not guilty of arson, which is the crime of causing criminal damage by fire.

For a short while in the years following *Caldwell* objective recklessness was taken to apply to all offences of recklessness unless Parliament had otherwise ordained: *Seymour* [1983] 2 AC 493 (HL) *per* Lord Roskill. Offences committed maliciously, which means as *Cunningham* held, 'intentionally or recklessly', constituted the main example of offences where Parliament had otherwise ordained, and subjective recklessness continued to apply to such offences: see *Savage* [1992] 1 AC 699 (HL). However, even crimes such as rape, which at that time included the mental element of committing sexual intercourse knowing that the victim did not consent or being reckless as to whether the victim consented or not, were held to be ones of objective recklessness: see the perhaps aptly named case of *Pigg* [1982] 1 WLR 762 (CA). However, the courts began what might be called a retreat from *Caldwell*, holding that certain offences including rape were not crimes of objective recklessness. Parliament also abolished two of the principal crimes of objective recklessness, reckless driving and causing death by reckless driving (on which see *Lawrence* [1982] AC 510 (HL) and *Reid* [1992] 1 WLR 793 (HL)). For further details of the retreat from *Caldwell* see M. Jefferson ('Recklessness: The objectivity of the *Caldwell* test' (1999) 63 JCL 57. By 2000 it was difficult to find a crime of objective recklessness other than criminal damage, but the astute knew of recklessly flying a microlight plane and recklessly misusing personal data contrary to the Data Protection Act 1984.

How far does G go?

All the Law Lords held that the interpretation by *Caldwell* of s 1 of the Criminal Damage Act was incorrect. Parliament did not intend to give a novel definition to recklessness when it replaced the crime of malicious damage with that of intentional or reckless criminal damage. Four of their Lordships also said that *Caldwell*, besides being legally wrong, was morally repugnant: as Lord Bingham put it, '. . . it is not clearly blameworthy to do something involving a risk of injury to another if . . . one genuinely does not perceive the risk'. Such a person may 'fairly be accused of stupidity or lack of imagination, but neither of those failings should expose him to conviction of serious crime or the risk of punishment . . . It is neither moral nor just to convict a defendant . . . on the strength of what someone else would have apprehended if the defendant himself had no such apprehension'. (Lord Bingham, however, cast no doubt on what is sometimes known as 'constructive recklessness', i.e. the deeming of the accused to be reckless when intoxicated by alcohol or drugs for crimes of basic intent in the defence of drunkenness: see *Majewski* [1977] AC 443 and the part of *Caldwell* which deals with intoxication). Lord Bingham also disapproved of *Elliott* v *C* [1983] 1 WLR 939 (DC, a case where a tired, hungry and 'backward' 14-year-old girl was convicted of arson): 'It is neither moral or just to convict a defendant (least of all a child) on the strength of what someone would have apprehended if the defendant had no such apprehension.' The House could have restricted their speeches to overruling *Elliott* v *C* because the defendants were children, thereby preserving *Caldwell* for adults or at least non-disabled ones, as suggested by the question certified by the Court of Appeal but they did not: both statutory interpretation and moral considerations required the overruling of *Caldwell*.

However, the doctrine of parliamentary supremacy should not be forgotten. At the time when the House of Lords in its judicial capacity was abolishing objective recklessness, the House of Lords in its legislative capacity and the House of Commons were passing the Sexual Offences Act 2003. Unreasonable belief in the victim's consent is no longer a defence. The statute is, depressingly but unsurprisingly, unclear about children as defendants. The first quote from Lord Bingham, above, continues: 'Such a person [i.e. an objectively reckless one] may fairly be accused of stupidity or lack of imagination, but neither of these failings should expose him to conviction of serious crime or the risk of punishment.' Rape is a serious crime; the maximum punishment is life imprisonment. Yet it can now be committed by a person who believed on unreasonable grounds in the consent of the victim. Parliament has not heeded *G*. The then Home Secretary was pleased with the revised definition of rape, and there is something, indeed quite a bit, to be said in favour of objective recklessness in sexual offences but it is disappointing to see the arguments of academic commentators not being taken into account by Parliament on such an important issue. It will be interesting to see how the courts deal with boys of 11 and 12 years of age who are charged with rape and who contend that they gave no thought as to whether or not the victim was consenting or believed that the victim was consenting when a reasonable person would not have so believed. *Elliott* v *C* produced a disastrous outcome; surely we should be able to prevent similar injustices to children. Let us recall that the extension of the perpetration of the crime of rape to boys under the age of 14 was enacted as recently as 1993 and it was as recent as 1998 that the doctrine of mischievous discretion was abolished.

Outstanding issues

(a) Lord Bingham said: 'I wish to make it as plain as I can that I am not addressing the meaning of "reckless" in any other statutory or common law context.' This proposition is very much akin to that of Lord Steyn in *Woollin* [1999] 1 AC 82 (HL) that the definition he gave for intent in murder was not necessarily the one which applied throughout criminal law. This method of proceeding is unacceptable in a mature system of law. Can it really be true that *Caldwell* is abolished for criminal damage but not for other offences of objective recklessness such as recklessly flying a microlight? Lord Bingham stated that a person was reckless as to a circumstance when 'he is aware of a risk that it exists or will exist' and that a person is reckless as to a consequence if 'he is aware of a risk that it will occur'. These are standard definitions of subjective recklessness as to a circumstance and as to a consequence and are generalisable throughout criminal law but he prefaced these definitions by saying that they applied for the purposes of the Criminal Damage Act. In *B* [2000] 2 AC 428 (HL) in the context of strict liability a different formulation was made. In the context of sexual offences at least, if the accused has not thought about a circumstance, such as the consent of the victim, then he is guilty unless he believes that the circumstance does not exist. It is, it must be said, difficult to envisage someone who is not thinking about a circumstance but who at the same time genuinely believes that it does not exist. Perhaps an example might be this: Y and Z have been lovers for several years; Y does not on this occasion think about whether Z is consenting or not but, if asked, would say that he believes that his partner is consenting because he or she has always consented before. If this example is correct, Y is not guilty of rape as it was then defined under both *G* and *B*. If, however, Y and Z have not been in a long-term relationship but this is the first occasion of sexual intercourse, then if Y gave no thought to whether Z was consenting or not, he is not guilty under *G* but is under *B*.

Five Law Lords dealt with statutory interpretation, four of them with the lack of moral culpability of inadvertent recklessness. That leaves one Lord who did not treat of the moral dimension. This was Lord Rodger. He said that objective recklessness was a possible ground of liability for some offences. If *Caldwell* is overruled in relation to criminal damage but *Caldwell* is so morally repugnant that four Law Lords say that it should not be part of a civilised system of law, what scope is there for Lord Rodger's exception? It is highly tentatively suggested that what he may have had in mind was the previous offence of reckless driving. Here the recklessness is not as to a consequence or as to a circumstance but as to the *manner* in which the act, driving, was performed. Lord Bingham said: '. . . I would wish to throw no doubt on the decisions of this House in *Lawrence* and *Reid*.' If there are offences where recklessness is as to the way in which the act is done, it may be that the mental element is one of objective recklessness. This issue will have to be settled in the future.

It would seem that the lower courts take *G* to apply to all defences. In *A-G's Reference (No. 3 of 2003)* [2004] EWCA Crim 868 the subjective test was applied to the common law crime of misfeasance in a public office. However, the House did not in *G* overrule cases which had held that *Caldwell* applied to various offences such as recklessly flying a microlight plane.

(b) Cases like *G* and *B* indicate a return to subjective *mens rea*. It should be noted that nothing in *G* affects gross negligence manslaughter. Of course, that offence was according to *Seymour* replaced by reckless manslaughter but the House of Lords in *Adomako* [1995] 1 AC 171 returned to manslaughter by gross negligence, reviving the pre-*Caldwell* law (see Chapter 12). Similarly, nothing in *G* affects duress, whether by threats or circumstances. The Court of Appeal in *Graham* [1982] 1 WLR 294, which was approved by the House of Lords in *Howe* [1987] AC 417, held that in duress the accused's belief in the existence of the threat had to be based on reasonable grounds. Lord Steyn in **G** opined that **Graham** and **Howe** were correct. There is some contrary authority, **Martin** [2000] 2 Cr App R 42 (CA): see this book for further details. **Martin**, as is demonstrated, is incorrect. **G** also does not affect the law of intoxication. A drunken accused is guilty of recklessly causing the *actus reus* if he was very drunk, even though he did not foresee the outcome. This type of recklessness is sometimes known as 'constructive recklessness'. For more on intoxication, see Chapter 8.

(c) In both subjective and objective recklessness there exists the prerequisite that the accused's behaviour must not be justifiable. If the conduct is justified, there is no recklessness. For example, if a car driver swerves to avoid a child and as a result crashes into a van, on a charge of criminal damage to the van the driver is not reckless because his action was justified, even if he foresaw that some criminal damage might be caused to the van. At this stage the test is objective even in subjective recklessness: whether the accused thought his conduct was justified is irrelevant.

Some criticisms of objective recklessness

(a) *The viewpoint of legal authority.* When Parliament enacted the Criminal Damage Act 1971 it did not intend to change the law. It simply intended to replace the old-fashioned term of 'maliciously' with the modern term of 'recklessly'. Lord Diplock thought otherwise, but was wrong. The Act is based on a Report by the Law Commission, *Offences of Damage to Property*, Report No. 29, 1970, which wished the Act to do the same. The Court of Appeal in **Briggs** [1977] 1 WLR 605, **Parker** [1977] Crim LR 102 and **Stephenson** [1979] QB 695 did not attempt to state the law of recklessness in criminal damage in any way other than that underlying the proposals of the Law Commission and the 1971 Act. Criminal law previously drew the line for most serious offences between advertently taking a risk (guilty) and inadvertently doing so (innocent). **Caldwell** runs these morally different states of mind together. There is little support for **Caldwell** in the earlier law. For example, the House of Lords in **Andrews v DPP** [1937] AC 576 equated recklessness and gross negligence, postulating an objective standard of behaviour, but that case occurred before the law's terms were settled. (In tort recklessness is subjective, at least in relation to fencing out child trespassers: the law looks the wrong way round.)

(b) It is often said that criminal law is based on choice. An accused should be guilty only if he had a choice to commit the crime. Choice includes a conscious decision to run the risk of causing harm. In other words, subjective recklessness is acceptable. However, if the accused does not consider whether harm may be caused, he had not chosen to break the law.

(c) **Caldwell** made people guilty who previously were not guilty because they were careless but now are reckless. (Incidentally the job of the prosecution is thereby facilitated.) The Supreme Court of Canada in **Sansregret v R** (1985) 17 DLR (4th) 577 said that negligence should not be confused with recklessness.

> Negligence is tested by the objective standard of the reasonable man. A departure from his accustomed sober behaviour by an act or omission which reveals less than reasonable care will involve liability at civil law but forms no basis for the imposition of criminal penalties . . . [R]ecklessness, to form part of the criminal *mens rea*, must have an element

of the subjective. It is found in the attitude of one who, aware that there is danger that his conduct could bring about the result prohibited by the criminal law, nevertheless persists, despite the risk. . . . It is in this sense that the term 'recklessness' is used in the criminal law and it is clearly distinct from the concept of civil negligence.

(d) One of the theories of punishment is specific deterrence: an accused must be deterred by punishment from committing an offence. However, if he does not advert to the risk of harm, he cannot be deterred.

It is an issue of policy whether people who gave no thought to a risk should be criminally liable. Lord Diplock did not think that the law should distinguish between the two states of mind, being aware and taking a chance on the one hand and not being aware on the other. In his view both were equally culpable frames of mind. People are blamed for not taking care. If a scaffolder drops a piece of equipment carelessly, he would be blamed if the equipment hit someone in the street on the head. After all, punishment of such careless people may make them take care next time. The House of Lords in *Reid* [1992] 1 WLR 793 adopted this view too. Indeed, Lord Keith said that *Cunningham* recklessness was hard to apply. His proposition is difficult to accept, for thousands of juries have over the years used the subjective definition without question. Academic commentators have, on the whole, rejected his approach. S. France 'Reckless approach to liability' (1988) 18 VUWLR 141 at 152–153 made the point:

> The real dangers of *Caldwell* lie in its potential to bring the might of the criminal law into the ordinary situations of life by equating acts of negligence with deliberate wilful acts of malice . . . Such acts do not involve consciously dangerous antisocial activity.

Do we really want the accused guilty of arson in *Elliott v C* [1983] 1 WLR 939 (DC)? The accused was 14, tired, hungry and had learning difficulties. She set fire to a shed after sprinkling a flammable liquid around; and was found guilty of arson. She did not choose to break the law, and she lacked the capacity to realise that what she was doing was dangerous. It was not that her actions showed an indifference to the harm she caused but that she was not capable of foreseeing any risk because of her learning difficulties.

Legal policy also comes to the fore when one considers the thrusts of *Caldwell* and *B v DPP* [2000] 2 AC 428 (HL). The latter states that a person is not liable for an offence which for many years had been a crime of strict liability: *mens rea* in the sense of knowledge as to the age of the victim is needed; however, *Caldwell* stated that for offences of objective recklessness knowledge is not needed.

Reform

Both before and after *Caldwell* law reform bodies have recommended continuing with the *Cunningham* definition. The Law Commission in *The Mental Element in Crime*, Report No. 89, 1978, the Criminal Law Revision Committee's Fourteenth Report, *Offences Against the Person*, Cmnd 7844, 1980, and the draft Criminal Code (Law Com. No. 177, 1989), all adopted the *Cunningham* approach. Lord Diplock did not refer to any English proposals. The sole law reform matter he looked at was the US Model Penal Code, and even then he did so selectively. Academic comment supported a return to *Cunningham*, which is thought to be easy to apply, instead of *Caldwell*, which was thought to be hard for juries and judges to understand. Recklessness would need a definition because without one a jury might think that recklessness and negligence were the same. The draft Code, cl 18(c), defines 'recklessly' in relation to offences contained in the Code thus:

> A person acts 'recklessly' with respect to –
> (i)   a circumstance when he is aware of a risk that it exists or will exist;
> (ii) a result when he is aware of a risk that it will occur;
> and it is, in the circumstances known to him, unreasonable to take the risk . . .

(The same definition occurs in *Legislating the Criminal Code – Offences Against the Person and General Principles*, Law Com. No. 218, 1993, and is the one adopted by the House of Lords in *G*.) Recklessness defined in this way will be the minimum level of fault in Code offences, unless otherwise provided (cl 20(1)). The Law Commission stated that cl 8(c) is to the same effect as the definition it proposed in its 1978 Report, *The Mental Element in Crime* (p. 193). The Law Commission thought that a person should be liable only if he consciously took a risk, and it preferred to adopt the subjectivist approach, while leaving it open to Parliament to enact *Caldwell*, should it so wish. If the accused is unaware of the risk, the inadvertence is negligence and not part of the Code.

There are two or three distinctions between *Cunningham* and the draft Code. First, there is no reference in *Cunningham* to the justifiability of the risk, but that omission is soon remedied. If the risk is justified, it remained the case that the accused was not reckless under the *Cunningham* definition. Secondly, *Cunningham* did not refer to risks as to circumstances but the draft Code does. Thirdly, *Cunningham* refers to foresight of this *type* of harm whereas the draft Code refers to the actual harm caused, and in this respect the *Cunningham* definition appears wider than that in the draft Code.

The House of Lords in *Reid* [1992] 1 WLR 793 spoke to the effect that the person who gave no thought to the possibility of harm or substantial damage when driving a car was just as blameworthy as someone who did consider the risk. The reader is invited to consider whether she or he agrees. The House of Lords stated also that the former (lack of a) state of mind constituted *mens rea*. Lord Keith said: 'Inadvertence to risk is no less a state of mind than is disregard of a recognised risk.' Lord Diplock in *Caldwell* stated that it required 'meticulous analysis' to distinguish between an accused who foresees a risk and one who ought to have foreseen one. Do you agree?

'Knowingly'

Parliament sometimes uses this word to impose a requirement of *mens rea*. For example, a person is guilty of handling only if he knows or believes the goods to be stolen. Where the definition of the offence does not include 'knowing', the courts sometimes read it in (see Chapter 4 on strict offences).

The criminal courts recognise several degrees of knowledge.

(a) *Actual knowledge*. The principal authority is *Roper v Taylor's Central Garages (Exeter) Ltd* [1951] 2 TLR 284 (DC). Devlin J said that this type of knowledge is when the accused knows for a fact that something exists or is true.

(b) *Wilful blindness*. Devlin J in *Roper* called this state of mind 'knowledge in the second degree'. Lord Bridge in *Westminster CC v Croyalgrange Ltd* [1986] 1 WLR 674 said that knowledge could be based 'on evidence that the defendant had deliberately shut his eyes to the obvious or refrained from enquiring because he suspected the truth but did not want to have his suspicions confirmed'. Although Lord Bridge spoke of 'inference', it is arguable that the rule is one of law: *Roper*, above.

(c) *Constructive knowledge.* Again this term was expanded in **Roper**. This degree of knowledge occurs when the accused ought as a reasonable person to have made inquiries.
This is negligence (see below).

The first type is always covered by 'knowing' or 'knowingly'. The second type is usually
covered, but not always. In handling, wilful blindness is not sufficient (see Chapter 17).
The third is rare in traditional criminal law but arises when Parliament creates an offence
where the accused had reasonable cause to believe. An example comes from s 25 of the
Firearms Act 1968. A person is guilty of an offence if he sells a firearm or ammunition to
anyone who he knows or has reasonable cause to believe is drunk. A more recent example
comes from the Protection from Harassment Act (1997). A person is guilty if he ought to
have known that his conduct would harass the victim.

A person does not know that he has something if he has forgotten about it: **Russell**
(1984) 81 Cr App R 315. It may be, however, that an accused continues to know something if he has the capacity to remember the relevant information: **Bello** (1978) 67 Cr
App R 288 (CA).

Under the draft Criminal Code, cl 18:

> A person acts . . . knowingly with respect to a circumstance not only when he is aware that
> it exists or will exist, but also when he avoids taking steps that might confirm his belief that
> it exists or will exist.

'Wilful blindness' is therefore to be covered by 'knowingly'.

'Wilfully'

Like 'knowingly', 'wilfully' is a term which normally gives rise to *mens rea*. The principal
authority is **Sheppard** [1981] AC 394 (HL). By s 1(1) of the Children and Young Persons
Act 1933:

> [I]f any person who has attained the age of sixteen years and has custody, charge, or care
> of any child or young person under that age, wilfully assaults, ill-treats, neglects, abandons,
> or exposes him . . . in a manner likely to cause him unnecessary suffering or injury to
> health . . . that person shall be guilty . . .

Lord Diplock said that 'wilfully' connoted usually intention or recklessness in relation to
'assaults, ill-treats . . . , abandons or exposes'. It did not simply mean that the accused
had to act voluntarily. Cases which are to the effect that 'wilfully' is simply a synonym
for 'voluntarily' may need revision after **Sheppard**. Since voluntary conduct is implied
into offences, saying that 'wilfully' means 'voluntarily' leads to the proposition that
'wilfully' means nothing or perhaps Parliament was expressing what was already implied.
However, in relation to neglect, which was in issue in **Sheppard**, he held that the failure
to summon a doctor with the result that the child died

> . . . could not be properly described as 'wilful' unless the parent either (1) had directed his
> mind to the question whether there was some risk . . . that the child's health might suffer
> unless he were examined by a doctor . . . , and had made a conscious decision . . . to refrain
> from arranging for such medical examination, or (2) had so refrained because he did not
> care whether the child might be in need of medical treatment or not.

This explanation is the equivalent of recklessness **Caldwell**-style in the era before **G**
[2004] 1 AC 1034. Unlike in **Caldwell**, however, Lord Diplock stated that defendants who

acted 'through ignorance or lack of intelligence' were not wilful. 'Wilfully' is not a 'fault term' within the draft Criminal Code. Therefore, it is not defined therein.

While normally 'wilfully' is a *mens rea* word, the courts have at times held that 'wilfully' governs one part of the *actus reus* but not another part. If one wilfully destroys an oak which is subject to a tree preservation order, one is guilty if one knows that one is chopping down a tree; one need not know that there is a preservation order attached to it: **Maidstone BC v Mortimer** [1980] 3 All ER 502 (DC). One need not, therefore, in this crime be wilful as to all parts of the *actus reus*. For this reason the offence is one of strict liability, a topic discussed in the next chapter. A contrasting case is **Willmott v Atack** [1977] QB 498 (DC). An accused is guilty of wilfully obstructing a constable only if he knows he is obstructing the officer. It is not sufficient that he performs an act which in part obstructs her.

Negligence

Offences of negligence such as careless driving are not seen by all academics as pukka. Professor Hogan wrote: 'Stupidity does not seem . . . to be an adequate basis for offences which society regards very seriously' ('Strict liability' ([1978] Crim LR 593). Glanville Williams in *Criminal Law: The General Part*, 2nd edn (Stevens, 1961) 122, added: 'Some people are born feckless, clumsy, thoughtless, inattentive, irresponsible, with a bad memory and a slow "reaction time". With the best will in the world, we all of us at some times in our lives make negligent mistakes. It is hard to see how justice (as distinct from some utilitarian reason) requires mistakes to be punished.' These defects are not morally blameworthy. Moreover, criminal law is the state's most serious methods of obliging people not to do things, yet, if they cannot stop themselves doing so because, for example, they are careless, how will the penalties of the law stop them? Nevertheless, the utilitarians reason that crimes of negligence may oblige persons to think before acting. Unreasonable behaviour should be subject to penal sanctions. There are indeed many statutory offences of negligence, most of which are minor, just as there are many statutory crimes of strict liability. George Fletcher wrote: 'Negligence is suspect as a deviation from the paradigm of intentional criminality' ('The theory of criminal negligence: a comparative analysis' (1971) 119 U Pa LR 401 at 403).

(a) When one moves from intention and subjective recklessness to negligence the focus moves from conscious activity to inadvertence. Few authorities discuss the definition of negligence, but what it means is this. The accused has failed to attain the objective standard required by the criminal law. One argument against negligence as a basis for imposing criminal law liability is that the accused is judged by an objective criterion, not by his state of mind. In the context of manslaughter by gross negligence the Court of Appeal in **Attorney-General's Reference (No. 2 of 1999)** [2000] QB 796 emphasised in a passage approved by the Divisional Court in **DPP ex p Jones** [2000] IRLR 373 that the test for negligence was objective and no evidence need be led of the accused's state of mind. Negligence as a standard of liability is not built on individual culpability. Therefore it should not be used to impose criminal sanctions. The contrary argument is that negligence connotes that the accused ought to have been aware of an unjustifiable risk of harm. In England it is accepted that liability for negligence imposes an objective standard: did this accused fall short of the standard required of a reasonable person?

'The underlying rationale of subjectivism appears to be that it allows punishment only where a person exercised some choice and that it prevents the natural converse, the punishment of those who had no choice' (C. Wells 'Swatting the subjectivist bug' [1982] Crim LR 209 at 212). A subjectivist would say that a person should not be convicted if she was not capable of changing her behaviour to stop committing an offence. Criticism of negligence might be reduced if a variable standard were adopted. A higher standard of liability might be imposed on a local authority or large firm than on a backward, tired and hungry 14-year-old. Even where the general standard is that of a reasonable person, a higher, i.e. variable, standard is already imposed on a person who has special knowledge. Since the standard is variable upwards, why is it not variable downwards in relation to age, size, intelligence and the like? It might be asked whether a backward, tired and hungry 14-year-old deserved punishment even if a reasonable person would have deserved it. Furthermore, it is sometimes argued that liability should not be imposed where the accused did not have a fair opportunity to become aware of the risk. Did a backward, tired and hungry girl of 14 have such an opportunity? Nevertheless, one may not always wish to exculpate some defendants despite their personal characteristics. Would one want to find a person not guilty of driving without due care and attention because she was young, tired and hungry and lacking in intelligence? Similarly one might wish, as the law does at present, to keep learner and experienced drivers to the same standard. It seems strange that the civil law should be more reflective of personal characteristics in this regard than criminal law (see ***BRB*** v ***Herrington*** [1972] AC 877, on child trespassers). It should be remembered that the usual defences apply to offences of negligence, including ones based on mental capacity such as insanity and infancy. Even in relation to these offences the insane person is not treated as a sane one. The child of nine or eleven is not treated as a person of 35.

One of the strongest supporters of subjectivism in English law, J. C. Smith, wrote in 'Subjective or objective? The ups and downs of the test of criminal liability in England' [1981–82] Villanova LR 1179 at 1214 (spelling anglicised):

> [T]o support the subjectivist theory of criminal liability is not to deny that there is a place for offences where an objective test is justified, as with offences of negligence. For example, negligence is the appropriate criterion of liability in many regulatory offences, the very purpose of which is to ensure a high degree of care in the carrying out of certain activities like the sale of food and drugs, where negligence can be extremely harmful to the parties . . . Negligence is, of course, by definition, fault; but not every fault should entail liability. The process of the enforcement of the criminal law is costly and produces much pain . . . The onus of proof should be on the objectivist to show that we need criminal liability for negligence.

However, since Parliament may make new laws it may make new offences of negligence. Rape, a serious offence, is defined in part under the Sexual Offences Act 2003 as a crime where the accused 'does not reasonably believe' that the victim consents. This makes a serious offence into the crime of negligence. Similar is the crime of causing or allowing the death of a child or vulnerable adult contrary to s 5 of the Domestic Violence, Crime and Victims Act 2004.

(b) Some commentators argue that *mens rea* denotes the accused's own state of mind. Falling short of a standard is not a state of mind. Therefore, negligence is not *mens rea*. This argument, however, is a definitional one: if one defined *mens rea* negatively as the offence less the *actus reus*, negligence would fall within this definition. It is also sometimes said that *mens rea* is a state of mind. If, however, one is acting negligently, by definition one does not have a state of mind or one has a blank state of mind. If one's mind is empty with regard to a risk, how can one be grossly negligent? When a mind is empty, it cannot be more empty. This criticism is met by the response that negligence is a failure to comply with an objective norm. One can fail to a greater or lesser extent.

The Court of Appeal in **Misra** [2005] 1 WLR 1 touched on the definitions of *mens rea* in the context of gross negligence manslaughter. It was said that *mens rea* meant either the accused's state of mind or 'the ingredient of fault or culpability required'. In the former sense negligence is not *mens rea*; in the latter sense it is. For the purposes of this crime negligence was the mental element.

(c) Some commentators go further. They believe that the criminal law should punish only those who act knowingly, that is intentionally or subjectively recklessly. Negligence ought not to be *mens rea* because one does not advert to the consequences of one's behaviour. Perhaps the proposition may be differently put as: 'How can one have a wrongful state of mind, a *mens rea*, if one has no frame of mind at all?' One's mind is blank to the consequences when one acts negligently. Contrariwise negligence can be seen as liability based on fault just as intention and conscious recklessness are. The accused has not performed his duty because he was careless. He is at fault and is to be blamed. Ordinary people would, it is thought, hold a person to be at fault when he was driving without lights in the middle of the night down an unlit portion of a motorway. It would not always be inquired whether he knew his lights had not been turned on. It may be socially useful to punish such a person. Furthermore, circumstances alter cases. G. Fletcher in *Rethinking Criminal Law* (Little, Brown & Co, 1978) uses this illustration: would one call negligent a person who threw a lighted match into a bucket containing liquid? Presumably one would if the bucket were at a petrol station, but not if it were under a drainpipe in a garden.

Another argument against negligence is that punishing people for acting carelessly would not deter them, though the issue is in doubt. Moreover, to say that people who are negligent are dangerous is over-inclusive. If that is so, why not abolish *mens rea* totally?

(d) H. L. A. Hart argued that it was not unjust to individuals to convict them when they had acted negligently. Contrary to the view of most English academics, no line should be drawn between a person who foresaw the forbidden consequence and one who did not advert to it. The accused should be punished when he failed to pay attention to what he was doing or to examine the circumstances in which he found himself. Provided that his carelessness was unreasonable, he should be criminally liable. However, criminal law should not cover persons who could not have prevented the occurrence of the harm by reasonable care. Neither should the law cover people who because of mental deficiency could not take care in what they were doing (cf. **Elliott v C**, above). Children would be exculpated if they could not understand the consequences of their behaviour. Where the accused is guilty, he is criminally liable for failing to examine the situation in which he is and to assess the risk, and not for his state of mind in failing to advert to the consequences of his behaviour. In Hart's words 'negligence does not consist in [a] blank state of mind but in . . . failure to take precautions against harm by examining the situation' (*Punishment and*

Responsibility (Clarendon Press, 1968) 148). Accordingly Hart postulated a duty to take reasonable care against harm, and criminal law should be directed at careless people, not for their states of mind, but for getting into such mental states. The accused is therefore punished for failing to use his mental faculties such as judgment, which, if used, would have avoided harm.

Hart's thesis has been criticised on several grounds: (i) It does not explain why we punish those who intend more than those who are reckless, and those who are reckless more than those who are careless. (ii) The law does not look at whether the accused himself should have examined the situation, though perhaps it should. (iii) The negligent person, it is argued, does not deserve to be punished. There may, however, be other reasons for imposing liability.

(e) One can argue that since the police and prosecuting authorities cannot cope with crimes of intention and recklessness, negligence should not be a basis of liability, at least until those authorities are given more resources.

(f) Many offences can be committed intentionally or recklessly but not negligently. The wider the scope of recklessness, the less ground there is for negligence. When *Caldwell*, above, and *Lawrence* [1982] AC 510 expanded liability into part of the area previously covered by negligence, academic criticism focused on this extension. Lord Diplock's argument in *Caldwell* was that the person who acted without thinking was just as blameworthy as someone who thought about the risk but went ahead. In a modern society there is something to be said for penalising the careless, but to determine that they are just as culpable as those who advert to the risk is not a just assessment of the different states of mind, though reasonable people may disagree. *Caldwell* was 'departed from' by the House of Lords in *G* [2004] 1 AC 1034.

(g) There is a type of manslaughter called manslaughter by gross negligence. It is one of two common law offences of negligence, albeit that the jury has to hold that the accused was not merely negligent but grossly so: *Large* [1939] 1 All ER 753 (CCA). The principal authority was *Andrews v DPP* [1937] AC 576 and is now *Adomako* [1995] 1 AC 171. Terminology in cases such as *Andrews*, where the House of Lords spoke of 'reckless' conduct as a synonym for grossly negligent behaviour, was inexact and not settled, but emphasis was laid on the grossness of the carelessness. Mere civil law negligence is insufficient. See Chapter 12 for this type of manslaughter. It should be noted that there is no crime of causing harm, even serious harm, in a grossly negligent manner.

The second common law defence of negligence is public nuisance. Employers are liable for the acts of their employees which have created a public nuisance. They need not know of those acts: it is sufficient that they ought reasonably to be aware of them. The House of Lords in *Rimmington* [2006] 1 AC 459 ruled that this definition stood after *G*. In other words the *mens rea* of negligence survived the revival of subjective recklessness.

(h) Under statute there are offences where the accused is guilty if he inadvertently takes a risk. One such crime is selling a firearm to a person who the accused has reasonable cause to believe is drunk. Therefore, if the accused ought to have been aware that the accused was drunk, he is guilty.

The most common negligence offence is driving without due care and attention or without reasonable consideration for other road users (s 3 of the Road Traffic Act

1988 as substituted by s 2 of the Road Traffic Act 1991). It differs from the former offence of reckless driving ('reckless' then having its *Caldwell* definition) in that the accused is guilty even though the risk of harm was not serious. A similar offence is causing death by careless or inconsiderate driving contrary to s 28 of the Road Traffic Act 1988, inserted by the Road Safety Act 2006, s 20 (not in force at the time of writing). The offence of bigamy is treated as an offence of negligence because the alleged bigamist who makes a mistake that his former marriage was annulled or dissolved has a defence only if that mistake was based on reasonable grounds.

(i) Where the offence is one of negligence, Parliament may give a special defence. The principal illustration is unlawful sexual intercourse with a mental defective, contrary to the now repealed s 7(1) of the Sexual Offences Act 1956. By s 7(2):

> [A] man is not guilty of an offence under this section, . . . if he does not know and has no reason to suspect her to be defective.

The defence is one of 'no negligence'. If the accused himself did not know and a person with his characteristics including mental ones would not have known that the woman was a defective, he has a defence. The test is therefore not a purely objective one, as can be seen from the words of s 7(2).

The wording of the defence defines what has to be shown. The Food Safety Act 1990, s 21(2), gives the accused a defence if he can prove both due diligence (i.e. no negligence) and that the defect was due to the act or default of a third party such as the manufacturer. The Trade Descriptions Act 1968, s 24(1)(b), gives a defence when 'he took all reasonable precautions and exercised all due diligence to avoid the commission of' one of several offences of strict liability. The Misuse of Drugs Act 1971, s 28(2), provides a defence for the accused to prove that 'he neither knew of nor suspected nor had reason to suspect the existence of some fact alleged by the prosecution', proof of the fact being necessary for conviction. The House of Lords ruled in *Lambert* [2002] 2 AC 545 that s 28(2) imposed only an evidential burden on the accused. It did so in reliance on the presumption of innocence found in Article 6(2) of the European Convention of Human Rights. However, not all reverse onus provisions are now to be interpreted in a similar fashion. See Chapter 1 for further details.

It might also be that there is a defence at least to careless driving when the accused relied on instructions from someone else who was at fault in telling the driver to proceed. In *Thornton v Mitchell* [1940] 1 All ER 339 a bus driver was acquitted of careless driving when he reversed his bus over a pedestrian, relying on signals from the conductor. Martin Wasik 'A learner's careless driving' [1982] Crim LR 411 argued that the same applied to a learner who obeyed the instructor's order.

(j) *Reform.* The Law Commission in *Offences of Damage to Property*, Report No. 29, 1970, 44, stated that 'in the area of serious crime . . . the elements of intention, knowledge or recklessness have always been required as a basis of liability. The tendency is to extend this basis to a wider range of offences and to limit the area of offences where a lesser mental element [e.g. negligence] is required.' The Law Commission was in sympathy with this view. The efforts of law reform bodies over the last 40 years have been to promote a subjectivist approach in relation to serious offences. The draft Criminal Code, Law Com. No. 177, 1989, continues this process. Unless Parliament determines differently, recklessness in its subjective state will be the lowest culpable mental state for Code offences. Parliament, however, has chosen to follow a different route. In 2003 it made rape into an offence of negligence. Since rape is such a serious crime, the route is open to making more offences into ones of negligence, even very serious ones.

Some problems of *mens rea*

This section brings together difficulties in relation to the mental element which can be gleaned from this chapter and Chapter 2.

(a) There is no set terminology. Is gross negligence the same as recklessness?

(b) The boundaries of concepts may be highly imprecise. Is oblique intent part of intention or foresight? And what exactly is oblique intent? It is amazing that fundamental notions such as intention cannot be defined after hundreds of years.

(c) Terms may cover more than one mental state. *Caldwell* recklessness used to be the obvious example in that it covered both advertence and inadvertence. And is wilful blindness *Caldwell* recklessness?

(d) Older terms may require different definitions for each offence. There may be no set definition throughout criminal law. Stephen J in *Tolson* (1889) 23 QBD 168 at 187, said: 'Malice means one thing in relation to murder, another in relation to the Malicious Mischief Act, and a third in relation to libel, and so of fraud and negligence.'

(e) Some terms may be 'bent' to catch persons who ought to be caught but who are not caught under the usual width of the concept. The class of persons most obviously fitting within this kink in the law is terrorists.

(f) Where the accused has a defence such as prevention of crime it is difficult to describe his state of mind as a *mens rea*.

The draft Criminal Code, Law Com. No. 177, 1989, seeks to avoid some of these difficulties by having consistent usage and certainty of meaning. *Mens rea*, to be called the fault element, consists of intention, knowledge and recklessness, unless Parliament ordains differently. By cl 19(1) '[A]n allegation in an indictment or information of knowledge or intention includes an allegation of recklessness.' The element of recklessness is satisfied by intention or knowledge (cl 19(2)). The minimum fault element is recklessness (cl 20(1)).

Transferred malice

In *Latimer* (1886) 17 QBD 359 the accused quarrelled with a person in a pub. He removed his belt and aimed a blow at him. The blow struck the victim, who was standing nearby. She was badly injured. The court held that the accused was guilty of unlawfully and maliciously wounding the victim. He had the *mens rea* and *actus reus* of the crime. He did not expect what occurred and in that sense the outcome was accidental, but the law holds him guilty under the doctrine of transferred malice. His mental state ('malice') is transferred. The doctrine is not restricted to crimes of malice or intent but extends to the transfer of the mental element however defined. In *McBride* v *Turnock*

[1964] Crim LR 456 the accused struck at a person but hit a constable in the execution of his duty. He was guilty of the offence of assaulting a constable in the execution of his duty, an aggravated battery, even though his 'malice' was only as to common assault. Both crimes have the same *mens rea* because the accused is guilty of the aggravated offence even though he does not know that the person assaulted was a constable. The same principle applies to the crime of assaulting an officer of the court in the execution of his duty. Similarly if in ***Latimer*** it had been a father aiming at his daughter with his hand intending to effect reasonable chastisement and his hand hit her friend standing next to her, his defence would be transferred.

For the so-called doctrine to apply, the *mens rea* and *actus reus* must coincide (subject to the point in **McBride v Turnock**, above). In **Pembliton** (1876) LR 2 CCR 119, the accused was in a fight outside a pub. He broke a window with a stone. He was held by the Court for Crown Cases Reserved not to be guilty of malicious damage, the precursor of criminal damage. The accused did not have the *mens rea* of this offence. One could also charge attempted actual or grievous bodily harm, which captures what the accused meant to do better than criminal damage, which is the chance result of his actions. The basic point remained, that *mens rea* cannot be transferred across crimes.

Another restriction has been best stated by (ed. D. Ormerod) Smith and Hogan, *Criminal Law*, 12th edn (OUP, 2008) 127 (footnote omitted):

> The intent which is transferred must be a *mens rea*, whether intention or recklessness. If D [the accused] shoots X with intent to kill because X is making a murderous attack on him and this is the only way in which he can preserve his own life, he does not intend an *actus reus* . . . for to kill in these circumstances is justified. If, however, D misses X and inadvertently kills V, an innocent bystander, he does so cause an *actus reus* . . . to transfer; the result which he intended was a perfectly lawful one.

It should be realised that in many instances one need not refer to this doctrine. One is guilty of recklessly damaging property if one throws a stone at a window of a pub belonging to the victim and the stone goes through the window, which is open, and breaks an optic belonging to the victim. If the stone happens to break a valuable vase left by a starving potter in payment for a meal, one is still guilty of criminal damage because property belonging to another has been destroyed or damaged. In murder one is guilty if one kills a human being. If one sets out to kill one person and accidentally kills another, one is guilty of murder. Malice aforethought covers intentionally killing a victim. It does not matter who the victim is, provided that the victim is in being at the time of the attack. For example, the stabbing of the accused's girlfriend caused the death of a baby which was born alive prematurely in ***Attorney-General's Reference (No. 3 of 1994)*** [1998] AC 245 (HL). The accused was not guilty of murder of the child. A foetus was held not to be part of the mother. Lord Mustill said:

> The defendant intended to commit and did commit an immediate crime of violence to the mother. He committed no relevant violence to the foetus, which was not a person, either at the time or in the future, and intended no harm to the foetus or to the human person which it would become. . . . I would not overstrain the idea of transferred malice by trying to make it fit the present case.

Malice was not to be transferred from the mother to the foetus and then from the foetus to the child (who would be a person in being for the purposes of the law of homicide only at some time in the future). It seems strange that there could be no transferred malice to make the accused guilty of murder, a homicide offence, yet he was convicted of manslaughter. An alternative approach is to say that the accused has a 'general intent' in relation to the property and the person. For these reasons the use of the doctrine is rare. Moreover, if the accused killed a victim, it does not matter in which way he killed him. If they are in an opera house and the accused shoots at the victim intending to kill him but the bullet hits a chandelier, which falls on the victim and kills him, the accused is guilty.

Transferred malice is restricted in participatory offences. If the acts of the principal offender go beyond the agreed plan, the accessory is not guilty to the offence which takes place. In *Leahy* [1985] Crim LR 99, the accused told the principal offender to 'glass' X; the principal deliberately glassed Y. The accused was not guilty of counselling grievous bodily harm. The result is in accord with the ancient case of *Saunders and Archer* (1573) 75 ER 706. On the advice of the 'accessory', the principal gave his wife a poisoned apple intending to kill her. He stood by while his wife gave the apple to their child, who ate it and died. It was held that the 'accessory' was not guilty of being the secondary offender to the murder. There was a deliberate change from the plan agreed on. The case would have been one of transferred malice with the accessory now guilty if the killing of the child had been accidental in the sense that the principal could not have prevented it.

The Law Commission's draft Criminal Code (Law Com. No. 177, 1989) proposed to retain transferred malice for 'an attempt charge may be impossible (when it is not known until trial that the defendant claims to have X [the intended victim] and not Y [the actual victim] in contemplation); or inappropriate (as not describing the harm done adequately for labelling or sentencing purposes). Moreover, recklessness with respect to Y may be insufficient to establish the offence or incapable of being proved' (para 8.57). Clause 24(1) of the draft Criminal Code provides:

> [I]n determining whether a person is guilty of an offence, his intention to cause, or his recklessness whether he causes, a result in relation to a person or thing capable of being the victim or subject matter of the offence shall be treated as an intention to cause or, as the case may be, recklessness whether he causes that result in relation to any person or thing affected by his conduct.

This clause is repeated in the Criminal Law Bill attached to the Law Commission Report No. 218, *Legislating the Criminal Code – Offences against the Person and General Principles*, 1993, with the replacement of 'recklessness' by 'awareness of a risk': cl 32(1). The change is because 'recklessness' in the Bill bears a specific meaning, but the Bill applies to other *mens rea* words. Clause 24(2) of the draft Criminal Code codifies the point made by Smith and Hogan quoted above:

> Any defence on which a person might have relied in relation to a person or thing within his contemplation is open to him on a charge of the same offence in relation to a person or thing not within his contemplation.

This provision is now cl 32(3) of the Criminal Law Bill.

The term chosen by the Law Commission for this so-called doctrine is 'transferred fault', 'fault' being the Law Commission's term for *mens rea* or the mental element. The terminology is better chosen than the usual current one of transferred malice because it demonstrates that the law is not restricted to crimes in which the mental element is malice. Lord Mustill in *Attorney-General's Reference (No. 3 of 1994)*, above, called the doctrine of transferred malice a fiction and said that it had a misleading title, but 'one which is too firmly entrenched to be discarded'. Nevertheless, it has to be said that *Latimer*, above, reflects good sense. Surely one would not want the accused in that case to be not guilty. If a defendant kills or injures a human being, why should it matter that the human being so harmed was not the one aimed at? It is suggested that 'transferred fault' could in fact quite easily supplant 'transferred malice'. Perhaps a more modern name for the doctrine would make transferred malice more acceptable to Lord Mustill.

Contemporaneity

Consider this fact situation. The accused has decided to get rid of her partner. Before she can kill him intentionally, she accidentally runs him over and kills him. She has the *mens rea* for murder and she has caused his death. However, the *mens rea* and *actus reus* are not simultaneous and it would be unjust to convict her of murder. There are, however, situations where it is not unjust to convict. The principle is one of contemporaneity or, as some Americans call it, the union of *actus reus* and *mens rea*. Another example is the crime of burglary. One form of this offence is entry into a building or part of one with intent to commit one of four crimes. If the accused performs the *actus reus* and later decides to steal etc., he is not guilty of this type of burglary. One could say that the principle is a flexible requirement or the number of exceptions has been growing.

(a) *The Dutch courage rule.* The accused who decides to commit a crime and gets into a drunken state to do so is guilty of the crime even though at the time of committing it he was so dead drunk that he was mindless, and without a '*mens*' one cannot have a *mens rea*. The House of Lords in **Attorney-General for Northern Ireland v Gallagher** [1963] AC 349 so decided.

See pp 311–12 for an in-depth discussion of *Majewski* in relation to the defence of intoxication.

(b) Under **DPP v Majewski** [1977] AC 443 one is guilty of a crime of recklessly doing something if one commits the crime while under the influence of alcohol or drugs. The House of Lords decided as a matter of policy that recklessly getting drunk supplied the recklessness for the crime later committed. After **MPC v Caldwell**, above, there is no need for the **Majewski** approach for the defendant is deemed to be unaware of the risk of which ordinary people would have been aware at the time of the *actus reus*. On this view the mental element and the *actus reus* coincide. However, the use of the word 'deemed' should alert us to the fact that something strange is going on.

(c) *Continuing state of affairs.* In **Fagan v MPC** [1969] 1 QB 439, the accused accidentally drove onto a police officer's boot. The police officer pointed out what the accused had done. The accused deliberately left the wheel on the foot for a short while. There were various imprecations. The accused was convicted of a battery. *Fagan* demonstrates the strength of police boots – the constable suffered only two bruised toes after having a Mini parked on his foot – and the way in which the courts can stretch the law to catch the accused. The problem was that battery was thought (at that time) to be an offence which could not be committed by an omission, and leaving a car on a foot looks like an omission. The court held that the *actus reus* of battery can be a continuing act. That continuing act lasted until the accused realised what he had done and decided not to drive off. The accused continued to apply force by not removing the car, and he acted intentionally. In this way the *actus reus* and *mens rea* coincided. There is therefore no need for the mental element to accompany the *actus* *reus* throughout the sequence of events. Contemporaneity for a moment is sufficient. Moreover, since the *actus reus* is held to be continuing it is not difficult to hold that the two overlap in time at some point.

If **Fagan** is accepted as laying down a rule of law, there are extensive problems with its width. D. Husak, *Philosophy of Criminal Law* (Rowman & Littlefield, 1987) 178, suggests the following:

> Suppose the defendant manufactures cars and deliberately cuts corners by installing defective emergency brakes. A year later he notices one of his cars parked on a hill. Because the emergency brake is defective it rolls backwards and comes to rest on a policeman's foot. The defendant fails to assist the policeman for several moments, revelling in his suffering. Here the defendant initiated a causal chain culminating in harm. Is the sequence 'deemed' a 'single act' comparable to **Fagan**? There is no fact of the matter about how this question should be answered. [Spelling anglicised and footnote omitted.]

Fagan was said to have been decided on its own facts according to the House of Lords in **Miller** [1983] 2 AC 161, which is equivalent to saying that **Fagan** should not be followed. **Fagan** now falls within (d) below, causing a danger and intentionally not remedying it. **Fagan**, said the Lords, should be seen as a case in which the accused adopted his previous conduct. It is suggested that the *ratio* of **Fagan** should now be used only where the *actus reus* is of a continuing nature. By using the 'duty' approach courts can avoid the question of whether an *actus reus* is a continuing one or whether it is complete by the time there is *mens rea*.

(d) *The Miller principle*. In **Miller**, above, the House of Lords decided that a person who created a dangerous situation unwittingly and then realised what he had done was guilty if he failed to avert the prohibited consequence. This case is discussed above and in Chapter 2. It could have been treated as one of the exceptions to contemporaneity but instead was dealt with as a case where the common law imposed liability for omissions. The accused had a duty to act. The **Miller** principle is preserved in the draft Criminal Code, cl 23.

(e) *The principle established in* **Thabo Meli v R** [1954] 1 WLR 228. This situation is the opposite to **Fagan**. In **Thabo Meli** the *mens rea* preceded the *actus reus*. In **Fagan** the start of the *actus reus* preceded the *mens rea*. The facts of **Thabo Meli** were that the victim was beaten up and left for dead. His supposed corpse was thrown over a cliff, and he died of exposure. The Privy Council upheld the appellants' conviction for murder on the basis that the sequence of events constituted a series which could not be split into separate acts: 'It is too refined a ground of judgment to say that, because they were under a misapprehension at one stage and thought that their guilty purpose had been achieved before in fact it was achieved, therefore they are to escape the penalties of the law.' Although the defendants' plan to kill was completed at the time when they believed the victim to be dead and pushing what they believed to be a corpse over the cliff was part of the plan to get rid of the body, the whole sequence was deemed to be one act. The appellants could have been found guilty of attempted murder, but by holding as the Privy Council did, they were guilty of murder.

Thabo Meli was followed in **Church** [1966] 1 QB 59 by the Court of Criminal Appeal. There was no plan to kill but the accused thought he had killed his victim. He put her into a river, where she drowned. The conviction for manslaughter was upheld. The latest authority is **Le Brun** [1992] QB 61, which confirmed that the principle in **Thabo Meli v R** applied to manslaughter (where there was no plan to kill) just as it did to murder (where there was).

Le Brun [1992] QB 61

The accused struck his victim on the chin. She fell. In an attempt to conceal the battery he moved her. Her head accidentally struck the pavement. Her skull was fractured and she died. Lord Lane CJ in the Court of Appeal ruled that the unlawful application of force and the act which caused death were part of the same transaction. It did not matter that there was an appreciable time between the two events. The position was even more certain where the accused's subsequent actions were designed to conceal his earlier attack and the chain of causation (see Chapter 2) was unbroken.

The outcome would have been different if a passer-by had broken the chain of causation by the act of dropping the still-living victim's head onto the pavement. Perhaps it might be the law that the accused would not be guilty if he had been trying to drag the victim to hospital when she hit her head. The Court of Appeal in **Attorney-General's Reference (No. 4 of 1980)** [1981] 1 WLR 705 had previously some doubts whether the court was correct in **Church** to extend **Thabo Meli** to manslaughter. In the case the accused hit the victim. She fell down some steps and banged her head. The accused dragged her upstairs with a rope, drained off her blood, and dissected her. The problem was that it was impossible to state which act caused death. If it was uncertain to say which act caused death, it was impossible to say whether the accused had *mens rea* at the time of death. On the facts the accused had *mens rea* for manslaughter both (on normal principles) at the time of knocking her downstairs and (following **Thabo Meli**) when he cut her throat. There was a series of acts which could be viewed as one transaction; the accused had *mens rea* at some time in the transaction; therefore he was guilty. All cases on this topic have as yet concerned homicide but it is thought that the principle is not so restricted.

(f) *The rule in automatism.* As with regard to drunkenness there is a principle in the defence of automatism that the accused will not receive the defence if he brought about the condition. It is as if the rule of contemporaneity applies to this defence. The principle was laid down in **Quick** [1973] QB 910, with the proviso that the condition had to be reasonably foreseeable. If it is reasonably foreseeable that the accused would fall into a state of automatism through failing to take prescribed drugs or regular meals, he could not have this defence. In **Bailey** [1983] 2 All ER 503, the Court of Appeal resiled from its position in **Quick**. The accused was not guilty if the accused himself did not foresee the consequences of his inaction, even if a reasonable person would have. **Quick** and **Bailey** should be compared with **Kay v Butterworth** (1945) 173 LT 191, where the problem was avoided. The accused fell asleep at the wheel and mowed down soldiers. He was held guilty of careless driving, not for crashing into the soldiers when he was asleep but for not stopping to recover from tiredness after working in a munitions factory when he was still awake. This case is useful authority but useful to prosecutors only when the act can be described as a continuing one, as driving can be.

(g) An accused is guilty if he with *mens rea* sets in train a course of events which will lead to the *actus reus* even though he no longer has *mens rea* when the *actus reus* occurs.

Where these exceptions do not apply, there must be contemporaneity. In **Edwards v Ddin** [1976] 1 WLR 942, the accused asked a garage attendant to fill up his tank. He intended to pay. When the petrol was in the tank, he dishonestly drove off without paying. By that time, under civil law, the petrol was his. He had not appropriated property belonging to another at the time when he had the *mens rea* because the property belonged to him. Therefore, he was not guilty of theft. There was no *actus reus* at the time of the *mens rea*. (Parliament intervened to create an offence to cover this situation. The offence is called making off without payment in s 3 of the Theft Act 1978.)

Summary

This is the second chapter concerned with the 'building blocks' of criminal law. This time the concentration is not on the physical side but on the mental side. What state of mind did the accused have when he or she was committing the *actus reus*? Each crime is composed of an *actus reus* and usually of a *mens rea* but not just does the *actus reus* differ from offence to offence, but so does the *mens rea*. For example, the *mens rea* of murder is either the intent to kill or the intent to cause grievous bodily harm, but the *mens rea* of theft is dishonesty and the intent permanently to deprive. The student has to know both the *actus reus* and the *mens rea* for the crimes taught on his or her course. The discussion then concentrates on the major *mens rea* words in criminal law: intent, recklessness, knowledge, wilfulness and negligence, though with regard to the last there is debate whether or not a lack of a state of mind ('I didn't think') may be regarded as a state of mind, a *mens rea*. The chapter concludes with an explanation of various issues surrounding *mens rea*, including the need for contemporaneity of *actus reus* and *mens rea* and the doctrine usually known as transferred malice.

- Definition of *mens rea*: *Mens rea* may be defined as 'the mental state which is required by the definition of the offence to accompany the act which produces or threatens harm' (S. H. Kadish).

- Examples of *mens rea*: The *mens rea* of murder, also known as malice aforethought, is in part composed of an intent to kill or commit grievous bodily harm. In theft, the mental element is 'dishonesty' and 'intention permanently to deprive'. The *mens rea*, like the *actus reus*, differs from crime to crime.

- Motive: In general the motive of the accused is irrelevant in criminal law. For instance, it does not matter if I kill you to get your money or your lover or if I do so in order to save you from a life filled with pain. Some offences do, however, make motive relevant in the sense that they are defined in such a way that the triers of fact have to consider the reason why the defendant behaved as she did. An illustration is blackmail. If the accused believed she was warranted in acting as she did, there is no offence and 'warranted' covers the accused's motive.

  Modern statutes sometimes make crimes more serious when the accused acted out of a certain motive, e.g. racially motivated crimes.

- Intent: The definition of intention is one basic to English criminal law, partly because some offences may be committed only intentionally but more fundamentally because intent is morally the worst state of mind with which one can act: e.g. murder is more serious than manslaughter, not because of the *actus reus* (which is the same), but because murder is committable only where the accused intends to kill or cause grievous bodily harm. It is usually very easy to decide whether or not the accused intended a certain consequence. If she decided to kill, if her aim or purpose was to kill, if she made her mind up to kill, she intended to kill. This state of mind is sometimes known as 'direct intent'. If the accused did not decide to kill but foresaw death as a virtually certain consequence (and death actually was virtually certain), then the jury may but need not find that the accused intended to kill. Therefore, the fact that she did foresee death as virtually certain does not mean that she intended to kill; it means that she may have intended to kill, but the question is one of fact for the jury. After all, the law that a jury may find intent has as its corollary that the jury may decide not to find intent. This state of mind is often called 'oblique intent'.

It is thought but not expressly determined that the definition of intent given in the previous paragraph applies throughout criminal law.

The Law Commission proposes to define intent as covering both direct and oblique intent. In that event foresight by the accused that something would virtually certainly occur would definitely be intent, unlike now when it is just evidence of intent.

- Recklessness: Some crimes such as criminal damage may be committed intentionally and recklessly but not carelessly. Therefore, recklessness is distinguished from both intent and carelessness. The House of Lords has in the quite recent past returned to having one definition of recklessness for (at least most) crimes. If an accused foresees an outcome as possible, she is said to be reckless. This frame of mind is often known as 'subjective recklessness'. For twenty or so years until the early years of this millennium there was a second, competing definition: did the accused pay no heed to an obvious and serious risk of a consequence's occurring? This definition, sometimes called 'objective recklessness', did not replace the subjective test: some crimes were defined in terms of objective recklessness, and some in terms of subjective recklessness. Current law is, therefore, that subjective recklessness applies in all crimes, unless Parliament otherwise ordains.

- Knowingly: 'Actual' knowledge is when the accused knows for a fact that something is true. Sometimes the law extends to 'wilful blindness': the accused shuts her eyes to the obvious. 'Constructive knowledge' is when a reasonable person would have known certain facts but the accused did not: sometimes the law stretches thus far.

- Wilfully: This term normally means 'intentionally or recklessly'.

- Negligence: Few serious crimes may be committed carelessly, the exception being manslaughter by gross negligence. Lesser crimes such as careless driving may be committed negligently. What negligence connotes is that the accused has fallen short of the standards of a reasonable person. Whether a person should be convicted for acting negligently remains contested, and with some exceptions the Law Commission strives to hold to the position that the minimum level for conviction for a serious offence is recklessness.

- Transferred malice: If one attacks one person but strikes another, one's intention ('malice') to assault the first is 'transferred' to the second. Similarly, an attack on one piece of property is transferable to other property. However, intent against a person is not transferable against property or vice versa.

- Contemporaneity: The general rule is that *actus reus* and *mens rea* must coincide in point of time. If I decide to kill you and then change my mind but then by chance I do kill you, perhaps by running you over, I am not guilty of murder. My *mens rea* and *actus reus* did not occur simultaneously. Sometimes the law regards not just a single point in time but the whole transaction, which may take place over a period. For example, I attack you and leave you for dead; you are not dead but you later die of exposure. Here, the attack and the death are seen in law as being indivisible and I will be guilty of murder or manslaughter depending on my *mens rea*.

References

Reports

Criminal Law Revision Committee Report no. 14, *Offences against the Person* (1980) Cmnd 7844

Law Commission Consultation Paper no. 177, *A new Homicide Act for England & Wales?* (2005)

Law Commission Report no. 29, *Offences of Damage to Property* (1970)

Law Commission Report no. 89, *The Mental Element in Crime* (1978)

Law Commission Report no. 177, *A Criminal Code for England and Wales* (1989)

Law Commission Report no. 218, *Legislating the Criminal Code – Offences against the Person and General Principles* (1993)

Law Commission Report no. 306, *Murder, Manslaughter and Infanticide* (2006)

Report of the Select Committee of the House of Lords on Murder and Life Imprisonment (Nathan) (1989), HL Paper 78-1

Books

Clarkson, C. M. V. *Understanding Criminal Law* 4th edn (Thomson, 2005)

Clarkson, C. M. V. and Keating, H. *Criminal Law: Text and Materials* 5th edn (Sweet & Maxwell, 2003)

Fletcher, G. *Rethinking Criminal Law* (Little, Brown & Co., 1978)

Hall, J. *General Principles of Criminal Law* 2nd edn (Bobbs-Merrill, 1968)

Hart, H. L. A. *Punishment and Responsibility* (Clarendon Press, 1968)

Husak, D. N. *Philosophy of Criminal Law* (Rowman & Littlefield, 1989)

Smith, J. C. and Hogan, B. *Criminal Law* 10th edn (Butterworths, 2002)

Smith, J. C. and Hogan, B. *Criminal Law* (ed. D. Ormerod) 11th edn (Oxford University Press, 2005)

Stannard, J. *Recent Developments in Criminal Law* (SLS, 1988)

Williams, G. *Criminal Law: The General Part* 2nd edn (Stevens, 1961)

Yeo, S. *Fault in Homicide* (Federation Press, 1997)

Journals

Fennell, C. 'Intention in murder' (1990) 41 NILQ 325

Fletcher, G. 'The theory of criminal negligence' (1971) 119 U Pa LR 401

France, S. 'Reckless approach to liability' (1988) 18 VUWLR 141

Hogan, B. 'Strict liability' [1978] Crim LR 593

Jefferson, M. 'Reckless: the objectivity of the *Caldwell* test' (1999) 63 JCL 57

Kadish, S. 'The decline of innocence' [1968] CLJ 273

Packer, H. '*Mens rea* and the Supreme Court' [1962] Sup Ct Rev 107

Smith, J. C. 'Subjective or objective?' [1981–82] Villanova LR 1179

Williams, G. 'Oblique intention' [1987] CLJ 417

Further reading

Arlidge, A. 'The trial of Dr David Moor' [2000] Crim LR 31. (See also response by Sir John Smith, 'A comment on Dr Moor's case' [2000] Crim LR 41.)

Ashworth, A. 'Reform of the law of murder' [1990] Crim LR 75

Ashworth, A. and Mitchell, B. *Rethinking English Homicide Law* (Clarendon Press, 2000)

Bingham, Lord http://www.open.gov.uk/lcd/judicial/speeches/mansent.htm

Brudner, A. 'Subjective fault for crime: a reinterpretation' (2008) 14 *Legal Theory* 1

Buxton, R. 'Some simple thoughts on intention' [1988] Crim LR 484

Chiu E. M. 'The challenge of motive in criminal law' (2005) 8 Buff Crim LR 653

Ferzan, K. K. 'Beyond intention' (2008) 29 Cardozo L Rev 1147

Gledhill, K. 'Criminal carelessness' [2007] 157 NLJ 41

Horder, J. 'Intention in criminal law: a rejoinder' (1995) 58 MLR 678

Horder, J. 'Transferred malice and the remoteness of unexpected outcomes' [2006] Crim LR 383

Kaveny, M. C. 'Inferring intention from foresight' (2004) 120 LQR 81

Keating, H. 'Reckless children' [2007] Crim LR 546

Kugler, I. 'Conditional oblique intention' [2004] Crim LR 284

Mitchell, B. 'Culpably indifferent murder' (1996) 25 A-ALR 64

Norrie, A. 'After Woollin' [1999] Crim LR 532

Norrie, A. 'Between orthodox subjectivism and moral contextualism' [2006] Crim LR 486

Patient, I. H. E. 'Transferred Malice – a misleading misnomer' (1990) 54 JCL 116

Pedain, A. 'Intention and the terrorist example' [2003] Crim LR 579

Rubin, G. R. 'New light on Steane's case' (2003) 24 *Journal of Legal History* 143

Simester, A. P. 'Can negligence be culpable?', in J. Horder (ed.) *Oxford Essays in Jurisprudence*, 4th series (Oxford University Press, 2000)

Simons K. W. 'Dimensions of negligence in criminal and tort law' (2002) *Theoretical Inquiries L* 283

Smith, Sir John 'A comment on Dr Moor's case' [2000] Crim LR 41 (in response to A. Arlidge [2000] Crim LR 31)

Stannard, J. E. 'Stretching out the *actus reus*' (1993–5) xxviii–xxx IJ 200

Wasik, M. 'A learner's careless driving' [1982] Crim LR 411

Williams, G. 'Oblique intent' [1987] CLJ 417

Williams, G. 'The *mens rea* for murder: leave it alone' (1989) 105 LQR 387

Wilson, W. 'A plea for rationality in the law of murder' (1991) 10 LS 307

Wilson, W. 'Doctrinal rationality after *Woollin*' (1999) 62 MLR 447

Yeo, S. *Fault in Homicide*, Federation Press, Annandale, New South Wales (1997)

For a full-length treatment of fatal and non-fatal offences and the defences thereto, see B. Mitchell, *Law Relating to Violent Crime* (CLT Publishing, 1997). For an academic approach to *mens rea* see V. Tadros, *Criminal Responsibility* (Oxford University Press, 2005). For an attempt to define intent see I. Kugler, *Direct and Oblique Intention in the Criminal Law* (Ashgate, 2002). For a theoretical approach to intent see W. Wilson, *Central Issues in Criminal Theory* (Hart, 2002), ch. 5, and for good motives see A. J. Ashworth in A. P. Simester and A. T. H. Smith, *Harm and Culpability* (Clarendon Press, 1996). For a comment on carelessness in criminal law, see A. P. Simester in J. Horder (ed.), *Oxford Essays in Jurisprudence* (Clarendon Press, 2000).

Visit **www.mylawchamber.co.uk/jefferson** to access
exam-style questions with answer guidance, multiple
choice quizzes, live weblinks, an online glossary,
and regular updates to the law.

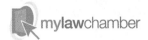

Use **Case Navigator** to read in full some of the key cases referenced in
this chapter:

DPP v *Majewski* [1976] 2 All ER 142
Fagan v *Metropolitan Police Commissioner* [1968] 3 All ER 442
R v *Adomako* [1994] 3 All ER 79
R v *Cunningham* [1957] 2 All ER 412
R v *G* [2003] 4 All ER 765
R v *Quick* [1973] 3 All ER 347
R v *Woollin* [1998] 4 All ER 103

4

Strict liability

> The contention that an injury can amount to a crime only when inflicted by intention is no provincial or transient notion. It is as universal and persistent in mature systems of law as belief in freedom of the human will and a consequent ability and duty of the normal individual to choose between good and evil. (US Supreme Court, **Morissette** v **United States** (1952) 342 US 246, 250)

In some offences the prosecution need not prove *mens rea* as to one or more elements of the *actus reus*. These crimes are known as ones of strict liability. Therefore, though there must always be an *actus reus*, there need not always be a mental element in relation to each part of the *actus reus*. For example, suppose that a statute forbids butchers to sell meat unfit for human consumption. If one does, the court may say that he or she is guilty even though he or she does not know that the meat is bad. There is then no *mens rea*, knowledge, as to the unfitness. However, presumably the butcher must know that the act being done is 'selling' and that what is being sold is meat. Accordingly, strict offences may well require *mens rea* as to some elements of the *actus reus*, and that is why strict liability means that there is no *mens rea* as to one (or more) elements of the *actus reus*. It does not mean that the prosecution is totally released from the duty of proving *mens rea*. This definition seems to be accepted by the courts: see Lord Edmund-Davies in **Lemon** [1979] AC 617 (HL).

There are thought to be perhaps 11,000 offences in English law. About half of these are strict ones. They are not strange interlopers but a large part of the fabric of criminal law. Strict offences committed feature largely in criminal prosecutions, and in magistrates' courts. More than half of the offences are strict. This surprising number is partly because many motoring crimes are strict, e.g. in speeding one is guilty even though one does not know one is breaking the speed limit. Many strict offences are concerned with regulating behaviour, and for this reason strict offences are often known as 'regulatory offences'. It must not be thought, however, that the harm resulting from strict offences is minor. An individual or company may have been guilty of such an offence after causing the death of dozens of people in a transport disaster.

The previous paragraph demonstrates that there is nothing peculiar in English law about strict offences. There are also some offences which are sometimes called 'half strict' or 'half *mens rea*' crimes. These are crimes in which the fault element does not or need not correspond to the external element. In assault occasioning actual bodily harm, the accused is guilty if he is reckless as to applying force (*mens rea*) but causes actual bodily harm (*actus reus*). In murder, death must be caused but the accused need intend only grievous bodily harm. Offences of strict liability are not isolated in the law. Indeed it may be said that few crimes can be defined in terms only of intentionally or recklessly committing the *actus reus*.

The effect of the Human Rights Act 1998 is somewhat uncertain. One possibility is that offences of strict liability violate Article 3 of the European Convention on Human Rights, the right not to be punished in an inhuman or degrading manner, and Article 6(2), minimum rights in a criminal trial. If placing the burden on the accused is contrary to the Convention so should strict offences be. In that event a court might write in a defence of due diligence. The European Court held in *Salabiaku v France* (1988) 13 EHRR 379 that strict offences were not forbidden by Article 6(2), though evidential presumptions may be, particularly if they are irrebuttable. Currently the law is in a state of flux because of two recent House of Lords decisions. The effect that they will have is not clear, but it appears that as a result (one cannot be precise because English courts have a tendency not to apply principles in the area of strict offences) and because of the Convention courts will more rarely hold that an offence is strict than they have in the past, but that a crime can be held to be strict despite the enactment of the Human Rights Act 1998 and the two Lords cases: *Muhamad* [2003] QB 1031 (CA), which concerned the offence of materially contributing to, or increasing the extent of, insolvency by gambling. The court cited *Salabiaku*: '. . . the Contracting States may . . . penalise a simple or objective fact as such, irrespective of whether it results from criminal intent or from negligence.' In *Gemmell* [2003] Cr App R 23, Dyson LJ in the Court of Appeal said: 'So far as Article 6 is concerned, the fairness of the substantive law of the Contracting States is not a matter for investigation. The content and interpretation of domestic substantive law is not engaged by Article 6.' The Divisional Court in *Barnfather v London Borough of Islington* [2003] 1 WLR 2318 held that Article 6(2) did not restrict the creation of strict offences by Parliament, and the same court in *R (on the Application of Grundy & Co. Excavations Ltd) v Halton Division Magistrates Court* [2003] EWHC 272 (Admin) similarly held that Article 6(2) did not affect substantive law. The most recent authority is *G* [2006] 1 WLR 2052 (CA). The accused was charged with rape of a child under 13 contrary to s 5 of the Sexual Offences Act 2003. The court held that this offence was strict as to the age of the victim but that in this instance strict liability did not contravene the presumption of innocence found in Article 6(2). Again the court said that Article 6(2) was concerned with procedural fairness, not with substantive criminal law. The House of Lords gave leave to appeal: [2006] 1 WLR 3181. The House [2008] UKHL 37 unanimously confirmed the lower court's decision on Article 6(2). It is suggested that these courts acted too dismissively and the arguments will be raised again. It seems absurd that Article 6(2) comes into play when the burden of proving an element is on the accused but not when that element is totally removed in a strict liability offence!

Strict and absolute offences

In the past strict liability was often called absolute liability. This phraseology is still sometimes used both in England and Wales and in the Commonwealth: see e.g. the High Court of New Zealand in *Jackson v Attorney-General for and on behalf of the Department for Corrections* [2005] NZHC 377 and the Court of Appeal in *G*, above. Nowadays, however, it is common to say that strict offences are not absolute ones. Absolute liability means that the accused is guilty without any mental element at all and that he has no defence either at common law or under statute. Strict offences do need some type of mental state, as we have seen, and all the defences are available. For instance, a child under 10 cannot be convicted of a strict offence, just as he cannot be convicted of a crime of full *mens rea*. Sometimes a special defence may be created by the statute which lays down the strict offence. In s 3 of the Food Act 1984 it is a defence for the accused to show that the adulteration of food was an 'unavoidable consequence of the process of . . . preparation'. The House of Lords in **Smedleys Ltd v Breed** [1974] AC 839, a case on the predecessor to the 1984 Act, the Food and Drugs Act 1955, held that the accused had no defence where they had taken all practicable precautions. The presence of a caterpillar in a tin of peas was not 'unavoidable'. This ruling would seem to accord with what Parliament wanted to happen. If Parliament knowingly creates a strict offence and then provides a defence, presumably it wants the defence to be narrowly construed so that it does not swallow the offence. Moreover, if it had wanted a defence of taking all practicable precautions, it would have said so. It did not. The word used was 'unavoidable' and it was not unavoidable to put a caterpillar into a tin.

Besides defences, the accused will not be convicted unless it can be shown that he was acting voluntarily. Sometimes this requirement is thought to be a separate defence, that of automatism, and it will be dealt with as such. Sometimes it is thought that the requirement of voluntary action is a part of a crime separate from *actus reus* and *mens rea*. Whichever it is, if the accused is not acting voluntarily in the sense that he has no control over his bodily movements, there can be no conviction. Three cases will make the point clearer:

Hill v Baxter [1958] 1 QB 277: *obiter*, a person who while driving is stung by a bee is not 'driving' for the purposes of the Road Traffic Acts when he crashes, and so cannot be found guilty of a crime involving driving, whether strict or otherwise.

Watmore v Jenkins [1962] 2 QB 572: a person who is unconscious during a diabetic episode is not acting voluntarily.

Bratty v Attorney-General for Northern Ireland [1963] AC 386: the House of Lords held that a man is not acting voluntarily when he is undergoing an epileptic fit, or at least those types of convulsions which involve jerky movements.

In those cases the accused cannot be said to have control over his actions, and the law does not permit a conviction in such circumstances. This proposition applies to strict offences. In the butcher illustration, the butcher would not be guilty of selling contaminated meat, a strict offence, if someone had clobbered him over the head with a blunt instrument and as a 'robot' the accused had 'sold' the meat. Just as the driver who is stung by a bee is not 'driving', so the butcher suffering from concussion is not 'selling'. For details of automatism as a general defence, see Chapter 9. This section merely makes the point that strict offences do require some mental activity. Therefore, even in strict offences, the prosecution must do more than simply prove that the defendant contrived the forbidden act, omission or state of affairs. And do not forget, as stated above, that the butcher will not be guilty of a strict offence if he has a defence. So if you threaten to shoot a butcher unless he sells bad meat to the next customer, he will have a defence even to a strict offence, that of duress.

Offences are therefore divided into three types: (a) *mens rea* ones; (b) strict ones; and (c) absolute ones: **City of Sault Ste Marie** [1978] 2 SCR 1299 (SCC). Absolute offences are discussed next.

The exceptional cases

The principal exception to the statement that the prosecution must show more than the *actus reus* even in strict offences is **Larsonneur**, a decision of the Court of Criminal Appeal.

Larsonneur (1993) 24 Cr App R 74

The accused, Mme Larsonneur, came from France to England and was deported to Dublin. The Irish police sent her back. On arrival at Holyhead she was charged with being an illegal immigrant contrary to the Aliens Order 1920, which has since been repealed, in that she had been found in the UK and her presence there was illegal. Her appeal from conviction was dismissed.

She was guilty even though she had no choice as to whether she should come into the UK: she was guilty though faultless. The full facts disclose that the accused was partly to blame for her predicament, but the court did not take any fault into account.

This case has been constantly criticised by commentators.

(a) On the reasoning of the court, it would not have mattered whether the accused was drugged and taken to Wales, or forced to parachute into Holyhead. She would be guilty even though by no exercise of her will could she avoid entering the country. It is hard to see that she had any state of mind at all. She was liable for what she did, but her acts were done under the control of other people. One might compare her position with that of a farmer who sells adulterated milk, a strict offence. That person has a choice whether to sell any milk or not; Mme Larsonneur had no choice.

(b) The prosecution did not need to charge her with any offence. It is hard to see what benefit the UK derived from having her found guilty.

(c) It is arguable that there was no need to define the crime as one which did not require a blameworthy act. The crime could easily have been defined as being found in the UK, having willingly or knowingly entered the UK, and as the Order put it, being an alien to whom leave to land in the UK has been refused.

(d) The main judge in the case is generally reckoned to be the worst or second-worst criminal law judge of the twentieth century.

(e) Judges still continue to call strict offences 'absolute' ones, e.g. Auld LJ in **Loukes** [1996] 1 Cr App R 444 (CA). Where, however, the distinction has been noted, judges have strongly castigated absolute liability. In **Mayer v Marchant** (1973) 5 SASR 567 Zelling J called it a 'throwback to a highly primitive form of concept'.

For these reasons it is suggested that **Larsonneur** may not survive direct challenge in the House of Lords.

It should be noted that Mme Larsonneur was sent to prison, unlike most strictly liable offenders, and that the conviction concerned a matter of her private life. Most strict crimes result in fines and are concerned with matters of business or motoring. For an academic comment supporting **Larsonneur**, see D. Lanham '*Larsonneur* revisited' [1976] Crim LR 276, an article which gives more facts about the case, enabling the reader to understand the outcome somewhat more easily than if one just considers the briefly reported case itself. He argues that the accused brought about the situation she found herself in but could have not been guilty had she been physically compelled to enter the UK if she did not culpably bring about the facts giving rise to the alleged offence.

Despite criticism of **Larsonneur**, which seemed to be highly exceptional and not to be followed, it was followed by the Divisional Court in **Winzar v Chief Constable of Kent** (1983) *The Times*, 28 March. The criminal responsibility in these cases is sometimes known as 'situational liability', an alternative name is '**status offences**'.

Winzar v *Chief Constable of Kent* (1983) *The Times*, 28 March

The accused was found guilty of being found drunk on the highway, despite being removed from a hospital to where he had been brought on a stretcher, the bearers believing that he was ill, and gently placed on the pavement by the police, contrary to s 12 of the Licensing Act 1872. He argued that he had not been found drunk on the highway because the police had carried him there. The court held that 'found drunk' meant 'perceived to be drunk'. The police perceived him to be drunk on the highway. Therefore, he was found drunk on the highway, and was accordingly guilty.

However, even if one accepts that 'found drunk' means 'perceived to be drunk' and does not involve *mens rea* on the part of the accused, surely he was perceived to be drunk in the hospital corridor, to which the police had been summoned. He was not on these facts perceived to be drunk at the later stage when he had been put onto the pavement. Accordingly he was not, contrary to the view of the court, perceived to be drunk when he was lying on the pavement, and even on the court's reasoning he ought not to have been guilty of being found drunk on a highway. He would have been guilty apparently if he had been thrown out of a speeding car onto the pavement! Alternatively, one might argue that he is really being punished for getting drunk, but that is no crime. If the accused is really being punished for getting drunk (what is sometimes known as 'preceding fault') or for not leaving the hospital despite numerous requests to do so, the law should say so. One can also blame Parliament for enacting a law which can be read as the court did in **Winzar**. As Smith and Hogan (D. Ormerod, ed.), *Criminal Law*, 12th edn (OUP, 2008) 59 comment:

> Larsonneur and Winzar were convicted of offences the conviction of which was in fact procured by the police; and this seems peculiarly offensive (footnote omitted).

As might be expected, the police were not prosecuted for procuring the commission of the offences but this is what really happened. C. M. V. Clarkson, *Understanding Criminal Law*, 4th edn (Thomson, 2005) 47 takes a similar view:

> Our sense of justice would be outraged by a law that made it a crime to have measles – a condition one is powerless to prevent.

It is the 'impossible-to-prevent' point which goes against these two cases. Compulsion is no defence. The defendants were guilty even though they had no control over their actions at the time of the arrest. Despite the criticism of **Larsonneur** that the accused would have been guilty even if drugged and brought into the UK, it is suggested that even a court bound by **Larsonneur** and **Winzar** would distinguish those authorities when faced with a situation where at the barrel of a gun a person has been forced to enter the UK or has been forced out of one's home and to lie down drunk on the pavement. Moreover, a court could hold the cases restricted to their particular facts and the House of Lords of course is not bound by either case. Defences such as duress and, *a fortiori*, infancy apply even to absolute offences.

It remains to be seen whether such cases will survive testing under the European Convention on Human Rights.

Strict liability: the basics

Having clarified some issues, we can proceed to a discussion of strict offences.

Although there is some dispute as to which is the first crime of strict liability (see Singer 'The resurgence of *mens rea*: the rise and fall of strict criminal liability' (1989) 30 Boston College LR 377), **Woodrow** (1846) 153 ER 907 is generally treated as being the first one dealing with a statutory offence (certainly the common law crime of criminal libel was held to be strict before **Woodrow**). The accused was found guilty of possessing adulterated tobacco contrary to the Tobacco Act 1842, s 3, even though he did not know that there was something in the tobacco. **Woodrow** exemplifies one view of strict offences: that they form a sort of 'administrative criminal law', as Professor Leigh put it in his book *Strict and Vicarious Liability* (Sweet & Maxwell, 1982) 101. On this approach strict offences are not true crimes like murder but part of a system of regulation of activities, and this is why strict offences are sometimes called 'regulatory offences': they regulate enterprises for the public good. It should be mentioned that the legal thinking behind **Woodrow** seems to have been that in 1846 it had not been settled where the burden of proof should lie, and it did not seem unjust to place it on the accused, who after all had the tobacco in his possession.

Though regulation of undertakings sounds like a good thing, criticism of strict offences is strong. The basic argument is that strict liability sometimes punishes people who are not morally wrong. An example is **Sweet v Parsley**, a case which eventually reached the House of Lords, but the magistrates' court's decision is being considered here.

Sweet v Parsley [1970] AC 132

Ms Sweet was a young teacher who worked in Oxford. She rented a farmhouse seven miles away in the countryside. She sublet the house to what the judges called 'beatniks' while she stayed in a flat in Oxford because her car (nicknamed 'Young Maiden's Misery', because of its registration letters of YMM) had broken down. The beatniks smoked cannabis. She was found guilty of managing premises used for the purpose of smoking cannabis. She lost her job, even though she did not know that the sub-lessees were breaking the law and even though she had no control over them.

This case demonstrates that where one is convicted of a strict offence, one still suffers the social stigma of being branded a criminal and having one's name in the local newspaper. We shall see later what happened when Ms Sweet appealed.

Crimes which require *mens rea* and crimes which do not

We come to the difficult problem of determining which crimes are strict as to one or more elements of the *actus reus* and which are crimes of full *mens rea*. There is no simple rule, but the law is not totally unpredictable.

(a) Generally speaking, all major crimes, especially those involving breaches of morality, require *mens rea*, e.g. rape, murder and theft. However, it must be said that the outcome of a violation of a rule in a strict offence may be extremely serious. A victim may be killed as a result of speeding, a strict offence.

(b) All common law crimes require *mens rea* except those listed below. Since no new common law offences can be created, this list is definitive.

    (i) *Public nuisance.* The case usually cited is **Stephens** (1866) LR 1 QB 702, but that case is really an authority on vicarious liability, and it may be that in modern times *mens rea* is needed for this offence. In the most recent authority, **Shorrock** [1993] 3 All ER 917 (CA), the court held that the accused need not know of the offence he had caused. It was sufficient that he ought to have known that a nuisance would result from his activity on the land.

    (ii) *Contempt of court.* The authority is **Evening Standard Co. Ltd** [1954] 1 QB 578. Parliament expressly recognised the 'strict liability rule', as it called this principle, when it created the Contempt of Court Act 1981.

    (iii) *The various forms of criminal libel.* All forms were said by Lord Salmon in **Lemon**, above, to be strict. Certainly **Lemon** decided, Lords Diplock and Edmund-Davies dissenting, that in blasphemous libel there was no requirement of an intention to outrage Christians when publishing a poem depicting Christ as a homosexual, though there remained some *mens rea*, an intent to publish. Blasphemous libel was abolished by s 79 of the Criminal Justice and Immigration Act 2008, which came into force on 8 July 2008. However, seditious libel may require *mens rea*: **Bow Street Magistrates Court ex parte Choudhury** [1991] 1 QB 429 (CA).

    (iv) *Outraging public decency.* The Court of Appeal in **Gibson** [1990] 2 QB 619 applied **Lemon** from the cognate offence of blasphemous libel to this common law crime. A person is guilty whether or not he intends to corrupt or outrage public decency or is reckless as to whether he is corrupting or is outraging public decency.

(c) Under statute much turns on the individual offence. One cannot state that if Parliament has omitted to mention *mens rea*, the court will or will not read it in. There is no authoritative guidance as to which factors are important. Lord Nicholls in **B v DPP** [2000] 2 AC 428 (HL) gave examples of these factors: 'the language used, the nature of the offence, the mischief sought to be prevented and any other circumstances that might assist in determining what intention was properly to be attributed to Parliament'. **B v DPP** reemphasised that there is a presumption of *mens rea*. It may take some years before the full effect of this authority is felt. Certainly it is less likely than before that a sex crime will be held to be a strict offence, but exceptions still arise, as in **Doring** [2002] Crim LR 817 (see below).

Many offences dealing with the welfare of the public do not require a mental element. Wright J in **Sherras v de Rutzen** [1895] 1 QB 918 said that such offences criminalised persons whose acts 'are not criminal in any real sense but are acts which in the public interest are prohibited under a penalty'. He instanced the possession of adulterated tobacco. This phrase continues to be used, e.g. by Lord Scarman and Viscount Dilhorne in **Alphacell Ltd v Woodward** [1972] AC 824. Another term is 'regulatory' offences. Unfortunately terms such as 'public interest' and 'regulatory' are conclusory rather than explanatory. They do not tell us which crimes are strict, which are not. The two other categories Wright J mentioned were public nuisance and 'cases in which, although the proceeding is criminal in form, it is really only a summary mode of enforcing a civil right' such as an unintentional trespass in pursuit of game.

These types of offences are sometimes called 'quasi-criminal', as, e.g., Lord Reid put it in **Warner v MPC** [1969] 2 AC 256. However, the term is not very helpful: is selling bad meat a crime or a quasi-crime? Keeping to the point about public welfare offences, one can, however, state that the subject matter of some offences attracts strict liability more than do others. The selling of tainted food may well not require *mens rea*; e.g. *Parker* v *Alder* [1899] 1 QB 20, where the crime was one of selling bad milk, whereas bigamy is a crime requiring mental element: *Gould* [1968] 2 QB 65 overruling *Wheat and Stocks* [1921] 2 KB 119. Lord Diplock was to similar effect in *Sweet* v *Parsley* above, when he spoke of activities involving 'potential danger to public health, safety or morals'. The citizen had a choice whether or not to participate in these activities. If he did, he was subject to a higher duty of care than normal. 'An obligation to take whatever measure may be necessary to prevent the prohibited act, without regard to those considerations of cost or business practicability which play a part in the determination of what would be required of them in order to fulfil the ordinary common law duty of care.' In Lord Diplock's mind there were probably thoughts of butchers, pharmacists, milkmen. It should be mentioned that bigamy is sometimes seen as an offence contrary to morality, yet it is not a strict offence and, furthermore, murder involves actual danger to public health and safety, yet is not strict. What Lord Diplock seems to have meant is that there is a wide span of possible victims in strict crimes; e.g., any one of a million customers might suffer if milk is contaminated.

(d) At least outside the area of food and drugs, the courts are often not willing to impose an unreasonable burden on the accused. In *Sherras* v *de Rutzen*, above, a pub landlord was held not to be guilty of supplying liquor to a constable on duty, contrary to s 16(2) of the Licensing Act 1872, because in the view of one of the two judges he had no easy way of checking whether the police constable was on or off duty. The contrasting case to *Sherras* is always *Cundy* v *Le Cocq* (1884) 13 QBD 207, where a landlord was convicted under s 13 of the same Act of selling liquor to a drunk. One distinction between the two cases may be that a landlord can be expected to know that a drunk is indeed drunk. Accordingly, it can be said that the courts are generally reluctant to punish people when there is nothing they could have done to prevent it occurring: how can one report a road accident, when one does not know there has been one? In the Privy Council case of *Lim Chin Aik* v *R* [1963] AC 160, the accused could not easily find out that it was illegal for him to enter Singapore, punishment would serve no purpose, and so was not guilty. He was not to be expected to check whether he was permitted to enter at all times. This reasoning has not always been followed; often persons are convicted despite their having taken all possible precautions.

This attempted reconciliation of the famous cases of *Sherras* and *Cundy* does not explain everything. Two equally well-known cases are *Prince* (1875) LR 2 CCR 154 and *Hibbert* (1869) LR 1 CCR 184. Both cases are concerned with what became s 20 of the Sexual Offences Act 1956:

> It is an offence for a person acting without lawful authority or excuse to take an unmarried girl under the age of sixteen out of the possession of her parent or guardian against her will.

In *Prince* the accused believed the girl to be 18; she was in fact under 16 and he was found guilty (the majority, eight judges, said that the words of the statute were to be read literally, others (a minority of six) that taking the girl was immoral and wrongful and the accused (who in the words of Stephen J in *Tolson* (1889) 23 QBD 168 could be likened to 'seducers and abductors', which it has to be said Mr Prince was not) acted at his peril, and one judge dissented), yet only six years earlier the same court, the Court for Crown Cases Reserved, had decided in *Hibbert* that an accused was not guilty when he did not know that the girl whom he had taken away was in the possession of her parents. Accordingly, s 20 had to be read in this way: the accused was guilty if he takes a girl, knowing her to be a girl, who is unmarried, knowing her to be unmarried, out of the possession of her parent or guardian, knowing her to have a parent or guardian, and she happened to be under 16. A solid distinction between these two cases has not been found. Perhaps the difference is that in **Hibbert** the accused did not intend to take the girl out of anyone's possession, whereas the accused in **Prince** did. Surely, though, the crime was not so defined. The age of the girl was a most material element. Mr Prince would not have been guilty if the girl was over 16. Moreover, if the accused was guilty even though he did not know the age, why was he not guilty when he had not even checked whether the girl had a father? It should be noted that the accused in **Prince** was guilty no matter how deeply he had inquired into the girl's age and no matter how reasonable his error as to her age was. **Prince** was trenchantly criticised (*obiter*) in **B v DPP**, above, but it was not overruled and until it is, it remains authoritative on what was s 20 of the 1956 Act. **B v DPP** was not a case on s 20. However, as a result of the next two cases mentioned it is difficult to see **Prince** continuing to exist for much longer. Both decisions were made unanimously by the House of Lords.

B v *DPP* [2000] 2 AC 428 (HL)

The accused pressed a girl who was 13 to perform oral sex on him. She refused. He was charged with inciting a girl under 14 to commit an act of gross indecency contrary to the Indecency with Children Act 1960, an offence which was repealed and replaced by the Sexual Offences Act 2003. His defence was that he believed the girl to be over 14. The Divisional Court held that, as in **Prince** (above), liability as to the age of the girl was strict, and the conviction was affirmed. The Divisional Court reasoned that the purpose of the 1960 statute was to protect children under 14; therefore, it was immaterial that the accused was mistaken as to the age of the girl. (The age was raised to 16 by the Criminal Justice and Court Services Act 2000, s 39.)

The 1960 Act was enacted because a defendant was not guilty of indecent assault on a child when he did not use threats (assault) or force (battery). This aim would be undermined if the accused had a defence when he was mistaken as to age. Moreover, Parliament did sometimes provide defences based on such errors, but it did not do so for the offence of indecency with children. It should be noted that the 1960 Act created an offence of grave social stigma and with a maximum sentence of 10 years' imprisonment: the offence was not a regulatory one. Brooke LJ stated: 'Parliament continues to legislate in this area on an *ad hoc* piecemeal basis, and declines to set aside the time to make the necessary policy choices as to the *mens rea* requirement in relation to the changes in the law it enacts, let alone the many parts of the law it leaves unaltered. Hour after expensive hour has to be spent in the courts and elsewhere puzzling over these matters.' The court certified that a point of law of general public importance was involved, but refused leave to appeal.

The House of Lords overruled the Divisional Court and decided that the offence was not one of strict liability. It was held that the accused was not guilty if he made an honest mistake as to the girl's age. There was no special rule relating to age: the presumption of *mens rea* applied to all elements of offences. The mistake need not be one based on reasonable grounds. Lord Steyn spoke of the 'constitutional principle' that *mens rea* was to be presumed in a statute. Lord Nicholls applied the common law presumption that *mens rea* is part of a statutory offence unless Parliament has indicated otherwise, whether expressly or by necessary implication. Implication on reasonable grounds was not enough. The implication had to be 'compellingly clear'. This is a high hurdle to jump, and if correct, many of the other authorities were wrongly decided. (The other Law Lords spoke to similar effect. For example, Lord Hutton said that the implication that the statute ruled out *mens rea* had to be a '*necessary*' one (his emphasis).) The fact that the offence was serious reinforced that presumption, as did the fact that the crime covered a wide range of facts from 'predatory approaches by a much older paedophile' to 'consensual sexual experimentation between precocious teenagers of whom the offender may be the younger of the two'. The fact that sometimes the offence was used to protect vulnerable children was not of itself sufficient to make the crime one of strict liability. Furthermore, it was uncertain whether or not strict liability would lead to better enforcement of the crime. He added that insofar as the reasoning in *Prince* was inconsistent with the *mens rea* principle, it was wrong; the presumption applied even when the accused's act was immoral; the displacement of the presumption must be made clearly; and it is not displaced by comparing two badly drafted sections. Lord Nicholls stressed that the decision was not restricted to cases where the age of the victim is an ingredient of the offence. Lord Steyn said that the House of Lords in *Sweet* v *Parsley* may have expected that their decision would have overruled *Prince*. He said that that authority was 'was out of line with the modern trend in criminal law which is that a defendant should be judged on the facts as he believes them to be'. He added that *Prince* 'is a relic from an age dead and gone'. Any reform of the law was for Parliament, which despite the expert advice of the Criminal Law Revision Committee and the Law Commission over the years, had not acted decisively. In criticism it should be said that when Parliament re-enacted the crime which was at issue in *Prince*, it did so on the basis that *Prince* was authoritative.

B v *DPP* was applied in *K* [2002] 1 AC 462 (HL). There was no necessary implication that an accused was guilty of indecent assault on a victim aged under 16 when he honestly believed her to be over 16; she had also told him that she was 16. Both cases are concerned with mistakes as to age, as *Prince* was, but neither's *ratio* is so restricted. In criticism it must be said that when Parliament enacted the Sexual Offences Act 1956 it did not intend to affect *Prince*. Both *B* v *DPP* and *K* are now subject to the Sexual Offences Act 2003 which provides that a mistake as to the age of a child is irrelevant if he is under 13 and, if the child is between 13 and 16, only mistakes made on reasonable grounds suffice. In relation to a child under 13, liability is now strict. Liability for those 13–16 is arguably not strict because of the general rule in *B* v *DPP* and *K*. It would have been better for Parliament to have stated the law clearly in the 2003 Act. However, the cases remain authoritative as general statements on the law of strict liability. Both Lords Steyn and Bingham in *K* said that the presumption of *mens rea* was a constitutional principle.

A stronger case than *Hibbert* and *Sherras* v *de Rutzen* exemplifying the courts' implying a *mens rea* word into the statutory definition of a crime is *Harding* v *Price* [1948] 1 KB 695. The Divisional Court held that the accused was guilty of failing to report a road accident only if he knew that there had been one. The ruling is surprising when one realises that the statute at issue was the Road Traffic Act 1930. Parliament omitted 'knowingly' in that Act, whereas in the first statute dealing with the matter, the Motor Car Act 1903, the statute did contain this *mens rea* word. It would not be difficult for a court to hold that the omission was deliberate and that Parliament intended the offence to be strict. See also *Tolson* (1889) 23 QBD 168 where, as in *Prince*, there was no *mens rea* word, yet the accused was not guilty. Wills J spoke to the effect that circumstances alter cases.

(e) Another helpful guide is that where the punishment for the crime is severe, there is at times a presumption that *mens rea* is required. Lord Nicholls in *B v DPP* said: 'The more serious the offence, the greater was the weight to be attached to the presumption, because the more severe was the punishment and the greater the stigma that accompanied a conviction.' Originally the crime discussed in *B v DPP* had a maximum sentence of two years but that was raised to 10. But this presumption does not always take effect, e.g. on a second conviction for polluting a river, a strict offence, the accused may be sentenced to prison; similarly s 5(b) of the Dangerous Drugs Act 1965 created an offence with a maximum of 10 years' imprisonment, yet it was held to be strict. In *Howells* [1977] QB 614, the Court of Appeal held the crime of possessing a firearm to be strict, yet the penalty was a maximum of five years. Inconsistencies continue to flourish. In *Blake* [1997] 1 WLR 1167 (CA) a maximum sentence of two years made the offence 'truly criminal', whereas in *Harrow London Borough Council v Shah* [1999] 2 Cr App R 457 (DC) it was said that the same maximum did *not* make the offences truly criminal. (Both cases are further discussed below.) Accordingly, the mere fact that imprisonment is the sentence does not mean that the crime is a *mens rea* one: *Wells St Magistrates* [1986] 1 WLR 1046. This conclusion may not survive challenge under the Human Rights Act 1998. For example, as stated the maximum penalty in *Howells* was quite high, yet Parliament had not provided a due diligence defence. It is suggested that *Howells* may fall foul of Article 3 (inhuman or degrading treatment) or Article 6 (presumption of innocence) or both.

Too much should not be read into the severity of the maximum penalty. Since strict offences can also be committed intentionally, recklessly and negligently, the maximum is reserved for intentionally bringing about the *actus reus*. The sentence for a strict liability breach of the same offence may be minor: *Matudi* [2003] EWCA Crim 697.

(f) The words of the statute are sometimes interpreted as giving rise to strict liability. The following offer illustrations. Humphreys J in *Grade v DPP* [1942] 2 All ER 118 (DC) said that 'sell' does not require knowledge, but 'permit' does. In *Grade* the accused was charged with unlawfully presenting part of a new stage play before that part had been passed by the Lord Chamberlain, contrary to s 15 of the Theatres Act 1843, since abolished. A joke had been inserted into a music-hall revue *To See Such Fun* without the accused's knowledge, while he was away from the venue, and contrary to his instructions. Nevertheless, he was guilty. In *James & Son Ltd v Smee* [1955] 1 QB 78 the offence of permitting someone to use a vehicle which had defective brakes was held not to be a strict offence. The accused was guilty only if he knew that the brakes were faulty. However, the crime of permitting the use of a vehicle without insurance is a strict one: see e.g. *Braugh v Crago* [1975] RTR 453 and *Chief Constable of Norfolk v Fisher* [1992] RTR 6 (DC). In the latter case, which is also known as *DPP v Fisher*, *Newbury v Davies* [1974] RTR 367 (DC) was distinguished. In *Newbury v Davies* the owner was found not guilty of the offence when he permitted use of a vehicle only on the express condition that the daughter arranged insurance cover. Since, subject to the obtaining of the licence, use was not permitted, use of the car without a licence was not permitted. In *Fisher*, which involved the same offence, the accused knew that a person was disqualified and allowed him to have the car only if he got someone else to drive. He did so, but that other was not insured. The owner was convicted. The distinction between the cases is weak. Surely it should be immaterial whether the condition not to drive without insurance was imposed directly as in *Newbury* or indirectly as in *Fisher*. At present therefore some 'permitting' offences are strict but others are not, a not very helpful conclusion but one based on the cases. 'Uses' has been held to give rise to strict liability: ***Green v Burnett*** [1955] 1 QB 78. Therefore using a vehicle with defective brakes is a strict offence but permitting or allowing a person to drive a car with defective brakes is not!

Even 'wilfully' has been read as not importing knowledge in relation to s 86(3) of the Police Act 1996, wilful obstruction of a police officer: ***Rice v Connolly*** [1966] 2 QB 414 and ***Lewis v Cox*** [1985] QB 509. However, the House of Lords held in ***Sheppard*** [1981] AC 394 that 'wilfully' in s 1 of the Children and Young Persons Act 1933, which creates the crime of wilful neglect, meant both wilfully neglecting the child and knowing of the risk that the child's health might suffer or not knowing of the risk because the accused did not care whether or not the child needed medical treatment. Therefore, the crime was not one of strict liability but of objective recklessness. Moreover, 'permit' requires *mens rea*, per Lord Diplock in ***Sweet v Parsley***, above, as does 'procure' and probably 'suffer'. In all cases except one (***Brooks v Mason*** [1902] 2 KB 743), 'knowingly' has been held to require *mens rea*. One cannot imagine that ***Brooks v Mason*** would ever be followed, particularly not after ***B v DPP*** and ***K***.

(g) The fact that *mens rea* is required in one section of a statute but not in another does not mean that *mens rea* is not required in the latter: ***Sherras*** and ***Lim Chin Aik***, ***B v DPP***, all above. A similar case is one from New South Wales. In ***Turnbull*** (1944) 44 NSWLR 108, the phrase 'knowingly suffering' a girl under 18 to be in a house of ill-fame contrary to s 91D of the Crimes Act 1900 was read so that the accused was guilty only if he knew that the girl was under 18 (cf. ***Prince*** above). Contrary cases include ***Cundy***, above, which was approved in ***Hobbs v Winchester Corp*** [1910] 2 KB 471, and ***Neville v Mavroghenis*** [1984] Crim LR 42: in the latter case, which turned on s 13(4) of the Housing Act 1961, the court held that the subsection could be divided into two parts, one having 'knowingly' in it, the other not: the second part was held to be strict. Somewhat similar is the statement of Lord Goff in ***PSGB v Storkwain Ltd*** [1986] 1 WLR 903 (HL) that in the Medicines Act 1968 Parliament had made it plain by the use or omission of a *mens rea* word which offence was strict and which was not. It must be said, however, that the presence or absence of a *mens rea* word is more dependent on the vagaries of draftsmanship than on forethought. For example, Lords Steyn and Hutton in ***B v DPP*** said that, while it can be said that the Sexual Offences Act 1956 was aimed in part at protecting the vulnerable, that consolidation statute contained such a disparate mixture of crimes, that the fact that *mens rea* was stated in some sections but not in others did not mean that the latter were offences of strict liability.

(h) The fact that there is a defence of due diligence is a good indication that the offence is strict. If the offence is not strict, there is no need for a 'no negligence' offence because the prosecution has to prove fault, negligence. Section 7(1) of the Children and Young Persons Act 1933 provides a defence of taking all reasonable precautions and exercising due diligence to the crime of selling tobacco to a child under 16.

The above guidelines are just that – guidelines, though subject to what the House of Lords said in ***B v DPP*** and ***K***. It is easy to point to cases which are inconsistent. In the case of a crime created by Parliament, one has to look both at the words of the statute and at the intention of Parliament, as the courts put it. The words are important, e.g. if the Act says 'knowingly' it has to be proved that the accused acted knowingly: ***Westminster CC v Croyalgrange Ltd*** [1986] 1 WLR 674 (HL), knowingly permitting premises to be used as a sex establishment. Some judges have gone further and said that the requirement of *mens rea* is to be presumed when Parliament has omitted to state any. Brett MR in ***Attorney-General* v *Bradlaugh*** (1885) 14 QBD 689 said:

> It is contrary to the whole established law of England (unless the legislation on the subject has clearly enacted it) to say that a person can be guilty of a crime in England without a wrongful intent.

Similar sentiments abound, e.g. Cave J in ***Tolson***, above, stated that the elimination of *mens rea* was:

> . . . so revolting to the moral sense that we ought to require the clearest and most indisputable evidence that such is the meaning of the Act.

In one of the most important cases on this topic, ***Sweet* v *Parsley***, above, Lord Diplock went so far as to say that:

> The mere fact that Parliament has made the conduct a criminal offence gives rise to *some* implication about the mental element.

It is not difficult to find contrary sentiments. In ***Mallinson* v *Carr*** [1891] 1 QB 48, just two years after ***Tolson***, the court held that a criminal statute was to be read literally and if no *mens rea* was stated, none was to be implied. Nevertheless, the strong modern trend as exemplified by ***Sweet* v *Parsley***, ***B* v *DPP*** and ***K*** is that in the words of Lord Nicholls in the second case the presumption of *mens rea* in statutory offences could be displaced only by 'necessary implication' using 'compellingly clear evidence'. That evidence may sometimes be easy to find. The Sexual Offences (Amendment) Act 2000, s 3(1) (see now the Sexual Offences Act 2003), made it an offence to have sexual activity with a person under 18 if the accused was in a position of trust in relation to him. He had a defence if he proved that he did not know and could not reasonably have been expected to know that he was under 18. This defence would have no effect unless the offence were a strict one as to the age. Here is an example that Parliament on compellingly clear evidence intended this offence to be strict.

How the courts apply these guidelines

The reader, having grasped what has been said in the previous section, may be in some doubt as to how the law there stated is to be applied. This section examines several cases in order to show how the courts deal with this issue.

A relevant authority is ***Bradish*** [1990] 1 QB 981. The accused was found in possession of a canister which contained CS gas. He was charged with possessing a prohibited weapon contrary to s 5(1)(b) of the Firearms Act 1968. Did the accused have to know that what he was carrying was a CS gas canister? No mental element was stated in the paragraph. Auld J, giving the judgment of the Court of Appeal, referred to ***Warner* v *MPC*** [1969] 2 AC 256 for the proposition that the dangerous subject matter of the crime, coupled with the plain words used, might well rebut the presumption of *mens rea*. In the Firearms Act 1968 there was no exception which gave the accused a defence if he could prove that he did not believe that the thing was dangerous as the defendant had under s 28(3) of the Misuse of Drugs Act 1971. Previous cases had held other parts of the 1968 Act to be strict. In ***Howells*** [1977] QB 614 and ***Hussain*** [1981] 1 WLR 416, s 1, possessing a firearm without a certificate was held to create a strict offence; in ***Harrison*** [1996] Crim

LR 200 (CA) s 19, possessing a loaded shotgun in a public place was held to be a crime of strict liability; while in *Pierre* [1963] Crim LR 513, s 17, using a firearm to resist arrest was held to be strict. Auld J said:

> The clear purpose of the firearms legislation is to impose a tight control on the use of highly dangerous weapons. To achieve effective control and to prevent the potentially disastrous consequences of their misuse strict liability is necessary, just as it is in the equally dangerous field of drugs . . . Given that s 1 has been held to create an offence of strict liability, this consideration applies *a fortiori* to s 5 which is concerned with more serious weapons, such as automatic handguns and machine guns, and imposes a higher maximum penalty.

He added: '. . . the possibilities and consequences of evasion would be too great for effective control' if the offence were other than one of strict liability, and 'to the argument that the innocent possessor or carrier of firearms or prohibited weapons . . . is at risk of unfair conviction . . . there has to be balanced the important public policy behind the legislation of protecting the public from the misuse of such dangerous weapons'.

Therefore, the court referred to decisions on other sections of the 1968 Act and to another dangerous matter, drugs. What is interesting in the light of other cases is that the court ruled that the severe penalty was a factor in treating the offence as strict, whereas in other cases judges have said that since the penalty was low the offence was a regulatory offence and so strict! A case for comparison is *Berry (No. 3)* [1995] 1 WLR 7. The accused was charged with making an explosive substance, electronic timers, contrary to s 4(1) of the Explosive Substances Act 1883. That section penalises a 'person who makes or knowingly has in his possession or under his control any explosive substance . . .' The word 'knowingly' was not placed before 'makes' but the word was implied by the Court of Appeal. The court did not give a reason for not following the successful contentions in the firearms authorities. The court reasoned that the maker of the substance could be in no doubt that he had made it. In Lord Taylor CJ's judgment the addition of 'knowingly' '. . . simply emphasises that where possession or control is relied upon, the defendant must know the substance is in his possession, for example in his house or his car. No person who makes the substance can be unaware that he had done so.' The sentence, a maximum of 14 years, was not mentioned, and there was no reference to the need for 'tight control' of explosive devices.

A second illustration of judicial activity in this field is *Miller* [1975] 1 WLR 1222. The accused was charged with driving a vehicle on a road while disqualified. The defence was that he did not know that the place where he was driving was a 'road' within the meaning of the Road Traffic Acts. The Court of Appeal rejected his contention. First, while noting that the absence of the words 'knowingly' or 'negligently' in the relevant section was not conclusive, it was a factor; secondly, the crime was not a 'truly criminal' one, but rather the crime existed 'for safeguarding the safety of the public by prohibiting an act under sanction of a penalty'; and thirdly, previous authorities had treated the section as imposing strict liability. Accordingly the offence was strict in the light both of principle and precedent. A contrasting case is *Phekoo* [1981] 1 WLR 1117, where the Court of Appeal sifted through similar factors and reached the opposite conclusion. The accused had to believe that the persons to whom he was doing 'acts calculated to interfere with the peace or comfort of the residential occupier' with intent to cause them to give up occupation of the premises contrary to s 1(3) of the Protection from Eviction Act 1977 were indeed residential occupiers and not, e.g., squatters.

Another example of the court's inconsistency, this time at the House of Lords level, is provided by the contrast between *Warner v MPC* and *Sweet v Parsley*, both above. In

Warner their Lordships, Lord Reid dissenting, held that possession of drugs contrary to the Drugs (Prevention of Misuse) Act 1964 was a partly strict offence. Lords Morris and Guest simply followed the wording of the Act. Lord Pearce considered the gravity of the evil, while he and Lord Wilberforce said that the offence was not really strict because the accused must know that he is possessing something, i.e. the prosecution must prove that the accused knows that he is in possession of something, and if that matter turns out to be a forbidden drug, the crime is proved. (There has been since *Warner* a conviction for possessing cannabis resin when the accused had put it into his wallet two years earlier and had forgotten it: *Martindale* [1986] 1 WLR 1042 (CA).) The dissentient also looked at the seriousness of the offence but determined that because the crime was a grave one, *mens rea* was needed. *Warner* looks like a policy decision against drugs.

The arguments in *Warner* were in people's minds when *Sweet v Parsley* reached the House of Lords. The House persuaded itself that Ms Sweet was not concerned in the management of the farmhouse which was used for smoking cannabis. The case involved drugs, yet the Lords did not convict. Lord Reid repeated his stigma point from *Warner*: the crime was not strict because a person guilty of it suffered social stigma. *Mens rea* was to be presumed but that presumption could be rebutted. Whether it was not depended in part on whether the act was truly criminal or was criminal merely because public welfare so demanded. Lord Pearce said that the accused had no control over the people at the farmhouse and therefore should not be guilty. The House of Lords decided that, for the purposes of s 5(b) of the Dangerous Drugs Act 1965, the purpose mentioned had to be that of the manager of the premises. Here her purpose was not to provide premises to be used for the purpose of smoking cannabis. Her purpose was to provide a dwelling house for the 'beatniks'. It is unclear whether Parliament really wished s 5(b) to be interpreted as their Lordships did. One reading of the statute was that Ms Sweet was concerned in the management of premises and those premises were used for the purpose of smoking cannabis. If that construction is correct Ms Sweet should have been found guilty. If you are a student in a hall of residence, imagine what your college authorities would think about that result! Certainly the House of Lords was anxious to exonerate Ms Sweet, and despite the strong vocabulary of the judgments, the case does not provide definite guidance for the future. *Sweet v Parsley* was seen as marking a change in attitude by the judges. If Parliament enacts legislation and is silent as to *mens rea*, that silence is presumed to mean that liability is not strict. The House of Lords did not overrule cases where liability had been held to be strict, so the presumption was rebuttable. As we shall see, later cases continue to impose strict liability, and indeed *Bradish* [1990] 1 QB 981 demonstrates the Court of Appeal's upholding strict liability post-*Sweet v Parsley*. Perhaps *Sweet* is authority for the proposition that since that decision the courts scrutinise all factors to see whether or not strict liability is justified: they do not impose strict liability without thinking, as they have sometimes appeared to have done in the past. Parliament enacted the result in *Sweet* in s 8(d) of the Misuse of Drugs Act 1971, which requires the prosecution to prove that the defendant acted knowingly.

The law elsewhere has, however, not been clarified by Parliament, and the courts have been left to their own devices. The Law Commission in *The Mental Element in Crime*, Report No. 89, 1978, said the following about *Sweet* and *Warner*:

> [T]hese cases strikingly illustrate the difference of view and emphasis which can occur even in the highest judicial tribunal when dealing with the general problem of attributing an intention to Parliament with regard to the mental element (if any) in an offence when . . . Parliament has given no express indication of that intent.

Strict liability continues to pose questions in the highest judicial tribunal. In **Sheppard**, above, a bare majority determined that in wilful neglect the accused must realise that the child is in need of medical attention. The House of Lords was of the opinion that the courts were nowadays less likely to hold that an offence was a strict one than it had been in earlier years. Yet in the first case to reach their Lordships after **Sweet**, **Alphacell Ltd v Woodward** [1972] AC 842, the appellants were found guilty of causing effluent to enter a river from their factory, contrary to s 2(1)(a) of the Rivers (Prevention of Pollution) Act 1951, thereby showing that the House of Lords was still willing to impose strict liability. The appellants had caused the pollution through the design of the system for dealing with effluent. By building an overflow from their system to the river, they caused the effluent to enter this river when their system could not cope. Lords Wilberforce and Cross simply looked at the wording of the statute and gave a common-sense meaning to 'cause', a term which does not require *mens rea*. Viscount Dilhorne took into account the nature of the offence, but unlike Lord Wilberforce he emphasised that the section said 'causes or knowingly permits': it does not say 'knowingly causes or permits', i.e. the position of the *mens rea* term was vital. If the paragraph had stated 'knowingly causes or permits', 'permits' would be otiose, because 'knowingly causes' includes 'knowingly permits'. Lord Salmon – a good name for a judge dealing with pollution – pointed out the grave social consequences which would follow if the offence were not one of strict liability: pollution would be unchecked if negligence had to be proved. He stated that if the defendant had not acted with *mens rea*, only a small fine need be imposed. He added: 'This [outcome] may be regarded as a not unfair hazard of carrying on a business which may cause pollution on the banks of a river.' In other words, firms who build factories on riversides act at their peril. As M. Cremona and J. Herring put it in *Criminal Law* 2nd edn (Macmillan, 1998) 83 (not in 5th edn (Palgrave, 2007, by J. Herring):

> [I]t is a question, then, of weighing up different aspects of the public interest: in **Sweet v Parsley** the stigma of conviction was regarded as crucial: in **Alphacell Ltd v Woodward** the evidence of pollution was given greater weight. This was then reinforced by characterising the offence in the former case as 'truly criminal', and in the latter as 'quasi-criminal' . . .

Though the accused were found guilty in **Alphacell**, the House of Lords went out of its way to stress that other accused charged with the same offence were not totally defenceless. Lord Wilberforce stated that a defendant would have a defence if the act causing the pollution was that of a third party, Lord Pearson would have given a defence if the discharge of effluent was an Act of God or the result of interference by a trespasser, and Lord Cross said that there was a defence if the event was out of the defendants' control or beyond their foresight. There are cases showing that riparian factory owners are not guilty of causing pollution if the harm was caused by a vandal or by a lorry-driver spilling diesel oil.

In **B v DPP**, above, the House of Lords was divided whether or not interpreting the words of a statute so as to read in *mens rea* was effective in preventing the sexual abuse of children. Lord Hutton said: 'This purpose may be impeded if the happiness and stability of a child under 14 is harmed by the violation of his or her innocence by some act of gross indecency or incitement to gross indecency committed by a person who honestly believes that the child is older than 14', whereas Lord Nicholls stated: 'There is no general agreement that strict liability is necessary to the enforcement of the law protecting children in sexual matters.' Certainly **B v DPP** and **K** have been trenchantly criticised by commentators for not protecting children. Among the less condemnatory critiques is that of (Please replace by) C. M. V. Clarkson, H. Keating and S. R. Cunningham, *Criminal Law: Text and Materials*,

6th edn (Thomson, 2007) at 200: '. . . the basis of . . . **K** is flawed. The effect of this case is that a middle-aged paedophile can escape liability for [the then existing crime of] an indecent assault on a girl under the age of 16 on the basis that he genuinely believed, albeit unreasonably, that she was 16. Surely, if older men want to have sex with "children" they should be under a duty to ensure that the person is at least 16 . . .'

Even in relation to sex crimes the courts still sometimes construe statutes to provide for strict liability. An example is **G** [2006] 1 WLR 2052. The Court of Appeal said that s 5 of the Sexual Offences Act 2003, rape of a child under 16, created an offence which was strict as to the age of the victim. The court said with reference to other sections of the Act that this was so 'by necessary implication', to use the words of Lord Steyn in **K**. Other nearby sections referred to a reasonable belief as to age, whereas s 5 did not. Therefore, the accused is guilty of this offence even if he believes on reasonable grounds that the child is older than 13. The HL [2008] UKHL 37 concentrated on the effect of the European Convention on Human Rights.

Doring [2002] Crim LR 817 (CA) distinguished **B v DPP** and **K** in effect. The Court of Appeal held, *obiter*, the offence of acting as a director of a company as an undischarged bankrupt and being concerned in the management of a company known by a prohibited name. Lord Steyn in **K** had said: '. . . the presumption [of *mens rea*] can only be displaced by specific language, i.e. an express provision or a necessary implication.' Yet the court looked beyond the language to the public interest, which after **B v DPP** and **K** they should not be doing. Buxton LJ said that **B v DPP** did not offset pre-existing jurisprudence which was to the effect that 'social policy and prudence' could displace the presumption of *mens rea*.

Brief mention should also be made of **Wings Ltd v Ellis** [1985] AC 272. The accused were charged with making a false statement which they knew to be untrue, contrary to s 14(1)(a) of the Trade Descriptions Act 1968. The accused had published a false description in a travel brochure, realised their error, and corrected it, but someone had read an uncorrected brochure. The House of Lords decided that they were guilty, holding that the outcome was in accord with the purpose of the statute. Accordingly strict liability was imposed, despite the accused doing their best to prevent anyone relying on the brochure to book a holiday.

Summary

One may agree with Wright J in **Sherras v de Rutzen**, above: 'There are many cases on the subject and it is not very easy to reconcile them.'

One cannot always predict whether *mens rea* will be imported. It would be a good idea for Parliament to settle the law. The House of Lords in **B v DPP** and **K** has been placing the ball firmly in Parliament's court: offences will only be strict if Parliament expressly says so or if such is the necessary implication. One attempt at pulling together the considerations which may affect the courts was put forward by Lord Pearce in **Sweet v Parsley**, above:

> The nature of the crime, the punishment, the absence of social obloquy, the particular mischief and the field of activity in which it occurs, and the wording of the particular section and its context may show that Parliament intended that the act should be prevented by punishment regardless of intent or knowledge.

This *dictum* has been influential and was applied in, e.g., **Phekoo** [1981] 1 WLR 1117, see above. Such considerations may override the presumption in **Sweet** that Parliament does not intend to create strict offences. A case illustrating the rebuttal of the presumption of *mens rea* is **PSGB v Logan** [1982] Crim LR 443 (Croydon Crown Court). The accused was charged with selling a medicinal product not on the general sale list without the transaction being supervised by a pharmacist, contrary to s 52 of the Medicines Act 1968. The judge said: Parliament intended to restrict sales of medicinal products in the interests of safety; the product could be locked away or the shop closed when the pharmacist was absent; the offence was not a truly criminal one: therefore, the crime was strict. Moreover, to say that strict offences involve matters of social concern is not to the point. Rape and murder, both *mens rea* crimes, are of social concern.

It should be noted that when the courts declare that they are seeking the intention of Parliament they are not really doing so, for as a result of a self-denying ordinance they cannot readily have access to the best available material, *Hansard*, the reports of proceedings in Parliament, to discover what the true intention of Parliament is, unless the words creating the offence are ambiguous (**Pepper v Hart** [1993] AC 593); that is always provided that a body can have a state of mind. Often *Hansard* is not helpful. In **B v DPP**, above, Rougier J in the Divisional Court said that the need for *mens rea* was not discussed in either House and Lord Steyn in the House of Lords noted that the Report of the Criminal Law Revision Committee which led to the creation of the crime at issue also did not discuss it.

Reasons for strict liability

(a) If a person runs a business properly, the law should not be broken. If he commits the *actus reus* of a crime, he is running the business improperly. (However, not all strict offences involve businesses. The crime in **Prince** can be seen as one of public morality.)

(b) Certain activities must be prohibited in the interests of public well-being. Activities which harm society must be stopped. Some of these are regulatory offences (called in the USA 'trader' offences), but some are not, especially drug offences. A utilitarian argument is sometimes advanced: there is a greater good in raising standards than in not convicting faultless people. **Yeandel v Fisher** [1966] 1 QB 440 illustrates the principle. Lord Parker said: 'Drugs are a great danger today and legislation has been tightening up the control of drugs.' The courts are looking for socially dangerous activities when they implement the doctrine of strict liability. So in **Searle v Randolph** [1972] Crim LR 779 the accused was guilty of possessing cannabis when he knew that he had a cigarette end, but not that it contained cannabis. Moreover, a regulatory offence may be more serious than a 'standard' crime. Leonard Leigh gave this example in his book *Strict and Vicarious Liability* (Sweet & Maxwell, 1982): '. . . is it clear that theft necessarily poses a graver violation of a basic rule than does the pollution of a beach in a resort which depends upon its summer trade for prosperity?'

As stated above, certain types of behaviour attract strict liability more than others, e.g. pollution (**Alphacell**, above), some licensee offences, e.g. serving alcohol to drunks (**Cundy v Le Cocq**, above), and anti-inflation crimes (**St Margaret's Trust** [1958] 2 All ER 289). As Donovan J put it in the last case:

> There would be little point in enacting that no one should breach the defences against a flood, and at the same time excusing anyone who did it innocently.

He said that there was no presumption of *mens rea*.

Similarly food legislation is often strict, e.g. ***Pearks Gunston and Tee v Ward***
[1902] 2 KB 1: selling food not of the quality demanded. Some road traffic offences
are strict, such as driving on a road while disqualified (***Miller*** [1975] 1 WLR 1222,
above), but not all are. One has to know that there has been an accident before one
can fail to report it: ***Harding v Price***, above, and the crime of dangerous driving,
which was abolished in 1977, was not strict: ***Gosney*** [1971] 2 QB 674.

The following cases provide a selection of regulatory offences which have been
held to be strict: being concerned in the organisation of a public musical entertain-
ment (an acid house party) at a place for which no licence had been obtained:
Chichester DC v Silvester (1992) *The Times*, 6 May (DC), the court so holding in view
of the public mischief to be avoided, of risk to health and safety and of the lack of a
mens rea word in the relevant sub-sub-paragraph when its sister sub-paragraph contained *mens rea* words; cutting trees in contravention of a preservation order, even
though the statute contained the word 'wilfully': ***Maidstone BC v Mortimer*** [1980]
3 All ER 502; not sending a child to school regularly: ***Crump v Gilmore*** [1970] Crim
LR 28; failing to give 28 days' notice of working with blue asbestos and failing to
provide workers with protection against asbestos: ***Atkinson v Sir Alfred McAlpine &***
Son Ltd (1974) 16 KIR 220; executing unauthorised work on a listed building: ***Wells***
St Magistrates [1986] 1 WLR 1046: the accused need not know that the building was
listed. Public concern over attacks by Rottweilers and pit bull terriers was one reason
for deciding that the crime of being the owner of a dog which was dangerously out
of control in a public place was a strict one: ***Bezzina*** [1994] 1 WLR 1057 (CA). The
owner did not have to know that the dog might behave dangerously. Similarly, the
accused need not know that he has allowed a dangerous dog to enter a prohibited
place: ***Greener*** (1996) 160 JP 265. The Divisional Court held that if *mens rea* had
to be proved, convictions would be almost impossible if the accused was not accom-
panying the dog. In both of the last two offences the courts did not accept the
argument that a crime punishable by imprisonment could not be a strict offence.
This principle extends beyond regulatory offences. In ***Densu*** [1998] 1 Cr App R 400
(CA) the accused was convicted of having with him an offensive weapon, even
though he did not know its purpose. The article was a telescopic baton, but he
thought it was an aerial.

As can be seen from the drugs cases, the principle in this section is not limited to
what laypeople might not think of as being crimes, but extends to possessing an
altered passport (***Chajutin v Whitehead*** [1938] 1 KB 306) and advertising for the
return of goods 'no questions asked' (***Denham v Scott*** (1983) 77 Cr App R 210). The
courts state that in relation to these offences they are not trying to penalise certain
conduct but to prohibit it. For example, in the last-named decision the court said
that no stigma attached to the accused who committed the crime: he had not read
the advertisement; the deed was against public policy: the offence was not truly
criminal, and the law would be impossible to enforce if the offence were a *mens rea*
one. It was accordingly justifiable to impose strict liability.

(c) Difficulties of proof can be got round if the prosecution does not have to prove *mens*
rea. Guilty people will not escape through lack of evidence. This factor has been mentioned in several cases, e.g. ***Maidstone BC v Mortimer***, above. This rationale applies
especially to companies. One does not have to show, for instance, that one of the
directors, the directing mind of the company, knew that his company was pouring
effluent into a river.

(d) It is easier to enforce the law when *mens rea* is irrelevant than when the prosecution have to prove it. This reasoning was mentioned by the Privy Council in **Lim Chin Aik** [1963] AC 160, see above, and was approved by Lord Diplock in **Sweet v Parsley** above. A fairly recent illustration of this way of thinking occurs in the following Privy Council case.

Gammon (Hong Kong) Ltd v *Attorney-General of Hong Kong* [1985] AC 1

The defendants were charged with deviating in a material way from approved plans for a building, contrary to the Hong Kong Building Ordinance. They contended that they were not guilty because they did not know that the deviation was a material one. The Judicial Committee held that the offence did not require knowledge if the deviation was a material one and that the offence did not require knowledge of the materiality of the deviation from the plans. To make the offence strict meant that persons in the position of the accused would be obliged to exercise control and vigilance to stop the occurrence of the prohibited act. The purpose of the Ordinance was to regulate building sites which were dangerous to workers and the public. The public's protection would be seriously weakened if the offence were not strict. The aim of the offence was, *therefore*, to keep up standards and *mens rea* was irrelevant to that objective.

Gammon provides a good example of the present approach of English judges to analysing whether a crime is strict or not. First, Lord Scarman stated that there was a presumption of *mens rea*; secondly, this presumption may be displaced by considering the words and subject matter of the statute (in this case there was a 'social concern' in 'public safety'), and by investigating whether the act was 'truly criminal' (a tendentious phrase, it must be said) and whether strict liability would assist in preventing the forbidden act; thirdly, the maximum penalty was substantial, but that fact showed only the seriousness with which Hong Kong viewed lack of supervision on building sites. **Gammon**, which is a Privy Council case, is subject to the House of Lords rulings in **B v DPP** and **K** that the presumption of *mens rea* can be displaced only when Parliament has expressly said so or if the presumption is excluded by necessary implication. Moreover, do not all statutes reflect a 'social concern'? **Gammon** is often cited in the cases, e.g. **Bezzina**, above. An example is **Collett** [1994] Crim LR 607. Using land in contravention of a planning enforcement notice was a strict liability crime because the aim behind the relevant statute was to encourage users of land to check whether such notices were in force. Another example is **Brockley** (1994) 99 Cr App R 385 (CA). The law which prevented an undischarged bankrupt from being a company director was a matter of social concern. Otherwise he could escape the consequences of his insolvency by turning himself into a company. If the prosecution had to prove that the accused knew he was undischarged this would undermine Parliament's will. **Gammon** was applied on the basis that, in the words of Lord Scarman, 'the creation of strict liability will be effective to promote the objects of the statute by encouraging greater vigilance to prevent the commission of the prohibited acts'. Henry LJ said that it was 'unacceptable' for an irresponsible bankrupt to bury his head in the sand and thereby fail to establish his true status. In **Blake** [1997] 1 WLR 1167 the Court of Appeal held that the crime of using apparatus for wireless telegraphy was a strict offence because to so hold would encourage radio operators to avoid committing the offence, and interfering with the emergency services and air traffic control was a matter of public safety, despite the fact that the offence was a truly criminal one because of the possibility of imprisonment. ***Gammon*** was applied. The most recent illustration of the application of ***Gammon*** is ***Jackson*** [2006] EWCA Crim 2386, where it was held that flying a military plane below 100 feet is an offence of strict liability.

An application of ***Gammon*** is ***Harrow London Borough Council v Shah*** [1999] 2 Cr App R 457 (DC). The defendants were charged with selling National Lottery tickets to children under 16 contrary to s 13 of the National Lottery Act 1993. They believed on reasonable grounds that the purchaser was over 16 but he was in fact 13. In holding that this offence was strict as to the age, Mitchell J held that the offence was not a truly criminal offence (using the language of Wright J in ***Sherras v de Rutzen*** [1895] 1 QB 918 and of Lord Reid in ***Sweet v Parsley*** [1970] AC 132), that gambling was an issue of social concern particularly in respect of those under 16, that the maximum penalty, two years, though severe, was not conclusive (it was three years in ***Gammon***), and that attaching strict liability to this crime 'will unquestionably encourage greater vigilance in preventing the commission of the prohibited act'. He added that no stigma attached to the offence, and that the defendants' belief could be taken into account when determining the sentence. In criticism surely Parliament intended this offence to be 'truly criminal' when it attached a maximum penalty of two years' imprisonment.

Even after ***B v DPP*** and ***K*** English courts are applying ***Gammon***. In ***Muhamad***, above, the Court of Appeal cited ***Gammon*** when dealing with whether the offence of materially contributing to insolvency by gambling was strict. The maximum sentence was two years' imprisonment whereas the maximum for some other offences under the statute was ten years, and because of that the court was uncertain whether the offence was 'truly criminal'. (As we have seen, in ***Blake*** the court decided that a maximum imprisonment of two years made the offence strict, whereas in ***Harrow London Borough Council v Shah*** the court held that the same maximum did not make the offence strict.) The court then discussed ***B v DPP***, holding that the language, maximum sentence and social concern led to the conclusion that the offence was strict.

Lord Scarman took a similar view of 'social concern' in ***Wings Ltd v Ellis***, above. His approach was followed in ***PSGB v Storkwain Ltd*** and ***Wells St Magistrates***, both above. In the former case, the accused supplied drugs on prescriptions purportedly signed by a doctor. In fact the prescriptions were forged. The defendants were found guilty by the Divisional Court, even though they were deceived, for the reasons advanced by Lord Scarman. On appeal the House of Lords confirmed the decision without mentioning ***Gammon***. Indeed the House of Lords in ***Storkwain*** did not give much weight to the fact that the maximum penalty was two years' imprisonment or that the principle in favour of *mens rea* should have been weighed in the balance. It must be admitted that many traditional areas of criminal law, such as murder and rape, are also matters of social concern, yet they are not strict offences. The same applies to non-traditional areas, such as planning. Parliament is hardly likely to enact legislation which is not a matter of some social concern.

(e) Public disapproval of various forms of behaviour may be marked by the use of sanctions without proof of fault. Business people ought not to pollute rivers, and if they do, they should be made to pay.

(f) Strict liability deters others from committing the same offence.

(g) The doctrine obliges people to adopt high standards of care in their trades and other activities. Beldam LJ said in ***Hallett Silberman Ltd v Cheshire CC*** [1993] RTR 32:

'The reason for the creation of offences of strict liability is to put pressure on the thoughtless and inefficient to do their whole duty in the interests of public health or safety.' People do not like their names in the paper, so they will try hard to avoid contravening the public good. The fact that some people are convicted when they are blameless is outbalanced by the raising of standards generally. For example, in *Bezzina* the imposition of strict liability was justified by the court as a spur to owners taking more care of their dangerous dogs than before.

(h) Because of strict liability, courts are not overburdened with prosecutions seeking to prove petty violations.

(i) If a person creates a risk and takes a profit from that risk, he ought to be liable if the happening of that risk creates problems. This rationale was first advanced by Kennedy LJ in *Hobbs* v *Winchester Corp* [1910] 2 KB 471, above. The pollution case of *Alphacell*, above, may provide an illustration of this principle. The accused could have established a back-up system for disposing of the effluent, but did not do so to save money. (This argument cannot be taken too far. It assumes that all business activities are run for profit, which is not necessarily so.)

These reasons demonstrate to some that strict offences are not always morally repugnant, and that it may sometimes be better to convict the innocent in order to prevent a large number undermining well-being than to let the blameless go. Some of these arguments do, however, prove too much. Surely convenience of lawyers in argument (h) ought not to outweigh the *mens rea* principle. If it did, why does murder have a *mens rea*? It would be easier to convict people of murder if the prosecution did not have to prove malice aforethought, but murder is a crime which does require a mental element. Such arguments lead us into the next section.

Reasons why there should not be offences of strict liability

(a) As Dickson J said in the Supreme Court of Canada in *City of Sault Ste Marie* (1978) 85 DLR (3rd) 161, there is no evidence that standards are raised by strict liability. Similarly in *B* v *DPP*, above, Lord Nicholls stated that there was no general agreement whether strict liability was of use in preventing the sexual abuse of children. Moreoover, a series of small fines is hardly a deterrent. Bad publicity may be a better method than strict liability for improving standards.

(b) It is morally wrong to punish people who have not voluntarily broken the law. These people are not blameworthy and should not be. Not all strict offences are so minor that it may be said that a small punishment for a violation of a law was ethically acceptable. For example, in *Prince*, above, the maximum sentence was two years' imprisonment, while in *Chajutin* v *Whitehead*, above, the accused was deported.

(c) Even if a person has taken all reasonable care, he is guilty, yet he does not deserve punishment. For example, in *Callow* v *Tillstone* (1900) 83 LT 411 (DC) a butcher was guilty of exposing for sale meat which was unfit for human consumption despite a veterinary surgeon's certifying it as sound. In *PSGB* v *Storkwain*, above, a pharmacist was guilty even though the prescription contained a forgery. He would have been guilty even if he had checked with the doctor.

(d) The laws on strict liability are not always vigorously enforced. Factory inspectors rarely prosecute until they have warned owners about breaches. Surely this type of rule is best enforced by a mechanism which is not the criminal law. In any event there should be controls over the discretion to prosecute. The argument that prosecutions are rarely brought unless the accused is at fault was said to be a weak one by the High Court in **Barnfather v London Borough of Islington**, above.

(e) Respect for the law is lessened because people who are not at fault are punished. A. A. Cuomo said in (1967) 40 S Cal LR 463, 518, strict liability 'can only breed frustration and disrespect for the law . . .'. The accused has a conviction, though not blameworthy.

(f) People (e.g. butchers, perhaps) would be put out of business if strict liability laws were always enforced. Such may not be what the public want. A person should not be forced to do something unreasonable. Making strict offences into cases of negligence would ensure that reasonable standards are maintained. However, as J. Brady put it 'Strict liability offences: a justification' (1972) 8 Crim L Bull 217:

> First, there is little evidence to show that the effect of strict liability offences has been to make these socially beneficent enterprises less attractive. [Secondly], . . . a person who does not have the capacity to run (for example) a dairy in such a manner as to prevent the adulteration of milk is not to be protected on the sole ground that he is engaged in a 'socially beneficial' enterprise. An incompetent carrying on an enterprise in which there is the danger of widespread harm . . . is *not* engaged in a 'socially beneficial' enterprise.

(g) When a judge deals with a strict offence, he or she excludes from the jury all arguments about intention, recklessness and carelessness, yet such arguments are relevant to sentence. They are made to the judge after conviction. The judge decides as a matter of fact what the accused's state of mind was. It is, therefore, not true to say that strict liability saves time.

(h) Authorities tend not to prosecute for strict offences unless the accused, intentionally or subjectively, acted recklessly. Since *mens rea* is considered at the stage of the decision to prosecute, it should also be taken into account when crimes are created and defendants are tried.

(i) If one considers the theories of punishment, a person who breaks a rule of strict liability is not deterable individually and there is no general deterrence. He will not be reformed by a conviction, and he will not be incapacitated unless he is put into prison or his licence withdrawn, sanctions which may be disproportionate to the breach of the law.

The arguments for and against strict liability have to be balanced. The courts have not placed these arguments in any order of priority.

Suggestions for reform of the law relating to strict liability

(a) The fiction that Parliament intends offences to be strict or not is not helpful and should be abolished. As Jordan CJ put it in the New South Wales case of **Turnbull** (1944) 44 NSWLR 108, see above, if legislators knew that the courts would always read in *mens rea*, they would soon become accustomed to stating whether the offence was strict or not. The present situation leads to litigation and a multitude of reported cases, many of them irreconcilable. The Law Commission, in *The Mental Element in Crime*, Report No. 89, 1978, recommended the abolition of the fiction.

(b) One suggested reform is that all regulatory offences should be dealt with by tribunals, not courts. The accused would know that he was being tried for a public welfare violation, not for a crime. However, the effect of a tribunal appearance might be the same as court proceedings for the accused would be held up to public display, and certainly some offences, especially drugs ones, cannot be taken out of the criminal law.

(c) In Report No. 89, 1978 (see above), the Law Commission recommended that strict offences should remain within the criminal law, but treated as crimes of negligence. This proposal is similar to the 'half-way house' idea of Lord Diplock in **Sweet v Parsley**, above. The burden of proof would be on the prosecution. For example, in **PSGB v Storkwain**, the pharmacist would not be guilty unless the prosecution proved that he did not check the doctor's signature on the prescription. One possible drawback of this suggestion is that the courts might impose a very high standard of care. In **Evans** [1963] 1 QB 412 the accused, a learner driver, was charged with the offence of causing death by dangerous driving, an offence which has been repealed. Though he had been doing his best, he knocked a man down and killed him. The court found him guilty because he fell short of the standard expected of a good driver. This approach makes negligence little different from strict liability, though the charge would allow the accused to adduce evidence that he was not at fault.

(d) The onus of proof could be placed on the accused. The accused to have a defence would have to show that he or she did not have the *mens rea* for the offence and was not negligent. Lord Reid hinted at this reform in **Tesco Supermarkets Ltd v Nattrass** [1972] AC 153. This reasoning has some historical support. In **Grade v DPP** [1942] 2 All ER 118, Humphreys J treated **Sherras v de Rutzen** [1895] 1 QB 918 as a case where the accused had to show that he did not know that the constable was on duty. Day J in **Sherras** said that the omission of 'knowingly' shifted the burden. The same view was taken in **Harding v Price**, above, but was doubted in **Roper v Taylor's Central Garages (Exeter) Ltd** [1951] 2 TLR 284 and **Lim Chin Aik**, above, and was rejected by Lord Pearce in **Warner v MPC** [1969] 2 AC 256. More recently the House of Lords in **B v DPP**, above, also rejected this version of the 'half-way house'.

(e) One should look at each crime to see whether adequate reasons exist for retaining that offence as one of strict liability.

(f) Lord Reid in **Warner** was prepared to tolerate strict liability where people set themselves up in certain businesses such as pub landlords and butchers and where the penalties were minor and the stigma small. He thought that the doctrine could be tolerated only in order to protect the public, and he advocated a defence where 'the defect was truly latent so that no one could have discovered it'.

(g) Other commentators have proposed an exception for persons who are not careless (a 'no-negligence' defence). Such provisions are becoming common. In the Food Act 1984, ss 2–3, it is a defence to a charge of possessing contaminated food if the accused can show that the adulteration was unavoidable.

(h) One of the most interesting proposals is that of David Tench in his pamphlet *Towards a Middle System of Law*, Consumers' Association, 1981. He contends that it is not always necessary to make a crime of something that has to be forbidden or controlled. Some forms of conduct such as murder and theft must remain offences, but others – not displaying a car licence, parking on a yellow line and the like – should become subject to a so-called 'civil penalty' and not subject to imprisonment or a fine. He writes:

> It surely is ridiculous for Parliament to go on legislating to make things criminal which no civilised individual really regards as criminal.

The proposal would save time and money. There would be no investigation and no need to go to court, and penalties could be fixed. He suggests that people may become more ready to obey the criminal law which remains. Into this middle system Tench would also put regulatory offences such as the one which affected the butcher in *Hobbs* v *Winchester Corp*, above, sexual and racial discrimination, tax penalties, picketing, and a new law on privacy. Tench would like the middle system of law to be dealt with by magistrates, who now try most strict offences. His idea has not been taken up. However, civil penalties are now used in the fields of direct taxation and VAT.

(i) Baroness Wootton of Abinger wrote in *Crime and the Criminal Law*, 2nd edn (Stevens, 1981), that crimes should contain no *mens rea*. The accused should be guilty not because he was at fault but because the accused had acted in a criminal way. She wanted strict offences to replace *mens rea* ones, leaving the fault element to become relevant only after conviction for sentencing purposes. In her view (at 46):

> If . . . the primary function of the Courts is conceived as the prevention of forbidden acts, there is little cause to be disturbed by the multiplication of offences of strict liability. If the law says that certain things are not to be done, it is illogical to confine this prohibition to occasions on which they are done from malice aforethought . . . A man is equally dead . . . whether he was stabbed or run over by a drunken motorist or an incompetent one.

In her view offenders should be treated (e.g. taught to drive better), not punished. The rejoinder to this attempted destruction of *mens rea* comes from the doyen of English criminal lawyers, J. C. Smith, in his essay 'Responsibility in Criminal Law' in P. Bean and B. Whynes (eds), *Barbara Wootton* (Tavistock, 1986). Smith retorted:

(i)   Blameless people who kill by accident deserve sympathy not stigma.

(ii)   Wootton's view would stigmatise the blameless and place them in the same category as those who intentionally broke the law. People who have drugs planted on them should not be treated in the same way as those who intentionally hold large quantities of drugs.

(iii) If one looks at matters of fault at the sentencing stage, one does not get rid of the difficulty of determining degrees of fault.

(iv)   Strict liability leads to the conviction of people like Mrs Tolson who was prosecuted for bigamy even though she thought that her husband was dead. She was found guilty by the trial judge and five out of 14 judges in the Court for Crown Cases Reserved ((1889) 23 QBD 168). She should not have been prosecuted at all, never mind convicted of a crime for which the maximum penalty was seven years' imprisonment.

(v)   Wootton wanted the criminal law to prevent the recurrence of forbidden acts, but Mrs Tolson would not do what she had done again.

(vi) The work of the police and courts would be multiplied if all non-intentional breaches of the criminal law had to be prosecuted.

(vii) 'To remove the element of fault is to empty the law of moral content' (at 154).

It should be added that no amount of re-education could change the behaviour of some people convicted of strict offences. Would re-education help the landlord in **Cundy v Le Cocq** (1884) 13 QBD 207, above? To all appearances the drunk did not look drunk.

(j) The 1985 version of the draft Criminal Code, Law Commission, Report No. 143, provided in cl 24(1):

> Unless a contrary intention appears, a person does not commit a Code offence unless he acts intentionally, knowingly or recklessly in respect of each of its elements other than fault elements.

Therefore, if Parliament did indicate that an offence was strict that interpretation was to be adopted, but if Parliament did not so enact, the offence was to be a *mens rea* crime. The courts would be permitted to look only at 'the terms of enactment'. A similar provision appears in the 1989 version (Law Com. No. 177):

> Every offence requires a fault element of recklessness with respect to each of its elements, other than fault elements, unless otherwise provided (cl 20(1)).

Like the 1985 version, the 1989 one would not apply to offences existing before the Code ('pre-Code offences'). The examples given by the Law Commission are these (Law Com. No. 177, 157):

> Under clause 147 a person commits burglary if he enters a building as a trespasser intending to steal in the building. Nothing is said as to any fault required in respect of the fact that the entrant is a trespasser. The offence is committed only if the entrant knows that, or is reckless whether, he is trespassing.

The second example would reverse **Alphacell Ltd v Woodward**, above, prospectively:

> An offence of causing polluting matter to enter a watercourse is created after the Code comes into force. In the absence of provision to the contrary the offence requires (a) an intention to cause the matter to enter the watercourse or recklessness whether it will do so, and (b) knowledge that the matter is a pollutant or recklessness whether it is.

The Law Commission opined that cl 20 would clarify the 'regrettable' state of uncertainty in the law. It should be noted that cl 20 does not apply where Parliament has *expressly* or *impliedly* provided to the contrary. The rationale is that courts are constitutionally obliged to apply the law Parliament has decided whether that law is expressly or impliedly stated. The possibility of impliedly strict offences may still leave room for uncertainty.

Conclusions

Strict offences have been dealt with at length for several reasons.

(a) The mere fact that such crimes exist shows that the criminal law is not based on breaches of a moral code. A crime is what Parliament or in strict offences the judges say is a crime.

(b) From this proposition one can deduce that *mens rea* does not mean a malicious or guilty frame of mind. Morals and law form different sets of rules.

(c) Many crimes exist without there being any intentionally or recklessly caused act. *Mens rea* therefore need not exist in every crime in relation to each element of the *actus reus*. Such indeed is the definition of strict liability.

(d) The topic makes one look at the rationale of certain laws and of law in general. Should people be punished who are not consciously at fault? Can the criminal law be used to improve standards? Why are murder and polluting a river both crimes? Is the criminal law addressed to the citizen to make him or her change behaviour or is it addressed to the police, the Crown Prosecution Service and the judiciary to catch, prosecute and punish those breaching standards?

(e) The topic has links with other law subjects. For instance, if Parliament enacts that doing X is an offence, how can the courts say that only doing X knowingly is a crime in the light of the doctrine of Parliamentary sovereignty? If one argues that Parliament passes statutes against the background of the common law, which has a presumption of *mens rea*, why does it often not state what the mental element is, and why does not the common law always introduce *mens rea*? Glanville Williams put it in this way in *Criminal Law: The General Part*, 2nd edn (Stevens, 1961) 260: 'The law of *mens rea* belongs to the general part of the criminal law, and it is not reasonable to expect Parliament every time it creates a new crime to enact it . . .'.

(f) The law is not a set of rules to be learned by rote. Some matters are certain but at times law consists of principles to which differing weight is attached according to the circumstances. On particular facts it may be difficult to predict whether a court would decide that the offence was strict or not. Yet people are convicted and imprisoned on those decisions. The criminal law is not a game; nor is it an exact science. It constitutes part of everyday life, e.g. speeding, and affects people's lives and jobs. Indeed, for some people it *is* their job.

(g) Studies of the effects of strict liability laws do not affirmatively support those academics who wish to abolish the doctrine. Those involved in enforcing such rules do not always use the law as their first mode of attack. For example, in dealing with accidents at work the Health and Safety Inspectorate relies largely on persuasion, but the availability of strict offences helps inspectors to enforce the law when other means have failed. One can conclude from this illustration that there is a gap between law in theory and law in practice.

(h) The criminal law is only one way of controlling harmful activities. There are others such as warnings, supervision, inspection, seizure of equipment, persuasion, and giving no effect to the wrongful behaviour.

Finally, a comment from N. Lacey *et al.*, *Reconstructing Criminal Law*, 3rd edn (LexisNexis, 2003) 50: 'Instances of strict liability are . . . marginalised as exceptional, relatively non-serious and calling for special justification.' Yet as we have seen, about half of the criminal calendar consists of strict offences, and most crimes are strict. There is nothing marginal about strict liability. Some are grave, and as for justification, what do you think?

Summary

This chapter deals with the doctrine of strict liability; that is, with crimes where, to use Smith and Hogan's definition, there is no *mens rea* as to one or more elements in the *actus reus*. Take, for instance, a crime of a butcher selling bad meat. The *mens rea* can be analysed as: (1) the butcher must know that what she is doing is 'selling'; (2) she must know that what she is selling is 'meat'; (3) however, if she is guilty even though she does not know that the meat she is selling is 'bad', the offence is one of strict liability. The distinction is drawn between the crimes of absolute (see **Larsonneur** (1933) and **Winzar** (1983)) and strict liability. There are few common law crimes of strict liability and these are noted. The courts have over time differed in their approach to offences of strict liability where the source of the crime is statute. The current approach is that adopted by the House of Lords in two recent cases and the difference between the present law and earlier approaches is drawn. The chapter terminates with an extensive discussion of the arguments for and against the doctrine, including various suggestions for reform (e.g. introducing a due diligence defence).

- Strict and absolute offences: Strict offences must be distinguished from absolute offences, which are ones where *mens rea* is lacking and to which there is no defence. However, the older cases use 'absolute liability' as a synonym for strict liability. Examples of absolute offences found by the courts are the former crime of being found in the UK illegally and the offence of being found drunk on the highway. A term used in the literature to mean absolute liability is 'situational liability'.

- Strict liability and common law crimes: Rarely at common law are crimes strict but the following are: public nuisance, contempt of court, criminal libel and outraging public decency.

- Strict liability and statutory crimes: Courts interpret statutes and often Parliament does not state the requisite *mens rea*. In that event, the judges look to 'the language used, the nature of the offence, the mischief sought to be prevented and any other circumstances that might assist in determining what intention was properly to be attributed to Parliament' (per Lord Nicholls in *B v DPP* [2000] 2 AC 428 (HL). Also considered are whether the accused could have avoided committing the crime and whether the maximum sentence is severe. The fact that these considerations form guidelines only means that it is not always predictable how the courts will apply them. While the courts' views on strict offences have varied across the years, the current position is that there is quite a strong presumption that an offence is strict and usually *mens rea* is read in.

- The arguments for and against strict liability: There has been debate over the years as to whether strict liability is justified or not. Among arguments in favour are the ease of proof and the 'gadfly' contention, i.e. that strict liability forces people to adopt high standards. The contrary approach includes the arguments that the criminal law should not apply to those who are not at fault and it should not apply to those who cannot be deterred.

- Suggestions for reform: Several proposals have been made for reform of the law. These include converting all strict offences into negligence-based ones and providing a defence of due diligence to all strict offences.

References

Reports

Law Commission Report no. 89, *The Mental Element in Crime* (1978)

Law Commission Report no. 143, *Criminal Law: Codification of the Criminal Law – A Report to the Law Commission* (1985)

Law Commission Report no. 177, *A Criminal Code for England & Wales* (1989)

Books

Bean, P. and Whynes, B., (eds.) *Barbara Wootton* (Tavistock, 1986)

Clarkson, C. M. V. *Understanding Criminal Law* 4th edn (Thomson, 2005)

Clarkson, C. M. V. and Keating, H. *Criminal Law: Text and Materials* 5th edn (Thomson, 2003)

Cremona, M. and Herring, J. *Criminal Law* 2nd edn (Macmillan, 1998)

Lacey, N., Wells, C. and Quick, O. *Reconstructing Criminal Law* 3rd edn (LexisNexis, 2003)

Leigh, L. *Strict and Vicarious Liability* (Sweet & Maxwell, 1982)

Smith, J. C. and Hogan, B. *Criminal Law* (ed. D. Ormerod) 11th edn (Oxford University Press, 2005)

Tench, D. *Towards a Middle System of Law* (Consumers' Association, 1981)

Wootton, Baroness *Crime and the Criminal Law* 2nd edn (Stevens, 1981)

Journals

Brady, J. 'Strict liability offences: a justification' (1972) 8 Crim L Bull 217

Further reading

Brudner, A. 'Imprisonment and strict liability' (1990) 40 UTLJ 73

Fitzpatrick, B. 'Strict liability: reverse burden and Article 6(2) of the European Convention on Human Rights' (2003) 67 JCL 363

Fitzpatrick, B. 'Strict liability and Article 6(2) of the European Convention on Human Rights' (2004) 68 JCL 11

Hamdani, A. 'Mens rea and the cost of ignorance' (2007) 93 Va L Rev 415

Horder, J. 'Strict liability, statutory construction and the spirit of liberty' (2002) 118 LQR 459

Horder, J. *Excusing Crime* (Oxford University Press, 2004) ch. 6

Jackson, B. S. '*Storkwain*: a case study in strict liability and self-regulation' [1991] Crim LR 892

Lanham, D. '*Larsonneur* revisited' [1976] Crim LR 276

Levenson, L. L. 'Good faith defenses: reshaping strict liability crimes' (1993) 78 Cornell LR 401

Manchester, C. 'Knowledge, due diligence and strict liability in regulatory offences' [2006] Crim LR 213

Moodie, R. A. 'Refulgent *mens rea* eclipsed' (1974–5) 6 NZULR 230

Parker, J. S. 'The economics of *mens rea*' (1993) 79 Virg LR 741

Richardson, G. 'Strict liability for regulatory crime: the empirical research' [1987] Crim LR 295

Simons, K. W. 'Criminal law: when is strict liability just?' (1997) 87 JCL & Crim 1075

Smith, J. and Pearson, A. 'The value of strict liability' [1969] Crim LR 5

Stanton-Ife, J. 'Strict liability: stigma and regret' (2007) 27 OJLS 151

The principal theoretical work is the series of essays in A. P. Simester (ed.), *Appraising Strict Liability* (Oxford University Press, 2005). An older account is L. Leigh, *Strict and Vicarious Liability* (Sweet & Maxwell, 1982).

Visit **www.mylawchamber.co.uk/jefferson** to access exam-style questions with answer guidance, multiple choice quizzes, live weblinks, an online glossary, and regular updates to the law.

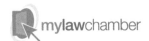

5

Principal parties and secondary offenders

Introduction

The Judicial Studies Board's Specimen Direction on Joint Responsibility reads in part:

> Where a criminal offence is committed by two or more persons, each of them may play a different part, but if they are in it together as part of a joint plan or agreement to commit it, they are each guilty. The words 'plan' and 'agreement' do not mean that there has to be any formality about it. An agreement may arise on the spur of the moment. Nothing need be said at all. It can be made with a nod and a wink, or a knowing look. An agreement can be inferred from the behaviour of the parties.

The Judicial Studies Board provides trial judges with specimen instructions on the law to be given to juries. This area of law is often known as 'secondary participation'.

Grundy is an illustration of this topic.

Grundy [1989] Crim LR 502 (CA)

Two accused were beating up a constable on the stairs up to an Indian restaurant. The first accused joined in after a few seconds. The constable suffered a broken nose and other injuries. All three were charged. The first accused was convicted of aiding (see below for definition) that offence.

The court held that the whole of the injuries suffered by the constable amounted to grievous bodily harm. The first accused was aiding the commission of the offence as soon as he joined in. It was therefore immaterial that he had joined in after the other defendants had begun to inflict the injuries and had already broken the officer's nose. The two other defendants were the principal offenders. Both were striking the officer. They perpetrated the harm. The first accused was the secondary offender or accessory to the injuries other than the broken nose. In *Grundy* the people who inflicted the harm were joint principals. A principal is defined as a person who commits or contributes to the *actus reus*. A secondary party or accessory is someone who encourages or helps the principal. These definitions, which are explained below, are subject to various exceptions such as the doctrine of innocent agency but in the general run of fact situations these definitions suffice.

In the general run of cases the secondary party is guilty only if a principal committed an offence with the requisite *actus reus* and *mens rea*, though no principal offender need have been identified, let alone tried and convicted. The principle is called 'derivative liability'. Modern law is moving away from this form of liability (see *Howe* [1987] AC 417, discussed below, and *DPP* v *K&B* [1997] 1 Cr App R 36 (DC), though the latter case may be explained as being an authority on procedure to which different principles may apply) but normally it still applies. As the Supreme Court of Victoria in *Demirian* [1989] VR 97, 116, said: 'The accessory may play a dominant, an equal or a subsidiary role in respect of the commission of the crime.' Mafia godfathers, for instance, may be worse than their minions who perform the act of killing.

Lord Goddard CJ in *Abbott* [1955] 2 QB 497, which was distinguished in *Grundy*, noted the problem with persons jointly charged.

> If two people are jointly indicted for the commission of a crime and the evidence does not point to one rather than the other, and there is no evidence that they were acting in concert, the jury ought to return a verdict of not guilty in the case of both because the prosecution have not proved the case.

In *Aston* (1991) 94 Cr App R 180 the Court of Appeal quashed the appellants' convictions for cruelty and manslaughter because it could not be proved whether the victim's mother or a person who treated the victim as his own daughter caused the harm. Both of these persons, the appellants, had the opportunity of inflicting the fatal injury, but it could not be proved that this one rather than the other killed, that the two were acting in concert, that they had expressly or tacitly agreed that the victim should be injured, or that either had encouraged the other to inflict harm. There are several similar cases involving parents, such as *Lane* (1986) 82 Cr App R 5 and *Strudwick* (1994) 99 Cr App R 326 (CA) which followed both *Abbott* and *Lane*, and spouses or cohabitees: *Collins* v *Chief Constable of Merseyside* [1988] Crim LR 247 (DC), which also followed *Abbott* and *Lane*. Either of the appellants could have disconnected the meter from the electricity supply. There was no joint enterprise in these cases, and either could have acted without the other knowing. The law was neatly summarised in *Collins* thus: 'where two people were jointly indicted and the evidence did not point to one rather than the other, they both ought to be acquitted because the prosecution had not proved its case. The uncertainty could not be resolved by convicting both. (See now the Domestic Violence, Crime and Victims Act 2004, s 5, mentioned on the next page.) In summary, if the prosecution can prove that one of two persons was guilty, but cannot prove which one committed the offence, neither is guilty, unless it is shown that one was the principal, the other the accessory. In that situation it does not matter which was the principal, which the accessory.

If the triers of fact find that of the defendants one must be the principal and the other must be the accessory, the Accessories and Abettors Act 1861, s 8, deems the accessory to be the principal and so both are guilty. *Mohan* v *R* [1967] 2 AC 187 (PC) illustrates this proposition. Two defendants attacked their victim with cutlasses. It could not be proved who struck the fatal blow. Both were guilty of murder. Each had been encouraging the other. They both intended (at least) grievous bodily harm. It did not matter that they did not kill as a result of any agreement between them. In *Fitzgerald* [1992] Crim LR 660, which is similar to *Mohan* v *R*, either the accused set fire to a scooter by flicking matches out of the car he was driving or his passenger did so. He was either the principal offender or engaged in a joint unlawful enterprise. He could be convicted on either basis, similarly if he was either the principal or the accessory. In *Swindall* & *Osborne* (1846) 2 Cox CC

141 either the first defendant killed the victim by running him over, with the second accused being the accessory, or the second accused killed him, the first defendant being the accessory. Both parties were guilty where it was proved that each must be liable either as principal or accessory. This authority was applied in *Giannetto* [1997] 1 Cr App R 1 (CA). The accused had either killed his wife himself or he had hired another to do so. He was guilty of murder. Whether he participated as principal or as accessory was irrelevant. Provided he had the *mens rea* of murder or of being a secondary party to murder, he was guilty. This principle can apply to parents. In strict offences in such circumstances neither party is guilty unless the prosecution can show that he had the *mens rea* of being a secondary party: *Smith v Mellors* (1987) 84 Cr App R 279. On the facts each accused had to know that the other was over the limit when it could not be proved who was driving.

The Domestic Violence Crime and Victims Act 2004 provides a partial solution to the difficulty of proving which of two or more defendants attacked a child. The Act differs from the Law Commission Reports, *Children: Their Non-Accidental Death or Serious Injury (Criminal Trials)*, Law Com. Nos 279 and 282, 2003. It creates an offence of causing the death of a child or other vulnerable person. The offence may be committed by killing or failing to protect a member of the accused's household from a known threat or from a threat which ought to have been known of from another person in that household, and the accused did not take such steps as could reasonably be expected to protect the victim. The killing of the victim must occur in circumstances which the accused did foresee or ought to have foreseen. Although this is a serious offence akin to manslaughter, negligence (and not even gross negligence) suffices as the mental element. The maximum sentence is 14 years' imprisonment.

This chapter deals with participatory offences deriving from the common law. There are similar statutory provisions such as s 28(1) of the Sexual Offences Act 1956: encouraging unlawful sexual intercourse with a girl under 16 for whom he is responsible. Unless Parliament excludes the possibility, one can be a secondary party to any offence: *Jefferson* [1994] 1 All ER 270 (CA). One can, for example, be an accomplice to an attempted offence, for an attempt is itself an offence.

Under the draft Criminal Code, Law Com. No. 177, 1989, a person may be liable as principal or accessory, and defences apply to both, unless in relation to both propositions Parliament provides otherwise (cl 25). The principal is the person who does the act or acts with the requisite fault element, or 'does at least one such act and procures, assists or encourages any other such acts done by another; or (c) . . . procures, assists or encourages any other such acts done by another who is not himself guilty of the offence because – (i) he is under 10 years of age; or (ii) he does the act or acts without the fault required for the offence; or (iii) he has a defence' (cl 26(1)). Sub-clause (1)(c):

> applies notwithstanding that the definition of the offence – (a) implies that the specified act or acts must be done by the offender personally; or (b) indicates that the offender must comply with a description which applies only to the other person referred to in sub-cl (1)(c).

By cl 28(2)(a) a person may be convicted as an accessory even though the principal has not been identified, charged or convicted. To a large extent both present law and the draft Criminal Code are based on 'derivative liability'. The criminal culpability of the secondary offender derives from the liability of the principal. Not until the primary offence has been committed is the secondary party liable. Inroads have been made into the doctrine and it may be that an accomplice can be found guilty where only the *actus reus* of the principal offence has been committed (see below) and therefore the alleged perpetrator is not guilty.

The Law Commission's proposals outlined below would make assisting and encouraging crimes into inchoate offences like those discussed in Chapter 10, thereby abolishing the principle of derivative liability.

This Chapter considers the *actus reus* and then the *mens rea* of accomplices.

Definitions and terminology

The principal is the person who commits the crime. The secondary party is the one who in some sense assists or encourages the principal. One must be a secondary party of an offence charged. One is, for example, an accomplice to murder and not simply an accomplice.

By the Accessories and Abettors Act 1861, s 8, as amended,

> [W]hosoever shall aid, abet, counsel or procure the commission of any indictable offence shall be liable to be tried indicted and punished as a principal offender.

There is a similar provision for summary crimes: Magistrates' Courts Act 1980, s 44. Therefore, the accessory may be charged as a principal. The effect is stark. The person who encourages the principal offender to kill is guilty of the same crime as the killer. The practice should be to charge as an accessory in order to give the defendant detail of the accusation: **DPP for NI v Maxwell** [1978] 1 WLR 1350 (HL). However, this practice seems to be rarely adopted, and accessories are charged as principals. The practice was held not to be a breach of Article 6(3) of the European Convention of Human Rights in **Mercer** [2001] EWCA Crim 638, despite the Article's wording that an accused is entitled to be told 'in detail of the nature and cause of the accusation against him'. It was sufficient for the accused to be charged as one of three persons engaged in a joint enterprise (see below) when in fact he was the getaway driver.

The accomplice is subject to the same penalty as the principal, though the degree of participation may affect sentence. Exceptionally, the Road Traffic Offenders Act 1988, s 34(5), provides that disqualification of accessories is discretionary but disqualification of principals is mandatory. In the well-known case of **Craig and Bentley** (1952) *The Times*, 10–13 December, the accused who killed could not be hanged because he was under age. However, the secondary party is by s 8 liable to be punished as principal and was hanged, even though he did not fire the shot. (Bentley received a posthumous pardon in 1998.) It is arguable that while sometimes the accessory is worse than the principal (as when he is a 'godfather'), on the facts of this case – and perhaps of most – the accessory should not be punishable to the same extent as the principal, for he may be less culpable than the latter.

There is nowadays very little distinction between principals and accessories. 'The law no longer concerns itself with niceties of degrees of participation in crime' is how the Court of Appeal put it in **Cogan and Leak** [1976] QB 217. The chief differences of substantive law are that one cannot be an accessory to an attempted crime, there are differences in the *mens rea* of principals and accessories, only a principal can be liable vicariously, sometimes only certain people can be guilty as principals (only a man may be convicted of rape as a principal but a woman may be convicted as an accessory), and the law on strict liability does not apply to accessories (see below). Beyond these matters the capacity in which the accused acted is irrelevant. Whether a person acted as accessory or joint principal is immaterial.

Terminology has changed since the older cases were reported. A principal in the first degree is nowadays the principal. A principal in the second degree is an aider, abettor and perhaps procurer. He assisted at the time when the offence was committed. An accessory before the fact was not present at the scene of the crime. He is now a counsellor, procurer or aider. An accessory after the fact, a person who assisted after the crime, was guilty of a crime now abolished. That offence has been partly replaced by s 4(1) ('impeding') and s 5(1) ('concealing and giving false information') of the Criminal Law Act 1967 (see below). Even though some terminology has been modernised, not all has been updated. The person in the street may have difficulty in defining 'abet'.

For more on impeding and concealing, see pp 204–5 in Chapter 5.

An accessory can be liable as a secondary party to a greater crime than that committed by the principal. The House of Lords so ruled in *Howe* [1987] AC 417, overruling a previous authority to the contrary. What the accused is guilty of depends on his state of mind, not on the offence the principal committed. Accordingly a person may be guilty of aiding murder when the principal is guilty only of grievous bodily harm. *Howe* represents a break from the orthodox English theory of derivative liability: there is no single principal offence to which the accused is a party. The intended more serious offence did not take place. By s 2(4) of the Homicide Act 1957 the defence of diminished responsibility for one party does not affect the liability of others. The same, it is suggested, applies to other forms of voluntary manslaughter.

To be liable as an accomplice, the principal offence must have been committed. That is why secondary liability is sometimes said to be based on the principle of 'derivative liability'. The accomplice is not, generally speaking, liable unless the principal offender is. The secondary's liability derives from the principal's liability. The ancient authority for this proposition is *Vaux* (1591) 76 ER 992. If it has not, there may still be conviction for one of the inchoate offences: incitement, attempt and conspiracy. If, therefore, a person advises on an offence, but the principal does not commit the offence, the person is not a counsellor, but an inciter. Both abetting and incitement are based on one party's persuading another to do something. Current law has been criticised on the ground that basing liability of the secondary offender on the liability of the principal fails to support the policy of intervening before crimes have been committed.

Being an accomplice is not in itself an offence. There has to be a principal offence to which one is an accomplice. The charge is not, e.g., 'aiding and abetting' but 'aiding and abetting murder' (or theft, and so on).

'Aid, abet, counsel or procure'

A secondary party is one who aids, abets, counsels or procures the commission of the offence. In *Bryce* [2004] 2 Cr App R 35 (CA) it was said that 'the shades of difference between them are far from clear.' For that reason the charge often involves all four terms. These terms are said (wrongly in the light of history) to mean different things on the ground that 'Parliament would be wasting time in using four words where two or three would do': *Attorney-General's Reference (No. 1 of 1975)* [1975] QB 773 (CA). Unfortunately the court did not state in which respects the verbs differ and it is difficult to see how abetting adds anything not already covered by the other three terms.

(a) Aiding and abetting

In *Bentley v Mullen* [1986] RTR 7 the Divisional Court stated:

As was pointed out in *A-G's Reference (No. 1 of 1975)* . . . , the words 'aiding' and 'abetting' have to be given their ordinary natural meaning. The natural meaning of 'aid' is to give help, support or assistance to and the natural meaning of 'abet' is to incite, instigate or encourage.

It was held that the accused, a driving instructor, aided and abetted the crime of failing to stop after an accident when he walked away with the driver and then both of them returned, hoping that the mess had been cleared away and that they could drive away with no trouble. It is suggested that 'abet' does not have an ordinary meaning because it is no longer used in ordinary language and the definition given in *Bentley v Mullen* also applies to 'counsel'. However, in *NCB v Gamble* [1959] 1 QB 11 and *Lynch v DPP for NI* [1975] AC 653, 'aid' and 'abet' were thought to be synonymous. In *NCB v Gamble* Devlin J said that counselling took place before the crime, whereas abetting occurred at the time of the offence, but this distinction seems to have disappeared over the last half-century. In *Lynch* 'aid and abet' were thought to be the same concept: 'aid' was the *actus reus* of that concept; 'abet' was the *mens rea*. No authority was supplied for this proposition. Under present law an aider is an accused who assists the principal offender, e.g. by supplying a gun or metal-cutting equipment, and an abettor is the person who acts to incite, instigate or encourage the principal at the time of the offence. The Court of Appeal in *Giannetto* (above) both stated that abetting covered 'any involvement from mere encouragement upwards' and approved the trial judge's statement that patting a person on the back and saying 'oh, goody' constituted abetting if done and said in response to the principal saying 'I am going to murder your wife'.

The definition of abetting looks very much like counselling. The aider gives help or support to the principal such as occurs where the accused drives the principal to the scene of the crime. Aiding can take place before or during the crime. Devlin J in *NCB v Gamble* and Lord Lowry in the Northern Ireland Court of Criminal Appeal in *DPP for NI v Maxwell*, above, adopted similar definitions.

(b) Counselling

A counsellor is a person who before the commission of the offence (and often not at the scene of the offence) conspires to commit it, advises its commission or knowingly gives assistance to the principal: *DPP for NI v Maxwell* (HL). Giving information to and urging the principal also fall within 'counselling'. The accused must be in contact with the principal.

The old distinction between abetting and counselling was that abetting took place at the time of the offence, whereas counselling occurred before. The requirement of presence at the crime seems to have disappeared, though it is still sometimes mentioned in the cases. In *Attorney-General v Able* [1984] 1 QB 795, a civil case, there was discussion of whether a person aided and abetted suicide by publishing a booklet about the various methods. Under old law the appropriate charge would have been counselling suicide, not aiding and abetting, because the writer would not have been present at the self-killing. Similarly in the civil case of *Gillick v West Norfolk and Wisbech AHA* [1986] AC 112 the House of Lords discussed whether a doctor would be aiding and abetting sexual intercourse with a girl under 16, which is a crime, by prescribing contraceptives to her. If aiding and abetting are restricted to events at the time of the offence, it is very difficult to envisage a doctor being present at the time of the illegal sexual intercourse. Either the House of Lords should have been discussing counselling and procuring or the rule has disappeared. In *Rook* [1993] 1 WLR 1005 the accused arranged the killing of the wife of one of his co-defendants. The Court of Appeal applied the same law on joint principals (see below) whether he was present or not. If presence at the scene of the crime is required, as it was at the time of *Bowker v Premier Drug Co Ltd* [1928] 1 KB 217, the 'scene' is construed broadly to include the place where the lookout man was. The suggestion remains, however, that this former rule no longer exists. (Cf. *Lynch* where the accused, who was guilty as aider and abettor, drove a terrorist gang to the scene of the offence.) If abetting means assistance at the time of the offence, it is likely that the accused is at the scene but he need not be. In abetting the accused and principal need not have agreed beforehand that the abettor should join in: *Mohan v R*, above.

(c) Procuring

Lord Widgery CJ in *Attorney-General's Reference (No. 1 of 1975)* said that 'procure' meant 'produce by endeavour'. (It is uncertain whether 'by endeavour' adds anything to 'produce'.) In other words, a procurer instigates or causes the crime. The instigation may take the form of persuasion or even threats. Despite this narrow ruling the Divisional Court in *Blakely v DPP* [1991] Crim LR 763 gave a wider meaning to 'procure'. The accused procures if he foresees something as a possible consequence of his behaviour. If this is so, in procuring there is, contrary to previous authority, no need for the accused to cause the principal party to commit an offence. However, in *Marchant* [2004] 1 WLR 442 (CA) the accused, who directed the driver to drive on the road, was held to be not guilty of procuring death by dangerous driving when a motor cyclist drove on to a spike on the grab unit at the front of his agricultural vehicle. Driving the vehicle on a public road did not cause the death of the victim and the accused did not procure the driver to cause death. The next case illustrates the thrust of the law. In *Attorney-General's Reference (No. 1 of 1975)*, the Lord Chief Justice held the accused guilty of procuring the principal (who did not realise what was happening) to drive with a blood-alcohol concentration above the legal limit when he had laced his drink with alcohol. Hosts who give their guests lots of alcohol should be aware of this decision. Lord Widgery considered that if the principal was aware that his drinks were being laced, the alleged accessory would probably not be guilty of procuring this offence because the principal's knowledge and his 'free, deliberate and informed' decision to drive off would break the chain of causation. It used to be said that procuring takes place before the commission of the principal offence, but there seems no reason why it cannot cover producing by endeavour at the time of the offence.

(d) 'Causal link'

In abetting and counselling it seems that there must be consensus between secondary party and principal; that is, the principal must be aware that he is being assisted or encouraged, though it need not be proved that he would not have committed the offence without the assistance or encouragement: *Calhaem* [1985] 1 QB 808. The Court of Appeal held that the accused was guilty of being a secondary party to murder when she hired a man to kill her rival in love, even though he had decided not to kill her but changed his mind when she screamed and he killed her. In aiding there need be no consensus. The principal need not be (but can be) aware that he is being assisted. In procuring the secondary party must be proved to have caused the offence. For example, in *Attorney-General's Reference (No. 1 of 1975)* the accused was guilty of procuring the principal to drive with excess alcohol in his body when he surreptitiously laced his drinks. Lord Widgery CJ said: 'You cannot procure an offence unless there is a causal link between what you do and the commission of the offence.' Accordingly, the accused would not have been guilty of procuring driving with excess alcohol if the principal was already over the limit when he supplied him with alcohol. There need, however, be no communication, no consensus, between the parties. There is a statement in this case that usually in aiding, abetting and counselling the parties will have met, but a meeting is not a requirement of these offences. In procuring the parties need never have known each other and, as the facts show, the principal need not know that he is being helped to break the law, nor need he make up his mind to break the criminal law. It is suggested that whatever the mental element in the other forms of accomplice liability, one can procure an outcome only intentionally ('by endeavour').

In *Bryce* [2004] 2 Cr App R 35 the court held that in respect of all for types of secondary participation the accused had to have what Lord Widgery CJ called a 'causal link' with the principal. The accused drove the principal offender to a caravan near where the victim lived. The principal the next day killed the victim. It was held that there was a causal link with the effect that the accused was guilty of counselling the principal. It had been argued, particularly by Sir John Smith, that there did not need to be a causal link for counselling but this case holds that for all forms of participation there must be a causal nexus. That link, however, is broken only by an 'overwhelming supervening event', relegating the accused's conduct to the mere setting for the offence.

(e) Framing the charge

The charge is generally one of 'aiding, abetting, counselling or procuring'. The accused is convicted if he participated in any of those ways: *Ferguson v Weaving* [1951] 1 KB 814. This is done because 'the shades of difference between [these terms] are far from clear': *Bryce*, above. One is a secondary party to the principal offence. One does not 'aid' in general but one aids a particular crime. Aiding (etc.) is not in itself a crime but a way in which a crime is committed.

Failure to act

Omission is described in Chapter 2 on p 70.

The basic rule, as elsewhere in criminal law, is that an omission does not give rise to liability unless there is a duty to act. Presence at the scene of the principal offence does not necessarily mean that the accused is an accessory, though it may be evidence of encouragement. The old-established authority is *Coney* (1882) 8 QBD 534, where standing watching a prize fight did not mean that the spectators were aiding an illegal boxing match. Hawkins J said that 'some active steps must be taken by word or action'. The accused would have been guilty had he cheered or applauded. Another old case is *Atkinson* (1869) 11 Cox CC 330. An employer was not guilty of being a secondary party to a riot by his employees when he did nothing to stop it. More recent is *Clarkson* [1971] 3 All ER 344 (CMAC) where drunken soldiers stood around while a girl was raped in a barracks. A perhaps worse case is the Ontario one of *Salajko* [1970] 1 Can CC 352 where the accused, who had his trousers around his ankles, watched a gang rape. There are several similar cases such as *Bland* [1988] Crim LR 41 (CA): the accused was not guilty of being a secondary party to the crime of unlawfully possessing controlled drugs by continuing to share a room with the principal offender after she found out about the drugs. It could not be inferred that she assisted him in his possession of the drugs. She would be guilty if she encouraged the principal or if she had a right of control (see below). Presence at a crime is some evidence that the accused did encourage the principals: e.g. *Allen v Ireland* [1984] 1 WLR 903 (CA). A secret resolve to help one's friend in a fight is not sufficient: *Allan* [1965] 1 QB 130 (CCA). Accordingly there must be an act of encouragement or assistance (but see below for duty situations). A case drawing the line is *Wilcox v Jeffery* [1951] 1 All ER 464 (CCA) where the accused invited an alien saxophonist, Coleman Hawkins, into the UK contrary to the Aliens Order, met him at the airport, clapped his performance and wrote about him. He was guilty of aiding and abetting the breach of the Order by encouraging the principal party. Similar is **Ellis** [2008] EWCA Crim 886. Encouraging attackers is participating in crime; it would have been different if, as in **Clarkson**, the accused had simply stood around while the victim was being beaten up. There is, moreover, no need for the accused to be present at the scene of the principal offence: **JF Alford Transport Ltd** [1997] 2 Cr App R 326 (CA). In this case the accused, a company and its managers, were guilty of aiding and abetting employees to make false entries on tachograph records (which state how many miles the driver has driven in the day). They knew what the employees were doing. They had the legal right to stop them, but they had done nothing.

Where there is a duty to act in order to control the behaviour of the principal, the accused is guilty of being an accessory (provided the other elements are fulfilled) if he does nothing to prevent the occurrence of the crime. The accused must know that he had an opportunity of intervening to prevent the commission of the substantive crime: **Webster** [2006] EWCA Crim 415. In **Rubie v Faulkner** [1940] 1 KB 571, an instructor of a learner driver was convicted of aiding and abetting driving without due care and attention. There was no need for direct control over the steering wheel. Hilbery J said: '. . . the supervisor could see the driver was about to do the unlawful act of which he was convicted [careless driving] and the magistrates found that the supervisor remained passive . . . For him to refrain from doing anything when he could see that an unlawful act was about to be done, and his duty was to prevent an unlawful act, if he could, was for him to aid and abet.' In **Tuck v Robson** [1970] 1 All ER 1171, a pub landlord did not make his customers leave. He was convicted of aiding their consumption of alcohol after time. Simply calling 'Time, glasses please' and turning off the main lights did not serve to exonerate the landlord. Failure to prevent was also taken to be assistance or encouragement (that is, one need not prove that the accused's omission did in fact encourage or assist the principal) in **Du Cros v Lambourne** [1907] 1 KB 40, where the owner of the car, who was at the time of the principal offence a passenger, did not stop the driver from driving at a dangerous speed. (In fact it could not be proved who was driving. If the owner was driving, he was the principal offender. If he was the passenger, he had a right of control. Whichever seat he was in, he was guilty.) The same result occurs where, e.g., a mother watches her husband killing their child. She has a duty to intervene. (A stranger has no such duty: see Chapter 2.) Similarly a police officer is under a duty to prevent another officer hitting a suspect: **Forman** [1988] Crim LR 677.

The outcome in these cases would have been different if the accused had no right of control or duty to act. In that eventuality inactivity would not constitute being a secondary party. To secure a conviction, the prosecution would have to prove that the accused encouraged or assisted. For example, in **Du Cros v Lambourne** if the car had belonged to the other party, the accused would have had no right of control over it. As a passenger he would not have been guilty unless he authorised or encouraged the dangerous driving. Cases such as **Tuck v Robson** are getting a bit long in the tooth. Modern authorities are necessary to determine the scope of this exception to the general rule of non-liability for omissions.

The Law Commission's draft Criminal Code, Law Com. No. 177, 1989, rationalises present law in cl 27(3) by creating a general principle. Assistance or encouragement includes assistance or encouragement arising from a failure by a person to take reasonable steps to exercise any authority or discharge any duty he has to control the relevant acts of the principal in order to prevent the commission of the offence.

Mens rea

A person is not liable as an accessory unless he has the required mental elements. These elements apply to all principal offences, including strict liability ones. There is therefore a difference between the *mens rea* of the secondary offence and that of the principal party. The Court of Appeal in **Rook**, above, which was approved in **Bryce**, above, stated that the mental element is the same for aiding, abetting, counselling and procuring. The law is relatively underdeveloped. The following strives to encapsulate it.

The accused must intend to do the act which constitutes the encouraging, advising or assisting. One authority among several is **Bryce**.

Intention to encourage, advise or assist

An accessory is guilty only if he did acts which he knew were capable of encouraging and assisting: **JF Alford Transport Ltd** (above). There is no need to prove that the accused intended that the crime be committed: **Rook**, above, which was endorsed in **Bryce**, above. Potter LJ said in **Bryce**: '. . . it is sufficient if the secondary party at the time of his actions . . . contemplates the commission of the offence, that is knows that it will be committed or realises that it is a real possibility that it will be committed'. As elsewhere in the criminal law motive is irrelevant. The principal authority is **NCB v Gamble**.

NCB v Gamble [1959] QB 11

An employee of the National Coal Board, the precursor of British Coal, was the weighbridge operator. He told a driver that his lorry was overladen. Driving an overladen vehicle is an offence. The driver said that he was prepared to take the risk of being caught and the employee gave him a weighbridge ticket, without which the driver could not have left the pit. Was the employee guilty of being a secondary party to the principal offence of driving an over-laden lorry?

The Divisional Court held that he was. Devlin J said:

> An indifference to the result of the crime does not of itself negative abetting. If one man deliberately sells to another a gun to be used for murdering a third, he may be indifferent about whether the third man lives or dies and interested only in the cash profit to be made out of the sale, but he can still be an aider and abettor. To hold otherwise would be to negative the rule that *mens rea* is a matter of intent only and does not depend on desire or motive.

Since the employee had intentionally assisted the principal he was liable as accessory. The effect of **NCB v Gamble** should be noted. If the accused knows that the bag of sugar he has just sold to the principal may be used by him to cosh an old lady in a house in which the principal will be rummaging for money to steal, he will be guilty of being an accessory to aggravated burglary. His intention is not that the principal will cosh the old lady. He is happy to have made the sale and does not care how the principal will use the sugar. The principle also catches the landlord who sells alcohol to a man who he knows intends to drive.

There is no need for the accused's *purpose* to be the commission of the crime; oblique intent suffices, as was said in **JF Alford Transport Ltd**, above. It is the intent to aid, abet,

173

counsel or procure which counts, and it has indeed at times been suggested that knowledge that acts may assist is sufficient for liability, though cases such as *Gamble* reject this approach. There is earlier authority for the proposition that it is not counselling or procuring when the accused hopes that the offence will not be committed, at least if the accused tries to stop the principal party committing the offence (cf. *Lynch* v *DPP for NI*, above, where the accused, who drove terrorists to a place where they murdered their victim, was guilty but it has to be said that he did not make strenuous efforts to prevent the killing). In *Fretwell* (1862) 9 Cox CC 471 (CCR), a lover gave his woman a drug to cause an abortion under threats of her suicide. He hoped that she would not take it but she did. She died. He was held not to be a secondary party to her suicide, which at that time was an offence. The case appears to be wrongly decided in the light of *NCB* v *Gamble* because it is one in which motive exonerated the accused: he did not wish to see her dead. It has been said in the civil case of *Attorney-General* v *Able* [1984] QB 795 to be restricted to its own facts. However, *Fretwell* was cited approvingly in *Gamble* for the proposition that knowingly supplying an article does not amount to an intent to aid, and it has not been overruled. In *Bryce*, above, the Court of Appeal reiterated the law that one could intend to assist a principal even though one intended to hinder his plans. The same was true in *Lynch*. In *Rook*, above, the court said that the accused was guilty even though it was not his intention that the principal offence was committed.

There is a statement in *NCB* v *Gamble* that an accessory is not liable if before delivery ownership passed and the accused was not aware of the illegal purpose until after ownership passed. (On the facts ownership of the coal passed when the employee gave the driver the ticket.) If this *dictum* were correct, and the law remains uncertain, then if the alleged accessory sold a gun to the principal but before handing it over found out that it was to be used to kill someone, he would not be guilty, whereas he would be guilty if he knew from the start of the transaction that the gun would be used to kill. Similarly, to use the facts of an early case, if the accused handed over the principal's jemmy to him, he would not be liable, for he was doing what in law he was obliged to do. It is suggested that this distinction does not serve any purpose. It is also not soundly based on civil law, as the Divisional Court seemed to think. An illegal contract is unenforceable no matter when the seller, the accessory, comes to know of the illegality. More recent is *Garrett* v *Arthur Churchill (Glass) Ltd* [1970] 1 QB 92 (CA). Lord Parker CJ said that the legal duty to hand the item over is subordinated to the public interest in preventing a crime being committed with the item. This issue is dealt with in cl 27(6)(c) of the draft Criminal Code, where the accused is not guilty if he believes that he is under a legal obligation to do the act and acts 'without the purpose of furthering the commission of the offence'. A person supplying an article in the ordinary course of business would, therefore, not be liable.

Knowledge of 'the essential matters'

Lord Goddard CJ said in *Johnson* v *Youden* [1950] 1 KB 544 (which was approved in *Churchill* v *Walton* [1967] 2 AC 224 (HL), a case on conspiracy, by the Privy Council in *Mok Wai Tak* v *R* [1990] 2 AC 333 and by the Court of Appeal in *Roberts* [1997] Crim LR 209) that:

> [B]efore a person can be convicted of aiding and abetting the commission of an offence he must at least know the essential matters which constitute that offence. He need not actually know that an offence has been committed, because he may not know that the facts constitute an offence and ignorance of the law is not a defence.

Solicitors were not guilty of conveying a house at a price above the maximum, when they did not know the price. While not pellucid, the phrase 'essential matters' seems to include the circumstances of the *actus reus*, any relevant consequences and perhaps the principal's fault element. The circumstances are the facts which give rise to the offence. If a person supplies a ladder, he is not guilty of aiding burglary unless he knows 'the facts [which] constitute the offence'. However, the accused, as Lord Goddard CJ put it, 'need not actually know that an offence has been committed, because he may not know that the facts constitute an offence and ignorance of the law is no defence'. 'Wilful blindness' is sufficient: *D Stanton & Sons Ltd* v *Webber* [1973] RTR 86 (DC) and *Roberts*, above.

It was said in *Carter* v *Richardson* [1976] Crim LR 190 that 'know the essential matters' extends to recklessness as to circumstances and wilful blindness as to a risk that the facts constituting the principal offence probably would occur (see Chapter 3). The supervisor of a learner driver was held to be guilty of abetting the learner to drive with a blood-alcohol concentration above the limit. He knew that the learner was above the limit, but *obiter* the court said that he would have been guilty if he thought that the driver was probably over the limit, the state of mind known as subjective recklessness. In *Blakely* v *DPP*, above, the accused's conviction for procuring a person to drive above that limit was quashed because the justices had used the *Caldwell* definition. The accused were the principal's mistress and a friend. They spiked his non-alcoholic drink with vodka in an attempt to prevent him driving back to his wife. In fact he drove off before they could tell him the truth. The Divisional Court said that the accused's knowledge that his act might help the commission of the principal offence was sufficient for aiding, abetting and counselling and probably for procuring. *Blakely* v *DPP* was approved in *Webster* [2006] EWCA Crim 415. 'It is the defendant's foresight that the principal was likely to commit the offence which must be proved and not merely that he ought to have foreseen that the principal was likely to commit the offence.'

It may be that *Blakely* is wider than *Carter* v *Richardson*. In the latter case the secondary party was reckless as to circumstances, namely, the amount of alcohol in the blood, but was intentional as to encouraging this principal's driving, whereas in the former case she was reckless as to both and would have been convicted on a proper direction. If so, the spectre of liability of hosts at parties resurrects itself. He will be guilty of aiding drunk driving if he was aware that his conduct might encourage the commission of this offence. By definition, however, procuring requires that the accused must intend to bring about the principal offence. As the court said in *Blakely* v *DPP*: '. . . mere awareness that [the principal offence] might result would not suffice'. Nevertheless, while stating that *Caldwell* recklessness, which existed at that time, would also not suffice, it did not rule subjective recklessness out. The draft Criminal Code does not permit *Caldwell* recklessness and would confirm the court's view in *Blakely* v *DPP* that recklessness is defined in *Cunningham* terms. Clause 27(1)(b), quoted below, would preserve recklessness as to circumstances, an outcome in accord with the present law of attempt, but there must be intent as to the principal's conduct: *Carter* v *Richardson* would be overruled. If *Carter* v *Richardson* is correct it may apply only to strict offences.

The Divisional Court in *Blakely* v *DPP* said that in procuring and perhaps counselling and commanding it must be shown that the accused intended to bring about the principal offence and that the position might be different in relation to other forms of participation where the accused assisted the principal. In relation to forms of secondary participation such as counselling where the accused is encouraging the principal before the commission of the offence, the accused can hardly be said to 'know' the facts surrounding the crime. It is better to say that the accused must believe that action will occur

Caldwell recklessness is described in Chapter 3 on pp 110–16. Compare with *Cunningham* recklessness.

which will give rise to an offence. It is difficult to square these authorities with the definition of procuring as 'produce by endeavour'. Procuring would seem to require intent alone.

An example of the requirement of knowledge is *Ferguson* v *Weaving* [1951] 1 KB 814. A pub landlady was not guilty of aiding and abetting the offence of consuming alcohol after hours when she did not know that the customers were so doing. This rule even applies to strict offences. In *Callow* v *Tillstone* (1900) 19 Cox CC 576, a butcher was convicted of the strict offence of exposing unsound meat for sale. The vet who had examined the heifer at the butcher's request was not guilty of aiding and abetting the offence because he did not know of the unsoundness of the meat. He was not guilty even though he had performed his inspection carelessly. In terms of justice, the case looks topsy-turvy. The butcher who had done his best not to expose unsound meat for sale was guilty, while the vet, who was careless over such an important matter, was not guilty.

As stated above, knowledge of the 'essential matters' includes knowledge of the principal's *mens rea*. The accused does not aid murder if the principal does not possess malice aforethought.

Both intention to encourage or assist and knowledge (subject to *Carter* v *Richardson*) of the essential facts are necessary for conviction as an accessory. The width of these rules should be noted. If a person provides the principal with a room, turning a blind eye to the fact that the principal is going to set up girls in a brothel, he is guilty of being an accessory to living off the earnings of prostitutes. The question of whether a doctor who prescribes contraceptives to a girl under the age of 16 intends to aid and abet unlawful sexual intercourse has exercised minds. The House of Lords thought not in *Gillick* v *West Norfolk and Wisbech AHA* [1986] AC 112, a civil case, but the decision looks incorrect. It has been suggested that doctors are not guilty because of their good motive, despite the fact that elsewhere in the criminal law motive provides no defence. Another idea is that the defence of necessity applies. An alternative view is that 'intent' in this area of law means 'direct intent'. Since it was not the doctors' purpose to encourage unlawful sex, they are not accessories. Other authorities, however, do not restrict intent to purpose. If *Gillick* is correct, *Fretwell* (discussed above) may also be correct. In respect of secondary participation, where the *actus reus* is an omission, as in *Tuck* v *Robson* (above), the *mens rea* was stated in *JF Alford Transport Ltd* (above) as being: (i) knowledge that the principal was committing a crime; (ii) deliberately turning a blind eye to that crime; and (iii) knowledge that the principal was being encouraged to commit the crime.

The external and fault elements of accessorial liability are restated in cl 27(1) of the draft Criminal Code:

> A person is guilty of an offence as an accessory if –
> (a) he intentionally procures, assists or encourages the act which constitutes or results in the commission of the offence by the principal; and
> (b) he knows, or (where recklessness suffices in the case of the principal) is reckless with respect to, any circumstance that is an element of the offence; and
> (c) he intends that the principal shall act, or is aware that he is or may be acting, or that he may act, with the fault (if any) required for the offence.

By sub-cl (2), '[I]n determining whether a person is guilty of an offence as an accessory it is immaterial that the principal is unaware of that person's act of procurement or assistance.' Clause 27(1)(b) preserves the result in *Carter* v *Richardson*, above. The accused intentionally assisted or encouraged the act (driving) being reckless as to a circumstance (excess alcohol). The mistress in **Blakely v DPP**, above, would, however, not be guilty because she did not procure a circumstance. Driving is not a circumstance but an act. The circumstance was the excess of alcohol, but she intended that circumstance: she was in a state of mind which falls under 'know', not under 'reckless'. Therefore, the phrase in brackets was irrelevant. She did not intentionally procure an act, driving, since her intention was to prevent the principal from driving.

Therefore, 'aid, abet, counsel or procure' are replaced by 'procures, assists, or encourages'. These terms are to be given their everyday meaning, and it does not matter that the accessory was not present at the scene of the offence. The word 'encouragement' is omitted from cl 27(2). The effect is that in relation to that type of secondary participation the principal must know of the encouragement. **Carter v Richardson** is expanded to cover not just crimes where the fault element is satisfied by strict liability, but recklessness. The Law Commission states that the enactment of **Carter v Richardson** merely clarifies the law. The accused intentionally assisted the act (driving) and was reckless as to whether the driver had excess alcohol in his blood.

The result in **Gillick** is preserved by cl 27(6)(b), which states that a person is not liable as an accessory if he acted to prevent harmful consequences provided that he did so 'without the purpose of furthering' the commission of the offence. The Law Commission instances (p. 209) the supply of hypodermic needles to drug users to prevent the spread of AIDS. It is extremely doubtful that such a defence exists at present.

Contemplation of a range of offences

It does not matter that the accessory does not know when and how the principal offence will take place: **Bullock** [1955] 1 WLR 1. On the other hand, it is not sufficient that the principal is going to break the law *simpliciter*. In **Bainbridge** [1960] 1 QB 129 the accused thought that oxyacetylene equipment was to be used to cut up stolen goods. In fact it was used to break into the Midland Bank, Stoke Newington, London. The accused was not guilty. He would have been guilty if he knew that a burglary would take place but he did not know when or in which building (following **Bullock**).

After **Bainbridge** it was thought that the accused was guilty if he knew, in the words of Lord Parker CJ, that 'a crime of the type in question was intended'. This requirement is additional to 'knowledge of the essential matters'. The principal authority despite **Bainbridge** never being overruled and being an English case now is **DPP for NI v Maxwell**, above. Four Law Lords held that the same type of case test was to be widened. Lord Scarman adopted the formulation of Lord Lowry CJ in the Northern Irish Appeal Court. The guilt of the accessory springs 'from the fact that he contemplates the commission of one (or more) of a number of crimes by the principal and he intentionally lends his assistance in order that such a crime will be committed'. The accused is convicted of counselling the offence which actually occurs if he contemplated a range of offences and the actual offence which took place was one of those. **Maxwell** differs from **Bainbridge**, which it did not overrule, because (a) there is no need for knowledge; (b) the accused must foresee the offence committed; (c) the 'type' of offence is not relevant: one looks at the contemplated range of offences. The fifth Law Lord, Lord Hailsham, said 'bullet, bomb or incendiary device, indeed most if not all types of terrorist violence' gave rise to offences of the same type within **Bainbridge**. 'The fact that, in the event, the offence committed by the principals crystallised into one rather than the other of the possible alternatives within his contemplation only means that in the event he was an accessory to that specific offence rather than one of the others.'

As a result of the majority in **Maxwell**, the law can be stated thus:

(a) if the accused knows of the offence, he is liable as accessory;

(b) if the accused knows that one or more of a range of offences will take place, he is guilty if one or more of those offences occur;

(c) if the accused contemplated that one offence was to be committed, but another similar crime took place, he is not guilty. The result would have been different under **Bainbridge**;

(d) if the accused knows only the general class of offence, not the specific offence, it appears that he is guilty.

One issue raised but not resolved in **Maxwell** was: how far into the future does liability stretch? Is the accused guilty as an accessory to an offence 60 years in the future? It is suggested that criminal liability ought not to stretch so far, but the policy under-lying accomplice liability, that of deterring those who encourage crime, may support a conviction. Another problem with **Maxwell** was well put by P. Seago, *Criminal Law*, 4th edn (Sweet & Maxwell, 1994) 127 (the words slightly differ in A. Reed and B. Fitzpatrick, *Criminal Law*, 3rd edn (Thomson, 2006) 113):

> If B suspects A is about to commit burglary and the equipment he has supplied will be used to force open the windows of the premises, will he be liable if A's plan, which he carried out, is to rape a girl who lives there? Your immediate reaction will be to say that this is an entirely different crime from the one B contemplated. However, where A enters the house as a trespasser with intent to rape someone this is burglary . . . and burglary is the very crime B contemplated. Perhaps the courts will take the common sense view . . . and hold B should not be convicted as a party to a particular crime he . . . would not have supported. [The accused will not be an accessory to the rape itself.]

Contrariwise, it might be argued that 'supported' involves motive and it is sufficient if the accused knowingly assisted or encouraged the burglary and accordingly he is guilty.

The principle in **Bullock** is rendered in the draft Criminal Code in this way. By cl 27(4) '. . . a person may be guilty of an offence as an accessory although he does not foresee, or is not aware of, a circumstance of the offence which is not an element of it (for ex-ample, the identity of the victim or the time or place of its commission, where this is not an element of the offence).' Sub-clause (4) is made subject to sub-clause (5).

> Notwithstanding s 24(1) [transferred fault], where a person's act of procurement, assistance or encouragement is done with a view to the commission of an offence only in respect of a specified person or thing, he is not guilty as an accessory to an offence intentionally com-mitted by the principal in respect of some other person or thing.

This sub-clause preserves the rule in **Saunders and Archer** (1573) 75 ER 706, discussed in Chapter 3. **Maxwell** is to be enacted by cl 27(1)(a), quoted above.

Summary of the conduct and fault elements

In **Bryce**, above, the Court of Appeal summarised the law thus. To be guilty of aiding, abetting, counselling or procuring the accused must be proved to have done:

(a) an act . . . which in fact assisted the later commission of the offence;

(b) . . . [the accused] did the act deliberately realising that it was capable of assisting the offence;

(c) . . . [the accused] at the time of doing the act contemplated the commission of the offence by . . . [the principal] i.e. he foresaw it as a 'real or substantial risk' or 'real possibility'; and

(d) . . . [the accused] when doing the act intended to assist the [principal] in what he was doing.

Joint enterprise liability

If two or more persons agree to carry out a common purpose, a joint venture or **joint enterprise**, the secondary party is liable for crimes committed by the principal in executing that purpose, even unforeseen ones, provided that there is not a 'fundamental difference' between the act agreed on and the act carried out. Such crimes are sometimes known as 'collateral offences'. He is guilty irrespective of the actual part he played in the venture. This doctrine means that where a member of an unlawful enterprise kills, members of the group can also be found guilty of murder even though they did not commit the *actus reus* of murder. This point marks a distinction between this form of liability and ordinary accessorial responsibility. In the latter the accused must have encouraged or assisted the principal in the commission of the offence. In the former the accused is guilty without encouragement of assistance. In *Baldessare* (1930) 29 Cox CC 193, two defendants took a car. The first accused drove so recklessly that he killed someone. He was guilty of manslaughter. It was held that the common purpose was reckless driving. The second defendant was convicted of abetting manslaughter, even though the killing was not foreseen by him. Often cases involve two parties who set out to burgle a house. One kills the occupier. The other is guilty of the murder if that crime was committed in pursuance of their common intent, the burglary. The violence need not be contemplated at the start of their venture. It does not matter that the principal cannot be identified: *Conroy*, unreported, 10 February 2000 (CA). Similarly, if there is spontaneous violence, that is, violence about which there was no plan (as distinguished from where there was a plan but one accused went beyond what was agreed), the question for the jury is whether the actions of the participants and what they knew led to the inference of a joint enterprise: *O'Flaherty* [2004] 2 Cr App R 315 (CA). On the facts there was evidence that one of the accused pursued the victim as part of a joint enterprise with others. When the others attacked and killed the victim, he was holding a cricket bat at the scene of the killing and was, it seems, encouraging them. The others, however, did not form part of the joint enterprise. They had originally been part of the group which attacked the victim but they did not join in the pursuit of him to a different place. That pursuit was not part of the joint plan. Therefore, there was no evidence that these two defendants were at the time of the killing part of the joint enterprise.

If, however, there was no joint enterprise, but one of only two persons could have committed the offence, as we have seen neither is guilty if it cannot be proved which one did it. For example, in *Swallow v DPP* [1991] Crim LR 610 (DC), where the preventing of the recording of electricity by means of a black box had to have been done either by the landlord or by his wife, neither was to be convicted. Both would have been liable if both knew of the black box and the rest of the *mens rea* and *actus reus* existed. Similarly in *Petters* [1995] Crim LR 501 (CA) there was no joint enterprise where two persons had come separately to a car park and one of them had kicked the victim to death. They had not communicated to one another the fact that they had a common objective. Therefore, their conviction for manslaughter was quashed. The law is that separate actions by two defendants do not constitute a joint enterprise. They had to share a common purpose.

Joint enterprise differs from joint principalship liability. In the latter both defendants had the external and fault element for the principal offence. In the former only one accused did. It is the liability of the other accused which is at issue in this section. There is a debate, which is noted below, as to whether joint enterprise is merely one part of the law of accessorial liability or whether it constitutes a separate area. If the law is separate, the joint enterprise principle is that the accused is liable according to his own *mens rea*. Therefore, the principal may be a murderer, but the accused may be guilty only of manslaughter. If the accused is a true secondary party, he is liable as an accessory of the principal's actual offence. An example of this point is this: if two defendants have a common purpose, they are engaged in a joint enterprise; if, however, one accused spontaneously comes to the other's aid, there is no such venture but there could be a conviction in the ordinary way for secondary participation.

If, however, there is a joint enterprise, but one party intentionally goes beyond what was agreed, the accessory is not liable for the unforeseen circumstances. A blow with a knife is not within the contemplation of an accessory who expected a blow with a fist. Whether the principal exceeded the scope of the agreement is a question of fact. In **Davies v DPP** [1954] AC 378, there was a gang-fight on Clapham Common, London. The first accused stabbed the victim to death. The second accused, though a member of the same gang, did not know of the knife. The first accused was guilty of murder, but the second was not an accomplice to that offence. The use of the knife was not within his contemplation. Similarly, the abandonment of a car by the driver who has joy-ridden in it and left it in gear with the result that it mounted the pavement and killed a baby in a pram were not within the contemplation of the accused; the grossly negligent acts were not in pursuance of the joint enterprise (joy-riding) but beyond anything the accused contemplated as a real possibility: **Mahmood** [1994] Crim LR 368 (CA).

If the accused knows that the principal *will* commit an offence if need be to carry out their joint enterprise, he will be liable if the principal does carry out that offence: **Betts and Ridley** (1930) 22 Cr App R 148.

Powell; English now forms the landmark authorities on joint enterprise. Two appeals were heard together by the House of Lords.

Powell; English [1998] AC 147

In **Powell** the two defendants went to the home of a drug dealer in order to buy drugs. The dealer was shot dead, apparently by a third party. The defendants were convicted of murder on the basis that they knew that the third party was armed with a gun and foresaw that he might use it to kill or cause serious harm to the dealer. The House of Lords dismissed their appeals. In **English** the two defendants jointly attacked a police sergeant with wooden posts. A third person killed him with a knife. The defendants did not know that he had a knife. The first accused appealed against the judge's direction that he was guilty of murder if he had taken part in a joint unlawful enterprise, knowing that there was a substantial risk that the third person might kill or cause grievous bodily harm. The appeal was allowed.

The following propositions can be drawn from the speeches and later developments.

(a) 'A secondary party to a criminal enterprise may be criminally liable for a greater criminal offence committed by the primary offender of a type which the former foresaw but did not necessarily intend' (Lord Steyn). The Privy Council advice in **Chan Wing-siu v R** [1985] AC 168 and **Hui Chi-ming v R** [1992] 1 AC 34 was approved. For this reason the defendants in **Powell** were guilty of murder. It should be noted that the secondary party has to be reckless both as to the *actus reus* of the principal crime and as to whether that *actus reus* would be caused by the principal with *mens rea*. Earlier cases seem to have required recklessness only as to the *actus reus*.

Why was the accessory liable for murder when he did not intend to kill or cause grievous bodily harm?

- First, the House of Lords in **Moloney** [1985] AC 905 and **Hancock and Shankland** [1986] AC 455 (which are discussed in Chapter 3) did not lay down any rule as to accessories. Therefore, they are not authoritative on the law of what Lord Steyn called the 'accessory principle', namely that 'criminal liability is dependent on proof of subjective foresight on the part of a participant in the criminal enterprise that the primary offender might commit a greater offence'.

See Figure 12.3 in Chapter 12 for a diagram illustrating constructive (unlawful act) manslaughter.

- Secondly, if the secondary party has a lesser *mens rea* than the principal offender, his liability is not a form of constructive liability. The House of Lords did not explain what it meant by 'constructive liability', but the best current illustration is constructive manslaughter. The accused is liable even though he did not foresee death or grievous bodily harm: it suffices that he foresaw a lesser crime such as battery.

- Thirdly, while it was accepted that it was anomalous that an accessory could be guilty of murder even though he was merely reckless as to death or grievous bodily harm, 'practical and policy considerations', as Lord Steyn put it, militate against the secondary party's not being convicted of murder. If intent was needed, it would be hard to prove, thereby undermining 'the utility of the accessory principle'. 'Experience has shown that joint criminal enterprises only too readily escalate into the commission of greater offences. In order to deal with this important social problem the accessory principle is needed and cannot be abolished or relaxed' (Lord Steyn). The public must be protected against gangs. Sir John Smith 'Criminal liability of accessories: law and law reform' (1997) 113 LQR 453 added: 'The accessory to murder . . . must be proved to have been reckless, not merely whether death might be caused, but whether murder might be committed; he must have been aware, not merely that death or grievous bodily harm might be caused, but that it might be caused intentionally . . .' Lord Steyn approved this passage in **Powell; English**, above. The argument to the contrary is that an accused who did not intend to kill or commit GBH is by definition not guilty of murder. He may have been reckless as to death or GBH but that is not sufficient *mens rea* for murder as a principal offender. Therefore, he should be convicted of manslaughter, because he has foreseen the risk that the principal might kill or commit GBH.

  There is a strong dissent by Kirby J in **Clayton v R** [2006] HCA 58 on the point that accessories may be murderers without their having malice aforethought. He wished to 'restore greater concurrence between moral culpability and criminal responsibility' by replacing the 'seriously unprincipled' law that a secondary offender is liable for murder 'merely on the foresight of a possibility'.

(b) Lord Hutton stated in relation to the degree of foresight necessary for conviction: 'the secondary party is subject to criminal liability if he contemplated the act causing the death as a possible incident of the joint venture, unless the risk was so remote that the jury take the view that the secondary party genuinely dismissed it as altogether negligible'.

(c) As Lord Parker CJ said in **Anderson and Morris** [1966] 2 QB 110, 'if one of the adventurers goes beyond what has been tacitly agreed as part of the common enterprise, his co-adventurer is not liable for the consequences of that unauthorised act'. There need be no tacit agreement; foresight suffices: *Hyde* [1991] 1 QB 134 (CA) was approved. It remains a question of fact whether the principal offender has acted in a fundamentally different manner from what was agreed: *Attorney-General's Reference (No. 3 of 2004)* [2006] Crim LR 63 (CA).

The appellant in *English* fell within this principle. The use of the knife was in the words of Lord Hutton 'fundamentally different to the use of a wooden post', despite the fact that both could be used to cause serious injuries. The accused was not guilty of murder or manslaughter. Whether the principal acted beyond the scope of the joint enterprise is 'an issue of fact for the common sense of the jury' (Lord Hutton). Later Court of Appeal decisions including *Rafferty* [2007] EWCA Crim 1846 have uniformly applied this 'substantial deviation' law. Some authorities before *Powell; English* had taken the view that if the principal offender had exceeded the limits as foreseen by the accused, the secondary party, the latter was guilty of a less serious offence than a principal. For example, if the principal went beyond the plan and killed, he was guilty of murder: the accessory was guilty of manslaughter. These earlier authorities must now be taken to be wrong. In *Mitchell* [1999] Crim LR 496 the Court of Appeal said *obiter* that a secondary party can no longer be convicted of manslaughter when the principal goes beyond the scope of the joint enterprise and is guilty of murder. However, if the principal intends a serious offence but the accessory contemplates only a minor one, then if the victim dies, the principal is guilty of murder but the accessory only of manslaughter. An example given by the Northern Ireland Court of Criminal Appeal in *Gilmour* [2000] 2 Cr App R 407 was of two parties agreeing to carry out a conspiracy to post an incendiary bomb through a letter box. The principal intends death or serious injury; the accessory foresees superficial harm. The victim dies. The accessory is guilty of (being a secondary party to) manslaughter, not to murder. Lord Carswell CJ saw no 'convincing reason why a person acting as an accessory to a principal who carries out the very deed contemplated by both should not be guilty of the degree of offence appropriate to the interest with which he so acted. This is not a deviation case (as in *Anderson and Morris*) but one of differing *mens rea*. The outcome is one which aligns the defendant's *mens rea* with the crime, which is praiseworthy, but one strange result should be noted. The accused in *English* foresaw grievous bodily harm but was not guilty; the accused in *Gilmour* did not foresee such harm, yet he is guilty! It may be that *Gilmour* and *Powell; English* are irreconcilable. *Powell; English* appears to hold that an accused can be guilty of the same crime as the principal or of nothing, whereas *Gilmour* permits the conviction for an offence lesser than the one committed by the principal.

There are different streams of authority. Cases such as *Day* [2001] Crim LR 984, *Gilmour*, *Stewart and Schofield* [1995] 3 All ER 159 and *Reid* (1975) 62 Cr App R 109 support the view that a secondary party can be guilty of (being an accessory to) a lesser offence such as manslaughter when the principal party is guilty of a more serious crime such as murder. In *Gilmour*, for example, the court distinguished cases such as *Anderson and Morris* and *English* as being ones where 'the principal departs from the contemplated joint enterprise and perpetrates a more serious act of a different kind unforeseen by the accessory. In such cases . . . the accessory is not liable at all for such unforeseen acts. It does not follow that the same result should follow where the principal carries out the very act contemplated by the accessory, though the latter does not realise that the principal intends a more serious consequence . . .' In such an event the accessory may be convicted of a lesser offence than that committed by the principal. Clarification from the House of Lords would be helpful.

(d) In respect of a deviation from the venture Lord Hutton opined: 'if the weapon used by the primary party is different to, but as dangerous as, the weapon which the secondary party contemplated he might use, the secondary party should not escape liability for murder because of the difference in the weapon, for example, if he foresaw that the primary party might use a gun to kill and the latter used a knife to kill, or vice versa'.

Powell; English was applied by the Court of Appeal in *Uddin* [1999] QB 431. The accused had joined in an attack on another man who was having an argument with the driver of a car in which friends of the accused were. Six men in total had attacked the victim with poles or bars. The deceased was killed by a flick-knife wielded by one of the co-defendants. Apparently the accused did not know of the knife. He was convicted at first instance. The Court of Appeal allowed the appeal on the ground that the conviction was unsafe. The flick-knife's use was 'of a completely different type' from the use of poles. However, it ordered a retrial because the jury had not been directed as to the use of the knife by the killer and whether the accused was aware that the killer might use it. The reserved judgment of the court was delivered by Beldam LJ. He considered that *Powell; English* could not be directly applied to cases where there was 'spontaneous behaviour of a group of irrational individuals who jointly attack a common victim, each intending severally to inflict serious harm by any means at their disposal and giving no thought to the means by which the others will individually commit similar offences on the same person'. *Powell; English* was an authority on conduct performed as a result of a plan.

Beldam LJ laid down seven principles governing the type of case with which he was concerned. It must be stressed that the seven principles are just that: they are not rules of law (*O'Flaherty* [2004] 2 Cr App R 315 (CA)). They are matters of evidence, not substantive law. The court stressed that they aimed to avoid 'the creation of a complex body of doctrine as to whether one weapon (for instance a knife) differs in character from another (for example a claw hammer) and which weapons are more likely to inflict fatal injury'.

(i) Where several persons join to attack a victim in circumstances which show that they intend to inflict serious harm and as a result of the attack the victim sustains fatal injury, they are jointly liable for murder, but if such injury inflicted with that intent is shown to have been caused solely by the actions of one participant of a type entirely different from actions which the others foresaw as part of the attack, only that participant is guilty of murder.

(ii) In deciding whether the actions are of such a different type the use by that party of a weapon is a significant factor. If the character of the weapon, e.g. its propensity to cause death, is different from any weapon used or contemplated by the others and if it is used with a specific intent to kill, the others are not responsible for the death unless it is proved that they knew or foresaw the likelihood of the use of such a weapon.

(iii) If some or all of the others are using weapons which could be regarded as equally likely to inflict fatal injury, the mere fact that a different weapon was used is immaterial.

(iv) If the jury conclude that the death of the victim was caused by the actions of one participant which can be said to be of a completely different type to those contemplated by the others, that are not to be regarded as parties to the death whether it amounts to murder or manslaughter. They may nevertheless be guilty of offences of wounding or inflicting grievous bodily harm with intent which they individually commit.

(v) If in the course of the concerted attack a weapon is produced by one of the participants and the others knowing that he has it in circumstances where he may use it in the course of the attack participate or continue to participate in the attack, they will be guilty of murder if the weapon is used to inflict a fatal wound.

(vi) In a case in which after a concerted attack it is proved that the victim died as a result of a wound with a lethal weapon, e.g. a stab wound, but the evidence does not establish which of the participants used the weapon, then if its use was foreseen by the participants in the attack they will all be guilty of murder notwithstanding that the particular participant who administered the fatal blow cannot be identified (see *Powell*). If, however, the circumstances do not show that the participants foresaw the use of a weapon of this type, none of them will be guilty of murder, though they may individually have committed offences in the course of the attack.

(vii) The mere fact that by attacking the victim together each of them had the intention to inflict serious harm on the victim is insufficient to make them responsible for the death of the victim caused by the use of a lethal weapon used by one of the participants with the same or shared intention.

The Court of Appeal in *O'Flaherty*, above, stated that whether weapons were of the same type was a matter for the jury. Therefore, the trial judge was correct in leaving to the jury whether a claw hammer, cricket bat and broken bottles were of the same type of weapon as a knife, with which the principal offender killed.

Powell; English, above, was also applied in *Greatrex* [1998] Crim LR 733. At least six men attacked the victim. One of them killed him with a metal bar. None of the others knew of the bar. The others were not guilty of murder because the principal had acted in a way fundamentally different than what was foreseen by the others. They foresaw the use of kicking but not of the metal bar. Therefore, despite the others' intent to cause serious injury, they were not guilty of murder or manslaughter, just as in *Mitchell*, above. A retrial was ordered so that the jury could determine whether the hitting with the bar was fundamentally different from the kicking.

As *Greatrex* illustrates, the issue whether the principal acted in a 'fundamentally different' war is one for the jury. Assume that in *Greatrex* the potential accessories agreed to kick the victim to death but before they could do so the principal shot and killed him. All the defendants intended to kill and one did kill. Why should it matter if the mode of killing was fundamentally different from that agreed on by the non-perpetrators of the killing?

The House of Lords reconsidered the 'fundamental difference' rule in *Rahman* [2008] UKHL 45. A gang armed with wooden and metal poles set out to attack the victim. One participant killed the victim with a knife. Were the other members of the gang guilty as secondary parties to murder or was there a fundamental difference between what they intended and the principal's stabbing? The House held that the doctrine of 'fundamental difference' did not come into play simply because the accessories had a different state of mind from the killer at the time of the killing. Therefore, the secondary participants were guilty of murder in the normal way of accessories just as much as the person who knifed the victim to death. There is a helpful summary of the law provided by Lord Brown (at [68]):

> If B [the accessory] realises without agreeing to such conduct being used that A [the principal offender] may kill or intentionally inflict serious injury, but nevertheless continues to participate with A in the venture, that will amount to a sufficient mental element for B to be guilty of murder if A with the requisite intent, kills in the course of the venture unless (i) A suddenly produces and uses a weapon of which B knows nothing and which is more lethal than any weapon which B contemplates that A or any other participant may be carrying

and (ii) for that reason A's act is to be regarded as fundamentally different from anything foreseen by B.

The first part of the quote is based on *Hyde*, above, and the second part (after 'unless') is derived from *Powell; English*, above.

The accused may be convicted of being an accessory even though he does not approve of the action. In *Day* [2001] Crim LR 984 (CA) the accused contended that he did not approve of his co-defendants' kicking the deceased in the head. The court held that this lack of approval was irrelevant. He was guilty if he foresaw that the kicking might occur. Moreover, it was not necessary for him to foresee that death or GBH might occur from the kicking. His co-defendants were convicted of murder; he was convicted of manslaughter on the grounds that there was a 'joint enterprise at least to inflict some harm' and it did not matter that his co-defendants intended to inflict at least GBH.

Throughout this law the secondary party is not liable if he ought to have been aware of the risk. This principle applies even where the crime is one of negligence: *Reid* (1975) 62 Cr App R 109, *obiter*. The Court of Appeal considered that the secondary party seemed to have known of the intention of the principal and so he was rightly convicted.

For an explanation of negligence, see Chapter 3.

In *McKechnie* (1992) 94 Cr App R 51 one accused was acting in pursuance of a joint enterprise. He was provoked by the victim, whom he killed. It was held that his outburst meant that the other joint principals were not liable. The act of the killer was outside the common purpose of the others. However, the law is not clearly stated and appears irreconcilable with *Calhaem* [1985] 1 QB 808. One party went berserk and killed. Nevertheless, the accused was guilty of counselling the offence. Why did not the running amok break the chain of causation?

Is joint enterprise part of secondary liability?

There is debate whether the law of joint enterprise is separate from secondary liability. This paragraph considers the arguments and the authorities. Most cases do not refer to any distinction. *Rook* [1993] 1 WLR 1005 expressly stated that the doctrine of joint enterprise applies whether the accused is present or not. It does not matter whether the assistance is given before or after the principal offence. In *Bryce*, above the Court of Appeal applied the law on the *mens rea* on joint enterprise liability to a person who was not part of a joint enterprise. There are other authorities to this effect.

However, there are contrary authorities. In *Stewart* [1995] 3 All ER 159 the Court of Appeal said that whereas an accessory is liable only for the secondary offence though he may be charged as a principal, a person who takes part in a joint enterprise does participate in the primary offence. The doctrine 'renders each of the parties to a joint enterprise liable for the acts done in the course of carrying out the joint enterprise.' The outcome is that counsellors and procurers are not engaged in a joint enterprise because they are not present when the principal offence is committed. The same court spoke to similar effect in *O'Brien* [1995] 2 Cr App R 649, which also held that on a charge of being an accessory to attempted murder, it was sufficient that the accused knew the principal *might* kill; it did not have to be proved that he knew the principal *would* kill. The latest authority is *Bryce*, above. The Court of Appeal said that the joint enterprise doctrine differed from secondary participation because in the latter it was necessary to show an intent to assist the principal whereas in the former such an intent is not required. The court also said that those who assist at a 'preliminary stage' are accessories, whereas those who assist at the time of the offence are joint enterprise participants. While the cases do not descend to details, one difference seems to be in the *mens rea*. In a joint enterprise scenario the accused is guilty if he foresees that the principal may commit an offence, whereas in secondary participation he is guilty only if he knows the 'essential facts'. It is, however, suggested that the Court of Appeal's view is erroneous. The law on joint enterprise is truly part of accessorial liability. The joint venturer participates as an aider, etc. What distinguishes it from the law on secondary parties is that proof of guilt is easier when two or more persons are engaged in a joint enterprise than if they are not. Joint participation supplies the evidence of assisting and encouraging. In **Reardon** [1999] Crim LR 392 the Court of Appeal approved the trial judge's direction that in a joint enterprise the accused was liable as secondary if he foresaw the principal offence 'as a strong possibility'. This statement is very much a direction used in the law of secondary participation without a joint enterprise. The court's mind was not on the current issues. But the law as stated in **Reardon** is inconsistent with **Stewart** and **O'Brien**. One criticism of **Reardon** is that there was no joint enterprise between the parties. Therefore, the court should not have been discussing joint enterprise. The High Court of Australia considered that the doctrine was separate in **McAuliffe v R** (1995) 69 ALJR 621 because to be liable in a joint enterprise one did not have to aid, abet, counsel or procure, but this proposition is wrong. This issue was not considered in **Powell; English**, but since all the speeches treat parties to a joint venture as accessories, it is suggested that they are against the principle stated in **Stewart**. Clarification is needed.

The argument that joint enterprise and liability as secondary parties are discrete doctrines is best put by A. P. Simester 'The mental element in complicity' (2006) 122 LQR 578. This article is well worth studying.

Joint enterprise and the ECHR

The Court of Appeal in **Concannon** [2002] Crim LR 213 held that joint enterprise liability did not breach Article 6 of the European Convention on Human Rights, the provision on the right to a fair trial. The accused and the killer went to the flat of a drug-dealer, intending to rob him. The killer used a knife to kill the dealer. The jury convicted the accused of (being an accessory to) murder. The defence contended that the accused should not be guilty of murder when he did not intend to kill or commit GBH. The court held that Article 6 applied to procedural, and not to substantive, matters. The law of joint enterprise may be unfair, but any change was for Parliament. Laws may be unfair. The doctrine of joint enterprise may be unfair, as may be the law of murder, but unfairness is not a ground for determining that a criminal law breaches Article 6.

The reform of joint enterprise

Liability in a joint enterprise is preserved in the draft Criminal Code, by means of cl 27(1)(a) and (c). Present law is difficult, has moved on since 1989 when the draft Code was promulgated and is in need of streamlining. For later reform proposals, see below.

Non-conviction of the principal offender

No *actus reus* and acquittal of principal

If the principal offender is not guilty because he did not perform the *actus reus*, the accessory is also not guilty. The authority is **Thornton v Mitchell** [1940] 1 All ER 339. A bus conductor signalled to the driver to back up. Two pedestrians were knocked down. The driver was held not guilty of careless driving. He had driven with due care and attention because he had relied on the conductor's signals. There was therefore no *actus reus*. The conductor was held by the Divisional Court not to be guilty of aiding and abetting. There was no offence to which the alleged secondary party could be accessory. The law was pithily put by Avory J in *Morris v Tolman* [1923] 1 KB 166: 'A person cannot aid another in doing something which that other has not done.' The doctrine of innocent agency cannot apply because again there was no *actus reus* of which the conductor could be guilty (see below).

If, however, a principal is acquitted because evidence is not admissible against him (e.g. because it is hearsay), the accomplice may be guilty where evidence is admissible against him (e.g. he has confessed).

Exemption from liability

A person may be convicted as accessory even though he cannot be guilty as principal. Even when a boy under 14 could not be guilty of rape, he could be guilty as accessory: *Eldershaw* (1828) 172 ER 472. A woman cannot be guilty as a rapist but she can as a secondary offender: *Ram and Ram* (1893) 17 Cox CC 609. More up to date was the charge of being an accessory to rape made against Rosemary West of 25 Cromwell Street, Gloucester, notoriety. She helped her husband Fred to kill women who stayed at their house.

So far the position of accessories where the principal is guilty has been dealt with. What if the principal is not guilty not because there is no *actus reus* but because he is exempt? In those circumstances the accessory is guilty. At one time a father could not be guilty of child-stealing. However, the accessory who helped the father in the snatch was guilty as a secondary party: *Austin* [1981] 1 All ER 374. The Court of Appeal held that the father had committed the offence but was exempt from prosecution. Thus, there was a crime to which the accused could be a secondary party. The wording of the statute was that a person who claimed a right to possession of the child should not 'be liable to be prosecuted'. The decision illustrates the principle of derivative liability.

Can a 'victim' be an accessory?

There is no general rule that a 'victim' cannot be an accessory to a crime. For instance, if the 'victim' encourages the accused to cause him serious harm, the victim is guilty of a participatory offence. Sometimes judges have held that when a statute is intended to protect persons, members of that class cannot be convicted as accessories. A girl under 16 could not be convicted of an offence involving unlawful sexual intercourse because the statute penalising such behaviour was passed to protect girls from themselves: *Tyrrell* [1894] 1 QB 710. It is irrelevant whether she initiated the act. A similar case is *Whitehouse* [1977] QB 868. A girl of 15 was held to belong to a class protected by ss 10 and 11 of the then existing Sexual Offences Act 1956, which punished men for committing incest with their daughters. The outcome in *Whitehouse* was quickly changed by statute but the principle stands, as *Pickford* [1995] 1 Cr App R 420 (CA), discussed in the chapter on incitement, demonstrates. *Tyrrell* was applied. A boy under 14 was the victim of the crime of incest with his mother. The stepfather was guilty of inciting his wife to commit incest with his stepson but at that time could not have been found guilty of inciting his stepson to commit incest with his wife. He also could not have been found guilty of aiding and abetting his stepson to commit the crime of incest. At that time Parliament protected boys under 14 by ruling that such boys could not be guilty of committing crimes of sexual intercourse, a category which included incest. The rule has since been abolished but the principle stands. There was no *actus reus*. In *Congdon* (1990) 140 NLJ 1221 (Crown Court), it was held that a prostitute could not be convicted of abetting her husband (or any other pimp) to live on her earnings, an offence which could be committed only by a man. She was to be protected from his exploitation of her. The law applies whether or not the woman egged the man on. In other words, the woman need not in fact be the victim of the principal. It is sufficient that she fell within a class expressly or impliedly protected by Parliament. The offence of living off immoral earnings was abolished by the Sexual Offences Act 2003 but the principle remains.

It is uncertain how far this 'victim' doctrine goes. Sometimes it is said that it applies only to sexual offences. The decision in *Tyrrell* arguably turns very much on statutory interpretation but the principle has become a general one. Mental defectives form a protected class. It has been held that the immunity does not extend to a woman on whom an unlawful abortion is performed even though the woman cannot be convicted of using an instrument to procure her own abortion: *Sockett* (1908) 1 Cr App R 101 (CCA). If the argument is that the statute is not designed to protect women, the outcome is sound. If, however, the statute is aimed at backstreet abortionists, women do fall within the protected class, and the accused in *Sockett* ought not to have been found guilty as accessory. In *Brown* [1994] AC 212 sado-masochists were convicted of aiding and abetting assaults on themselves. They were not 'victims' for the purpose of this rule. The persons who perpetrated what were held to be offences on them were guilty of committing crimes against the 'victims'. The same persons were not victims for one purpose but were for another!

The Law Commission's draft Criminal Code, cl 27(7), retains the victim rule.

> Where the purpose of an enactment creating an offence is the protection of a class of persons no member of that class who is a victim of such an offence can be guilty of that offence as an accessory.

The offence must be directed against the victim (at 210).

It should be remembered that this exemption applies only to the statutorily protected victim, e.g. of the unlawful sexual intercourse. If a 15-year-old girl assists a man to have sexual intercourse with a girl aged 14, she is the secondary party, because she is not the victim. It is the girl aged 14 who is the victim – she is not guilty as accessory. (A prostitute can be convicted of living on the earnings of another prostitute.)

Innocent agency

Where the 'principal' performed the *actus reus* of an offence with the accused's assistance or encouragement, but where the 'principal' has a defence or lacks *mens rea*, the accused who would otherwise be the accessory is treated at times as if he were the principal. He stands in the shoes of the person who would otherwise be the principal offender. (A straightforward application of the principle of derivative liability would render the person who would otherwise be the secondary party not guilty.) If a postman delivers a parcel bomb, he is not guilty and no doubt most of us would not even think of charging him, but the person who sent the parcel will be liable as a principal offender. A simple example is *Tyler and Price* (1838) 172 ER 643. The person who told an insane person to kill someone was deemed to be the principal offender when he did so. A similar case is *Michael* (1840) 169 ER 487. The accused gave a childminder a bottle of laudanum, a poison, intending her to give it to her child. She said it was medicine. In fact the childminder's child, aged five, gave it to the child, not knowing what the contents were. The child died. It was held that the childminder's child was the innocent agent. The accused was convicted of murder. (Had the otherwise innocent agent, the child, been over 10 and had that child known of the poison, the minor would have been the principal offender and the adult who provided the poison would have been the accessory.) In *Manley* (1844) 1 Cox CC 104, the accused was the principal offender when he told a nine-year-old child to take money out of the father's till. The principle is not restricted to situations where the 'principal' has a defence such as insanity or infancy. It applies where the 'principal' does not have the *mens rea*. In *Stringer* (1991) 94 Cr App R 13, the accused dishonestly sent bogus invoices through a firm's accounting system with the result that money was transferred from the firm to him. It was held that it was he who had appropriated for the purposes of theft because he was responsible for the accounts staff appropriating what he intended to steal. The staff were innocent agents. He was the principal offender. *Stringer* accords with the older case of *Butt* (1884) 15 Cox CC 564. The accused is not liable as accessory because the alleged principal has committed no crime. A final illustration is where the accused persuaded another to steal a car from a garage. The person who innocently took the car is not guilty but the one who induced him to take it is guilty of burglary as a principal offender. A modern Australian authority is *Pinkstone v R* (2004) 219 CLR 444 (HCA). The accused sent prohibited drugs via an air courier. Kirby J quoted from Brooking JA in *Franklin* [2001] 3 VR 9, 21: 'The law regards the puppet master as causing the mischief done by the puppet.' The courier was the innocent agent: the firm delivered the drugs but the accused 'supplied' them within the meaning of the legislation.

As stated above, the doctrine of innocent agency does not apply where the accused cannot be said to have done the *actus reus*. In *Thornton v Mitchell*, above, the conductor could not be said to have committed the act of careless driving through the innocent agency of the actual driver because he was not driving at all. 'Driving' requires the accused himself personally to do the act. One does not drive a car when someone else's hands are on the wheel and feet are busy on the pedals. The problem is even clearer in bigamy. Take this situation. A man believes that his wife is dead but she is in fact alive. A woman knows that the wife is alive but persuades the man to re-marry. The husband is not guilty of bigamy because he does not have *mens rea*. Is he an innocent agent? If he were, the woman would be the principal. However, to hold so would mean that the woman had 'married' the man's second 'wife', but one woman cannot 'marry' another. The position is exacerbated if the woman is not already married. Bigamy requires the *actus reus* of 'being married, marries again', but on these facts the woman is not married. It is not possible to say that she, being married, married again. For a person to be liable as an accessory, moreover, the principal offence must have been committed. In the cases discussed in this paragraph there was no principal offender and under the derivative liability rule the accused should not have been convicted.

To this exception to the doctrine of innocent agency there is a sub-exception, which might be called the doctrine of 'semi-innocent agency'. It is uncertain how far this doctrine extends and whether it is restricted to sexual offences. It derives from two cases which the Law Commission in 1993 called 'lurid' and 'unforgettable'. In *Bourne* (1952) 36 Cr App R 125, the accused forced his wife to have sexual intercourse with a dog. She probably had the defence of duress. There was therefore no principal offender. The husband was convicted of aiding and abetting, even though he was not physically capable of committing the offence as charged. The line between this case and ***Thornton v Mitchell*** seems to be that in ***Bourne*** there was an *actus reus*, bestiality, whereas in ***Thornton v Mitchell*** it was not an *actus reus* to drive a bus. In ***Bourne*** there was a perpetrator; in ***Thornton v Mitchell*** there was not. In ***Bourne*** there was a principal crime on which the secondary offence could be parasitic. In ***Cogan and Leak*** [1976] QB 217, the husband compelled his wife to have sexual intercourse with the accused who believed that the wife was consenting. The accused's conviction for rape was quashed on appeal: there was no *mens rea* (cf. ***Bourne*** where there was an *actus reus*). The Court of Appeal held that the husband's conviction as a secondary party could stand. The derivative theory of secondary participation was not applied in this case. This part of ***Cogan and Leak*** can continue even though the part discussed next is incorrect. A husband could not until recently be guilty of rape as principal. In ***Cogan and Leak***, however, Lawton LJ went beyond ***Bourne***. He also said that the husband became the principal to the crime of rape, an offence which he could then not commit as principal. If this case is correct, ***Bourne*** could have been decided similarly, notwithstanding the difficulty of finding a person guilty of an offence which he cannot physically commit. Moreover, the reasoning in ***Cogan and Leak*** could be applied to women. If one woman forces another to have intercourse with a man who does not know that the second woman was not consenting, is the first woman guilty of rape through the innocent agency of the second, even though only a man, because of the definition of the crime of rape (see Chapter 14), can be guilty as principal? Lawton LJ said in ***Cogan and Leak*** that 'convictions should not be upset because of mere technicalities of pleading', but what occurred in the law seems to be more than technical. The decision in ***Cogan and Leak*** that the accused can rape through the genitals of someone else does not seem correct in principle. If one cannot 'drive' through another, how can one have vaginal sex through another? It is hard to say that a person who stands around is engaged in intercourse. This is not to say that the husband should not be guilty of something. It is only by altering the derivative liability doctrine underlying secondary offences that the accused could be found guilty. Neither judgment provides much in the way of theoretical justification for liability. Take another illustration, provided by B. Mitchell, *Law Relating to Violent Crime* (CLT Publishing, 1997) 313:

> . . . A woman deceives another woman into visiting a man's house and, pointing a gun at both of them, orders him to rape the other woman. The man has a good defence to the charge of rape on the ground of duress . . . , and the woman cannot be convicted of rape as a principal (with the man being treated as the innocent agent) because of her sex. . . . It seems unsatisfactory that the woman can escape criminal liability because of these 'technicalities'.

In a footnote Mitchell adds: 'Obviously, she cannot be convicted as an accessory to rape because no offence of rape has been committed.'

In ***Millward*** (1994) 158 JP 1091 (CA) the accused had given his employee instructions to tow his trailer. The trailer's hitch was poorly maintained. The trailer became detached, hit a car and killed a passenger. The employee was acquitted of causing death by reckless driving (a crime now abolished). The accused was charged with procuring the crime. He argued that he could not be convicted of a secondary offence when there was no principal offence, since the employee's acquittal meant that there was no crime to which he could be a party. The court, however, rejected his appeal. Since in procuring there need be no joint intention between the parties, the accessory can be liable when the principal is acquitted because he does not have the mental element for the crime or because he has a defence personal to him, provided that there is an *actus reus*. The employee did not have the *mens rea* for the offence charged and was therefore not guilty. The *actus reus* was taking a defective vehicle on to a road so as to cause death. The accused had procured that *actus reus*. (However, it may be doubted that the accused had the *mens rea* of procuring.) The court distinguished **Thornton v Mitchell**, above. The driver was not guilty of careless driving when he reversed his bus on the accused's instructions and killed a pedestrian. He had no *actus reus*. Therefore, there was no *actus reus* which the accused could abet. In other words, the driving was not careless; there was no principal crime and the defendant could not be convicted of abetting something which was not a crime.

The court ruled that the case was on all fours with **Cogan and Leak**, above. Scott Baker J said:

> . . . it is the authority of **Cogan & Leak** that is relevant to the decision that we have to make. In this court's view, the *actus reus* in the present case was the taking of the vehicle in the defective condition on to the road so as to cause the death of the little boy. It was procured by this appellant. The requisite *mens rea* was . . . present . . . The appellant caused [the employee] to drive that vehicle in that condition just as Leak had caused Cogan to have sexual intercourse with his wife.

Mr Cogan believed that Mrs Leak was consenting to sex when she was not. Mr Leak was convicted of aiding and abetting rape. The court in **Cogan and Leak** said that the offence of rape had occurred, not just the *actus reus*, and the accused was an accessory to that offence, though the alleged perpetrator was not liable. In **Millward** the court said that the offence had not taken place but the *actus reus* had. (This is the same situation in theft as seen in **Cogan and Leak**, but the court in **Cogan and Leak** said that an offence and not merely the *actus reus* had occurred.) In this sense the cases are different and the rule is new. This development has been criticised for creating crimes where none existed before.

The court said in **Millward** that its new rule was one applying to procuring (and it may be that the rule is restricted to procuring) and that **Cogan and Leak** was essentially a case on procuring. The question may be asked whether the accused did procure at all. He did not produce the victim's death by endeavour. He was not trying to kill anyone. He was reckless as to whether death might occur, but recklessness is insufficient *mens rea* for procuring. Furthermore, it is uncertain whether the principle enunciated in this case applies to other modes of participation. The court emphasised that in procuring the minds of the parties need not be as one. This distinction may place procuring in a different category from the others. It should be emphasised that **Millward** breaks away from the doctrine of derivative liability underlying the present law. A person can now definitely procure an offence where the principal is not liable in situations where it can be said that the *actus reus* of a crime has occurred. **Millward** was approved *obiter* by the Court of Appeal in **Wheelhouse** [1994] Crim LR 756. The court said that the accused's use of a dupe to remove a car from a garage was an instance of **Millward**. Actually the case is one of innocent agency. There is no difficulty in saying the accused burgled, whereas in **Cogan and Leak** and **Millward** one cannot hold the accused to have raped or driven. It is, however, arguable that the accused can rape and drive through an agent. It seems that the doctrine of innocent agency was not discussed in **Millward**. It might also be inquired whether the accused in **Millward** had the *mens rea* to be an accessory. Did he know the essential matter that the hitch was poorly maintained? If not, he should not have been found guilty. Another criticism of **Millward** is that the rule is stated as one of procuring the *actus reus* of a crime. In the former crime of reckless driving the principal had to drive in such a way as to create an obvious and serious risk of causing physical injury. This element is part of the *actus reus*. Since the principal did not drive in such a manner, there was no *actus reus* to which the accused could be attached. Therefore, he should have been found not guilty. The same analysis, it is suggested, applies to dangerous driving.

Millward was applied in *DPP* v *K & B* [1997] 1 Cr App R 36 (DC). Two girls, the defendants, procured an unidentified boy who was older than 10 but younger than 14 and who may have had the then-existing defence of infancy to have sexual intercourse with a girl of 14 without her consent, i.e. subject to the defence of infancy he raped her. The Court held that the defendants were guilty of rape, even if the boy was not. The Court thought it possible that a woman who deceived a man into having sexual intercourse with another person could be convicted of the offence of rape despite the offence being restricted by Parliament to male offenders. As stated above, *DPP* v *K & B* is a breach of the derivative theory of liability for secondary participation.

It may be that cases like *Millward* and *DPP* v *K & B* are irreconcilable with the House of Lords decision in *Powell; English*, above. The Lords said that the accused was guilty only if he realised that the principal may commit an offence with the appropriate *mens rea*. However, the defendants in *Millward* and *DPP* v *K & B* did not realise that. Possibly the cases may be reconciled by holding that *Millward* and *DPP* v *K & B* are cases on procuring to which different principles may apply.

In *Pickford* [1995] 1 Cr App R 420 the Court of Appeal distinguished *Bourne* and *Cogan and Leak*. The court considered *obiter* what would have happened if a person had been charged with aiding and abetting a boy to commit incest with his mother. At that time boys under 14 were irrebuttably presumed not to be capable of committing crimes involving sexual intercourse. Laws J said that in *Bourne* and *Cogan and Leak* 'the person who committed the act said to constitute the principal offence . . . was fully capable at law of committing the offence in question, but had a complete defence on the facts. These authorities do not support the proposition that where the principal offender lacks all legal capacity to commit the crime in question another may nevertheless be guilty of aiding and abetting him.'

Subject to the doctrine of innocent agency and cases such as *Cogan and Leak*, the principal offence must have been committed before the accused is guilty as an accessory, though the perpetrator need not have been convicted. Without a principal offender, the accused is not guilty: see *Morris* v *Tolman* [1923] 1 KB 166, where the employer was not guilty of using a commercial van for private purposes for only the licensee could be guilty of this offence but it was the employee of the licensee who had used the vehicle for a purpose not covered by the licence, and accordingly the employee was not guilty of aiding. There was no *actus reus*. The Court of Appeal in *Loukes* [1996] 1 Cr App R 444 applied *Thornton* v *Mitchell* and distinguished *Millward*. The accused was charged with being a secondary party to an offence of causing death by dangerous driving. The trial judge directed the jury to acquit the driver. The Court of Appeal held that since there was no primary offence, the accused could not be guilty of procuring that offence. There was no *actus reus* (obviousness to a competent driver that the car was dangerous) which the accused had procured (cf. *Millward*). The position would have been different, had the alleged principal offender been found not guilty on the ground that he lacked *mens rea*. In that event *Millward* would have applied, and the accused could have been found guilty of procuring the *actus reus*. As it was, the principal crime was a strict offence and *mens rea* was irrelevant. The court asked for Parliament to change the law. It could be argued that this principle hinders crime prevention, for the reason why the principal offence does not take place may be fortuitous.

The statutory crime of abetting suicide should be noted. There is no crime of suicide, but a person may be guilty of abetting suicide. Perhaps in reality 'abetting suicide' is best described as the principal offence and the abettor is in truth the principal. Similarly there is a crime of procuring the execution of a valuable security. In this context 'procuring' is the principal offence. The accessory would be guilty of procuring the procuring [*sic*] of the execution of a valuable security!

The doctrine of innocent (and 'semi-innocent') agency forms part of the draft Criminal Code, cl 26(1)(c), quoted near the start of the Chapter, which deems the person acting through the agent to be the principal. The accused in **Bourne** would be guilty as principal, not as accessory. The Law Commission (at 205–206) expressed doubt whether their draft would lead to the conviction of the conductor in **Thornton v Mitchell** as principal (he would not be liable as accessory because of cl 27(1)(a), which preserves the law that there must be a guilty principal). Surprisingly the Law Commission passed responsibility for deciding this point to the courts.

Withdrawal

English law grants a defence to secondary parties who withdraw before the commission of the full offence. One possible rationale is that the accused is given an incentive to prevent the crime; another is that the accused is less blameworthy than one who continues. For a modern view on the possible rationales see A. J. Ashworth's commentary on **O'Flaherty** [2004] Crim LR 751 (CA). If in a case involving pre-planned violence the accused assists or encourages a person to commit an offence but withdraws before the crime takes place, he is not liable as a secondary party, provided that he expressly or impliedly communicates his repentance or revocation to, it is thought, all the principals, but may remain liable for conspiracy or incitement or both. The accused must give 'clear warning' that he has withdrawn from the criminal enterprise: **Becerra** (1976) 62 Cr App R 212 (CA), which remains the leading case, and **Whitefield** (1984) 79 Cr App R 36. In the latter case the Court of Appeal allowed the accused's appeal when he had told his co-conspirators that he had decided to play no more part in the burglary of an adjoining flat. The accused must give 'unequivocal communication' of withdrawal. It is not enough to avoid culpability that the accused has said to himself that he will withdraw (**Rook** [1993] 1 WLR 1005, following **Whitefield**, where the Court of Appeal said: 'If . . . participation is confined to advice or encouragement [the alleged accessory] must at least communicate his change of mind to the other'), and according to **Becerra** it is insufficient to say 'let's go'. In **Rook** it was said that the accused had to communicate his withdrawal unequivocally. In **Baker** [1994] Crim LR 444 (CA) the words 'I'm not doing it' were held to be equivocal. They could mean, 'I will stay but not do anything after having struck my blows'. The accused had not demonstrated an effective withdrawal by his deeds or words. Similarly in **Nawaz** (1999) *Independent*, 19 May, simply saying that he had withdrawn from the joint enterprise was insufficient. His withdrawal had to be unequivocal, notified to the other participants and included some effort at dissuading the others from proceeding. Perhaps in **Becerra** and **Baker** withdrawal would have been effective only if the accused had sought to restrain the other defendants. If communication is possible, there is no need to go to the police. If no communication is possible, presumably the accused must contact the police. Glanville Williams, *Textbook of Criminal Law*, 2nd edn (Stevens, 1983) 127, quotes from a US case: 'A declared intent to withdraw from a conspiracy to dynamite a building is not enough if the fuse has been set. He must step on the fuse.' Lloyd LJ in *Rook* said, *obiter*, that it was perhaps an effective withdrawal when the accused had done his best to step on the fuses. In other words, the accused must go beyond effectively communicating withdrawal: there must be a negating of the assistance. The question whether the accused has withdrawn is one for the jury: *Grundy* [1977] Crim LR 543. In that case the accused gave two men information about a house which they later burgled. Two weeks before the commission of the crime, he had been trying to stop them. There was evidence of an effective withdrawal. It is arguable that on the facts of *Grundy*, as well as some other cases such as *Whitefield*, there should not have been a defence, since the information continued to be valuable after withdrawal. Nevertheless, the Court of Appeal in *O'Flaherty* approved both *Grundy* and *Whitefield*.

The Court of Appeal in *Perman* [1996] 1 Cr App R 24 thought that in a joint enterprise scenario the accused could not withdraw once the criminal activity had begun. The statement was *obiter*. The court postulated that what was thought to be withdrawal in such circumstances was in truth the principal's exceeding the scope of the joint enterprises so that the accused was no longer liable. The Northern Ireland Court of Appeal faced a similar problem in *Graham* [1996] NI 157. In a joint enterprise case it was insufficient to urge that the victim should not be killed. The court did not wish to state what was needed, so the case's value as a precedent is somewhat limited, but it was said *obiter* that even informing the police would probably not be a withdrawal if the perpetrators of the crime, here terrorist murderers, were close to committing the offence.

The Court of Appeal in *Mitchell* [1999] Crim LR 496 said without citing authority that communication of withdrawal, while necessary when violence was planned, was not a requirement for withdrawal when the violence was spontaneous. On the facts the court said that the accused had withdrawn when he stopped fighting, threw down the stick he was carrying and walked away. *Mitchell* may be criticised on the grounds that the accused did not seek to put an end to the encouragement he had previously given and that the law of joint enterprise is not based on distinguishing planned and spontaneous violence. In the Court of Appeal in *Robinson*, unreported, 3 February 2000 Otton LJ said that *Mitchell*, in which he had also given the leading judgment, was exceptional. Even when violence was spontaneous, withdrawal must be communicated to give the other the opportunity to desist 'unless it is not practicable or reasonable so to communicate as in . . . *Mitchell* where the accused threw down his weapon and moved away before the final and fatal blows were inflicted'. *Mitchell* was not a joint enterprise case but was applied to a joint enterprise in *O'Flaherty*, above. Two of the defendants who originally attacked the victim did not pursue him with the others in to the next street. They did not communicate their withdrawal but simply did not pursue him. The Court of Appeal held, where there was spontaneous violence, there was no need to communicate withdrawal to the others. On this point *O'Flaherty* is contrary to *Robinson*.

Mantell LJ summarised the law in *O'Flaherty*:

> . . . mere repentance does not suffice. To disengage from an incident a person must do enough to demonstrate that he or she is withdrawing from the joint enterprise. This is ultimately a question of fact and degree for the jury. Account will be taken of *inter alia* the nature of the assistance and encouragement already given and how imminent the infliction or the fatal injury or injuries is, as well as the nature of the action said to constitute withdrawal.

If the accused's repentance is not sincere, as when he has been caught by the police, he is still liable as a counsellor, and even as an abettor if he is still encouraging his partner, as was said to have occurred in the famous case of *Craig and Bentley* (1952)

The Times, 10–13 December, above. (An alternative is to say that the first defendant went beyond the scope of their joint enterprise by killing a police officer and, therefore, the second defendant was not an accessory to murder.) If the accused is in police custody, he will remain liable for encouragement or assistance previously given: *Johnson and Jones* (1841) 174 ER 479. It is uncertain whether the defence is available when the accused is physically not in a position to countermand his help. Perhaps it should not be, for the help given to the principal remains of use to him.

The previous paragraph spoke of 'repentance', and some English cases do the same. All that that term means is that the accused has to withdraw effectively. There need be no true repentance.

If there is more than one principal offender, it is uncertain whether the accused can withdraw only by unequivocally notifying all of them or whether notice to one is sufficient. Case law on this point would be helpful.

Under the draft Criminal Code, Law Com. No. 177, 1989, there is a defence of withdrawal (cl 27(8)). However, unlike present law there is a requirement in cl 27(8)(a) that the withdrawal must be done with a view to preventing the full offence. In fact *Whitefield* rejected that precondition. The Law Commission is also of the view that communication of withdrawal to one of the several principals would suffice, for this is 'a sufficient earnest of the accessory's desire to withdraw'. See the next section for the Law Commission's 1993 proposals.

Proposals for reform: encouraging and assisting crime

Reform proposals are contained in a lengthy Law Commission Consultation Paper, No. 131, *Assisting and Encouraging Crime*, 1993. In this substantial and radical document the Law Commission recommended:

(a) the abolition of the present law of participation including s 8 of the Accessories and Abettors Act 1861 and *Attorney-General's Reference (No. 1 of 1975)* and of incitement, and

(b) the creation of two new offences, assisting crime and encouraging it.

Both offences, unlike the current forms of accomplice liability, are to be inchoate offences just as incitement is, i.e. the principal offence need not be committed. The line between abetting and incitement would disappear for the concept behind them is the same, the encouragement of crime. The principle of derivative liability would be abolished.

The crime of assisting is defined as follows.

A person commits the offence of assisting crime if he –
(a) knows or believes that another ('the principal') is doing, or causing to be done, acts that do or will involve the commission of an offence by the principal; and
(b) knows or believes that the principal, in so acting, does or will do so with the fault required for the offence in question; and
(c) does any act that he knows or believes assists or will assist the principal in committing that offence.

The following comments on assisting are offered.

(a) Assistance covers supplying tools, giving advice, driving the principal to the scene of the crime, and positively misleading the police.

(b) The principal crime must be identifiable at the time of assisting but the accused need not know the time, place, or victim, e.g. he must know that burglary is to take place but not that it is burglary at the Midland Bank, Stoke Newington. The law in **Bainbridge** dealing with knowledge of the type of crime is abolished. The Law Commission said that **Bainbridge** was an 'evasion' of the requirement that the accused had to know the 'essential matters' (**Johnson v Youden**, above) (para 3.22).

(c) Currently assistance given in advance of the crime gives rise to no liability until the principal offence is committed. The Law Commission argues that 'it may be thought unsatisfactory that the law enforcement agencies have to wait until that crime is actually committed before they can intervene to control the conduct of assisters' (para 4.20). The commission of the full offence may also be fortuitous. Even at present there is no requirement that the accused cause the principal offender to commit the crime, and his culpability is judged by his fault in assisting: it is not dependent on whether the principal did or did not commit *his* offence. Incitement and attempt are already inchoate offences. The Law Commission's view is that the switch to inchoate responsibility would not in practice greatly extend the law for usually 'the act of assistance will only come to light, or be thought worth prosecuting, where the principal crime has in fact been committed' (para 4.26). It would, however, catch the social host where the principal, who had been intending to drive, in fact leaves his car and walks home, but such an offence would be unlikely to be prosecuted. The move to inchoate form will cut the law of accomplices from its present base, derivative liability.

(d) Assisting should apply to all offences, whether common law or statutory.

(e) An omission to act should not be assisting. **Tuck v Robson** would be reversed.

(f) There should be no *de minimis* defence.

(g) The mental element covers situations where the accused is indifferent to the commission of the full offence but not suspicion that the principal may commit an offence. Belief that the offence will take place is one aspect of the *mens rea*. This test will exculpate those who sell items as part of their business, even when the sale is to 'suspect customers' (para 4.85).

(h) The situation which arose in **DPP for Northern Ireland v Maxwell**, contemplation of a range of possible offences, is met by a provision that an accused is guilty 'if he knows or believes that the principal intends to commit one of a number of offences and does any act that he knows or believes will assist the principal in committing whichever of those offences the principal in fact intends'. The basic rule that knowledge is required replaces the lower threshold in **Maxwell**, contemplation of possible offences from a 'shopping list', but the basic **Maxwell** principle is retained.

(i) The law in **Callow v Tillstone**, where the vet was not liable as abettor, when he negligently certified a heifer as sound, but the butcher was liable as principal for exposing unsound meat for sale, is confirmed.

(j) The 'victim' exception in **Tyrrell** is widened in para 4.103: 'a person is not guilty of complicity by assisting an offence if the offence is so defined that his conduct is inevitably incidental to its commission and that conduct is not made criminal by that offence'. This defence would not be granted where the assister's purpose was the commission of the full offence.

(k) Employees would not be liable for assisting in a summary offence committed by their employers in the course of their employment. They would be liable for assisting indictable offences for then the policy of crime prevention outweighs that of putting 'undue burdens' on workers (para 4.111). The employment defence would not be available at all where it was the employee's purpose to assist (para 4.138).

(l) There should be no defence that the person assisting acted in the course of their ordinary business such as supplying the coal which led to the overloaded lorry in **NCB v Gamble**. 'Indeed, from the point of view of discouraging or inhibiting the commission of the principal crime, it might be thought desirable that "business" suppliers, above all others, should be deterred from providing the means of crime' (para 4.116).

(m) 'Social assisters' such as the host who gives alcohol to a person who becomes unfit through drink to drive should continue to be liable.

(n) A good motive should not affect liability (cf. **Gillick v West Norfolk and Wisbech Health Authority**).

(o) There should be a defence covering a person who assists but with the purpose of preventing the commission of a crime such as an undercover agent.

(p) Another defence would be assistance done 'with the purpose of avoiding or limiting any harmful consequences of the offence and without the purpose of furthering its commission', such as supplying condoms to male prisoners to prevent the spread of AIDS through buggery. Neither defence in (o) or (p) would be available when the assister's purpose was the commission of the principal offence.

(q) A defence of withdrawal should be afforded to assisters when they take all reasonable steps to prevent the commission of the full offence. The continuance of this defence is, however, hard to square with not basing assisting on the commission of the principal offence.

The following comments are addressed to the proposed offence of encouraging crime.

(a) The definition suggested is:
  (1) A person commits the offence of encouraging crime if he –
    (a) solicits, commands or encourages another ('the principal') to do or cause to be done an act or acts which, if done, will involve the commission of an offence by the principal; and
    (b) intends that that act or those acts should be done by the principal; and
    (c) knows or believes that the principal, in so acting, will do so with the fault required for the offence in question.
  (2) The solicitation, command or encouragement must be brought to the attention of the principal, but it is irrelevant to the person's guilt whether or not the principal reacts to or is influenced by the solicitation, command or encouragement.
  (3) The defendant need not know the identity of the principal, nor have any particular principal or group of principals in mind, provided that he intends his communication to be acted on by any person to whose attention it comes.
  (Fortunately or not, no definition is provided of 'intends' but the Commission expects 'knows or believes' to be interpreted as in handling.)

(b) This offence will replace incitement, counselling and abetting.

(c) It will be an inchoate offence.

(d) It may be committed by omission. The law stated above would continue to apply.

(e) The new *mens rea* will abrogate the rule in **Curr** [1968] 2 QB 944 (knowledge of principal's *mens rea*).

(f) Defences to assisting such as employment, law enforcement and limitation of harm, noted above, should not apply to encouraging for in this offence the accused's purpose is to get the principal to break the law.

(g) There might be a defence where the 'victim' encouraged the crime such as when a girl under 16 encouraged a boy to have sexual intercourse with her.

(h) Withdrawal should be a defence but it is 'arguable that where it is possible for him to do so, the encourager should not only countermand his encouragement but also take steps to prevent the offence . . .'. The defence is therefore differently formulated for assisters and encouragers.

(i) The accused need to know the identity of the victim or other details.

See Chapter 10 for an explanation of impossibility.

The Commission opens for discussion the issue of whether the proposed offences should apply in relation to summary offences. There should be no defence of impossibility: *Fitzmaurice* [1983] QB 1083 (CA) on incitement would be overturned. It will not be possible to assist or encourage attempt or conspiracy; the crime may be attempted and persons can conspire to commit them. The maximum sentence for the new crimes should be the same as that for the principal offence. It proposes a crime of procurement where the accused does an act with intent that a strict offence is committed or being reckless whether the act will bring about the commission of the offence. The Commission was unsure whether the law of joint enterprise should be retained or abolished with the crime of assisting taking its place. It is suggested that it should be retained. If the defendants act together and one of them kills the victim but the jury is not sure which one, neither could be convicted of murder and neither could be convicted of assisting. Innocent agency is retained. To retain convictions in *Bourne* and *Cogan and Leak* there will be liability in the accused where the principal party has a defence of duress or is acting under a mistake intentionally brought about by the accused. The Commission was sceptical about the doctrine which since the Paper was published has come to be associated with *Millward* (1994) 158 JP 1091, that of procuring the *actus reus*. It thought that the doctrine 'in its anxiety to meet cases' such as *Bourne* and *Cogan and Leak* 'will reach too far'.

For comment see K. J. M. Smith 'The Law Commission Consultation Paper on complicity: (1) A blueprint for reform' [1994] Crim LR 239, G. R. Sullivan 'Fault elements and joint enterprise' [1994] Crim LR 252 and Sir John Smith 'Secondary participation in crime – can we do without it?' [1994] NLJ 679. One major criticism is that the proposed offence of assisting crime would lump together those who set the crime in motion and those who helped once the crime had begun. Is the person who drives a hit-man to the scene as blameworthy as one who hires the killer? One difference between the proposed law and current law is this. At present the accused is guilty of an offence if the prosecution can prove that he took part in an offence either as a principal or as an accessory. This advantage would be lost under these proposals. The law has developed in a haphazard fashion, which has led to complexity, and policy and analytical issues have not been addressed. Reform is overdue.

The Law Commission's 2006 recommendations on complicity in murder and manslaughter

The Law Commission published its Report No. 304 *Murder, Manslaughter and Infanticide* in late 2006. In it it proposed that the accused would be liable as an accomplice to first or second degree murder (for details of these two recommended tiers of murder see Chapter 11) if:

> he or she (D) intended to assist or encourage the principal offender (P) to commit the relevant type of murder, (for example, D would be liable for a first degree murder committed by P if D intended that P should or foresaw that he or she might commit the conduct element of first degree murder with the required fault element of first degree murder) or D was engaged in a joint criminal venture with P and realised that P might commit the relevant offence of murder.

There would be no need for a common purpose agreed on by D and P beforehand to fall within the 'joint criminal venture' proposal; it would be sufficient that D was encouraging or assisting P to commit a crime. In this regard the statutory reformulation would be the same as currently exists at common law. The Commission opines (at para. 4.11) that 'D carries the additional fault of being involved in a joint venture with P to commit a crime. Individuals who perform a criminal act in groups have been shown to be more disposed to act violently than those who act alone, and this can be taken to be common knowledge.' It should also be noted that D would be liable as an accomplice to first degree murder, even though he or she did not intend to kill or did not intend to cause serious injury being aware that there was a serious risk of death, the proposed mental states for first degree murder. In this respect D would as now be liable for first degree murder even though he or she did not have the *mens rea* for it whereas the perpetrator (P) would of course have to have the requisite *mens rea*. The Law Commission foreshadowed in the 2006 Report its 2007 Report *Participating in Crime* which recommended defences of acting in order to prevent the commission of the crime and acting in order to prevent or limit the occurrence of harm and these defences will apply to fatal offences as well as other crimes. In this respect the harshness of the current and proposed rule about complicity as a joint venturer in a first degree murder would be mitigated. Similarly, there may be circumstances in which the murder came to be committed which are 'too remote from what D anticipated to make it right to regard the murder as within the foreseen scope of the joint venture. The question will be a matter of fact and degree for the jury to decide.' (para. 4.30, footnote omitted) The sentence for first degree murder whether committed by the principal or the secondary offender would be mandatory life imprisonment; for second degree murder it would be a discretionary life sentence.

This proposal would rectify the anomaly whereby if D and P were involved in a joint venture and P committed a murder which D did not foresee, D would escape all criminal liability. In the words of the Law Commission (para. 4.5), 'This treats D too generously if D was aware that P meant to do *some* harm to V [the victim], even if D did not realise that P might commit murder.'

In relation to manslaughter, the third tier of non-fatal offences, the Commission proposed that D should be liable for manslaughter if:

> D and P were parties to a joint venture,
>
> P committed the crime of first degree or second degree murder when fulfilling that common purpose,
>
> D intended or foresaw that (non-serious) harm or the fear of harm might be caused by P, and
>
> 'a reasonable person in D's position, with D's knowledge of the relevant facts, would have foreseen an obvious risk of death or serious injury being caused by a party to the venture.' (para. 4.6)

This offence would be called 'manslaughter'. There was some argument in the Consultation Paper No. 177 *A New Homicide Act for England and Wales?* (2005) which preceded this Report that the crime should be called 'complicity in an unlawful killing' but in its Report the Commission settled on manslaughter. The concept of a 'reasonable person in D's position' in the proposed definition would include D's age, but which other factors would be taken into account by the jury would be determined on a case-by-case basis.

The Law Commission's Report No. 306 *Participating in Crime*

The Commission's proposals in Report No. 306 are not intended to replace but to supplement those in the 2006 Report on complicity in murder. The 2007 Report may be seen as a partner to the Law Commission Report No. 300, *Inchoate Liability for Assisting and Encouraging Crime*, 2006. The relationship between inchoate offences and secondary offences forms the crux of the Report: without the recommendations on inchoate liability the proposals on secondary offences would not have seen the light of day. For that reason, the two Reports must be read together, and the Law Commission's view was that they stood together. The government seems to have taken the view that they do not. It has already enacted the Serious Crime Act 2007, which replaces the common law inchoate offence of incitement. The Act is based on, but does not completely follow, Report No. 300.

Introduction

The Law Commission's Report focuses on the situation where one party assists or encourages another to commit a crime, the principal offence, and that offence is completed. Where the principal offence is not completed, there is the possibility of inchoate liability at present for incitement to commit the principal offence, but when the principal offence is completed, secondary liability occurs, and the secondary offender is liable to be prosecuted as if she were a principal offender and is subject to the same potential punishment as the principal offender. Also included, at least arguably within secondary offending, is the doctrine of joint enterprise which occurs when the secondary party agrees to commit an offence with the principal party. These are the areas covered by the Report.

The starting point is the proposal in the 2006 Report to extend the law of inchoate liability. At present there is such liability for encouraging the principal offender to commit the principal offence when that offence is not committed but none such for assisting her to do so. The 2006 Report recommended that inchoate liability be extended to assistance. As the Law Commission puts it in para. 1.3 of the 2007 Report.

> This recommendation now enables the problem of secondary liability's scope to be addressed along with problems that have arisen in relation to the very nature of such liability, without the distraction of a simultaneous concern with the nature and scope of inchoate liability.

The effect of enacting both Reports, the Commission opined at para. 1.4 would result in 'a scheme whereby inchoate and secondary liability will support and supplement each other in a way that is rational and fair'.

The defects of current law

The Report begins with a critique of current law, in particular how the secondary party may be liable for the crime the principal party has committed even though she did not personally commit that offence but merely aided, abetted, counselled or procured it, yet she is liable as if she did personally commit the offence. For example, the principal offender's *mens rea* for murder is the intent to kill or cause grievous bodily harm but the secondary party is liable for murder with a lesser *mens rea*, the belief that the principal may commit the offence. The Commission recommends that in order for there to be 'parity of culpability' between the principal and secondary offenders the latter should be convicted as a secondary offender only if she intended that the principal would commit the offence; otherwise, the person who is now the secondary offender would become guilty of the recommended offence of assisting or encouraging the principal offence. However, where there is a joint venture, the Commission's view is that the secondary party should be liable as such because she has agreed or did intend to join in the criminal venture, and that agreement or intent constitutes 'parity of culpability' with the principal offender: if, for example, the secondary party in a joint enterprise foresaw that the principal offender might kill, she is appropriately labelled as a murderer just as much as is the principal offender who did kill and did intend to kill. The Commission says at para. 1.23 that:

> . . . the mere fact of agreement is sufficient to render D [the accused] liable for the agreed offence, with no requirement that D does anything further by way of encouragement or assistance. By contrast, where D and P [the principal offender] are not parties to a joint criminal venture, there must be a discrete act of encouragement or assistance.

For this reason, the draft Bill attached to the Report deals with joint ventures separately from other instances of secondary participation.

A second criticism the Commission has of secondary liability is the definition of the *mens rea* and the defences possibly available to the accused. The Commission does not comment on the law in depth in the main part of the Report, but it does in Annexe B when discussing the present law and comment on the position is picked up below when the recommendations are discussed. In summary, there is debate as to whether or not the accused is guilty if she foresaw that the principal *may* (rather than *would*) commit the principal offence; there is also controversy as to when the accused is guilty or not guilty when the principal commits an offence which is different from that agreed, a so-called 'collateral' offence: is the collateral offence 'fundamentally different' from the crime agreed?; also debatable is the liability of the secondary party for a string of offences, for example, if she loans the principal a gun for use on one occasion, is she liable on each occasion the principal uses it to kill others? The Commission refers to other points of difficulty: when is the accused liable as a secondary offender when she stands by and omits to control the principal's commission of the principal offence? Is the accused not guilty if she performs a duty imposed on her by law? For example, in **NCB v Gamble** [1959] QB 11, Devlin J said that the accused was not criminally liable if she returned the jemmy in the following circumstances (Law Commission Report, para. 1.19): 'P [the principal offender] lends D [the potential secondary party] a jemmy. Later P demands the jemmy back. D knows that P intends to use the jemmy to burgle V's [the victim's] premises. D, who hates V, returns the jemmy so that P can commit the burglary. P commits the burglary.' Further issues are noted by the Commission. One is the scope of the doctrine of innocent agency when the vagaries of the English language can lead to difficulties. This problem is well put by the Commission at para. 1.29:

> The problem, actual or perceived, has arisen when the principal offence can be committed only by a person who meets a particular description and D [the person who would normally be the secondary offender] does not meet that description. For example, where D, who is not married, causes X [the person who normally would be the principal party], who is

married, to 'marry' V [the victim] by falsely telling X that his wife has died. On one view, convicting D as a principal [as the doctrine of innocent agency would normally lead to] is illogical because the definition of bigamy stipulates that a principal offender can commit the offence only if he or she is already married.

Finally, and again to quote the Law Commission (para. 1.30):

> if D 'procures' the commission of a no-fault [strict liability] offence by P, P is guilty of the offence as a principal party and D is guilty as a secondary party. However, in our view, holding D liable for the offence as a secondary party does not accurately reflect the nature of D's wrongdoing. This is because in reality D commits the offence through P.

The Law Commission proposes a new offence to deal with this situation.

The proposals

The question than becomes one of how to deal with these issues. The 1993 Law Commission Consultation Paper recommended the abolition of secondary offences. However, the Commission now proposes to retain the area of law but in a modified form, as it had already said in its 2006 Report. There are (para. 1.38):

> cases where D's culpability was such that D would be insufficiently condemned and labelled if he or she was convicted of merely assisting or encouraging the commission of the principal offence rather than convicted of the offence itself. The obvious case, particularly it is D who is the instigator, is where D assists or encourages P with the intention that P should commit the principal offence.

The other advantage of retaining secondary liability occurs when it is not possible to prove which party was the principal offender and which the secondary one: at present it is irrelevant if the accused was the principal or secondary offender provided she must be one or the other. Abolishing secondary liability in favour of (mere) assisting or encouraging would abrogate this forensic advantage.

The Commission's solutions to the problems around secondary liability are to be found in one of the draft Bills attached to the Report. The proposals are:

- a crime of assisting or encouraging the principal party: the accused's *mens rea* would be that she intended (as defined in Chapter 3: see **Woollin** [1999] 1 AC 82 (HL)) the principal offence to be committed (clause 1);

- a crime whereby the accused would be liable for any crime, agreed or collateral, carried out during a criminal venture: the mens rea would be that the accused foresaw that the offence might be committed (clause 2).

There would also be a clause dealing with innocent agency and the current doctrine would be abolished. The Commission states (para. 1.52):

> D would be liable for an offence as a principal offender if he or she intentionally caused P, an innocent agent, to commit the conduct element [i.e. the *actus reus*] of an offence but P does not commit the offence because P:
> 1. is under the age of 10 years;
> 2. has a defence of insanity; or
> 3. acts without the fault required to be convicted of the offence.

The Commission adds in the next paragraph that the recommendations 'would ensure that D could be convicted of a principal offence as a principal offender even if the offence can only be committed by a person who meets a particular description and D does not fit that description'. In this way the Commission deals with the illustration of the bachelor boy and bigamy mentioned above. The Commission also proposes to address the issue also mentioned above of the accused who currently is guilty of being a secondary party to a strict offence committed by the principal. Instead the accused will be guilty as a principal offender. One effect of the scheme is that procuring in the sense of intentionally *causing* the principal to commit the crime will no longer form part of *secondary* liability. Instead, the accused will be guilty as *principal*.

The Commission next proposes to refine the defences to the new offences. First, the **Tyrrell** exception is preserved. Clause 6 of the draft Bill will exculpate the accused (whether as a secondary party or as a principal offender through the doctrine of innocent agency) if the principal offence is aimed at protecting a class of persons and she falls within that class and she is the victim of the offence. Secondly, the Commission proposes a defence when the accused acts to prevent the commission of an offence or to prevent or limit the harm. The burden of proof in respect of this defence would lie on the accused, and it would be question for the jury as to whether the accused did act reasonably. The Commission provides the following example of the application of this defence in para. 1.59:

> D and P are at a pub after a football match and meet a rival gang of supporters. P, along with some others, plan to attack the rival gang and stab their most vocal member (V). D, who does not want V to be harmed, manages to persuade P and the others to damage an item of V's property instead. D is charged with encouraging P to commit criminal damage.

It would be for the jury to take all the facts into account e.g. how serious was the harm prevented? Should the accused have called the police?

Summary

Reading Reports Nos. 300 and 306 together would result in the following proposed state of the law:

(a) Where the principal offender does not commit the offence assisted or encouraged, the accused who assisted or encouraged the principal would be guilty of an inchoate offence. She will be guilty if she does an act capable of encouraging or assisting the person who would be the principal offender ('P') if the principal offence had been committed, and intends to assist or encourage P to perpetrate the *actus reus* of the principal offence OR believes that her act will encourage or assist P to commit the actus reus; and where in all cases the principal crime is not a strict offence, the accused must also believe that P will commit the *actus reus* with the *mens rea* required for that offence and the accused's 'own state of mind is such that were [s]he to perpetrate the conduct element, [s]he would do so with the requisite [mens rea].' (para. 1.61]

(b) Where the principal offender [P] does commit the principal offence, the accused ['D']:

would be liable for P's offence as a secondary party provided that D intended P to engage in the [*actus reus*] of the offence and:
  (1) D believed that P would perpetrate the [*actus reus*] with the fault required to be convicted of the offence; or
  (2) D's state of mind was such that, had he or she perpetrated the [*actus reus*], it would have been with the [mens rea] required for conviction for the offence. (para. 1.63]

One effect of the enactment of the new offences is that the accused would no longer be guilty as a secondary party if she assisted or encouraged but was indifferent as to whether the principal offence took place; if, however, the accused believed that the principal would commit the principal offence, she would be guilty of the offence in (a) above of assisting or encouraging in the belief that the principal offender will be assisted or encouraged in committing the actus reus. In other words, the accused may be guilty of an *inchoate* offence, even though the principal has *committed* the principal offence!

In respect of joint venturers, the accused would be guilty of any offence within the scope of the venture. It will be for the jury to determine whether the principal offence was within the ambit of the venture. Even if the accused opposed the collateral offence, there can still be liability.

In respect of both the new forms of inchoate and secondary liability there would, according to the Report, be the two defences outlined above. The Serious Crime Act 2007 ran these two defences into one and the Commission now proposes to do the same with regard to secondary participation to keep these two areas of law consistent: Consultation Paper No. 183, *Conspiracy and Attempts*, 2007.

Assisting an offender and compounding an arrestable offence

By s 4(1) of the Criminal Law Act 1967:

> [w]here a person has committed an arrestable offence, any other person who, knowing or believing him to be guilty of the offence or of some other arrestable offence, does without lawful authority or reasonable excuse any act with intent to impede his apprehension or prosecution shall be guilty of an offence . . .

It does not matter that the alleged principal offender has been acquitted (*Donald* (1986) 83 Cr App R 49 (DC)), provided that in the accused's trial it can be proved that the accused was guilty. It is uncertain whether the opening words refer solely to the perpetrator of the offence or whether the phrase covers an accessory.

The *actus reus* includes 'any act'. Obvious examples include shielding the principal, destroying evidence, telling lies to the police about the whereabouts of the principal and providing a getaway car or a passport. The accused need not in fact do something which assists the offender. It is sufficient that the act is done with the intent required. Since an act is required, an omission to inform the police of the whereabouts of the principal offender does not give rise to liability. The *mens rea* comprises the intention to impede and knowledge or belief. The phrase 'with intent to' may mean that only direct intent is included (see Chapter 2) and not even foresight that the act is a (virtually) certain consequence is sufficient. 'Knowing or believing' may cover wilful blindness but not, it is thought, recklessness (see further Chapter 3 for knowledge and wilful blindness). The same phrase occurs in the crime of handling and precedents from that offence may be relevant to the interpretation of s 4(1). The accused need not know the identity of the principal: *Brindley* [1971] 2 QB 300 (CA). The defence of lawful authority will cover a decision by the Crown Prosecution Service to abandon a prosecution. It has been suggested that 'reasonable excuse' may include a wife helping her husband: see D. Ormerod (ed.), Smith and Hogan, *Criminal Law*, 12th edn (OUP, 2008) 240, n. 29. There is no liability for attempting this offence: Criminal Attempts Act 1981, s 1(4)(c).

By s 5(1) of the same Act:

> [w]here a person has committed an arrestable offence, any other person who, knowing or believing that the offence or some other arrestable offence has been committed, and that he has information which might be of material assistance in securing the prosecution or conviction of an offender for it, accepts or agrees to accept for not disclosing that information any consideration other than the making good of loss or injury caused by the offence, or the making of reasonable compensation for that loss or injury shall be liable . . .

The word 'consideration' is well known in the law of contract. It will certainly include money and benefits in kind. 'Knowing or believing' bears the same meaning as in s 4(1). There is no requirement of 'with intent to' in s 5(1). Like s 4(1) this offence cannot be attempted: Criminal Attempts Act 1981, s 1(4)(c). A person is not guilty of the s 5(1) offence simply by not reporting an arrestable offence but there is a common law offence, misprision of treason, for failing to report treason. No prosecution may be brought for this offence without the DPP's consent.

Summary

Not just is the perpetrator guilty of an offence but the people who assist may be too. The perpetrator is the principal (offender); the helper is the secondary offender or accomplice. For example, if I help you to kill your enemy by handing over the gun, you, the killer, are the principal offender. In law those who assist are called aiders, abettors, counsellors, and procurers. The law is complicated and is broken down into problem areas such as the mental element of the secondary party, whether the accused can aid by doing nothing, and what happens where the person who would otherwise be the principal party is exempted from liability, whether a victim of the offence may also be an accomplice. The doctrine of innocent agency is considered. There is an explanation of the Law Commission's plans for reform. The chapter ends with the offences of assisting offenders and compounding an arrestable offence.

- Definitions: The principal offender is the one who commits the principal offence: he or she stabs the victim, burns the house down, rapes the complainant. Other people, accessories, accomplices, or secondary parties, may in various ways encourage or assist the principal. For example, they may hand over the knife, shout words of encouragement to the perpetrator of the arson on the house, or hold the victim down in the crime of rape. The accomplice is liable to the same maximum sentence as the principal, but his or her culpability will affect the sentence; and the accomplice may be liable for being a secondary party to an offence more serious than that committed by the principal. The theory behind secondary offences is that the principal offence must have been committed before there can be a secondary offence: this is the doctrine of 'derivative liability'. For example, one cannot be an accessory to murder until the killing has taken place. (One may be guilty of conspiring to murder, incitement to murder or attempted murder if the killing has not yet taken place.) However, the theory of derivative liability is sometimes not followed.

The law states that aiders, abettors, counsellors and procurers are the ways in which accomplices are criminally liable.

An aider is one who assists, helps or supports the principal party, as when he or she supplies a gun.

An abettor would seem to be the same but perhaps the term is more apt to cover those who encourage, incite or instigate the commission of the principal offence.

A counsellor is one who gives advice or assistance.

It has to be said that the distinctions between these forms of secondary liability are hard to find or non-existent. However, there is one form of secondary liability which is more certainly defined than the other three and that is 'procuring'. A procurer is one who produces an outcome by 'endeavour', as the cases put it.

Whatever the form of the secondary participation there must be some 'causal link' between the assistance or encouragement and the principal offence but that link may be an attenuated one, e.g. one can be guilty of being an accessory although the primary accused would have committed the crime in any case. Procuring would seem to be an exception in that there must be a strong causal link between the procuring and the act procured.

- Failure to act: Normally, as we saw in Chapter 2, there is no criminal responsibility for omissions, subject to the imposition of duties to act. One exception is where the accused, the secondary offender, has control over the perpetrator, as occurs when a driving instructor fails to control his or her learner.

- *Mens rea*: The mental element for accessories is complex but it may be stated as: (i) the intent to advise, assist or encourage; and (ii) knowledge of the 'essential matters' of the principal offence (though recklessness would also seem to suffice); and (iii) in cases where there is more than one offence within the accused's contemplation, knowledge that that offence may take place.

- Joint enterprise liability: In recent years some judges have taken the view that where two or more set out to commit a crime (e.g. burglary) and one of them goes further (and, for example, kills), there is a doctrine of joint enterprise separate from that of liability of accessories which governs the liability of the party who did not commit the principal offence (here, murder). The stance taken in this book is that there are not two separate doctrines but that joint enterprise is a subset of secondary liability, but differences reside, not in the substantive law, but in ease of proof.

- Non-conviction of the principal: Because secondary liability is based on the theory of derivative liability, difficulties are faced when the person who would otherwise be the principal is acquitted, is exempt from liability or did not commit the *actus reus*. If there is no *actus reus*, there can be no accessorial liability; if, however, the person who would otherwise be the principal party is exempt, there is an *actus reus* – it's just that the accused cannot be convicted of it – and therefore the accessory may be convicted.

- May the victim be an accessory? In general there is no problem. For example, if a masochist incites a sadist to perform sadistic acts on him or her, the masochist can be guilty of being an accomplice to the principal's crime. However, statutory crimes may be interpreted as protecting members of a certain class. In that event the person who would otherwise be the secondary offender is not liable because he or she is protected. The usual illustration is that of girls under 16 who encourage boys over 16 to have sexual intercourse with them; the girls form a specially protected class and are not liable as accessories to boys' crimes.

- Innocent agency: If the person who would otherwise be the principal is a child under 10 or insane, the accessory is deemed to be the principal. For example, if Peter helps Queenie to commit burglary, normally Peter is the accessory to Queenie's principal; if, however, she is insane, Peter as it were steps into her shoes and he becomes principal. In law Queenie is said to be the innocent agent.

- Withdrawal: There is a defence if the accused withdraws before the commission of the principal offence. The boundaries of the defence seem to vary with the facts. It may consist of simply communicating the fact of withdrawal, stopping the offence or informing the police.

- Reform of the law: The Law Commission has treated of this area in recent consultation papers. These are outlined.

- Assisting an offender and compounding an arrestable offence: The crime of being an accessory after the fact was abolished in 1967 and partly replaced by assisting an offender (to avoid apprehension or prosecution for an arrestable offence) and by not revealing information 'which might be of material assistance in securing the prosecution or conviction of an offender' for an arrestable offence in return for consideration such as money. The latter crime is known as 'compounding' or 'compounding an arrestable offence'.

References

Reports

Judicial Studies Board, *Specimen Direction on Joint Responsibility*

Law Commission Consultation Paper no. 131, *Assisting and Encouraging Crime* (1993)

Law Commission Consultation Paper no. 177, *A new Homicide Act for England & Wales?* (2005)

Law Commission Report no. 177, *A Criminal Code for England & Wales* (1989)

Law Commission Report nos. 279 and 282, *Children: Their Non-accidental Death or Serious Injury (Criminal Trials)* (2003)

Law Commission Report no. 304, *Murder, Manslaughter and Infanticide* (2006)

Law Commission Report no. 305, *Participating in Crime* (2007)

Books

Mitchell, B. *Law Relating to Violent Crime* (CLT Publishing, 1997)

Reed, A. and Fitzpatrick, B. *Criminal Law* 3rd edn (Thomson, 2006)

Seago, P. *Criminal Law* 4th edn (Sweet & Maxwell, 1994)

Smith, J. C. and Hogan, B. *Criminal Law* (ed. D. Ormerod) 11th edn (Oxford University Press, 2005)

Williams, G. *Textbook of Criminal Law* 2nd edn (Stevens, 1983)

Journals

Smith, J. C. 'Criminal liability of accessories' [1997] 113 LQR 453

Smith, J. C. 'Secondary participation in crime' [1994] NLJ 679

Smith, K. J. M. 'The Law Commission Consultation Paper on complicity' [1994] Crim LR 239

Sullivan G. R. 'Fault elements and joint enterprise' [1994] Crim LR 252

Further reading

Beaumont, J. 'Abetting without a principal' (1977) 30 NILQ 1

Bohlander, M. 'The Sexual Offences Act 2003 – The *Tyrrell* principle – criminalizing the victims' [2005] Crim LR 701

Buxton, R. 'Complicity in the Criminal Code' (1969) 85 LQR 252

Clarkson, C. M. V. 'Complicity, *Powell* and manslaughter' [1998] Crim LR 556

Giles, M. 'Complicity – the problem of joint enterprise' [1990] Crim LR 383

Kadish, S. H. 'Reckless complicity' (1997) 87 JCL & Crim 369

Lanham, D. 'Accomplices and withdrawal' (1981) 97 LQR 575

Lanham, D. 'Primary and derivative criminal liability – an Australian perspective' [2000] Crim LR 707

Ormerod, D. 'Joint enterprise: in course of a joint enterprise to inflict unlawful violence the principal kills with an intention to kill which is unknown and unforeseen by a secondary party' [2007] Crim LR 721

Simester, A. P. 'The mental element in complicity' (2006) 122 LQR 578

Smith, J. C. Commentary on *Wan* [1995] Crim LR 297

Smith, J. C. 'Joint enterprise and secondary liability' (1999) 50 NILQ 153

Smith, K. J. M. 'Complicity and causation' [1986] Crim LR 663

Smith, K. J. M. 'The Law Commission's Consultation Paper on complicity: a blueprint for rationalisation' [1994] Crim LR 239

Smith, K. J. M. 'Withdrawal in complicity: A restatement of principles' [2001] Crim LR 769

Sullivan, G. R. 'Fault element and joint enterprise' [1994] Crim LR 252

Sullivan, G. R. 'Complicity for first degree murder and complicity in an unlawful killing' [2006] Crim LR 502

Sullivan, G. R. 'Inchoate liability for assisting and encouraging crime' [2006] Crim LR 1047

Sullivan G. R. 'Participation in Crime: Law Crim No. 305 – joint enterprise' [2008] Crim LR 19

Taylor, R. 'Procuring, causation, innocent agency and the Law Commission' [2008] Crim LR 32

Williams, G. 'Which of you did it?' (1989) 52 MLR 179

Williams, G. 'Letting offences happen' [1990] Crim LR 780

Williams, G. 'Victims and other exempt parties in crime' (1990) 10 LS 245

Wilson, W. 'A rational sentence of liability for participating in crime' [2008] Crim LR 3

The principal work is K. J. M. Smith, *A Modern Treatise on the Law of Criminal Complicity* (Clarendon, 1991). A more theoretical approach is found in W. Wilson, *Central Issues in Criminal Theory* (Hart, 2002), ch. 7.

For the problem of parents and the like killing children, see the Law Commission's Report, *Children: Their Non-accidental Death or Serious Injury (Criminal Trials)*, Law Com. No. 282, 2003, which was preceded by a Consultative Report, Law Com. No. 279, 2003. The government did not faithfully carry out the Commission's recommendations in the Domestic Violence, Crime and Victims Act 2004.

For an Australian view, see New South Wales Law Reform Commission Report Paper 2, *Complicity* (2008)

Visit **www.mylawchamber.co.uk/jefferson** to access
exam-style questions with answer guidance, multiple
choice quizzes, live weblinks, an online glossary,
and regular updates to the law.

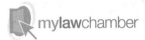

Use **Case Navigator** to read in full some of the key cases referenced in
this chapter:

R v *Brown* [1993] 2 All ER 75
R v *Cunningham* [1957] 2 All ER 412

6

Vicarious and corporate liability

Introduction to vicarious liability

In criminal law one person is not generally speaking liable for the crimes of another. This accords with Judaeo-Christian morality: why should a person be guilty of another's crimes? Normally only one person is criminally liable for acts or omissions. A recent example is the decision of the House of Lords in **Seaboard Offshore Ltd v Secretary of State for Transport** [1994] 2 All ER 99. After the Zeebrugge ferry disaster, in which almost 200 were killed when a roll-on roll-off ferry sank off the Belgian coast, a new crime was introduced, failure by the owner or charterer of a ship to take all reasonable steps to ensure that it is operated in a safe manner. 'Reasonable' is defined as 'reasonable for him to take in the circumstances of the case'. The House of Lords held that the crime did not permit vicarious liability, emphasis being put on the phrase 'for him'. Therefore, the shipowner or charterer was not guilty when the crew or officers of the company operated the ship in an unsafe way. The duty was personal to the owner or charterer. Lord Keith noted that it would have been strange if Parliament had imposed liability on owners and charterers for all actions of their subordinates including failures by cabin stewards to close portholes. There are exceptions, and those exceptions form the topic of vicarious liability.

There is a doctrine of the same name in the law of tort, but the width of the two sets of law is different. In tort employers are usually liable for the tort of their employees committed in the course of their employment. In criminal law liability is exceptional because as a general rule liability and therefore the stigma of being convicted of an offence is personal to the accused. The old case of **Huggins** (1730) 92 ER 518, where the accused, warden of the Fleet prison, London, was acquitted of murder when the victim's death had been caused by his incarceration in an unhealthy cell by a gaoler, exemplifies the distinction. The warden did not know of the facts. In tort he would be liable; in criminal law he was not guilty. The gaoler and the warden, in the words of the court, 'must each answer for their own acts and stand or fall by their own behaviour'. The next section deals with the exceptions where a person is vicariously liable.

The exceptions are aimed at obliging the accused to exercise control over others, but it may be unfair to penalise someone for what another has done and the accused may not be deterred in the future. The perpetrator will also be guilty of the offence either as a principal or as an accessory.

The exceptions

(a) At common law two offences give rise to vicarious liability. The exception of public nuisance was established in **Stephens** (1866) LR 1 QB 702. Since the aim of the prosecution was not to punish the accused but to prevent the continuation of the nuisance, the accused was guilty when his servants had dumped rubbish into a river and thereby obstructed navigation. The court argued that the proceedings were in substance civil in character: it was as if the civil law doctrine of vicarious liability applied. It is assumed that if the proceedings are in truth criminal, the doctrine may not apply. It is difficult to distinguish criminal and civil objectives. Certainly **Stephens** is not applicable to statutory nuisances, where the accused is guilty only when the words of the statute so demand. The other common law crime importing vicarious liability is criminal libel: see **Holbrook** (1878) 4 QBD 42. The accused is liable for the acts of his employees in publishing a criminal libel only if he acted negligently: Libel Act 1843, s 7.

(b) Some statutes expressly make one party liable for the acts of another. For example, the Transport Act 1982, s 31, conclusively presumes that the owner of a vehicle was the driver at the time of the commission of certain offences, but the owner can avoid liability by proving that another person was driving without his consent. An accused, the licensee of premises, is guilty of a crime if either he or his servant sells intoxicating liquor to a person out of permitted hours.

(c) Sometimes Acts of Parliament are construed so as to make one person liable for the acts of another. For this reason the principle is sometimes known as 'extensive construction'. The Law Commission in its Consultation Paper No. 135, *Involuntary Manslaughter*, 1994, called it 'extended construction'. There is no need for the relationship to be that of employer and employee (see below). This type of liability arises where the duty is said to be absolute, i.e. personal to the accused. He cannot escape responsibility for delegating the obligation to another. In this sense the liability of the accused is personal, not vicarious. This type of vicarious liability works only when the statute creates a strict offence. (If the offence is not strict, the fourth exception, below, may be applicable.) The principal is liable for the physical acts of his agent, but not for his mental element. In order to see whether this principle applies, the court in **Mousell Bros v LNWR** [1917] 2 KB 836 held that the aim of the Act, its words, and the nature of the duty had to be investigated as well as 'the person upon whom it is imposed, the person for whom it would in ordinary circumstances be performed, and the person upon whom the penalty is imposed'. This is an example.

Duke of Leinster [1924] 1 KB 311

An undisclosed bankrupt was convicted under s 155 of the Bankruptcy Act 1914 of obtaining credit of more than £10 without disclosing his financial situation. He was guilty, even though he had told his agent not to obtain such credit.

Among words which have given rise to this form of vicarious liability is 'use'. Employers 'use' a vehicle when an employee or independent contractor drives it: **Green v Burnett** [1955] 1 QB 78 and **Hallett Silberman Ltd v Cheshire CC** [1993] RTR 32 (DC). Both the employers and the driver 'use' the vehicle. Another word so interpreted is 'sell'. Employers are guilty of selling something which it is unlawful to sell (such as cigarettes to a person under 16) when the actual sale is made by an employee: *Coppen* v *Moore (No. 2)* [1898] 2 QB 306. It does not matter that the employers did not know of the sale (or use) and were not even in the country at the time. An alternative approach to cases such as this is to say that the employers are the legal owners of the items sold; only they can sell them; they sell through the medium of the sales assistants; therefore, they are directly, not vicariously, liable. Employers also possess an item though it is their employee who controls it in fact. They supply a video to under-age persons and possess goods through their employees. The accused is deemed to have done the unlawful act despite not having been physically the actor. For example, a person, including a company, can cause pollution to enter a river, even though the individual who actually did pollute the river was an employee. Some activities, however, cannot be interpreted as making the employers or principals liable. It is thought that such persons do not 'drive' when it is their employee's or agent's hands which are on the steering wheel. (Compare *Thornton* v *Mitchell* [1940] 1 All ER 339.) There has been little discussion in the courts as to why some words are interpreted to impose liability and some not.

Besides the restriction that the verb must as a matter of English language be referable to the accused, the act must be within the course of employment or agency. For example, if the employee of an estate agency takes an illegal premium for a tenancy, the employer is not liable because the employee has no authority to take one: *Barker* v *Levinson* [1951] 1 KB 342. Cf. cases such as *Coppen* v *Moore (No. 2)*, above, which involve doing an authorised act, selling, in an unauthorised manner. The taking of the premium was not a way of doing the job, whereas using a car is a way of doing it. As in tort law a defendant is liable even though the delegate acted contrary to instructions, as *Coppen* v *Moore (No. 2)* illustrates. Employers would not be using a vehicle when the accused was on a frolic of his own such as when he is driving his family to the seaside on a summer Sunday. It should be noted that this extensive construction principle has been said not to apply to licensing offences: *McKenna* v *Harding* (1905) 69 JP 354. Also under this principle the verb or adverb must not import *mens rea* as, e.g., 'allowing' (see *DPP* v *Kellet* [1994] Crim LR 916 (DC) but cf. *Greener* (1996) 160 JP 265 (DC) which is *contra*) and 'knowingly' usually do. As *Coppen* v *Moore (No. 2)* demonstrates, the accused remains liable even though he has forbidden the employee to do the forbidden act, in this case to sell American ham as 'Scotch ham'. The House of Lords approved this principle in *Director General of Fair Trading* v *Pioneer Concrete (UK) Ltd* [1995] 1 AC 456, a case on contempt of court.

The ability to get at the owner is especially useful where there are several branches. Since the accused is not in direct control of each branch, he would not be liable if the prosecution had to prove that he knew of the wrongdoing. However, the view of Card, Cross and Jones, *Criminal Law*, 17th edn (OUP, 2006), 854, should be mentioned.

> It seems that under the extensive construction principle only the act of the employee etc., and not his *mens rea*, can be imputed to the employer etc. The result is that the principle is limited to offences of strict liability. Where . . . a strict liability offence requires *mens rea* as to [some] elements, the employer . . . must have *mens rea* as to those elements before [he] can be vicariously liable.

It should be noted that this exception is not restricted to the employer/employee relationship but includes, e.g., the co-licensee of a refreshment house: *Linnett* v *MPC* [1946] KB 290. Other instances include club committee members for bar staff, employers for sub-contractors, partners for partners, and principals for agents. The issue is whether one person had control over another.

It should also be noted that extensive construction is not in truth an instance of vicarious liability but of personal liability. The act of one person is treated as if it were the act of the accused.

(d) The fourth exception is the delegation principle, which may make the accused vicariously liable when the offence is a *mens rea* one. Unlike in the third exception *mens rea* is attributed to the employers, or principals, or other delegators. The employer is liable for breach of a duty which statute has placed on him. Without this doctrine defendants could escape criminal liability by delegating their duties and the criminal law would be rendered unenforceable. The main use of this doctrine is in relation to licensees and the principle appears to be restricted to those such as licensees who possess a particular status. An authority is *Allen v Whitehead*.

Allen v *Whitehead* [1930] 1 KB 211

The accused employed a manager to run a cafe in London. He instructed him not to allow prostitutes to gather on the premises, and visited the cafe once or twice daily. On eight consecutive days prostitutes stayed there from 8 p.m. to 4 a.m. He was held to be guilty of knowingly permitting prostitutes to remain in a place of refreshment, contrary to s 44 of the Metropolitan Police Act 1839. He was guilty even though his manager had flouted his instructions, even though he had put up notices telling prostitutes not to sit in the cafe, and even though he did not know that prostitutes had gathered together. (The manager could be convicted of being an accessory.)

The delegator is convicted for not doing anything (an omission), and even if he forbade the act. Lord Hewart CJ said that if the accused was not guilty, 'this statute would be rendered nugatory'. If there is delegation the accused is guilty whether he is in the next room or in the next county. The accused is liable vicariously even for the acts of employees low in the hierarchy and even though he is well away from the premises.

The doctrine ensures that natural and juristic persons do not escape liability when they have delegated a duty to low-level workers but it should be noted that the doctrine applies even though the accused has taken great care in selecting his employees. Most cases in this area, including *Allen v Whitehead*, are concerned with keeping certain premises or licensing offences.

Sopp v *Long* [1970] 1 QB 518

The accused was secretary to a firm which ran the station buffet at Windsor. The manageress gave a short measure of whisky. The accused was convicted under s 24(1) of the Weights and Measures Act 1963. He 'sold' the whisky, which was served by the person on the spot, to whom the running of the premises had been delegated.

If the third exception, extensive construction, applied to licensing offences, the position would have been that the licence-holder 'sold' within the meaning of the statute. *Sopp v Long* illustrates that the delegation principle applies to subdelegates. If one person, the licensee, delegates the running of a restaurant to another who sub-delegates it to a third party, the licensee is liable by means of this principle for the acts of the third party.

To the delegation principle there are three restrictions.

(i) *The delegation must be complete.* The landmark case is the House of Lords authority of **Vane v Yiannopoullos**.

Vane v Yiannopoullos [1965] AC 486

The accused, a restaurateur, held a licence under which he could serve alcohol only to persons taking meals. He ordered his staff to stick to the terms of the licence. One waitress did not follow his instructions. By a three to two majority and with little enthusiasm for the doctrine, the House of Lords held that there was only a partial delegation, which was not sufficient for conviction. The accused was not on the floor where the alcohol was served, but was on the premises.

Power must be generally delegated: **Winson** [1969] 1 QB 371, following *dicta* of Lords Reid and Evershed, two of the majority in **Vane**. Accordingly, on the facts of **Allen v Whitehead**, above, if the accused has not delegated control fully, he will not be guilty of allowing prostitutes to gather, even if he ought to have known of their presence and even if he was in control.

The line between 'complete' or 'general' and 'partial' delegation may not be easy to draw on the facts of cases. The case to compare with **Vane** is **Howker v Robinson** [1972] 2 All ER 786. A licensee, the accused, delegated the running of the lounge bar to a barman, but kept control of the public bar. Alcohol was served to a person under 18. The licensee was held to be guilty. The facts do not look like complete delegation and the outcome appears inconsistent with **Vane**. **Howker** can be supported on the ground that the question of delegation is one of fact, and since the magistrates had held there to be full delegation, the Divisional Court simply confirmed that decision. Nevertheless, on the facts **Howker** looks like a case of partial delegation at best, with the barman in the lounge being exactly that, the barman and not the delegate with full authority, and so the licensee should not have been guilty vicariously. Moreover, even accepting that there had been only partial delegation would not have exculpated the accused. The sub-section under which the accused was charged did not only catch the 'servant' who sold alcohol to someone under age. It also applied to 'the holder of the licence', i.e. to the accused in **Howker**. There was no need to stretch the facts to fit the doctrine because the accused was liable personally anyway. **Howker v Robinson** demonstrates that the delegation principle applies even when the employee himself would be liable and the purpose of the legislation thereby promoted.

While the court did not reason in this way, **Howker** was distinguished in **Bradshaw v Ewart-James** [1983] QB 671 (DC). The master of a ship set a course which complied with the Collision Regulations. He handed over the watch to the chief officer and left the bridge. While under that officer's charge the vessel was navigated in such a way that the Regulations were violated. The ship's master was held to be not guilty. One way of justifying that result is to say that a temporary delegation (as here where the accused was asleep) is not a complete delegation. Similarly, the court in **Howker** should not have held that there was a complete delegation.

(ii) *The delegation principle applies only to* mens rea *offences.* Lord Parker CJ in **Winson**, above, decided that the delegation principle did not apply where the principal offence was a strict one. If the offence is strict (where there is no *mens rea* attached to any element of the *actus reus*: see Chapter 4), the accused may be liable under the third exception. Accordingly, where there is full delegation, the defendant is liable for *mens rea* crimes. If there is only partial delegation, the accused who did not know of the facts is not liable under this principle but can be liable where the statute can be interpreted in such a way that it covers what he did.

(iii) *The delegate must have acted within the scope of his authority.* As with extensive construction the delegator is not liable if the delegate acted on an unauthorised project. He remains liable for the doing of an authorised act in an unauthorised manner.

Under the fourth exception, where the licensee is guilty (as the principal offender), the person who did the act is liable as an accessory. If the third exception applies, both parties may be liable as joint principals. For example, both the driver and his employers 'use' a vehicle or 'sell' hams.

The delegation doctrine applies only to natural persons. Therefore, a company cannot be liable under this principle.

One final point on the delegation doctrine is this. If there is full delegation, the employer is liable no matter how well he has chosen his subordinates. However, if the delegation is not complete, he is not liable no matter how badly he supervises his subordinates.

Vicarious liability and attempts: vicarious liability and secondary participation

See p 422 for a definition of a crime of attempt. See pp 168–9 for an explanation of aiding and abetting.

Gardner v *Ackroyd* [1952] 2 QB 743 held that there can be no vicarious liability for attempting an offence even when that crime is one which imposes vicarious liability when completed. Similarly, *Ferguson* v *Weaving* [1951] 1 KB 814 decided that the doctrine did not apply to aiding and abetting an offence, even though that offence imposed vicarious liability on the principal offender. To be guilty as a secondary offender the accused must know the essential facts constituting the offence, even a crime of strict liability. He would not know them if he were liable vicariously.

The rationale of vicarious liability

This section considers the arguments for and against vicarious liability.

The justification for this doctrine is social policy. The statute is made effective by vicarious liability. As Lord Reid said in *Vane* v *Yiannopoullos*, above:

> If there was no provision making the servant liable to prosecution it would be impossible to enforce the law adequately if it was necessary in every case to prove *mens rea* in the licence holder.

Lord Reid considered that the effect was to oblige employers to choose employees who took care. However, employers are liable whether or not they themselves took care in the selection of employees, where the delegation has been total. Defendants are guilty even if they have instructed their agents to comply with the law. A second reason is illustrated thus: if one makes the owner of the car liable to pay excess parking charges even though someone else left it too long at the meter, the police are saved time and money in getting the right person. A third reason is that the employers may have financially benefited from the wrongdoing.

The rationale of the law and a statement of doctrine of delegation were brought together by Lord Evershed in **Vane**.

> Where the scope and purpose of the relevant Act is the maintenance of proper and accepted standards of public order in licensed premises or other comparable establishments, there arises under the legislation what Channell J in **Emary v Nolloth** [1903] 2 KB 264, called a 'quasi-criminal offence' which renders the licensee or proprietor criminally liable for the acts of his servants, though there may be no *mens rea* on his part. On the other hand, where the relevant legislation imports the word 'knowingly' . . . the result will be different . . . In the absence of proof of actual knowledge, nevertheless, the licensee or proprietor may be held liable if he is shown . . . effectively to have 'delegated' his proprietary or managerial functions.

The phrase 'quasi-criminal' offence was a popular one around the end of the nineteenth century in vicarious and corporate liability cases. The justification used by J. Edwards, *Mens Rea in Statutory Offences* (Macmillan, 1955) 243 is:

> [s]o long as the criminal law is used as a means to securing the legislative standard of correct trading, business and social welfare behaviour, it is legitimate to have recourse to the principle of vicarious liability.

For example, polluting streams is deleterious. It is beneficial to prevent effluent entering water. If employers were not liable for the acts of their employees in letting a stream become polluted, pollution would not be controlled – with disastrous consequences for life. The effectiveness of legislation is increased by vicarious liability and defendants are obliged to increase training, numbers of supervisory personnel and the checking of machinery. Similarly sales of adult videos to children would not be prevented if it had to be proved that directors knew the child's age: **Tesco Stores Ltd v Brent LBC** [1993] 2 All ER 718 (DC). It was held that the company 'supplied' a video to an under-age child when it was sold by a shop assistant. She had reasonable grounds to believe that the child was under age. Her state of mind was imputed to her employers who therefore had no defence that they neither knew nor had reasonable grounds for believing that the child was over age.

The contrary arguments may be summarised thus.

(a) It is a fundamental principle that criminal responsibility should be personal. Why should a blameless person be punished for something another has done? Devlin J put this well in **Reynolds v GH Austin & Sons Ltd** [1951] 2 KB 135: 'If a man is punished because of an act done by another, whom he cannot reasonably be expected to influence or control, the law is engaged, not in punishing thoughtlessness or inefficiency, and thereby promoting the welfare of the community, but in pouncing upon the most convenient victim.'

(b) The accused may be guilty despite his not knowing that any offence has been committed.

(c) He is guilty even though he has done his best to prevent the offence. For example, he may have told the employee not to do as he did.

(d) The argument that the effect of the statute would be minimised if the courts did not read in vicarious liability is a weak one. It is certainly not proved. It should be for

Parliament, not the courts, to decide when a person is guilty of a crime. Another way of making the same point is that the doctrine is an invention of the courts. It is not for the judiciary to create new crimes. If Parliament did not state that an accused was guilty, the courts should not interfere. If Parliamentary drafting is poor, the remedy does not lie in the hands of the courts. The reader may care to compare strict liability where sometimes the judges read in *mens rea* when Parliament has (perhaps at times through poor drafting) not expressly stated the requisite fault element.

(e) The doctrine of delegation has come in for particular criticism. If the accused remains on the premises and there is no complete delegation, he is not liable no matter how careless he has been in selecting the delegate. However, if the accused is off the premises and has completely delegated, he is liable even though he took all due care in appointing a subordinate. One effect of this argument is that restaurateurs and the like should delegate only partly. However, surely liability should not turn on whether delegation is complete or not because the restaurateur may be performing other jobs as an employer which call for his attention and one would not want him to stop doing these tasks in order to provide complete supervision at all times.

The strength of these arguments both pro and con turns on the facts of individual cases unless one believes that criminal law should apply only where the accused committed the *actus reus* and had the *mens rea* of the offence charged.

The Human Rights Act 1998 may in time affect the law of vicarious liability. Article 3 of the European Convention on Human Rights forbids inhuman or degrading punishment and here the accused is penalised for another's actions.

The draft Criminal Code

The Law Commission's draft Criminal Code, Law Com. No. 177, 1989, cl 29, would allow vicarious liability only for the acts of the agent and not for his state of mind. The *mens rea* in the statute would have to be proved against the accused (cl 29(2)). One effect would be to abolish the delegation principle for the future (cl 29(3)). Otherwise, cl 29(2) provides:

> . . . an element of an offence (other than a fault element) may be attributed to a person by reason of an act done by another only if that other is –
> (a) specified in the definition of the offence as a person whose act may be so attributed, or
> (b) acting within the scope of his employment or authority and the definition of the offence specifies the element in terms which apply to both persons.

Situations where the statute expressly makes one person liable for the acts of another are dealt with in (a); (b) deals with exception; (c) (see p 211, above), extensive construction. Clause 29(1)(b) would preserve the results of cases such as *Coppen v Moore (No. 2)*, above, and the accused would still be guilty even if he ordered the perpetrator not to do the forbidden act, as the example given by the Law Commission illustrates (the example, 29(ii), gives the facts of *Coppen*).

> A statute provides that it is an offence for a person to sell goods to which a false trade description is applied. No fault is required for this offence. E, an assistant employed in D's shop, sells a ham as a 'Scotch' ham. D had previously given instructions that such hams are not to be sold under any specific name of place or origin. The ham is in fact an American ham. Both D and E are guilty of the offence as principals.

An express statutory version of vicarious liability is found in example 29(i):

> A statute provides that it is an offence for the holder of a justices' licence whether by himself, his servant or agent to supply intoxicating liquor on licensed premises outside permitted hours. No fault is required for this offence. D is the licensee of a public house. E, his barman, serves a drink to a friend outside the permitted hours . . . D is guilty of the offence as a principal. Assuming fault on E's part, E is guilty as an accessory.

The draft Criminal Code, like the present law, is not limited to employers and employees but covers independent contractors. The Law Commission thought (at 212) that the law should be left for judicial interpretation, but it considered that a householder would not 'use' a removal van owned by removers when he was moving house, whereas a person might 'use' a lorry when he has contracted out deliveries to someone else.

Corporate liability

This section deals with situations in which a company is liable criminally (corporate liability). Only companies can be liable in these ways, not partnerships or unincorporated associations. However, an association is liable if the statute punishes a 'person', unless the contrary intention appears.

For many years companies were not criminally liable. Part of the problem was that criminal law was designed for individual defendants. For example, companies cannot be brought before the court and could not be hanged or put into prison. Over time most of these restrictions were abolished but companies still cannot be found guilty of murder because the sole sanction is life imprisonment and one cannot imprison an intangible entity. Problems did remain. *Mens rea* is the doctrine which deals with the fault of human beings, not artificial entities. The problem of affixing a company with *mens rea* is considered below. Reform in respect of killings (only) came about in the Corporate Manslaughter and Corporate Homicide Act 2007, which, except for some provisions not relevant here, came into force on 6 April 2008.

Corporate liability is particularly important because most defective products are put onto the market by, most pollution is caused by, most crashes occur in transport run by, and most accidents at work take place at sites occupied by companies. Lord Hoffmann in the Privy Council in a civil case (but the same principles apply in criminal law) *Meridian Global Funds Asia Ltd* v *Securities Commission* [1995] 2 AC 500 advised that whether a company was liable for a statutory offence depended on the terms of the enactment, its content and its policy. The issue was whether a company was liable for the acts of its senior investment managers done without its knowledge. The Judicial Committee decided that it was, after investigating the policy of the statute, which was to compel disclosure of the identity of persons who had acquired substantial security. In a company those persons were those who had the company's authority to acquire the security. Therefore, the company was liable. This case marked a break from earlier law.

There are several ways in which a company may be made liable. Each mode has separate rules. The person in the company who actually committed the offence is guilty as joint principal.

(a) A statute may impose liability on a company just as on anyone. If a statute penalises the occupier of premises, and a company is the occupier, the company is guilty. Statute imposes a duty on companies to ensure the health and safety of employees and sub-contractors, and a breach of this duty renders the company criminally liable. For example, in ***Gateway Foodmarkets Ltd*** [1997] 2 Cr App R 40 (CA) a company was liable when it failed to ensure the safety of a lift and an employee was killed. The statute may impose liability either expressly or by necessary implication. Similarly, the corporation as owner of the vehicle is guilty of various offences committed by the driver: Transport Act 1982, s 31 (see under vicarious liability). There used to be several difficulties facing a prosecution. A company could not be personally present in court; a company could not be committed for trial; and a company could not be hanged. These difficulties were in time evaded, and none poses a problem nowadays.

(b) If the offence is a strict one, such as public nuisance and criminal libel, there is no problem in imposing liability: ***Great North of England Railway Co*** (1846) 2 Cox CC 70. The company was liable for obstructing the highway while building a railway. Liability was therefore imposed for doing an act, not merely for omitting to act. Denman CJ said liability was imposed to deter the company.

(c) A company is liable for omissions. While there may be a conceptual difficulty in understanding how it is that a company can act, there is none in punishing a company for failing to act.

(d) A company is vicariously liable in the same way as a person. Corporate vicarious liability is of the same width as the vicarious liability of natural persons. At least in a small company there is a good deal of supervision over employees. Vicarious liability punishes failures to exercise care. The human actor (the employee) is seen as the company's agent. However, it should be noted that the company, just like a natural person, is liable even though it has not been at fault.

The company can be liable for crimes of *mens rea*. In ***Mousell Bros*** v ***LNWR***, above, a company was guilty of fraudulently evading freight charges. A company will be liable for tax evasion, fencing machinery, not holding a car licence, selling contaminated food, and so on. In ***Chuter*** v ***Freeth & Pocock Ltd*** [1911] 2 KB 832, it was held that a company 'believes' through its agents. The rule applies even though the company has told the employee not to do the act: ***Griffiths*** v ***Studebakers Ltd*** [1924] 1 KB 103. However, if it requires a natural person to perform the prohibited activity, a corporation will not be vicariously liable even though a natural person would be so liable. For example, a company cannot drive a vehicle, though a natural person can. Therefore, a company cannot be found guilty of an offence which has 'drives' as part of the *actus reus*: see ***Richmond-upon-Thames LBC*** v ***Pinn & Wheeler Ltd*** [1989] Crim LR 510 (DC).

As in vicarious liability there is an exception to liability. The company is not liable vicariously for aiding and abetting. The corporation must have knowledge of the facts out of which the offence arises through a responsible agent, though it need not know that a crime has been committed: ***John Henshall (Quarries) Ltd*** v ***Harvey*** [1965] 2 QB 233.

It cannot be too strongly emphasised that when vicarious liability applies, the master (whether a natural or juristic person) is liable for the activities of all employees, even subordinate ones. The doctrine, unlike the identification doctrine, below, is not limited to controlling officers: see ***National Rivers Authority*** v ***Alfred McAlpine Homes (East) Ltd*** (1994) 158 JP 628 (DC) and ***Tesco Stores Ltd*** v ***Brent LBC***, above. In the former case a company was liable for causing polluted matter, wet cement, to enter controlled water, a stream, even though the pollution was actually caused by employees and the site manager who were not directing minds of the company. This point received the approval of the Lords in ***Director General of Fair Trading*** v ***Pioneer Concrete (UK) Ltd***, above.

One might have expected cases such as ***Tesco Stores Ltd*** v ***Brent LBC*** to be resolved using the identification doctrine. As a result it cannot be said with any certainty whether a company will be liable for all employees vicariously as in this case or only where the individual is part of the directing mind and will of the company.

(e) There is a *dictum* in ***Seaboard***, above, that a company would be liable for the crime of failing to ensure that a ship is operated safely if it had not provided a system for ensuring the safe operation. If this *dictum* is correct, a company would be liable even though the prosecution could not prove that any one natural person was at fault. If followed, the *dictum* would swallow up the identification doctrine, which is discussed next.

(f) Under the doctrine of identification (which is also known as the *alter ego* doctrine) the company is personally liable. It is not liable vicariously. It is deemed to have committed the offence by itself. A term which is coming to be used in this context is direct liability. The doctrine makes a company liable for *mens rea* offences. The knowledge of the person to whom full delegation is made is treated as being the knowledge of the company. Under this doctrine a company is liable even when a natural person would not be liable. The methods of founding corporate liability in (a)–(d) are the same as for natural persons but this head marks a break from orthodox theory and penalises companies as companies, not as substitutes for natural persons. Where vicarious liability applies, the company is liable no matter what the status of the employee but the identification thesis governs only when the employee is a controlling officer. This doctrine applies to both common law and statutory offences. It is dependent on statutory interpretation when the crime is statutory: ***Meridian***, above (cf. extensive construction, discussed above).

In what was until ***Meridian*** the principal authority, ***Tesco Supermarkets Ltd*** v ***Nattrass*** [1972] AC 153, Lord Reid stated the basis of the doctrine in this way:

> A living person has a mind which can have knowledge or intention or be negligent and has hands to carry out his intentions. A corporation has none of these: it must act through living persons. Then the person who acts is not speaking or acting for the company. He is acting as the company . . . He is not acting as a servant, representative, agent or delegate . . . If [his mind] is a guilty mind, then that guilt is the guilt of the company.

A company, being a legal institution, cannot operate without human intervention. It cannot take action or have a state of mind. The principle, which is sometimes known as the *alter ego* doctrine, was established in a trilogy of cases from 1944. In ***DPP*** v ***Kent & Sussex Contractors Ltd*** [1944] KB 146 Macnaghten J said:

> If a responsible agent of the company puts forward on its behalf a document which he knows to be false and by which he intends to deceive, . . . his intention and belief must be imputed to the company.

That is, the acts of the controlling officer of the company are deemed to be those of the company. The same is true of the officer's state of mind. A company not being a natural person has no mind but others' states of mind are attributed to it. In ***Meridian***, above, Lord Hoffmann called the methods by which acts and states of mind are imputed to the company 'rules of attribution'. The decision in ***Kent & Sussex*** was approved in ***ICR Haulage Ltd*** [1944] KB 551 (CCA). A company was held liable for conspiracy, then a common law offence. A natural person cannot in general be liable vicariously for a common law crime (the exceptions are criminal libel and public nuisance), yet the company was liable. The court adopted the test of identification. The acts and state of mind of the managing director were held to be those of the company. Unlike the doctrine of delegation, there is no need for an absolute or personal duty to be delegated before the company is liable. The next case was *Moore v I Bresler Ltd* [1944] 2 All ER 515. False returns were made to purchase tax forms. The Divisional Court held that the acts of the company secretary and branch managers were to be treated as those of the company. In *Meridian* Lord Hoffmann advised that the question whose act and state of mind was to be attributed to the company was answered 'by applying the usual canons of interpretation, taking into account the language of the rule (if it is a statute) and its content and policy'. This response was especially problematic in respect of common law crimes but later authority on corporate manslaughter (see below) is to the effect that common law crimes are still governed by *Tesco v Nattrass* and are not affected by *Meridian*, though there is civil law authority that *Meridian* is of general application. The law is now more uncertain than it was after *Tesco v Nattrass*.

Moore raises the issue of whether the activities of all employees are deemed to be those of the company. Modern law used to stress that only acts of controlling officers were taken to be those of the company. The question was: how far down the chain of command do the courts go? The metaphor often used was 'brain' and 'hands', terms which derive from the civil law judgment of Denning LJ in *HL Bolton (Engineering) Co Ltd v TJ Graham & Sons Ltd* [1957] 1 QB 159. Under this anthropomorphic distinction, which Y Z Stern in 'Corporate criminal personal liability: who is the corporation?' (1987–88) 13 *Journal of Corporation Law* 125 at 130 called 'another plastic and useless description', the company was liable only for the forbidden acts or omissions of its 'brain', and not for those of its 'hands'. Leigh wrote ('By whom does a company permit?' (1966) 29 MLR 568): 'The "brains" and "hands" dichotomy essentially represents vivid journalism. It is not a substitute for analysis.' The cases, however, depend very much on the facts: one role in one company may be a 'brain' but a 'hand' in another. This point was emphasised in *Meridian* where Lord Hoffmann advised that the policy behind the statute had to be investigated to determine whether a certain person's acts and state of mind were to be attributed to the company. The use of the terms 'hand' and 'brain' is a distraction from this task. For example, in *Moore v I Bresler Ltd* the court was right in attributing the *mens rea* of the servant authorised to complete the returns to the company, but that ruling did not automatically apply to other crimes such as manslaughter, while *Tesco v Nattrass* turned on the words of the relevant statute and did not lay down a general rule. In *Worthy v Gordon Plant (Services) Ltd* [1989] RTR 7 (DC) the *actus reus* and *mens rea* of a traffic manager were imputed to a company. This case demonstrates that the identification doctrine is not limited to directors (as Lord Diplock thought in *Tesco v Nattrass*: see below) nor to employees of the company: the manager was self-employed; nevertheless, the company was liable. The following are examples of 'hands' on the facts of the case:

Depot manager: *Magna Plant v Mitchell* [1966] Crim LR 394.

Weighbridge manager: *John Henshall*, above.

Shop manager: *Tesco v Nattrass*, above.

Transport manager: *Readhead Freight Ltd v Shulman* [1988] Crim LR 696 (DC).

Ship's master: *P & O Ferries (Dover) Ltd* (1991) 93 Cr App R 72.

European Sales Manager of a company's aircraft division: *Redfern* [1993] Crim LR 43 (CA). The court said that the doctrine depended on the delegation of the true power of management, not of administrative or executive functions, no matter how important those functions were. The manager was four ranks below the chief executive.

In *Tesco v Nattrass* the manager was simply one manager out of some 800. The larger a company is, the easier it will be to say that a person is a 'hand'. It does seem unfair that a large company would escape liability when a smaller one would not. Lord Reid postulated that the test of identification applied where there was a substantial delegation of the functions of management. Only a few people such as the managing director and the members of the board are in such positions. The majority looked for those who 'represent the directing mind and will of the company and control what it does'. The phrase 'directing mind and will', which is often used nowadays, comes from a civil case, *Lennard's Carrying Co Ltd v Asiatic Petroleum Co Ltd* [1915] AC 705. Lord Hoffmann in *Meridian* advised that courts should not place too much emphasis on this phrase. Instead they should ask whether an individual's acts and state of mind were to be attributed to the company for the purpose of the relevant statute. Viscount Dilhorne in *Tesco v Nattrass* looked for someone 'in actual control of the operations of the company . . . and who is not responsible to another person . . . for the manner in which he discharges his duties . . .'. Lord Reid looked for the substance of the transaction, not just at the form as Lord Diplock did. He instanced 'the board of directors, the managing director and perhaps other superior officers . . . [who] . . . speak and act as the company'. Lord Diplock laid down an even narrower test, a mechanical one. Companies with so-called 'Table A' articles of association were liable only when the acts were performed by those persons mentioned in Table A, i.e. the directors. Whichever test is adopted, *Kent & Sussex* looks wrong in relation to the transport manager. And it may be that *Moore v I Bresler Ltd* was incorrect before *Meridian* in respect of the branch managers. It is now correct as a matter of statutory construction. *Tesco v Nattrass* must now be seen as a case of statutory interpretation: *Meridian*. The manager was not a 'brain', for the purpose of the relevant statute. A manager may be a 'brain' for another purpose. *Tesco v Nattrass* is a poor decision in terms of controlling wrongdoing: perhaps *Meridian* heralds a new era. However, in criticism of *Meridian* it may be said that until a decision by the court one will not know whether a person's activities are to be attributed to the company.

One observation about *Tesco v Nattrass* should be made. The offence was a regulatory one. Corporate liability could have been based upon vicarious liability: there was no need to investigate the identification doctrine. Applying vicarious liability the company would have been liable for the acts of any of its employees including the store manager. It should not have made any difference that the offence was phrased in terms of an offence coupled with a defence that the accused had taken all due diligence to prevent the occurrence of the crime. (C. Wells 'Corporate liability for crime – *Tesco v Nattrass* on the danger list?' [1996] 1 *Archbold News* 5 at 6, called the decision 'bizarre'.)

An important application of the identification doctrine took place in *P & O European Ferries (Dover) Ltd*, above, but which is unreported on this point. The case arose out of the sinking of the *Herald of Free Enterprise* at Zeebrugge. The assistant bosun, who was asleep when the ship was leaving the harbour, and chief officer, who should have checked whether the bow doors were closed but could not because he was on the bridge, were not senior enough for their alleged carelessness to be deemed to be the carelessness of the company. The failure to prove carelessness against senior management despite the fact that the directors were warned of the dangers of sailing with the bow doors open meant that the trial of the company for manslaughter collapsed. The case makes one think about the reasoning behind the identification test and its width. If Lord Diplock's rule were adopted, companies would rarely be liable. Yet it could easily be said that the failures of the bosun and the chief officer demonstrated the company's failure to execute the performance of its duty not to kill or injure passengers and crew. Moreover, the Board of Directors did not wish to fit lights showing that the doors were open because they employed a man to check, but he was asleep and no cover was provided by the company. Indeed, the Board seemed complacent. In other words, the company was negligent. Furthermore, if the rationale of the doctrine is to deprive companies of profits made out of breaches of law, why is it that the doctrine is not applied to middle managers and below who have made profits for the company? It might be better to speak of control of the company rather than management, depending on how far one wanted the law to apply, as Woolf J did in *Essendon Engineering Co Ltd v Maile* [1982] RTR 260. It is the judge who decides whether a person is 'brain' or 'hand'.

P & O European Ferries (Dover) Ltd was a case on manslaughter, which is a common law crime. Therefore, *Meridian*, which talks about statutory interpretation, is not directly applicable. A recent exploration of corporate manslaughter occurred in *Attorney-General's Reference (No. 2 of 1999)* [2000] QB 796 (CA), a case on a railway crash in which seven people died. It was held that a company (and, as the Divisional Court held in *Rowley v DPP* [2003] EWHC 693 (Admin), a local authority) could not be liable for manslaughter by gross negligence unless a human defendant had been convicted of it. The identification doctrine remained the rule of attribution for this common law offence. The person who was the 'directing mind and will' within *Tesco v Nattrass* had to be liable first. The effect of adhering to *Tesco v Nattrass* is easy to uncover. If that doctrine requires a director to be criminally liable, in a larger company it will be almost impossible to make a director guilty. A director does not drive a train, a train driver does; but the gross negligence of the driver cannot be attributed to the company – he is too low in the hierarchy. However, it would be hard to show that a decision of a director had caused the death of passengers when the immediate cause was, for example, a driver passing a signal at red. Furthermore, Rose LJ in *Attorney-General's Reference (No. 2 of 1999)* said that 'it would bring the laws into disrepute if every act and state of mind of an individual employee was attributed to a company which was entirely blameless'; however, that is the doctrine in the English tort law of vicarious liability and it is the general rule of criminal liability in the USA.

There are two restrictions on the identification doctrine. First, it has been suggested that it applies only when a 'brain' is performing a managerial function. A company would not be liable in criminal law (even though it may be liable in tort) when its managing director ran someone over, because driving is not a managerial function. It is uncertain whether this proposition represents the law or not but it is hard to believe that judges would find a company liable if its managing director stole an ashtray even if he was on a business trip. Secondly, the doctrine applies only where one or more 'brains' are individually liable. One cannot aggregate several directing minds and activities to make the company liable: *R v HM Coroner for East Kent, ex parte Spooner* (1989) 88 Cr App R 10 (DC). Each individual 'brain' has to be liable before the company can be convicted under the identification doctrine. In a large company, where decisions are often jointly made, it is unlikely that one controlling officer will have the requisite knowledge. In an era of large multinational companies neither the identification principle nor the delegation doctrine takes effect because of the need to delegate further and further down the corporate hierarchy to make the company work in a competitive marketplace. It is suggested that even if the aggregation doctrine were adopted, the law would not stretch to finding guilty a corporation which did not have a corporate policy on the relevant issue, such as safety at work. For this reason the defendant company in *P & O European Ferries (Dover) Ltd* (above) may still not have been guilty.

Limitations on liability

A company is not liable in certain situations.

(a) A company may be convicted only of offences punishable by a fine. It cannot be imprisoned or hanged. Therefore, it cannot be guilty of treason or murder, for how can one put a legal construct into prison? Since most offences are punishable nowadays by a fine or some other non-corporal method, this restriction is minimal. This exception was accepted in *ICR Haulage* and *P & O European Ferries (Dover) Ltd*, above, as was the second exception, though perjury was said to be arguable. The argument contrary to the view that a company can be convicted of only those offences which are punishable by fines is that there should be other sentences available, such as 'corporate probation' and dissolution of the company. Where the company cannot be found guilty of an offence because no sanction is available other defendants may be guilty in the normal way. However, this chapter is devoted to corporate liability.

(b) It seems that there are several offences which cannot be committed by an employee within the scope of his employment. There is a *dictum* of Finlay J in *Cory Bros & Co* [1927] 1 KB 810 to the effect that perjury is one of those offences. However, this *dictum* may be wrong, for a director who perjures can be identified with the company. The argument to the contrary is, however, strong. Only the person who has been lawfully sworn can be guilty of perjury, and a company cannot lawfully be sworn. Other such offences include being a rogue and a vagabond, bigamy, incest and rape. These crimes may be called personal offences. A company cannot, for example, have sexual intercourse. However, a company can be liable as a company to those offences. An illustration is given by A. Reed and B. Fitzpatrick, *Criminal Law*, 3rd edn (Thomson, 2006) 168: 'If Z, the managing director of X Company Ltd, a film company, supervises the filming of intercourse between M, an 18-year-old male, with N, a 15-year-old girl, there is no reason why Z and hence the film company should not be convicted as secondary parties to the unlawful sexual intercourse.' For most crimes such as theft and burglary there is no problem in finding the company liable. Lord Steyn in *Deutsche Genossenschaftsbank v Burnhope* [1995] 1 WLR 1580 gave an example: '. . . If the chairman of a company dishonestly instructs an innocent employee to enter [a] warehouse and remove a bag containing valuables, the company may be guilty of burglary.'

(c) In *Cory Bros*, above, it was said at Assizes that a corporation could not be tried for a crime of personal violence including manslaughter. That case was criticised in *ICR Haulage*, above. In *Northern Strip Mining Construction Co Ltd*, unreported, 1965, a company was tried for manslaughter but the issue of the propriety of the indictment was not discussed and the firm was acquitted; in *ex parte Spooner*, above, Bingham LJ tentatively accepted that a company could be guilty of manslaughter.

The final breakthrough came in *P & O European Ferries (Dover) Ltd*, above; the Court of Appeal accepted this change in the law in *Attorney-General's Reference (No. 2 of 1999)*, above. This part is reported. The successor company of the firm which owned the *Herald of Free Enterprise* was held to be properly tried for manslaughter. However, in the unreported portion of the trial the prosecution case collapsed because it could not be proved that the actions of the controlling officers were objectively reckless. No reasonably prudent person occupying the positions of the individual members of senior staff would have recognised the risk to a ship leaving port as 'obvious and serious'. (See also the discussion of reckless and gross negligence manslaughter in Chapter 12, where it is pointed out that objective reckless manslaughter has been abolished.) This point was reached despite the inquiry of Sheen J into the capsize, which stated that managers should have been aware that there was a real risk of ferries leaving port with their door open and that there were no standing orders to cover closure of the bow doors. The directors had not applied their mind to the type of instructions they should give in order for the ship safely to leave the harbour. However, each person's 'sloppiness' as Sheen J called it could not be aggregated to make the company liable. There was no recklessness. The system of the ship had worked on over 60,000 sailings. The ship's officers testified that they had not thought about the risk; therefore, it could not have been an obvious one. The ferry had left harbour several times with its doors open, but there had been no incidents and neither the Department of Transport nor the insurers required a system of reporting to the captain that the doors were closed or the installation of lights in the bridge to show that they were. It is thought that the resurgence of gross negligence manslaughter would make no difference to the outcome. A reasonably skilled ship's officer would not have operated a different mode of sailing from a harbour. The case also illustrates the importance of corporate liability. Each year there are some 600–800 homicides. The sinking of the *Herald of Free Enterprise* caused some 30 per cent of those in 1988.

Despite the collapse of the case, *P & O European Ferries (Dover) Ltd* signified that a company may be liable for crimes of violence. The third exception has disappeared. Difficulties of proof will not arise in every case. The first company convicted of manslaughter was the one accused of causing the Lyme Bay canoe tragedy: *OLL Ltd*, unreported, 9 December 1994. It was fined £60,000. The company was found guilty of manslaughter by gross negligence. The managing director, the controlling mind of the company, knew that safety standards were low. His knowledge was imputed to the company. The effect of the fine was to put the company into liquidation. The difference from *P & O European Ferries (Dover) Ltd* seems to consist in the difference in size of the company. The second company to be convicted of manslaughter was *Jackson Transport (Ossett) Ltd*, unreported, 19 September 1996 (Bradford Crown Court). The former managing director was the company's 'directing mind' and ran the business personally. The victim had died while cleaning chemicals from a road tanker. The company was convicted of gross negligence manslaughter (and the individual accused received a sentence of 12 months' imprisonment). The sole other convictions have been of *Jackson Transport (Ossett) Ltd* (1996), *English Brothers Ltd* (2001), *Teglgaard Hardwood Ltd* (2003), *Dennis Clothier and Sons Ltd* (2003), *Nationwide Heating Services Ltd* (2004) and *Keymark Services* (2006). The fines, respectively, were: £15,000, £25,000, £25,000, £4,000, £90,000 (including for Health and Safety offences) and unknown. To use the first of these cases as an example: an employee was killed after a toxic chemical was sprayed in his face while he was cleaning chemical residues from a road tanker. He had not been supervised or trained and he was not provided with protective equipment. At the same time fines have been increasing for health and safety offences, undermining the arguments in favour of reforming the whole law of corporate liability.

In 1989 there were 143 deaths and 4,010 serious injuries on building sites. Many of these were caused in the same way, such as by the collapse of trenches or scaffolding. Therefore, persons in charge of such construction companies ought to foresee such occurrences. Companies can accordingly be made liable. A similar point can be made about the King's Cross Underground fire. Between 1956 and 1988 there were 46 escalator fires on the tube, of which 32 had been caused by smoking. These figures are taken from D. Bergman 'Recklessness in the boardroom' (1990) 140 NLJ 1496 at 1501. He adds:

> The tangle of the common law of manslaughter could be avoided in these situations if a new crime were created, whereby a director faced large fines and possible imprisonment if his failure to abide by his duties caused a person to die.

Bergman estimated in 'Weak on crime – weak on the causes of crime' [1997] NLJ 1652 that there had been more than 10,000 workplace deaths in the previous 10 years and G. Slapper and S. Tombs, *Corporate Crime* (Longman, 1999) 69, estimated 1,316 in 1994, a substantial increase on the number, 376, reported by the Health and Safety Executive. The Health and Safety Commission reported 212 deaths and 28,605 serious injuries at work (*Health and Safety Statistics 2005/06*, 2006).

The conviction in the Lyme Bay case occurred because of the small size of the company. The managing director *was* the company. The salient point is that no medium or large company has yet been convicted.

It should be noted that the *ultra vires* doctrine does not operate in criminal law and that directors may be disqualified by a court under the Company Directors Disqualification Act 1986, s 2, if they mismanage the health and safety matters of a company. In an unreported trial at Lewes Crown Court, R. J. Chapman was banned for two years after exposing employees to danger from falling rocks. The first director to be imprisoned for manslaughter in relation to his business was Peter Kite, the managing director in **OLL Ltd**. He was sentenced to three years' imprisonment on four counts, to run concurrently but the sentence was reduced to two years on appeal.

Critique of the law

After transport and industrial disasters corporate liability reform is on the agenda, and the law is in a state of flux. The public perceives companies to be at fault in failing to prevent such incidents. No longer are these disasters seen as accidents (cf. the Aberfan disaster of over 40 years ago): they are viewed as foreseeable and preventable. Companies are seen to be culpable and there is a desire to transmute moral blameworthiness into criminal liability. The phrase 'corporate manslaughter' is now known to the man in the street.

One difficulty with making companies criminally responsible for their acts or omissions is that criminal law is founded on personal liability, another is that prosecuting authorities are slow to act on 'crime in the suites'. For example, deaths on construction sites rarely came in the past to the attention of the police, but were dealt with solely by the Health and Safety Executive. This attitude was criticised for failing to take seriously deaths at work. The position is changing. There are several reasons for imposing criminal liability on corporations. Companies would escape regulation by the criminal law if they were not liable, and regulation is at times a good thing. It obliges companies to adopt policies which lead to careful procedures. Only the company can remedy some of the things which led to the deaths. For example, only P & O could install lights to signify that the bow doors were closed. The assistant bosun could not. It may be procedurally convenient to prosecute the company. The company is more likely to be able to pay a fine than an individual. Shareholders may be encouraged to exercise control, and the company may be deprived of unjust enrichment through fines. Fines, however, must be set high enough to be more than the profit gained from the violation of the law; otherwise there would be no deterrence and fines could be seen as a business expense. Punishing only natural persons would not strike at the cause of the wrongdoing: natural persons may be merely minions. Indeed the fault may be that of the company, not that of an individual. It is possible that the existence of corporate liability can help to prevent companies placing pressure on employees to break the law. Adverse publicity and fines may act as a deterrent. Indeed, bad publicity is likely to be more of a deterrent than fines, which are often paltry. Nevertheless, it must be admitted that the effect of adverse publicity on consumers is uncertain, though it must be stronger than would occur if only the individual wrongdoer were prosecuted. Public opinion may be in favour of imposing liability on a company the activities of which have led to a disaster. It is not in favour of imposing liability only on employees at the base of the corporate hierarchy, and where people are killed there is a growing feeling that corporations ought to be convicted of 'normal' crimes such as manslaughter and not just of health and safety offences. Companies are seen as the cause of deaths and injuries. They could have prevented the harm. It is often said that the police and Health and Safety Executive do not treat corporate offending as 'real' crime. The name of the offence may not reflect the wrongdoing, there may be inaction by the prosecuting authorities, and the fine may be derisory.

However, not all these arguments are strong. The amount of a fine is not proportionate to the amount of enrichment; fines affect companies differently from individuals; shareholders very rarely exercise control over firms; and the fine may be too paltry to deter. It is thought that corporate policy in large firms is not affected by the imposition of fines: Anon 'Increasing community control over corporate crime – problem of sanctions' (1961) 71 Yale LJ 280 at 290. Of course, the fact that fines are incorrectly calibrated does not mean that corporations should go unpunished. Some corporations such as universities do not have shareholders. A. M. Polinsky and S. Shavell argue 'Should employees be subject to fines and imprisonment given the existence of corporate liability?' (1993) 13 *International Review of Law and Economics* 239 at 255, that (a) a company's control over its employees will not be increased by the imposition of corporate liability because control is already executed to the socially optimal level, and (b) a company should not be liable to a greater extent than the harm it has caused because otherwise its production costs will increase, thereby depressing the optimal level of consumption. Certainly these arguments do not differentiate between 'brain' and 'hands' as the identification doctrine does. Despite the weakness of some arguments, J. A. Andrews made a sensible comment in [1973] Crim LR 91 at 94:

> Where we use the penal law to support fiscal, health and safety and other regulations, corporations must be brought within the system. On the other hand when we use the penal process to deter delinquency, we should recognise that companies are not delinquents, only people are.

Moreover, there are some states, such as Italy, which do not have corporate liability law. The argument is that corporations have no morality, no personality in that sense, which criminal law and punishment can change. Prosecuting the company alone may miss the individuals who caused the harm.

The draft Criminal Code

The Law Commission's draft Criminal Code, Law Com. No. 177, 1989, cl 30, proposed several reforms.

(a) A company will not be liable where the controlling officer was acting against the interests of the company. This recommendation reverses *Moore* v *I Bresler*, above. As the Law Commission's Working Paper No. 44, 1972, para 39, had it:

> [T]he principle established in *Moore* v *I Bresler* is clearly inequitable since it penalises a corporation and its shareholders for something done in fraud of the corporation and to the detriment of its shareholders.

(b) Corporations will continue to be liable vicariously: cl 30(1).

(c) The identification principle is retained. The acts and states of mind of controlling officers acting within the scope of their offices are those of the company: cl 30(2). A controlling officer is 'a person participating in the control of the corporation in the capacity of a director, manager, secretary or other similar officer (whether or not he was, or was validly appointed to any such office)' (cl 30(3)). This sub-clause is meant to be an enactment of the various definitions of the Law Lords in *Tesco* v *Nattrass*, above. At least one of the controlling officers must have the whole of the mental element of the offence.

(d) The rule that a company cannot be guilty of a crime which is not punishable by a fine is retained: cl 30(7).

(e) By cl 30(8):

> A corporation has a defence consisting of or including:
> (a) a state of mind only if –
>   (i) all controlling officers who are concerned in the offence; or
>   (ii) where no controlling officer is so concerned, all other employees or agents who are so concerned, have that state of mind;
> (b) the absence of a state of mind only if no controlling officer with responsibility for the subject matter of the offence has that state of mind;
> (c) compliance with a standard of conduct required of the corporation itself only if it is complied with by the controlling officers with responsibility for the subject matter of the offence.

Except for proposal (a), these proposals reflect current law.

Non-governmental proposals for reform

Other reforms have been suggested. Rodger Pannone, England's chief disaster lawyer, thought that a company should be made civilly liable for punitive damages. N. J. Reville 'Corporate manslaughter' [1989] LSG No. 37, 17 at 19, proposed massive fines. However, a massive fine may lead to liquidation, an outcome which may not be appropriate. At present fines may not deprive the company of its ill-gotten profits, and they may not be pitched high enough to deter. Gary Slapper in 'A safe place to work' [1992] LSG No. 37, 24, pointed out that when BP Ltd was fined £750,000 by a Scottish court in 1987, that sum was 0.05 per cent of the company's after-tax profits and was the equivalent of a fine of £7.50 on a person earning £15,000 per year. The system of 'unit fines', introduced by the Criminal Justice Act 1991 but since repealed, did not apply to companies. Nevertheless, post-2000 fines for health and safety offences may be substantial. Although the Court of Appeal reduced the fine on Balfour Beatty for the Hatfield rail crash by £2.5m, the fine was still £7.5m: ***Balfour Beatty Rail Infrastructure Services Ltd*** [2006] EWCA Crim 1586. It is the shareholders (and the customers) who suffer from fines. Shareholders simply do not exercise their company law rights to control corporate officers. Moreover, heavy fines may leave the company with not enough money to remedy the situation. Employees may have to be dismissed when no fault is attached to them.

David Bergman in his *Deaths at Work: Accidents or Corporate Crime* (WEA, 1991) suggested that prosecutions for death at the workplace should be tried only on indictment and that courts should be able to impose imprisonment on a director or manager by whose ineptitude a worker was killed or seriously injured. He has on several occasions over the years criticised the Health and Safety Executive for failing to pursue what in reality are cases of corporate manslaughter. Other sanctions have been suggested, e.g. the dissolution of the company, nationalisation, monitoring its activities, corporate probation (which means that professionals, such as accountants, supervise and monitor the company's activities), community service, preventing it from working in certain areas of business, prohibiting it performing government contracts, publicising the breach of the law in some official way. The last method has been tried in the USA, but experience in that country demonstrates that close control over such advertising has to be exercised, otherwise the company publishes only in rarely read journals. As early as 1948 Sir Roland Burrows wrote in 'The responsibility of corporations under English law' (1948) 1 *Journal of Criminal Science* 1 at 19, 'Restriction of activities and even extinction by forfeiture are neither impossible nor absurd.'

Research work would have to be done to see whether these methods would be effective. Prevention, such as training in health and safety or an increase in the numbers of Health and Safety Inspectors, may be more helpful than criminal law, and criminal laws should be utilised to prevent harm. Laws made for individuals cannot always be easily applied to companies. Certainly at present there is an imbalance between prosecutions by the Crown Prosecution Service for minor shoplifting and non-prosecution by arms of the government for breaches of health and safety at work subordinate legislation and for pollution, where prosecution is seen as very much a last measure after various admonitions. If the criminal law has a part to play in tackling modern social problems such as pollution and food hygiene, the principles of corporate liability must be clear and enforced. Reform of both corporate liability and involuntary manslaughter is necessary. The difficulties in one are exacerbated by those in the other.

Despite the arguments outlined in this section, it is sometimes said that corporate liability serves no purpose. The authors of a well-known textbook, Smith and Hogan, *Criminal Law*, 10th edn (Butterworths, 2002) 206, wrote, as they did in previous editions: 'The necessity for corporate criminal liability awaits demonstration.' (This comment does not appear in the twelfth edition, 2008, OUP, the second to be edited by D. Ormerod.) G. R. Sullivan commented 'Expressing corporate guilt' (1995) 15 OJLS 281 at 289:

> If we were to follow Smith and Hogan, the myriad of regulatory laws relating to safety, pollution, hygiene etc. would be lifted off the backs of companies and confined to individuals. It would be a deregulation beyond the imaginings of the most doctrinaire free-marketeer . . . It is in the enforcement of regulatory criminal law against limited companies that we must continue to seek the major improvements in standards of safety. [footnote omitted]

The Law Commission's proposals

The Law Commission published its Report No. 237, *Legislating the Criminal Code: Involuntary Manslaughter*, in 1996. It suggested the continuation of the identification principle, but did not recommend the extension of vicarious liability to corporate manslaughter or the introduction of the doctrine of aggregation. *OLL Ltd*, above, would therefore not be affected by any change in the law. The main proposal is a new offence of corporate killing, a specific offence applying only to companies. A company would be guilty of the offence if '(a) a management failure by the corporation is the cause or one of the causes of a person's death; and (b) that failure constitutes conduct falling far below what can reasonably be expected of the corporation in the circumstances'. Management failure is in turn defined as a failure of the management or organisation to ensure the health and safety of persons employed in or affected by its activities. Management failure may be 'a cause of a person's death notwithstanding that the immediate cause is the act or omission of an individual'. The emphasis on management demonstrates the shift from imposing corporate liability based on identifying the directing mind and will of a superior agency with the company. The penalty is to be a fine with the possibility of a novel sanction, a remedial order. This order would be one by which the court would direct the company 'to take such steps, within such time as the order specified, for remedying the failure in question and any matter which appears to the court to have resulted from the failure and been the cause or one of the causes of death'.

The definition of corporate killing is the same as the proposed offence of killing by gross carelessness noted in Chapter 12, with the difference that with regard to a natural person the risk of death or serious injury has to be obvious to a reasonable person in his position and he must have been capable of appreciating the risk. In this respect the Report differs from Consultation Paper No. 135, *Involuntary Manslaughter*, in which the Law Commission had recommended that there should be no distinction in this regard between natural and corporate persons. The Law Commission comments (at para 8.1) that corporate killing is 'modelled on our proposed offence of killing by gross carelessness, but with such adaptation as is dictated by the peculiar characteristics of corporations'. Such traits include the fact that a risk cannot be obvious to a company because it is not sentient and that for the same reason it is incapable of appreciating a risk. The Law Commission excludes these characteristics as irrelevant to corporate liability for death: 'In judging the conduct of an individual defendant, the law must in fairness take account of such personal characteristics as may make it harder for her to appreciate risks that another person would appreciate; but the same considerations scarcely apply to a corporate defendant' (para 8.3, emphasis omitted). One effect of the removal of the requirements of obviousness to a reasonable person in the position of the accused and of his capacity to appreciate the risk is that there will be no necessity that a person in the company should be aware that the company's conduct fell far below the required standard.

The condition that the company's conduct fall far below the standard which could reasonably be expected of it in the circumstances means both that the offence is only available when the negligence was gross and that the jury may take into account the practicability of reducing or eliminating the risk of death or serious injury, the social utility of the activity and whether there was any deviation from the norms of the industry concerned. Management failure is to be distinguished from casual negligence by an employee (the Law Commission could have explained the concept in more depth) but, while causation will remain a question for the jury, death may still be attributable to the company even though an employee's carelessness was the immediate cause of death: 'Management failure may have consisted in a failure to take precautions against the very kind of failure that in fact occurred. . . . The company's fault lies in its failure to anticipate such foreseeable negligence of its employee, and any consequence of such negligence should therefore be treated as a consequence of the company's fault' (para 8.37). Otherwise the company would escape liability by arguing that it provided merely the setting for the death and not the legal cause of it. This proposal, which deviates from the normal law of causation discussed in Chapter 2, is illustrated by reference to the Zeebrugge disaster: 'Even if the immediate cause of the deaths was the conduct of the assistant bosun and the Chief Officer or both, another of the causes was the failure of the company to devise a safe system for the operation of its ferries; and . . . that failure fell far below what could reasonably have been expected' (para 8.50). Therefore, the company could be found guilty of corporate killing. Only if the act or omission of an individual completely broke the chain of causation would the company escape liability. It should also be noted that the company and the individual employees could be convicted of the proposed crimes of killing by gross carelessness and reckless killing. For example, a company could be convicted of the latter where its employees knew of serious risks but proceeded nevertheless. The principal criticism from business of the proposal to base liability on 'management failure' is that companies would not know what they had to do to avoid liability.

The definition of corporate killing would, it was thought, make it easier for prosecutions to be more successful than they are at present, as the Zeebrugge illustration shows. This revision would be in line with public perceptions of the deadly behaviour of companies. What has previously been treated as an accident, tragedy or disaster is now viewed as manslaughter, and there is irritation that companies have not been convicted in the past. The removal of obstacles to conviction may go some way towards satisfying the public but the reforms still need to be enacted and then fully implemented. There is, however, an argument that the recommendations could not give a different result in the Zeebrugge scenario. If the company acted as an experienced company in the same line of business would have acted, it did not fall far below what reasonably could be expected.

The Law Commission proposed a new sanction, the remedial order, in addition to, or in substitution for, a fine. The company may be required to remove the matter which caused death. The prosecution, the Health and Safety Executive or a body designated by the Secretary of State will have to apply for the order and both sides may adduce evidence as to its wording. The sanction for failure to comply would be a fine. Therefore, if the company disobeys the order, the law will not ensure the removal of the death-dealing matter.

Corporate killing would be a crime with no requirement of intent or subjective recklessness, of choice or capability to foresee results. In terms of the modern English approach to *mens rea* it would not be a crime of *mens rea*. It would be based on gross carelessness. Accordingly, there would be no difficulty in proving intention or foresight. Corporate responsibility would have a structure of its own separate from that of natural persons. This decoupling of individual and corporate criminal responsibility would mean that it would be possible to convict large companies of a serious offence, for there would be no need to refer to the state of mind and the act of a directing mind. The Commission considered that public confidence in the law would be improved if perpetrators were not allowed to escape, that the deficiencies of the identification doctrine would no longer be a bar to conviction, and that companies would be deterred from irresponsible conduct which might result in death or serious injury. The restriction of the recommendations to killings is a consequence of the Report's being concerned with manslaughter but there is nothing to stop the creation of new offences of corporate injury and serious injury. It would be invidious if a company were convicted of a crime if the victim happened to die but of no offence if he happened to live. It is also worthy of note that the Report does not deal with the fundamental problem, that of preventing employees and others from being killed or injured. The recommendation on remedial orders applies only after the event. Corporate killing may deter companies from engaging in egregious mismanagement but the suggested cure may not work. Training and supervision in this area of endeavour are of better value than the criminal law.

The reforms of the Law Commission were timid in comparison with those found in the Australian Criminal Code Act 1995, which applies to federal offences. Besides the identification doctrine (which is extended to 'high managerial agents') liability is imposed where the corporate culture has led to situations in which offences have taken place. Corporate culture is to be derived from the company's (or department of a company's) attitude, course of conduct, policy, practice or rule. The aim is to catch large companies which at present are not liable because they have delegated their powers to low-level employees. The reforms come nowhere near the idea of Fisse and Braithwaite 'The allocation of responsibility for corporate crime' (1988) 11 Sydney LR 468 to infer corporate guilt from the efficacy of the company in remedying the harm it caused. This idea would abrogate the present requirement of fault at the time of the *actus reus*. The approach is sometimes called 'reactive fault'. The difficulty with it is to find the correct offence with which a company could be charged. If the deceased was killed at work by the company's negligence, manslaughter would be appropriate because reactive fault is aimed at conduct after the crime. If a new offence is created, it could be argued that this would marginalise the company's failure to take care.

The government's proposals

In 2000 the Home Office issued a Consultation Paper, *Reforming the Law of Involuntary Manslaughter: The Government's Proposals*. The government accepted the Law Commission's recommendation that there should be an offence of corporate killing in order to 'restore public confidence that companies responsible for loss of life can properly be held accountable in law' (para 3.1.9). However, it proposed to extend the possible defendants from companies alone to 'undertakings' such as schools, partnerships, voluntary organisations, charities, and hospital trusts (yet keeping the title 'corporate killing'). Prosecutions could be brought not just by the Crown Prosecution Service and the Health and Safety Executive but also by bodies such as the Civil Aviation Authority. The government also took the view that company officers who had contributed to the management failure should be subjected to disqualification from acting in a managerial role in any undertaking in Great Britain, though in a letter of 10 September 2002 to private sector industries with a fatal/ major injuries rate of over 250 per 100,000 employees, the Criminal Policy Group of the Home Office stated that reform would not include a separate law on disqualification. This recommendation may be contrary to the European Convention on Human Rights if the officers were not aware of the failing. There is in addition a proposal that corporate killing proceedings would continue against insolvent companies. The Home Office further proposed that company managers and directors should be guilty of an offence if they significantly contributed to the offence which the company committed. To prevent evasion of fines, the Home Office wondered whether the court should have the power to freeze corporate assets. For a review of the government's proposals, see Bob Sullivan 'Corporate killing – some government proposals' [2001] Crim LR 31.

In October 1997 the then Home Secretary, Jack Straw, promised that the offence of corporate killing would be enacted. The Labour manifesto of 2001 promised 'to make provisions against corporate manslaughter. Finally the Corporate Manslaughter and Corporate Homicide Act 2007 came into force on 6 April 2008. The Law Commission intends to publish a consultation paper on general corporate liability in late 2009.

Corporate Manslaughter and Corporate Homicide Act 2007

This statute deals in England and Wales with corporate liability for death. It replaces the common law, which is abolished. The offence is called corporate manslaughter in England and Wales (s 2(5)). Most provisions came into force on 6 April 2008. However, since it deals only with corporate liability for deaths, and not with corporate liability for example for injuries, to which the common law remains, there is the possibility of dual forms of liability. If a company causes the death of one person and injury to another through the same act of gross negligence, the death falls under the Act but the injury is subject to he common law, and then applies even the injured person would have died, had he not been saved by immediate paramedic intervention. According to the Health & Safety Commission's website there were 241 work-related deaths in 2006–07 (note that this figure excludes deaths by industrial diseases such as asbestosis and it is unclear how many work-related road traffic deaths are contained in the figures) but 141,350 injuries. The Act will reach only the deaths. It should be added that the Act is not limited to work-related deaths and goes beyond firms killing their workers, extending to killing members of the public.

The Act is focused on the liabilities of bodies which fall within its scope. There is no liability imposed on directors and senior managers by the Act, and they remain liable for common law manslaughter by gross negligence. Indeed, every criminal statute imposes secondary liability unless Parliament otherwise ordains and in the Act Parliament has so ordained. These exclusions may be surprising, for it is directors and senior executives who conceive and implement policies, not the incorporeal organisation.

Section 1 of the Act reads in part:

(1) An organisation to which this section applies is guilty of an offence if the way in which its activities are managed or organised –
   (a) causes a person's death, and
   (b) amounts to a gross breach of a relevant duty of care owed by the organisation to the deceased.

The government anticipated that the widening of the concept of causation through *Environment Agency* v *Empress Car Co. (Abertillery) Ltd* [1999] 2 AC 22 and in the period leading up to the House of Lords' decision in *Kennedy (No. 2)* [2008] AC 269 (see Chapter 2) would obviate the need to refer to the doctrine of *novus actus interveniens* but the House has reverted to the previous law in *Kennedy (No. 2)*. The problem is this: if the death is caused by the gross negligence of a junior employee, does the organisation also cause that death within s 1(1)(a)? If the act of the employee is voluntary, on normal principles she is liable and her act or failure to act breaks the chain of causation, unless the organisation's conduct also is a significant contribution to the killing. It would have been better to rephrase by adding 'and the organisation remains guilty despite the fact that the act or omission of an individual was the immediate cause of death'.

Section 1 continues:

(2) The organisations to which this section applies are –
   (a) a corporation;
   (b) a department or other body listed in Schedule 1;
   (c) a police force;
   (d) a partnership, or a trade union or employers' association, that is an employer.

It should be noted that while the Act's title refers to 'corporate' manslaughter, the statute is not restricted to companies. This is in line with the Home Office's Consultation Document, *Reforming the Law on Involuntary Manslaughter: The Government's Proposals*, 2000.

Section 1 goes on to provide:

(3) An organisation is guilty of an offence under this section only if the way in which its activities are managed or organised by its senior management is a substantial element in the breach referred to in subsection (1).

(4) For the purposes of this Act –

   (a) 'relevant duty of care' has the meaning given by section 2, read with sections 3 to 7;

   (b) a breach of a duty of care by an organisation is a 'gross' breach if the conduct alleged to amount to a breach of that duty falls far below what can reasonably be expected of the organisation in the circumstances;

   (c) 'senior management', in relation to an organisation, means the persons who play significant roles in –

      (i) the making of decisions about how the whole or a substantial part of its activities are to be managed or organised, or

      (ii) the actual managing or organising of the whole or a substantial part of those activities.

The use of the concept of 'senior management' calls into question how far the 2007 Act breaks, as it should do, from the previous law of identification, to which reference should be made. Certainly there is no requirement as at common law for one specific senior person to be at fault; in this sense aggregation is permissible under the 2007 Act. The concept ensures that the acts of lesser employees are not attributed to the organisation but it must be appreciated that it is senior management who lay down general policies on, for instance, recruitment of staff. In respect of the requirement of 'gross' breach, the question whether the organisation's behaviour fell far below that which could reasonably be expected in the circumstances is a question for the jury and it is uncertain just how far below the standard the body must go to be criminally liable. It is also unclear what 'in the circumstances' means: surely it cannot mean that an organisation is not grossly in breach of a duty when it decides not to comply with it because it is short of money and as a result someone is killed:

(6) An organisation that is guilty of corporate manslaughter . . . is liable on conviction on indictment to a fine.

Section 2 reads in part:

(1) A 'relevant duty of care', in relation to an organisation, means any of the following duties owed by it under the law of negligence –

   (a) a duty owed to its employees or to other persons working for the organisation or performing services for it;

   (b) a duty owed as occupier of premises;

   (c) a duty owed in connection with –

      (i) the supply by the organisation of goods or services (whether for consideration or not),

      (ii) the carrying on by the organisation of any construction or maintenance operations,

      (iii) the carrying on by the organisation of any other activity on a commercial basis, or

      (iv) the use or keeping by the organisation of any plant, vehicle or other thing;

(d) a duty owed to a person who, by reason of being a person within subsection (2), is someone for whose safety the organisation is responsible.

(2) A person is within this subsection if –
   (a) he is detained at a custodial institution or in a custody area at a court or police station;
   (b) he is detained at a removal centre or short-term holding facility;
   (c) he is being transported in a vehicle, or being held in any premises, in pursuance of prison escort arrangements or immigration escort arrangements;
   (d) he is living in secure accommodation in which he has been placed;
   (e) he is a detained patient.

(3) Subsection (1) is subject to sections 3 to 7.

(4) A reference in subsection (1) to a duty owed under the law of negligence includes a reference to a duty that would be owed under the law of negligence but for any statutory provision under which liability is imposed in place of liability under that law.

(5) For the purposes of this Act, whether a particular organisation owes a duty of care to a particular individual is a question of law.
   The judge must make any findings of fact necessary to decide that question.

(6) For the purposes of this Act there is to be disregarded –
   (a) any rule of the common law that has the effect of preventing a duty of care from being owed by one person to another by reason of the fact that they are jointly engaged in unlawful conduct;
   (b) any such rule that has the effect of preventing a duty of care from being owed to a person by reason of his acceptance of a risk of harm.

(7) In this section –

'construction or maintenance operations' means operations of any of the following descriptions –
   (a) construction, installation, alteration, extension, improvement, repair, maintenance, decoration, cleaning, demolition or dismantling of –
      (i) any building or structure,
      (ii) anything else that forms, or is to form, part of the land, or
      (iii) any plant, vehicle or other thing;
   (b) operations that form an integral part of, or are preparatory to, or are for rendering complete, any operations within paragraph (a);

'custodial institution' means a prison, a young offender institution, a secure training centre, a young offenders institution, a young offenders centre, a juvenile justice centre or a remand centre;
'detained patient' means –
   (a) a person who is detained in any premises under –
      (i) Part 2 or 3 of the Mental Health Act 1983 . . . ('the 1983 Act'), or . . .
   (b) a person who (otherwise than by reason of being detained as mentioned in paragraph (a)) is deemed to be in legal custody by –
      (i) section 137 of the 1983 Act . . .
'immigration escort arrangements' means arrangements made under section 156 of the Immigration and Asylum Act 1999 . . . ;
'the law of negligence' includes –
   (a) in relation to England and Wales, the Occupiers' Liability Act 1957 . . .), the Defective Premises Act 1972 . . . and the Occupiers' Liability Act 1984 . . .); . . .

'prison escort arrangements' means arrangements made under section 80 of the Criminal Justice Act 1991 . . . or under section 102 or 118 of the Criminal Justice and Public Order Act 1994 . . . ;

'removal centre' and 'short-term holding facility' have the meaning given by section 147 of the Immigration and Asylum Act 1999;

'secure accommodation' means accommodation, not consisting of or forming part of a custodial institution, provided for the purpose of restricting the liberty of persons under the age of 18.

The restriction to pre-existing duties of care was not foreshadowed by the Home Office Consultation Document, mentioned above, or any Law Commission consultation paper or report. It may be questioned whether the use of civil law doctrines in criminal law serves any useful purpose: the House of Lords in **Hinks** [2001] 2 AC 241 and the Court of Appeal in **Wacker** [2003] QB 1207 may be cited as authorities to that effect. It is uncertain what purpose it saves: after all, persons, natural and juristic, are under a duty not to kill.

Section 3 exempts certain public functions from the coverage of the Act. It reads:

(1) Any duty of care owed by a public authority in respect of a decision as to matters of public policy (including in particular the allocation of public resources or the weighing of competing public interests) is not a 'relevant duty of care'.

(2) Any duty of care owed in respect of things done in the exercise of an exclusively public function is not a 'relevant duty of care' unless it falls within section 2(1)(a), (b) or (d).

(3) Any duty of care owed by a public authority in respect of inspections carried out in the exercise of a statutory function is not a 'relevant duty of care' unless it falls within section 2(1)(a) or (b).

(4) In this section –

'exclusively public function' means a function that falls within the prerogative of the Crown or is, by its nature, exercisable only with authority conferred –

(a) by the exercise of that prerogative, or

(b) by or under a statutory provision;

'statutory function' means a function conferred by or under a statutory provision.

Sections 4, 5 and 7 relate to military and police activities and child protection respectively, which do not fall within the ambit of this book. Section 6, which deals with emergencies, may, however, be of relevance.

(1) Any duty of care owed by an organisation within subsection (2) in respect of the way in which it responds to emergency circumstances is not a 'relevant duty of care' unless it falls within section 2(1)(a) or (b).

(2) The organisations within this subsection are –

(a) a fire and rescue authority in England and Wales . . .

(d) any other organisation providing a service of responding to emergency circumstances either –

(i) in pursuance of arrangements made with an organisation within paragraph (a) . . . or

(ii) (if not in pursuance of such arrangements) otherwise than on a commercial basis;

(e) a relevant NHS body;

(f) an organisation providing ambulance services in pursuance of arrangements –
  (i) made by, or at the request of, a relevant NHS body, or
  (ii) made with the Secretary of State or with the Welsh Ministers;

(g) an organisation providing services for the transport of organs, blood, equipment or personnel in pursuance of arrangements of the kind mentioned in paragraph (f);

(h) an organisation providing a rescue service;
  (i) the armed forces.

(3) For the purposes of subsection (1), the way in which an organisation responds to emergency circumstances does not include the way in which –
  (a) medical treatment is carried out, or
  (b) decisions within subsection (4) are made.

(4) The decisions within this subsection are decisions as to the carrying out of medical treatment, other than decisions as to the order in which persons are to be given such treatment.

(5) Any duty of care owed in respect of the carrying out, or attempted carrying out, of a rescue operation at sea in emergency circumstances is not a 'relevant duty of care' unless it falls within section 2(1)(a) or (b).

(6) Any duty of care owed in respect of action taken –
  (a) in order to comply with a direction under Schedule 3A to the Merchant Shipping Act 1995 . . . (safety directions), or
  (b) by virtue of paragraph 4 of that Schedule (action in lieu of direction),
  is not a 'relevant duty of care' unless it falls within section 2(1)(a) or (b).

(7) In this section –
  'emergency circumstances' means circumstances that are present or imminent and –
  (a) are causing, or are likely to cause, serious harm or a worsening of such harm, or
  (b) are likely to cause the death of a person;
  'medical treatment' includes any treatment or procedure of a medical or similar nature;
  'relevant NHS body' means –
  (a) a Strategic Health Authority, Primary Care Trust, NHS trust, Special Health Authority or NHS foundation trust in England . . .
  'serious harm' means –
  (a) serious injury to or the serious illness (including mental illness) of a person;
  (b) serious harm to the environment (including the life and health of plants and animals);
  (c) serious harm to any building or other property.

(8) A reference in this section to emergency circumstances includes a reference to circumstances that are believed to be emergency circumstances.

Section 8(1) defines gross breach for the jury:

This section applies where –

(a) it is established that an organisation owed a relevant duty of care to a person, and
(b) it falls to the jury to decide whether there was a gross breach of that duty.

(2) The jury must consider whether the evidence shows that the organisation failed to comply with any health and safety legislation that relates to the alleged breach, and if so –
  (a) how serious that failure was;
  (b) how much of a risk of death it posed.

(3) The jury may also –

    (a) consider the extent to which the evidence shows that there were attitudes, policies, systems or accepted practices within the organisation that were likely to have encouraged any such failure as is mentioned in subsection (2), or to have produced tolerance of it;

    (b) have regard to any health and safety guidance that relates to the alleged breach.

It is unclear why a jury *may* refer to policies and the like but *must* refer to health and safety legislation.

Section 8 continues:

(4) This section does not prevent the jury from having regard to any other matters they consider relevant.

(5) In this section 'health and safety guidance' means any code, guidance, manual or similar publication that is concerned with health and safety matters and is made or issued (under a statutory provision or otherwise) by an authority responsible for the enforcement of any health and safety legislation.

Section 9 adds to the usual sanction of a fine the power to issue a remedial order:

(1) A court before which an organisation is convicted of corporate manslaughter . . . may make an order (a 'remedial order') requiring the organisation to take specified steps to remedy –

    (a) the breach mentioned in section 1(1) ('the relevant breach');

    (b) any matter that appears to the court to have resulted from the relevant breach and to have been a cause of the death;

    (c) any deficiency, as regards health and safety matters, in the organisation's policies, systems or practices of which the relevant breach appears to the court to be an indication.

(2) A remedial order may be made only on an application by the prosecution specifying the terms of the proposed order.

    Any such order must be on such terms (whether those proposed or others) as the court considers appropriate having regard to any representations made, and any evidence adduced, in relation to that matter by the prosecution or on behalf of the organisation.

(3) Before making an application for a remedial order the prosecution must consult such enforcement authority or authorities as it considers appropriate having regard to the nature of the relevant breach.

(4) A remedial order –

    (a) must specify a period within which the steps referred to in subsection (1) are to be taken;

    (b) may require the organisation to supply to an enforcement authority consulted under subsection (3), within a specified period, evidence that those steps have been taken.

    A period specified under this subsection may be extended or further extended by order of the court on an application made before the end of that period or extended period.

(5) An organisation that fails to comply with a remedial order is guilty of an offence, and liable on conviction on indictment to a fine.

Section 10 is new. It provides the court with a power to issue a publicity order:

(1) A court before which an organisation is convicted of corporate manslaughter or corporate homicide may make an order (a 'publicity order') requiring the organisation to publicise in a specified manner –

(a) the fact that it has been convicted of the offence;

(b) specified particulars of the offence;

(c) the amount of any fine imposed;

(d) the terms of any remedial order made.

(2) In deciding on the terms of a publicity order that it is proposing to make, the court must –

(a) ascertain the views of such enforcement authority or authorities (if any) as it considers appropriate, and

(b) have regard to any representations made by the prosecution or on behalf of the organisation.

(3) A publicity order –

(a) must specify a period within which the requirements referred to in subsection (1) are to be complied with;

(b) may require the organisation to supply to any enforcement authority whose views have been ascertained under subsection (2), within a specified period, evidence that those requirements have been complied with.

(4) An organisation that fails to comply with a publicity order is guilty of an offence, and liable on conviction on indictment to a fine.

At the time of writing s 10 had not been brought into force.

Section 17 provides that prosecutions for corporate manslaughter cannot be brought without the consent of the DPP. This provision has been criticised for putting prosecutions into the hands of a government-appointed official. It is contrary to the recommendation of the Home Consultation Document, mentioned above, and the Law Commission Report No. 237, *Legislating the Criminal Code: Involuntary Manslaughter*, 1996, which is the basis for much of the statute.

The Act may not lead to many more prosecutions per year than there were before the Act but it is the culmination of public concern over corporate failings that lead to death.

Summary

This chapter examines the law relating to the doctrines of vicarious and corporate liability. With regard to vicarious liability, the doctrine gives rise to one party being liable for the acts of another: this is rare in criminal law and if the reader has done Tort Law, he or she must not assume that the tort law applies in criminal law where vicarious liability is the exception to the principle that one person is not criminally liable for the conduct of another. The exceptional liability in criminal law is outlined. There follow two aspects of vicarious liability which can occasion difficulties: how the doctrine applies to attempts and secondary offenders. The next topic is corporate liability: that is, when may companies be criminally liable? For some offences such as murder a company cannot be liable: the sole sentence for murder is imprisonment for life but companies cannot be imprisoned. Vicarious liability for corporate conduct and the doctrine of extensive construction of statutes are examined before there is treatment of the main bone of contention, the doctrine of identification. This doctrine is based on the theory that certain high-ranking officials in the company such as members of the board *are* the company: what they do is what the company does. There is then a discussion of matters such as sanctions for corporate misbehaviour, which leads into the reform of the law, in particular the Law Commission's and the government's attempts to revise the law of corporate manslaughter, which at long last led to the Corporate Manslaughter and Corporate Homicide Act 2007.

● Vicarious liability: Rarely in criminal law is one person liable for the crimes of another. The exceptions are:
1 public nuisance and publishing a criminal libel;
2 where Parliament expressly makes one person liable for another's conduct;
3 where statutes are construed to the same effect through the doctrine of extensive construction, the most famous authority being ***Coppen v Moore (No. 2)*** [1898] 2 QB 306;
4 the delegation principle. This doctrine is subject to the restriction that the delegation must be complete (see ***Vane v Yiannopoullos*** [1965] AC 486 (HL)), the principle applies only to *mens rea* offences, and the delegate must have acted within the scope of his or her authority.

It should be noted that there can be no vicarious liability for attempted crimes or for secondary participation in crimes.

There has been a long-standing debate on whether it is acceptable to make one person liable for what another has done. The principal argument in favour is that without it criminal behaviour would occur unpunished; the principal argument to the contrary is that criminal liability should be *personal* to the accused.

● Corporate liability: Companies may be criminally liable:
1 statute may impose liability;
2 companies are liable for strict liability offences;
3 companies are liable for omissions in the normal way (see Chapter 2);
4 vicarious liability applies to companies as it applies to natural persons;
5 controversially, the doctrine of identification makes companies liable for the conduct and states of mind of high corporate officers: see ***Tesco Supermarkets Ltd v Nattrass*** [1972] AC 153 (HL) and for statutory offences see ***Meridian Global Funds Asia Ltd v Securities Commission*** [1995] 2 AC 500 (PC). There is debate how far down the corporate hierarchy one can go to make the company liable and one of the main criticisms of this form of liability is that because more can be delegated down the chain of command in larger than in smaller companies, it is much more likely that smaller enterprises will be held criminally liable than larger ones.

There are some offences for which companies cannot be criminally liable. One such is murder. The sentence for murder must be life imprisonment and companies not being natural persons cannot be imprisoned. Rape is another example: a corporation cannot insert its penis into one or more of the victim's anus, mouth or vagina.

Arguments in favour of and against corporate criminal liability have raged in recent years and further reform is on the cards.

References

Reports

Home Office Consultation Paper, *Reforming the Law of Involuntary Manslaughter* (2000)
Law Commission Consultation Paper no. 135, *Involuntary Manslaughter* (1994)
Law Commission Report no. 177, *A Criminal Code for England & Wales* (1989)
Law Commission Report no. 237, *Legislating the Criminal Code: Involuntary Manslaughter* (1996)

Books

Bergman, D. *Deaths at Work: Accidents or Corporate Crime?* (WEA, 1991)

Card, R., Cross, P. and Jones, P. A. *Criminal Law* 17th edn (Oxford University Press, 2005)

Slapper, G. and Tombs, S. *Corporate Crime* (Longman, 1999)

Smith, J. C. and Hogan, B. *Criminal Law* 10th edn (Butterworths, 2002)

Smith, J. C. and Hogan, B. *Criminal Law* (ed. D. Ormerod) 11th edn (Oxford University Press, 2005)

Journals

Andrews, J. A. 'Reform in the law of corporate liability' [1973] Crim LR 91

Anon. 'Increasing community control over corporate crime' (1961) 71 Yale LJ 280

Bergman, D. 'Recklessness in the boardroom' [1990] NLJ 1496

Polinsky, A. M. and Shavell, S. 'Should employees be subject to fines and imprisonment given the existence of corporate liability?' (1993) 13 IRLE 239

Burrows, R. 'The responsibility of corporation under English law' (1948) 1 *Journal of Criminal Science* 1

Reville, N. 'Corporate manslaughter' (1989) LSG no. 37, 17

Slapper, G. 'A safe place to work' [1992] LSG no. 37, 27

Stern, Y. Z. 'Corporate criminal personal liability' (1987–88) 13 Journal of Corporation Law 125

Sullivan, G. R. 'Expressing corporate guilt' (1995) 15 OJLS 281

Wells, C. 'Corporate liability for crime' [1996] 1 *Archbold News* 5

Further reading

Belcher, A. 'Corporate killing as a corporate governance issue' (2002) 10 *Corporate Governance* 47

Bergman, D. 'Recklessness in the boardroom' (1990) 140 NLJ 1496

Bergman, D. 'Weak on crime – weak on the causes of crime' [1997] NLJ 1652

Bergman, D. *Deaths at Work: Accident or Corporate Crime*, WEA (1991) (See also the website www.corporateaccountability.org.)

Centre for Corporate Accountability / Disaster Action / Trades Union Congress *Why we Need a New Corporate Killing Law* (2003)

Clarkson, C. M. V. 'Kicking corporate bodies and damning their souls' (1996) 59 MLR 557

Clarkson, C. M. V. 'Corporate culpability' [1998] 2 Web JCLI

Clarkson, C. M. V. 'Corporate manslaughter: yet more government proposals' [2005] Crim LR 677

Clough, J. 'Sentencing the corporate offender: the neglected dimension of corporate criminal liability' (2003) *Corporate Misconduct Ezine*

Clough J. 'Bridging the theoretical gap: the search for a realist model of corporate criminal liability' (2007) 18 Crim LF 267

Colvin, E. 'Corporate personality and criminal responsibility' (1995) 6 *Criminal Law Forum* 1

Field, S. and Jorg, N. 'Corporate liability and manslaughter: should we be going Dutch?' [1991] Crim LR 156

Glasbeek, M. 'Shielded by law: why corporate wrongs and wrongdoers are priviledged' [2002] UWSL Rev 1

Glazebrook, P. 'A better way of convicting businesses of avoidable deaths and injuries' (2002) 61 CLJ 405

Gobert, J. 'Corporate criminality: four models of fault' (1994) 14 LS 393

Gobert, J. 'Corporate criminality: new crimes for the times' [1994] Crim LR 722

Gobert, J. 'Controlling corporate criminality: penal sanctions and beyond' [1998] 2 Web JCLI

Gobert, J. 'Corporate killing at home and abroad – reflections on the government's proposals' (2002) 118 LQR 72

Gobert, J. and Punch, M. *Rethinking Corporate Crime* (Butterworths, 2003)

Griffin, S. 'Corporate manslaughter: a radical reform?' (2007) 71 JCL 151

Hill, J. 'Corporate criminal liability in Australia' [2003] JBL 1

Jefferson, M. 'Corporate criminal liability in the 1990s' (2000) 64 JCL 106

Jefferson, M. 'Corporate criminal liability: the problem of sanctions' (2001) 65 JCL 235

Mays, R. 'The criminal liability of corporations and Scots law: learning the lessons of Anglo-American jurisprudence', [2000] Edin LR 46

Ormerod, D. and Taylor, R. 'The Corporate Manslaughter and Corporate Homicide Act 2007' [2008] Crim LR 589

Pace, P. J. 'Delegation – A doctrine in search of a definition'[1982] Crim LR 627

Punch, M. '(g.b.h.) Grievous Business Harm: exploring corporate violence' (1995) 3 EJCPR 92

Reville, N. J. 'Corporate manslaughter' [1989] LSG 17

Slapper, G. 'Corporate manslaughter: an examination of the determinants of prosecutorial policy' (1993) 2 *Social and Legal Studies* 423

Stessens, G. 'Corporate criminal liability – a comparative perspective' (1994) 43 ICLQ 493

Sullivan, G. R. 'Expressing corporate guilt' (1995) 15 OJLS 281

Sullivan, G. R. 'The attribution of culpability to limited companies' [1996] CLJ 515

Sullivan, G. R. 'Corporate killing – some government proposals' [2001] Crim LR 31

Swigert, V. L. and Farrell, R. A. 'Corporate homicide' (1980–81) 15 *Law Society Review* 161

Tombs, S. 'Law, resistance and reform: 'regulating' safety crimes in the UK' (1995) 4 *Social and Legal Studies* 343

Wells, C. 'The decline and rise of English murder: Corporate crime and individual responsibility' [1988] Crim LR 788

Wells, C. 'The criminal liability of corporations and their officers' (1990) 2 *Law for Business* 120

Wells, C. 'Culture, risk and criminal liability' [1993] Crim LR 551

Wells, C. 'Corporate manslaughter: a cultural and legal form' (1995) 6 *Criminal Law Forum* 45

Wells, C. 'Corporations and the risk of criminal liability' (1996) 10 *The Whistle* (Bulletin of Freedom to Care, available on www.freedomtocare.org/page165.htm)

Wells, C. 'The corporate manslaughter proposals: pragmatism, paradox and peninsularity' [1996] Crim LR 545

Wenham, D. 'Recent developments in corporate homicide' (2000) 29 ILJ 378

Wickens, R. J. and Wong, C. A. 'Confusion worse confounded: the end of the directing mind theory' [1997] JBL 524

Williams, G. '*Mens rea* and vicarious liability' [1956] CLP 57

Celia Wells has also had a book published, *Corporations and Criminal Responsibility* (Clarendon, 2nd edn, 2001). In it she argues that companies should be punished if they exhibit practical indifference to a risk. For some of her other work see I. Loveland (ed.), *Frontiers of Criminality* (Sweet & Maxwell, 1995). See also B. Fisse and J. Braithwaite, *Corporations, Crime and Responsibility* (CUP, 1993). Fisse's (and Braithwaite's) articles are legion and include 'Reconstructing corporate criminal law: deterrence, retribution, fault and sanction' (1983) 56 S Cal LR 1141; 'Corporate criminal responsibility' (1991) 15 Crim LJ 166; 'The attribution of criminal liability to corporations' (1991) 13 Syd LJ 277. For a practitioner text see A. Pinto and M. Evans, *Corporate Criminal Liability* (Sweet & Maxwell, 2003).

There are many excellent American articles which discuss corporate liability; the following is a selection from the 1990s and early 2000s.

Barnard, J. 'Reintegrating shaming in corporate sentencing' (1999) 5 Cal L Rev 959

Beale, S. S. and Safwat, A. G. 'What developments in Western Europe tell us about American critiques of corporate criminal liability' (2004) 8 Buff Crim L Rev 89

Forschler, A. 'Corporate criminal intent – toward a better understanding of corporate misconduct' (1990) 78 Cal LR 1287

Hall, J. S. 'Corporate criminal liability' (1998) 35 Am Crim L Rev 549

Khanna, V. S. 'Corporate criminal liability: what purpose does it serve?' (1996) 109 Harv LR 1477

Khanna, V. S. 'Corporate crime liability: a political economy analysis', John M. Olin Centre for Law & Economics, University of Michigan, Paper no. 3–012

Laufer, W. S. 'Corporate bodies and guilty minds' (1994) 43 Emory LJ 647

Lederman, E. 'Models for imposing corporate criminal liability' (2000) 4 *Buffalo Criminal Law Review* 642

Lott, J. R. 'Corporate criminal penalties' (1996) 17 *Managerial and Decision Economics* 349

Parker, J. S. 'Doctrine for construction: the case of corporate criminal liability' (1996) 17 *Managerial and Decision Economics* 381

Ragozino, A. 'Replacing the collective knowledge doctrine with a better theory for attributing corporate *mens rea*' (1995) 24 Southwestern LR 423

Ulen, T. S. 'The economics of corporate criminal liability' (1996) 17 *Managerial and Decision Economics* 351

Walsh, C. and Pyrich, A. 'Corporate compliance programs as a defense to corporate criminal liability: can a corporation save its soul?' (1995) 47 Rutgers LJ 605

For a lobbying and advice organisation see the Centre for Corporate Accountability at www.corporateaccountability.org

For an Irish view see Law Reform Commission, *Consultation Paper on Corporate Killing*, LRC CP 26, 2003

For an Australian view see Tasmania Law Reform Institute, *Criminal Liability of Organizations*, Issues Paper No. 9, 2005 and the Report No. 9 of the same name, 2007

Visit **www.mylawchamber.co.uk/jefferson** to access exam-style questions with answer guidance, multiple choice quizzes, live weblinks, an online glossary, and regular updates to the law.

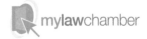

7

Infancy, duress, coercion, necessity, duress of circumstances

Introduction to Chapters 7–9

This chapter and the next two deal with what are normally called 'general defences' which apply to most if not all offences. The exception is diminished responsibility, which is a defence only to murder but is treated in the way that it is because of its affinity with insanity. The defences in the present chapter are often known as true defences in that they do not negate the *actus reus* or *mens rea* but act as a third element. Other so-called defences such as automatism and mistake are seen as operating differently. They do negate the external or fault element.

Introduction to defences

The criminal law is not based solely on a series of offences, which are concerned with preventing harms on pain of sanctions, but also on a number of defences which qualify the offences. As will be seen, some defences (such as self-defence) apply to all offences, while some defences apply only to some offences (e.g. diminished responsibility applies only to murder and reduces the offence to manslaughter; duress does *not* apply to murder, attempted murder and some forms of treason). One could analyse all offences into *actus reus* and *mens rea*, leaving no room for defences. Murder would become an unlawful killing with malice aforethought. If the accused killed in self-defence, it would not be murder because the killing was not unlawful. For the purposes of exposition, the style adopted in this book is that defences form a separate element. A killing in self-defence is not murder because even though the accused did kill and did intend to do so, he has a defence. This method facilitates learning for there is no need to say whether a certain defence obviates *actus reus* or *mens rea* (or both) and there is no difficulty with stating the burden of proof. One can therefore look at offences and defences in this way: is there an *actus reus*? If so, is there the relevant *mens rea*? If so, does the accused have a defence? Some defences are specific to certain offences, the obvious one being pro-vocation, which is a defence only to murder. Sometimes it may be difficult to state whether some matter is a failure by the prosecution to prove part of the offence or whether it is a defence. In rape the consent of the woman is part of the definition of the crime. If the woman consents to sexual intercourse, the offence of rape has not taken place. If, however, one consents to what would otherwise be a battery when one is engaged in a sport, the consent of the victim seems more appropriately to be a defence and not a failure by the prosecution to prove all the elements of the crime. Seeing consent as a separate defence enables us to consider it as a whole and not independently in each offence.

Each defence has its own rules and should not be confused with any other. If there is a common theme, it is that there has to be some kind of aberration of mind, such as the chemical change in drunkenness, the lack of mental responsibility in infancy and perhaps in duress, or the falling below a mental level as in insanity. It appears common sense to say for instance that a person forced to commit a crime should have a defence and that a young child should not suffer punishment for having broken the criminal law when he did not know that what he was doing was morally wrong. Why punish people who cannot change?

As Jordan CJ put it in *Turnbull* (1944) 44 NSWLR 108:

> A person is never regarded as criminally liable for an act which, although physically the act of his body, was done while his mind was in so abnormal a state that it cannot be regarded as his act at all, e.g. if he was sleep-walking, or so young, or so insane, as to be incapable of knowing that he was acting or the nature and quality of his act.

It should be noted that although the matters in this and the next two chapters are called 'defences', the burden of proof in most of them lies on the prosecution, which must disprove the defence beyond reasonable doubt. The exceptions are insanity and diminished responsibility, where the defence must prove them affirmatively but only on the balance of probabilities.

Until recently defences were not categorised: they either applied or they did not. Nowadays various attempts have been made to classify defences. The chief modern classification or taxonomy distinguishes between justifications and excuses.

Justification and excuse

English law used to distinguish between justification and excuse in relation to killings. Some homicides were justified, some others were excused. The distinction came to have no relevance to the accused for, whichever class of killing took place, he was not guilty. Until the early nineteenth century the distinction had some importance. An excusable killing led to the murderer's goods being forfeited to the Crown. Forfeiture did not take place when the killing was justifiable. Recently, however, it has become usual in the USA to divide defences into those which provide a justification and those which excuse. The division is a tool of analysis. It could be used to see how defences should be extended or reduced. The principal commentator is G. Fletcher, *Rethinking Criminal Law* (Little, Brown & Co, 1978). Readers who find difficulty with the concepts of justification and excuse should look at the individual defences first and then return to this section.

Justification means that the defendant's action is not disapproved of, e.g. in self-defence, in the use of force to effect a lawful arrest, in consent, and in the lawful chastisement of a child. The accused is not blameworthy because it has been decided that what he did was permissible. The otherwise wrongful conduct is legitimised. The law does not seek to deter such behaviour: it does not seek to punish persons who engage in such conduct. Joshua Dressler put it this way ('Provocation: Partial justification or partial excuse' (1988) 51 MLR 467, 468): 'There is a considerable moral difference between saying that an intentional killing is warranted (partially or fully), and saying that it is entirely wrong but that the actor is partially or wholly morally blameless for his wrongful conduct.' Perhaps another way of making the same point is to say that the accused when he is acting in, say, the prevention of crime, does not commit the *actus reus*. If the accused killed an assailant in the lawful prevention of the attack, he is not guilty of murder because there was no unlawful killing. He is not guilty because he does not fall within the prohibition when the crime is fully defined. Therefore, criminal law does not condemn what he has done. One does not look at this particular accused's state of mind. In justification defences, since the accused is seen not to have acted wrongly, rules on justification provide guidance for citizens. A person who has a defence of self-defence was not acting in breach of the criminal law. Therefore, others will not be in breach if they do as he did. In excuse defences, however, the behaviour of the defendant himself is investigated. He is not guilty because of some lack of blame attaching to him. Perhaps he has misperceived reality, and accordingly he is not fully responsible for his actions. He has acted wrongfully but his position was such that he is excused. An insane person is not blameworthy. On this basis, these defences would provide only an excuse: duress both by threats and of circumstances, intoxication, mistake, insanity, diminished responsibility, automatism, infancy and provocation. Defences such as provocation and diminished responsibility do not totally exculpate the accused. They are sometimes called 'partial excuses'. For discussion of duress, provocation and mistake, see below. Judges have spoken similarly. In **Harding** [1976] VR 129 Gowans J stated that duress 'is properly to be classed as a matter of excuse for what otherwise would be criminal conduct on account of the will or intent with which it was done'.

One omission from those lists is necessity. That defence could be treated either as justification or as excuse. It is suggested that it is a justification when the harm which the accused is threatened with is greater than the harm which he does. When the harm to be caused is equal to the crime which results one might say that the actor is excused but the action is not justified. Perhaps the same should be said of duress both by threats and of circumstances, provided that the offence committed was a lesser evil than the act threatened. It must be stated that at least with regard to duress and necessity their place in this scheme is not secure and may depend on the object to be achieved. If one says that the accused when under threat did what a reasonable person would have done because neither he nor that paragon could have resisted, the defence is excusatory. If one says that the defence is based on the accused's choosing the lesser evil, breaking a legal rule, it is justification. Killing two to save one may be excused; it cannot be justified. English law sees duress as excusatory. Dickson J said in the Supreme Court of Canada in **Perka v R** (1984) 13 DLR (4th) 1: 'praise is indeed not bestowed, but pardon is, when one does a wrongful act under pressure.' The present view of necessity is not always accepted. L. Vandervort 'Social justice in the modern regulatory state: duress, necessity and the consensual model in law' (1987) 6 Law & Phil 205 treats it as a defence of justification. The Law Commission in its 1993 Report No. 218 noted in this chapter seems to have viewed duress as excusatory (the mind was overcome) but necessity as justificatory (the choice was permissible). The difference between the two forms of necessity is that when it operates as a justification there has to be a choice of evils; there is no such requirement when it operates as an excuse. In turn, when it operates as an excuse the accused has acted or failed to act because of pressure exerted on him, but, when it operates as a justification, there is no such requirement: the accused then may act calmly and rationally. If duress were justificatory, many of the limitations on its application, such as duress is not a defence to murder, would disappear. One difficulty would be that politics would become part of the law because one would have to weigh up evils to determine which was the lesser one.

A similar problem arises in respect of provocation. One possible rationale of this defence is that the accused has lost his self-control and did not plan to kill; therefore, he did not in truth choose to kill; the blame attached to him is reduced; therefore, he has an excuse. This excuse rationale explains the first limb, but what about the 'reasonable person' test? An accused who has for reasonable reasons lost his self-control has the defence but so does a person who did not have a reasonable reason. In either case the accused has responded in a reasonable manner. One explanation is that of policy: the rule that the accused must exercise reasonable control is one which promotes self-restraint in the face of provocation. If the defence is a justification, it is accepted that some killings, e.g. of domestic abusers, are justified. The anger was justified. If this is the true rationale, the decision in **Smith** [2001] 1 AC 146, now overruled, was contentious. If a person is justified in doing as he did, the accused's personal characteristics should not be considered. Fortunately the law has reverted to its pre-**Smith** position. Mistake also poses a problem. If one accepts that mistake negatives *mens rea*, it is not truly a defence but a failure to prove all elements of the offence. If mistake is in some fashion a defence, the argument runs that the defendant is to be excused because he made a mistake. Professor Williams [1982] Crim LR 33 considered self-defence to be justified if the facts allowing force exist, but only excused if the accused wrongly believes that such facts exist. It is suggested that where the accused believes he is acting in self-defence but in fact is not, one may wish to say that if the mistake was reasonably made, he should have a defence, but if it was unreasonably made, he should not, for a person who makes an unreasonable mistake is still blameworthy. Present law, however, exculpates both: **Williams** [1987] 3 All ER 411 (CA). The theory could explain the difference between the need according to most authorities for a reasonable mistake in duress (an excuse) but the fact that an honest mistake suffices in self-defence (a justification), but if it is not certain whether a defence is an excuse or a justification, the distinction loses its basis as a tool of analysis.

Academics, particularly US ones, trying to utilise this division have come up with a small number of reasons why the dichotomy is helpful.

(a) Where the assailant's defence is a justificatory one, a person threatened by the conduct is not entitled to resist because the accused who is using or threatening force is acting in accordance with law, whereas if the defence is excusatory, he is entitled to resist. For example, one is not entitled to resist a constable's making a lawful arrest but one is entitled to resist an attack by an insane person, an automaton or a child because that person acts wrongly.

(b) Where the principal has a defence which is justificatory in nature, a party who assists the principal is entitled to give that help. The person who assists is behaving appropriately. It should not be criminal to act acceptably. However, if the defence is excusatory, the secondary party is liable. The fact that the defendant's act is excused does not necessitate that the helper's assistance is also excused. A person who helps another to batter a victim should be liable as accessory even when the other has a defence of automatism. A 'crime' has been committed; therefore, applying the theory of derivative liability (see Chapter 5) the secondary party can aid and abet that 'crime'. However, if the principal is justified in acting as he did, there is no principal offence to which an accessory can be a party.

(c) Where the accused has a justificatory defence, the courts do not have to prevent the behaviour recurring. Excusatory defences should lead to attempts to stop the behaviour recurring. This rationale would support the use of some kind of court-ordered supervision of those excused. This outcome may not be what an accused who is at present acquitted totally, say by reason of automatism, would desire. This third distinction may be only a definitional one, though it looks consequential.

Another distinction may be that the accused only has an excusatory defence when he is aware of the facts which give rise to the excuse, whereas in a justificatory defence the accused is relieved of responsibility even though he did not know the facts giving rise to the justification. One might add that if a defence is classified as justificatory, it should be available to all offences; however, one might argue that public policy might be to the effect that one may be excused from culpability for some offences but not for others. One may be excused from assault occasioning actual bodily harm but not from murder, for instance. Certainly it is difficult to understand the concept that one can be only partially justified in committing a crime. Therefore, if one kills, one should be acquitted, and not just guilty of manslaughter, when one's defence is justificatory. It has also been said that if the accused makes a mistake in respect of a justification, he has a defence if his error was honestly made, whereas in relation to an excuse the mistake must be one made on reasonable grounds.

The difference between justification and excuse is, it is suggested, most vital when considering reform of the law. In respect of one defence the (Irish) Law Reform Commission, *Homicide: The Plea of Provocation*, Consultation Paper 27 (2003) 105, put this very well:

> The contrasting rationales of justification and excuse . . . reflect competing policy object-ives. On the one hand, there is a feeling that the criminal law should make allowance for the infirmities of human nature. On the other, there is the general expectation that members of society should exercise a minimum standard of self-control. The aspiration for set standards inspired by this expectation does not sit easily with the sense of empathy aroused by a concern for human weakness. . . . The defence of provocation represents a compromise between these competing policy goals; indeed elements of both justification and excuse are often intermingled in the plea. The recent history of the defence has however been shaped by excusatory considerations, with the result that the issue of justification has . . . been pushed to the background.

The principal English discussion occurs in Chapter 1 of J. C. Smith's *Justification and Excuse in the Criminal Law* (Stevens, 1989). He believes that the theory is helpful in relation to resistance by a person threatened by an attack. One can resist an attack by a nine-year-old (infancy is an excuse), but one cannot resist a lawful arrest because that arrest is justified. If the arrest is, however, taking place with force, surely one is entitled to resist the force when the police have made a mistake as to the identity of the person they are arresting. The outcome is the same whether the behaviour of the police is described as justified or excused. The second distinction, assisting the person who has a defence, works well, says Smith, at the extremes. A person who helps a nine-year-old child to kill is guilty through the doctrine of innocent agency, whereas a person who helps the police in making an arrest is not guilty of an offence even though the arrest is unlawful because no crime has taken place. However, in other cases the division into excuse and justification is unhelpful. If it is held that police who shot in order to effect an arrest are excused but not justified in their action, why should a person who assists them in making the arrest be guilty because the police were mistaken in thinking that the person they were arresting was a violent criminal? One should look at what he believed, not at what the police believed.

With regard to the distinction in relation to the awareness of the circumstances, Smith argues that whether the defendant must know of the circumstances which justify or excuse his conduct, as was ruled in **Dadson** (1850) 4 Cox CC 358 in relation to the shooting of an escaping felon, is a matter of policy, and is not to be determined by inquiry whether the defence is justificatory or excusatory. **Dadson** is incorrect according to the theory, as the constable was preventing crime, a justificatory defence. He illustrates the point through the defence of infancy, which is excusatory. If a nine-year-old thinks he is 10, surely he is not to be convicted because he did not know of the excusatory circumstance that he is only nine. The outcome is a matter of law, and what the child believes is irrelevant. A similar argument demonstrates that even in a justificatory defence the accused must know of the circumstances which give rise to the defence. If Alf assists Beth in breaking into the Post Office which he runs, he is surely guilty even though Beth has unknown to him threatened his family that she will kill them unless he helps her.

The basic thrust of the late Professor Smith's comment seems to be that the distinction is at times useful but should not be allowed to dictate a result which is contrary to common sense or policy. Where the outcome would be 'pernicious' or 'outrageous' the dichotomy must not be applied. As Smith wrote elsewhere, [1991] Crim LR 151, he is 'not persuaded that the reception of the theory into English law is either practicable or desirable . . .'. Another difficulty is knowing whether an accused has an excuse or whether the prosecution has failed to prove the *mens rea*. For example, there is recent authority holding that insanity is no defence to strict offences because it affects the *mens rea*. If so, insanity is in truth a failure by the prosecution to prove all the elements of the offence, and the distinction between excuse and justification is inapplicable. There are many American critiques of the dichotomy. A book of this nature cannot deal with all of them. A way into the literature is via T. Morawetz 'Reconstructing the criminal defenses: the significance of justification' (1986) 77 JCL & Crim 277. Despite such criticisms the terms are infiltrating into English criminal law discourse and were espoused by the Law Commission in the 1989 draft Criminal Code. Clause 45 (1) refers to 'Acts justified or excused by' law.

A one-sentence summary of the distinction is that the accused who has a justification has acted rightly; he who has an excuse acted under some kind of disability. Another one-sentence summary of the law is: 'English criminal law does not make any clear-cut distinction between a justification and an excuse.' (Per Brooke LJ in *Re A (Children) (Conjoined Twins: Surgical Separation)* [2001] Fam 147.) Whether it should is for a book on criminal law theory.

Infancy

The law absolves infants under the age of 10 from responsibility for what would otherwise be criminal acts or omissions. The defence of infancy (sometimes called nonage) applies to all crimes including strict liability offences. Therefore, this defence is not based on the absence of the mental capacity to commit an offence. The policy appears to be that children cannot distinguish between (moral) right and wrong. It might be added that punishment would serve little purpose, for some minors would not be able to link the penalty with breach of the law and so would not be deterred for the future. However, since 1998, children aged 10 and upwards are treated as if they were adults for the purposes of criminal liability.

(a) *Up to 10 (i.e. nine and below)*: A child cannot be convicted of any offence: Children and Young Persons Act 1933, s 50, as amended by the Act of the same name from 1963, s 16. Such person may, however, be subject to care proceedings in the youth court.

One effect of infancy follows from the child's not being guilty. If an adult encourages a child to commit a crime and the child does perform the *actus reus*, the child is the innocent agent and the adult is deemed to be the principal offender. See Chapter 5. Moreover, since the child is not guilty of theft, the person who would otherwise be guilty of handling stolen goods is not guilty because the goods have not been stolen. In **Walters v Lunt** (1951) 35 Cr App R 94 (DC) a child of seven took another child's tricycle in circumstances in which, had he been adult, the act would have amounted to theft. Since he could not be convicted, the tricycle was not stolen and his parents could not be found guilty of the offence which is now called handling.

(b) *10 to 13 (inclusive)*: There was until 1998 a rebuttable presumption that the child cannot form *mens rea*. This presumption was rebutted by the prosecution showing that the accused had a 'mischievous discretion', i.e. that the child knew that what he was doing was morally or seriously wrong. This law was approved in the White Paper, *Crime, Justice and Protecting the Public*, Cm 965, 1990. 'The Government does not intend to change these arrangements which make proper allowance for the fact that children's understanding, knowledge and ability to reason are still developing.' The presumption no longer saved children from being hanged, but it remained as a protection for children. Each child had to be looked at individually.

The doctrine had been under attack for some time because of its differential application to children from good homes, who – knowing the difference between right and wrong – were more likely to be convicted than children from bad homes, and because – in an era of education for all – children did know when they were doing wrong. It has to be said, however, that in the words of Lord Lowry in *C v DPP* [1996] 1 AC 1 'better formal education, and earlier sophistication, do not guarantee that the child will more readily distinguish right from wrong'. The House of Lords reinstated the law that proof that the child committed the *actus reus* did not in itself prove that he knew that his act was seriously wrong, no matter whether his act was horrifying or appraised as seriously wrong by ordinary people, and that proof that the child knew that what he was doing was naughty did not demonstrate that he knew that it was seriously wrong. However, the then-existing law was condemned *obiter* by several of their Lordships. Lord Jauncey is representative: 'It is almost an affront to common sense to presume that a boy of 12 or 13 who steals a high-powered motor car, damages other cars while driving it, knocks down a uniformed police officer and then runs away when stopped is unaware that he is doing wrong.' He (a Scottish judge) also noted that the presumption did not apply in Scotland.

The House of Lords in *C v DPP* called for parliamentary revision of the law, which happened with the Crime and Disorder Act 1998. The Law Commission in its draft Criminal Code, 1989, had earlier recommended no change because it did not wish to see the extension of the use of the criminal law to deal with children. European countries vary tremendously in the minimum age of criminal responsibility. It is seven in Cyprus, Ireland, Liechtenstein and Switzerland, and in Northern Ireland and Scotland, but 16 in Andorra, Poland, Portugal and Spain, and 18 in Belgium and Luxembourg. This call was taken up by the Labour government.

The Crime and Disorder Act 1998, s 34, abolished the rebuttable presumption that children aged 10–13 inclusive were not guilty of crimes unless, in addition to the *actus reus* and *mens rea*, the prosecution proved that they knew that what they were doing was seriously wrong. The Home Office's Consultation Paper, *Tackling Youth Crime*, 1997, proposed to abolish the presumption because:

(i) a child over 10 can distinguish right from wrong in an age of universal compulsory education;

(ii) such a child no longer needs protection from state punishment because the youth court has many sentencing options;

(iii) the presumption was illogical in that it could be rebutted by showing that the accused was of normal mental development for a child of that age, yet it was presumed that the accused did not know right from wrong;

(iv) the interests of justice and the victim are not served by not convicting children;

(v) discontinuance of prosecution is not in the young offender's interests if it means that the opportunity is missed to take appropriate action to prevent reoffending; and

(vi) 'justice is best served by allowing courts to take account of the child's age and maturity at the point of sentence, not by binding them to presume that normal children are incapable of the most basic moral judgments'.

The White Paper, *No More Excuses*, Cm 3809, 1997, stressed that children 10–14 do know the difference between naughtiness and serious wrongdoing and, therefore, the presumption was contrary to common sense. Moreover, excuses were not to be made for children who offend.

The general view is that the criminal liability of children aged 10–13 is now assimilated with that of older people. There is, however, a different view put forward by N. Walker 'The end of an old song' (1999) 149 NLJ 64. This holds that while the presumption is abolished, children can still have a defence if they can show that they do not know that what they did was seriously wrong. It has to be said that this is exactly what the White Paper rejected. For a case supporting Walker's views see *Crown Prosecution Service* v *P* [2007] EWHC 946 (Admin). However, in *T* [2008] EWCA Crim 815 the court rejected *CPS* v *P*, holding that s 34 of the Crime and Disorder Act 1998 abolished not just the rebuttable presumption of incapacity but the whole concept that a child aged 10–13 inclusive could not be guilty of any crime.

Infancy and human rights

Setting the minimum age of criminal responsibility at 10 does not offend the European Convention on Human Rights. In *T v UK* [2000] Crim LR 187 the ECHR held there was no 'common standard amongst the member states of the Council of Europe as to the minimum age of criminal responsibility. Even if England and Wales is among the few European jurisdictions to retain a low age of criminal responsibility, the age of ten cannot be said to be so young as to differ disproportionately from the age-limit followed by other European States.' Therefore, there was no breach of Article 3, which prohibits torture and inhuman or degrading treatment. The age of criminal responsibility is 8 in Scotland. The Court in *T v UK* did, however, say that: '. . . it is essential that a child charged with an offence is dealt with in a manner which takes full account of his age, level of maturity and intellectual and emotional capacities, and that steps are taken to promote his ability to understand and participate in the proceedings.' The Court held that the trial of the defendants in *T v UK* did breach Article 6 because the state had failed to ensure that the boys understood the nature of the criminal proceedings against them.

Duress

Introduction

The law of **duress** may be seen as the outcome of two conflicting principles. The first was put by Sir James Fitzjames Stephen in his *History of the Criminal Law of England* (Sweet & Maxwell, 1883) 107:

> It is, of course, a misfortune for a man that he should be placed between two fires but it would be a much greater misfortune for society at large if criminals could confer impunity upon their agents by threatening them with death or violence if they refused to execute their commands.

This sentiment was approved by the Court of Appeal in **Gotts** [1991] 2 All ER 1. The law is there as a deterrent to people surrendering to threats. The contrasting rationale was adopted by another Court of Appeal in **Ortiz** (1986) 83 Cr App R 173:

> The essence of [this] defence is that the will of the subject of the threats is no longer entirely under his own control because of the fear engendered by those threats.

To convict persons in situations of duress would be inhumane. These people are blameless. Punishment would serve no purpose. A phrase sometimes used in this context is that the act of the accused was 'morally involuntary'. He could not help doing as he did, although his conduct was not truly involuntary because he had control over his limbs: indeed, he may well have both the *actus reus* and *mens rea* of the offence.

The second rationale was adopted by the Law Commission in its Report No. 83, *Defences of General Application*, 1978. Duress was to be seen as a concession to human weakness: the accused had chosen one evil, the apparent breaking of the law, when faced with a choice of two evils, the second one being to suffer serious injury or death either personally or to a third party (see later for a possible qualification of this proposition). The Court of Appeal rephrased the 'choice-of-evils' rationale in **Abdul-Hussain** [1999] Crim LR 570 as the alleged crime must be 'a reasonable and proportionate response' to the threat. The Law Commission's view was accepted by the House of Lords in **Howe** [1987] AC 417. However, as the Court of Appeal pointed out in **Shepherd** (1988) 86 Cr App R 47, this rationale fails to reveal why duress is a defence, rather than a factor in mitigating sentence. It also does not explain why duress is not a defence to all crimes. (Compare provocation which to all crimes except murder is an element in mitigation of sentence, not a defence to the offence.)

Duress and reasonableness

In the important case of **Graham** [1982] 1 WLR 294 the accused, a homosexual, lived with his wife and a man. He was taking drugs for anxiety. The other man, a violent person, was jealous of the wife. At that man's suggestion, the accused and that man killed the wife. The defendant's conviction for murder was upheld. The Court of Appeal determined that it did not matter that his fortitude had been weakened by drugs. A sober person would not have given way. The court held that the test of human weakness was: how would a sober and reasonable person with the accused's characteristics (race, sex, age, etc.) have reacted? (The reference to 'sober' is omitted when there is no evidence of intoxication. In fact in provocation, from where this test derives, the accused has a defence if because of intoxication he believes that there is provocation but in fact there is none.) A reasonable, frail old person would not be expected to reach the standard of fortitude of a reasonable, strong young person. On the facts of *Graham*, the question was: how would a reasonable bisexual man have reacted? This test was imported from the defence of provocation as it then was formulated and approved by the House of Lords in *Howe*, above. As in provocation there is a subjective and an objective test. Did he succumb? Might a reasonable person with his legally relevant characteristics have succumbed? The argument in favour of *Graham* runs thus. The accused has committed what would otherwise be an offence but has acted under duress. If a person of reasonable fortitude may have capitulated to the threat, and this accused did, then the accused is excused from liability.

In *Bowen* [1996] 2 Cr App R 157 the Court of Appeal garnered the following propositions in relation to the second issue from the cases (Stuart-Smith LJ at 166–167):

(1) The mere fact that the accused is more pliable, vulnerable, timid or susceptible to threats than a normal person are not characteristics with which it is legitimate to invest the reasonable/ordinary person for the purpose of considering the objective test.

(2) The defendant may be in a category of persons who the jury may think less able to resist pressure than people not within that category. Obvious examples are age, where a young person may well not be so robust as a mature one; possibly sex, though many women would doubtless consider they had as much moral courage to resist pressure as men; pregnancy, where there is added fear for the unborn child; serious physical disability, which may inhibit self-protection; recognised mental illness or psychiatric condition, such as post-traumatic stress disorder leading to learned helplessness.

(3) Characteristics which may be relevant in considering provocation, because they relate to the nature of the provocation itself will not necessarily be relevant in cases of duress. Thus homosexuality may be relevant to provocation if the provocative words or conduct are related to this characteristic; it cannot be relevant in duress, since there is no reason to think that homosexuals are less robust in resisting threats of the kind that are relevant in duress cases.

(4) Characteristics due to self-induced abuse, such as alcohol, drugs or glue-sniffing, cannot be relevant.

It is uncertain why the court took the view that a 'recognised mental illness or psychiatric condition' was needed. This dictum was approved by the Court of Appeal in *Moseley*, unreported, 21 April 1999. One should focus on whether this accused was capable of resisting the threat. It is also uncertain why some characteristics listed in (2) may affect the standard of fortitude. Is a person suffering from 'serious physical disability', even one which may 'inhibit self-protection', to be expected to be able to resist pressure less than an able-bodied person? Furthermore, addictions, for example to alcohol, are excluded even though they constitute recognised mental illnesses. The reference, however, does ensure that abused people can adduce evidence as mitigation of sentence to show that their wills have been crushed: *Emery* (1993) 14 Cr App R (S) 394. Similarly, in *Antar* [2006] EWCA Crim 2708 evidence that the accused was suffering from learning difficulties was admissible in determining whether the objective test as to reasonable steadfastness was satisfied.

Contrary to what had been assumed in *Howe*, the law as to this objective test does not totally incorporate the law of provocation. This point is made clear by the court in (3) but (4) is also different from provocation; see Chapter 12 where glue-sniffing is discussed. The court opined that low IQ was not a characteristic which makes those with it less courageous than an ordinary person. Therefore, it could not be attributed to the person of reasonable firmness used in this test. The court did, however, consider that mental impairment and mental defectiveness were relevant characteristics. The line between such conditions and low IQ may not be clear. The court in **Bowen** held that mental disabilities which reduced the capacity of the accused to resist the threat could be imputed to the reasonable person for the purpose of duress, but this prohibition is inconsistent with the law stated in the next paragraph. It should be noted that as in provocation the phraseology is shifting from 'reasonable persons' to 'ordinary persons', and that as in provocation in a usual case the sole relevant characteristics will be age and sex. Since the decisions in **Howe** and **Bowen** the Lords diluted the 'reasonable person' test in provocation: **Smith** [2001] 1 AC 146; however, the Privy Council in **Holley** [2005] 2 AC 580 restored the pre-**Smith** law. For details of provocation see Chapter 13.

The court in **Graham** stated that its test conformed with public policy. One might, however, say that the same threat may be more compelling when used against a weak person than a normal one. If the conceptual basis of duress is that individuals are not expected to resist extremely compelling threats, some persons are not as able to resist threats as others are. Yet the law demands that even timid persons conform to a high standard of behaviour: the law makes no concession to the weakness of timid persons. The fact that the accused was vulnerable (**Horne** [1994] Crim LR 584 (CA)), had a weak personality because of sexual abuse as a child (**Hurst** [1995] 1 Cr App R 82 (CA)), had suffered ill-treatment and violence (**Moseley**, unreported, 21 April 1999 (CA), which confirmed that for a mental characteristic to be included it had to be a medically recognised illness) or is unstable (**Hegarty** [1994] Crim LR 353 (CA) 'grossly elevated neurotic state') is irrelevant. If these characteristics were to be included in the reasonable firmness test, they would undermine it. A person of reasonable firmness is by definition not one of little firmness. As the court said in **Horne**: 'A person of reasonable firmness is an average member of the public; not a hero necessarily, not a coward, just an average person.' It is fascinating to note that the mental instability of the accused in **Hegarty** had earlier provided him with a defence of diminished responsibility on a charge of murdering his wife. Omitting the reasonable steadfastness point in relation to duress is a misdirection.

Since the reasonable person is not drunk, the accused who is drunk is to be judged against the standards of the reasonable sober person. In **Graham** the accused had been taking valium and alcohol. The Court of Appeal held that the jury should disregard the fact that drugs or drink or both had reduced the accused's ability to resist the threats. His intoxicated state was not to be attributed to the reasonable person when judging how a reasonable person with his legally relevant characteristics might have reacted. The case of **Kingston** [1995] 2 AC 355 (HL) is a reminder of the possibility of involuntary intoxication. It could be that an accused whose drink has been spiked is to be judged against the standards of the reasonable involuntarily intoxicated person. Self-induced drug addiction was rejected as a relevant characteristic in **Flatt** [1996] Crim LR 576 (CA). The accused was addicted to crack cocaine. His addiction was not to be attributed to the 'person of reasonable firmness' when judging his resistance to a drug-dealer. The addiction was a self-induced state, not a characteristic. As a result, all self-induced characteristics are irrelevant. **Flatt** should be compared with **Morhall** [1996] 1 AC 90, wherein the House of Lords held that glue-sniffing could be a characteristic of the ordinary person for the purposes of the defence of provocation. Triers of fact may have difficulty envisaging what they are being asked to do, and they are not helped by the exclusion of evidence which would tend to show that the accused was not a person of reasonable firmness such as that he was weak, vulnerable or susceptible to threats. It is uncertain whether changes in the law of provocation affect the defence of duress.

Because duress is on most arguments an excuse and not a justification, one might expect the 'reasonable person' test to play a part and the theory is partly reflected in the case law. In *Graham* the court also ruled that the accused must have good cause for his belief, and that his belief must have been based on reasonable grounds. The accused would have no good cause for his belief if he did not think that the threat would be carried out. These objective tests were also approved in *Howe* and followed in *DPP v Davis* [1994] Crim LR 600 (DC) and *Abdul-Hussain* [1999] Crim LR 570 (CA). However, there is a contrary view, namely that in light of the onward march of subjectivism in the House of Lords (*K* [2002] 1 AC 462, *B v DPP* [2000] 2 AC 428, and *G* [2004] 1 AC 1034) there is no room for an objective element, the reasonableness of the mistake. Even before these authorities, in *Martin* [2000] 2 Cr App R 42 the Court of Appeal ruled that in relation to duress by threats the test of belief was subjective. The accused is to be judged according to the facts as they appeared to him. Mantell LJ noted the analogy between duress and mistake which Lord Lane CJ had mentioned in *Graham*. Since the test in mistake is subjective, so should it be in respect of both forms of duress. An alternative view is that this case is simply wrong! Part of the reasoning against *Martin* is this: duress is an excuse; therefore, what the accused had done under duress was wrong; therefore, he should have a defence only if he has a reasonable explanation for committing what would otherwise be a crime. In *Martin* Mantell LJ purported to follow his previous judgment in the duress of circumstances case of *Cairns* [1999] 2 Cr App R 137 (Court of Appeal) but in fact he had used the objective test in that decision ('reasonably believed'). The Court of Appeal in *Safi* [2004] 1 Cr App R 14 certified a question for the House of Lords whether the accused's belief was based on reasonable or (only) genuine grounds, but the House refused leave to appeal. However, in *Hasan* [2005] 2 AC 467 the Lords held that the objective approach was correct. Lord Bingham said: '. . . there is no warrant for relaxing the requirement that the belief must be reasonable as well as genuine.' Therefore, *Martin* is wrong. It should be noted that, provided the accused reasonably believes that there is a threat, there need not actually be one.

If the accused has a reasonable belief in the threat, it need not be proved that the threat actually existed: *Cairns*. There are, however, authorities to the contrary. In *Abdul-Hussain* it was said that the danger must 'objectively' exist and this statement was approved by the Court of Appeal in *S* [2001] 1 WLR 2206. Unfortunately all these cases were heard in the same court, and the authorities are inconsistent.

If enacted the draft Criminal Code, Law Com. No. 177, 1989, cl 41(1), would reverse *Graham* by holding that any mistake, reasonable or not, would give rise to the defence ('a person who acts in the belief that a circumstance exists has any defence that he would have if the circumstance existed'), while cl 42(3) would take into account the accused's own capacity to resist. The Law Commission continues to approve of this reform: Report No. 218, *Legislating The Criminal Law – Offences against the Person and General Principles*, 1993. The argument is that reasonableness relates to evidence, not to substantive law. Certainly the objective test as to belief in *Graham* and *Howe* looks frail after the House of Lords' decision in *B v DPP* [2000] 2 AC 428, *K* [2002] 1 AC 462 and *G* [2004] 1 AC 1034 which strongly supported the subjective test of mistaken belief.

The question of reasonableness is sensible in provocation because one is comparing the accused with a person of reasonable firmness sharing the accused's characteristics to see whether the hypothetical person would have done as the accused did. In duress, however, the events are not connected with the defendant's characteristics. They are foisted on him. On this approach the reasonableness test in duress does not bear the same function as in provocation, and one might ask whether it is needed. It perhaps serves no purpose except to deny the defence to persons who ought to have it. Certainly provocation and duress are not directly comparable defences. Provocation is a defence only to murder, whereas duress is not a defence to that crime, and provocation is based on the loss of self-control, whereas the modern English view of duress is that it is based on a choice of evils, the accused breaking the law in order to escape a greater evil (the concession-to-human-frailty argument).

For a list of most of the limitations on the defence of duress see the judgment of Smith J in *Hurley and Murray* [1967] VR 526 and *Abdul-Hussain* [1999] Crim LR 570 (CA). The accused must know of the facts which give rise to this defence.

The effect of a successful plea of duress

The accused escapes conviction if the prosecution fail to disprove duress beyond reasonable doubt. There are *dicta* to the contrary in the dissenting speech of Lord Simon in *Lynch* v *DPP for Northern Ireland* [1975] AC 653 but they are wrong: see the House of Lords, *Howe*, above. The burden of proof for all defences lies on the prosecution, with one common law exception (insanity). Parliament may place the onus on the accused but has not done so in respect of duress (cf. diminished responsibility).

The burden of proof

There are several cases, such as *Gill* [1963] 1 WLR 841, which state that the prosecution must disprove duress. For an Australian authority see *Smyth* [1963] VR 737. The judge must instruct the jury that the prosecution bears the burden. Contrary *dicta* in *Steane* [1947] KB 997 are incorrect. *Lynch* finally settled the issue. The defendant, however, bears the evidential burden. He must lead evidence that his mind was affected by duress.

Duress, *actus reus and mens rea*

There are three theories as to how duress fits in with *actus reus* and *mens rea*.

(a) The accused had no *mens rea*. This approach would mean that duress would not be a defence to strict liability offences, contrary to the Divisional Court's ruling in *Eden DC* v *Braid* [1998] 12 May. This approach was rejected by Lords Edmund-Davies and Kilbrandon in *Lynch*, above, the Northern Ireland Court of Criminal Appeal in *Fitzpatrick* [1977] NI 20, and the House of Lords in *Howe* [1987] AC 417, refusing to follow *dicta* of Lord Goddard CJ in *Bourne* (1952) 36 Cr App R 125. A person acting under duress does nevertheless intend to act, knowing of the consequences, although his freedom of action is constrained by the coercive power of the duressor.

(b) The defendant did not act voluntarily because his will was overborne. But for the duress, he would not have committed the crime. Therefore, there is no *actus reus*. This viewpoint was rejected in *Lynch*. (Compare automatism where the accused does not act voluntarily, but in a different sense. The accused is not unconscious when he acts under duress.) The defendant acts under pressure but he is not forced by someone's hand to do as he did. He had a choice. Nevertheless, it is arguable contrary to *Lynch* that when he acts under duress, he is compelled to do so in a way not dissimilar from involuntary action. In relation to the 'overborne will' theory, it is suggested that there are pressures which overbear the will just as much as duress but which do not constitute duress or any other defence. For example, financial pressures may overbear the will but it is not a defence to say that the accused stole because his will was overborne by worries about the mortgage.

(c) The accused had both *actus reus* and *mens rea* but duress is the reason why he escapes conviction. This stance was seemingly accepted in *Lynch*, *Fitzpatrick* and *Howe*. In *Lynch* Lord Wilberforce said that the accused 'completes the act and knows that he is doing so; but the addition of the element of duress prevents the law from treating what he has done as a crime'. Lord Simon said: 'There are both *actus reus* and *mens rea* . . . duress is not inconsistent with act and will . . .'. The accused's conduct is excused, even though he intended harm, because society stipulates that he could not have been expected to act otherwise: faced with a choice of two evils, he chose to break the law.

Whichever theory is correct, there must be an evidential basis for duress. In *O'Too*, unreported, 4 March 2004, the accused said that he associated with members of a criminal gang but not that he was a member of it. Since he was not a member of a gang, there was no room for duress based on the law stated in the next section. In *Giaquinto* [2001] EWCA Crim 2696 it was said that the judge should not leave the defence to the jury if the accused's evidence contradicted it.

Associating with criminals

In the mid-1970s the Northern Ireland Court of Criminal Appeal held that duress was not a defence where the accused voluntarily joined up with violent criminals and thereby exposed himself to the risk of being compelled by pressure of a violent kind to commit an offence: *Fitzpatrick*, above. The accused had joined a terrorist organisation, the IRA. The court held that he had no defence to a charge of robbery. The House of Lords refused leave to appeal; so the assumption was that the law was as the Northern Irish Court had stated. In *Howe*, above, Lord Hailsham approved *Fitzpatrick*. Since then English courts have adopted the doctrine: *Sharp* [1987] QB 853, *Shepherd*, above, and *Ali* [1995] Crim LR 303 (all CA). There is no need for the defendant to join an organisation: it is sufficient if he joins a one-off conspiracy. *Hasan* [2005] 2 AC 467 (L) is the most authoritative supporting case. In *Ali* the accused, a heroin addict, was a dealer for the duressor. He used all of one batch for himself, thereby placing himself in debt to the duressor, who gave him a gun and told him to rob a bank or a building society: otherwise he would be killed. The court held that he could not rely on duress because he had voluntarily joined himself to a violent individual. A similar case is *Heath* [2000] Crim LR 109 where the accused became indebted to a drugs dealer and thereby accepted the risk that he might be threatened with violence if he did not act as a drugs carrier. The Court of Appeal held in *Lewis* (1993) 96 Cr App R 412 that for this rule to apply the criminal enterprise and the threat must not be too remote from each other. The accused took part in a robbery with the duressor. Both were imprisoned and the latter attacked the former while they were both in prison. The accused refused to give evidence against the duressor. The court held that he was not guilty of contempt of court. The robbery was too remote from the alleged offence. The Court of Appeal in *Sharp* stated that the accused must be an active member of the organisation at the time of the pressure for this rule to apply.

The pressure on the accused must be one which took the form of violence or the threat of violence either to the accused or to a member of his immediate family: *Baker* [1999] 2 Cr App R 335 (CA). It may be that pressure on the accused via a threat to a third party is sufficient. This would make the law consistent with that on duress and duress of circumstances generally. *Baker* also illustrates the point that this exception is not limited to joining a criminal gang; it is sufficient to associate with violent people. The House of Lords in **Hasan** held that the accused was not afforded the defence when he voluntarily associated himself with violent people: there was no need for the prosecutor to prove that he knew he would be coerced to commit offences, much less that he knew he would be coerced to commit offences of the type which in fact occurred. Any suggestion to that effect in **Baker** was incorrect. The accused, held the House, had no defence when he knew or ought reasonably to have known, that he may be subject to threats.

Sometimes the judge can rule that the accused cannot rely on duress, as when he joins a terrorist organisation or a violent gang: **Baker**. Otherwise it is a question for the jury whether the accused accepted the risk of violence on joining the gang or criminal activity (**Baker**). In **Ali** the court said that this rule applied whenever the accused knew he would become part of a crime. He did not need to know which specific crime (e.g. robbery) he would be ordered to commit. The House of Lords approved this principle in **Hasan**.

The law on joining violent gangs ceases to apply when the accused has served his sentence and abandons a life of crime. A subsequent threat by a former conspirator will now lead to the accused's regaining the defence of duress.

The Court of Appeal in **Harmer** [2002] Crim LR 401 rejected an argument that the accused should have a defence of duress when he did not foresee that he might be asked to commit crimes, though he had foreseen that he might be subjected to violence. It was sufficient that he had voluntarily exposed himself to threats by becoming indebted to a drugs supplier. **Heath**, above, is similar.

One might argue that this limitation ought not to be part of the law. If the basis of the defence is that the accused's will was overborne, his will was overborne when he was obliged to commit a crime by the gang he had joined. Moreover, the behaviour the courts are aiming at is membership of bodies which carry out illegal actions. The defence of duress is not an apt place for the courts to punish this conduct. In **Lynch**, above, Lord Morris said that defendants must not put themselves under the sway of gangster tyrants. It is doubtful whether this restriction does in fact help to dissolve the subjugation of those who are under the sway of such tyrants. Should there be no concession to frailty if the accused has voluntarily assumed the risk of duress? Nevertheless, the Law Commission in its Report No. 218, *Legislating the Criminal Code: Offences against the Person and General Principles* of 1993 proposed that this rule should continue to apply.

The types of threat sufficient to raise this defence

(a) Threats of death or serious physical violence are sufficient. For example, a threat to cut up two girls on the streets of Salford was a sufficient menace in **Hudson and Taylor** [1971] 2 QB 202 (CA). The Privy Council in **Sephakela v R** [1954] Crim LR 723 restricted duress to these types of threat and the Court of Appeal in **A**, unreported, 12 May 2003, doubted whether the threat of a punch in the face was sufficient to give rise to this defence. 'Serious harm' has not been much discussed in the cases. In **Quayle** [2006] 1 WLR 3642 it was held that pain was insufficient: death or serious injury was required. The avoidance of severe pain was not to be treated as the avoidance of a threat to life or serious injury. The Count of Appeal noted that pain involves 'a large element of subjectivity.' Therefore, taking cannabis to avoid pain remains an offence. It ought to bear the same meaning as grievous bodily harm, discussed in Chapter 13, a phrase which includes serious psychiatric injury but see (f) below. Where the threat is insufficient to give this defence, it is a mitigating factor in punishment.

(b) A threat to expose someone to a charge involving immorality is not enough; e.g. *Valderrama-Vega* [1985] Crim LR 220 (CA) involving homosexuality. Similarly, as occurred in that case a threat to make the accused lose money must be disregarded.

(c) Threats to property would seem not to be enough. In *M'Growther* (1746) 18 State Tr 391 the accused was guilty when friends of Bonnie Prince Charlie compelled him to join their rebellion under a threat among other things to steal his cattle. The Divisional Court held in *DPP v Milcoy* [1993] Crown Office Digest 200 that a threat by a cohabitee to his partner's pony and dogs did not give rise to a defence of duress.

(d) Threats of imprisonment are almost certainly not enough, but there is a contrary *dictum* of Lord Goddard CJ in *Steane* [1947] KB 997. Modern cases refer only to death and serious injury.

(e) A threat to reveal the accused's financial position is insufficient: *Valderrama-Vega*, above. In *Lynch* Lord Simon said that a threat to bankrupt the accused's son was not a defence, for the law had to draw a line somewhere and this type of threat fell below that line.

(f) A threat of serious psychological harm is insufficient: *Baker* [1999] 2 Cr App R 335 (CA). This is an authority on duress of circumstances, but in this respect the same principles apply. The decision is out of line with those on the law of non-fatal offences. See *Ireland; Burstow* [1998] AC 147 (HL). It is suggested that *Baker* is incorrect for what difference is there between physical and psychological harm if both are severe? The Court of Appeal in *Shayler* [2001] 1 WLR 2206 said that duress existed to protect 'the physical and mental well-being of a person' but it cannot be said that the court was thinking of this issue when it did so. (The case is one of duress of circumstances but the same principle applies.)

(g) There has to be a threat. Committing a crime because one believes one has no choice is not sufficient.

(h) Outside circumstances prompting suicidal tendencies were held in *Rodger* [1998] 1 Cr App R 143 (CA) not to constitute grounds giving rise to duress of circumstances. The law was that the threat had to be extraneous to the accused. The court said that to allow a defence of duress based on suicidal tendencies would give people a licence to commit crimes if they were vulnerable. The test for duress was an objective standard, not a subjective one. *Rodger* may be criticised on the ground that the reason why the defendants had such tendencies was because the Home Secretary had increased their sentences, an external cause, but the court said that the circumstances were 'solely' ones subjective to the defendants. The Home Secretary's decision was the background to the suicidal tendencies, not the legal cause of the desire to escape from prison.

It seems strange that if duress is based on the overborne-will theory, only one type of threat is considered sufficient to overbear the will, despite the fact that another type of threat has actually caused the accused to act as he did. If fear of force is the motivating factor, why are not other fears taken into account? If I steal to avoid bankruptcy, I have no defence. If I drive dangerously to avoid being raped, I have no defence.

In *Graham*, above, the Court of Appeal restricted its model direction to threats of death or serious physical injury. In *Abdul-Hussain*, above, the Court of Appeal spoke of 'death or serious injury'. Two cases on the analogous defence of duress of circumstances call for 'death or serious injury'/'death or serious bodily injury' (*Conway* [1989] QB 290

(CA)) and 'death or serious injury'/'death or serious physical injury' (*Martin* [1989] 1 All ER 652). It is unclear whether the court definitely meant to exclude serious mental injury, a point not raised on the facts. The Law Commission in its 1993 Report No. 218 recommended that the restriction to death and serious injury should continue.

The threat that the accused perceived need not be one which in fact exists. It is sufficient that the accused believed on reasonable grounds that he had good cause to fear death or serious harm. In *Cairns*, above, a driver drove off with a youth on his car bonnet. He was frightened both of the youth who had his face against the windscreen and of the youth's friends who followed the car shouting and gesticulating. In fact they were trying to get the youth to climb off the car. The court held that it did not matter that there was in truth no threat: it was the accused's perception of the situation that counted.

The threat need not be the sole cause of the accused's acting as he did. The defence applies if he would not have committed the offence but for the threat: *Valderrama-Vega, Ortiz* (both above).

Threats to whom?

Successful applications of the defence in England have involved the accused or his close family. In *K* (1984) 78 Cr App R 82 (CA), the threat involved the defendant's mother. In *Wright* [2000] Crim LR 510 (CA) the threat was to the accused's boyfriend. The court held that the accused must reasonably regard herself responsible for the person threatened, and the Court of Appeal approved this limitation in *S* [2001] 1 WLR 2206, which is also known as *Shayler*. In *Ortiz*, above, the court assumed that a threat to a wife and child was sufficient, while in *Shepherd*, above, Mustill LJ did not refer to the fact that the threat was to the accused and her family. Lord Mackay in *Howe*, above, mentioned a close relation such as a 'well-loved child'. Rose LJ in *Abdul-Hussain*, above, spoke of 'imminent peril or death or serious injury to the defendant or those to whom he has responsibility'. This restriction comes from a specimen direction provided by the Judicial Studies Board ('person for whom [the accused] would reasonably regard himself as responsible'). Lord Bingham spoke to the same effect in *Hasan*, above. It is suggested that English law does not recognise such a restriction. The Supreme Court of Victoria went further in *Hurley and Murray* [1967] VR 526 to hold that the defence was available when the threat was to a mistress. In *DPP v Milcoy* the court did not question that a threat to a cohabitee was sufficient. There would seem to be no stopping place despite the restriction in *Wright* and *S* to, as the latter case put it, 'a person or persons for whom he has responsibility or . . . persons for whom the situation makes him responsible'. As the Court of Appeal noted in *S*, *Pommell* [1995] 2 Cr App R 607 (CA) is at variance, because the threat was to kill various people not connected with the accused. A threat to a hostage unrelated to the accused would be sufficient. In duress of circumstances a threat to the accused or some other person is sufficient (*Conway* – threat to passenger in the accused's car, the parties not being related by blood, marriage or sex – *Martin*, both above). If such a threat is sufficient in duress of circumstances, which applies the rules from duress, it should also be sufficient in duress itself. Moreover, as one of the doyens of US criminal law, R. M. Perkins, wrote: 'Impelled perpetration restated' (1981) 33 Hastings LJ 403:

> [a] person might be willing to chance that a threat to kill, if directed at that person, was only a bluff, but may not be willing to chance it if it was a threat to kill his or her spouse or child.

This argument may also apply to strangers. Surely reasonable people are concerned for the safety of others. Under the draft Criminal Code, cl 42(3)(a)(i) states that the threat may be to another (Law Com. No. 177, 1989). The same proposal occurs in the latest recommendations: see 'Reform proposals' below. The relationship between the accused and the person threatened can be taken into account when determining whether or not he could reasonably have resisted the threat. A threat to kill one's children may be more overwhelming than one to a stranger. It might be added that it is arguable whether an accused should be allowed to say that he injured a stranger in order to prevent injury to another stranger.

Opportunity to escape

Duress is not available if the accused could have avoided the threat without harm to himself or to others: **Heath** [2000] Crim LR 1011 (CA). The accused was ordered to help to transport drugs the next day or he would be harmed. It was held that he was given enough time to go to the police for protection or he could have moved into his relatives' house in Scotland. The court also said that the fact that the accused was a drug user and therefore unlikely to go to the police did not affect the law that he could have turned to the police in this situation. Similar is **Hasan**. Lord Bingham said: '. . . if the retribution threatened against the defendant or his family or a person for whom he reasonably feels responsible is not such as he reasonably expects to follow immediately or almost immediately . . . there may be little if any room for doubt that he could have taken evasive action, whether by going to the police or in some other way, to avoid the crime'. There must be no opportunity of putting oneself under effective (as **Baker** shows: police protection may not have stopped the duressors to whom the duressees owed money for cannabis) official protection, such as that provided by the police and prison warders: **Lynch, Sharp**, both above. In **Gill**, above, the court considered that the accused would not have this defence if the threat was not to be carried out immediately because he could have sought police protection. The law seems to be that the accused is judged according to how a person of the same age and sex as him with his relevant characteristics would have reacted: **Baker** [1999] 2 Cr App R 335 (CA).

The modern view is that the accused may be afforded the defence if the threat is imminent; the threat need not be one which can be executed immediately: **Abdul-Hussain**, above. The defendants hijacked a plane to escape from Iraq. The rule now seems to be that it is sufficient that the threat was one which would probably be carried out in the near future; it does not matter that it was not one which could be carried out there and then. The defendants could successfully plead duress at a time earlier than a request for extradition from the state whose aircraft they hijacked. In **Eden DC v Braid**, above, Lord Bingham CJ spoke of the accused's having 'no other viable options'. In the well-known Irish case of **Attorney-General v Whelan** [1934] IR 518 Murnaghan J said: '. . . if there were reasonable opportunity for the will to reassert itself, no justification can be found in antecedent threat'. The Court of Appeal spoke to similar effect in **Abdul-Hussain**: 'The peril must operate on the mind of the defendant when he commits the otherwise criminal act, so as to overbear his will . . .'. The Court of Appeal in **Hudson and Taylor**, however, held that the accused had the defence because police could not provide protection on all occasions. Girls in **Hudson** committed perjury 'by immediate and unavoidable pressure'. Lord Parker CJ said that it did not matter that the threat could not be carried out 'instantly, but after an interval'. As Lord Griffiths put it in **Howe**: 'If duress is introduced as a merciful concession to human frailty it seems hard to deny it to a man who knows full well that any official protection he may seek will not be effective to save him from the threat of death under which he has acted.' This statement is quite a strong one. It is not sufficient that the accused believes official protection will be ineffective: he must know 'full well' that it is so. It seems strange that the judiciary, one arm of the state, is saying that another arm of the state, the police, cannot protect the state's citizens. All the circumstances including the age of the accused have to be taken into account. On the facts it might be doubted that the threat would be put into place immediately.

Hudson and Taylor may require reconsideration in the light of *Cole* [1994] Crim LR 582 (CA) and *Hasan* (HL). The court in *Cole* held that there had to be a direct and immediate link between the threat and the crime. On the facts the crimes committed by the accused, robberies at building societies, in order to obtain money to repay lenders, were not closely enough linked to threats to himself, his girlfriend and their child. The threat was not specific enough. The court spoke of duress only applying when the duressor had nominated the crime. (This area of law may be one where duress of circumstances is different.) The concept of nomination may be difficult to apply: if I tell you to steal money, have I nominated the crime if you obtain the money by fraud?

The court is looking for a much more spontaneous reaction than occurred in *Hudson and Taylor*. Lord Bingham in *Hasan* stated that *Hudson and Taylor* was wrong: 'I cannot, consistently with principle, accept that a witness testifying in the Crown Court at Manchester has no opportunity to avoid complying with a threat incapable of execution then or there.' *Hudson and Taylor* was, however, applied by the Court of Appeal in *Abdul-Hussain*. Rose LJ said in chilling words: 'If Anne Frank had stolen a car to escape from Amsterdam and been charged with theft, the tenets of English law would not . . . have denied her a defence of duress of circumstances, on the ground that she should have waited for the Gestapo's knock on the door.' *Cole* was doubted: a spontaneous reaction was not needed. The same rule occurs in necessity: the threat need not be one which forced the accused to act immediately, as the facts of *Re A* [2001] Fam 147, discussed below, illustrate. One twin would not cause the death of the other unless the surgeons operated immediately. It was sufficient that without separation fairly soon one twin would cause the other's death.

Once the threat is over, the accused must desist, e.g. *DPP v Davis*, above, where driving two miles to escape unwanted sexual advances with excess alcohol in the accused's blood ruled out the defence. Similar is the New South Wales case of *Lawrence* [1980] NSWLR 122. The navigator of a ship was threatened with violence if he did not continue navigating. He had a reasonable opportunity to escape. Therefore, the threat no longer operated. In one of the latest English cases, *DPP v Tomkinson* [2001] RTR 583 (DC), the accused drove 72 miles to escape from her abusive husband. Her defence of duress of circumstances to a charge of driving with excess alcohol failed because she had driven further than necessary to escape the danger. A more recent authority is *DPP v Mullally* [2006] EWHC 3448 (Admin). The accused lost her defence of duress on a charge of driving with excess alcohol in her blood because she was being followed by the police.

Offences to which duress is not a defence

Duress does provide a defence to most crimes, e.g. perjury (*Hudson and Taylor*, above), contempt of court (*K*, above, and *Lewis*, above), what is now theft (*Gill*, above), possessing ammunition (*Subramaniam* [1956] 1 WLR 965 (PC)), hijacking (*Abdul-Hussain*) and what is now handling (*Attorney-General v Whelan*, above). Note that one does not use gradations. One does not say that a threat of death alone is sufficient to give rise to a defence in a case of contempt, but one of serious harm suffices for, say, perjury. There are statements in the cases that duress is no defence to all felonies and no defence to robbery. This section considers those exceptions which are recognised in modern English law, though the fourth one has not been definitively established.

(a) According to **Abbott v R** [1977] AC 755, where the Privy Council split three to two, duress is no defence to the perpetrator of murder. The accused killed a British woman on the orders of a wicked individual. The victim among other things had a cutlass rammed down her throat and was buried alive. The Privy Council ruled that the accused had no defence even though he acted under pressure from a person who in English terms was a gangland boss. Lord Salmon bolstered his conclusion by reference to war criminals: they were not allowed to rely on duress or superior orders even though they might or would be shot if they disobeyed. He also referred to the speech in **Lynch**, above, of Lord Simon, who stated that if the defence were afforded, it would provide a charter for terrorists, gangleaders and kidnappers. Lord Simon's argument has since been undermined by the development of the rule relating to voluntary membership of criminal gangs: see above. **Abbott** was approved by the House of Lords in **Howe** (above). The accused had acted under the malign influence of one Murray. They had assaulted one person whom another killed; they were participants in that murder and actually killed another victim at Murray's order. The result is that the accused has no defence to murder even though he would have been killed had he not killed. The law that duress is no defence to murder remains as true today as it did 30 years ago: **Wilson** [2007] *The Times*, 6 June.

(b) **Howe** ruled that duress is no defence for accessories to murder. **Lynch**, above, was departed from. Lord Hailsham LC said:
(i) the law had to protect the innocent;
(ii) a person of ordinary fortitude was capable of heroism, i.e. would sacrifice his life rather than take innocent life (Lord Hailsham noted that if the accused did kill, he could not rely on the principle that he was choosing the lesser evil, but as we have seen the English law of duress is not predicated on the 'lesser evil' principle);
(iii) the law should not protect cowards and poltroons;
(iv) conviction could be mitigated by administrative remedies, such as occurred in **Dudley and Stephens** (1884) 14 QBD 273, on which see below. The prerogative of mercy could be used; the judge need not recommend a minimum length of life sentence; and the Parole Board could recommend release.

Lord Mackay emphasised that the law should not give anyone the power to choose who would survive. Lord Griffiths spoke of 'the special sanctity that the law attaches to human life'. Innocent life was to be protected even at the cost of the life of the accused or another. There are cases in other jurisdictions where duress has been held not to be a defence to secondary parties to murder such as **Brown** [1968] SASR 467 and **Harding** [1976] VR 129, and English institutional writers in the main supported the rule.

The House of Lords in **Howe** and law which fails to provide for a defence to murder may be criticised on several grounds.
(i) Circumstances may occur when a person of ordinary firmness would submit to threats. Why should a person suffer life imprisonment for not acting as a hero?
(ii) If the accused is ordered under threat of death to injure someone seriously, e.g., to kneecap him, and the victim dies, he is guilty of murder. The threat was: injure someone or be killed, and the accused has no defence. On a

choice-of-evils approach the accused chose the lesser evil. What if the threat is to the accused's family? Is it really the legal position that the law encourages a person to stand by while his family is killed? The accused remains guilty of murder even if the victim refused a blood transfusion because he was a Jehovah's Witness. It seems harsh to convict the accused of murder in these circumstances.

(iii) The discretion not to prosecute does not always save the law from absurdity. The accused was prosecuted in **Anderton v Ryan** [1985] AC 560 (HL) even in circumstances in which the Law Commission predicted no prosecution would take place. The same could apply in duress.

(iv) The sole penalty for murder is life imprisonment. Duress cannot be taken into account in the sentence as it can in other offences. Surely it should be for the courts, and not for the executive, to decide the penalty?

(v) It is harsh to call a person who yielded to a threat to kill his family a coward and a poltroon. Would only a coward choose to kill a third party?

(vi) Lord Griffiths said that the Law Commission Report No. 83, *Defences of General Application*, 1978, had not been acted on by Parliament. Therefore, he thought Parliament did not wish to change the law. Yet if that were so, Parliament's inactivity must have shown also that it did not wish to abrogate **Lynch**, above, which only 12 years earlier had decided in the opposite manner to **Howe**.

(vii) The two cases relied on by the House of Lords are not strong. **Tyler** (1839) 172 ER 643 is out of date because it was considered at that time that duress was no defence at all. **Dudley and Stephens** concerned necessity not duress. The two defences are linked but not the same. For example, necessity is not a defence to theft but duress is. In a third case, **Kray** (1969) 53 Cr App R 569, the Court of Appeal had considered that duress was a defence to an accessory to murder but the relevant passage was omitted in the major series of law reports.

(viii) In **Howe** no one asked the question: if the would-be accused refused to kill and was killed, what is there to prevent the duressor from threatening someone else with death and so on? The law encourages the killing of two or more persons and discourages the killing of one. Not a happy outcome!

A useful comparison is with the IRA's use of 'proxy bombers' in Northern Ireland. The organisation might have gone on killing people until someone yielded and drove the explosives to a checkpoint. In fact the proxy bombers were not prosecuted. If they had been, they would have had no defence to murder.

(ix) The law is brought into disrepute in such circumstances. In the words of Lord Morris in **Lynch**, above, 'The law would be censorious and inhumane which did not recognise the appalling plight of a person who perhaps suddenly finds his life in jeopardy unless he submits and obeys.'

(x) The House of Lords in **Howe** referred to authorities on provocation when approving the proposition that a duressee must act as a person of reasonable firmness might act. Yet provocation is a defence to murder but duress is not. Is a person who kills under provocation less morally blameworthy than a person who kills under duress? It is suggested indeed that a person who kills under duress is *less* blameworthy than a person who kills as a result of provocation.

(xi) The majority in **Abbott v R** refused to afford the accused a defence to a charge of murder on the ground that concerned citizens might believe that a 'not guilty' verdict implied that what the accused had done was the morally correct thing to do, but since duress is an excuse, a concession to human weakness, and not a justification, this argument is inappropriate. The accused is excused because of his weakness; his killing is not justified.

(xii) The departing from **Abbott v R** is a breach of Article 7 of the European Convention on Human Rights, the principle of non-retroactivity. The accused is guilty of an offence when he would not have been guilty before **Howe**.

(c) Lord Griffiths in **Howe** went further than his brethren. He suggested that duress was no defence not just to murder, being an accessory to murder and some forms of treason (see (d) below), but also to attempted murder. Lord Hailsham thought the law required reconsideration. Until 1996 the law was that, if the accused intended to kill and the victim died within a year and a day, the offence was murder. However, if the victim survived for longer but still died, a charge of murder was not possible, only a charge of attempted murder. Why should the date of death of the victim affect the position whether duress was available? The House of Lords by a three to two majority in **Gotts** [1992] 2 AC 412 accepted that duress was not a defence to attempted murder. (The case does not discuss s 18, but for the sake of elegance the law should be the same.) The accused's father threatened that unless the accused killed his mother, he would be shot. He stabbed but did not kill his mother. She might have died but for prompt treatment. Lord Lane CJ in the Court of Appeal rejected the argument that there was a distinction between murder and attempted murder with regard to duress. Early commentators did not distinguish the two, and there was no common law rule on the matter. The law ought to intervene. The Lord Chief Justice said in the Court of Appeal:

> One can imagine a situation where a man under duress fires a shotgun in order to kill two men standing together. He kills one and maims the other. It would seem strange if he were convicted as to one victim and acquitted altogether in relation to the other when the death of the one victim and the maiming of the other were caused by the very same act committed with the very same intent.

Innocence or guilt should not depend on chance. He suggested that the rule of attempted murder did not apply to conspiracy and incitement to murder because such offences were 'generally speaking' further away from the full offence than attempt; anyway, wherever the line was drawn anomalies would arise. Lord Jauncey in the House of Lords said: '[a] man shooting to kill but missing a vital organ by a hair's breadth can justify his action no more than can the man who hits that organ. It is pure chance that the attempted murderer is not a murderer.' He added: 'The law regards the sanctity of human life and the protection thereof as of paramount importance.' He left open for future discussion whether the defence should be available for any serious crime. Duress would, however, mitigate the sentence. The minority, led by Lord Lowry, thought that duress was available. He argued that, wherever the line was drawn between offences to which duress is or is not a defence (e.g. is duress a defence to conspiracy or incitement to murder?), there would be anomalies. He said:

> Attempted murder, however heinous we consider it, was a misdemeanour . . . [w]hen attempted murder became a felony, that crime, like many other serious felonies, continued to have available the defence of duress.

Gotts is open to criticism on several counts.

(i) There are problems with other offences. Incitement and conspiracy are, like attempt, inchoate offences. Why should the defence apply to two but not to the third? What about other crimes such as arson with intent to endanger life? Lord

Jauncey suggested that duress should not be available for 'all very serious crimes', a term which he did not define. Certainly before the abolition of the year-and-a-day rule it would have been anomalous if the accused who attacked the victim was guilty of murder if the victim died within a year and a day but not guilty of inflicting grievous bodily harm with intent if she survived longer. If duress is a defence to s 18 of the Offences Against the Person Act 1861, but not to murder, there is an inconsistency. Both offences have the mental element of an intent to commit grievous bodily harm. To rule out the defence for murder, but not for s 18 would be strange. Moreover, the difference between murder and s 18 may be fortuitous. Assume that the accused stabs his victim intending to kill. If the victim dies, that is murder: if, however, by the purest good fortune a superb surgeon is at hand and the victim does not die, that is not murder. Why should the distinction between conviction and acquittal depend on luck?

(ii) The defence of coercion (see next section) found in s 47 of the Criminal Justice Act 1925 is restricted. It does not apply to treason and murder, but is a defence to attempted murder. It is said that the draughtsman of the statute adopted the common law position for duress. Since coercion and duress are parallel defences, the same rule should apply in duress.

(iii) Nowhere is it suggested that attempted murder does not give rise to the defence, except for a Royal Commission of 1879 (C 2345).

(iv) Murder has a mandatory sentence. This penalty marks murder off from other crimes. Therefore, a line can be drawn between murder and other offences, and this line can separate murder and attempted murder in duress.

(v) The dissentients expressed the view that if the accused formed an intent to kill under duress, he was not so immoral that the law should withdraw the defence from him.

(vi) Should a person who kills to save others be treated differently from one who kills to save himself? Arguably there is a moral distinction.

(vii) In criminal law chance does play a part in the definition of offences. If one drives badly but by luck kills no one, one is guilty of dangerous driving; if one by mischance happens to kill somebody, one is guilty of causing death by dangerous driving. The sentence for the latter crime is more serious than that for the former, but luck may be the factor which differentiates them. The same is true in ordinary life: I carelessly fall and no injury is caused; I carelessly fall and by ill luck I knock someone over. Only in the latter situation is a passer-by likely to think me at fault, but what I did and did carelessly is exactly the same. There is therefore no reason for treating murder and attempted murder in the same way. There is a whole literature on the part so-called 'moral luck' plays in criminal law. A way into the literature is A. Ashworth, 'Taking the consequences', in S. Shute, S. Gardner and J. Horder (eds), *Action and Value in the Criminal Law* (OUP, 1993).

(d) There is doubt whether duress is a defence to treason. Lord Goddard CJ in **Steane**, above, said *obiter* that duress was not a defence but his statement may be *per incuriam*. **M'Growther**, above, and **Purdy** (1946) 10 JCL 182 (*obiter*) are *contra*, **Purdy** was not cited in **Steane** (and this despite the factual similarities), and Lord Morris in **Lynch** accepted that the *dictum* was incorrect. The phrasing of this exception has remained fairly constant: duress is a defence to 'some forms of treason'. The phrase was used in **Abdul-Hussain**, above. This phrase means that minor acts of treason do attract the defence. It may, however, be difficult to distinguish major and minor acts of assistance, and Nelson J in the Full Court of Victoria rejected the distinction in relation to those who help in a major way in a murder and those who act in a minor way: *Harding*, above. If duress is a defence, it will apply only if the accused escapes at the first opportunity: *Oldcastle* (1419) noted in 3 Co Inst 10, and apparently only if the accused does not engage in battle: *Axtell* (1660) 84 ER 1060.

As the Court of Appeal put it in *Abdul-Hussain*, above, which the same court approved in *S* [2001] 1 WLR 2206, a case also known as *Shayler*: '. . . the defence of duress, whether by threats or from circumstances, is generally available in relation to all substantive crimes, except murder, attempted murder and some forms of treason . . .'. For suggested reform of this topic, see below. Present law is a prime illustration of illogicality. Some judges, such as Lord Hailsham in *Howe*, are content to reject logic and consistency in favour of precedent but law reformers need not work within common law constraints. Law reforming should be on the side of Lord Bingham, who in *Hasan*, above, said that the argument for extending duress to murder was irresistible.

Should there be a general defence of duress?

Duress is much more commonly pleaded than it was at the time of *Hudson and Taylor* (1971) and the courts have taken a tough stance in recent years on the width of the defence: see the speeches of the House of Lords in *Hasan*. If the basis of duress is that the law regards self-preservation as excusing an otherwise criminal deed, duress should be a defence to all offences, and the exceptions abolished. This rationale has been given full rein in self-defence, which is a defence to all crimes including murder. (One difference is that in duress the victim is an innocent person but he is not in self-defence.) The law should not condemn people who act under a compulsion which they are unable to resist and should not demand standards of heroism from ordinary people such as the accused in *Gotts*. It is suggested that if persons act reasonably under pressure exerted by threats they should have a defence. A comparison with diminished responsibility, which is a defence to murder, is instructive. An abnormal person can rely on this defence, but a person, even a normal reasonable one, cannot have a defence of duress if he kills. To say that they are guilty but their sentences would be reduced, as Lords Keith and Templeman did in *Gotts*, does not meet this argument. And the sentence for murder, life imprisonment, is mandatory. Duress as mitigation not as exculpation has no effect. Moreover, the law's penalties do not work whether as retribution or deterrence in situations where the defence is potentially applicable.

The Law Commission, which has always been in favour of duress being a general defence and not merely a mitigating factor, in Report No. 83, *Defences of General Application*, 1978 (see above), put the following arguments against duress as a general defence:

(a) It is never justifiable to do wrong.

(b) It is not for the individual to balance the doing of wrong against the avoidance of harm to himself or others.

(c) Duress could be classified as merely the motive for committing a crime, and the criminal law does not take motive into account.

(d) The criminal law is itself a system of threats, and that structure would be undermined if some other system of threats were permitted.

(e) To allow the defence is to provide a charter for terrorists, kidnappers and others of that ilk.

Further arguments against duress may be advanced. Lord Morris in **Lynch** said that 'Duress must never be allowed to be the easy answer of those who can devise no other explanation of their conduct . . .'. It might be said that a person is at fault and worthy of punishment if he yields to a threat. Moreover, arguments in favour of duress may be false. The law would not act as a deterrent if duress were available for all offences including murder.

The 1978 Law Commission Report took into account these arguments and recommended as follows:

(a) Duress should be a defence available generally, i.e. it should apply to the then exceptions of treason and murder. The Law Commission did, however, recognise the sanctity of human life. (The 1989 version, below, preferred this recommendation but in the light of present law did not give the defence to murder and attempted murder. The Select Committee of the House of Lords on Murder and Life Imprisonment (HL Paper 78–1, 1989) recommended the abolition of the mandatory sentence for murder. Duress could then be taken into account in the sentence. This Committee under the chairmanship of Lord Nathan rejected the view that duress should reduce murder to manslaughter.)

See p 446 in Chapter 11 for an explanation of the mandatory sentence for murder.

(b) A threat of harm to the accused or another should be sufficient, but a threat to property would not.

(c) The mental element was to be that the accused believed:

> . . . whether or not on reasonable grounds –
> (a) that the harm threatened was death or serious personal injury (physical or mental);
> (b) that the threat would be carried out immediately if he did not take the action in question or, if not immediately, before he could have any real opportunity of seeking official protection; and
> (c) that there was no other way of avoiding or preventing the harm threatened.

This recommendation would reverse **Graham**, above, on reasonable belief. The Law Commission accepted this recommendation in the 1989 draft Criminal Code.

(d) The threat must be such that 'in all the circumstances of the case . . . he could not reasonably have been expected to resist'. See also the section 'proposed reform of duress by threats', below.

The Law Commission also recommended the abolition of the defence of marital coercion (see next section). These proposals formed part of cl 42 of the 1989 draft Criminal Code and cl 36(2)(b) of the Criminal Code Bill attached to Law Commission Paper No. 218, 1993. Parliament has not acted on either set of recommendations. The Law Commission in its 1993 Report considered that after the House of Lords in **Howe** and **Gotts** had called for parliamentary intervention the time was ripe for Parliament to clarify the width of duress.

It should be noted that the proposals leave for the jury the odious task of balancing one harm against another, and juries might hold that murder is always so heinous that duress is no defence, so stultifying the first proposed reform. The jury will also have to put themselves in the position of a defendant with certain long-term characteristics. In provocation this approach can lead to difficulties. Presumably the same can happen in duress. One suggested reform which was not proposed was to link the gravity of the threat with the heinousness of the crime: the greater the harm caused under duress, the greater the threat must be. In the 1970s in **Lynch v DPP for Northern Ireland** [1975] AC 653 and **Abbott v R** [1977] AC 755, both discussed above, there were *dicta* in favour of such an approach. If accepted, one effect would presumably be that there would be no restriction as to the nature of the evil threatened. A threat to imprison would be sufficient if the matter demanded were small. Such reform would bring duress into line with self-defence where there is no limit on the type of threat uttered or used. There could still be restrictions on the type of harm threatened (e.g. no defence where the harm was to be the loss of the accused's job) or the crime to be committed (e.g. no defence to treason). The accused under the draft Criminal Code would not have the defence if he brought the circumstances of duress on himself.

Reform proposals

The Law Commission investigated duress in its Report No. 218, *Legislating the Criminal Code – Offences against the Person and General Principles*, Cm 2370, 1993. Clause 25 reads:

(1) No act of a person constitutes an offence if the act is done under duress by threats.
(2) A person does an act under duress by threats if he does it because he knows or believes –
    (a) that a threat has been made to cause death or serious injury to himself or another if the act is not done, and
    (b) that the threat will be carried out immediately if he does not do the act or, if not immediately, before he or that other can obtain effective official protection, and
    (c) that there is no other way of preventing the threat being carried out, and the threat is one which in all the circumstances (including any of his personal characteristics that affect its gravity) he cannot reasonably be expected to resist. It is for the defendant to show that the reason for his act was such knowledge or belief as is mentioned in paragraphs (a) to (c).
(3) This section applies in relation to omissions as it applies in relation to acts.
(4) This section does not apply to a person who knowingly and without reasonable excuse exposed himself to the risk of the threat made or believed to have been made.
    If the question arises whether a person knowingly and without reasonable excuse exposed himself to such a risk, it is for him to show that he did not.

Clause 26, which is in similar terms, deals with duress of circumstances. Because the clauses are so similarly phrased, they will not be separately discussed. The definition of duress of circumstances found in cl 26(2) was approved by the Court of Appeal in *Baker* [1999] 2 Cr App R 335. One development which occurred after the publication of the Report is *Cole* [1994] Crim LR 582, in which the court distinguished between the two types of duress by reference to whether the duressor nominated the crimes (threats) or not (circumstances). It is uncertain how far the duressor must nominate the crime. Certainly he need not specify any particular building society branch to hold up: *Ali* [1995] Crim LR 303 (CA). It is hard to believe that this distinction truly represents the law. Why is it duress by threats if I say 'Steal from shops', but duress by circumstances if I say 'Get me some money'? The proposals partly amend and partly encapsulate present law. For example, cl 25(2)(a) states that a threat to any third party (e.g. a hostage) will suffice. The Law Commission had been of the opinion in the Consultation Paper No. 122 which preceded the Report (they bear the same name) that the accused would not have the defence if he believed that official protection would not avail him (such as in *Hudson and Taylor* [1971] 2 QB 202). This recommendation finds no place in the Report. There is no definition of 'effective'. Moreover, cl 25(2)(c) does not address the issue of a belief that official protection is not available (rather than that it is available but ineffective). The proposal, while presented as one which mirrors current law, may be in truth a widening of it in the accused's favour. No longer need he know full well, as Lord Griffiths put it in *Howe* [1987] AC 417, that protection is ineffective but he has the defence if he knows *or believes* it is.

One difference from present law is the extension of the defence to all offences including murder. This is a long-standing Law Commission commitment, and the House of Lords in *Hasan*, above, thought the extension to all crimes was 'irresistible'. If Parliament did not like this proposal, the Law Commission suggested that duress should reduce the crime to manslaughter. The Commonwealth of Australia in the Criminal Code Act 1995 allowed duress as a defence to murder.

Another change is the proposed abolition of the objective elements in *Graham* [1982] 1 WLR 294: was the accused compelled to act because, as a result of what he *reasonably* believed the other to have said or done, he had *good cause* to fear death or serious injury? The *Graham* test of reasonable steadfastness is to be abolished. Timidity can be considered. The accused is still, however, to be judged against a standard of a reasonable person. Therefore, a timid accused is judged according to the standard of a reasonable timid person. The Court of Appeal in *Baker* did not notice that the terms of reasonable belief and good cause to believe were not to be found in the proposed definition of duress of circumstances.

The Law Commission proposed a shift in the burden of proof in relation to cl 25(2) and (4) and considered that the shift would not breach Article 6(2) of the European Convention of Human Rights. The Law Commission seemed to have taken this view in order to make Parliament accept that duress should be available to murder. The reasons advanced for the amendment were that the facts giving rise to the duress were peculiarly within the ken of the accused and members of a violent gang could escape guilt if they concocted a story of compulsion. The law on violent gangs has not caused problems in the past and the 'peculiar knowledge' doctrine was exploded long ago in murder, and if it were to apply to duress, it should also apply to, say, provocation; the person who besides the accused had an inkling about what happened is dead. There is no stopping place with regard to the doctrine. If the accused kills, even in the absence of provocation, there may be no one else present as witness. The deceased had peculiar knowledge of the events, and the victim is dead. The Court of Criminal Appeal in *Spurge* [1961] 2 QB 205 strongly rejected the 'peculiar knowledge' doctrine in relation to provocation and self-defence. Duress is no different. The Law Commission opined that where the defence is part of one incident, the prosecution should shoulder the burden. So in self-defence the onus is on the Crown because the accused is reacting to the use or threat of force immediately, whereas in duress there is a gap between the threat and the otherwise wrongful action. However, in self-defence one can strike pre-emptively, and in duress the threat may be immediately linked with the act: 'do this now or I shall kill you now'. Furthermore, in duress of circumstances the threat will almost always be immediately linked to the act: 'unless I knock this person off the ladder, all of us will die in seconds'. The Law Commission has since resiled from its recommendation and it no longer wishes to place the legal burden on the accused. It is suggested that contrary to the Commission's view the proposal would breach Article 6(2), the presumption of innocence, because Article 6(2) does not permit legal burdens on the accused when to shift the onus is disproportionate. See also *Lambert* [2002] 2 AC 545 (HL), discussed in Chapter 1.

One aspect of the proposed definition should be noted. The recommendation confirms current law that only threats of death or serious injury suffice for duress. Some lesser threats, however, can overwhelm an ordinary mortal. Lord Simon, dissenting, in *Lynch v DPP for Northern Ireland* [1975] AC 653 stated:

. . . a threat to property may, in certain circumstances, be as potent in overbearing the actor's wish not to perform the prohibited act as a threat of physical harm. For example, the threat may be to burn down his house unless the householder merely keeps watch against interruption while a crime is committed. Or a fugitive from justice may say, 'I have it in my power to make your son bankrupt. You can avoid that merely by driving me to the airport.' Would not many ordinary people yield to such threats, and act contrary to their wish not to perform an action prohibited by law?

The concession-to-human-frailty rationale would support such a rule though it has to be admitted that that basis has been undermined by the later House of Lords authorities, *Howe*, above, and *Gotts* [1992] 2 AC 412. Nevertheless, there is statutory support for a defence in such circumstances. The Criminal Damage Act 1971, s 5(2)(b), stipulates that if a person destroys or damages property 'in order to protect property belonging to another' he has a lawful excuse to the offence of criminal damage.

In *Hurley and Murray* [1967] VR 526, the Full Court of Victoria said that 'The whole body of law relating to duress is in a very vague and unsatisfactory state . . .'. The law has since firmed up but it remains controversial. We have not heard the last of the reform of duress, but calls for changes, in *Hurst* [1995] 1 Cr App R 82, *Cole* [1994] Crim LR 582, *Baker*, and *Abdul-Hussain* [1999] Crim LR 570, remain unheeded by the government. The Court of Appeal noted in *Safi*, above, that Parliament seemed content to leave the development of the law to the judges.

The Law Commission's 2006 proposals

The Law Commission issued its Report No. 306 on *Murder, Manslaughter and Infanticide* in late 2006. In it it proposed that contrary to current law duress whether by threats or of circumstances should be a defence to first and second degree murder and to attempted murder. For first and second degree murders, see Chapter 11. The proposals are different from that contained in the Consultation Paper *A New Homicide Act for England and Wales?* of December 2005, which had proposed that a successful defence of duress would reduce first to second degree murder, while also recommending that duress should be a full defence to second degree murder and attempted murder. It noted (para. 6.60) that current law provided a strange outcome in relation to excuses: '. . . in cases of provocation and diminished responsibility, D has not killed in order to preserve innocent life and yet he or she has a partial excuse. By contrast, a person who pleads duress is one who sought to avoid the death of or serious physical harm to an innocent person (not necessarily him or herself) by doing no more than is required to avert the harm. Yet, provocation and diminished responsibility excuse murder while duress does not.' (footnote omitted) The Commission strongly endorsed the rules as to the width of duress as a defence laid down in *Z* [2005] 1 WLR 1269 (CA), which is known as *Hasan* in the House of Lords, as to the risk of threat with the rider that the threat believed to exist would have to be one of death or life-threatening harm: at present it is sufficient that the threat was one of 'serious harm', whether the accused believed the threat to be life-threatening or not. It should be noted that whether harm is life-threatening or not turns in part on the victim's age and vulnerability; the Law Commission provides this example: '. . . a jury might well conclude that D reasonably believed that a threat of torture to his or her five-year-old child involved a risk of life-threatening harm while taking a different view if the threat of torture was directed at D's spouse' (para. 6.75). What is different from present law is the recommendation that in respect of these three offences the legal burden of proof should be on the accused (the standard of proof would be on the balance of probabilities).

The Law Commission rejected the proposal for a partial defence of duress in respect to first degree murder but a full defence as to second degree and attempted murder because of (1) the wide difference in outcome dependent on whether the accused had the fault element for first degree murder, (2) the element of chance, which is illustrated by the following example (para. 6.26–7):

> D, under duress, shoots both V1 and V2 with intent to kill, killing V1 but not V2.... [If the Consultation Paper's recommendation had been adopted,] D would have a partial defence in relation to the killing of V1 but a full defence in relation to the attempted killing of V2. The element of chance in whether the full defence is or is not available, depending on whether D is successful in carrying out his instructions, makes this option an unattractive one.

(3) The Commission is also strongly of the view that 'as a matter of principle' (para 6.28) duress should be a complete defence to first degree murder. To quote the Law Commission's Report No. 83 on *Defences of General Application*, 1977, para 2.43,

> where duress is so compelling that the defendant could not reasonably have been expected to resist it, ... it would be ... unjust that the defendant should suffer the stigma of a conviction even for manslaughter. We do not think that any social purpose is served by requiring the law to prescribe such standards of determination and heroism.

Moreover, what would be gained by punishing an accused in these circumstances? The Commission quoted the view of the Criminal Bar Association (para 6.51): '. . . if duress were not a complete defence to first degree murder, it would give the impression that, in law, "it is better to prevent the death of a stranger than to prevent the death of one's children."'

The Commission rejected any analogy with provocation and diminished responsibility, which under the proposed scheme would be a defence only to first degree murder and would lead to a conviction for second degree murder. The Commission noted that sometimes duress but not provocation or diminished responsibility came close to a justificatory defence and it gave the example, drawn from duress of circumstances, where one roped mountaineer cuts the rope to save his or her own life when had he or she not cut it, both would have died. It rejected the argument that a person who intentionally killed should not have a complete defence. It also rejected the proposition that killing in defence of self was in itself morally worse than killing in defence of others. It gave (para. 6.56) several examples in favour of not differentiating, including: 'An uncle threatened with death commits murder so that he can donate a kidney to his desperately ill nephew.' It rejected the argument that principal and secondary parties could be distinguished because an accomplice acting under duress may be just as culpable as a perpetrator. 'For example, a husband and his wife are told that their child will be killed unless they kill V who is the husband's brother. They agree that the wife will perpetrate the killing and the husband will keep watch. It would be wrong to afford the husband but not the wife a complete defence.' (para 6.57)

The Law Commission also proposed to retain the 'reasonable belief' limitation; that is, that the accused has to believe on reasonable grounds that a threat exists and that the threat will be put into effect: *Graham* above approved by the House of Lords in *Howe*, above. The 1989 draft Criminal Code and the Law Commission's Report No. 218, *Legislating the Criminal Code: Offences against the Person and General Principles*, 1993, had previously called for a subjective test, as is the law in self-defence and provocation, but the 2006 Report distinguished those defences: in duress the accused would normally have time to think about the threat, whereas he or she would not in self-defence and provocation; further-more, since in respect of theft and other offences the law is that there has to be reason-able belief, it would be anomalous if a subjective test were used in first and second degree murder and in attempted murder. However, 'we see no reason why the particular char-acteristics of D should not be capable of being taken into account in determining whether or not his or her belief was reasonably held. This would enable account to be taken of the age and vulnerability of D.' (para 6.81) It was further proposed that the law on duress should be brought into line with that on provocation (see **A-G for Jersey v Holley** [2005] 2 AC 580 (PC) discussed in Chapter 12) in respect of the 'reasonable firmness' criterion: 'the jury should be entitled to take into account all of the circum-stances of D, including his or her age, other than those which bear on his or her capa-city to withstand duress.' (para 6.84) This recommendation will lead to the reversal of **Bowen** above in relation to the three crimes of first degree murder, second degree murder and attempted murder: for the others **Bowen** would remain.

Coercion

Coercion is a (rarely used) defence akin to duress but available only to a married woman. For that reason it may be called 'marital coercion' to distinguish it from the defences of duress. Before 1925 such a person had a defence if she committed a crime other than treason or murder in her husband's presence. One argument for this defence was that if the husband was convicted of a felony he would not be hanged for a first offence because, if he could read a certain verse from the Bible, he would not be executed (he received 'benefit of clergy') whereas a woman not being able to be a cleric would be hanged. The argument against the existence of this defence was put with force in the American case of **US v de Quilfeldt** (1881) 5 F 276. Coercion was the 'relic of a belief in the ignorance and pusillanimity of women'. The law is now stated in s 47 of the Criminal Justice Act 1925, which, however, does not define coercion.

> Any presumption of law that an offence committed by a wife in the presence of her husband is committed under the coercion of the husband is hereby abolished, but on a charge against a wife for any offence other than treason or murder, it shall be a good defence to prove that the offence was committed in the presence of, and under the coer-cion of, the husband.

The reversal of the burden of proof may be the sole reason why s 47 was enacted. It has been suggested that only the evidential burden was placed on the wife, but the cases do not so hold. The burden is on the balance of probabilities: **Richman** [1982] Crim LR 507 (Crown Court).

It is unknown which fact situations would give rise to this defence. It was at one time thought that coercion was simply the name for the defence of duress where the accused was a married woman. In other words, the boundaries of duress were the boundaries of coercion. The modern view is that coercion is wider than duress and would cover matters such as a threat by the husband not to buy food for his wife and children, a threat to desert the wife and a threat to bring a mistress into the matrimonial home. Since neither Parliament nor the common law had defined the term, Lord Simon in **Lynch v DPP for Northern Ireland** [1975] AC 653, above, said that coercion was 'used in its ordinary sense . . .'. It is not limited to threats. **Richman** held that there was no need for physical force. The Court of Appeal in **Ditta** [1988] Crim LR 43 rejected the defence when the wife was acting out of loyalty. The test for coercion in **Richman** was: did she act willingly?

Coercion could be an overbearing of the will by moral means not amounting to physical force or the threat of such force. This test was approved by the Court of Appeal in **Shortland** [1996] 1 Cr App R 116. In **Ditta** the test was: 'Was she forced by her husband either by physical, moral, psychological or mental processes, to do what she would not otherwise have done?' In duress a threat to expose the accused's homosexuality is insufficient. Is a threat to reveal one's wife's lesbianism to the tabloid press such a threat as to fall within 'moral, psychological or mental' pressure? If the threat is of death or serious injury, both coercion and duress may be available, but it should be noted that coercion is narrower than duress in one respect: the 'crime' must take place in her husband's presence. The term 'presence' has not been the subject of authoritative guidance. In **Caroubi** (1912) 7 Cr App R 149 it was held that it was sufficient that the wife was within sight of the husband. Presence was not restricted to being next to the husband. In **Whelan** [1937] SASR 237 the court held that 'it is sufficient if the husband is in a situation where he is close enough to influence the wife in doing what he wants done, even if he is not physically present in the room'.

Ditta is an authoritative case. The third defendant was charged with being concerned in the importation of heroin. She contended that the second defendant, to whom she believed she was married, had prevailed upon her to strap the drug round her body while in a plane which was to land at Heathrow. The court held that the statute, which was in straightforward terms, did not provide a defence in such a situation. She had to prove that she was married to the coercer. The fact that she believed, even on reasonable grounds, that she was married to him was insufficient. (Compare duress where the accused has a defence if he believes on reasonable grounds that he was obliged to do as he did.) The court did not deal with the question whether a polygamous marriage would give rise to this defence, but the hint was that it would not. The court distinguished the defence of mistake to bigamy, which is available only when the accused erred on reasonable grounds, as being concerned with mistake as to a vital element of the offence, whereas in coercion the mistake was one to a defence. Therefore, if one believes on reasonable grounds that one's husband is dead, one is not guilty of the offence of bigamy, but if one believes on reasonable grounds that one is married one does not have the defence of coercion. Certainly a mistress does not have this defence.

As stated above, the Law Commission in 1978, 1989 and 1993 proposed the abolition of coercion. It does not accord with modern views of marriage and is gender-based. It might be thought surprising that it has survived for so long.

One matter of which readers should be aware is that judicial and academic terminology vary. Sometimes coercion like compulsion is used as a synonym for duress. Usually in modern times coercion means the separate defence under the 1925 statute.

Necessity and duress of circumstances

Introduction

If terrorists aim a plane at Canary Wharf in London, may the Army shoot it down?

Lord Goff in **Richards**, unreported, 10 July 1986 (HL) said: 'That there exists a defence of necessity at common law, which may . . . be invoked to justify what would otherwise be a trespass to land, is not in doubt. But the scope of the defence is by no means clear.' This statement was *obiter*, but gives a flavour of this topic. Lord Goff had developed his views by **Re F** [1990] 2 AC 1, a civil case. He stated that the defence did exist at common law to render lawful what would otherwise be criminal: (1) public necessity (e.g. to create a firebreak in the Great Fire of London); (2) private necessity (e.g. to cause criminal damage to a neighbour's property to save oneself from harm); and (3) 'Action taken as a matter of necessity to assist another person without his consent.' His example of the third category was the dragging of a person from the path of an oncoming vehicle. He confined category (3) to cases where it was not practicable to communicate with the assisted person and the action was 'such as a reasonable person would in all the circumstances take, acting in the best interests of the assisted person'. The facts of *Re F* fell within the third category. A mentally ill patient could be sterilised when she lacked the capacity to consent provided that the operation was in her best interests. It is uncertain whether Lord Goff's classification is exhaustive.

Modern cases tend to assume that there is a defence. In *Hutchinson v Newbury Magistrates Court*, unreported, 9 October 2002, the Queen's Bench Division Administrative Court said that a successful plea required a reasonable and proportionate response to present danger and there had to be no other means of avoiding it. A similar formula was adopted by the same court in *DPP v Hicks*, unreported, 19 July 2002. There was no defence of necessity where the accused drove with excess alcohol in his blood to get a bottle of medicine from the chemist's because either there was no risk of serious harm to the child or using the medicine would not have alleviated the risk of harm. In *S* [2001] 1 WLR 2206 the Court of Appeal held the following to be the requirements for the defence: 'the act must be done only to prevent an act of greater evil: the evil must be directed towards the defendant or a person . . . for whom he has responsibility . . . ; the act must be reasonable and proportionate to the evil avoided.'

Recent cases have focused on necessity as a possible defence to taking illegal drugs such as marijuana to relieve the effects of debilitating injuries. In *Altham* [2006] EWCA Crim 7 it was held that the accused could not rely on Article 3 of the European Convention on Human Rights (no inhuman or degrading treatment) to bolster a defence of necessity because the accused's condition was not worsened by any state act. In *Quayle* [2006] 1 WLR 3642 (CA) it was held that there was no defence of necessity to taking cannabis to relieve pain. To allow the defence was incompatible with the statutory scheme for regulating illegal drugs. The court did not rule on what the law would have been, had there been no statute in the field. The court stressed that there was no overarching doctrine of necessity but only a wilderness of single instances. Those single cases were decided on their particular facts. Insofar as the defence existed it was akin to duress and was to be kept within the same boundaries as that defence as laid down in *Hasan* (above). The court certified a point of law of general public importance but refused leave to appeal. The court in *Quayle* also held that denying a defence on these facts was not in breach of Article 8 of the Convention.

In one of the latest cases on necessity as a choice-of-evils defence, *Jones v Gloucestershire Crown Prosecution Service* [2005] QB 259 (CA) the court held that when the accused thought he had the choice between committing a less serious crime and committing a more serious one and he chose the former, the latter had to be a crime according to English law. Therefore, when the defendants committed various offences at RAF Fulford in order, they contended, to prevent aggression by the UK and the USA against Iraq, they had no defence of necessity because there was no crime of aggression in English law, even if it were an offence in international law. The House of Lords spoke to similar effect: *Jones* [2006] UKHL 16.

In duress the accused has the choice of breaking the law or having evil done to him or another by a person. In necessity the defendant is in a similar position except that the choice is imposed on him by natural events or by other situations not constituting a threat by a person in the form of 'do this or else' (I will kill you, etc.). In **Howe**, above, the House of Lords considered duress to be a species of necessity. Yet duress generally is a defence, while necessity generally is not, as the Court of Appeal recently reiterated in **Rodger** above. In **Cichon v DPP** [1994] Crim LR 918 the Divisional Court accepted the existence of this defence but held on the facts that Parliament had excluded it in relation to the crime of allowing a pit bull terrier to be in a public place without a muzzle by the wording of the offence. Parliament had created an offence for the safety of the public. That policy was not to be wrecked by an accused's reaching a decision that the removal of the muzzle outweighed the public's safety. It might be said that the muzzle's removal was the physical manifestation of the accused's good motive, the prevention of cruelty to the dog: the accused took it off because the dog had a cough. The reasoning of the court is weak. Necessity, when it exists, is a defence to all offences (except perhaps those to which duress is not a defence), including statutory offences. Parliament rarely states expressly that a certain defence applies to the crime it is creating. Perhaps the court would have allowed a defence of necessity if the accused had removed the muzzle so as to let the dog bite the arm of a person who was robbing a post office. Another way of reaching the same result would be to say that there was on the facts no defence of necessity because the crime was defined in terms of permitting a dangerous dog to be in a public place. The accused could have kept it in a private place until the cough was cured. In this way the possibility of the defence could have been accepted. **Cichon v DPP** also illustrated the difference between duress of circumstances and a true defence of necessity. The former defence applies only when the accused acts to prevent death or serious injury to a person, and a dog is not a person. Necessity is not so restricted and applies whenever a greater good is done, and on the facts there may have been a greater good. In **Rodger** the defendants broke out of prison because they had suicidal tendencies. The court treated duress of circumstances and necessity as being the same, but they are not. Even if breaking prison was a greater good than committing suicide, the defence was not one of necessity, but of duress of circumstances. They acted under a threat to their lives.

Accordingly, for example, a doctor cannot take blood from a non-consenting person in order to save someone's life. It is no defence, even though the action of the accused promoted a value higher than that which would be served by compliance with the law. The social cost may be less by providing a defence than by not so doing.

This section considers necessity and duress of circumstances. It is suggested that the rationales of these defences, if they are to be distinguished (case law as yet is unclear), differ. In necessity the accused chooses the lesser evil: the pressure need be irresistible. In duress of circumstances the accused acts because of pressure: he need not choose the lesser evil. Jeremy Horder in 'Self-defence, necessity and duress: understanding the relationship' (1998) 11 *Canadian Journal of Law and Jurisprudence* 143 put the distinction in this way:

> In necessity cases, the key issue is the *moral imperative* to act: what matters is whether in the circumstances it was morally imperative to act, even if this might involve the commission of wrongdoing, in order to negate or avoid some other evil. In duress cases, the key issue is the *personal sacrifice* [the accused] is being asked to make: should [the accused] be expected to make the personal sacrifice involved in refusing to give in to a coercive threat, rather than avoid implementation of the coercive threat by doing wrong?

It is suggested that contrary to the view of Lord Woolf CJ in *S*, above, there are differences. The juridical bases, threats in duress and choices of lesser evils in necessity, have been mentioned. As we shall see, the Court of Appeal in *Re A* [2001] Fam 147 permitted a defence of necessity to facts which constituted murder, had the case been a criminal one, at least on the particular facts of the case. Duress is not a defence to murder. Moreover, duress is restricted to threats of death or grievous bodily harm but it is suggested that necessity is not. Can one doubt that one may shoot down a plane seized by terrorists who intend to crash it into Canary Wharf? Finally, as *Re A* shows, necessity may create a duty to act; however, as the law currently stands, duress does not create such a duty. The House of Lords in *Shayler* [2003] 1 AC 247, which is the appeal from *S*, said that the Law Lords did not agree with all that was said in the Court of Appeal about necessity but unfortunately did not specify the precise points on which they disagreed.

Dudley and Stephens

The principal reason why necessity has not got off the ground as a defence is *Dudley and Stephens* (1884) 14 QBD 273, one of the most celebrated cases of English criminal law. Four men were adrift in a boat. Two, after some days without food and water, said a prayer (not Grace!) and killed the weakest, Parker, the cabin boy. After a reference to a court of five judges, the accused were found guilty of murder and sentenced to be hanged. The sentence was, however, commuted to six months' imprisonment. (For more details of this and other similar occurrences, see A. W. B. Simpson, *Cannibalism and the Common Law* (University of Chicago Press, 1984).)

Dudley and Stephens is a fascinating case. It is not certain whether the victim would have died anyway. Not long after he was killed, the survivors were rescued. The cabin boy was not bringing the accused nearer to death. The case was not one like the hypothetical one of two roped mountaineers; the lower one falls, dragging the upper one down; seconds before they both would have been killed, the upper one cuts the rope thereby accelerating the lower one's death. The lower person had no chance of surviving, come what may. On those facts the lower person was dragging the upper one to his death. Parker did not volunteer to die, and he might have lived, had he been allowed to eat one of the others. Furthermore, though the accused had no defence, it is not certain to what they had no defence. There are three views:

(a) *Dudley and Stephens* held that there is no general defence of necessity in criminal law. Lord Coleridge said that if necessity were allowed, it might become a smokescreen for 'unbridled passion and atrocious crime'. This approach constitutes the widest view of the *ratio*.

(b) Necessity is no defence to murder. This was the emphatic stance of the judge, Lord Coleridge. The House of Lords took this approach in *Howe*, above. This view allows *Dudley and Stephens* to be distinguished from cases shortly to be mentioned where necessity was a defence.

(c) The narrowest view is that on the facts necessity did not arise. Therefore, the court did not reject the defence either generally or specifically in relation to murder. Such was the approach of the Victoria Court in *Loughnan* [1981] VR 443. This case like many US ones dealt with a prisoner who escaped from jail to avoid being killed. The court held that in exceptional circumstances necessity afforded a defence. The conditions for the defence were: the crime must have been committed to avoid irreparable evil on the accused or on those he was under a duty to protect; the danger must be immediate; and the response must be proportionate to the danger. This approach derives support from the jury's special verdict that the accused would probably have died, had they not eaten the boy, but that verdict also stated that there was no real chance of surviving except by feasting on someone. If no necessity existed, everything said about the defence was *obiter*.

Whatever the true view of **Dudley and Stephens**, the case has impeded the rational development of the law. It should also be noted that:

(a) The facts of the case were peculiar. There was an emergency. Action was needed immediately on the facts as the defendants judged them to be. It is sometimes said that to give a defence of necessity would be dangerous because it could be used as an easy excuse. However, there was nothing bogus about the facts of **Dudley and Stephens**. Even the relatives of the cabin boy did not think that the defendants were to blame. The dreadfulness of the defendants' situation ought on this view to have given them an excuse. They were not arguing that the boy's life was of less value than theirs (a justificatory approach, if successful) but that they were not blameworthy because of the situation they found themselves in.

(b) The courts are reluctant to grant a defence where there is some immorality. Lord Coleridge, giving the principal judgment, noted that the weakest had been selected for being killed, and he said that in circumstances such as those at issue people were under a duty to sacrifice their lives.

(c) Because of the extremity of the situation, it was no deterrent to threaten punishment or, indeed, to hang the accused. By killing the victim, the accused gained at least several months of life, and on the facts they gained the rest of their natural lives. Had they not eaten the cabin boy, they might have died before they could have been rescued. 'The underlying rationale for permitting the necessity defence is that given the circumstances the usual purposes for meting punishment under the criminal law would not be served.' So wrote M.R. Conde (1981) 29 UCLA LR 409 (spelling anglicised). Even if the lack of a necessity defence is justifiable on the grounds that the criminal law exists to deter, that justification does not show why persons who acted as most would have done should be punished.

(d) To convict in **Dudley and Stephens** was to adopt a standard above that of reasonable people, as the court noted. Surely criminal law should not be based on saintliness. Lord Hailsham, however, in **Howe**, above, did think that in such circumstances reasonable people would die. Criminal law might also be seen as providing support for the Judaeo-Christian ethic: Thou shalt not kill. Intentional killing is unacceptable. To provide a defence might lead some members of the public to believe that some forms of intentional killing were acceptable.

(e) On the facts of **Dudley and Stephens** it might be argued that the two possible harms could not be balanced against each other. One cannot quantify a death. The accused made, in US jargon, an inexcusable choice. Different principles might apply where the defendant had brought about a lesser harm than the one threatened by natural occurrences.

(f) In a similar situation a US court, the Circuit Court for the Eastern District of Pennsylvania, held in **US v Holmes** (1846) 26 Fed Cas 360 that there should be selection by lot. Selecting by lot would exculpate sailors who threw overboard passengers on an overloaded lifeboat. **Dudley and Stephens** is distinguishable as a case involving no selection by chance. Presumably those to be thrown overboard would in law not have a right to fight against being cast into the sea, though one would not expect a person who resisted to be prosecuted whether his resistance was successful or not. Incidentally that court sentenced the accused to six months' imprisonment, the same end-result as in *Dudley and Stephens*.

Perhaps Lord Coleridge would not have argued as he did had he known that the accused would really be hanged, though in the opinion of the writer credence should not be given to such a view in the light of the phrasing of his speech. Nevertheless, it should be remembered that from the viewpoint of precedent the case is not a House of Lords one.

Though the three judges said different things, Ward LJ sitting in the Court of Appeal in *Re A*, above, a civil case, said that in some circumstances necessity was a defence to murder. On the facts surgeons who separated conjoined twins were not guilty of murder even though they knew it was certain that one of the twins would die. Brooke LJ distinguished *Dudley and Stephens*. First, he said, the decision to kill the cabin boy was arbitrary but in *Re A* it was certain which twin would die. Secondly, Lord Coleridge in *Dudley and Stephens* said that if the criminal law gave the defendants a defence, there would be a total divorce of law and morality; however, in *Re A* some people would say that it was *not* immoral to kill the weaker twin to save the stronger one rather than letting them both die. The case at least in part turns on its own facts: the twin which died was bringing the other twin closer to death but the latter could survive on her own. In other words, if necessity has a 'lesser evil' rationale, it was a lesser evil to kill one twin than to let both die.

It is difficult to reconcile the judgments of the three Lords Justices in *Re A*. Brooke LJ was prepared on the facts to allow a defence of necessity. Necessity had three conditions: the act was needed to avoid 'inevitable and irreparable evil,' the accused must do no more than was reasonably necessary to avoid the evil; and the evil done by him must not be disproportionate to the evil averted. What he failed to notice was that these three conditions were satisfied in *Dudley and Stephens*, who should therefore have had a defence. Instead he, along with his brethren, said that the sailors were rightly convicted. Walker LJ, *obiter*, thought that necessity should be extended to cover the present case but no further. Ward LJ permitted the defence but only in these circumstances: '. . . it must be impossible to preserve the life of X without bringing about the death of Y, . . . Y by his or her very continued existence will inevitably bring about the death of X within a short period of time, and . . . X is capable of living an independent life but Y is incapable under any circumstances . . . of viable independent existence.' Therefore, only Brooke LJ would have come to a conclusion different from Coleridge J in *Dudley and Stephens*.

Dudley and Stephens is also out of line with some Commonwealth authorities. In *Perka* v *R* (1984) 13 DLR (4th) 1 the Supreme Court of Canada ruled that the defendants had a defence, which the judges called an excuse, when they had taken their boat into the shelter of Canadian waters during a storm. They were charged with importing cannabis for the purposes of sale. It was in the words of Dickson J (later CJ) one of those 'urgent situations of clear and imminent peril when compliance with the law is demonstrably impossible'. There was no reasonable lawful alternative. The judge stated that it did not matter that the accused were doing something unlawful, but that it would not amount to necessity if the accused's fault contributed to the emergency. *Perka* v *R* was distinguished by the Supreme Court of Canada in *Latimer* v *R* [2001] SCR 1. A father had no defence when he killed his quadriplegic daughter. He was not in imminent peril; he did have a reasonable alternative to breaking the law; and the harm inflicted was disproportionate to the harm avoided. Somewhat similarly in one Scottish case, *Tudhope* v *Grubb* 1983 SCCR 350, a sheriff held that necessity was a defence where the accused drove with excess alcohol in his blood to avoid an assault. Perhaps this case could be explained nowadays as an example of duress of circumstances, on which see below.

Beyond **Dudley and Stephens**, when does necessity provide or not provide a defence? The law, as a result of **Re A**, is in a state of flux. Development will happen case by case.

Necessity is sometimes a defence in specific instances. The law has a 'pebble-dash' approach. These instances are pebbles of the defence in a wall of no defence. Surely, however, one would not charge a prisoner with escaping from a burning jail, never mind convict him. As a US court put it: 'He is not to be hanged because he would not stay to be burnt' (**US v Kirby** (1869) 7 Wall 482). Even before the Abortion Act 1967, preservation of the woman's life was a defence to abortion: **Bourne** [1939] 1 KB 687. **Bourne** may be seen as a case of what is sometimes called 'hidden necessity'. The accused, a surgeon, was charged with unlawfully using an instrument with intent to procure a miscarriage, contrary to s 58 of the Offences Against the Person Act 1861. The judge instructed the jury that the accused was not acting unlawfully if he acted bona fide to save the life of the woman, who was a 14-year-old rape victim. The use of the word 'unlawfully' allowed the judge, as it were, to smuggle in a defence. Other instances are jettisoning cargo (**Mouse's case** (1608) 77 ER 1341, a civil law authority) and taking an infected child through the streets to obtain medical advice (**Vantandillo** (1815) 105 ER 762). Cases such as **Bourne** could now be treated as ones of duress of circumstances (see below). Lord Goff's taxonomy in **Re F**, noted at the start of this section, does not cover **Bourne**.

Following **Buckoke v GLC** [1971] Ch 655, preservation of property or life is not a good defence to a charge of going through traffic lights at red brought against firefighters, though Lord Denning MR did say that the accused were to be congratulated. (The law has since been changed to allow fire officers, the police and paramedics to go through red lights and to exceed the speed limit in an emergency.) According to the same judge in **Southwark LBC v Williams** [1971] Ch 734 the defence does not extend to the homeless or the starving. Therefore, a homeless person cannot break into an empty house to squat, nor may a woman steal in order to feed her starving children. The common law of crime has always turned its back on a defence of 'economic necessity'. **Buckoke** and **Southwark LBC** would presumably now be subject to the defence of duress of circumstances. If, for instance, food was taken to prevent someone starving to death, the accused would have a defence; if, however, it was taken merely to cure hunger, the defence would not be available. To permit a defence of necessity in the circumstances noted in this paragraph would allow the accused to rely on motive. I took the food because my children were hungry. I stole; my motive, however, was good. If the court permitted motive to be impleaded, evidence such as the effect of capitalism would have to be adduced. It is also unclear why a shopkeeper should suffer for the consequences of the socio-economic milieu we live in.

Though no statute expressly provides a defence of necessity some statutes may be read as covering situations of necessity. The most obvious illustration is the Criminal Damage Act 1971, s 5. This section defines a defence of 'lawful excuse'. That phrase covers the protection of property. Accordingly knocking down a home to create a firebreak – a necessitous situation – gives rise to a defence under statute just as it would at law.

Section 34(3) of the Road Traffic Act 1988 exempts a person from conviction for driving a vehicle elsewhere than on roads 'if he proves to the satisfaction of the court that it was driven in contravention of this section for the purpose of saving life or extinguishing fire or meeting any other like emergency'. There are other sections of like nature. Professor Smith's comment on **Wood v Richards** [1977] Crim LR 295 (DC), where the accused was convicted, should also be noted. On a charge of driving without due care and attention, a police officer hurrying to an emergency should have a defence: 'due care' means 'due in the circumstances'. However, it would not provide a defence where the constable was rushing to the police ball, even though he performed exactly the same act. There may well be other circumstances of concealed necessity under statute.

Proposed reform of necessity in the 1970s

Looking at the law one might expect that necessity should be made consistent with duress by affording a defence in similar circumstances. It is, however, sometimes argued that it is better to consider and then mitigate the penalty as occurred in *Dudley and Stephens*. There are, however, several arguments against this view. The penalty for murder is the mandatory life sentence. That punishment cannot be reduced by the court. It is also wrong to convict someone when he has acted properly, and the possibility of conviction may be a disincentive to acting in a correct way: one is stigmatised by a conviction and has a criminal record even if one gets an absolute discharge. Such arguments lead to the suggestion that if necessity is to have any effect in criminal law, it ought to be as a defence, and not as a mitigating factor.

In the late 1970s, however, the Law Commission in its Report No. 83 on *Defences of General Application*, above, came out strongly against this reasoning. There were two major recommendations. First, there should be no attempt by Parliament to establish this defence; secondly, insofar as the defence existed at common law, it should be abolished. The Law Commission argued that there was no need for the defence because it would cover so few eventualities; that the discretion not to prosecute would cover necessitous situations; that necessity could be taken into account during sentencing; and that in some offences there always is a specific defence such as 'without lawful excuse' which includes facts which would otherwise fall within a defence of necessity. This approach was open to criticism. If all aspects of the defence were abolished, what would be done with those cases where most people would agree that some defence should be available, e.g. emergency operations on children?

Surely there must be some kind of a defence in circumstances such as those which occurred in *Kitson* (1955) 39 Cr App R 66, which is one of the more ludicrous cases in post-war English law. The passenger in a car, having taken drink, fell asleep. He awoke to find the driver gone and the car coasting downhill. He grabbed hold of the steering-wheel and in doing so prevented a crash. Surely he should be congratulated not prosecuted, in Lord Denning MR's terms quoted above. If prosecuted for driving while under the influence of drink, he should have a defence. Similarly, if a person breaks the speed limit to avoid an accident, a result which has been reached in New York: *People* v *Cataldo* (1970) 65 Misc 2d 286. It cannot be foreseen in which circumstances a plea of necessity will be raised. For this reason a general defence is needed. Surely it would be unjust to convict the prisoner who broke out of his burning cell. He is not acting of his own free will. Indeed, it would not be absurd to say that the policy of the law is to encourage conduct such as in *Kitson*. The arguments of the Law Commission may also be criticised. The lack of demand for a defence does not mean that the defence should not exist. A person who should not be convicted should not have to rely on executive discretion not to prosecute or on judicial discretion to impose a light sentence. The law should clearly state that he has a defence. Duress of circumstances which developed after the Law Commission's Report has partly but not completely answered this criticism. Finally, the fact that there are special defences tied to specific offences does not undermine the claim that there should be a general defence to fill in such gaps in the law as exist.

Duress of circumstances as a separate defence

These arguments suggest that there should be some defence. Recently – and the law is not yet completely settled – the courts have shown themselves more amenable than previously in creating a defence in the normal haphazard common law way. The Court of Appeal in *Conway* [1989] QB 290 established a defence called 'duress of circumstances' and subsequent cases have confirmed its existence. The defendant was charged with reckless driving. He said that he had driven recklessly because he feared that two men who approached his car were going to kill his passenger. The court allowed his appeal. The judges held that the facts amounted to duress of circumstances; that duress was an example of necessity; and that whether duress of circumstances was called duress or necessity did not matter. It should be noted that the threat came from a human agency, not from, say, starvation, a natural cause, as in *Dudley and Stephens*, above. In terms of justification and excuse, duress of circumstances looks like a justification, whereas normally at least duress is an excuse.

The defence is restricted in the same way as duress: the defendant must act to avoid a threat of death or serious physical injury, as was said, e.g., in *Abdul-Hussain* [1999] Crim LR 570 and *Quayle*. Therefore, a threat of psychological harm does not suffice: *Baker*, above; cf. the law of non-fatal offences, and it is uncertain whether the law on duress of circumstances should be brought into line with that of non-fatal offences: *DPP v Rogers* [1998] Crim LR 202 or he must act to avoid an honestly (see *Cairns*, above) imagined threat of the same; and he must act with the steadfastness reasonably to be expected of the ordinary citizen in the defendant's situation. That is, the tests in *Graham*, above, applied. The court certified that a point of law of general importance arose but the House of Lords refused leave to appeal. More recently, in *Hampshire County Council v E* [2007] EWHC 2584 (Admin) it was held that the objective tests were to be applied: may 'the failure of her son to attend regularly at school . . . be the result of reasonable fear on the respondent's part that if she tried to get him to school she or her daughter could be at risk of death or serious injury at his hands'? The objective requirement precludes the use of a subjective element, such as suicidal tendencies found in *Rodger* (above) and the pain supposed in *Quayle*. In *Quayle* one reason for the failure of the defence was that there was no imminent risk of death or serious injury from the pain. Another similarity is that duress of circumstances is not available when the accused could have done something other than break the law. In the Scottish case of *Moss v Howdle* 1997 SLT 782 the accused broke the speed limit in order to drive as quickly as possible to the nearest service station for medical attention for his passenger who had cried out in pain. The court denied the defence on the ground that there were alternatives such as stopping on the hard shoulder.

The law on duress by threats as laid down in *Hasan*, above, therefore lays down the limits of duress of circumstances. One difference, however, which the Court of Appeal laid down in *Cole*, above, is that duress by threats occurred when the threatener nominated the crime (e.g. perjury in *Hudson and Taylor*, above), whereas in duress by circumstances there was no such nomination. In *Cole* the moneylenders did not nominate robbery and therefore his defence could not be duress by threats. *Cole* holds that the two defences are related, but not overlapping. They should not be confused. The Court of Appeal in *Abdul-Hussain*, above, stated that *Cole* was wrong as to this distinction. Rose LJ said: 'We see no reason of principle or authority for distinguishing the two forms of duress . . . In particular, we do not read the court's judgment in *Cole* as seeking to draw any such distinction.' There must be, in his words, 'a close nexus between the threat and the criminal act' but there is no requirement of 'a virtually instantaneous reaction'. *Cole* laid down the rule that there had to be a direct and immediate connection between the peril and the crime. On the facts there was no such link because of a gap of one hour 50 minutes between the crime, robbery at a building society, and payment of the money stolen there to a moneylender. It is suggested that on this point *Cole* is incorrect. The threat was an immediate one, never mind an imminent one, when the accused committed the robbery. One interesting consideration is that the defence of duress of circumstances was being created at the same time that the defence of duress by threats was being restricted by the imposition of new limits on the crimes to which it applies and the use of the three objective tests in *Graham*.

The Court of Appeal in *Conway* believed themselves bound by their decision in *Willer* (1986) 83 Cr App R 225, a case definitely not one concerned with duress by threats. The term 'duress of circumstances' was not used. The first use was in *Conway*. The accused in *Willer* was charged with reckless driving. He had driven very slowly along a pavement to avoid a gang of youths. The court held he was driving under duress, but in fact he was not. The youths did not impliedly order him: drive on the pavement or we shall beat you up. Indeed, they very much wanted him to stay where he was. The case was really one of necessity. As Smith and Hogan, *Criminal Law*, 12th edn (OUP, 2008, ed. D. Ormerod) 343, wrote: 'the court was simply allowing the defence of necessity . . . It should surely make no difference whether D [the accused] drove on the pavement to escape from the youths, or a herd of charging bulls, a runaway lorry, or a flood, if he did so in order to escape death or serious bodily harm.' A similar phrase appears in (D. Ormerod, ed.) Smith and Hogan, *Criminal Law: Cases and Materials*, 9th edn (OUP, 2006) 431. Simon Brown J in *Martin* said that this defence arose from 'objective dangers' and only in 'extreme circumstances'.

These two cases, *Conway* and *Willer*, were followed in *Martin* [1989] 1 All ER 652, where the Court of Appeal drew the boundaries of the defence. The question to be asked was whether a person of reasonable firmness sharing the defendant's characteristics would have responded as the accused did. As in duress, the accused must reasonably believe that he has good cause to fear death or serious injury (the requirement of reasonableness as to belief was omitted by the Divisional Court in *DPP v Rogers* [1998] Crim LR 202, but is wrong in the light of *Howe* on duress and the earlier cases on duress of circumstances). These limits do not appear in necessity as a defence. The Divisional Court in *DPP v Harris* [1995] 1 Cr App R 170 said that the accused had to act reasonably and proportionately, as did the court in *Martin*. McCowan LJ thought *dubitante* that there did exist a defence of necessity but that it was not needed on a charge of driving without due care and attention because the term 'due' incorporated the span of the defence. The other judge considered that necessity was a defence to this crime. The court thought that it was not faced with a situation of necessity and considered that *Willer* was the same. Therefore, the case is not conclusive. However, if a disqualified driver takes his wife to hospital by car when she has had a heart attack in remote countryside the situation is not one of duress but of necessity. The Court of Appeal in *Backshall* [1998] 1 WLR 1506 held, contrary to McCowan LJ, that duress of circumstances (which the courts called 'necessity') was a defence to driving without due care and attention and not part of the analysis of whether there was *due* attention. In other words the facts gave rise to an excuse, duress of circumstances; they did not result in the accused's not having the fault element as defined by the offence. It should be noted that in *Martin* the threat was that the threatener would kill herself unless the accused, who was disqualified, drove her son (his stepson) to work, i.e. the threat was to harm the threatener herself and not as it always has been so far in duress to harm the accused or a third party. (A threat, 'I will blow myself up unless you commit perjury', ought, it is thought, to give rise to a defence of duress, provided of course that all the limits on duress are fulfilled.) Actually the facts of **Martin** would seem to constitute a situation of duress by threats. The accused's wife was making a threat in the classic duress formula: 'break the law or I shall do so-and-so'. (It did not matter that the wife's threat, to kill herself, was lawful.) Compare **Willer**: the accused was not ordered to drive on the pavement or else he would be killed. Indeed the gang did not want him to drive on the paved area for by doing so he escaped their threats. Another issue raised by **Martin** is whether the threat must be an unlawful one. Suicide is no longer a crime under English law. The point was not discussed by the Court of Appeal. If **Cole**, above, is correct, **Martin** should indeed be treated as a case on duress by threats.

While **Backshall** held that duress of circumstances is a defence available to careless driving, rather than part of the offence itself, there is a situation where the facts giving rise to what would otherwise be a defence of duress of circumstances are taken into account when determining whether or not there is an offence. In crimes of subjective recklessness it has to be proved that the accused took a risk which a reasonable person would not have taken. In examining the gravity of the risk the triers of fact could say that a reasonable person must have taken the risk of causing harm in order to prevent a greater harm. If so, the accused is not guilty because the prosecution has failed to prove all the elements of the offence; it is not the case that all the ingredients have been proved but there is a defence. The threat which is the subject of the defence must be one which objectively menaces the accused or others and makes him immediately fear a danger. The fact that one's conscience tells one to break the criminal law is not such a threat. In **Blake v DPP** [1993] Crim LR 586 the appellant believed that the voice of God instructed him to write a quotation from the Bible on a concrete pillar near the Houses of Parliament as a protest against the Gulf War. There was no immediate danger to himself or others, and his defence to a charge of criminal damage failed.

Willer was followed in **DPP v Bell** [1992] RTR 335 (DC), again a driving case. The accused was not guilty of driving with excess alcohol when he drove his car to escape a threat of serious injury to himself. A similar case was **DPP v Whittle** [1996] RTR 154 (CA). Once the threat is over, the accused must stop driving; if he does not, he will be guilty of this crime: **DPP v Jones** [1990] RTR 33 and **DPP v Mullally**, above.

The first cases on duress of circumstances involved motoring offences. There was never any real doubt that it applied to other crimes (such as hijacking: **Abdul-Hussain**, above, and cultivating cannabis: **Blythe** (1998) *The Independent*, 4 April (Warrington Crown Court)) and **Pommell** [1995] 2 Cr App R 607 (CA) confirmed the general application of the defence subject to the same exceptions found in duress by threats. Accordingly the defence was available on the facts of **Pommell** to an accused who took a sub-machine gun from a friend of his who intended to kill persons who had murdered a friend of the friend. There was no relationship between the accused and these third parties and after **Hasan**, **Pommell** may well be wrong on this point. The court also held that the objective limitations of duress by threats applied to this offence ('reasonable belief', 'good cause' and 'person of reasonable firmness') as well as the rules that the threat had to be one of death or serious injury and the accused had to go to the police as soon as he could: a delay could, however, be explained away. **Pommell** also illustrates the law that duress of circumstances need not come from natural circumstances but can arise from a human cause. The court stressed that necessity in its 'lesser evil' guise was not a defence, whereas duress of circumstances was. **Pommell** illustrates the difference between duress and necessity. There was no threat; therefore, the case could not have been one of duress, contrary to the thinking of the court. What the accused did was to take a weapon from the accused when the alternative was to allow the other to kill with it. These facts gave rise to a choice-of-evils defence. The accused had the choice of breaking the law, possessing a firearm without a licence, or allowing the other party to kill. He chose the lesser evil. Whether necessity should exist on these facts is a matter of policy, but a conviction on the facts may have sent wrong signals to the public.

As already stated, the accused must have a reasonable belief that he had good cause to fear the threat. The requirement of reasonable belief has at times been ignored, but to keep consistency with duress by threats, this condition must be retained. *Howe* and *Hasan* are after all House of Lords authorities.

Duress of circumstances and necessity

The present law was summed up in *Conway*: 'It appears that it is still not clear whether there is a general defence of necessity or, if there is, what circumstances in which it is available.' But there are indications that necessity may shortly be recognised as a defence. *Re A* is especially significant in this regard. However, the judiciary still displays confusion about the legal foundations of duress and necessity. For example, as stated above, Lord Hailsham in *Howe* regarded duress as a species of necessity. And some say 'duress of circumstances' is another name for necessity. In *Quayle* the defence of duress of circumstances was said to be one of 'necessity by circumstances'.

A different view was put by C. Gearty, 'Necessity: a necessary defence in criminal law?' [1989] CLJ 357:

> Well-meaning people who think the world is fair believe a defence of necessity would make it fairer still. The judges, who know better, realise that it would parade for public view the inequalities and iniquities inherent in our affluence, without ever threatening to remove them – the Crown Court is hardly the place, after all, to abolish the law of property.

For this reason the hungry are not permitted to steal, the homeless to squat. He continued:

> Where does the defence go from here? After *Martin*, duress of circumstances would appear to have a general application across the law (other than murder, one presumes). It remains to be seen whether the courts will be so eager to apply it where the crime said to have been necessary is more gruesome than the motoring infractions (a wounding or kidnapping for example). And nowhere is it suggested that [the accused] should be required to choose the lesser evil – yet such utilitarian calculus is the essence of necessity. We are still some way from a defence that might stimulate the needy into approved banditry.

Present law has not reached the stage of balancing evils which some see as the conceptual basis of necessity, which indeed in the USA is sometimes known as 'choice of evils'. However, since it is a defence to use reasonable force to injure a person damaging property, it seems absurd not to give a defence to someone who steals property to feed a starving child. *Pommell* has been taken to be the start of the opening of the floodgates to a full-scale defence of necessity. In the view of the present writer *Pommell* does not go so far. Duress of circumstances remains restricted to the same requirements as apply to duress by threats. Theft and squatting are rarely excused by duress of threats; similarly they will rarely be excused by duress of circumstances. Necessity is distinguished from duress of circumstances by its rationale of the balance of evils. Duress of circumstances does not have the rationale: the will of the accused is overridden by the threat. Necessity is a justificatory defence, whereas duress of both forms is an excuse. In terms of the distinction explored at the start of this chapter an accused who acts under duress of either variety is excused but one who acts under necessity is justified.

Conway and *Martin* do, however, suggest that some of the older cases requiring a defence ought to be reviewed. Interestingly cases at present except *Cole*, above, where the defence failed are concerned with victimless offences but it is assumed that the defence is not so restricted.

In one instance Parliament has ruled out a defence of duress of circumstances. The Human Fertilisation and Embryology Act 1990, s 37, amends s 5(2) of the Abortion Act 1967, which now provides that anything done with intent to perform a miscarriage is unlawful unless authorised by s 1, which requires a registered medical practitioner to perform the abortion.

The position taken in this book

(1) There is a defence of duress (by threats).

(2) While the defence is perhaps still in the process of emerging, there is a defence of duress of circumstances.

(3) Necessity, which is to be distinguished from duress of circumstances, is an embryo defence ripe for development.

Reform of duress of circumstances and necessity

This area of the law would receive the imprimatur of the Law Commission if its draft Criminal Code, Law Com. No. 177, 1989, were enacted. Clause 43 aptly restates present law:

(1) A person is not guilty of an offence . . . when he does an act under duress of circumstances.

(2) A person does an act under duress of circumstances if –
   (a) he does it because he knows or believes that it is immediately necessary to avoid death or serious personal harm to himself or another; and
   (b) the danger that he knows or believes to exist is such that in all the circumstances (including any of his personal characteristics that affect its gravity) he cannot reasonably be expected to act otherwise.

These recommendations find their most recent expression in the Law Commission Report No. 218, *Legislating the Criminal Code – Offences Against the Person and General Principles*, 1993, discussed under duress, above. The 1993 definition would leave to the jury the question of whether the defendants in *Dudley and Stephens* had an excuse for killing the cabin boy. Clause 43(3) denies the defence to murder and attempted murder in order to keep the law consistent with *Howe* on duress. The Law Commission would have preferred the defence to apply generally. There are provisions dealing with the overlap between this defence and others. Clause 43(3)(b)(iii) states that the defence does not apply if the person 'has knowingly and without reasonable excuse exposed himself to the danger'. That approach is also taken in the USA in the Model Penal Code Official Draft, 1985, s 3.02(2) and at common law, e.g. *State v Diana* (1979) 604 P 2d 1312, a decision of the Washington Court of Appeals. US law differs, however, from even the proposed

English law by balancing harms. The Model Penal Code, s 3.02(2), provides that 'the harm or evil sought to be avoided . . . is greater than that sought to be prevented', while **State v Diana** stipulated that 'necessity is available as a defence when the physical forces of nature or the pressure of circumstances cause the accused to take unlawful action to avoid a harm which social policy deems greater than the harm resulting from a violation of the law'. As Gearty, quoted above, wrote, English law has not adopted this utilitarian calculus. At present therefore the law of necessity is in a state of flux.

In the draft Criminal Code, 1989, the Law Commission did not define necessity but left it to judicial development. Similarly in the 1993 Report it did not propose to put necessity, if it existed, on a statutory footing. Case law had to develop before the defence could be encapsulated by Parliament. Necessity-as-justification is therefore not touched, whereas necessity-as-excuse (duress of circumstances) is to be encapsulated in a statute because of its resemblance to duress by threats. Who knows: before your exam the law may have changed again! The Australian states of Queensland and Western Australia provide a defence where a person acted or omitted to act 'under such circumstances of sudden or extraordinary emergency that an ordinary person possessing ordinary powers of self-control could not reasonably be expected to act otherwise' – and the sky has not fallen in.

Summary

The next three chapters deal with defences. It begins with an outline of 'defence theory', looking mainly at the attempts to divide defences into justifications (where the accused's behaviour is praiseworthy or at least permissible) and excuses (where the conduct remains a crime but where the accused is excused (because for instance he or she was acting under duress). It should be noted that of the defences treated of in this text only in respect of insanity and diminished responsibility is the burden of proof on the accused. Normally, despite 'defences' being so called, the burden is on the prosecution, and not just that but the prosecution must disprove the defence beyond reasonable doubt. This chapter concentrates on those defences which in a general sense relate to the voluntariness of possible criminal conduct. Children may be seen as not acting of their own free will because, for example, they are unable to foresee the consequences of their behaviour. The law has changed in the quite recent past so that children aged 10–13 are now as criminally liable as adults, and comment is made on that change. Duress (also known as duress *per minas*) occurs where the defendant is threatened that death or serious harm will be done to herself or another unless she commits a crime. The severe limits, especially after the House of Lords decision in **Hasan**, are scrutinised, as are the crimes to which at present duress cannot provide a defence (murder, attempted murder, and 'some forms of treason'). The next defence discussed is that of coercion, which is available only to married women. The nature and justification of this defence are scrutinised. There follows the alleged defence of necessity, which bears several definitions – here, the 'choice of evils' definition is advanced (partly in light of the next defence). **Re A** (2001), the civil case of the separation of conjoined twins, is considered. Duress of circumstances is a fairly recent development of the law where the threat does not come from a human source as in duress (*per minas*). The relationship between duress and duress of circumstances is one focus of the inquiry. Finally there is an extensive consideration of the long-standing attempts by the Law Commission to reform the law, culminating in the Consultation Paper of December 2005, *A New Homicide Act for England and Wales?* No. 177 and the Report *Murder, Manslaughter and Infanticide* No. 306 of November 2006.

- Infancy: Children under 10 may not be convicted of any offence; children above 10 may be convicted of any offence. The law or presumption that children aged 10–14 could not be convicted of any offence unless the prosecution could prove not just the *actus reus* and *mens rea* but also the fact that the child knew the conduct was seriously (or morally) wrong was abolished in 1998. However, it should be noted that the doctrine of *mens rea* will sometimes work in favour of children: they may not intend or foresee consequences when an adult in the same position would have so intended or foreseen.

- Duress: This defence, also known as duress by threats, is based on the thinking that people cannot be expected to resist threats of serious harm of death to themselves and their loved ones (and quite possibly strangers). The basis is: 'do this or else', e.g. 'unless you commit the crime of theft, I will kill you'. The defence is quite circumscribed and the House of Lords in **Hasan** has recently reemphasised that the defence is a narrow one. Its limits are:
  1 there is no defence of duress to murder, attempted murder, and some forms of treason;
  2 the threat must be one of death or serious personal injury;
  3 it seems that the threat must be one against the accused or his or her family or perhaps someone with whom the defendant has a special relationship: it is, however, arguable that the threat could be against a stranger;
  4 the threat must be one which can immediately (read fairly broadly) be carried out: if there is an opportunity to escape, the duressee must use it; and for a similar reason, once the duress is over, the accused must desist from the criminal behaviour;
  5 the accused must act reasonably to avoid the threat: he or she must have acted like a sober and reasonable person might have behaved;
  6 the belief that he or she is threatened with death or serious harm must be based on reasonable grounds;
  7 the accused must have 'good cause to fear that if he did not so act [the duressor] would kill him or cause him serious personal injury' (**Graham** (1982) CA, approved by the House of Lords in **Howe** (1987)); and
  8 no defence is available if the accused voluntarily joined a criminal organisation which he or she knew or ought to have known would expose him or her to the risk that duress would be used.

- Coercion: This defence is similar to duress but is available only to a married woman. The wife must prove that she acted under the coercion and in the presence of her husband: Criminal Justice Act 1925, s 47. Note that the burden of proof is placed on the accused. It is thought that coercion has a wider meaning than duress and includes, for example, a threat by the husband to leave his wife; 'presence' is not limited to the wife being in the same room as the husband but extends to being in the husband's sight. The husband and wife must actually be married: a reasonable belief by the alleged wife that they are is insufficient.

- Duress of circumstances: Cases over the last twenty years have established a defence of this name. The defence is similar to duress in that the restrictions noted above in respect of duress also apply to duress of circumstances but the basic formulation differs from duress which, as stated, is in the form of 'do this or else' (e.g. do this crime or we will kneecap you!') whereas duress of circumstances takes the form of: 'there is an emergency and the accused has to escape it by breaking the law'. An example occurs where the driver of a car drives on the pavement to avoid masked gunmen: the gunmen are not saying: 'we will shoot you unless you break the law by driving on the pavement'.

- Necessity: Sometimes duress of circumstances is called necessity and sometimes necessity is called duress of circumstances. The view taken here is that duress of circumstances is similar to the defence of duress: they share the same limitations, e.g. neither is a defence to murder. Necessity differs in that it is a choice-of-evils defence without such boundaries; it can, therefore, be a defence to all crimes including murder. The status of this defence remains uncertain but there is a modern view that it does exist.

References

Reports

Home Office Consultation Paper, *Tackling Youth Crime* (1997)

Irish Law Reform Commission Consultation Paper no. 27, *Homicide: the Plea of Provocation* (2003)

Law Commission Consultation Paper no. 122, *Legislating the Criminal Code: Offences against the Person and General Principles* (1992)

Law Commission Consultation Paper no. 177, *A new Homicide Act for England & Wales?* (2005)

Law Commission Report no. 83, *Defences of General Application* (1978)

Law Commission Report no. 177, *A Criminal Code for England & Wales* (1989)

Law Commission Report no. 218, *Legislating the Criminal Code: Offences against the Person and General Principles* (1993)

Law Commission Report no. 306, *Murder, Manslaughter and Infanticide* (2006)

Model Penal Code *Official Draft* (1985)

Report of the Select Committee of the House of Lords on Murder and Life Imprisonment (Nathan) (1989)

White Paper *Crime, Justice and Protecting the Public* (1990)

White Paper *No More Excuses*, Cm. 3809 (1997)

Books

Fletcher, G. *Rethinking Criminal Law* (Little, Brown & Co., 1978)

Smith, J. C. *Justification and Excuse in the Criminal Law* (Stevens, 1989)

Shute, S., Gardner, S. and Horder, J. *Action and Value in the Criminal Law* (Oxford University Press, 1993)

Simpson, A. W. B. *Cannibalism and the Common Law* (University of Chicago Press, 1984)

Smith, J. C. and Hogan, B. *Criminal Law* (ed. D. Ormerod) 11th edn (Oxford University Press, 2005)

Stephens, J. F. *History of the Criminal Law of England* (Sweet & Maxwell, 1883)

Journals

Dressler, J. 'Provocation: partial justification or partial excuse' (1988) 51 MLR 467

Gearty, C. 'Necessity: a necessary defence in criminal law [1989] CLJ 357

Horder, J. 'Self-defence, necessity and duress' (1998) 11 Can JLP 143

Morawetz, T. 'Reconstructing the criminal defences' (1986) 77 JCL & Crim 277

Perkins, R. M. 'Impelled perpetration revisited' (1981) 33 Hastings LJ 403

Vandervort, L. 'Social justice in the modern regulatory state' (1987) 6 Law & Phil 205

Walker, N. 'The end of an old song' (1999) NLJ 64

Further reading

Alexander, A. 'Lesser evils: a closer look at the paradigmatic justification' (2005) 24 *Law and Philosophy* 611

Ashworth, A. 'Murder: defence – young defendant – intention to kill – defendant's father instructing him to assist in murder [2008] Crim LR 138

Baron, M. 'Justifications and excuses' (2005) 2 Ohio St J Crim L 387

Baron, M. 'Excuses, excuses' (2007) 1 Crim Law and Philos 21

Berman, M. N. 'Justification and excuse, law and morality' (2003) 53 Duke LJ 1

Bohlander, M. *'In extremis*: hijacked airplanes, "collateral damage" and the limits of criminal law' [2006] Crim LR 579

Cavadino, P. 'Goodbye *Doli*, must we leave you?' (1997) 9 *Child and Family Law Quarterly* 165

Centre for Crime and Justice Studies *From Punishment to Problem Solving – A New Approach to Children in Trouble*, Centre for Crime and Justice Studies (2006)

Clarkson, C. M. V. 'Necessary action: A new defence?' [2004] Crim LR 81

Crofts, T. *'Doli incapax'* (2003) *E Law: Murdoch University Electronic Journal of Law*, Pt 3

Dennis, I. 'Developments in duress' (1987) 51 JCL 463

Dressler, J. 'Why keep the provocation defense? Some reflections on a difficult subject' (2002) 86 Minnesota LR 959

Duff, R. A. 'Rethinking justifications' (2004) 39 Tulsa L Rev 829

Duff, R. A. 'Excuses, moral and legal' (2007) 1 Crim Law and Philos 49

Elliott, D. W. 'Necessity, duress and self-defence' [1989] Crim LR 611

Gardner, J. 'The gist of excuses' (1998) 1 *Buffalo Criminal Law Review* 575

Horder, J. 'Occupying the moral high ground? The Law Commission on duress' [1994] Crim LR 334

Horder, J. *Excusing Crimes* (Oxford University Press, 2004)

Jefferson, M. 'Householders and the use of force against intruders' (2005) 69 JCL 405

Kugler, I. 'Necessity as a justification in *Re A (Children)*' (2004) 67 440

Maher, G. 'Age and criminal responsibility' (2005) 2 Ohio SE J Crim L 493

Ormerod, D. 'Necessity of circumstances' [2006] Crim LR 151 (comment on *Quayle*)

Padfield, N. 'Duress, necessity and the Law Commission' [1992] Crim LR 778

Peiris, G .L. 'Duress, volition and criminal responsibiity' [1998] A-ALR 182

Rogers, J. 'Necessity, private defence and the killing of Mary' [2001] Crim LR 515

Smith, J. C. 'Official secrets' [2001] Crim LR 987 (comment on *S*, also known as *Shayler*)

Smith, K. J. M. 'Duress and steadfastness; in pursuit of the unintelligible' [2001] Crim LR 363

Tadros, V. 'The character of excuses' (2001) 21 OJLS 495

Tadros, V. *Criminal Responsibility* (Oxford University Press, 2005)

Uniake, S. 'Emotional excuses' (2007) 26 Law and Phil 95

Urbas, G. *The Age of Criminal Responsibility* (2000) Australian Institute of Criminology, Trends and Issues in Crime and Criminal Justice, No. 181

Walsh, C. 'Irrational presumptions of rationality and comprehension' [1998] 3 Web JCLI

Westen, P. 'An attitudinal theory of excuse' (2006) 25 *Law and Philosophy* 289

Westen, P. 'Offences and defences again' (2008) 28 OJLS 563.

Westen, P. and Mangiafico, J. 'The criminal defense of duress: a justification, not an excuse – and why it matters' (2005) 6 Buff Crim L Rev 833

Williams, G. 'The theory of excuses' [1982] Crim LR 732

Wilson, W. 'The structure of criminal defences' [2005] Crim LR 108

For a symposium on *Re A (Children) (Conjoined Twins)* see (2001) 9 Medical LR 201

For a critique of excuses and justifications, see R. F. Schopp, *Justification: Defences and Just Convictions* (Cambridge University Press, 1998) or his article of the same name (1993) 24 Pacific LJ 1233. For an English approach to the same topic, see W. Wilson, *Central Issues in Criminal Theory* (Hart, 2002), chs. 10–11

For the Scottish Law Commission's approach, see their *Report on Age of Criminal Responsibility*, Scot. Law Com. no. 185, 2002. For an Irish view, see Law Reform Commission, *Duress and Necessity*, Consultation Paper no. 39, 2006.

Visit **www.mylawchamber.co.uk/jefferson** to access exam-style questions with answer guidance, multiple choice quizzes, live weblinks, an online glossary, and regular updates to the law.

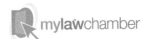

Use **Case Navigator** to read in full some of the key cases referenced in this chapter:

Atlorney General for Jersey v Holley for Jersey v Holley [2005] 2 AC 58
R v G [2003] 4 All ER 545

8

Mistake, intoxication, self-defence

Mistake

Introduction

English law divides mistake as a possible defence in criminal law into two parts: mistake of law and mistake of fact. The general rule is that if the accused makes a mistake of law, he is guilty, whereas if he makes a mistake of fact, he is not. Unfortunately the law is more complex than these propositions allow. A preliminary point is that if an accused because of a 'disease of the mind' makes a mistake of law, he may have a defence of insanity. This defence is discussed in the next chapter.

Mistake and ignorance of law

In *Esop* (1836) 173 ER 203 the accused was convicted of an offence under English law, buggery; under his personal law no such offence existed. Accordingly, where the accused has the relevant *actus reus* and *mens rea* for the crime, he is guilty even though he did not know that the *actus reus* was forbidden by the criminal law. He was mistaken as to the rules of English law. Moreover, ignorance of the law is no defence: *Bailey* (1800) 168 ER 657. The accused was convicted of a crime which Parliament had created while he was on the high seas, and there was no way of finding out that a law had been enacted. The case has been taken to hold that impossibility is no defence. However, it may be that *Bailey* should be read differently. The case was referred to all the judges. They recommended a pardon. Since at that time a pardon was the sole way of reversing the first instance decision, it may be that they disagreed with the proposition that ignorance of the law was no defence. *Bailey* has nevertheless been treated as deciding that, and the rule has been accepted in, e.g., *Carter v McLaren* (1871) LR 2 Sc & D 120. The rule was stated by the Court of Appeal in *Lightfoot* (1993) 97 Cr App R 24: '. . . Knowledge of the law . . . is irrelevant . . . The fact that a man does not know what is criminal and what is not . . . cannot save him from conviction if what he does, coupled with the state of his mind, satisfies all the elements of the crime of which he is accused.' An illustration is *Broad* [1997] Crim LR 666 (CA). The defendants were convicted even though they were ignorant of the law. They did not know that what they were making was a controlled drug proscribed by criminal law. Certainly it is not always easy to discover that a Bill has been enacted or that a statute has come into force. If the accused believes that he is using force to prevent a crime, but there is no such crime, he has made a mistake as to the law and has no defence.

A fairly recent illustration of a mistake of law is *Hipperson v DPP*, unreported, 3 July 1996 (DC). The defendants had used bolt-cutters to break through the perimeter fence of the Atomic Weapons Establishment, Aldermaston, where the UK's atomic deterrent is produced. They contended that they had a defence to criminal damage in that they were acting to prevent genocide or conspiracy to commit genocide. However, the definition of genocide in the UK is restricted to acting 'with intent to destroy in whole or in part a national, ethnical, social or religious group as such', and does not extend, as the defendants submitted, to the destruction in whole or in part of the human race. Therefore, the defendants had made a mistake of law and had no defence.

The rule that ignorance of the law is no defence is supported by the arguments that if it were a defence, the floodgates would open and the courts would be swamped by bogus claims of ignorance, people would not try and find out what the law is; 'floodgates' is a weak argument against justice and it would be impossible for the prosecution to show that the accused was truly ignorant of the law. However, it has to be said that no person could know all possible offences, and it may well be unjust to convict a person when only a few people would know of the crime. Judges, lawyers and law students in their professional lives are not expected to know all crimes. Surely ordinary citizens should not be!

There is no defence if the accused consulted a lawyer who stated that their activity was not a crime when it was: *Shaw v DPP* [1962] AC 220 (HL). The defendants wanted to know whether publishing a list of prostitutes and their services, *The Ladies' Directory*, was lawful. The Lords held they were guilty of conspiracy despite the legal advice that they had been given. *A fortiori* reliance on legal advice from a para-legal provides no answer: *Brockley* [1994] Crim LR 671 (CA). Reliance on local authority or police advice is also no defence: *Cambridgeshire and Isle of Ely CC v Rust* [1972] 2 QB 426. The Divisional Court directed magistrates to convict the accused of the crime of setting up a stall on a highway without lawful excuse, even though he had sought advice and had paid rates on the stall to the local council. It is arguable that mistake of law should be a defence if the accused tried to find out the law or relied on official advice. He attempted to comply with the law, but failed. It is doubtful whether convicting him serves any purpose other than preventing bogus defences, and the triers of fact could do that: finding flimsy defences to be untrue is part of their role. At present reliance on official advice does not exculpate, but only mitigates the sentence, e.g. *Howell v Falmouth Boat Construction Co* [1951] AC 837 (HL), *obiter*, and *Surrey CC v Battersby* [1965] 2 QB 194 (DC). The latter case involved a crime of undertaking childcare without informing the council that the children were to spend more than a month in the house. She had taken advice that she was not guilty of the offence because no one period extended beyond a month because the parents took the children away at certain weekends. She was held to be guilty. Breaks counted only if a fresh arrangement were made after the break. One might have thought that the Divisional Court might have held that penal statutes should be construed in favour of the accused. To grant her an absolute discharge does not resolve the issue. She had acted in good faith; she was a proper person to take care of the children; and she had taken the advice of the council, the same council which prosecuted her, and the council should have known the law it was administering. No advantage was gained from stigmatising the accused as a criminal, and the outcome may be to bring the legal system into disrepute. There has been some indication in the cases that where an accused relies on official advice, it is an abuse of authority for the body which gave the advice to prosecute, and while no defence is afforded, the criminal proceedings are stayed as being an abuse of process. In one case where the defendants relied on advice from the planning department of a local authority that they did not need planning permission to erect advertising boards but the authority prosecuted them for erecting hoardings, the Divisional Court stayed the proceedings. Trials which are an abuse of process may well breach Article 6 of the European Convention on Human Rights, which concerns the right to a fair trial.

The same rule applies to a reliance on a judicial decision which is later overruled: *Younger* (1793) 101 ER 253 (by inference). There is also no defence where the accused relies on *ultra vires* delegated legislation. No doubt with increasing EC legislation and judgments, reliance on UK law which is later found to be in conflict with EC norms will afford no defence. Such people are not at fault. Judges make mistakes of law: why do we have the doctrine of *per incuriam*, the Court of Appeal and House of Lords and the Practice Statement permitting the House of Lords to overrule its previous authorities? Yet they are not guilty of an offence. In *Campbell* (1972) 1 CRNS 273 Kearns DCJ thought that the outcome that if citizens relying on judgments make an error they are guilty but judges whose decisions are overturned on appeal are not was 'amusing'. Surely it cannot really be the law that ordinary people should be expected to know the law better than the judiciary. The heavens will not fall if mistake of law in reliance on official advice is accepted as a defence. South Africa does not have the rule: *S v de Blom* (1977) 3 SA 513 (A), and Canada has such a defence (*MacDougall* (1983) 1 CCC (3d) 65 (SCC)), and some US states have such a defence. For example, the New York Penal Code, s 15.20(2), relying on the Model Penal Code, provides a defence. Some states do not give a defence. In the Maryland case of *Hopkins v State* (1950) 69 A 2d 456 reliance on the State Attorney's advice was no defence. In summary P. Brett 'Mistake of law as a criminal defence' (1966) 5 Melb ULR 179 at 203, wrote:

> [i]f we are seeking to achieve respect for law, it is surely unwise to tell citizens that they must disregard the considered advice of the public officials whose duty it is to administer the law and who may therefore be expected to tell citizens in effect that the advice which they received bona fide from qualified lawyers is to be treated as worthless.

Brett called *Battersby* a 'glaring injustice'. It is unjust that the state through its courts can disregard the advice of its officials such as the Director of Public Prosecutions and convict defendants of offences on facts which the officials informed them were not offences.

It is not unknown for Parliament to afford a defence to a person who relies on official advice. In the Control of Pollution Act 1974, s 3(4), it is a defence to the offence of unlicensed waste disposal that the accused 'took care to inform himself from persons who were in a position to provide information'.

There are in fact a few stray cases where mistake of law was a defence. Parliament may give a defence to a person who has made a mistake of law. The obvious illustration is s 2(1)(a) of the Theft Act 1968, which provides that the accused is not dishonest for the purposes of theft if he believes, whether on reasonable grounds or not, that he had a legal right to deprive the victim of his property. If he believes he did but was mistaken, he is not guilty. In *Secretary of State for Trade and Industry v Hart* [1982] 1 All ER 817, the Divisional Court in relation to an offence under the companies legislation of acting as an auditor, knowing oneself to be disqualified, held that the accused was not guilty because he did not know that he was disqualified. It was not sufficient that he knew the *facts* which made him disqualified. His ignorance of the law was a defence. He did not have the requisite *mens rea*. He ought not to have acted as auditor because he was a director of the companies he was auditing. (If he knew he was disqualified but not that acting as an auditor when disqualified was an offence, he would not have a defence: he would have made a mistake of law.) Present law is stated in **Smith** [1974] QB 354, where a tenant destroyed property which had become his landlord's as a result of civil law in the belief that it was still his. The accused did intend to damage property, but he did not intend to damage property belonging to another. Indeed, he intended to damage property belonging to himself. He made a mistake as regards to whom the property belonged. Current law is sometimes stated as a mistake of civil law excuses. **Hart** could be explained as being a case on mistake of civil law.

One problem with having different effects depending on the type of mistake, civil or criminal, is that it may not be obvious whether the error is as to civil or criminal law, e.g. a mistake as to whether goods are 'stolen' for the purposes of handling is a mistake of criminal law. In **Grant v Borg** [1982] 1 WLR 638 the House of Lords held that an error as to whether leave has been granted to a visitor to remain in the UK was not a defence though 'leave' looks very much like a civil law concept. Either the House of Lords themselves made a mistake (and **Hart** is inconsistent with the decision) or **Smith** is a questionable decision if it lays down this rule that a mistake of civil law is a defence.

The basic rule that ignorance or mistake of law is no defence was preserved in the draft Criminal Code (Law Com. No. 177, *A Criminal Code for England and Wales*, 1989), cl 21. Parliament of course retains the power to create exceptions. Also preserved was the present rule that mistake of law provides a defence 'where it negatives a fault element of the offence'. The Law Commission (para 8.32) rephrases the exception as the accused's not having the fault element. The Law Commission did not feel able to provide a defence of reliance on official advice or court decision. The draft Criminal Code, cl 46, also restated current law that:

(1) A person is not guilty of an offence consisting of a contravention of a statutory instrument if –
   (a) at the time of his act the instrument has not been issued by Her Majesty's Stationery Office; and
   (b) by that time reasonable steps have not been taken to bring the purport of the instrument to the notice of the public, or of persons likely to be affected by it, or of that person.

The legal burden of proof in relation to (a) would be on the accused: cl 46(2).

Mistake of fact

Introduction

English law draws a sharp line between mistake of law (guilty) and mistake of fact (usually not guilty), yet the line is not always clear. According to the House of Lords in **Brutus v Cozens** [1973] AC 854, a case on the meaning of 'insulting' within s 5 of the Public Order Act 1936, which has since been repealed, the construction of an ordinary word in a statute is a matter of fact, not of law, though the rule seems to have been honoured in the breach more than in the observance. Two cases which are hard to reconcile are **Norton v Knowles** [1967] 3 All ER 1061 and **Phekoo** [1981] 1 WLR 1117, both of which concerned the term 'residential occupier'. In the former case whether the accused believed his victim to be a residential occupier was an issue of law and therefore he had no defence; in the latter the term was held to be a question of fact and accordingly the accused had a defence where he believed that the victim was a squatter and not a residential occupier. It is postulated that mistake of fact is a defence because as with some other defences punishing the accused would not deter him. This rationale is said to derive from J. Bentham, *An Introduction to the Principles of Morals and Legislation* (Methuen, 1982, first published 1789) Chapter 13, Section 3, though it can be argued that, while punishing a mistaken person would not deter him, it might deter others.

Logically mistake of fact should negate *mens rea*, i.e. the prosecution has not proved this element. There is nothing special about mistake. In this sense mistake is not a defence. The courts have, however, developed special restrictive rules. Three reasons might be hypothesised to explain this development. First, in the nineteenth century the current theory of subjective *mens rea* had not been formulated; therefore, the courts missed the opportunity of stating that mistake was incompatible with the fault element. Secondly, the judges were anxious not to let off an accused who, though telling the truth, had formed his opinion negligently. Thirdly, judges were worried that juries would accept bogus defences. Accordingly they laid down the rule that mistakes had to be reasonable. More recently the courts have brought mistake generally speaking more in line with *mens rea*. It should be remembered that while the courts have moved away from the requirement that a mistake had to be made on reasonable grounds, Parliament can stipulate that a mistake must be a reasonable one. An example was s 14(3) of the Sexual Offences Act 1956 (defence to a charge of the then existing crime of indecent assault when his marriage to a girl under 16 is invalid 'if he believes her to be his wife and has reasonable cause for the belief').

'Irrelevant mistakes'

Since mistake is intertwined with *mens rea*, if the offence is a strict one, the accused will not have the defence if his mistake is one as to the strict element. In **Prince** (1875) LR 2 CCR 154, s 55 of the Offences Against the Person Act 1861 was at issue: 'Whosoever shall unlawfully take . . . any unmarried girl, being under the age of 16 years, out of the possession of her father . . .' shall be guilty of an offence. The accused believed that the girl was over 16. He had no intention of doing what the law forbade. The court held that he was guilty. The abductee was a girl; she was unmarried; she was under 16; she was taken out of the possession of her parents. He knew that she was a girl, that she was unmarried, and that he was taking her out of the possession of her parents. He did not have to know that she was under 16. He was guilty because his mistake was an irrelevant one in that he was mistaken as to her age. Mistake is relevant only where the mistake is as to a *mens rea* element. In **Hibbert** (1869) LR 1 CCR 184 the accused was charged with the same offence. His conviction was quashed. He did not know that the girl had any parents. His mistake was a relevant one, because it related to a *mens rea* element. Before he could be convicted, he had to know that she had parents. He did not know that fact. Therefore, his conviction was quashed. The rule in **Prince** is not affected by developments in the next three sections but, as we have seen in Chapter 4, the doctrine of strict liability is in retreat: the fewer strict offences there are, the less scope there is for 'irrelevant mistakes'.

Tolson

Where there is a relevant mistake, it was stated for many years that the accused did not have a defence unless his mistake was made reasonably. If he made a mistake unreasonably in that he was careless, he had no defence. The principal authority was **Tolson** (1889) 23 QBD 168. The accused did not intend, being married, to marry again as required by the crime of bigamy, because she thought her husband was dead. The court gave her the defence of mistake. It argued that when Parliament gave a defence to bigamy that the spouse has been absent for seven years, it cannot have intended to penalise someone who believed on grounds other than seven years' absence that her spouse was dead. There was nothing in the statute about a defence for a person who believed on reasonable grounds that her spouse was dead. The reasonable grounds were that she thought he had been lost at sea.

Several comments may be made.

(a) Mrs Tolson did not intend to marry again; Mr Prince did not intend to elope with or abduct a girl under 16. She was not guilty; he was guilty. In legal terms she made a relevant mistake, he made an irrelevant one.

(b) The court decided that a mistaken belief was a defence only if reasonably held. Stephen J in *Tolson* had no doubt:

> It may be laid down as a general rule that an alleged offender is deemed to have acted under that state of facts which he in good faith and on reasonable grounds believed to exist when he did the act alleged to be an offence. I am unable to suggest any real exception to this rule, nor has one ever been suggested to me.

Saying that mistake is a defence only if reasonably made is equivalent to saying that the accused will not have the defence if he was careless. Bray CJ commented on the Australian law which is the same as *Tolson* that 'the criminal law is designed to punish the vicious, not the stupid or the credulous' (*Brown* (1975) 10 SASR 139) and that the rule was an 'anomalous and unwarrantable excrescence' (*Brambles Holdings Ltd v Carey* (1976) 15 SASR 270). In this respect the *Tolson* defence shifts the question from *mens rea* to negligence. Bigamy has in this sense become a crime of negligence. If the view is held that mistake ought to negate *mens rea*, what *Tolson* seems to have done is to mix up evidence and substantive law. A defendant who sets up a defence of unreasonable belief may well fail to put forward sufficient evidence to raise a reasonable doubt as to guilt in the minds of the triers of fact; yet even an unreasonable belief should as a matter of substance avail if the triers of fact accept the accused's evidence.

(c) The mistake in *Tolson* did not relate to a failure by the prosecution to prove an element of the offence of bigamy. The accused was given a defence. Her mistake related to that defence.

Diplock J followed *Tolson* in *Gould* [1968] 2 QB 65 where the accused believed that the first marriage had been dissolved. Only a reasonable mistake would afford a defence. Similarly, a belief that the first marriage was void exculpates the accused, provided that his mistake was reasonable: *King* [1964] 1 QB 285 (CA). On the *Tolson* approach the 'being married' element in bigamy is satisfied by carelessness. If bigamy is viewed as a serious offence, it is strange that one can commit it carelessly. The most important case in this area is *DPP v Morgan*.

 DPP v Morgan [1976] AC 182

One of the accused, a sergeant in the RAF, invited three men to have sexual intercourse with his wife. He told them that if she resisted or screamed, she was merely enjoying the sexual act. The men had intercourse with her by force. In fact she did not consent. The men were charged with rape as it was then defined. By a majority of three to two the House of Lords ruled that the men had a defence if they (honestly) believed that the woman was consenting. Their mistaken belief did not have to be reasonably held. (In fact the House of Lords determined that no reasonable jury would believe their story, and accordingly there was no miscarriage of justice. This procedure is called 'applying the proviso': on the law the men would not have been guilty had their evidence been believed, but it was not. By their verdict the jury believed the appellants' evidence to be 'a pack of lies' and that there was 'a multiple rape', not 'a sexual orgy' as Lord Cross put it.)

The House of Lords did not overrule **Tolson**. No good reason for retaining **Tolson** was provided by the majority. The House also had the opportunity to overrule **Tolson** in **B v DPP** [2000] 2 AC 428 but it did not take it. However, Lord Nicholls criticised the requirement of reasonableness found in **Tolson**. 'Considered as a matter of principle, the honest belief approach must be preferable. By definition the mental element in a crime is concerned with a subjective state of mind. . . . To the extent that an overriding objective limit ('on reasonable grounds') is introduced, the subjective element is displaced.' It could be that the element of the crime of bigamy, 'being married', has the *mens rea* of negligence attached to it. That is, if a person has the mental element of negligence as to the *actus reus* of being married, this element of the offence is satisfied. Since an unreasonable mistake demonstrates negligence, only a reasonable mistake will lead to an acquittal.

There are several ways of reconciling **Morgan** with **Tolson**.

(a) **Tolson** applies to statutory offences, **Morgan** to common law ones. This argument will not wash. **Morgan** has been applied to statutory offences and was itself put into statutory form for rape in the Sexual Offences (Amendment) Act 1976 which, however, was repealed by the Sexual Offences Act 2003. That statute provides for a test of belief in consent based on reasonable grounds.

(b) There may be a distinction between the mistake in **Tolson** which related to a defence and that in **Morgan** which related to the failure by the prosecution to prove part of the offence (or would have done so, had the men's evidence been believed). However, the line between offence and defence is hard if not impossible to draw, as can be argued from the discussion in Chapter 1 about the third exception to **Woolmington**. Parliament could easily have created a defence to bigamy of belief in the spouse's death but formulated as part of the offence: 'anyone without belief in the spouse's death who was married marries again . . .'. It should, however, be recalled that mistake in duress and duress of circumstances must be reasonably made. Is the mistake as to the unlawfulness of the act or is it one as to the defence? If one believes one is being subjected to duress when one is not, is one acting lawfully because one does not have the *mens rea* of the offence charged or does one have a defence? If the former, according to the distinction the mistake would exculpate, but under present law it does not because a reasonable mistake is needed.

(c) There is something peculiar about the layout of the offence of bigamy. The relevant section, the Offences Against the Person Act 1861, s 57, stipulates an offence followed by provisos. There is no such distinctiveness about the offence of rape. Lord Hailsham seemed to hint at this distinction when he held that **Tolson** was a narrow decision based on the interpretation of the statute.

(d) The House of Lords in **Morgan** said that it did not intend to upset the bigamy cases. Therefore, different rules apply to different offences. Obviously consistency was not seen as a virtue. However, in recent years the House of Lords has consistently taken a subjective view: *B v DPP* [2000] AC 428, *K* [2002] 1 AC 462 and *G* [2004] 1 AC 1034. It may nowadays be that *Tolson* would not survive challenge in the Lords.

(e) Lord Cross in *Morgan* apparently took the view that *Morgan* was confined to rape, but the others did not. Lord Cross did, however, draw another distinction: one between offences such as rape where the defining words expressly or impliedly provide that the accused is not guilty if he believes something to be true and ones such as bigamy where the definition is on its face one giving rise to strict liability.

(f) *Tolson* may apply beyond bigamy, but only to crimes of negligence. There may be other offences and defences of which this can be said. In relation to self-defence, e.g., take the situation of *Pagett* (1983) 76 Cr App R 279, discussed in Chapter 2. If the police had time to check what the victim was doing, surely only a reasonable mistake as to that conduct should exculpate: it is not far fetched to expect the police to check before shooting, provided that there is no danger to themselves or others.

(g) In situations involving the prevention of crime, there must, of course, be a crime to prevent. In *Baker* (CA), above, Brooke LJ, adopting counsel's argument, said: 'If a defendant honestly believes that somebody is eating fish and chips and that eating fish and chips is a crime, the law will not permit him to rely on s 3 [of the Criminal Law Act 1967] as a defence to a charge of assaulting the person eating fish and chips because as a matter of law no crime . . . is committed.' In other words, a mistake of law is no defence.

It was argued that the law in *Morgan* was unsatisfactory in relation to rape: the accused could easily have checked whether the victim was consenting. His carelessness should not exonerate him. Parliament took this view in the Sexual Offences Act 2003. The principle in *Morgan* was abrogated for sex crimes but it still remains authoritative elsewhere.

'The retreat from *Morgan*' and the ascendency of *Morgan*

For some time it was thought that the Court of Appeal was restricting *Morgan* to rape. In *Barrett* (1981) 72 Cr App R 212 the defendants thought that the court order which sent in the bailiffs had been obtained by fraud, and they used force to repel them. The court held that a mistake of civil law availed only if it was based on reasonable grounds. In *Phekoo* [1981] 1 WLR 1117 it was said, *obiter*, that a mistake that a residential occupier was a squatter provided a defence only when it was reasonably made. *Barrett* could be justified as being a case not concerned with mistake of fact. However that may be, *Morgan* came to prevail.

It came to prevail because of what Lord Hailsham in *Morgan* called 'inexorable logic'.

> Once one has accepted . . . that the prohibited act in rape is non-consensual sexual intercourse, and that the guilty state of mind is an intention to commit it, it seems . . . to follow as a matter of inexorable logic that there is no room either for a 'defence' of honest belief or mistake or a defence of honest and reasonable belief or mistake. Either the prosecution proves that the accused had the requisite intent or it does not. In the former case it succeeds, and in the latter it fails.

The Court of Appeal ruled in *Kimber* [1983] 1 WLR 1118 on the then existing crime of indecent assault that *Morgan* was not restricted to rape and that *dicta* to that effect in *Phekoo* were wrong. The accused was charged with indecent assault after he had sexually interfered with a mental patient. The court held that a mistaken belief that the woman was consenting was a defence, whether or not the mistake was based on reasonable grounds. It is now accepted that **Morgan** applies to all offences of subjective *mens rea*. The law is the same in Canada: **Pappajohn v R** (1980) 111 DLR (3d) 1. It may be that **Tolson** is restricted to bigamy.

Morgan is also applied to some defences. In **Williams** [1987] 3 All ER 411 the accused believed that a person was being attacked by X. In fact X was arresting him lawfully. It was said by the Court of Appeal that the accused was to be judged on the facts as he believed them to be. He believed that an assault was taking place. Therefore, he was not guilty of assault occasioning actual bodily harm on X when he attacked X. The accused did not intend to use unlawful force. He intended to use lawful force; that is, force to prevent a crime or in self-defence. His mistake negated his *mens rea*. **Williams** is thus an application of **Morgan**. (The conviction was overturned because the trial judge had misdirected the jury as to the burden of proof, so the above was *obiter*.) The court stressed that it was not dealing with any mental element necessary for a defence and the case could be distinguished on this basis. **Williams** was approved by the Privy Council in the following case.

Beckford v R [1988] AC 130

The accused, an armed police officer, was investigating a report that an armed man was terrorising his family. In fact the man was unarmed. The accused alleged that the man had been shooting and was killed when fire was returned. It was held that he had the defence of self-defence on the facts which he mistakenly thought existed.

The question to be asked in a case of mistaken self-defence is whether the accused's response was commensurate with the degree of risk which he believed to have been created by the attack under which he believed himself to be: **Oatridge** (1992) 94 Cr App R 367 (CA). The development of the law that in general both offences and defences require only an honest belief was approved by the House of Lords in **B v DPP** [2000] 2 AC 428. Lord Nicholls said:

> By definition the mental element in a crime is concerned with a subjective state of mind, such as intent or belief. To the extent that an overriding objective limit ('on reasonable grounds') is introduced, the subjective element is displaced. To that extent a person who lacks the necessary intent or belief may nevertheless commit the offence. When that occurs the defendant's 'fault' lies exclusively in falling short of an objective standard. His crime lies in his negligence. A statute may so provide expressly or by necessary implication. But this can have no place in a common law principle, of general application, which is concerned with the need for a mental element as an essential ingredient of a criminal offence.

B v DPP was followed by the House of Lords in **K** [2002] 1 AC 462. A mistake as to the victim's age in the then existing crime of indecent assault was a defence if the error was honestly made. The belief need not be on reasonable grounds.

The law is different in duress and presumably duress of circumstances. The accused must believe on reasonable grounds that he is under a threat. The line sometimes drawn between **Williams** and **Graham** [1982] 1 WLR 294 is that in the former case the mistake negated the mental element in respect of an element of the *actus reus* whereas in the latter the mistake related to a true defence, a concept separate from *actus reus* and *mens rea*. It is uncertain whether this distinction is the law. Certainly the mistake in duress does not negate the *mens rea*. A suggested reconciliation is that in respect of justificatory defences, such as prevention of crime, any mistake exculpates, but a reasonable mistake is needed in respect of excuses such as duress. Besides the line being difficult to draw it is hard to discern any reason for the distinction. Although the law is that outside bigamy and some defences a mistake, reasonable or not, as to a relevant element of an offence or defence grants a defence, the courts do not always apply the law correctly. In ***Brown*** (1985) 80 Cr App R 36 the court required reasonable grounds for a belief that a woman was not a common prostitute on a charge of attempting to procure a woman to become a common prostitute. Lord Nicholls in ***B v DPP*** did not advert to duress when he dealt with the common law presumption that an honest mistake exculpates. Lord Steyn spoke of the 'disharmony' which would occur if in respect of some offences only a reasonable mistake exculpated but again he made no attempt to overrule inconsistent authorities. ***Tolson*** is one of those authorities.

The rule in ***Morgan*** does not affect offences where Parliament provides a defence only where a mistake was reasonable. In relation to rape the Sexual Offences Act 2003 reversed ***Morgan***: a defence is now available only if the accused believed on reasonable grounds that the victim consented. Similarly ***Morgan*** does not affect the defences of duress by threats and duress of circumstances where the accused had to believe something on reasonable grounds (e.g. the existence of serious threats). This rule was indeed laid down after ***Morgan***. There seems to be no justification for treating duress and self-defence differently.

Mistake and crimes of recklessness and negligence

A person who makes an unreasonable mistake behaves negligently. Therefore he can be convicted of an offence of negligence. Only a defence based on reasonable grounds would exculpate. Crimes of ***Cunningham*** recklessness are treated under the principle in ***Morgan***.

Cunningham recklessness is described on pp. 110–16 in Chapter 3. Compare with *Caldwell* recklessness.

Intoxication and mistake

This topic is dealt with in the section on intoxication.

(a) Evidence of drunkenness to support a mistaken belief in the woman's consent to sexual intercourse was not admitted in ***Woods*** (1982) 74 Cr App R 312. Intoxication does not explain a mistake as to consent. Clause 88 of the draft Criminal Code, 1989, accepts the principle of ***Woods*** in sexual offences. However, for other offences evidence of intoxication causing a mistake will be admitted when intoxication is a defence to the crime charged.

(b) In ***Fotheringham*** (1988) 88 Cr App R 206 (CA), drunken sexual intercourse with a 14-year-old babysitter in the matrimonial bed in the mistaken belief that it was his wife did not give rise to a defence. A drunken mistake as to identity was irrelevant.

(c) Generally speaking a mistake brought about by drunkenness is no defence.

O'Grady [1987] QB 995 (CA)

The accused drank eight flagons of cider. He then killed his friend. He argued that if he had not killed his friend he would have been killed by him. The court held, seemingly by way of *dictum*, that where the defendant was mistaken in his belief that any force, or the force he used, was necessary, but that the mistake was caused by voluntary drunkenness, the defence failed. It did not matter whether the offence was one of basic or specific intent.

There was no drunkenness in **Williams**, above, so that case could be distinguished. Lord Lane CJ, who gave judgment in both authorities, said that the court was faced with two competing principles. The first was that the accused had acted only according to what he believed was necessary to protect himself. The second was that the victim was killed through the accused's drunken mistake and the public had to be protected. 'Reason recoils from the conclusion that in such circumstances a defendant is entitled to leave the court without a stain on his character.'

O'Grady was followed in **O'Connor** [1991] Crim LR 135 (CA). The accused had been drinking heavily. He got into an argument with the victim, whom he head-butted three times. It was held that where the defendant, due to self-induced intoxication, formed a mistaken belief that he was acting in self-defence, that plea failed. The trial judge was correct in not directing the jury how drunkenness affected self-defence. In **O'Connor** the court assumed that **O'Grady** was binding, but in fact the accused in **O'Grady** was convicted of manslaughter. Anything that court said about murder was *obiter*.

O'Grady is open to criticism. It creates an exception to the rule in **Williams** that a person has the defence of self-defence if he makes a mistake of fact. There is nothing in **Williams** to suggest that the court intended such an exception. One result of **O'Grady** is that if the accused is so drunk that he does not have the fault element, he will be acquitted of murder; however, if the accused was drunk and believed that the victim was attacking him, he cannot rely on self-defence. **O'Grady** is out of line with cases which give a defence to drunkenness for offences of specific intent.

The Law Commission, Report No. 177, *A Criminal Code for England and Wales*, 1989, recommended in para 8.42 that the **O'Grady** principle should be abolished because it was 'unthinkable to convict of murder a person who thought for whatever reason that he was acting to save his life and would have been acting reasonably if he had been right'. In the proposals drunkenness would be taken into account to determine whether the accused believed in the existence of exempting conditions such as self-defence. Another possibility suggested by J.C. Smith in [1994] CLP 101 is to convict the accused of gross negligence manslaughter.

Summary of the law of mistake of fact

If the accused makes a mistake of fact as to an element of the *actus reus*, the mistake is irrelevant if the offence is one of strict liability (**Prince**); if the offence is one of *mens rea*, the accused has a defence if he made the mistake honestly (**Morgan**), unless the offence is one of bigamy in which event the mistake must have been made on reasonable grounds (**Tolson**). Parliament can change any of these rules as it did in the Sexual Offences Act 2003.

Reform

The draft Criminal Code did not create a clause dealing with mistake of fact. The team of academics which drafted the precursor to the draft Criminal Code did provide a clause that 'ignorance or mistake . . . of fact . . . may negative a fault element of an offence'. In a footnote to para 8.32 the Law Commission commented:

> The real point of this statement was that even a mistake for which there are no reasonable grounds may be the reason why a person lacks the fault required for an offence. That this has not always been obvious is apparent from modern decisions in which it has had to be

pointed out that if, to constitute an offence, a person's conduct must be intentional with respect to a given circumstance, it is inconsistent to demand that, to exclude liability, a mistake with respect to the circumstance must be based on reasonable grounds.

By cl 41(1), 'unless otherwise provided, a person who acts in the belief that a circumstance exists has any defence that he would have if the circumstance existed'. There is no requirement of reasonableness, though the absence of reasonableness is a matter of evidence towards showing that the accused did not have the belief. Therefore, if enacted this clause would change the law relating to mistakes and some defences such as duress.

If the Law Commission's recommendations are implemented, the law will be that there will be no 'defence of mistake', the logic being that mistake is simply a failure by the prosecution to prove intention, knowledge, or recklessness. J. M. Williams wrote 'Mistake of fact: The legacy of *Pappajohn* v *The Queen*' (1985) 63 CBR 597 at 604–605 (footnote and emphasis omitted):

> Mistake of fact is not a 'defence' in the same sense that provocation, self-defence, duress, and necessity are defences. These latter defences justify or excuse, either partially or totally what would otherwise be criminal conduct. A mistake of fact which negates the *mens rea* renders the committed act innocent and thus there never arises any question of exonerating criminal conduct.

Mistake explains why the accused lacked *mens rea*. Clause 41 would override the present anomaly that a reasonable belief is needed in duress, but (only) an honest one in self-defence. That the present law's distinction is indefensible was well demonstrated by Professor D. W. Elliott 'Necessity, duress and self-defence' [1989] Crim LR 611. If a motorist drove his car at X in self-defence, he would have the defence of self-defence, if he unreasonably made an error that X was attacking him when X was not. However, if he unreasonably believed that X was attacking him when X was not, he cannot rely on the defence of duress of circumstances.

The reader is invited to speculate why the courts in **Tolson**, **Prince** and **Morgan** came to three different conclusions when they were faced by three crimes falling within the broad field of sexual offences.

Reform of mistake in rape

The Law Commission in its Policy Paper, *Consent in Sex Offences*, 2000, examined the arguments in favour of introducing the requirement of reasonable belief in the victim's consent. In favour of revising the law were the following:

(a) 'Belief in consent is an easy defence to raise but hard to disprove.'

(b) 'It encourages defences to run which pander to outmoded and offensive assumptions about the nature of sexual relationships. The more stupid and sexist the man and his attitudes, the better chance he has of being acquitted on this basis.'

(c) 'The damage is done to the woman [sic] by the act of rape. She is entitled to expect the protection of the criminal law where, on any view, the man has acted on an unreasonably held assumption about her consent.'

(d) 'The mistaken belief arises in a situation where the price of the man's (gross) neglect is very high, and paid by the woman, whereas the cost to him in time and effort of informing himself of the position is minimal by comparison.'

In favour of the subjective test are these arguments:

(a) 'A person should not be guilty of a serious sexual offence . . . on the basis of negligence.'

(b) 'The burden is on those who argue for a change . . . to demonstrate that persons are being inappropriately acquitted . . . No such evidence has been produced.'

(c) Whose reasonableness would apply? Would it be that of the accused, that of the jury, that of the hypothetical reasonable person?

(d) Juries can sort out fact from fiction.

(e) It would be rare for an accused to contend that he has a belief for which he had no reasonable grounds.

(f) The introduction of reasonableness might make juries convict of rape even less than they do now.

The Law Commission thought that the subjective approach should be retained. However, the accused would have no defence if he was intoxicated and in assessing whether the accused believed the victim did consent, the jury should take into account whether he availed himself of the opportunity to ascertain whether the victim was consenting or not.

The government refused to accept the Commission's recommendations and in the Sexual Offences Act 2003 only a reasonable mistake provides a defence. The result is, in the Law Commission's words, 'a person [is now] guilty of a serious sexual offence . . . on the basis of negligence.'

Intoxication

Introduction

> We confess that the doctrine touching cases of this character is not placed upon the clearest ground in the books (*Bishop's Criminal Law*, Vol 1, 9th edn (Little, Brown & Co, 1923) para 320).

This section discusses intoxication as a defence, not as an offence. It concentrates on situations where the accused did the prohibited act, does not have the required mental element, but is responsible for the fact that he does not possess it because of his self-induced intoxication. Drunkenness was a crime punishable by imprisonment in the stocks or a fine from 1607 (4 James 1, c 5) to 1828 (9 Geo 4, c 61, s 35) but the law seems not to have been enforced. There is now no offence of (simple) drunkenness, but some instances are punished, e.g. being drunk and disorderly and drink-driving. The connection between intoxication and criminality is not a causal one: being drunk does not mean that the accused will necessarily commit an offence. Some drugs such as alcohol do, however, release inhibitions, and many who commit crimes have taken drugs, whether dangerous ones or ones not classified in law as being dangerous, e.g. alcohol. It is thought that the majority of non-fatal offences are committed when the accused was drunk. The then Home Secretary, Jack Straw, was reported in *The Guardian*, 18 July 2000, as saying: 'Some 40% of violent crimes are committed when the offender is under the influence of alcohol, as are 78% of assaults and 88% of criminal damage incidents.' Over 50% of rapists are intoxicated, according to the website of Alcohol Concern, www.alcoholconcern.org.uk. Intoxication is considered here as a defence whether complete or in part, but it should be noted that intoxication sometimes makes the crime more serious than it otherwise would have been, as in drink-driving.

Involuntary intoxication

This section is largery restricted to voluntary intoxication. Where drunkenness was caused by a medically prescribed drug, the accused's mistaking an intoxicant for a non-intoxicant (such as thinking a recreational drug is a paracetamol), someone spiking the accused's drink (by, for example, putting LSD or Rohypnol into the accused's vodka), forcing him to drink alcohol, or perhaps an adult deceiving a young person into taking alcohol, the question whether the accused will be convicted of an offence was thought to depend on his state of mind. Authorities are rare but include *Pearson* (1835) 168 ER 131. The sole modern authority is the controversial one of *Kingston* [1995] 2 AC 355. A man enticed a 15-year-old boy to his flat and gave him some soporific drugs. The boy fell asleep. In order to blackmail him the man invited the appellant to his flat. He apparently also drugged him. The appellant sexually abused the boy. The man photographed and taped him so doing. The appellant admitted that he was a homosexual paedophile. The trial judge directed the jury that if the accused was so drugged that he did not intend to commit the crime, he was not guilty but if he did despite the drugs intend to commit it, he was guilty because a drugged intent is nevertheless an intent. The jury convicted but the conviction was quashed. The Court of Appeal held that if alcohol or drugs were surreptitiously given to the accused, he was not guilty if because of his intoxication he forms an intention which he would not have formed had he been sober. 'The intent itself arose out of circumstances for which he bears no blame.' Therefore, he was acquitted even though he had the *mens rea* of the crime. He was morally blameless. *Kingston* in the Court of Appeal was strongly criticised. The accused did intend to commit indecent assault. He had the *mens rea*. Accordingly, he should have been convicted. The fact that he could not resist his impulse is irrelevant (as in insanity), as is the fact that someone made him intoxicated. Contrary to the court's view his involuntary intoxication did not negate his *mens rea*. Certainly he was not responsible for getting into a drugged state, but he may be responsible for what he does in that state. If *Kingston* (CA) had been correct it would presumably apply where a rogue has forced alcohol down the accused's throat or threatened him or another with violence if he did not drink it, and perhaps when the accused has taken drugs by mistake. For an attempt to support *Kingston* (CA) if the accused was not a practising paedophile, see G. R. Sullivan 'Involuntary intoxication and beyond' [1994] Crim LR 272, who argues that: 'It is not a fair test of character to remove surreptitiously a person's inhibitions and confront him with a temptation he ordinarily seeks to avoid.'

On appeal [1995] 2 AC 355 Lord Mustill, with whom the other Lords agreed, said that there was no principle in English law, as the Court of Appeal thought there was, that if no blame was attached to the accused, he did not have the *mens rea* and therefore was not guilty of any offence. Moral judgments do not affect the criminality of the act though they may affect the sentence. '*Rea*' means criminally, not morally, wrong. Blame related to sentence, not to substantive law. It was no defence to argue that he would not have done what he did had he been sober, except for insanity where the accused did intend to commit the offence. Lord Mustill approved the views of academic commentators in relation to the Court of Appeal's ruling. If the defence existed on these facts, bogus claims as to involuntary intoxication might succeed. Whether the intoxication was voluntary or involuntary, 'a drunken intent is still an intent', as was stated in **Sheehan** [1975] 1 WLR 739 (CA). While the House of Lords was not bound by any authority, it considered that when the accused was so involuntarily intoxicated that he did not form an intent, there is a defence. However, in terms of principle there was no defence of irresistible impulse deriving from innate causes (an example might be kleptomania), and therefore there should be no defence for irresistible impulse arising from a mixture of innate forces and 'external disinhibition'. Accordingly, the appeal was allowed. It should be noted that the distinction between basic and specific intent offences does not apply to involuntary intoxication. In criticism of **Kingston** (HL) it can be said that excuse defences are not all predicated on the absence of *mens rea*.

Intoxication is not involuntary when the accused did not know that the wine drunk was of high alcohol content: **Allen** [1988] Crim LR 698 (CA). The outcome may be explained by saying that the effects of alcohol are in any case unpredictable. It is interesting to compare **Allen** with the law stated under preliminary point (e) below. Failure to foresee the consequences of wine led to guilt; failure to foresee the consequences of drugs led to acquittal! The law may be different where the accused thought that the wine was non-alcoholic, rather than low in alcohol. In **Shippam** [1971] Crim LR 434, it was held that spiking of drinks was a special reason not to disqualify a person for driving with a blood alcohol level above the prescribed limit, but the argument that he should not have been guilty at all does not appear to have been put. The successful argument in **Shippam** seems to have been that the accused was driving voluntarily. His involuntary drunkenness was irrelevant to that fact. It is uncertain whether intoxication is involuntary where the accused has a medical condition which he does not know about which predisposes him to becoming intoxicated more quickly than he otherwise would.

Drunkenness which is self-induced is also not a defence where the accused did possess the relevant *mens rea*. If a drunken person forms an intention to kill and does kill, he will be convicted of murder. If the accused killed his wife in a fit of temper, alcohol may explain why he was easily provoked. His inhibitions have been removed but the relaxation of inhibitions is not a defence. He is guilty of murder. Similarly, the fact that the accused would not have acted in the way that he did if he had not been drunk is no defence. The contrasting situation is where the accused while drunk stumbles against his wife, knocking her under a train. Drunkenness is relevant because he is claiming that he did not form malice aforethought. Intoxication is not a defence when the accused says that he did not foresee the consequence of his behaviour because of his intoxication.

Preliminary points

(a) The accused does not have this defence if he gets drunk to give himself Dutch courage. In **Attorney-General for Northern Ireland v Gallagher** [1963] AC 349 the accused formed the intent to kill his wife, drank most of a bottle of whiskey, and killed her. (See also Chapter 3 on contemporaneity.) He could not use drunkenness as a defence and was guilty of murder.

(b) Drunkenness must be 'very extreme' for the defence to apply: **Stubbs** (1989) 88 Cr App R 53. The Court of Appeal of New Zealand in **Kamipeli** [1975] 2 NZLR 610 seems to have approved the trial judge's direction that the accused must be 'blind drunk', though as that court held the prosecution need not go so far as to prove that the accused was 'acting as a sort of automaton without his mind functioning'. (If the evidence is not such that the accused's mind was not working because of alcohol, it may still be that the prosecution cannot prove that he intended to commit the offence.) The Supreme Court of Canada in *Daviault v R* (1995) 118 DLR (4th) 469 said that the accused had to be 'in such an extreme degree of intoxication that [he was] in a state akin to automatism or insanity'. Only rarely will a person be in such a condition. The court was relying on the judgment of Wilson J in *Bernard* [1988] 2 SCR 833. Accordingly, it is not enough to demonstrate that the accused has been drinking heavily for the effect of alcohol varies from person to person: *Broadhurst v R* [1964] AC 441. For example, in *Groark* [1999] Crim LR 669 the accused had drunk 10 pints of beer but was not drunk. English cases are to the effect that the accused must be so intoxicated that he did not form the requisite intent as laid down by the definition of the offence: see, e.g., *McKnight*, *The Times*, 5 May 2000 (CA), relying on the advice of Lord Hope in *Sooklal v State of Trinidad and Tobago* [1999] 1 WLR 2011 (PC). In *McKnight* the accused said that while she was drunk, she was not 'legless'. She gave a complete account of the incident in which she had killed the victim. The Court of Appeal held that her perceptions had not been altered by the alcohol and therefore she had no defence to a charge of murder. The trial judge was correct in not leaving the defence of intoxication to the jury. There is no need for the accused to be so drunk as to be almost unconscious: *Brown* [1998] Crim LR 485 (CA). Lord Denning in *Gallagher* said that the accused must be 'rendered so stupid by drinking that he does not know what he is doing . . . as where . . . a drunken man thought his friend was a theatrical dummy and stabbed him to death'. As we shall see, even if the accused is so drunk, he does not have a defence to all offences but only specific intent ones. In fact the amount of intoxication needed to afford a defence does not seem to have caused difficulties: Law Reform Commission of Ireland's Report on *Intoxication*, LRC 51, 1995, 2.

(c) If the accused's acts look involuntary, the defence is one of intoxication, not automatism, if the involuntariness was due to drunkenness. In legal terms the accused is acting voluntarily, and is so doing even though the imbibing and the deed are separated in time. However, if the intoxication is such that it falls within the *M'Naghten* rules, the defence is insanity, not intoxication. Since alcohol and other drugs are 'external' causes only rarely will intoxication amount to insanity. Delirium tremens ('DTs') is an example of a disease of the mind within *M'Naghten*. Normally even though the intoxication causes delusions there will not be a disease of the mind. In automatism and insanity basically the accused could not avoid the condition; in drunkenness he could. For the law on insanity, see Chapter 9. One issue which has arisen dealing with the borderline between insanity and intoxication is the following. A person is not insane if he cannot resist an impulse. If his irresolution in the face of an impulse is exacerbated by alcohol, he still cannot have the defence of insanity: *Gallagher*.

(d) The burden of proof is on the prosecution. *Dicta* to the contrary in *DPP v Beard* [1920] AC 479 are wrong: *Sheehan*. The Privy Council in *Broadhurst* accepted that *Woolmington v DPP* [1935] AC 462 had altered the burden of proof.

(e) The rules on intoxication as a defence apply to both alcohol and those drugs which are liable to make the user aggressive, dangerous or unpredictable. The definition of 'intoxicant' has not been a problem for the courts. Sedative drugs, however, such as valium are not to be classed with alcohol, according to *Bailey* [1983] 2 All ER 503 (see under automatism) and *Hardie* [1984] 3 All ER 848 (CA). In *Hardie* the accused was charged with damaging property with intent to endanger life or being reckless as to whether life would be endangered. He had taken valium (it had not been prescribed for him) and set fire to a bedroom. It was held that the effect of sedative drugs was not the same as intoxicating drugs or alcohol, which can produce aggression and unpredictable behaviour. Therefore, the accused is not (subjectively) reckless in taking his tablets, if the accused does not appreciate the risk of volatile behaviour. It may not be easy to decide which drugs have these dangerous effects and which do not. Presumably drugs like cocaine and LSD would be classified as dangerous ones; heroin, which is an opiate, should for that reason be categorised with valium, but it is doubtful whether a court would so hold. The court did, however, say that he would nevertheless be guilty of reckless driving. If so, he would nowadays be guilty of dangerous driving. Presumably the argument is that he should not take any drug not knowing of the consequences of so doing. If, however, he does realise that he might act aggressively, unpredictably or uncontrollably, his behaviour is reckless and he is liable for any crime of recklessness which he commits under the influence of the drug. He need not foresee the actual occurrence of any specific risk. These rules apply whether or not these drugs were medically prescribed. The line between drugs which sedate and drugs which cause aggression is not necessarily a clear-cut one. Indeed valium causes aggressive behaviour in some people. It is strange that the determination whether each drug is dangerous or not is left to the judge.

(f) Presumably the accused would have a defence if the alcohol were prescribed by a doctor. Alcohol given to a person after an accident would, it is thought, be treated similarly.

(g) Loss of memory caused by drunkenness does not excuse the accused's behaviour if he did what he did intentionally: **R v C** [1992] Crim LR 642 (CA).

The defence of intoxication is confused (Fig. 8.1). There is no easy way of stating the law. One reason for this mess is that drunkenness provides an arena for two conflicting principles. The first is the need to punish people who have acted wrongly. The second is that an accused who is intoxicated may not realise what he is doing and is not therefore deserving of punishment.

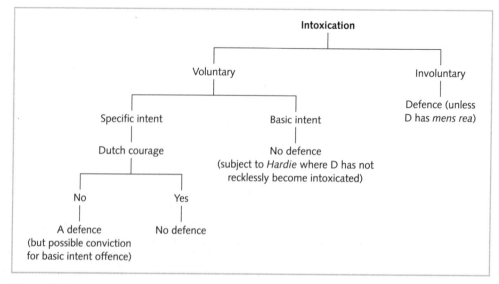

Figure 8.1 Intoxication

The special rules on intoxication

Note that 'specific intent' and 'basic intent' are not to be confused with 'intention' as defined in Chapter 3.

The law is that if the jury accepts the evidence of intoxication, the accused will not be convicted if the crime is one of 'specific intent', but will if the offence is one of 'basic intent'. For example, on a murder charge, murder being classified as a crime of specific intent, the accused's intoxication is relevant on the question whether he had malice aforethought. In other words, intention and intoxication are put together in a specific intent case. Where the accused is charged with murder and the accused either had direct intent or he did not, intoxication is taken into account at the point of determining whether he intended to kill or commit GBH. In an oblique intent case of murder, 'drink is relevant to the question whether the defendant appreciated that his actions were virtually certain to result in death or really serious bodily harm' (*Hayes* [2002] EWCA Crim 1945). Contrary to what was thought at the time of *Beard* – and contrary to what is still sometimes said by the Court of Appeal (see *McKnight*, above) – one does not inquire whether the accused was capable of forming the specific intent but whether he did actually have the intent: *Sheehan* and other cases including *O'Connor* [1991] Crim LR 135 (CA), *Horton*, unreported, 20 January 1992, *Cole* [1993] Crim LR 301 (CA), *Hawkins* [1993] Crim LR 888 and *Bowden* [1993] Crim LR 380 (CA). The law is the same in Australia: *O'Connor* (1980) 54 ALJR 349 (HCA). If the accused did have the necessary fault element, he is guilty whether or not he was intoxicated. One looks at the accused's mind, not at what a reasonable person might have thought. The term 'basic intent' covers all offences to which intoxication is not a defence including those which can be committed recklessly or negligently. If the crime is a basic intent one, the accused is convicted even though he did not know what he was doing. He is guilty even though he did not intend or advert to the consequences of his behaviour. The difficulty is to distinguish between basic and specific intent offences. As Lord Mustill said in *Kingston*, above: 'this area of law is controversial, as regards the content of the rules, their intellectual foundations, and their capacity to furnish a practical and just solution'.

The law was first authoritatively declared in *DPP v Beard* [1920] AC 479. Before 1957 there was a rule that a killing in the course of a felony was murder. This rule was called constructive murder or the felony/murder rule. Rape was a felony. The accused was committing a rape on a girl. He pressed his thumbs on her neck and killed her. Because of the doctrine of constructive murder, he was guilty of murder if the prosecution could show that he intended to rape and did kill. There was no need as nowadays to show that he intended to kill or commit grievous bodily harm. Lord Birkenhead stated that in those circumstances the accused had no defence unless he was so drunk as to be incapable of forming the intent to commit rape. (The question now is whether he did form the intent.) The accused could form this intent. Therefore, he was guilty of murder. Lord Birkenhead went on to utter *dicta* of high authority.

(1) If the accused is insane through drink, such as when he has delirium tremens, his defence is insanity, not intoxication.

The fact that the insanity was caused by drunkenness is irrelevant.

(2) Evidence of drunkenness which renders the accused incapable of forming the specific intent essential to constitute the crime should be taken into consideration with the other facts proved in order to determine whether or not he had this intent.

In *Beard* the accused did not make himself so drunk that he could not commit rape. The *dictum* is in terms of evidence. Therefore, the jury can reject the evidence and deal with the case in the usual fashion. Moreover, since intoxication relates to evidence in crimes of specific intent, it is a misnomer to call intoxication a defence; rather, it is a failure by the prosecution to prove all elements of the offence, namely the intent required is the definition of the offence. It should also be noted that intoxication does not negate *mens rea*; it is part of the evidence which is added to all the other evidence to determine whether the accused did have the *mens rea*.

> (3) Evidence of drunkenness falling short of a proved incapacity to form the intent necessary to constitute the crime, and merely establishing that his mind was affected by drink so that he more readily gave way to some violent passion, does not rebut the presumption that a man intends the natural consequences of his conduct.

Section 8 of the Criminal Justice Act 1967 qualifies the third proposition. A court or jury is no longer bound to infer from the facts that a person intends the natural consequences of his action. The triers of fact must look at the whole evidence to decide whether the accused did have the requisite intent or foresight. Section 8 does not make drunkenness purely a matter of evidence whether the accused did or did not have *mens rea*. It is still treated as a matter of substantive law: **DPP v Majewski** [1977] AC 443.

The second proposition is the difficult one. There is no restriction to crimes of intention, though it is likely that Lord Birkenhead simply meant 'specific intent' to be 'intent'. The necessity is to distinguish between specific and basic intent offences, though the term 'basic intent' occurs nowhere in Lord Birkenhead's speech. As M. Goode put it 'Some thoughts on the present state of the "defence" of intoxication' (1984) 8 Crim LJ 104 at 105: 'If there was no really coherent distinction, then the labels "specific" and "basic" intent were just that: labels. One might just as well have called murder a crime of "bacon" and manslaughter a crime of "eggs".' What has happened is that judges have thought that 'specific intent' bears a definite meaning in law different from 'intent' and they have sought to distinguish 'specific' from 'basic' intent. On the distinction rests English law.

The courts have struggled with defining the distinction. In **Gallagher**, Lord Denning followed **Beard** to hold that drunkenness was no defence unless it amounted to insanity or the crime was one of specific intent. He said that if drink impairs the accused's powers of perception so that he does not realise that what he is doing is dangerous, he has no defence if a sober and reasonable person in his place would appreciate the danger. This proposition does not occur in **Beard**, and if drunkenness is incompatible with specific intent, why is it not incompatible with foresight? Lord Denning stated that lack of self-control or moral sense induced by intoxication was no defence. In **Gallagher** the fact that the accused's psychomotor state was made worse by alcohol did not give him a defence of drunkenness if the effect of the alcohol made it harder for the accused to exercise self-control. Lord Denning relied on **Beard** and an anonymous case from 1748 (where a drunken nurse put a baby on a fire, thinking it was a log) to show that where the crime is one of specific intent, intoxication is a defence if the accused did not have that intent. It could be argued that the nurse's case is not one of specific intent because she had no *mens rea* at all. Lord Denning seems to have defined specific intent to mean crimes of ulterior intent (doing X with intent to do X or Y). Certainly all such crimes are specific intent ones, but the term 'specific intent' is wider. Lord Birkenhead may have meant 'specific intent' to mean the intent which forms part of the mental element in the offence. The mental element in murder is the intent to kill or commit grievous bodily harm. That intent is the 'specific' intent of murder. On this approach 'specific' adds nothing to 'intent'.

In *Gallagher* the earlier intention to kill was added to the *actus reus*, which took place after the accused had become drunk. This Dutch courage rule is at variance with the general principle of contemporaneity in criminal law. The argument is that such a breach is justified by catching dangerous people. *Lipman* [1970] 1 QB 152 exemplifies the continuing tendency of judges not to let defendants go free as they would if general principles of law were applied but to bend the law or create exceptions in order to convict 'manifestly guilty' persons of something, though it might be argued that the accused was not manifestly guilty.

Lipman [1970] 1 QB 152

The accused and his girlfriend took some LSD. Under the influence of the drug he hallucinated that he was being attacked by giant snakes. He awoke the next morning to find his girlfriend dead, eight inches of sheet having been pushed down her throat. Lord Widgery CJ held that intoxication through drugs formed part of the defence of drunkenness. Applying *Gallagher* manslaughter was a crime of basic intent. Intoxication was no defence to basic intent offences. Therefore, the accused was guilty of manslaughter. The House of Lords refused leave to appeal.

Criticism of *Lipman* has been strong. In *Beard* the accused, who was guilty, intended to rape. In *Lipman* the defendant, who did not intend any offence, was guilty of manslaughter. The accused had no 'mind' because he was under the influence of drugs; how could he have a *mens rea*? At the time of the killing he had no *mens rea*. At the time of taking the drug he had committed no *actus reus*. The contemporaneity rule was broken. Lord Birkenhead did say in *Beard* that drunkenness was no defence to manslaughter but did not relate his remarks to a distinction between specific and basic intent. Even in manslaughter the accused is guilty only if he did have some type of *mens rea*. The type of manslaughter at issue in *Lipman* was constructive or unlawful act manslaughter. There has to be an unlawful act, but the accused did not commit one because his mind did not accompany his act. If the unlawful act was the stuffing of the sheet into the victim's mouth, he was unconscious at that time. If the unlawful act was the taking of the drugs, that consumption did not cause her death and anyway taking drugs is not an offence: it is possession which is the crime. Possessing drugs did not kill the girlfriend. Lord Widgery CJ did not tackle this objection. It might be argued that the court could have relied on a different form of manslaughter, manslaughter by gross negligence, but if the accused was unconscious at the time, how could he be careless? There is still the separation in time between the grossly negligent taking of the drugs and the death. *Lipman* looks like the Court of Appeal's response to drugs, as in part does the next case.

Both *Lipman* and *Majewski*, above, punish really the act of becoming intoxicated, but the punishment is based on the outcome of the actions of the accused, whether the accused was acting consciously or not. Lord Salmon in *Majewski* approved both *Lipman* and *Beard*.

DPP v *Majewski* [1977] AC 443

A man spent 24 hours getting drugged and drunk. He smashed windows and attacked a police officer. The seven judgments in the House of Lords say different things but basically there was wide support for Lord Russell's analysis of Lord Birkenhead's speech in *Beard*.

Specific intent covered:

(a) ulterior or further intent such as wounding with intent to do grievous bodily harm;

(b) where the *mens rea* extends beyond the intent to do the act. On this approach assault is a basic intent crime. The *actus reus* includes the apprehension of force. The *mens rea* is intending or being reckless as to the victim's apprehension of force. The *mens rea* does not extend beyond the *actus reus*.

Lord Simon considered that 'specific intent' meant the 'purposive element' (i.e. direct intent) in a crime. He did not further define purposive element, and the term is difficult to fit in with present law. Rape is a crime involving a purpose, but it is a crime of basic intent, to which drunkenness is not a defence. All Law Lords agreed that **Beard** should stand and that to depart from **Beard** would be contrary to public policy because the rule punished persons who got drunk and misbehaved. The community needs protection from drunken violence, and if violent drunks were not convicted, the public would have contempt for the law. Therefore, this area of law is not based on logic. Lord Salmon stated:

> I accept that there is a degree of illogicality in the rule that intoxication may excuse . . . one type of intention and not another. This illogicality is, however, acceptable because the benevolent part of the rule removes undue harshness without imperilling safety and the stricter part of the rule works without imperilling justice. It would be just as ridiculous to remove the benevolent part of the rule . . . as it would be to adopt the alternative of removing the stricter part of the rule for the sake of preserving absolute logic.

As Lord Edmund-Davies said, 'It is unethical to convict a man of a crime requiring a guilty state of mind when *ex hypothesis* he lacked it.' Another way of putting this is to say that drunkenness is not in conformity with criminal law principles. For example, intoxication is a defence to grievous bodily harm with intent, but not to maliciously inflicting grievous bodily harm. Yet, if intoxication negates the *mens rea* of the former offence, why does it prove it in the latter? To say as Lord Simon did that performing a prohibited act when insensible through drink is as wrongful as *mens rea* does not mean that the insensible accused has *mens rea*. Before a person can be convicted of an offence where the mental element is subjective recklessness, the prosecution should have to prove that state of mind. They do not have to prove it when the accused is intoxicated. If the accused contends that he thought because of intoxication there was no risk, *Majewski* will convict him automatically of a 'subjective recklessness' offence. The presumption of innocence is not applied. The outcome of *Majewski* was that the highest court had decided that there was a distinction between basic and specific intent, but could not say what that difference was.

The public policy concerns in *Majewski* have come in for criticism. A drunken person is hardly likely to be deterred by the law, even if he knew what it was. In countries where intoxication is taken into account with the other evidence in determining *mens rea* there is not proportionally more crime than in England. Indeed intoxication by stripping away inhibitions may well show that the accused did have the requisite fault element for the crime charged. It is also argued that it is morally wrong to convict people of an offence when the form of behaviour which the law should penalise is that of getting into the intoxicated state. At present people are convicted of offences when they did not have the required *mens rea*.

For a full explanation of recklessness, see pp 110–16 in Chapter 3.

The most authoritative case at present is **MPC v Caldwell** [1982] AC 341, which in relation to intoxication is unaffected by the overruling in **G** [2004] 1 AC 1034 (HL) of Lord Diplock's definition of recklessness.

MPC v *Caldwell* [1982] AC 341

The accused did some work for the owner of a hotel. They quarrelled. The accused got drunk and set fire to the hotel. No one was injured, but there was some damage. He was charged, *inter alia*, with arson contrary to s 1(2) and (3) of the Criminal Damage Act 1971 in that he damaged property with intent to endanger life or being reckless whether life was endangered. He claimed he was so drunk that he never thought he was endangering life.

The majority's speech was delivered by Lord Diplock. He argued:

(a) 'If the only mental state capable of constituting the necessary *mens rea* for an offence under s 1(2) were that expressed in the words intending by the destruction or damage to endanger the life of another, it would have been necessary to consider whether the offence was to be classified as one of "specific" intent for the purposes of the rule of law which this House affirmed and applied in *DPP* v *Majewski* (1977); and plainly it is.' (That is, the *mens rea*, intent to endanger life, goes beyond the *actus reus*, criminal damage.)

(b) 'However, this is not . . . a relevant enquiry where "being reckless, as to whether the life of another should be thereby endangered" is an alternative mental state.'

(c) 'The speech of Lord Elwyn-Jones in *Majewski*, with which Lord Simon, Lord Kilbrandon and I agreed, is authority that self-induced intoxication is no defence to a crime in which recklessness is enough to constitute the necessary *mens rea*.'

(d) 'Reducing oneself by drink or drugs to a condition in which the restraints of reason and conscience are cast off was held to be a reckless course of conduct.' (There is a slippage in the reasoning between (c) and (d). 'Reckless' is used in two different senses. In (c) 'reckless' bears its *mens rea* meaning. In (d) it bears a non-criminal law meaning. By becoming drunk the accused does not become aware of the *actus reus* he may perform when he is drunk. The effect is that the accused is guilty of a crime of basic intent even though he did not have the *mens rea* of the crime.)

(e) 'In the instant case, the fact that the respondent was unaware of the risk of endangering the lives of residents in the hotel owing to his self-induced intoxication would be no defence if that risk would have been obvious to him had he been sober.'

The difference between the previous definition (*mens rea* goes beyond the *actus reus*) and the *Caldwell* recklessness one is seen from the crime charged in *Caldwell* itself. In s 1(2) of the 1971 Act the *mens rea* (intent to endanger life or recklessness thereto) goes beyond the *actus reus* (criminal damage). However, recklessness forms part of the *mens rea*, and therefore the crime is one of basic intent.

Accordingly where the defence was solely defined in terms of intention the distinction between basic and specific intent was relevant. If the offence were defined in terms of recklessness, getting drunk was reckless and the accused was guilty of the offence without the prosecution having to prove recklessness. Proof of intoxication amounted to proof of recklessness. The accused is deemed to be reckless. There is no need to show that at the time of getting intoxicated the accused foresaw the *actus reus* of the offence with which he is charged. In the words of the Law Commission in its Report No. 229, *Legislating the Criminal Code: Intoxication and Criminal Liability*, 1995, para 1.19, 'The intentional taking of an intoxicant without regard to its possible consequences is properly treated as a substitute for the mental element normally required.' Lord Mustill spoke to this effect in *Kingston*, above. The accused cannot rely on the absence of *mens rea* when that is caused by his own act of getting intoxicated. This approach, however, takes no account of the principle of concurrence stated at the start of Chapter 1. Once the accused has got intoxicated, he should no longer be regarded as reckless. Therefore, he is not reckless at the time of the *actus reus*. In **Cullen** [1993] Crim LR 936 (CA) the court laid down English law: once the prosecution proved that the accused started a fire, he was guilty of (aggravated) arson if there was an obvious and serious risk of damage to property and of danger to life. He did not have to foresee either risk. The position is even stronger with regard to strict offences and crimes of negligence. The accused is guilty without proof of recklessness. Intoxication shows that the accused was negligent, and in strict offences no state of mind is relevant. The rule applies despite the separation in time between getting drunk and the forbidden conduct.

This 'constructive recklessness' is also impossible to justify from the viewpoint of the principle of legality, also discussed in Chapter 1. It is not the fault element stated in the crime which is relevant but the fact that the accused got drunk. After **Caldwell** all crimes of recklessness are basic intent offences, to which intoxication supplies the mental element of recklessness, for the prosecution do not have to prove recklessness, only drunkenness. It is neither subjective nor objective recklessness. (What happened to the principle that the prosecution must prove all elements of the offence beyond reasonable doubt?) The result is a fiction. The accused is deemed to be reckless. As with all fictions current law is difficult to justify rationally. The House of Lords in **Caldwell** were adamant that whether there was recklessness was a matter for the jury, but that proposition is difficult to accept when intoxication is the recklessness element in an offence. The effect of **Caldwell** on drunkenness is this: the prosecution has to show that the accused gave no thought to an obvious and serious risk. It is irrelevant why no thought was given. Therefore, it is immaterial that it was intoxication which caused the accused not to give any thought. Accordingly, **Majewski** is not in point. The risk of harm from getting intoxicated need not relate to the actual injury or damage caused. The test for the obviousness of the risk under **Caldwell** is whether or not the risk would have been obvious to a reasonable prudent bystander. That paragon is not intoxicated by alcohol or drugs. The fact that the accused was intoxicated is irrelevant. That he was drunk merely explains why he gave no thought but does not excuse him. His drunkenness supplies the *mens rea* of recklessness. He is guilty of a basic intent crime if he would have been aware of the risk but for his intoxication.

The Supreme Court of Canada in **Daviault v R** (1995) 118 DLR (4th) 469 by a majority rejected the **Caldwell** approach as being contrary to the fundamental principle of justice that each element of the offence has to be proved by the prosecution. The present English law by which proof of intoxication substitutes for proof of recklessness was in breach of this principle. The dissentients argued that a person who commits the *actus reus* of a general intent offence (in England a basic intent crime) when intoxicated deserves to be stigmatised as an offender and that the requirements of fundamental justice were satisfied by proof of intoxication without proof of *mens rea*. Sopinka J said that 'the rules of fundamental justice are satisfied by showing that the drunken state was attained through the accused's own blameworthy conduct'. The same rule applies to a person who puts himself into a state of automatism through his own fault. 'Society is entitled to punish those who of their own free will render themselves so intoxicated as to pose a threat to other members of the community.' Sopinka J added: 'to allow generally an accused . . . to plead absence of *mens rea* where he has voluntarily caused himself to be incapable of *mens rea* would be to undermine, indeed negate, that very principle of moral responsibility which the requirement of *mens rea* is intended to give effect to.' Besides intoxication being deemed to be recklessness for crimes where the *mens rea* includes recklessness, the usual connection between *actus reus* and *mens rea* is rendered unnecessary. For example, the accused is guilty of reckless criminal damage if he is drunk and damage happens to occur as a result of what he did when drunk: he need not recklessly cause criminal damage, yet he is guilty of that offence.

Outstanding problems

(a) One result of **Caldwell** is that the defence has been narrowed. Lord Birkenhead in **Beard** in one passage noted that specific intent was not exceptional. The minority in **Caldwell** saw that when *mens rea* is defined in terms of 'intentionally or recklessly', as modern statutes often are, there is no need for the prosecution to prove recklessness, only drunkenness. Only where intention alone is charged is intoxication possibly a defence.

Anomalies are created. Intoxication can be considered in a crime of attempted rape, but not in rape itself. Rape is a basic intent crime. After the Sexual Offences Act 2003 the *mens rea* includes negligence as to the victim's consent. All attempts are specific intent offences. It is conceded, however, that the position is unclear and some academics have argued that since some attempts may be committed recklessly, these are now basic intent offences. The argument runs that after **Khan** [1990] 1 WLR 815 the *mens rea* of rape and attempted rape is the same when the attempt is based on the failure of the accused to achieve penetration. Therefore, attempted rape based on this missing element is also a crime of basic intent. However, if the missing element in attempted rape is the victim's lack of consent, the *mens rea* of attempted rape is different from that of the full offence. An intent to have sexual intercourse without the consent of the victim is required and this form of attempted rape is a specific intent crime.

In **Fotheringham** (1988) 88 Cr App R 206 (CA), the accused made a drunken mistake that the person with whom he was having sexual intercourse was his wife, whereas it was a 14-year-old babysitter, whom his wife had told to sleep in the matrimonial bed. He was guilty of the offence of rape as then defined. If, however, he had stopped just short of penetration, he would not have been guilty of attempted rape. The law looks the wrong way round. In rape the accused's *mens rea* is in part the intention to penetrate. Yet rape is always a basic intent offence.

Fotheringham may be criticised. On one view of **Majewski**, drunkenness supplies recklessness. Therefore, evidence other than that of intoxication, tending towards showing that the accused did not have the type of foresight required by the crime, is irrelevant: he is deemed to have the *mens rea* because he is intoxicated. In this case, however, the accused did not make a mistake as to a 'reckless' element, consent, but as to an element defined solely in terms of intent. The accused did not intend to have unlawful sexual intercourse, 'unlawful' being then understood as 'outside marriage'. He intended to have sexual intercourse with his wife. That was lawful. His mistake was as to the identity of the woman and drunkenness explained why he made the error. Drunkenness does not supply intention. Another way of putting this proposition is to say that rape was a crime of basic intent as to consent (the accused was guilty at that time if he was reckless as to the woman's consent: after 2003 only negligence as to consent is required), but was a crime of specific intent in relation to the victim not being his wife. It is unlikely that the courts will hold that the answer to a question whether rape is a specific or basic intent crime depends on which element of the offence the accused has made a mistake. If *Fotheringham* is correct in stating that an offence is one of basic intent if any element of it may be committed recklessly, the list of specific offences in the section 'The present position' will have to be revised. For example, in burglary not all the elements of the *actus reus* need to be performed intentionally. The court stated: 'In rape self-induced intoxication is no defence, whether the issue be intention, consent or . . . mistake as to the identity of the victim.'

In *Woods* (1982) 74 Cr App R 312, the accused had drunk a lot and said that he was not aware that the woman was not consenting. The Court of Appeal held that the accused was guilty of rape as then defined when he made a mistake as to the woman's consent. Griffiths LJ said: 'The law, as a matter of social policy, has declared that self-induced intoxication is not a legally relevant matter to be taken into account when deciding as to whether or not a woman consents to intercourse.' This statement does not explain why the social policy does not apply to attempted rape and all specific intent offences. *Woods* is a decision to the effect that intoxication is not a legally relevant matter when the jury is considering whether the woman was consenting. By the law as it then existed, s 1(2) of the Sexual Offences (Amendment) Act 1976 as amended (now repealed), the jury had to judge the man's belief that the woman (or man) was consenting and could take into account the reasonableness of his belief and 'any other relevant matters'. Drunkenness was, however, held to be excluded. It was not one of the 'relevant matters'. Therefore, the jury is invited to inquire whether the accused believed the alleged victim was consenting but to exclude his intoxication. Since the intoxication led him to believe that the woman was consenting, he cannot explain why he thought that the woman (or the man) was consenting. That is, he was guilty of rape, since had he not been in a state of intoxication, he would have known that she (or he) did not consent. In other words, since the accused would have realised that the alleged victim was not consenting if he had been sober, he is automatically guilty of rape. He was reckless as to consent, even though the jury has not taken drunkenness into account. There is a view that *Woods* is restricted to rape. In other offences being drunk takes away the requirement that the prosecution proves recklessness in offences of recklessness. In rape intoxication is excluded from consideration. Parliament surely did not have this distinction in mind when it enacted the 1976 Act. *Woods* is certainly inconsistent with the principle that in crimes of recklessness intoxication supplies recklessness, i.e. once intoxication is proved, so is recklessness. In *Woods*, however, the court said that the accused is to be acquitted if he would not have had the *mens rea* of the offence had he been sober. In other words, evidence other than that of intoxication is relevant if it shows that the accused did not have the foresight required by the offence. This is inconsistent with *Majewski*. Perhaps the ratio of *Woods* is restricted to rape for in other offences there is no such provision as s 1(2), and that sub-section was repealed by the Sexual Offences Act 2003. The difficulty with intoxication being proof of recklessness may have been resolved by *Heard* [2007] EWCA Crim 125. Instead of intoxication supplying recklessness, the two states were said to be of broad equivalence in terms of culpability.

A case to compare with *Woods* is *Richardson* [1999] 1 Cr App R 392 (CA) – a non-rape case. The two defendants and the victim had been drinking. While indulging in horseplay the former inadvertently dropped the latter over a balcony: the injuries to the victim were serious. The court said that the defendants were guilty if they would have foreseen the risk of harm, had they been sober. However, the defendants could lead evidence of intoxication to show any absence of belief in consent. This is a surprising judgment. The charge was one of inflicting GBH, a basic intent offence, yet intoxication was relevant to the proof of law of consent. However, since the charge was one of s 20 of the Offences Against the Person Act 1861 the defendants' drunkenness proved that they had the *mens rea*, foresight of some harm.

(b) It is sometimes said that drunkenness operates as a defence in relation to serious offences and there is a lesser 'fall-back' crime. This proposition is not true. Lord Salmon noted this point in **Majewski**, above, when he said that specific intent 'was not confined to cases in which, if the prosecution failed to prove [a specific] intent, the accused could still be convicted of a lesser offence'. One might have thought that rape would be a specific intent offence with indecent assault as the 'fall-back' crime but in fact rape is a crime of basic intent. The present law was best summarised and criticised on this point by C. M. V. Clarkson, *Understanding Criminal Law*, 4th edn (Thomson, 2005) 114–15.

> The whole concept of 'specific intent' was devised to enable drunkenness to operate as a substantive *mitigating* factor to certain crimes, particularly murder. But . . . drunkenness is sometimes a partial excuse (where there is a lesser included offence of basic intent) but sometimes a *complete defence* – as with theft where no lesser included offence exists. There is no rationale underlying such a distinction; the result is sheer chance. [Emphasis added.]

(c) It is sometimes thought that s 8 of the Criminal Justice Act 1967 creates a difficulty. By it the triers of fact are instructed to consider 'all the evidence'. It does not say 'all the evidence except drunkenness'. Lord Diplock did not mention s 8 in **Caldwell**. (In **Majewski** the House of Lords said that the law on drunkenness was a substantive, not evidential, matter: s 8 deals only with legally relevant evidence. Drunkenness is not legally relevant.) **Caldwell** demonstrates that evidence of recklessness is not required if there is sufficient evidence of drunkenness. It looks as if the House of Lords has disobeyed Parliament by creating a presumption of recklessness.

(d) The law on drunkenness in relation to other defences causes problems. In **O'Grady** [1987] QB 995 (CA), the court said *obiter* that intoxication was not a defence where it induced a mistake. It does not matter whether the offence was basic (where **Majewski** would apply) or specific. In either event drunkenness is no defence. The accused is guilty of murder although he did not intend to kill or cause grievous bodily harm unlawfully for he believed that he was acting to prevent a crime on himself. Compare **Williams** [1987] 3 All ER 411 (CA): the accused does have a defence of preventing crime when he makes a mistake which is not induced by intoxication. There is a failure to prove all the elements of the offence when a non-drunken error occurs. P. Seago, *Criminal Law*, 4th edn (Sweet & Maxwell, 1994) 178, commented:

> [a]lthough the case involved a manslaughter conviction, Lord Lane indicated *obiter* that the same [i.e. guilty] would be true of murder. If this is so, then it means that a man who, because of voluntary intoxication, mistakenly believes he is shooting at a gorilla will have a defence to murder if he kills a human being, whereas a defendant will have no defence if he mistakenly believes, because of voluntary intoxication, that he is about to be violently attacked by a man whom he consequently shoots. It is hard to justify such a distinction or see how you can keep the issues of mistake and intent apart since they are merely different ways of looking at the same issue.

For the use of the 'gorilla' example in the successor text, see A. Reed and B. Fitzpatrick, *Criminal Law*, 3rd edn (Thomson, 2006) 199–200. (See also the English case of *O'Connor*, above, where drunkenness was relevant to intent but not to self-defence. A reasonable juror may not be able to perform this mental contortion. The court also thought that the *dictum* in *O'Grady* was *ratio*. It was in fact *dictum* because the accused had been acquitted of murder. Anything said about specific intent offences such as murder was not *ratio*.) Despite criticism by academics of *O'Grady* it was followed by the Court of Appeal in *Hatton* [2006] 1 Cr App R 247. The accused, who had consumed over 20 pints of beer, killed the victim with a sledgehammer. He argued that he believed the accused was an SAS soldier armed with a sword. His appeal against a conviction for murder was dismissed. The court certified that a point of law of public importance was involved but refused leave to appeal. It is about time that this issue was resolved by the Lords. The policy argument against *O'Grady* is that if the reason for the rules on intoxication is that the public must be protected from the intoxicated, a conviction for manslaughter does that and there is no need to convict of murder.

The contrasting case is the controversial one of *Jaggard* v *Dickinson* [1981] QB 527 (DC) (see Chapter 18). Under the Criminal Damage Act 1971, s 5(2)(a), evidence of drunkenness was used to establish what the accused believed. The accused believed she was entering a friend's house; in fact she was entering someone else's. She was intoxicated and would not have made this mistake had she been sober. She was not guilty of criminal damage contrary to s 1(1) of the 1971 Act, a basic intent offence. She had the lawful excuse that the person, her friend, entitled to consent to the damage, would have done so, had the friend known of the circumstances. The decision of Lord Donaldson MR was based on the language of the statute. Mustill LJ spoke more generally. Drunkenness on the facts did not negative intention or recklessness. It explained why the accused had the belief she did. By s 5(2) Parliament had isolated belief from the general law of recklessness. However that may be, to allow drunkenness to a crime of belief but not to one of recklessness looks strange. This strangeness is exacerbated when one recalls s 8 of the Criminal Justice Act 1967 discussed in (c) above. Why is not s 5(2) of the 1971 Act read in the same way? If intoxication is not relevant in s 8, why is it in s 5(2)? The Courts-Martial Appeal Court in *Young* [1984] 1 WLR 654, 658 generalised *Jaggard* v *Dickinson*: 'Where there is an exculpatory statutory defence of honest belief, self-induced intoxication is a factor which must be considered in the context of a subjective consideration of the individual state of mind.' In *Young* it was held that self-induced intoxication was no defence where the accused, charged with possessing a controlled drug, seeks to prove within s 28(3)(b) of the Misuse of Drugs Act 1971 that he did not believe or suspect, nor had any reason to do so, that a substance or product was a controlled drug, when he would have done so when sober. The outcome of the interrelation between *Caldwell* and *Jaggard* v *Dickinson* is amazing. If the accused damages another's property believing the property to be his own, that belief being induced by intoxication, he is guilty of criminal damage. If, however, he damages another's property believing that it belongs to a third party who would consent to the damage, if he knew of the circumstances, he is not guilty. The point can be taken further. *Jaggard* v *Dickinson* makes the drunken accused not guilty of criminal damage if he believed in consent; however, a drunken accused is guilty of rape if he believed mistakenly in the woman's consent. Lawyers have taken leave of their senses! One possible difference between *O'Grady* and *Jaggard* v *Dickinson* is that the former applies to common law offences, the latter to statutory ones. This distinction does not reflect any policy value and if true is an unfortunate one dependent on chance.

(e) What about intoxication in relation to other defences? In provocation where the accused believes falsely because he is drunk that he is being provoked, a subjective view is taken. He is judged on the facts as he believed them to be: *Letenock* (1917) 12 Cr App R 221 (CCA). It is possible that *Letenock* would not be followed nowadays since the law on both intoxication and provocation have moved on since the First World War. However, in relation to duress and duress of circumstances, the law is that only a mistake made on reasonable grounds exculpates: *Graham* [1982] 1 WLR 294 (CA). A mistake occasioned by alcohol is not one which has been made reasonably. Therefore, in relation to these defences a drunken mistake does not avail.

In respect of consent to assaults the Court of Appeal ruled in *Richardson*, above, that an erroneous belief that the victim is consenting to rough horseplay is a defence to the offence of inflicting GBH contrary to s 20 of the Offences Against the Person Act 1861, even though the mistake was caused by intoxication. The law contrasts strongly with that in *O'Grady* where it was held that a drunken mistake as to self-defence did not provide the accused with a defence. The Court did not consider *O'Grady* or cases such as *Woods* and *Fotheringham*, above. Moreover, *Richardson* is inconsistent with the rule that intoxication is no defence to a crime of basic intent.

(f) The serious problem remains that lawyers have failed to provide an adequate statement of which offences are specific intent ones.

(i) As we have seen, Lord Simon in *Majewski* said that specific intent crimes have a purposive element. This definition has already been criticised.

(ii) Sometimes it has been said that specific intent crimes are those in which intention alone is the sole mental element in respect of one or more elements of the *actus reus*. Murder, however, for many years was not defined solely in terms of intention, yet it was never doubted that murder was a specific intent crime. Handling is a crime of specific intent yet intent is not part of the *mens rea*, which is dishonesty and knowledge or belief.

(iii) An accepted definition of specific intent is that the *mens rea* goes beyond the *actus reus*. This is a helpful tip but is not a definition. All ulterior intent offences are specific intent crimes, but the concept of specific intent crimes is not restricted to ulterior intent ones, as murder itself demonstrates. Another illustration is criminal damage with intent to endanger life or being reckless as to whether life is endangered. The crime is not solely defined in terms of intent but the *mens rea* does extend beyond the *actus reus*. One of the definitions must be wrong but it is unclear which one it is. Section 18 of the Offences Against the Person Act 1861 may be committed in several ways. One is by wounding with intent to do grievous bodily harm. On this definition this crime is one of specific intent. Another form is causing grievous bodily harm with intent to do grievous bodily harm. On this definition this crime is a basic intent one. *Davies* [1991] Crim LR 469, though not well reported, seems to hold that grievous bodily harm with intent to resist arrest is a specific intent crime. If this approach were correct, the defence of intoxication is dependent not on the distinction between basic and specific intent *crimes* but basic and specific intent *charges*. Some mental elements in offences such as s 18 are basic intent ones, some are specific intent ones. The problem is that offences have been held to be basic intent ones even though part of the *mens rea* is satisfied only by proof of intent. An example is rape. The accused must intend to have sexual intercourse and must intend to do so with a woman or a man, yet rape is classified as a crime of basic intent: see the discussion of **Fotheringham** above. One way of reconciling the authorities would be to say that rape is a crime of specific intent where the *charge* is one of rape knowing that the victim did not consent but one of basic intent where the *charge* is one of rape being negligent as to consent. The same reasoning could apply to all offences which are defined in terms of intentionally or recklessly misbehaving, such as criminal damage. The courts, however, classify by the *crime*, not by the *charge* or at least that was the majority view until **Heard** [2007] EWCA Crim 125, where Hughes LJ said: '. . . it should not be supposed that every offence can be categorised simply as either one of specific or of basic intent: the accused was charged with sexual assault contrary to s 3 of the Sexual Offences Act 2003. Section 3(1) reads:

A person (A) commits an offence if –
(a) he intentionally touches author person (B),
(b) the touching is sexual,
(c) B does not consent to the touching, and
(d) A does not reasonably believe that B consents.

The accused, who was extremely intoxicated, rubbed his penis on the thigh of a police officer. The court held that specific intent meant ulterior intent (as in burglary), a state of mind going beyond the act. Therefore, even though the touching had to be intentional, the crime was one of basic intent. Therefore, even crimes which can be committed only intentionally may be ones of basic intent. Where does that leave murder!?

The most acceptable categorisation of specific intent offences was provided by Sopinka J (dissenting, but not on this point) in **Daviault v R**, above. 'In addition to the ulterior intent offences there are certain offences which by reason of their serious nature and importance of the mental element are classed as specific intent offences notwithstanding that they do not fit the criteria usually associated with ulterior intent offences. The outstanding example is murder.'

None of these three definitions gives full weight to the precedents. The operation of the basic/specific dichotomy looks capricious. For some offences such as murder there is a 'fall-back' basic intent crime, manslaughter; but for other crimes such as theft there is no 'fall-back' offence. There is no policy which rationalises this distinction. It is safe to say that Lord Birkenhead did not mean to create this dichotomy.

The present position

One way out of this difficulty, though unsatisfactory from the viewpoint of principle, is to list those precedents. Table 8.1 does that for the more important offences.

It seems that all offences of dishonesty are specific intent crimes. Despite intoxication's being a defence to theft, an accused will appropriate when he sobers up by assuming the rights of the owner such as hiding the item away. Therefore, the drunken taker does not avoid liability for theft.

It may be helpful at this point to give a concrete illustration. In relation to s 20 of the Offences Against the Person Act 1861 the judge would direct the jury that they are to convict if they are sure that the accused foresaw that he might cause some injury or would have foreseen that his act might cause some injury had he not been intoxicated.

Table 8.1 Basic and specific intent – precedents

Basic intent	Authority (there are often others)
Manslaughter	*Lipman*
Rape	*Majewski* (Commonwealth courts are divided on this issue)
Section 20, Offences Against the Person Act	*Majewski*
Section 47, Offences Against the Person Act	*Bolton* v *Crawley* [1972] Crim LR 222 (DC)
Assault on constable	*Majewski*
Assault	
Joy-riding (s 12, Theft Act)	*MacPherson* [1973] RTR 157
Presumably removing articles from an exhibition is also a basic intent crime, though a precedent does not exist	
Reckless criminal damage	*Caldwell*
False imprisonment and kidnapping	*Hutchins* [1988] Crim LR 379
Allowing pitbull terrier to be in a public place without a muzzle and a lead	*DPP* v *Kellet* [1994] Crim LR 916 (DC), but see the commentary, which is to the effect that a sober accused is not guilty of this offence unless he knows and consents to ('allows') a dangerous dog to be in a public place whereas an intoxicated accused is guilty even though he or she does not permit the dog to be in such a place. How can one allow something if through drink or drugs one knows nothing about it?
Specific intent	*Authority*
Murder	*Beard*
Section 18, Offences Against the Person Act	*Pordage* [1975] Crim LR 575 (CA) (but see text)
Theft	*Ruse* v *Read* [1949] 1 KB 377 (DC)
Robbery	(Follows from theft)
Burglary with intent to steal	*Durante* [1972] 3 All ER 962 (CA)
Handling	Same case (though there is no mention of 'intent' in the definition)
Intentional criminal damage	*Caldwell*
Attempt	(Intention is sole *mens rea* subject to statement in text about reckless attempts in rape and possibly other offences)

For sexual assault, see *Heard*, above, where Hughes LJ said: 'sexual touching must be intentional . . . but voluntary intoxication cannot be relied upon as negating the necessary intention.'

Some suggestions for the reform of drunkenness

The difficulty in reforming the law was well stated by the Scottish Law Commission in its Discussion Paper, *Insanity and Diminished Responsibility*, No. 122, 2003: 'The problem . . . is that of reconciling the basic principle of *mens rea* . . . with conditions in which persons can hardly be said to have any mental capacity at all. At the same time the social consequences of recognising . . . intoxication as [a] complete defence [ ] in all circumstances would be extremely serious.'

Courts are reluctant to allow intoxicated persons to escape the consequences of their actions. *Lipman* and *Majewski* may be instanced. There is a feeling that these men should have been found guilty of something. There are few redeeming features of intoxication and drunkenness is the state in which many offences are committed. It could be said that in England and Wales people know the kind of events which can happen when a person becomes drunk or takes drugs. Nevertheless, as the High Court of Australia in *O'Connor*, above, demonstrated, the distinction between basic and specific intent makes no logical sense in *mens rea* terms. This breach of the fundamental principle of *mens rea*, the illogicality of the basic/specific intent distinction, and the lack of empirical support for the public policy concerns behind *Majewski* led to Australia's rejection of English law. If the accused had no *mens rea* because of intoxication, he cannot be guilty. This rule even applies to murder: *Martin* (1984) 58 ALJR 217, also a decision of the High Court of Australia. It does not matter that the lack of *mens rea* was caused by intoxication. An accused is guilty only if he had the mental element of the offence charged at the time of the *actus reus*. The fact that the accused got drunk recklessly does not prove that he had the fault element later. (Despite the logic of the situation the Australian Criminal Code Bill 1994 did revert to the specific/basic intent distinction, New South Wales, having accepted *O'Connor*, reverted to the *Majewski* position and Queensland did not adopt the *O'Connor* rule but applied English law.) On this approach there are no special rules applying to drunkenness. The normal principles of criminal law govern. The Criminal Law Reform Committee recommended in its Report on Intoxication, 1984, that New Zealand should adopt the Australian subjectivist approach and should also not enact a special offence dealing with intoxicated persons who commit the *actus reus* of crimes, as has been proposed for England (see below). See also *Kamipeli*, above. South Africa follows the *O'Connor* doctrine: *Chretien* 1981 (1) SA 1097 (AD). Empirical research by Judge G. Smith in 'Footnote to *O'Connor*'s case' (1981) 5 Crim LJ 270 has shown that the Australian approach has not led to the breakdown of law. The Australian approach should be contrasted with the former Canadian authorities which followed *Majewski*. In *Leary* (1977) 74 DLR (3rd) 103 (by a majority), which was overruled in *Daviault v R*, above, and *Bernard* [1988] 2 SCR 833, the Supreme Court approved the policy behind *Majewski*. That policy was expressed by P. Healy 'R v *Bernard*: difficulties with "voluntary intoxication"' (1990) 35 McGill LJ 610 at 612–613: 'Sodden people who do bad things deserve punishment.' A similar point was made over a century ago by Stephen J: 'It is almost trivial for me to observe that a man is not excused from crime by reason of his drunkenness. If it were so, you might as well shut up the criminal courts, because drink is the occasion of a large proportion of the crime which is committed' (*Doherty* (1887) 16 Cox CC 306). The contrary view is that endorsed by the majority in *Daviault* v *R*: 'The mental aspect of an offence, or *mens rea*, has long been recognised as an integral part of crime. The concept is fundamental to our criminal law. . . . However, the substituted *mens rea* cannot establish the *mens rea* to commit the offence' (*per* Cory J). The court rejected the Australian approach and retained the basic/specific intent distinction, but said that a person would be guilty of a basic intent offence if he had the minimum intent to do the prohibited act.

The Butler Committee on Mentally Abnormal Offences, Cmnd 6244, 1975, paras 18.51–18.59, suggested the creation of a new offence, being drunk and dangerous. The accused could be convicted of this offence if charged with a sexual assault, an offence against the person, and criminal damage endangering life. There are advantages in this proposal. The problem of distinguishing between basic and specific intent would disappear. Persons would not be totally acquitted as now happens when they are charged with a specific intent crime and there is no 'fall-back' basic intent offence. Moreover, if the mischief is truly one of intoxication, this proposed crime would focus on that mischief unlike present law. Three Lords in *Majewski* rejected this recommendation. One of its drawbacks is that it would be a status offence with little or no *mens rea* attached to it. Other proposals have included the creation of a crime of negligently causing injury, reforming offences so that there is always a 'fall-back' basic intent offence and treating drunken offenders outside the criminal law system. The present law is out of line with what judges thought was social policy in earlier years. In *Reniger* v *Fogossa* (1551) 75 ER 1 (KB), the court stated that drunkenness was no defence, and a drunken killer was sentenced to be hanged. This attitude seemed to be based on the thought that, since many crimes were committed when the accused was drunk, to provide a defence would mean that few would be convicted. If intoxication was a defence to murder (as it is now), 'there would be no safety for human life' (*Carroll* (1835) 173 ER 64 (NP)). There is some evidence for the view that in the seventeenth and eighteenth centuries drunkenness aggravated the crime, unlike nowadays where it mitigates the offence or provides exculpation.

Present reform proposals are largely based on the Criminal Law Revision Committee's Fourteenth Report, *Offences Against the Person*, Cmnd 7844, 1980. The recommendations were:

(a) The abolition of the basic/specific dichotomy and of the 'constructive recklessness' in *Majewski*.

(b) Intoxication which did not totally exclude *mens rea* should not be a defence.

(c) Involuntary drunkenness should remain a defence but only 'if it negates the mental element', and not if it loosens inhibitions.

(d) Self-induced intoxication was to be defined, as the Butler Committee did, as 'intoxication resulting from the intentional taking of drink or drugs knowing that it is capable in sufficient quantity of having an intoxicating effect, provided that intoxication is not voluntary if it results from a fact unknown to the accused that increases his sensibility to the drink or drug'.

(e) The majority advocated that evidence of voluntary intoxication should be capable of negating the mental element in murder (which at that time was wider than intent) and the intention required for the commission of other offences. In offences where recklessness was an element, if the accused did not appreciate a risk which he would have appreciated when sober, he would not have a defence. These recommendations would largely enact the common law. The minority would allow the defence where the accused was not aware of the risk of causing the *actus reus*, but would have been, were he sober. The dissentients comprised the two law professors on the Criminal Law Revision Committee.

(f) There should be no offence of being dangerously intoxicated, as the Butler Committee had proposed. That crime would lump together the drunken child-killer and the inebriated brawler. The Committee's majority thought that an offence in the area of intoxication should refer to the degree of harm so that, e.g., a drunken killer would still be convicted of manslaughter. The accused should not be labelled incorrectly. The majority opined that a drunken rapist should be guilty of rape, not of some general offence. The minority recommended a special verdict that the offence was committed while the defendant was intoxicated. He would be liable to the same potential penalty (except murder, where the penalty would be equivalent to manslaughter) as he would have been, had he been convicted. The sentence would reflect the harm. In this way the present 'constructive recklessness' rule would be abrogated.

The Law Commission's 1989, 1993 and 1995 proposals

Recommendations appeared in the draft Criminal Code, Law Com. No. 177, 1989, which if enacted would remove some of the difficulties and anomalies of present law. The draft Criminal Code was based on 1980 recommendations of the Criminal Law Revision Committee. As stated in Chapter 1 the draft Criminal Code would have enacted recent recommendations of law reform bodies without amendment. The main clause is cl 22(1), which would be the replacement for basic intent offences and applies to crimes in which part of the *actus reus* is recklessness. The whole of the *actus reus* need not be recklessness. In rape one part of the fault element is the intent to have sexual intercourse, but rape is an offence in which recklessness as to consent suffices. The draft Criminal Code contains the following clauses.

Clause 22(1)
Where an offence requires a fault element of recklessness (however described), a person who was voluntarily intoxicated shall be treated –
(a) as having been aware of any risk of which he would have been aware had he been sober;
(b) as not having believed in the existence of an exempting circumstance (where the existence of such belief is in issue) if he would not have so believed had he been sober.

Clause 22(2)
Where an offence requires a fault element of failure to comply with a standard of care, or requires no fault, a person who was voluntarily intoxicated shall be treated as not having believed in the existence of an exempting circumstance (where the existence of such belief is in issue) if a reasonable sober person would not have so believed.

Clause 22(3)
Where the definition of a fault element or of a defence refers, or requires reference, to the state of mind or conduct to be expected of a reasonable person, such persons shall be understood to be one who is not intoxicated.

Clause 22(4)
Subsection (1) does not apply –
(a) to murder (to which section 55 applies); or
(b) to the case (to which section 36 applies) where a person's unawareness or belief arises from a combination of mental disorder and voluntary intoxication.

Clause 55
A person is guilty of manslaughter if – . . .
(b) he is not guilty of murder by reason only of the fact that, because of voluntary intoxication, he is not aware that death may be caused or believes that an exempting circumstance exists; . . .

Clause 36
A mental disorder verdict shall be returned if –
(a) the defendant is acquitted of an offence only because, by reason of evidence of mental disorder or a combination of mental disorder and intoxication, it is found that he acted or may have acted in a state of automatism, or without the fault required for the offence, or believing that an exempting circumstance existed; . . .

Clause 56(3)
Where a person suffering from mental abnormality is also intoxicated, this section applies only where it would apply if he were not intoxicated. [Clause 56 concerns diminished responsibility.]

Since most offences in the draft Criminal Code would be defined in terms of intention *or* recklessness, intoxication would rarely be a defence.

By cl 22(5)(a) 'intoxicant' covers 'alcohol or any other thing which when taken into the body may impair awareness or control'. Therefore, dangerous drugs are included. By sub-cl (5)(b) a 'voluntary intoxication' covers taking something as an intoxicant (except properly for a medicinal purpose), knowing that it is or may be an intoxicant. By sub-cl (5)(c) a person is deemed to take an intoxicant if it is administered to him. By sub-cl (6) *Bailey* and *Hardie*, above, would be enacted. The legal burden would remain on the prosecution, but the defendant would bear the evidential burden (sub-cl (7)). There would be no special provision for the 'Dutch courage' rule.

By these proposals the Law Commission sought to accomplish the abolition of specific and basic intent and the replacement of the present recklessness liability. The accused would be guilty of an offence which may be committed recklessly if he was intoxicated. Clause 22 restated current law. There was no need to have a special rule for crimes of specific intent because intoxication is simply part of the evidence. If crimes committable 'maliciously' survived the enactment of the Criminal Code, they would be treated as recklessness offences. By cl 33(1)(b) a person who is unconscious through drink does not have the defence of automatism.

Clause 22(1)(b) would reverse *Jaggard v Dickinson*, above. The Law Commission commented (Report No. 177, para 8.41) that 'that decision created an anomalous distinction (between mistake as to the non-existence of an element of an offence and mistake as to the existence of a circumstance affording a defence) which it would be wrong to perpetrate in the Code'. The Law Commission also wished to reverse the *dictum* in *O'Grady*, above. The accused would be able to rely on a mistake brought about by intoxication in self-defence in offences where the sole mental element is intention, including murder. In the Law Commission's view, 'it would . . . be unthinkable to convict of murder a person who thought, for whatever reason, that he was acting to save his life and who would have been acting reasonably if he had been right'. This rule would bring self-defence into line with other defences when the accused was drunk. The law will be brought back into line with mistakes not based on intoxication (*Williams* [1987] 3 All ER 411). With regard to recklessness offences, the mistaken belief in self-defence will be irrelevant if that belief would not have been held if the accused had been sober. The Law Commission noted (Report No. 177, para 8.42) that the reversal of the *dictum* in *O'Grady* would not let the accused off scot-free: he would be convicted of manslaughter or the proposed offence of recklessly causing harm. The Law Commission was of the view that there should be no special rule for self-defence, or for public and private defence, defence of property, and self-defence.

It should be noted that the Law Commission had to provide a special rule for murder because by its recommendations murder would be in part an offence of recklessness to which cl 22(1) would otherwise apply. Murder is to contain the fault element of 'being aware that he may kill', a phrase of recklessness liability. The present law on intoxication and murder is preserved. As the Law Commission noted (Report No. 177, para 8.44) the accused is convicted of manslaughter, which has a maximum sentence of life imprisonment. Such a penalty was considered 'sufficient to protect the public interest'.

As restated the law remains complex. Intoxication still would not simply negative *mens rea*. Special rules would remain. The thinking of the Law Commission developed and changed between 1989 and 1995. In 1993 the Law Commission issued a Consultation Paper, *Intoxication and Criminal Liability*, LCCP No. 127. The Consultation Paper investigated the present law on intoxication and various alternatives. The issue was seen to be an arena for the conflict of two policies: the policy of not convicting persons who did not know what they were doing and the policy of safeguarding citizens from violence which resulted from drink or drugs. The current resolution of this clash of policies is the House of Lords decision in *Majewski*. However, *Majewski* is dependent on the distinction between basic and specific intent crimes. 'The differences between these two types of offence, the policy reasons for the distinction, and the basis on which the distinction is made, are all obscure' (LCCP No. 127, 3). The law is complex and it is possible that it is ignored by the triers of fact. It does not advance the policy of criminalising intoxicated individuals in a straightforward manner but through technical rules which do not always reflect that policy. English law is also out of step with that in other jurisdictions which have abolished the special rules on intoxication. There are also difficulties in knowing what *Majewski* decided. Is it that all offences are either basic or specific intent ones? On this view the offence found in s 18 of the Offences Against the Person Act 1861 is a specific intent crime. Or is the question whether an allegation is a specific or basic intent one? On this approach the allegation that the accused caused grievous bodily harm with intent to do so contrary to s 18 is a basic intent offence, but causing such harm with intent to resist or prevent apprehension is a specific intent crime. Whichever rule is adopted there is the difficulty of crimes which have intent as to one element but recklessness as to another one. Leaving aside intoxication the accused must intend to commit one of the offences listed in s 9(2) of the Theft Act 1968 if he is charged with a s 9(1)(a) type of burglary, but recklessness suffices in relation to the trespass. Applying *Majewski* intoxication is not to be taken into account in determining whether the accused knew he was entering as a trespasser but is considered with regard to the question whether he intended to commit an offence listed in s 9(2). Another question which arises in relation to *Majewski* is to say that the rule applies in relation to allegations of intent; i.e. 'basic intent offences' is a concept which is wider than crimes of recklessness for it covers some crimes of intention.

The Law Commission noted that most crimes have been allocated to the basic or specific intent category. However, there is difficulty with offences which have not been allocated, for the width of *Majewski* is uncertain. Moreover, the treatment of the distinction between the courts 'means that there is no necessary connection between the seriousness of the offence involved and its categorisation . . .'. Murder is a specific intent crime but manslaughter is a basic intent one, yet both are serious offences. Manslaughter is more serious than the crime of grievous bodily harm with intent, yet the former crime is a basic intent one, the latter is a specific intent one. Furthermore, there are problems in applying *Majewski* to some offences, as we have seen with respect to burglary. Some serious specific intent offences have a 'fall-back' basic intent offence attached to them. For example, s 18 is a specific intent crime; an accused can be convicted of the s 20 crime, which is a basic intent offence. However, the same is not true of all serious offences. Intoxication is a defence to burglary and theft; the accused is not guilty, however, of some lesser crime if he was intoxicated. The Law Commission also adverted to the problem of *O'Grady* [1987] QB 995. The defendant is guilty of an offence where he makes a mistake as to an element of it whether that offence is a basic or a specific intent one. The Law Commission in its 1995 Report noted below disagreed with the Consultation Paper's main recommendation but it did repeat these criticisms.

In the Consultation Paper, the Law Commission examined the options for reform of the defence. The first option is to leave the law as it is. The Law Commission rejected this proposal as failing to achieve the policy objectives of a law which was not complex, a law which was certain, and a law which fully implemented the aims of upholding public order while permitting intoxicated defendants to be acquitted of serious offences. A second option was to codify the *Majewski* approach but rectify inconsistencies. This approach would of course ensure that the law was certain but would otherwise meet none of the other policy objectives just mentioned. The Law Commission also rejected the 1980 recommendation of the Criminal Law Revision Committee that an accused should not have a defence of intoxication in relation to an element of a crime which was defined in terms of recklessness if he would have appreciated the risk had he been sober. The effect of that proposal would be that, e.g., in rape intoxication would be relevant to the intent to have sexual intercourse but not to recklessness as to consent. Why should the accused be exculpated on the first ground but not on the second? Moreover, it is thought that many believe that intoxication should not on policy grounds be a defence to rape at all. The Law Commission thought that the Criminal Law Revision Committee's proposal would be confusing to juries: they could for instance consider drunkenness in relation to the intent to have sexual intercourse but not in relation to recklessness as to consent. Moreover, the recommendation would lead to difficulties in sentencing. The drunken accused is to be treated as reckless. Should he be punished on the basis that he is reckless? The Law Commission opined that the offender should be penalised for what he was, not for what he was not, i.e. for being a reckless but sober individual.

The third option considered by the Law Commission was to disregard the effect of intoxication in any offence. The specific/basic intent rule would be abolished and the accused would not be able to rely on intoxication as negating the fault element in any offence – even ones nowadays categorised as specific intent ones. This option would be an undeniable deterrent, for drunken defendants would have no defence. The Law Commission considered that such a result would be 'draconian' in a society which tolerated alcohol. The effect would also be inappropriate in some crimes. In the type of burglary found in s 9(1)(a) of the Theft Act 1968 intoxication would not be relevant to the further or ulterior intent, the intent to commit one of the four offences listed in s 9(2). The result would be that the prosecution would have to prove only that the accused entered a building as a trespasser, but such an entry is not a crime: 'where the entrant's drunkenness prevents the formation of an ulterior intent, it is simply impossible to characterise the entry as a burglary, and thus similarly impossible to use a conviction for burglary as a sanction against such an entry.'

The fourth option outlined by the Law Commission was the same as the third but with the proviso that the accused would not be convicted if he could demonstrate that he did not have the *mens rea* required for the offence because he was voluntarily intoxicated. The Law Commission considered, however, that someone who caused harm in a drunken state should not go free, which would be the result if the accused established this defence.

The fifth option would be simply to abolish the *Majewski* approach. Intoxication would merely be part of the evidence of *mens rea*. The law would be simple. In view of jurisdictions such as the common law states of Australia which have adopted this solution, there is no need for special rules for drunken defendants. The *mens rea* principle should be supreme. The argument that *Majewski* deters the intoxicated is not supported by the facts. Victoria, which abolished the specific/basic intent rule, does not have a more serious problem with drunks who cause harm than states which have retained *Majewski*. The Law Commission, however, thought that public safety would suffer and respect for the law would diminish if a drunken accused would be completely acquitted. The Irish Law Reform Commission in its Report on *Intoxication* commented thus: 'the traditional *mens rea* doctrine is an appropriate one for the sane and sober criminal, but to adhere to it in an unbending and inflexible fashion enables the offender himself, voluntarily, not just to "move the goalposts" but to remove them altogether! The point was, neatly, couched in more traditional terms by Lord Mustill . . . in **Kingston**, when he held, first, that the intentional taking of an intoxicant without regard to its possible consequences is a substitute for the mental element normally required; and, secondly, that the defendant is "estopped" . . . from relying on the absence of a mental element if it is absent *because of his own acts*.' The Irish Law Reform Commission wanted voluntary intoxication never to be a defence.

The sixth option would be to abolish **Majewski** but replace it with a new offence of criminal intoxication. Criminal law should protect against drunken defendants. Such persons are at fault for committing harm. To acquit them would, it may be thought, be morally wrong and give an incorrect message to them, for they must be deterred. 'A new offence can be tailored by legislation to achieve more precisely the objective of the **Majewski's** approach without the faults of **Majewski** itself, and in particular without the practical difficulties that attend its present operation. A new offence can implement directly and overtly . . . policy considerations . . . by laying down clear rules in the light of that policy.' The Law Commission rejected the Butler Committee's proposal of an offence of dangerous intoxication and the idea of the minority of the Criminal Law Revision Committee of an offence of 'doing the act while in a state of voluntary intoxication', partly because in regard to the latter recommendation it required the jury to answer the hypothetical question: would this defendant have done what he did, had he been sober? The Law Commission proposed, first, that intoxication should be taken into account in determining whether the accused had the *mens rea* of an offence, whether he had made a mistake as to whether he was in a state of automatism; secondly, the creation of a new offence of criminal intoxication. The crime would be committed by an accused who, while substantially intoxicated, caused the harm proscribed by a so-called 'listed' offence. It would not be relevant that the accused did not have the mental element of the listed offence or that he was in a state of automatism. The Butler Committee's proposed offence would have applied only if the accused did not form the *mens rea* of an offence. A 'listed' offence is just that: one listed by the Law Commission. These were expressed as: homicide, bodily harm, criminal damage, rape, indecent assault, buggery, assaulting or obstructing a constable in the execution of his duty, violent disorder, affray, putting a person in fear of or provoking violence, and causing danger to road users. The offence would, therefore, not apply to other offences such as attempts, battery, theft and burglary. The maximum penalty would be less than for the substantive offence because a drunken defendant is less culpable than a person who intentionally or recklessly committed a crime. There should be no special maximum for the offence because having one maximum would not cater for punishment for the harm caused by an intoxicated accused. The Law Commission thought that there should be a maximum of two-thirds the maximum for the 'listed' offence but with a maximum of 10 years where the maximum for such offence was life. The Law Commission also recommended the abolition of the **O'Grady** principle, with the proviso that a drunken defendant would have the defence of mistake in a self-defence situation where a sober individual would have reasonably made the same mistake.

The Law Commission summarised the advantages of the proposed offence:

(i) Defendants will not be liable to be convicted of offences when, in law, they did not have the required mental state for guilt of that offence.

(ii) At the same time, the criminal law will be able to intervene in cases where the defendant, although not fulfilling the requirements for conviction of a specific crime, committed socially dangerous acts in a state of substantial intoxication.

(iii) This objective will be achieved by allowing the court and jury to apply a set of clear rules that require them to consider factual and not abstract or hypothetical questions; that clearly identify where the defendant has been convicted on grounds of intoxication rather than of actual intention or recklessness; and which accordingly give positive guidance to the sentencing tribunal as to the ground of his conviction. (LCCP No. 127, 93)

The Law Commission concluded by stating that the new offence could straightforwardly implement the policy of restraining intoxicated defendants, would concentrate on the damage or injury caused by them, and would abolish the complicated yet uncertain law found in *Majewski*.

One concern of commentators related to the sixth and favoured option. If the accused commits a listed offence when substantially intoxicated he has a defence. What, however, if despite his intoxication he intended to commit the offence? Surely as in *Kingston*, above, he should be liable for the (listed) offence, not just for the proposed offence. As *Kingston* confirmed, a drunken intent is nevertheless an intent.

The Law Commission published Report No. 229, *Intoxication and Criminal Liability*, 1995, which is noted below and which adopts a position very similar to that of the US Model Penal Code 1962, s 2.08(1), as the follow-up to LCCP No. 127. In the meantime it issued its Report No. 218, *Legislating the Criminal Code – Offences against the Person and General Principles*, 1993. Report No. 218 was restricted to non-fatal offences and three general defences. With regard to non-fatal offences, cl 21(1) provides that

a person who was voluntarily intoxicated at any material time shall be treated
(a) as having been aware of any risk of which he would have been aware had he not been intoxicated, and
(b) as not having believed in any circumstances which he would have believed in had he not been intoxicated.

The Home Office Consultation Document, *Violence: Reforming the Offences Against the Person Act 1861*, 1998, accepted this definition for the purposes of its draft Offences against the Person Bill. What should be noted is that the accused will no longer be deemed to be reckless if he is intoxicated. He can adduce evidence to show that despite being intoxicated he did not have the requisite *mens rea*. For purposes of the revised offences, 'a person who was voluntarily intoxicated at any material time shall be treated as not having believed in any circumstance which he would not then have believed in had he not been intoxicated' (cl 33).

The Law Commission opined that the current distinction between basic and specific intent crimes could not be 'expressed in statutory terms, because its limits are almost impossible to specify'. For convenience, the law was to be reformulated to apply 'only to allegations of or cognate to recklessness'. In other words *Majewski* was for the purposes of the Criminal Law Bill attached to Report No. 218 restricted to offences of recklessness, just as Lord Elwyn-Jones thought in *Majewski* and Lord Diplock did in *Caldwell*. Evidence of intoxication can, however, be considered in respect of intention crimes such as the proposed one of intentionally causing serious injury. The retention of the law on intoxication is not consonant with the Law Commission's insistence on subjective fault.

Clause 33 of the Criminal Law Bill was directed at preserving the rule in *O'Grady* pending the full Report on intoxication. It will be remembered that the Law Commission had previously called the effect of *O'Grady* 'unthinkable'. Schedule 3, para 13(3) to the Bill would revise s 5(2)(b) (protection of property) of the Criminal Damage Act 1971 to make it consistent with the restatement in cl 33. *Jaggard v Dickinson*, a case in s 5(2)(a), would not be affected.

The Law Commission surprisingly resiled from the chief recommendation contained in its Consultation Paper when it published *Legislating the Criminal Code: Intoxication and Criminal Liability*, Report No. 229, 1995. The Law Commission considered that 'prudent social policy' (para 1.14) overrode the general principle of criminal law that defendants were guilty only when as a minimum they were aware of the risk that their conduct might cause harm. They should not escape liability because they were intoxicated for the public must be protected from violence. It is reasonable to hold them liable for misbehaviour when drunk. Consultees responded to the recommendations in the Consultation Paper that the abolition of the rule in **Majewski** without replacement (option 5) was unacceptable because it would result in the acquittal of drunken defendants and that the creation of a new offence (option 6) was also unacceptable on the ground that more trials would take place, expert evidence would be needed as to whether the accused was substantially impaired, more police time would be spent on uncovering the extent of his intoxication and the prosecution would not know in advance of trial whether the proposed offence should be included in the indictment. Options 3 and 4 were not supported on consultation. That left option 1, doing nothing, and option 2, codifying and amending current law. These options were supported by the consultees: 'juries do not in fact experience as much difficulty with the present law as we had previously thought' (para 1.28). Option 1 was rejected because it did not deal with the problems of the law such as whether a crime was one of basic or specific intent. That left option 2. Among the recommendations flowing from that decision were, first, that in respect of allegations of purpose, intent, knowledge, belief, fraud and dishonesty evidence of intoxication should be considered along with all the other evidence to determine whether that allegation was proved; secondly, in respect of other mental elements such as recklessness the accused should be deemed to be aware of anything he would have been aware of, had he not been intoxicated; and thirdly, if the accused when intoxicated whether involuntarily or voluntarily held a belief which would have exculpated him if he had been sober, the belief will not exculpate him if he would not have held it but for his intoxication and the crime is not one of purpose, intent, knowedge, belief, fraud or dishonesty: cf. **Jaggard v Dickinson**, above. An example of the first two propositions is attempt. The accused to be guilty must intend the full offence and intoxication would be taken into account; however, recklessness as to the circumstances suffices for the attempt if it suffices for the full crime: the accused will not be able to rely on intoxication in relation to recklessness such as recklessness as to the victim's consent in rape. At least this is how the provision is expected to work. A court might say that where a crime consists of both allegations of intent and of recklessness, it is in fact a crime of recklessness. Therefore, the accused is guilty if sufficiently intoxicated. 'Intoxicated' would be defined as occurring when awareness, understanding or control was impaired by an intoxicant, which would be defined as 'alcohol, a drug or any other substance (of whatever nature) which, once taken into the body, has the capacity to impair awareness, understanding or control'. Involuntary intoxication would cover situations where the accused took the substance not knowing that it was an intoxicant, he was given it without consent, he took it under duress or had some other defence, he was particularly susceptible to it and did not know, or finally he took it solely for a medical reason and either did not know of its propensity to give rise to aggressive or uncontrollable behaviour or (if he was aware) he took it with medical advice. If in spite of the voluntary intoxication he did have the requisite mental element he would be guilty: **Kingston**, above, would be unaffected.

The proposals would abolish the basic/specific intent divide and replace it with one based on the mental element alleged (though the difference in practice may be minimal and the distinction seems to exist already: see above), would abrogate the rule in **Hardie**, above, and replace it with a rule about medical advice, would abolish the **O'Grady** principle and would tidy up the law of involuntary intoxication.

The proposals have been criticised for failing to conform with the general principles espoused in the draft Criminal Code. The recommendations are based on the workability, but they would lead to a complicated law.

The Home Office issued a Consultation Paper *Violence: Reforming the Offences against the Person Act 1861* in 1998. In it the government returned to the approach of the 1989 draft Criminal Code. Because of the nature of the document intoxication was restated only in relation to non-fatal offences but in its 2000 Consultation Paper on involuntary manslaughter the Home Office took the same view with regard to this offence. There has been no movement since by the government.

The Law Commission's 2006 recommendations

The Law Commission issued its Report No. 306 *Murder, Manslaughter and Infanticide* in November 2006. In it the Commission proposed a three-tier structure for fatal offences: first degree murder, second degree murder and manslaughter: see Chapter 11 for details. In respect of intoxication the Law Commission proposed that it should be a defence to first and second degree murder but not to manslaughter. The specific and basic intent formula would thus be mapped onto the new law. However, it should be noted that one form of the proposed mental element in first degree murder is 'intent to cause serious injury being aware that there is a serious risk of death'. This is therefore a crime partly defined in terms of (subjective) recklessness: awareness of a serious risk of death. Nevertheless, this type of murder will remain a crime of specific intent. Similar points may be made about second degree murder.

The Law Commission intended to publish a report in late 2008 but there was no sign of it in early January 2009.

Self-defence and the prevention of crime

Introduction

This section deals with the statutory defence of prevention of crime and effecting or assisting in an arrest found in s 3(1) of the Criminal Law Act 1967 and the common law defence of self-defence insofar as it survives the enactment of s 3(1). The Criminal Justice and Immigration Act 2008, s 76, came into force on 14 July 2008. It was presented by the Minister of Justice, Jack Straw, as a measure which would protect those charged with crimes who were seeking to prevent the commission of offences against themselves, others or property, particularly householders who used force against burglars, but in fact it is an enactment of the case law authorities. Section 76 may be outlined thus:

1 'The question whether the degree of force used by D [the accused] was reasonable in the circumstances is to be decided by reference to the circumstances as D believed them to be . . .' (s 76(3)).

2 Section 76(4) provides:
   If D claims to have held a particular belief as regards the existence of any circumstances –
   (a) the reasonableness or otherwise of that belief is relevant to the question whether D genuinely held it; but

    (b) if it is determined that D did genuinely hold it, D is entitled to rely on it for the purposes of subsection (3), whether or not –
      (i) it was mistaken, or
      (ii) (if it was mistaken) the mistake was a reasonable one to have made.

3 Section 76(5) stipulates: 'But subsection (4)(b) does not enable D to rely on any mistaken belief that was voluntarily induced.'

4 'The degree of force used by D is not to be regarded as having been reasonable in the circumstances as D believed them to be if it was disproportionate in the circumstances.' (s 76(6)).

5 Section 76(7) provides that:
In deciding the question mentioned in subsection (3) the following considerations are to be taken into account (so far as relevant in the circumstances of the case) –
    (a) that a person acting for a legitimate purpose may not be able to weigh to a nicety the exact measure of any necessary action; and
    (b) that evidence of a person's having done what the person instinctively thought was necessary for a legitimate purpose constitutes strong evidence that only reasonable action was taken by that person for that purpose.
Whether the accused has a legitimate purpose is determined by s 76(10)(a): common law self-defence and statutory prevention of crime and effecting or assisting in arrest under the 1967 Act.

6 The triers of fact are not restricted to these two pieces of evidence (s 76(8)).

7 Subsection (10) provides in part: '. . . (b) references to self-defence include acting in defence of another person; and (c) references to the degree of force used are to the type and amount of force used.'

All these points are dealt with below. For example, the point in s 76(5) about drunken mistakes is considered below in section (g) *Mistake of fact*. The reader will quickly find that the 2008 statute does not enact new law but codifies case law. Even the term 'weigh to a nicety' in s 76(7)(a) is taken from case precedents. However, s 76 is only a partial codification of self-defence and prevention of crime; moreover, to understand s 76 one needs to understand the law which it puts into statutory form.

The boundaries of self-defence and prevention of crime

It might be said that self-defence and the prevention of crime are not true defences but, like the defence of consent, are failures to prove that the accused did the act unlawfully. His act was justified and there is no *actus reus*. Therefore, there was no crime. The policy basis of the defence is to inhibit aggressive behaviour. The Court of Appeal in **Abraham** [1973] 1 WLR 1270 emphasised that a judge should point out to the jury that while a plea of self-defence is called a defence, the burden remains on the prosecution to disprove it. Other authorities are to similar effect, e.g. **Khan** [1995] Crim LR 78 (CA). A Privy Council authority is **Chan Kau v R** [1955] AC 206. For Australia see **Viro** (1978) 52 ALJR 418 (HCA). The judge must direct the jury on this defence if the facts raise it even though the accused did not seek to rely on it: **DPP v Bailey** [1995] 1 Cr App R 257 (PC).

By s 3(1) of the Criminal Law Act 1967:

A person may use such force as is reasonable in the circumstances in the prevention of crime, or in effecting or in assisting in the lawful arrest of offenders or suspected offenders or of persons unlawfully at large.

This rule replaced the common law. The defence of one's own person and others and of property is also a defence, this time at common law. This defence probably has the same bounds as s 3 except that possibly the common law defence is restricted to defence against the use of force whereas s 3 is not. The degree of force lawful in self-defence is the same as that under the Act: *McInnes* (1971) 55 Cr App R 551 and *Clegg* [1995] 1 AC 482 (HL). In the latter case Lord Lloyd rejected the view of Lord Diplock in *Reference under s 48A of the Criminal Appeal (Northern Ireland) Act 1968 (No. 1 of 1975)* [1977] AC 105 that a person who uses force in self-defence is more blameworthy than he who uses it to prevent crime. Self-defence could in many circumstances fall within s 3, and both defences are available on the same facts: *Cousins* [1982] QB 526 and *Clegg*. This is another reason for rejecting Lord Diplock's view. If the force used is not in the prevention of crime, such as where the accused is defending himself against an attack by a child under 10 or an insane person, s 3 cannot be used. Accordingly there is not a total overlap. It should be noted that to have a defence of self-defence the attack against which the accused defended himself need not be an unlawful one: *per* Ward LJ in *Re A (Children) (Conjoined Twins: Medical Treatment)* [2001] Fam 147 (CA), a civil case. The Court of Appeal (Criminal Division) in *Kelleher* [2003] EWCA Crim 3525, did say that there had to be an unlawful or criminal act against which the defendants were defending themselves, but it did not consider the position, for example, of children under 10. Since the planting of genetically modified maize seed was lawful, the defendants did not have the defence. ('Unlawful' here means tortious.)

The jury is entitled to take into account the physical characteristics of the accused in assessing whether his reaction was reasonable: *Martin* [2003] QB 1 (CA), the case of the Norfolk former who shot a fleeing burglar in the back, killing him. For example, the fact that the accused was weak or small or both when the victim was strong or tall or both can be taken into consideration. The court added that psychiatric conditions can 'in exceptional circumstances' be considered. What those circumstances are was left undefined. The accused in *Martin* suffered from paranoia but that psychiatric condition was not to be used. Therefore, the law is uncertain.

(a) *The interpretation of s 3.* The force must be used for the purposes specified. An example is *Renouf* [1986] 2 All ER 449 (CA). The accused was charged with reckless driving. He had forced a vehicle off the road and rammed it after the occupants had assaulted him and damaged his car. He was held to have been acting in order to assist in the lawful arrest of offenders. Whether the force was reasonable was a question for the jury. Another point of construction is that s 3 is limited to the use of force. There is no definition of 'force'. The term seems to require some sort of violent behaviour. Therefore, writing with a felt-tip on a concrete pillar is not force within s 3: *Blake v DPP* [1993] Crim LR 586. What about using something less than force? One answer is that such conduct falls within the common law and in principle if force is permitted, something less should be allowed too. An example given by Jeremy Horder in 'Self-defence, necessity and duress: understanding the relationship' (1998) 11 *Canadian Journal of Law and Jurisprudence* 143 at 144 is this: 'If the only way I can stop a would-be attacker killing me is to release a poisonous gas into a room through which he will pass to reach me, then I am entitled to have such a step considered as potentially necessary and proportionate, even though it does not involve the use of force.' In *Cousins*, above, Milmo J said: 'If force is permissible, something less, for example, a threat, must also be permissible . . .'. In *DPP v Bayer* [2004] 1 WLR 2856 (DC) the defendants chained themselves to tractors to prevent genetically modified maize being drilled. The court suggested *obiter* that they might have had a defence if the other elements of defence of property had been satisfied. However, it cannot be said that the law is settled.

(b) *The interpretation of self-defence.* Self-defence includes the protection of others: **Duffy** [1967] 1 QB 63 (CCA). It also covers protection of property: **Hussey** (1924) 18 Cr App R 160 (CCA): a trespasser may be killed in defence of one's home (but the force must be reasonable). The accused shot and wounded two of his landlady's friends, who were trying to break into his room to evict him illegally. Had the facts occurred today, the friends would have been guilty of at least two offences and therefore the accused would be acting in prevention of crime. For example, one may kill another's dog which is threatening other people or property. In **Workman v Cowper** [1961] 2 QB 143 (DC) the accused killed a foxhound which was running wild on common land where there were sheep. The dog was not worrying the sheep, but it was lambing season. In **Faraj** [2007] EWCA Crim 1033 it was held that a householder could rely on self-defence in order to detain a burglar. In fact the alleged burglar was a gas repair man. See (g) below for mistake of fact. Also included are preventing a trespass, breach of the peace and escaping from unlawful imprisonment. An act of self-defence need not be spontaneous: **Attorney-General's Reference (No. 2 of 1983)** [1984] QB 456, approved in **Beckford v R** [1998] AC 130. The accused therefore can prepare to repel an attack if that attack is about to start. This proposition could give a defence to a battered woman who is in fear of further violence provided, it is thought, that the attack is imminent. If, however, the abuser is asleep, no attack is imminent. Lord Griffiths in **Beckford** stressed the necessity for imminence. Northern Ireland law is the same. The requirement of imminence (or immediacy) means that people can 'get their blow in first' far in advance of any attack. The accused will not be acting in self-defence if he creates the dangerous situation for which he wished to use the defence. In other words, the defence is ruled out when the accused induces the victim to attack him. In **Malnik v DPP** [1989] Crim LR 451 the defendant was going to see a person who he believed had stolen cars belonging to his friend. Because the alleged thief was violent, the accused took with him a rice-flail, which is a weapon used in oriental martial arts. He was arrested before he reached the alleged thief's house. The court rejected his contention that he was justified in carrying the weapon because he feared being attacked. It was he who had created the situation of danger. This case was approved in **Salih** [2007] EWCA Crim 2750. Hooper LJ agreed with Bingham LJ in **Malnik v DPP** that 'the policy of the law' was against arming oneself with offensive weapons and that the exceptions were narrow. The requirement of imminence is one reason why battered wives may find difficulty in having this defence. Stabbing a sleeping partner does not suggest a situation of imminent danger. Another difficulty for such persons is that the degree of force may be excessive. This issue is discussed in (c) below.

(c) *The person attacked is under no duty to retreat:* **Julien** [1969] 1 WLR 839. In **Bird** [1985] 2 All ER 513, the Court of Appeal said that it was not necessary for the accused to have demonstrated an unwillingness to fight to have this defence. Whether the accused did retreat or show an unwillingness to fight is one factor to be taken into account: **Reference under s 48A of the Criminal Appeal (Northern Ireland) Act 1968 (No. 1 of 1975)**, above, and **Duffy v Chief Constable of Cleveland Police** [2007] EWHC 3169 (Admin). Trying to withdraw is therefore evidence of the accused's acting reasonably.

(d) *The burden of proof is on the prosecution:* **Lobell** [1957] 1 QB 547. The accused shoulders the evidential burden. Even if the accused does not rely on the defence, if the facts raise it the judge must put it to the jury.

(e) *The degree of force.* Under both s 3 and the common law the force used must (in fact) be reasonable in the circumstances. What is reasonable depends on the nature of the threat. It is common to say that the force used must be both necessary and proportionate. There is no need for exact proportionality: **Palmer v R** [1971] AC 814. The Court of Appeal in **Rivolta** [1994] Crim LR 694 followed **Palmer**, which is a Privy Council case. In **Oatridge** (1992) 94 Cr App R 367 the Court of Appeal stated that one of the questions to be answered was whether the accused's response was 'commensurate with the degree of danger created by the attack'. What the accused instinctively believed was necessary is evidence of the reasonableness of the force: **Whyte** [1987] 3 All ER 416. If the accused uses excessive force and kills when no reasonable person would have done so, he is guilty of murder (if he has malice aforethought): **Palmer v R**, above. A killing in excessive self-defence is sometimes thought not to be as serious as a true murder, but the outcome is not manslaughter but murder. There have been several calls for the reform of this law. The House of Lords in **Clegg** rejected the opportunity to declare that a killing in self-defence was manslaughter. The question of reasonableness is for the jury: **Reference under s 48A; Cousins**, above. In **Cousins** it was said that a threat of force may be reasonable, when force would not be. As was held in **Clegg**, once the danger is over there is no necessity to use force. Therefore, force used then is not in self-defence or in the prevention of crime but is illegal. On the facts of **Clegg** the danger had passed and the accused was not acting in defence of another or to prevent the crime of death by dangerous driving. Provided that the accused did use reasonable force, it does not matter whether the accused was in a state of funk or was calm.

See also the discussion of Article 2 of the European Convention on Human Rights in the 'Conclusion' below.

See p 282 in Chapter 7 for an explanation of duress of circumstances.

(f) *Self-defence and duress of circumstances.* Both defences are based on threats. If the accused grabs a knife and uses it to prevent himself being killed, he is acting in self-defence and under the influence of duress of circumstances. Self-defence is limited to the use of force, whereas duress is available for most offences. Therefore, if the accused does not use force, duress of circumstances is a possible defence. Self-defence is a defence to all crimes, though the Court of Appeal in **Symonds** [1998] Crim LR 280 had difficulty with the concept of self-defence applying beyond the realms of offences against the person (here, driving offences), but duress of circumstances is not a defence to murder. In duress the harm threatened must be of death or serious injury. In self-defence the accused has to use only reasonable force, whereas the test may be higher in duress of circumstances: did this accused fall short of the standard of a person of reasonable firmness? It is strange that the test where the accused need not use force (duress) is stricter than the test where he does use force (self-defence). This proposition applies also to the next point. The tests for mistake also differ. Duress of circumstances required reasonable belief. This difference can give rise to different verdicts. Take a variation on the facts of **Symonds**. Assume that the accused was mistaken as to what the victim was doing and to escape he drove his car at the victim. The defence is one of self-defence. The mistake, if honest, gives rise to a defence. If, however, in order to escape the accused drove away dangerously, the defence is one of duress of circumstances. An unreasonable mistake is not a defence. The outcome does differ depending on the defence. The Court of Appeal said that self-defence and duress of circumstances shared the same elements, but in relation to a mistaken belief they do not (though the law seems to be changing). Moreover, duress is no defence to murder, attempted murder, being an accessory to murder and some forms of treason; the threat in duress must be of death or serious injury; and there is no defence of duress when the accused has voluntarily put himself in a position where a criminal gang may exert violent pressure on him. Mistake in self-defence is discussed next.

(g) *Mistake of fact.* The accused is to be judged on the facts as he perceives them to be. The test is subjective. To omit this part of the law constitutes a misdirection: *Duffy*, above. If the accused used excessive force because he made a mistake of fact, he has a defence if he would have had a defence on the facts as he believed them to be. There is no need for a reasonable mistake: *Williams* [1987] 3 All ER 411, *Jackson* [1984] Crim LR 674, *Fisher* [1987] Crim LR 334 (CA), *Beckford*, above *Morrow* [1994] Crim LR 58, where the cases on self-defence were applied to the statutory defence of prevention of crime, and *Faraj*, above, where the law on mistake of fact was applied to the defence of property. Lord Griffiths in *Beckford* emphasised that basing the law of mistaken self-defence on honest belief rather than reasonable belief would not allow bogus defences to succeed, for juries were adept at distinguishing truth from falsity. The Court of Appeal ruled in *Oatridge*, above, that in cases of honest mistake of fact in self-defence (in this case the fact that the accused believed her partner was going to kill her – he had abused her previously) the judge should direct the jury on whether the victim's response was commensurate with the attack which he believed he faced. The force must still be (objectively) reasonable in the circumstances which the accused (subjectively) believed existed: *Owino* [1996] 2 Cr App R 128 (CA). Anything said by the Court of Appeal in *Scarlett* [1993] 4 All ER 629 to the effect that the accused was entitled to use such force as he believed reasonable was incorrect. *Owino* was followed in *Hughes* [1995] Crim LR 957 (CA). The court held that the trial judge must explain to the jury the effect of a mistaken belief. The law is that an accused who is mistaken that he is about to be attacked is entitled to be judged on the facts as he believed existed but he must use no more than reasonable force, reasonableness being assessed in the light of the circumstances the accused thought existed. Since Beldam LJ gave the judgment in *Scarlett* and in *Hughes*, *Scarlett* is now to be taken as incorrect. The Court of Appeal spoke to similar effect in *DPP* v *Armstrong-Braun* (1998) 163 JP 271. While the *facts* are to be judged as the accused honestly believed them to exist, the Court of Appeal in *Martin* [2003] QB 1 stated that his perception of the *danger* was to be assessed objectively. The fact that this accused because he had a paranoid personality saw danger when it did not exist was irrelevant. The court certified a question of law of general importance: 'Whether expert psychiatric evidence is admissible on the issue of a defendant's perception of the danger he faced . . . ?' Unfortunately leave to appeal was refused. However, the Privy Council advised in *Shaw* v *R* [2001] 1 WLR 1519 that the jury must take into account 'the circumstances and the danger as the [accused] honestly believed them to be . . .'. There is a clash of authority. It is suggested that the Privy Council is correct, for there is no distinction between 'facts' and 'danger'.

The contrast between *Williams* and *Clegg* should be noted. If the accused is mistaken as to whether there is a need for self-defence, he is acquitted: *Williams*. If, however, the accused is mistaken as to the degree of force, he is guilty, even of murder: *Clegg*. In respect of the latter situation, a comparison with provocation is instructive. In self-defence an overreaction leads to guilt, not an acquittal, whereas in provocation overreaction leads to acquittal on a charge of murder. Since a successful defence of provocation leads to a conviction for manslaughter, it is arguable that when the accused kills in defence of self or others but uses excessive force, this too should be manslaughter. However, it may well be that any killing in defence of property cannot be justified.

Four final points on mistake of fact should be made. First, 'If a defendant applies force to a police or court officer, which would be reasonable if that person were not a police or court officer, and the defendant believes that he is not, then even if his belief is unreasonable, he has a good plea of self-defence': **Blackburn v Bowering** [1994] 3 All ER 380 (CA, Civil Division). Secondly, if the mistake is caused by intoxication, the accused has no defence: **O'Grady** [1987] 3 All ER 420, which was approved in **Hatton** [2006] 1 Cr App R 247. Thirdly, if the accused does not believe that he is acting reasonably in preventing crime or in self-defence but circumstances in fact exist which would have given him a defence, had he known of them, he has no defence, for the principle in **Dadson** (1850) 4 Cox CC 358 explained in Chapter 2 applies. Fourthly, while the point has not been conclusively settled by the European Court of Human Rights, current English law laid down in **Williams** may be inconsistent with Article 2 of the European Convention, which the Court has interpreted as requiring the accused's belief to be based on reasonable grounds: see **McCann v UK** (1995) 21 EHRR 97, **Andronicou v Cyprus** (1998) 25 EHRR 491 and **Gul v Turkey** (2002) 34 EHRR 28. The European Court in **Brady v UK** (2001) 3 April had the opportunity to consider this issue but it seems that the Court failed to realise that a difference exists. The same must be said of **Caraher v UK** (2000) 11 January, an admissibility decision, and **Bubbins v UK**, 17 June 2005, where the requirement that force used by the police be 'absolutely necessary' was satisfied by a constable's honest belief that there was 'a real and immediate risk to his life and the lives of his colleagues'. Collins J in the Administrative Court said that English law and Article 2 were the same when it came to assessing the reasonableness of the force: **R (on the Application of Bennett) v H.M. Coroner for Inner South London** (2006) 170 JP 109. He added that Article 2 applies to both intentional and non-intentional killings. It should be noted that Article 2 is restricted to the use of fatal force in self-defence. It would be absurd if different rules applied to the use of non-fatal force.

(h) The same rules as apply to ordinary citizens govern the conduct of the security forces: **Clegg**. Lord Lloyd noted that there was no defence of superior orders in criminal law and that to create an exception for the armed services would be to make new law. Similarly, the High Court in **R (Bennett) v HM Coroner for Inner South London** held that Article 2 of the ECHR applied not just to agents of the state such as police officers but also to members of the public. Collins J suggested that the test of reasonableness in the English law of self-defence was the same as that found in Article 2 but as stated in (g), this *dictum* is questionable.

(i) The Court of Appeal held in **Jones v Gloucestershire Crown Prosecution Service** [2005] QB 259 that 'crime' in s 3 meant an act, omission or state of affairs and the mental element which constituted a crime in English domestic law. Therefore, the term did not include something which was a crime elsewhere or in international law but was not a crime in England and Wales. The international crime of aggression against a foreign country is not an offence in English law. Accordingly, aggression was not a 'crime' for the purposes of s 3, and the appellants could not use the defence against charges arising out of attempts to stop UK and US attacks on Iraq. The House of Lords dismissed the appeal on the same grounds [2006] UKHL 16. *Obiter* it was suggested that even if the crime of aggression existed in English domestic law, the defendants would not have been able to rely on the defence of prevention of crime because using force to obstruct military vehicles would not prevent the crime of aggression.

(j) In Australia a person, it seems, may defend himself, others and property against a lawful attack: *Zecevic* (1987) 71 ALR 641 (HCA). A similar rule exists in provocation. English law remains to be made. In *Re A* [2001] Fam 147 Ward LJ held that it was lawful to kill one of conjoined twins when her existence was dragging the other twin towards death: obviously the other twin's 'attack' was lawful. Ward LJ compared her with killing a six-year-old boy who was shooting people in the school playground. If English law were to demand an unlawful attack, one would not have a defence of self-defence against the type of persons mentioned earlier, the insane, automatons and those under 10. However, *DPP v Bayer* is to contrary effect. The defendants' claim of defence of property failed because they were not defending against unlawful behaviour. There was nothing criminal or tortious about drilling seeds of genetically modified maize.

(k) *Zecevic* also provided Australian authority for the proposition that an accused 'may not create a continuing situation of emergency and provoke a lawful attack upon himself and yet claim . . . the right to defend himself against that attack'. The law is different in provocation. Northern Irish law is the same as that stated in *Zecevic*: *Browne* [1983] NI 96. However, if the accused kills the victim in the course of a violent quarrel he (the accused) may rely on the defence if the victim's reaction was disproportionate to the accused's conduct: *Rashford* [2006] Crim LR 528 (CA). It is not certain whether *Rashford* has settled English law on this point but it seems to have done.

(l) The fact that an accused has a defence of self-defence does not prevent his losing a civil claim for damages in respect of the same act. See *Revill v Newbery* [1996] 2 WLR 239.

(m) The defendant's defence terminates when his victim is no longer threatening him. If there is a road rage incident, both drivers get out of their cars and one threatens the other with violence, the accused is entitled to use self-defence. If the first then drives off, the accused is not acting in self-defence if he follows him in order to drive him off the road.

(n) It does not matter whether the accused was acting calmly or in abject terror. The issue remains one of whether his action was reasonable.

(o) Section 3(1) affected both civil and criminal law. However, civil law is different not just as to the standard of proof but also the burden of proof. The defendant in civil law must prove that he has the defence: *Ashley v Chief Constable of Sussex Police* (2006) *The Times*, 30 August. The Court of Appeal also held, in distinction to criminal law, that a mistake as to whether the defendant had to act in prevention of crime had to be made on reasonable grounds. It is suggested that the civil law of mistake in self-defence is closer to the European Convention on Human Rights as interpreted in *McCann* than is the criminal law!

The present law and proposed reform of mistake of fact and intoxication are discussed under those headings.

As in necessity statutory words may conceal self-defence. By s 16 of the Firearms Act 1968 '[I]t is an offence for a person to have in his possession any firearm . . . with intent . . . to endanger life . . .'. While there is no express mention, counsel for the prosecution conceded in *Georgiades* [1989] 1 WLR 759 (CA) that it would be a defence for the accused to act to endanger life for a lawful purpose as when the accused raised a shortened shot-gun to waist level thinking he was about to be attacked. Note that force which causes the simple offence of criminal damage falls within the defence noted in Chapter 18, that of lawful excuse, whereas force causing the aggravated offence falls within self-defence.

The draft Criminal Code (Law Com. No. 177, 1989)

The Law Commission proposed to restate self-defence in the following fashion.

Clause 44(1)
A person does not commit an offence by using such force as, in the circumstances which exist or which he believes to exist, is immediately necessary and reasonable –
  (a) to prevent or terminate crime, or to effect or assist in the lawful arrest of an offender or suspected offender or of a person unlawfully at large;
  (b) to prevent or terminate a breach of the peace;
  (c) to protect himself or another from unlawful force or unlawful personal harm;
  (d) to prevent or terminate the unlawful detention of himself or another;
  (e) to protect property (whether belonging to himself or another) from unlawful appropriation, destruction or damage; or
  (f) to prevent or terminate a trespass to his person or property.

Law Commission Report No. 218, *Legislating the Criminal Code – Offences against the Person and General Principles*, 1993, on which see below, rejects a separate requirement that force is immediately necessary. If the requirement of imminence were abolished, battered persons who kill their sleeping or drunken partners might be afforded this defence. The 1993 Report also removed the reference in the opening words of cl 44(1) to 'circumstances which exist', thereby restoring the principle in *Dadson* (1850) 4 Cox CC 358.

Clause 44(2)
In this section, except where the context otherwise requires, 'force' includes, in addition to force against a person –
  (a) force against property;
  (b) a threat of force against person or property; and
  (c) the detention of a person without the use of force.

Clause 44(3)
For the purposes of this section, an act is 'unlawful' although a person charged with an offence in respect of it would be acquitted on the ground only that –
  (a) he was under ten years of age; or
  (b) he lacked the fault required for the offence or believed that an exempting circumstance existed; or
  (c) he acted in pursuance of a reasonable suspicion; or
  (d) he acted under duress, whether by threats or of circumstances; or
  (e) he was in a state of automatism or suffering from severe mental illness or severe mental handicap.

Clause 44(4)
Notwithstanding subsection (1), a person who believes circumstances to exist which would justify or excuse the use of force under that subsection has no defence if –

(a) he knows that the force is used against a constable or a person assisting a constable; and

(b) the constable is acting in the execution of his duty, unless he believes the force to be immediately necessary to prevent personal harm to himself or another.

(This is in accord with present law, the most recent authority being **Ball** (1990) 90 Cr App R 378 (CA). By putting the law into statutory form the Law Commission will give guidance to people on how to behave in a situation of potential or actual force.)

Clause 44(5)

A person does not commit an offence by doing an act immediately preparatory to the use of such force as is referred to in subsection (1).

Clause 44(6)

Subsection (1) does not apply where a person causes unlawful conduct or an unlawful state of affairs with a view to using force to resist or terminate it; but subsection (1) may apply although the occasion for the use of force arises only because he does anything he may lawfully do, knowing that such an occasion may arise.

Clause 44(7)

The fact that a person had an opportunity to retreat before using force shall be taken into account, in conjunction with other relevant evidence, in determining whether the use of force was immediately necessary and reasonable.

Clause 44(8)

A threat of force may be reasonable although the use of the force would not be.

Clause 44(9)

This section is without prejudice to the generality of section 185 (criminal damage: protection of person or property) or any other defence.

These provisions largely restate the law. However, one difference is found in cll 55 and 59. If the accused kills by using excessive force, the crime will no longer be murder but a new form of manslaughter. This was the position in Australia until the doctrine was abolished in 1987. The Australian direction was thought to be too complicated for juries. The English proposals, however, are not complex. This reform was also proposed by the Criminal Law Revision Committee in its Fourteenth Report, *Offences Against the Person*, Cmnd 7844, 1980, as well as the (Nathan) Select Committee on Murder and Life Imprisonment (HL Paper 78–1, 1989) para 89. The principal argument in favour of manslaughter is that the person who kills using excessive force is not as morally blameworthy as someone who kills and really intends to do so. Because of the stigma attached to murderers, those who have killed using unreasonable force should not be classified as murderers. The House of Lords in *Clegg* considered that this reform should not be achieved by the judiciary. Lord Lloyd said that the issue was one concerned with the mandatory life sentence for murder, which was one which only Parliament could resolve. There is certainly public concern that too many people who injure while acting in defence of property are prosecuted.

The Law Commission's 1993 proposals

In its Report No. 218, *Legislating the Criminal Code – Offences Against the Person and General Principles*, 1993, the Law Commission recommended a statutory restatement as to when the use of force is justified. Clause 27(1) of the Criminal Law Bill attached to the Report is in these terms.

The use of force by a person for any of the following purposes, if only such as is reasonable in the circumstances as he believes them to be, does not constitute an offence:

(a) to protect himself or another from injury, assault or detention caused by a criminal act;

(b) to protect himself or (with the authority of that other) another from trespass to the person;

(c) to protect his property from appropriation, destruction or damage caused by a criminal act or from trespass or infringement;

(d) to protect property belonging to another from appropriation, destruction or damage caused by a criminal act or (with the authority of the other) from trespass or infringement; or

(e) to prevent crime or a breach of the peace.

This clause incorporates the law in **Williams** [1987] 3 All ER 411, states expressly for the first time that force may be used against the property to protect the person, and revises s 5 of the Criminal Damage Act 1971 to bring it into line with the present s 3 of the Criminal Law Act 1967 with the effect that the force must be objectively reasonable and not merely reasonable from the accused's viewpoint. Clause 27(1)(a)–(e) lists the purposes for which the use of force is justifiable. It restates cl 44(1)(a)–(f) of the draft Criminal Code in slightly different words. It should be noted that the same act may fall within more than one of the categories, e.g. an accused who defends himself is preventing the commission of an offence and protecting against an assault. Clause 27(1)(e) is worth mentioning. The example given by the Law Commission is one where 'D restrains P, who is clearly dangerously intoxicated, from driving P's motor vehicle'. Here D is not protecting the person or property of himself or another but is preventing crime. There is special provision permitting defence against non-criminal acts done by persons under 10, acting under duress (of both kinds), acting involuntarily or in a state of intoxication and who are insane (cl 27(3)). This provision is needed only where the accused *knows* of the condition, for otherwise he is judged on the facts he believes to exist. There is another special provision dealing with the situation where the accused knows of the facts which make the other's acts non-criminal where the other has made a mistake. For example, the accused is making a lawful citizen's arrest; the other does not know this and thinks that the accused is attacking the victim; he intervenes; the accused uses force to resist the other; however, the accused knows that the other has made an error. By cl 27(6) the accused's reaction is lawful. The Law Commission argued that: 'P's act is lawful only because of a mistake or suspicion on the part of P that is in fact incorrect. D is nonetheless put in a position of potential peril that is not in any way lessened by P's error, and the fact that D knows of the error should not shut him out from the defence.'

There is no (separate) requirement that the accused is subject to or fears an immediate attack. The effect will be that more battered women who kill their sleeping or drunken abusers will have this defence. Clause 29(2) exempts from liability acts done immediately preparatory to the use of force such as the possession of firearms. Clause 27(7) takes away the defence from one who deliberately provokes an attack; however, an accused does have the defence where he is going about his lawful business as illustrated by **Beatty v Gillbanks** (1882) 9 QBD 308, the case of the Skeleton Army. As at present there is no rule that the accused is under a duty to retreat: cl 29(4). The **Dadson** (1850) 169 ER 407 principle is preserved by the Bill. In the words of the Law Commission:

It follows from the requirement that the defendant be judged according to circumstances as he believes them to be that he cannot rely on circumstances unknown to him that would in fact have justified acts on his part that were unreasonable on the facts as he perceived

341

them. . . . Citizens who react unreasonably to circumstances should not be exculpated by the accident of facts of which they were unaware.

Force to effect or assist in a lawful arrest receives separate treatment (cl 28). 'Force' in cll 27–29 is not defined. The restatement of the law of the justifiable use of force does not affect the defences of duress of circumstances or necessity. Therefore injury to a dog who is attacking one's children, and making a firebreak, will remain lawful.

Just as the defence of provocation has come in for criticism for being based on the male psyche with the result that few women are afforded it because they do not react in the same way as men, so too has the defence of self-defence been criticised. The Australian Law Reform Commission in its Report No. 69, *Equality before the Law: Justice for Women*, 1994, paras 12.2–3 put it this way.

> What is 'reasonable' has traditionally been assessed on men's experiences of a reasonable response to the circumstances. For example, in establishing self-defence, there must be an immediate threat and a proportionate response. The typical scenario is that of an isolated incident in a public place between two strangers of relatively equal size, strength and fighting ability, that is, a 'bar-room brawl' model. . . . The 'bar-room brawl' model bears little relation to the situation of a woman who has been subjected to prolonged physical, mental and emotional abuse within her home by her male partner. In her terrorised state and usually inferior physical size and strength, her only reasonable option may be to take action some time later when it is safe for her to do so. This may be during a lull in the violence, for example, when the aggressor is asleep or incapacitated by alcohol. However, the law may construct her act as a premeditated one arising out of a long held grudge rather than as a defensive response triggered by a particular incident. For this reason it is argued that defences should be revised to reflect women's experiences of violence and acts of self-preservation.
>
> . . . Where juries and judges lack an understanding of the dynamics and effect of violence in the home, they may not see the woman's response as 'reasonable'. They may see her use of a gun or knife as excessive force in relation to the physical assaults inflicted on her by her unarmed partner . . . They may ask why she did not simply leave. This approach ignores the disempowering effect of the violence on the woman, her practical difficulties, such as where to go and how to support herself and her children, and her fear of retaliation if she were to leave, particularly where police assistance has not been adequate in the past. [footnotes omitted]

Excessive force in self-defence: the Law Commission's 2004 Report

The Law Commission in its Report No. 290, *Partial Defences to Murder*, 2004, considered whether excessive force should reduce murder to manslaughter in the same way as diminished responsibility and provocation do. Currently self-defence operates as an 'all-or-nothing' defence; this is, either the accused succeeds in his defence, in which case he is acquitted, or he fails, in which case he is convicted of murder. Excessive force when some force would be reasonable in the context of the Report means that the accused is convicted of murder. This conclusion is to some degree mitigated by trial judges directing juries that they are to take all circumstances into account, including, for example, the size of the accused and victim, that they are not to use hindsight, and that where there is evidence of provocation, they should consider whether or not that defence succeeds with the effect that a verdict of voluntary manslaughter is reached.

The Commission rejected the provision of a defence of excessive force. In respect of householders who kill intruders, it considered that they could have a defence of provocation under the revised formula if these conditions were satisfied: if a person of ordinary tolerance and self-restraint acting in fear of serious physical violence to himself or another might have killed and the accused does kill, he will have a defence. In respect of battered adults or children who kill, fearing further abuse and not perceiving any route of escape and being aware of the mismatch in physique so that 'to respond directly and proportionately to an attack or an imminent attack will be futile and dangerous' (para 4.18), should they have a defence of self-defence if they use excessive force when, for example, their abuser is drunk or asleep? Again the Law Commission thought that such facts could fall within the revised definition of provocation: was the accused genuinely in fear of serious violence and might a person of ordinary tolerance and self-restraint have acted in the same or a similar way? In para 4.29 the Commission said that the revised definition of provocation will work 'through the acknowledgement that even a person of ordinary tolerance and self-restraint might, on occasion, respond in fear by using an excessive amount of force.'

In conclusion the Law Commission was strongly of the view that there should not be a defence of excessive self-defence because in situations where that defence might arise, householders and the abused, the reformulated defence of provocation would be available. However, the Commission in its Report No. 304 *Murder, Manslaughter and Infanticide*, 2006, concluded that there should be such a defence but that since self-defence was a general defence, it would not consider it further in this Report.

Conclusion

The Home Secretary announced in 1995 that, after the unsuccessful appeal of Private Lee Clegg, a Home Office group would review the law on excessive self-defence by members of the armed forces and the police. The Interdepartmental Steering Group on the Law on the Use of Lethal Force in Self-Defence or the Prevention of Crime did not come down firmly for any change in the law, including the creation of a partial defence available on a charge of murder of excessive self-defence and amendment to s 3 of the Criminal Law Act 1967 to flesh out the meaning of reasonable force, when it reported in 1996 because it favoured finer distinctions than murder or manslaughter and manslaughter or acquittal, but it rejected any difference between the armed forces and the police on the one hand and other citizens on the other. There is, however, an argument to the contrary. Experienced police marksmen should be judged against a higher standard than ordinary citizens because they are experts. Such an argument might lead to the law that members of the police force and the armed forces should have a defence only when they have made a reasonable mistake as to the amount of force. Furthermore, the use of force is a matter of political controversy, which it rarely is when force is used by private individuals. Since Parliament shows no inclination to define murder or to change the sentence for murder, any change to bring in a defence of excessive self-defence is just not going to happen.

The outcome in **Martin**, above, where a Norfolk farmer shot a burglar in the back, killing him, led to outcry in favour of the accused; listeners to the *Today* programme on Radio 4 voted the reform of self-defence as their top priority for a bill, and in 2005 the Conservatives pushed for a change to the law whereby force would be lawful unless it was 'grossly disproportionate', a higher threshold than 'unreasonable' or 'excessive'. Such strong feelings culminated in a bland (in the writer's view) and short Joint Statement from the Crown Prosecution Service and the Association of Chief Police Officers

'Householders and the Use of Force against Intruders', in February 2005. Among the statements are: 'So long as you only do what you honestly and instinctively believe is necessary in the heat of the moment, that would be the strongest evidence of you acting lawfully and in selfdefence [sic!]. This is still the case if you use something to hand as a weapon. As a general rule, the more extreme the circumstances and the fear felt, the more force you can lawfully use in self-defence' and '. . . if, for example: having knocked someone unconscious, you then decided to further hurt or kill them to punish them . . . you would be acting with very excessive and gratuitous force and could be prosecuted.' Interestingly, there is no mention of defence of property.

The European Convention on Human Rights does not permit the use of force to prevent harm to property. Therefore, a householder who killed a burglar in defence of property would not be able to rely on self-defence and the prevention of crime. However, the Convention provides an exception to the right to life only when 'the use of force . . . is no more than absolutely necessary'. See the decision of the European Court of Human Rights in **Andronicou v Cyprus** (1998) 25 EHRR 491 where it was held that force had to be strictly proportionate to the threat posed by the victim. On the facts police officers were justified in using sub-machine guns in an attempt to rescue a hostage. This is a more stringent test than current English law, which speaks of 'reasonable' force. Both statute and common law will have to be restricted to situations where only necessary force is used. The jurisprudence of the European Court of Human Rights may also lead to change. Present English law permits a defence based on mistaken belief. However, the European Court of Human Rights seems to look for an honest belief that is well founded ('good reason'), as it did in **McCann, Andronicou, Gul** and **Bubbins**. The reduction in scope of self-defence may lead to calls for the introduction of the defence of excessive self-defence. Another distinction is that the Convention, Article 2, applies only when the victim was using 'unlawful violence'. English law applies whether the victim was using unlawful or lawful violence. One would hope that two sets of rules would not emerge depending on whether the force was lawful or not. Finally, English law permits the use of force to prevent crime but no such purpose exists in Article 2(2), and Article 2(1) is restricted to the use of force to kill whereas English law is not: it includes situations where the victim is not killed.

Summary

The second chapter on defences considers three defences: mistake, intoxication and self-defence (which is nowadays sometimes called private defence). Mistakes of law and of fact are dealt with, as are mistakes as to an 'irrelevant' element of the offence definition. Intoxication, whether by alcohol or drugs, is a defence to certain offences only, the so-called crimes of specific intent, whereas it is not a defence to offences of basic intent. The various attempts by the judiciary to divide crimes into specific and basic intent ones are criticised. A helpful diagram of offences and their placing into the category of basic or specific intent is provided. The final defence examined in this chapter is here called self-defence, but the defence extends beyond defence of self to defence of others and even of property. It also covers the defence of prevention of crime found in s 3 of the Criminal Law Act 1967. The relationship between this defence and the common law one of self-defence is considered. There is discussion of whether current Anglo–Welsh law falls short of the standard demanded by the European Convention on Human Rights. Proposals for reform are discussed including those in the report *Partial Defences to Murder*, 2004.

- Mistake: The basic rule is that mistake as to law is no defence but that Parliament may create such a defence. Mistakes of fact may provide a defence but not if they are to the strict element (one to which no *mens rea* is attached) of an offence. The mistake of fact need usually only be one honestly made but bigamy provides the exception: the mistake must be one made on reasonable grounds. For mistakes caused by intoxication, see below.

- Intoxication: Involuntary intoxication is a defence to all offences but is no defence where the accused nevertheless had the *mens rea* for the offence; voluntary intoxication is a defence only to offences of specific intent (e.g. murder) but not to crimes of basic intent (e.g. manslaughter); and drunken mistake is no defence to all offences including ones of specific intent. Debate rages as to the definition of 'specific intent' and the position of soporific drugs is not crystal-clear. In relation to specific intent any suggested definition has a counterfactual argument, e.g. if a specific intent offence is one which involves a 'purposive element', why is rape a basic intent offence?; if specific intent means crimes which can be committed only intentionally (and not either intentionally or recklessly), why when malice aforethought in murder was defined wider than it is now because it included foresight of a highly probable consequence, was murder still a specific intent offence? While the law is not pellucid, it seems to be that a person does not have a defence of intoxication if she or he knew that soporific drugs would make her or him aggressive or violent: the law is not whether she or he ought to have known of the drugs' effects on him or her.

- Self-defence and the prevention of crime: Section 3 of the Criminal Law Act 1967 provides a defence to any offence where the accused uses reasonable force to prevent a crime; where that defence is not available, the common law provides a defence, self-defence, to all offences subject again to the force being reasonable. For example, if a child under 10 is proposing to kill the accused's child, and the accused kills the threatener, there is no crime to prevent because a child under 10 cannot be guilty of any offence; however, the common law steps in to provide a defence. For both defences the force used must be reasonable; that is, it must be necessary and proportionate. Excessive force does not provide a defence. If the accused honestly believes that he or she is under attack or others are, the defences apply on the facts as the accused believes exists. If the accused's mistake is, however, occasioned by alcohol, there is no defence.

  It should be noted that 'self-defence' is something of a misnomer because it applies to the defence of self, others and property.

References

Reports

Australian Law Reform Commission Report no. 69, *Equality before the Law: Justice for Women* (1994)

Criminal Law Revision Committee 14th Report, *Offences against the Person* (1980) Cmnd 7844

Interdepartmental Steering Group on the Law on the Use of Lethal Force in Self-Defence or the Prevention of Crime (1995)

Law Commission Consultation Paper no. 127, *Intoxication and Criminal Liability* (1993)

Law Commission Report no. 177, *A Criminal Code for England & Wales* (1989)

Law Commission Report no. 218, *Legislating the Criminal Code: Offences against the Person and General Principles* (1993)

Law Commission Report no. 229, *Legislating the Criminal Code: Intoxication and Criminal Liability* (1995)

Law Commission Report no. 290, *Partial Defences to Murder* (2004)

Law Commission Report no. 306, *Murder, Manslaughter and Infanticide* (2006)

Law Reform Commission of Ireland Report no. 51, *Intoxication* (1995)

Model Penal Code (1962)

Report of the Committee on *Mentally Abnormal Offenders* (Butler) (1975) Cmnd 6244

Report of the Select Committee on Murder and Life Imprisonment (Nathan) (1989) HL Paper 78-1

Scottish Law Commission Discussion Paper no. 122, *Insanity and Diminished Responsibility* (2003)

Books

Bentham, J. *An Introduction to the Principles of Morals and Legislation* (Methuen, 1932) (first published 1789)

Bishop's Criminal Law vol. 1, 9th edn (Little, Brown & Co, 1923)

Clarkson, C. M. V. *Understanding Criminal Law* 4th edn (Thomson, 2005)

Reed, A. and Fitzpatrick, B. *Criminal Law* 3th edn (Thomson, 2006)

Seago, P. *Criminal Law* 4th edn (Sweet & Maxwell, 1994)

Journals

Brett, P. 'Mistake of law as a criminal defence' (1966) 5 Melb ULR 179

Elliott, D. W. 'Necessity, duress and self-defence' [1989] Crim LR 611

Goode, M. 'Some thoughts on the present state of the "defence" of intoxication' (1984) 8 Crim LJ 104

Healy, P. '*R* v *Bernard*: difficulties with "voluntary intoxication"' (1990) 35 McGill LJ 610

Smith, G. 'Footnote to *O'Connor*'s case' (1981) 5 Crim LJ 270

Williams, J. M. 'Mistake of fact' (1985) 63 CBR 597

Further reading

Ashworth, A. 'Excusable mistake of law' [1974] Crim LR 652

Ashworth, A. 'Testing fidelity to legal values: Official involvement in criminal justice' (2000) 63 MLR 63

Ayyildiz, E. 'When battered women's syndrome does not go far enough: the battered women as vigilante' (1995) 4 Am U J Gender & L 141

Boyle, C. 'The battered wife syndrome and self-defence' (1990) 9 *Canadian Journal of Family Law* 171

Callaghan, A. R. 'Will the "real" battered woman please stand up?' (1994) 3 Am U J Gender & L 117

Dennis, I. 'What should be done about the law of self-defence?' [2000] Crim LR 417

Faigman, D. L. and Wright, A. J. 'The battered woman syndrome in the age of science' (1997) 39 Ariz LR 67

Gardner, S. 'The importance of *Majewski*' (1994) 14 OJLS 279

Getzler, J. 'Use of force in protecting property' (2006) *Theoretic Inquiries L*131

Gough, S. 'Intoxication and criminal liability' (1996) 112 LQR 335

Gough, S. 'Surviving without *Majewski*' [2000] Crim LR 719

Harlow, C. 'Self-defence: public right or private privilege' [1974] Crim LR 528

Horder, J. 'Cognition, emotion and criminal culpability' (1990) 106 LQR 469

Horder, J. 'Sobering up: The Law Commission on criminal intoxication' (1995) 58 MLR 534

Jefferson, M. 'Householders and the use of force against intruders' (2005) 69 JCL 405

Kaufman, W. R. P. 'Self-defense, imminence, and the battered woman' (2007) 10 New Crim L Rev 342

Lanham, D. 'Offensive weapons and self-defence' [2005] Crim LR 85

Leverick, F. 'Is English self-defence law incompatible with Article 2 of the ECHR?' [2002] Crim LR 347

Leverick, F. 'The use of force in public or private defence and Article 2' [2002] Crim LR 963

Leverick, F. *Killing in Self-Defence* (Oxford University Press, 2006)

Leverick, F. 'Defending self-defence' (2007) 27 OJLS 563

McAuley, F. 'The grammar of mistake in criminal law' (1996) xxxi IJ 56

McCord, D. 'The English and American history of voluntary intoxication to negate *mens rea*' (1990) 11 JLH 372

Macdonald, E. 'Reckless language and *Majewski*' (1986) 6 LS 239

Martinson, D. *et al.* '*Lavallee* v *R* 1 SCR 852 – the Supreme Court of Canada addresses the issue of gender bias in the court: Women and Self-Defence' (1991) 25 UBCLR 23

O'Leary, J. 'Lament for the intoxication defence' (1997) 48 NILQ 152

Ormerod, D. 'Voluntary intoxication: whether voluntary intoxication available on a charge of sexual assault' [2007] Crim LR 654

Orchard, G. 'Surviving without *Majewski*: A view from Down Under' [1993] Crim LR 426

Polsby, D. D. 'Reflections on violence, guns and the defensive use of reasonable force' (1986) 49 L & CP 89

Rogers, J. 'Justifying the use of firearms by policemen and soldiers' (1998) 18 LS 486

Rosman, J. B. 'The battered woman syndrome in Florida: junk science or admissible evidence?' (2003) 15 St Thomas L Rev 107

Segev, R. 'Justification, rationality and mistake' (2006) 25 *Law and Philosophy* 31

Shaffer, M. 'The battered woman syndrome revisited' (1997) 47 UTLJ 1

Simester, A. P. 'Intoxication is never a defence' [2009] Crim LR 3

Smith, J. C. 'The use of force in public or private defence and Article 2' [2002] Crim LR 958

Spencer, J. R. 'Drunken defence' [2006] CLJ 267

Virgo, G. 'Reconciling principle and policy' [1993] Crim LR 415

Wallerstein, S. 'Justifying the right to self-defense: a theory of forced consequences' (2005) 91 Virg LR 999

Ward, A. R. 'Making sense of self-induced intoxication' [1986] CLJ 247

White, S. 'Offences of basic and specific intent' [1989] Crim LR 271

Williams, R. 'Voluntary intoxication, sexual assault and the future of *Majewski*' [2007] CLJ 260

Yeo, S. 'Revisiting excessive self-defence' (2000) 12 *Current Issues in Criminal Justice* 39

Yeo, S. 'Killing in Defence of Property' [2000] NLJ 730

For an essay, see J. Horder in A. P. Simester and S. Shute (eds.), *Criminal Law: Doctrines of the General Part* (Oxford University Press, 2002), Chapter 12.

For a full-length study of self-defence, see S. Uniacke, *Permissible Killing: The Self-Defence Justification of Homicide* (Cambridge University Press, 1996). The principal English survey of excuses is J. Horder, *Excusing Crime* (Oxford University Press, 2003).

For Commonwealth reform proposals, see Tasmania Law Reform Institute, *Intoxication and Criminal Responsibility*, Issues Paper no. 7 (2005) and the Final Report no. 7 of the same name (2006), the principal recommendation being that intoxication should be relevant to all mental elements.

For a recent Irish approach, see Law Reform Commission, Commission Paper 41, *Legitimate Defence*, 2006.

For US law, which in general is similar to the law of intoxication in England and Wales, see M. Keiter, 'Just say no excuse' (1997) 87 JCL & Crim 482.

Visit **www.mylawchamber.co.uk/jefferson** to access exam-style questions with answer guidance, multiple choice quizzes, live weblinks, an online glossary, and regular updates to the law.

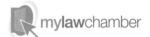

Use **Case Navigator** to read in full some of the key cases referenced in this chapter:

DPP v *Majewski* [1976] 2 All ER 142
DPP v *Morgan* [1975] 2 All ER 347
R v *Cunningham* [1957] 2 All ER 412
R v *G* [2003] 4 All ER 765
R v *Pagett* (1983) 76 Cr App Rep 279

9

Defences of mental disorder

Introduction

The accused does not necessarily have a defence if he is mentally disturbed through schizophrenia, paranoia, dementia or a myriad other upsets affecting the mind. To have a defence the defendant must fall within one of the recognised excuses: insanity, diminished responsibility, automatism. Each of these defences has a different definition from the others including burden of proof and outcome. They should not be confused. Moreover, the defences are legal ones: they should not be confused with medical diagnosis. However, these defences may overlap. When they do, the accused will be seeking the defence which is most favourable to him. For example, he will be acquitted on the grounds of automatism; however, if he successfully pleads insanity, until recently he would under the Criminal Procedure (Insanity) Act 1964, s 5, be detained in a hospital until the Home Secretary approved his release ('hospital order with restrictions'). This provision meant that he would be detained for a period longer than the norm for murderers, the 'life' sentence now being about 15 years' imprisonment plus the threat of recall. The result may have been that the accused would be kept longer away from the public if he was acquitted on the grounds of insanity than if he were guilty of murder. This way of thinking applies with even greater force to lesser offences. The effect is that the accused may be seeking to avoid succeeding on the defence! The accused may want to go to prison where he will not receive treatment for his ills. The interests of society, however, demand that mentally imbalanced persons who are 'dangerous' should be restrained and if possible treated. One major problem is to determine which people should be detained in hospital, which in prison, and which released. The law does not at present in all cases draw the most appropriate distinctions, as we shall see. The Criminal Procedure (Insanity and Unfitness to Plead) Act 1991 gives the judge discretion as to sentence. The outcome could be an absolute discharge, except for murder where the sentence must be a hospital order with restrictions on discharge.

Two principles may collide: individual responsibility for crime and the protection of society. A disordered person may not have the free will to control his actions and cannot be reformed by punishment. The law's commands are addressed to those who have the capacity to reason.

This chapter investigates mental aberration at the time of the offence or, in the case of unfitness to plead, at the time of trial. There are other ways of dealing with offenders, e.g. a person guilty of manslaughter may be given a hospital order under s 37 of the Mental Health Act 1983, if such is the most suitable way of disposing of his case.

Unfitness to plead

To stand trial the accused must be:

> . . . of sufficient intellect to comprehend the course of the proceedings in the trial so as to make a proper defence, to challenge a juror to whom he might wish to object and comprehend the details of the evidence.

So said Alderson B in *Pritchard* (1836) 173 ER 135, a case involving a deaf mute. This case is an illustration that the defence of unfitness to plead is available not just to the mentally incapable but also to others who cannot follow the proceedings. This test is the one still used as *Patel*, unreported, 7 August 1991 (CA) and *M*, unreported, 14 November 2003 (CA) demonstrate. The accused must also be able to plead to the indictment. He must be able to instruct counsel. A modern statement of the rule was given by Otton LJ in *Friend* [1997] 2 All ER 1012: 'The test of unfitness is whether the accused will be able to comprehend the course of the proceedings so as to make a proper defence. Whether he can understand and reply rationally to the indictment is obviously a relevant factor, but the jury must also consider whether he would be able to exercise his right to challenge juries, understand the details of the evidence as it is given, instruct his legal advisers and give evidence himself if he so desires.' However, it is irrelevant that the accused has a low mental age: *SC v UK* [2005] 1 FCR 347 (ECHR) (boy of 11 with the intellectual capacity of a six- or eight-year-old). The court said: 'The defendant should be able to follow what is said by prosecution witnesses and, if represented, to explain to his own lawyers his version of events, point out any statements with which he disagrees and make them aware of any facts which should be put forward in his defence.' There is a breach of Article 6(1) in relation to children if these criteria are not met. The conditions are generalisable. It is inhuman to try people who cannot understand anything of a trial, and it would reflect badly on the law if such persons were tried. The fact that he acts abnormally and cannot act in his own best interests is irrelevant, as is the fact that he can communicate with others on non-legal matters. Before 1992, if he could not perform these tasks, he was under the Criminal Procedure (Insanity) Act 1964 found unfit to plead at a Crown Court (i.e. this procedure does not apply to summary trial) by a specially empanelled jury (s 4(4)) and was hospitalised at a place specified by the Home Secretary (s 5(1)) for an indefinite period, a rather severe restriction when the charge was a petty one. The new procedure remains inapplicable to summary trials, as does the whole law of unfitness to plead. Magistrates instead have the power to make a hospital order. There is no jurisdiction to commit to the Crown Court for a jury to rule on fitness to stand trial.

The issue may be raised by the defendant, prosecution or judge. Where the accused raises the issue, the burden of proof is on him on the balance of probabilities: *Podola* [1960] 1 QB 325. This has been criticised on the ground that when the accused pleads unfitness to plead he is simply saying that the prosecution cannot prove all the elements of the crime alleged and it is for the prosecution to do so beyond reasonable doubt. If, however, the issue is raised by the prosecution, or presumably if it is raised by the judge, the burden is on the prosecution to show that the defendant is unfit beyond reasonable doubt: *Robertson* [1968] 1 WLR 1767 (CA). The judge could postpone the issue of unfitness to plead until the close of the prosecution case, so allowing the accused to submit that there was no case to answer. This discretion should be exercised if there is a decent chance that the prosecution case will not convince.

Criticism

D. Grubin wrote 'What constitutes fitness to plead?' [1993] Crim LR 748 at 755: '[T]here is a story, perhaps apocryphal, of a High Court judge who observed that if comprehension of court proceedings was a prerequisite for participation in a trial, then most of those in court, including members of the legal profession, would be considered unfit to plead.'

(a) In the words of the Butler Committee, *Report of the Committee on Mentally Abnormal Offenders*, Cmnd 6244, 1975, para 10.18:

> It is not in the interests of the defendant to seek the protection of a disability plea unless the charge is very serious. If the trial went ahead he might be acquitted altogether.

(b) The definition in **Pritchard** focuses on the accused's intellectual ability at quite a low level. It does not take into account whether he possesses an understanding of the consequences of conviction, or even why he is on trial. It is arguable that the trial is unfair if he cannot grasp the significance of the proceedings.

(c) There is no statutory definition of unfitness to plead.

(d) The criterion of being able to instruct counsel, which was not found in **Pritchard** but has come to be accepted, should be included.

(e) The definition of unfitness to plead covers deaf mutes, as **Pritchard** illustrates. This is inconsistent with Article 5 of the European Convention of Human Rights. The European Court in **Winterwerp v The Netherlands** (1979) 2 EHRR 387 demanded 'objective medical expertise' before a person could be detained as being 'of unsound mind,' but deaf mutes are not of unsound mind as a matter of objective medical expertise. The court emphasised that the term 'of unsound mind' could not be given a definitive definition because its meaning is 'continually evolving as research in psychiatry progresses . . .'.

Empirical research

R. D. Mackay examined the statistics for 1979–89 in 'The decline of disability in relation to the trial' [1991] Crim LR 87. There were 229 findings of unfitness to plead. Most of the accused were male, and most were aged between 20 and 39; 71 per cent had criminal records and 81 per cent had a psychiatric history. The number of trials for unfitness per year declined by half from the early to late 1980s (e.g. 28 in 1981, 13 in 1988). Offences against the person accounted for almost a quarter. Some defendants were back for up to their fourth unfitness-to-plead determination. Contrary to expectation the plea did not always involve serious crimes such as rape and murder. 'This was found to be particularly true of Theft Act offences which in many cases were accounted for by destitute and mentally ill defendants being unable to pay for meals or services' (at 90). A similar phrase occurs in his book (Mackay, *Mental Condition Defences in the Criminal Law* (Clarendon, 1995) 223). There were 28 pleas in 1994 and 27 in 1995. In 2001 there were 76 successful pleas. Numbers rose rapidly in the late 1990s.

Over half of the accused were diagnosed as schizophrenic, with a small number suffering from other mental illnesses such as dementia and psychosis. The Court of Criminal Appeal in **Podola**, above, held that hysterical amnesia was not within the definition of unfitness to plead because the accused was normal at the time of the hearing, but three of the defendants in the sample were suffering from amnesia. Moreover, the criteria in **Pritchard** were not always fulfilled: each aspect seems to be treated individually, not cumulatively, with emphasis being placed on the ability to instruct a lawyer and follow proceedings.

A second study by D. Grubin for 1975–88 found 285 persons dealt with under the unfitness to plead provisions. About one-quarter of the crimes alleged were minor, such as shoplifting. He noted that as a result of Home Office policy about 15 per cent of those found unfit were later tried in the early years of the survey but in the later years the percentage went up to 60 per cent ('Unfit to plead in England and Wales 1976–88 – A survey' (1991) 158 BJ Psych 540). He considered that the law worked only because psychiatrists and judges sometimes disregard **Pritchard**. The effect, however, is arbitrary: some persons suffering from the same disorder are found unfit, some are found fit ('What constitutes unfitness to plead?' [1993] Crim LR 748). As a minimum this finding is worrying.

A third survey published in 'An upturn in unfitness to plead?' [2000] Crim LR 532 by R. D. Mackay and Gerry Kearns found that in the five years after the coming into force of the 1991 Act the number of successful pleas of unfitness to plead had doubled. The largest proportion of those who were successful were schizophrenics. Those suffering from dementia, psychosis, brain damage and depressive states featured among the diagnostic groups. Two persons had 'deafness/communication difficulties'. Some 90 per cent of those found unfit to plead were male.

Criminal Procedure (Insanity and Unfitness to Plead) Act 1991

This Act, the first to be promoted by the Law Society, is directed at abolishing the mandatory commitment to a psychiatric hospital even though the accused has not been convicted of an offence. The procedure under the Act, which came into force on 1 January 1992, as amended by the Domestic Violence, Crime and Victims Act 2004, is:

(a) A judge decides whether the accused is fit to plead. The judge hears two doctors, one of whom was approved by the Home Secretary as experienced in this field.

(b) If the judge determines that the accused was unfit on his arraignment a jury decides whether he committed the *actus reus* of the offence. Where the issue falls for consideration after arraignment it may be tried by the same or a different jury. This process is sometimes known as 'trial of the facts'. The prosecution must prove that the accused committed the *actus reus* beyond reasonable doubt. Section 4A(2) of the Criminal Procedure (Insanity) Act 1964, as inserted by the 1991 Act, does not say this expressly but it is consistent with criminal law principles. If the accused did not do the act alleged, there is no reason to subject him to the rigours of the criminal law. There is support in **Attorney-General's Reference (No. 3 of 1998)** [1999] 2 Cr App R 214 for the view that any defence, such as prevention of crime, must be considered by the jury. The mental element would not be considered according to the generally accepted view, but the Court of Appeal in **Egan** [1997] Crim LR 225 said that the *mens rea* must be proved too, and counsel did not argue the point. **Egan** had some support, for the Butler Committee on Mentally Abnormal Offenders referred to proof of the mental state (Cmnd 6244, 1975, para 10.24). If the jury found that he did the act, the judge has a range of sentencing options, including detention in a psychiatric hospital with or without restrictions, an absolute discharge, a supervision and training order under the 1991 Act, and a guardianship order under the Mental Health Act

1983. As Stephen White wrote in 'Acts and facts' (1998) 62 JCL 360, *Egan* was wrong because if 'act' is not limited to *actus reus*, 'a successful defence of insanity could preclude a jury finding that the defendant had done the act charged as an offence, and the powers of restraint and control under the 1991 Act . . . could hardly ever – perhaps never – be exercised'.

The Court of Appeal held in *Attorney-General's Reference (No. 3 of 1998)* that *Egan* was wrongly decided. The determination was in the context of insanity where the jury has to say whether the accused 'did the act or made the omission charged' (Trial of Lunatics Act 1883, s 2). What was said about unfitness to plead was *obiter*, but the court stated that *Egan* was decided *per incuriam*. If the court was wrong on this point, *Egan* was restricted to unfitness to plead. The House of Lords ruled in *Antoine* [2001] 1 AC 340 that *Egan* was incorrect even in relation to unfitness to plead. *Antoine* also held that 'act' in s 4A(2) of the 1964 Act includes complete defences such as self-defence (it is often said that self-defence negates the *actus reus*). It left open the position as to provocation. However, in *Grant* [2002] 1 Cr App R 528 (CA) it was held that provocation, which depends on the accused's state of mind, does not fall within s 4A. Therefore, the defence of provocation cannot be raised at this stage. (If the issue of unfitness to plead arises during the trial, the same jury which determined fitness determines whether the accused performed the *actus reus*.) If the jury finds that the accused did not commit the *actus reus*, he is acquitted. The Court of Appeal laid down these steps in *O'Donnell* [1996] 1 Cr App R 286. There is one situation where *mens rea* is investigated and that is where the accused is charged as an accomplice. He will have to know of the acts of the principal before it can be said that he did 'the act or omission charged': *Martin* [2003] EWCA Crim 357.

Under previous law the sole outcome was a hospital order without limit of time. That remains the outcome under the 1991 Act only when the sentence is fixed by law, i.e. for murder. The Domestic Violence, Crime and Victims Act 2004 provides that such hospitalisation may take place only when the medical evidence as to the accused's mental state justifies a hospital order. The same applies to a restriction order. (After the 1991 Act the likelihood is that persons who would otherwise have pleaded unfitness to plead or insanity on a charge of murder are now opting for diminished responsibility as the defence because, if successful, they may receive a determinate sentence.) The Home Secretary may (not must) remit for trial when the accused has recovered. On conviction all the usual sentences including probation are available. Because of the broader range of disposal options, it is likely that more people will plead unfitness to plead and insanity than previously, and this seems to be happening. With this broadened range of sentences comes a new sentence of a supervision and treatment order, whereby a person found insane can be placed under the supervision of a social worker or probation officer for not more than two years and subject to medical treatment. The possibility of a guardianship order was abolished by the 2004 Act. Research is demonstrating that judges are alert to the sentencing options under the 1991 Act. If the accused has been found unfit to plead, the trial even for murder ends. Therefore, an accused found unfit to plead cannot use the defence of diminished responsibility to avoid the mandatory commitment for murder on a successful plea of unfitness to plead: *Antoine*.

It may be thought that a trial on the facts breaches Article 6 of the European Convention on Human Rights. Article 6 guarantees the right to a fair trial. It would seem not to be a fair trial if the accused cannot fully participate in it, as occurs when he cannot understand the charges against him. As the European Court held in

Winterwerp the person who is of unsound mind must not be deprived of the right to a fair trial. However, the House of Lords held in *H* [2003] 1 WLR 411 that there was no incompatibility between s 4A and Article 6, because the determination of fitness to plead does not involve a criminal trial. For comment on *H* and its compatibility with Strasbourg jurisprudence see A. Ashworth in his case comment on *H* [2003] Crim LR 818. It is certainly possible that the criteria for assessing unfitness to plead do not conflict with Article 6. See also the discussion of *Grant* below in relation to Article 5(1).

Appeal lies in both instances to the Court of Appeal.

Mental Health Act 1983, ss 47–48

There is a second way in which the Home Secretary can order an accused to be detained in a hospital. The power is found in the Mental Health Act 1983, ss 47–48, and is available only if the Home Secretary thinks it expedient to send a person who is committed in custody for trial to a hospital in the public interest. This order is called a 'transfer direction'. He must be satisfied by reports from two or more medical practitioners that the accused is suffering from mental illness or severe mental impairment and the accused must be in urgent need of treatment. Section 1(1) of the 1983 Act defines the latter term as:

> A state of arrested or incomplete development of mind which includes severe impairment of intelligence and social functioning and is associated with abnormally aggressive or seriously irresponsible conduct . . .

The accused is remitted for trial when he has recovered. It should be noted that this definition is by no means the same as that of insanity. A person can fall within s (1) but still not have the defence of insanity.

The 1983 Act applies where the accused is committed in custody for trial. Unfitness to plead arises when he is brought up for trial.

When the Mental Health Act 2007, Sch 1, comes into force, a judge will be able to make a hospital order whenever a convicted person is suffering from any disorder or disability of mind.

Insanity

In the defence of insanity (which applies only in the Crown Court; in a magistrates' court insanity results in a total acquittal, not a verdict of 'not guilty by reason of insanity', though there exist post-acquittal procedures) the accused was insane at the time of the offence but is fit to plead at the time of the trial. It is not often raised today. For example, there were two successful pleas in 1974, three in 1978, three in 1981, none in 1988, one in 1990, two in 1991, three in 1992 and 11 in 1996. Comparable figures for the companion defence of diminished responsibility are 78 in 1978, 75 in 1981 and 50 in 1988. It is suggested that many more people are legally insane than these figures suggest. Reasons why insanity is rarely used include:

(a) The accused is contending that he was insane, but now is sane: the defence looks hard to prove to a jury.

(b) Some people who formerly might have used this defence are now charged with infanticide or have the defence of diminished responsibility where the charge is one of murder. For example, in *Tickell* (1958) *The Times*, 24 January, the accused, a schizophrenic, successfully pleaded diminished responsibility but was sentenced to life imprisonment. Before the defence was instituted, he would have had a defence of insanity.

(c) If the punishment is less than life imprisonment it is better for the accused to spend time in prison for a few years than to go to a mental hospital for a longer time. Therefore, if the defence realises that the judge is going to rule that the defence is one of insanity, it is better for the accused to plead guilty than to be acquitted on the grounds of insanity. The effect may be that the public are not protected. Doctors may believe the accused to be legally insane but knowing the consequences of a verdict of insanity may not tell the court of their view. Moreover, the accused may succeed on diminished responsibility when the argument for it may not be very strong in order to avoid the life sentence for murder. Of the 49 insanity verdicts in the period 1975–88, 14 were in murder cases and 23 in non-fatal offences.

In practice, therefore, insanity is not important in terms of numbers, but it bulks large in lawyerly writing because of the need to distinguish insanity (where the outcome may be that the accused is sent to a secure hospital) and automatism (where the outcome is a complete acquittal). The insane person was detained until the Home Secretary or a Mental Health Review Tribunal ordered release. Some were released swiftly, some were not: R. D. Mackay 'Fact and fiction about the insanity defence' [1990] Crim LR 247. The Criminal Procedure (Insanity and Unfitness to Plead) Act 1991 gives the judge the same powers of disposal as he has when the accused is found unfit to plead (see above). As with unfitness to plead, no hospital or restriction order may be made except when medical evidence justifies such an order. The possibility of a guardianship order, supervision and treatment order or absolute discharge makes insanity a more attractive plea than previously. The new methods of disposal may over time undermine the argument in (c) above.

The definition of insanity is not laid down by statute but has to be gathered from the cases. The law was laid down in 1843 and according to the House of Lords in *Sullivan* [1984] AC 156 it is not necessary to go further back. Lord Diplock in that case said that the law on insanity was 'to protect society against recurrence of the dangerous conduct'. He argued that the purpose of the test for insanity was to identify the dangerous. Unfortunately he did not explain why on that test epileptics were dangerous but some diabetics not. The result in *Sullivan* is not affected by the 1991 Act.

The test for insanity

In the discussion in this section it must be remembered that the definition of insanity (Fig. 9.1) is a legal, not a medical one, as was shown by *Sullivan*, above, and confirmed by the Court of Appeal in *Hennessy* [1989] 1 WLR 287. It should also be noted that this section is limited to discussion of insanity on indictment. If the accused successfully pleads insanity in a summary trial, he is simply acquitted. It was said in *DPP v H* [1997] 1 WLR 1406 by the Divisional Court that insanity is available in magistrates' courts only if the offence is one of *mens rea*. This proposition is criticised below. Lord Hutton, delivering the sole speech in *Antoine* above, said that when insanity is successfully pleaded, the accused does not have the *mens rea* of the offence charged.

The principle governing insanity was laid down in *M'Naghten's Case* (1843) [1843–60] All ER Rep 229. The accused, believing he was being persecuted by the Tories, fired his gun at the Prime Minister, Peel, but killed Peel's secretary, Edward Drummond. Medical opinion showed that M'Naghten was suffering from morbid delusions which might have

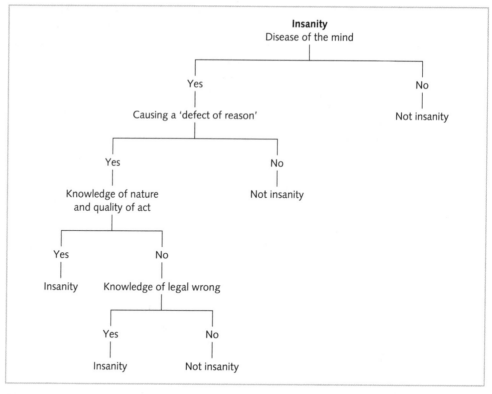

Figure 9.1 Insanity

affected his perceptions of right and wrong. The jury returned a verdict of not guilty by reason of insanity. The case came to the House of Lords, who asked a series of questions to the judges of England. The main response was delivered by Tindal CJ, who seems to have striven to state the law so that an accused would not be blamed for what he had done through lack of intelligence or reasoning power or the ability to foresee consequences where punishment would deter neither the accused nor others.

The main part of Tindal CJ's statement in response to the hypothetical questions is:

> the jurors ought to be told in all cases that every man is presumed to be sane and [to] possess a sufficient degree of reason to be responsible for his crimes, until the contrary is proved to their satisfaction; and that to establish a defence on the grounds of insanity it must clearly be proved that, at the time of the committing of the offence, the accused was labouring under such a defect of reason from disease of the mind as not to know the nature and quality of the act he was doing; or if he did know it, he did not know he was doing what was wrong.

This definition is not affected by the Criminal Procedure (Insanity and Unfitness to Plead) Act 1991.

From the viewpoint of precedent it must be remembered that these words were not spoken in a 'live' case; however, the words, while not *ratio*, have come to be accepted as stating the law. Moreover, as Tindal CJ said himself, one should not make 'minute application' of the quoted words, but those words have been treated as if they appeared in a statute. The procedure for summoning judges to the House of Lords to give answers to questions was last used in 1898 and will presumably not be used again because since the mid-nineteenth century there is a lot more expertise in the House of Lords. Despite the above it should be said that when all the judges of England state that the law is so-and-so (the exception in *M'Naghten* was Maule J) their opinion is entitled to respect even if it is not authoritative for the purposes of the doctrine of precedent. The argument from precedent is not overwhelming because the *M'Naghten* Rules have been applied in cases of the highest authority. Despite the criticism that the Rules should not be read like a statute, the words have been used as if they were and the following discussion looks at the concepts in the definition.

(a) Disease of the mind

Lord Denning in *Bratty v Attorney-General for Northern Ireland* [1963] AC 386 said that a disease of the mind was 'any mental disorder which has manifested itself in violence and is prone to recur'. The definition is quite broad and gives effect to the policy that dangerous people should not be on the street. It would be strange that insanity should be restricted to violence and the courts have not so restricted it. The principal judgment of the High Court of Australia in *Falconer* (1990) 65 ALJR 20 ran that a temporary mental disorder had to be prone to recur if it was to be classified as a disease of the mind. The likelihood of recurrence showed 'an underlying pathological infirmity'. This criterion was emphasised by Lord Lane CJ in *Hennessy*, above. Stress, anxiety and depression can be diseases of the mind even if caused by external factors, if they were prone to recur. The element of likelihood of recurrence is a frail basis for distinguishing between insanity and automatism. However, the Court of Appeal somewhat tentatively placed less emphasis on the possibility of recurrence in *Burgess* [1991] 2 QB 92. Lord Lane CJ said that the danger of recurrence was an extra reason for categorising the condition as a disease of the mind but 'the absence of the danger of recurrence is not a reason for saying that it cannot be a disease of the mind'. (It should be noted that the danger of recurrence of criminal behaviour in sane people is arguably not a reason for imprisoning them for a lengthy period.) That court otherwise accepted Lord Denning's proposition. In criticism of Lord Lane CJ's statement it may be said that the recurrence of a disease of the mind does not necessarily signify that the accused is dangerous. He may have been *very* dangerous at the time of the offences.

One criticism of the definition is that it is dependent on the nature of the accused's conduct and not on the nature of the disease. For this reason epilepsy as in *Bratty* and *Sullivan*, both above, is a disease of the mind, yet not all epileptics should be detained. In *Sullivan* the defendant suffered from a rare form of epilepsy which manifested itself in violence. The House of Lords investigated the cause, thereby demonstrating at the highest judicial level that Lord Denning's *dictum* is not fully accepted but the Court of Appeal in *Burgess* breathed new life into it. There are at present two streams of authority, though the courts do not seem to have noticed the definitional issue. Lord Diplock noted that it might seem harsh to call epileptics insane, but any reform was for Parliament.

Another problem with 'disease of the mind' is its uncertainty. Two cases are always contrasted. In *Charlson* [1955] 1 All ER 859 a father invited his son to look out of the window at the river below to see a rat swimming in it. When the boy did so the father hit the boy over the head with a mallet and threw him out of the window. The father said that he knew that he was killing the boy but did not know why. He was suffering from a brain tumour. Barry J directed the jury that the tumour was a physical disease, not a disease of the mind within *M'Naghten*. Lord Denning considered that *Charlson* was wrongly decided in *Bratty*. The companion case to *Charlson* is *Kemp* [1957] 1 QB 399.

The accused suffered from hardening of the arteries (arteriosclerosis) which led to a congestion of blood in the brain, causing a temporary loss of consciousness. While in this state he hit his wife over the head with a hammer. Devlin J said that the 'mind' in the definition covered the faculties of reason, memory and understanding, a phrase which gained Lord Diplock's approval in *Sullivan*, and that, while arteriosclerosis was a physical disease, the condition of the mind may be affected by it and if the mind is affected, there is a disease of the mind. Therefore, the physical cause of the mental disorder is not relevant. The general view is that *Charlson* and *Kemp* are indistinguishable, but *Kemp* is to be preferred because violent people should be detained. If *Kemp* is correct, insanity is defined broadly and covers forms of automatism which would not be included if *Charlson* were correct. If one wished, one could distinguish those cases by saying that in *Charlson* there was no medical evidence, whereas in *Kemp* there was. Nevertheless, the width of *Kemp* remains unclear. Would it cover a heart attack? The cause is the same as in arteriosclerosis: the brain's supply of blood is cut. In criticism of *Kemp*, one might inquire what the cause of the arteriosclerosis was. If the answer is high cholesterol food, the food is external, and the defence should not have been insanity but automatism. Cases such as *Kemp* illustrate that 'physical' diseases are included, and this is so despite such causes of 'disease of the mind' not being the concern of psychiatrists. The same may be said of diabetes and epilepsy.

Among the diseases which insanity would seem to cover are senility, traumatic brain injury, organic psychosis (as, e.g., caused by syphilis), drug-induced psychosis, post-traumatic stress disorder, some forms of epilepsy, melancholia, manic depression and schizophrenia. 'Disease of the mind' can be read widely. Indeed, no 'disease' is required. In *Bell* [1984] 3 All ER 842 voices from God were said to be a disease of the mind. In practice about half of those held to be insane are schizophrenics. However, disease of the mind does not cover a temporary malfunction caused by something external: *Quick* [1973] QB 910 where Lawton CJ criticised Lord Denning's definition as leading to a diabetic being classified as insane. *Quick* demonstrates that though the accused has a mental aberration which manifests itself in violence, the accused is not always insane. The defendant in *Quick* had the defence of automatism. (The main accused in *Quick* had in fact been admitted to hospital on a dozen occasions in a semi-conscious or unconscious state: automatism as a defence is a complete one, yet surely he needed help with the containment of his diabetes.) In Australia it has been held that a temporary malfunctioning of the mind caused by an external factor such as a blow to the head or alcohol is not a disease of the mind: *Carter* [1959] VR 105. The same position is taken in New Zealand: *Cottle* [1958] NZLR 999 (CA). Such factors, and the court added hypnotism in *Cottle*, cannot be called 'diseases'. In *Bailey* [1983] 2 All ER 503, a failure to take food to counteract the effect of insulin was categorised as an external factor and accordingly the resulting coma was not a disease of the mind. (For more on this see automatism, below.) Similarly, it was said by the House of Lords in *Attorney-General for Northern Ireland* v *Gallagher* [1963] AC 349 that a psychopathic state exacerbated by alcohol was not a disease of the mind.

The cases are not always easy to reconcile, especially those which lead to different results for epileptics and diabetics. Is it true that epileptics are more of a social danger than diabetics in a hypoglycaemic condition? Certainly there was no reason for keeping epileptics in mental hospitals in the era before additional methods of disposal were given in 1992. Moreover, very rarely do epileptics perform the sort of act which occurred in *Sullivan*. What should be borne in mind is that, as Lord Diplock said in *Sullivan*, the cause, if internal, of the disease is irrelevant, as is whether it is permanent or transient.

Similarly the fact that the medical profession would not call something a disease of the mind is immaterial. The difficulty is one of distinguishing in the light of policy if the **M'Naghten** Rules are to be retained. In the Australian case of **Porter** (1933) 55 CLR 182, Dixon CJ said that disease of the mind did not include 'mere excitability of a normal man, passion, even stupidity, obtuseness, lack of self-control, and impulsiveness'. He emphasised that there need be no physical deterioration to the brain cells. Two recent cases throw the subject into relief by showing the width of the term.

In **Sullivan** the accused kicked a friend's head and body while he was recovering from an epileptic fit. The House of Lords held that despite his state of mind being temporary, he was insane. His defence was not automatism because the cause of his mental aberration was not external, but internal. This decision has been severely criticised. C. M. V. Clarkson, *Understanding Criminal Law* (Fontana, 1987) 44–5, wrote:

> One can, perhaps, understand the thinking behind the judgment. If the involuntary conduct has an internal cause then it is likely to recur; society needs protection against the recurrence of such dangerous conduct . . . ; the insanity verdict allows control to be maintained over the defendant. However, it seems absurd as well as highly insulting to utilise the insanity verdict here.

The fourth edition (Thomson, 2005) makes the same points but in slightly different words (pp. 39–42). He adds (p. 42 in the 4th edition) that: 'Nothing can be achieved by any of the orders that can be imposed pursuant to a finding of "not guilty by reason of insanity"'. The reality is that most such persons will simply plead guilty to the charge, as Sullivan did, and will often receive a non-custodial sentence.

If, as Lord Diplock suggested, the **M'Naghten** Rules are meant to differentiate between dangerous and non-dangerous individuals, why are epileptics dangerous but some diabetics not? The line between internal and external causes does not divide dangerous from non-dangerous people. Moreover, even if the accused is insane, he can change his plea to guilty, yet he is still dangerous; after serving perhaps a short sentence, he is released on to the streets. Indeed, a custodial sentence need not be given. The classification of some epileptics as insane led a Crown Court judge in **McFarlane**, *The Guardian*, 11 September 1990, to refuse to follow **Sullivan**. The brief report does not give the reason for not following precedent. But the judge seems to have directed the jury that the accused was not guilty if she was undergoing a fit when she occasioned actual bodily harm on a police constable searching her home for stolen goods. (He said that psychiatrists did not consider epilepsy to be a disease of the mind and therefore epilepsy is not part of the law of insanity. Once it is realised that whether a condition amounts to a disease of the mind is a question of law, one can appreciate the fallacy of this argument.) Furthermore as Lawton LJ put it in **Quick**, above, the law of 'disease of the mind' should not cause incredulity to laypeople.

An important case is **Burgess**, above. The accused attacked a friend with a video recorder and tried to strangle her. He had been sleepwalking. Lord Lane CJ said that the accused's 'mind was to some extent controlling his actions rather than the result simply of muscular spasm, but without his being consciously aware of what he was doing'. He rejected earlier authorities which had consistently held that sleepwalking was automatism. There was no external cause. Lord Lane applied part of Lord Denning's definition ('any mental disorder which has manifested itself in violence') but said that the latter part ('and was prone to recur') was simply an added reason for classifying the disease as one of the mind. On the facts, sleepwalking demonstrated 'an abnormality or disorder, albeit transitory, due to an internal factor, whether functional or organic, which had manifested itself in violence'. Therefore, the accused, the sleepwalker, was legally insane, since 'a purely temporary and intermittent suspension of the mental faculties of reason, memory and understanding' could be insanity. Any reform was for Parliament. It seems strange that a person who is sleepwalking should be treated in the same way as if he were a psychopath or otherwise mentally disturbed. This comment is underlined by the fact that the accused's violent behaviour was likely to recur. It can hardly be said that the public needed protection from him. On the other hand, it can be argued that a somnambulist can be treated in hospital and so an acquittal pure and simple would be inappropriate. Certainly labelling a sleepwalker as 'insane' is even more inappropriate. And it is sometimes said that a sleepwalker does only acts which he would like to do when conscious. He can avoid objects and climb stairs even though he does not have full consciousness. In criticism of **Burgess** it can be said that sleep is a natural condition. Sleepwalking is a consequence of that natural condition; therefore, sleepwalking is not a disease of the mind. Furthermore, as F. Boland put it in *Anglo-American Insanity Defence Reform* (Dartmouth, 1999) 11: 'If caused by cheese [sleepwalking] will qualify for the defence of automatism as cheese would probably be considered to be an external cause' [footnotes omitted]. The Supreme Court of Canada decided in **Parks** (1993) 95 DLR (4th) 27 that sleepwalking was not a disease of the mind. Sleepwalking arose from sleep, a socially acceptable cause. The 'internal cause' theory in **Quick** was rejected. The draft Criminal Code, 1989, would have classified sleepwalking as automatism. This outcome would be better than the current one, insanity, but a successful plea of automatism means that the accused is acquitted, and no treatment is provided. A better solution would be to acquit the accused but then to oblige him to undergo an appropriate form of medical treatment such as a course of drugs.

(b) Defect of reason

This term is defined as a complete deprivation of the powers of reason, as distinguished from the failure to exercise those powers to the full, as the Court of Appeal held in **Clarke** [1972] 1 All ER 219. A depressed woman entered a supermarket and absentmindedly put goods into her basket. She was charged with theft. Her counsel counselled her to plead insanity – bad advice! A doctor in evidence said that depression was a (minor) mental illness. She had previously done things like putting sugar into her refrigerator. Thankfully for her, the court held her not to have a defect of reason. Failure to concentrate did not constitute a defect of reason. Looking at the **M'Naghten** Rules it might be said that her failure to understand what she was doing was a defect of reason. Even though the defect was only temporary, applying **Kemp**, above, her true 'defence' was insanity, and looking at **Burgess**, above, her movements were not simply muscular spasms. In fact the accused's appeal was allowed because she lacked *mens rea* in that she was not dishonest. An alternative way of reaching the same result is to hold that she did not have a disease of the mind. Non-severe depression is not such a disease. The defect of reason may be temporary or permanent, as the cases on epilepsy demonstrate. A defect of reason does not cover stupidity: **Kemp**.

(c)(i) Knowledge of the nature and quality of the act

Codere (1916) 12 Cr App R 21 (CCA) held that this phrase refers to the act's physical elements and not to the legal or moral constitution, i.e. the accused must not know that he was doing the act at all, that he was incapable of foreseeing the result, or that he was incapable of appreciating the circumstances. In **Cottle**, above, Gresson P in the New

Zealand Court of Appeal stated that: 'not to know at all is not to understand the nature and quality of the act'. A famous example is where a madman cuts a woman's throat under the delusion that he is cutting a loaf of bread. He may know that he is using a knife but he does not know the effect of using it and therefore does not know the nature and quality of his act. The accused in **Sullivan** did not know the nature of what he was doing. It is possible for the accused to fall under both this heading and the next. An irresistible impulse is not a lack of knowledge of the nature and quality of the act.

(c)(ii) Knowledge that the act was wrong

This phrase is the alternative to knowledge of the nature and quality of the act. It inquires of the accused whether he knew that what he was doing was contrary to law: **Windle** [1952] 2 QB 826, contrary to previous authorities. It is irrelevant whether he thought that what he did was morally wrong. The wife in **Windle** was certifiably insane. The husband had, as it were, caught a mental illness from her (*folie à deux*, a form of communicated mental disorder). He fed her 100 aspirins. When arrested he said: 'I suppose they will hang me for this?' The Court of Criminal Appeal ruled that his words meant that he knew that what he did was legally wrong, and he was indeed hanged. It should be noted that the sane adult has no defence of lack of knowledge that the act was legally wrong, at least if the act was criminally wrong (see the opening section of Chapter 8). A psychopath may well know that what he is doing is legally wrong and, therefore, he is not insane. In **Bell**, above, the accused heard what he thought were voices from God, which told him to ram the gates of a holiday camp with his van. He knew that what he did was legally wrong. It was irrelevant that he thought he was acting in a morally right way. A recent authority confirming that **Windle** remains good law is **Johnson** [2007] EWCA Crim 1978.

It would appear that the judges in **M'Naghten** intended 'wrong' to mean morally wrong. In **Codere**, above, the test was said to be that of 'the ordinary standard adopted by reasonable men', a moral not legal test. For those reasons **Windle** was not followed in Australia in **Stapleton v R** (1952) 86 CLR 358. If the Australian courts are correct, the accused in **Windle** may have had a defence. If he thought that mercy killing was morally proper, he did not know that his act was (morally) wrong. Canada has adopted the Australian approach: **Chaulk** (1990) 2 CR (4th) 1 (SCC). The accused is insane even though he knows that his act was illegal if he believes he was acting in a morally acceptable way. However, the Court of Appeal in **Johnson**, above, rejected **Stapleton** as being part of English law.

Summarising the effect of **Windle**, one may say that if the accused thought that what he did was right and believed that the law and public opinion agreed with him, he has a defence under this part of the **M'Naghten** Rules. (He may still know the nature and quality of his act.) If one of these beliefs is missing, he has no defence under this limb of the Rules – and let it not be forgotten that the question whether he knew that his act was legally wrong is being asked of a person who has suffered from a defect of reason from disease of the mind! Most murderers know that murder is a crime. The effect of **Windle** is to narrow the defence and under this limb of the Rules only those who are severely affected by a lack of intelligence will fall within it. Despite the above, research by Mackay demonstrates that Crown Court judges were not adhering to the principle in **Windle** but were instructing juries that an accused had the defence even though he thought he was doing something morally right but legally wrong. Psychiatrists giving evidence of insanity often took the same approach. **Johnson** recognised that this was happening.

Five procedural matters

(a) Since under the **M'Naghten** Rules every person is presumed to be sane, the accused bears the burden of disproving that he is sane. The burden, however, is the civil law one of the balance of probabilities: **Sodeman v R** [1936] 2 All ER 1138. See, however, point (c) below. The fact that the burden of proof is on the accused may be contrary to the European Convention on Human Rights. The Court of Appeal rejected this convention in **M** [2002] Crim LR 57, holding that findings that defendants are insane do not constitute criminal proceedings within Article 6(2) of the Convention. No one is convicted and no punishment is imposed. (This case is also called **Moore**.) For further discussion of the Convention see the next section.

(b) If the defence is successful, the verdict is 'not guilty by reason of insanity'. Formerly the verdict was 'guilty but insane'. Technically nowadays the outcome is an acquittal but there is an appeal against this verdict under the Criminal Procedure (Insanity) Act 1964, s 2.

(c) It is sometimes said the prosecution cannot raise the insanity issue. But in **Bratty**, above, the decision of highest authority, Lord Denning said that it was the prosecution's duty to raise the issue of insanity in order to prevent a dangerous person being free to roam the streets. It must, however, make available to the defence evidence supporting insanity: **Dickie** [1984] 3 All ER 173 (CA). The prosecution may, however, definitely raise the issue where the accused has led evidence of diminished responsibility (Criminal Procedure (Insanity) Act 1964, s 6), and where he has adduced evidence of mental incapacity. There is conflict whether in these circumstances the prosecution bears the burden of proof and, if so, how high that onus is. It is thought that the burden is on the prosecution, and the standard of proof is beyond reasonable doubt. However, with regard to cases where the accused has adduced evidence of mental capacity there is a *dictum* of Lord Denning in **Bratty** that the standard is on the balance of probabilities. This *dictum* seems incorrect. Only in exceptional cases such as on a charge of murder the accused raises the defence of diminished responsibility may the judge *sua sponte* (of his or her own accord) raise the issue of insanity: **Dickie**, above, and **Thomas** [1995] Crim LR 314 (CA). An exceptional case occurs when all the medical evidence is in favour of insanity, but the defence does not raise the issue.

(d) Under the Criminal Procedure (Insanity and Unfitness to Plead) Act 1991, s 1, a jury cannot return a verdict of not guilty by reason of insanity unless evidence of two medical practitioners, one of whom has been approved by the Home Secretary as having experience in mental disorder, has been adduced. It would seem that if the medical evidence is all one way, the jury must rely on it; if, however, the evidence is not all to the same effect, the jury has to choose which testimony is to be believed.

(e) Usually evidence of insanity is undisputed and both the Crown and the defence psychiatrists agree on the 'disease of the mind'. Nevertheless, a judge cannot dispose of the accused until the jury has delivered the special verdict of not guilty by reason of insanity.

Criticisms of the M'Naghten Rules

(a) An old criticism of the **M'Naghten** Rules is that no one is mad enough to be legally insane and have this defence. However, after the cases on epilepsy and sleepwalking, the force of this criticism has been reduced. A psychotic may not have this defence as the definition may not be satisfied. For example, the Yorkshire Ripper, Peter Sutcliffe, knew both the nature of his acts and the wrongfulness of them. This criticism should nowadays be phrased as this: in some respects the Rules are too narrow, while in others they are too wide.

(b) Key phrases in the definition are unclear: what is a disease of the mind? Until recently sleepwalking was not such an illness but was treated as an illustration of the defence of automatism. The width of this phrase, therefore, needs clarification.

(c) Under the Rules there is no defence for irresistible impulse: ***True*** (1922) 27 Cox CC 287, ***Kopsch*** (1925) 19 Cr App R 50, ***Sodeman v R***, above, and ***Attorney-General for South Australia v Brown*** [1960] AC 432, though it is evidence towards showing both of the third 'limbs' of the ***M'Naghten*** test. The test ignores self-control. Similarly the defence does not cater for emotional factors. The accused is guilty if he knew what he was doing and that what he was doing was legally wrong, even if he did not have the emotional development to give meaning to this knowledge. Some of this criticism has been mitigated by the introduction of diminished responsibility. See below.

(d) It is immaterial whether the insanity was permanent or temporary, and even whether the disease of the mind is curable.

(e) The test is unscientific. The jury is the body which decides whether a person is insane, not the doctors, after the judge has ruled where there is evidence of insanity. Juries may find difficulty in applying the law to the facts, and there is some anecdotal evidence that the ***M'Naghten*** Rules are disregarded: juries ask themselves whether or not the accused is mad. The jury may reject medical evidence, as occurred in, e.g., ***True***, above. It has been suggested that this law is in breach of Article 5 of the European Convention on Human Rights which provides that the mentally ill can be detained only after medical evidence has been used. Under the Criminal Procedure (Insanity and Unfitness to Plead) Act 1991, evidence of at least two medical practitioners, one of whom has been approved by the Home Secretary, is needed before a jury can return a verdict of not guilty by reason of insanity. One anomaly is that though the definition of insanity is a *legal* one, the accused may be committed to an institution which deals with conditions that are medical. Article 5(1) requires 'objective medical evidence' according to ***Winterwerp v Netherlands*** (1979) 2 EHRR 387. Since the jury has to apply a legal, not a medical, definition, it looks likely that Article 5(1) is breached. Hyperglycaemia, epilepsy and sleepwalking would not appear to make the sufferers of them 'persons of unsound mind' within Article 5(1). Moreover, ***Winterwerp*** demanded that the mental disorder must be of a type which warrants compulsory confinement; however, English law is that a person who is acquitted of murder by reason of insanity must be detained in a hospital. The Court of Appeal in ***Grant*** [2002] 1 Cr App R 528 said that it was a point 'of some difficulty' that 'no-one is required specifically to address, prior to the person's detention, the question whether he suffers from a mental disorder sufficiently serious to warrant detention'. The detention may be 'arbitrary' and fall foul of Article 5(1)(e), which, however, did not happen on the facts of ***Grant*** because the accused was mentally impaired in any case. She was therefore 'of unsound mind'. She also had the right to apply to the Mental Health Review Tribunal. ***Grant*** was itself a case of unfitness to plead but it applies generally. Mental illnesses and disabilities are not the proper subject for criminal law courts. In murder such commitment remains mandatory, yet the offender may not be medically mentally ill. Many of the illnesses discussed in this section are ones which can be controlled by drugs. It is inappropriate to label such conditions as 'insanity'. If the accused has not taken the drugs prescribed, the issue should perhaps be whether he was forgetful on one occasion or whether he was for some reason against taking drugs. Current law does not take into account such issues.

The issue was well put by the Scottish Law Commission in its Discussion Paper No. 122, *Insanity and Diminished Responsibility*, 2003. The **M'Naghten** Rules may be incompatible with

> 'the **Winterwerp** criteria (that there must be (i) a mental condition *at the time of disposal* [emphasis in original], (ii) established by medical evidence, which (iii) requires compulsory detention). The **M'Naghten** Rules do not necessarily fulfil these criteria, as they are concerned with insanity at the time of the offence . . . , and use a specialised definition of disease of the mind which does not coincide with the approach of medical science. . . . However it is far from obvious that a breach of the Convention is the result of the test used to establish insanity. If anything any breach is brought about by the provisions which deal with the disposal consequences of the defence. Article 5(1)(e) and the **Winterwerp** decision are not concerned with insanity as an issue of criminal responsibility but about limits on the power of the state to detain people on the basis of their mental disorder . . . It follows, as far as the Convention is concerned, that the test for the defence can be drawn up widely or narrowly and can take into account a whole range of policy considerations.

(f) The application of the Rules may cause problems. An old illustration is that a deluded person will not escape liability if his delusions do not relate to legal guilt. Accordingly if a person believes himself to be Napoleon, he will not have this defence because Napoleon was not allowed to kill.

(g) The burden of proof is anomalous. Insanity forms the sole common law defence where the burden is on the accused, and the position is hard to justify except historically. There may be a clash with the prosecutor's duty to prove *mens rea*. Proof of *mens rea* means that the accused knew the nature and quality of his act. However, the special rule for insanity means that he must prove that he did not know the nature and quality of his act. If the prosecution have proved *mens rea*, insanity calls for the accused to disprove what has been proved! This issue awaits judicial resolution. This conflict does not occur when the accused seeks to show that he did not know that what he was doing was wrong. The relationship between insanity and *mens rea* has not been satisfactorily resolved. In **DPP v H** [1997] 1 WLR 1406 the Divisional Court held that insanity, on the facts manic depression coupled with distorted judgment and impairments to the accused's moral sense and understanding of time, was not a defence to strict liability offences because insanity meant that the accused did not have the *mens rea* of the offence charged, whereas by definition strict liability offences lack *mens rea* as to one or more elements of the *actus reus*. **DPP v H** would appear to be incorrect. *Mens rea* is not inconsistent with insanity. A person may intend to kill, for example, but still be insane. Indeed, the part of the **M'Naghten** Rules which deals with the accused's knowledge that he has acted wrongly in law concerns persons who have *mens rea*. If the accused does not appreciate the nature and quality of his act, it could be said that the accused is not acting voluntarily and, therefore, there is no *actus reus*. The lack of *mens rea* is irrelevant in these circumstances. (**DPP v H** is also known as **DPP v Harper**.) There have been cases where insanity had been a defence to strict offence. A well-known example is

Hennessy [1989] 1 WLR 287 (CA), a case of driving while disqualified. This case was not referred to in *DPP v H*.

(h) The defence of insanity is the sole defence where the judge cannot accept the accused's plea. He or she can do so in the 'partner' defence of diminished responsibility.

(i) Psychiatrists lack reliable means of telling whether a person was insane at the time of the offence. They can rely only on what the accused said and did. A shrewd accused might lie. On this basis he might escape punishment for his crimes.

(j) It is apparently difficult to persuade an 'insane' person to plead insanity.

(k) The test is all-or-nothing. Either the accused is insane or he is not. There is no verdict of 'partially insane'.

(l) Some persons put into mental hospitals may be more dangerous when they come out than when they go in.

(m) Why should answers to hypothetical questions be legally binding? The judges in *M'Naghten* never intended their Rules to be read as if they were words in a statute.

(n) As stated above, it may be better to plead guilty than to attempt to prove insanity because of the problem of disposal. It may be more acceptable except in murder for the accused to take the punishment than to go to a hospital specified by the Home Secretary, as occurred before 1992. Even now a guilty verdict may be more to the accused's liking than one of insanity.

(o) A disease of the mind is partly defined in terms of the likelihood of recurrence. This prediction may be wrong, but people are classified as insane because of it.

(p) It cannot be said that arguments about a person's sanity are best heard in the criminal courts.

Summarising, perhaps the principal criticisms are the first and third. The Rules are too wide in that they cover epilepsy (*Sullivan*, above) but too narrow in that they do not cover lack of control arising out of a mental condition. If the Rules were based on a sound theory, application to the facts would not be difficult. The present quick release of some persons does not justify the law.

Reform

The Royal Commission on Capital Punishment, Cmd 8932, 1953, recommended that the whole set of *M'Naghten* Rules should be abolished. The jury (not, it should be noted, the doctors) should inquire whether the accused was suffering from a disease of the mind 'to such a degree that he ought not to be held responsible'. If that policy was not acceptable, the members wanted two new defences, irresistible impulse and diminished responsibility. Only the last proposal was partly put into effect in the Homicide Act 1957 (see below). The question of insanity was to remain in the hands of the jurors because it was seen as a matter of morality, not of medicine. The Criminal Law Revision Committee proposed in its Eleventh Report, *Evidence (General)*, Cmnd 4991, 1972, 88, to place the legal burden of proof on the prosecution, leaving only the evidential burden on the accused. The Butler Committee (*Report of the Committee on Mentally Abnormal Offenders*, Cmnd 6244, 1975) also proposed that the burden of proof should lie on the prosecution and recommended that mentally disordered persons should continue to be exempt from criminal liability. The question was 'whether the offender, as a result of insanity . . . , is so much less responsible than a normal person that it is just to treat him as wholly irresponsible'. Irrational people should not be criminally liable. There would not need to be a link between the mental disorder and the crime. The **M'Naghten** Rules were unsatisfactory and should be abrogated. A new verdict of 'not guilty on evidence of mental disorder' was proposed. The accused would have this defence if he either did not know what he was doing or was suffering from severe mental illness or severe subnormality. On the first limb the burden of proof would be on the prosecution, and the defence would not include transient states arising from intoxication or physical injury. The Butler Committee thought that their definition would be wider than the **M'Naghten** Rules in that it would cover persons such as the mentally subnormal who at present have no defence. On the second limb:

A mental illness is severe when it has one or more of the following characteristics:
(a) lasting impairment of intellectual functions shown by failure of memory, orientation, comprehension and learning capacity;
(b) lasting alteration of mood of such degree as to give rise to delusional appraisal of the patient's situation, his past or his future, or that of others or to lack of any appraisal;
(c) delusional beliefs, persecutory, jealous or grandiose;
(d) abnormal perceptions associated with delusional misinterpretation of events;
(e) thinking so disordered as to prevent reasonable appraisal of the patient's situation or reasonable communication with others.

The definition of mental disorder would therefore not include diabetics, sleepwalkers and epileptics as the present law does. The verdict would not automatically lead to the accused's being committed to hospital: the judge would have full powers of disposal, including the grant of an absolute discharge. The Butler Committee proposed that the burden of proof should lie on the prosecution but cl 35 of the draft Criminal Code provides that either the prosecution or the defence should be permitted to prove mental disorder on the balance of probabilities.

These proposals remain unimplemented. The Criminal Law Revision Committee in 1980, Fourteenth Report, *Offences against the Person* Cmnd 7844, recommended their adoption. They received a new lease of life in 1985 when the draft Criminal Code contained them (Law Com. No. 143) and in 1989 when the Law Commission proposed their enactment (Law Com. Report No. 177): *A Criminal Code for England and Wales*. Clauses 35–36 would abolish the insanity defence, thereby removing the stigma of being labelled insane, an appellation that the Law Commission found 'offensive', replace it by a defence of not guilty on evidence of mental disorder if the mental disorder negated the *mens rea* and by a verdict of 'mental disorder' whether it did negate the *mens rea* or not (in other words even though the accused did not have the mental element for the offence charged, he could still be subject to restraint by the criminal justice system), and to have this defence the accused would have to suffer from 'severe mental illness or severe mental handicap'. Uncontrollable impulses would not fall within the term 'severe mental illness'. There need be no causal link between the mental disorder and the crime. Either the prosecution or the defence could prove that the accused was suffering from mental disorder. However, the Law Commission did not propose the full implementation of the Butler Report. 'Mental disorder' would no longer cover temporary depression, but would cover a diabetic who did not take insulin and an epileptic, and a person with a 'severe mental disorder' would be punished whether or not the crime is ascribable to the illness. The Yorkshire Ripper would no doubt have a defence if these proposals were implemented. The 1991 Act retains mandatory commitment where the accused has committed murder.

The Law Commission's view on this is not known. Either the prosecution or the defence would be entitled to raise this defence, whereas the Butler Report placed the burden of proof firmly on the prosecution. The Commission at the time of writing intends to consider insanity and unfitness to plead.

The enactment of the Criminal Procedure (Insanity and Unfitness to Plead) Act 1991 may have reduced pressure for reform. That Act reforms procedure and sentencing but not the substance. It would be a pity if the reforms prevented the amendment of the law to prevent persons like the accused in *Burgess* being stigmatised as insane.

Many other reforms have been suggested especially in the USA after the acquittal of John Hinckley of the attempted assassination of the then President, Ronald Reagan. Some states totally abolished the insanity defence.

It is thought that the enforcement of the Human Rights Act 1998 will lead to changes in the law. One suggested is that the application of the *M'Naghten* Rules in cases such as *Burgess* can no longer be justified. *Burgess* was decided, at least in part, in the way that it was because the accused was dangerous. The European Convention on Human Rights provides for the lawful detention of those 'of unsound mind' but it does not allow that detention on grounds of dangerousness. See also the discussion of *Winterwerp* and *Grant*, above.

Diminished responsibility

This defence 'does something to compensate for the lack of an insanity defence that can be used' (E. Griew 'The future of diminished responsibility' [1988] Crim LR 75 at 87). Certainly pressure to reform the law of insanity declined after 1957. One statistic from before the coming into force of the Homicide Act demonstrates the justness of the quote: in 1990 there were 49 successful diminished responsibility pleas but only one of insanity. Similar figures occurred throughout the 1990s. There were 46 in 1997 but only 15 in 2001–02. Most pleas are successful. The main academic treatment is S. Dell, *Murder into Manslaughter* (OUP, 1984). She noted that in most cases the judge accepted the accused's plea (and the position remains the same today with fewer than 15 per cent of pleas leading to a trial). If the judge did not, most defendants were convicted of murder.

It is arguable that a person whose mental responsibility is impaired should not be found guilty at all and that he should have a defence to all crimes, but a special defence applying only to murder (Fig. 9.2) has been created by s 2(1) of the Homicide Act 1957:

> Where a person kills or is party to the killing of another, he shall not be convicted of murder if he was suffering from such abnormality of mind (whether arising from a condition of arrested or retarded development of mind or any inherent causes or induced by disease or injury) as substantially impaired his mental responsibility for his acts or omissions in doing or being a party to the killing.

Diminished responsibility is, therefore, a specific defence: that is, it applies only to murder or being a secondary party (aider etc.) to murder. It is not even a defence to attempted murder: *Campbell* [1997] Crim LR 495 (Crown Court). Therefore, if the victim dies, the accused will be guilty of manslaughter but if the victim lives, the accused will be guilty of attempted murder. In this regard it is different from insanity which potentially applies to all offences. In respect of other offences, diminished responsibility can be taken into account in the sentencing. Furthermore, diminished responsibility applies even though the accused knew the nature and quality of the act and knew that what he was

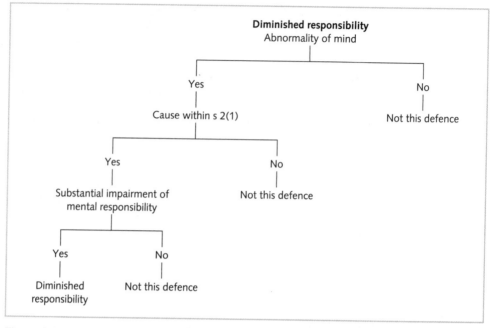

Figure 9.2 Diminished responsibility

doing was legally wrong. There is no need to prove that the diminished responsibility caused the death. Like insanity, however, the burden of proof is on the accused: s 2(2). The judge must direct the jury that this is so: **Dunbar** [1958] 1 QB 1. He must also tell them that the burden is on the balance of probabilities. The reverse onus found in s 2(2) is not incompatible with Article 6 of the European Convention because the defence is not an element in the crime of murder: **Lambert** [2002] 2 AC 545 (HL), discussed in Chapter 1. If the accused is represented by counsel, only the defence may raise this defence: **Campbell** (1987) 84 Cr App R 255 (CA, *obiter*). The court said that this ruling followed from s 2(2). If there is evidence of diminished responsibility, the judge can only point out the evidence to the defendant's counsel: the defence is in this sense optional. Compare provocation, where the burden of proof is on the prosecution: the judge must direct the jury on provocation even when the accused did not wish it to be considered. If the defence contends that the accused is suffering from diminished responsibility, the prosecution may lead evidence that he is insane: Criminal Procedure (Insanity) Act 1964, s 6. For the contrary situation see 'Points to note' below.

Discussion of the width of the defence

'Abnormality of mind', 'substantial impairment' and 'mental responsibility' have no settled legal or medical definition. The principal consideration of this defence took place in **Byrne** [1960] 2 QB 396, where the accused had irresistible urges and demonstrated them by mutilating the body of his victim. He was aware of what he was doing and did not fall within the **M'Naghten** rules on insanity. Instead he found it impossible or virtually impossible to resist his impulses. Lord Parker CJ in the Court of Criminal Appeal made three points.

(a) 'Abnormality of mind' includes the inability to form a rational judgment or to exercise will-power to control one's acts. There need not be a total inability to control one's impulses. Therefore, irresistible impulse falls within 'abnormality of mind'. It covers 'the mind's activities in all its aspects'. It will, for example, include not being able to distinguish right from wrong. 'Mind' includes understanding, perception and judgment. No limit has been placed on the types of mental disorder which may qualify, but the mental abnormality must stem from one of the causes in the brackets in s 2(1). For example, a psychopathic state is included, as is an abnormal craving for drink, and no doubt some cases of irresistible impulse: see *Spriggs* [1958] 1 All ER 300 (CCA): psychopath with emotional disturbances. In *Ahluwalia* [1992] 4 All ER 889 the Court of Appeal held that a major depressive illness may give rise to diminished responsibility. Dissociation is also an abnormality of mind. In *Sanderson* (1994) 98 Cr App R 325 (CA) a paranoid psychosis was said to arise from an inherent cause within s 2(1) of the Homicide Act 1957. Here then are three ways in which diminished responsibility differs from insanity: the *M'Naghten* Rules do not cover irresistible impulse; they are restricted to the defendant's knowledge; and they do not cover an inability to control one's actions.

Lord Parker thought that the phrase means something 'bordering on insanity'. However, in *Rose* v *R* [1961] AC 496 Lord Tucker thought that this explanation was unhelpful as did the Court of Appeal which quashed a conviction when the trial judge had directed the jury that the accused's mental state had to border on insanity in *Seers* (1984) 79 Cr App R 261, at least where the illness is a chronic depressive one. Depression is an abnormality of mind, but may not amount to a disease of the mind within the definition of insanity. The court in *Seers* quashed the conviction because the trial judge had not directed the jury in the terms laid down in *Byrne*, but had used the phrase 'partial insanity'. Diminished responsibility need not be partial insanity and is not when the cause is chronic depression. Similarly in *Brown* [1993] Crim LR 961 the court held that abnormality of mind was wider than insanity and mental disorder. It included aberrations of perception, understanding and judgment. In *Adams*, unreported, 29 January 1985, the court said that it was best to omit reference to insanity when the defence was diminished responsibility. Certainly the reader must not visualise the two defences as separate in terms of mental disorder: the same facts can give rise to either defence. The illness need not be one which is a disease of the mind.

(b) Abnormality means 'a state of mind so different from that of ordinary human beings that a reasonable man could term it abnormal'. Lord Parker CJ's definition seems to be merely another way of stating what the statute says. It does not in itself distinguish abnormal from normal states of mind. The phrase covers psychopaths, as in *Byrne* itself, depressives (but not a person who has become depressed as a response to external influences for there were no 'inherent causes', though battered women and at least one man who were depressed have succeeded in this defence on the ground that the battered persons' syndrome is caused by injury: see especially *Ahluwalia* [1992] 4 All ER 889) and persons suffering from irresistible impulses. Tony Martin, the accused who shot dead a burglar at his isolated farmhouse, suffered from a long-standing paranoid personality disorder and depression. The Court of Appeal held that he was entitled to this defence: *Martin* [2003] QB 1. It has included a person who killed in a fit of jealousy: *Miller* (1972) *The Times*, 16 May; and a woman suffering from PMT: among other cases, *Smith* [1982] Crim LR 531, but note that she was later found guilty of attempting to kill a police constable. Morbid jealousy falls within 'inherent causes': *Vinagre* (1979) 69 Cr App R 104 (CA). Paranoia was held to be an 'inherent cause' within s 2(1) in *Simcox* [1964] Crim LR 402. However, the Yorkshire Ripper *Sutcliffe* (1981) *The Times*, 23 May, and the north London homosexual killer *Neilson*, unreported, 1983, were both found guilty of murder even though there was much evidence of abnormality. Sutcliffe seemed a paranoid schizophrenic but the judge refused to accept the agreement between the prosecution and the defence that he had this defence. To the untutored eye a paranoid schizophrenic would appear more likely to have his responsibility diminished by his mental condition than a woman with PMT, but the cases are to opposite effects. A reported case where the Court of Appeal held that there was no injury to mind is *O'Connell* [1997] Crim LR 683. The accused's abnormality of mind was caused by taking prescribed drugs, not by an 'injury'. Where medical evidence is disputed, the jury is instructed to approach this causation point in a common-sense fashion. See also point (d) of *Points to note*, below. It is thought that the jury uses its moral sense, rather than applies the law. In other words, if the jurors think that the accused should bear the stigma of being convicted of murder, they do so convict despite the substantial evidence of mental abnormality. As we shall see, sometimes weak evidence leads to the opposite conclusion: see (f) under *Points to note*, below. Should it do so? It is suggested that this part of *Byrne* is not very helpful. What if some jurors think that the state of mind is abnormal and some do not? This is not a satisfactory basis on which to find a person guilty.

(c) The questions whether the accused was suffering from abnormality of mind and whether that substantially impaired his 'mental responsibility' (an ill-chosen phrase: presumably legal responsibility is meant, though there is no case law construing it) are for the jury using common sense, not for psychiatrists. There is to be no 'trial by psychiatrists': *Roberts* [2005] EWCA Crim 199. For example, in *Tulloch*, unreported, 25 February 2000 (CA) the accused with others had planned the killing, gone home for a hammer, clubbed the victim with it repeatedly, and concocted a false story for the police. It was held that even though he had a personality disorder brought about by physical and sexual abuse by his stepfather, his mental responsibility was not substantially impaired. Discussion of mental responsibility according to Lord Parker CJ in *Byrne* involves a consideration of the accused's 'ability to exercise will-power to control his physical acts'. The Court of Appeal confirmed this approach in *Tandy* [1989] 1 All ER 267. The jury forms the 'reasonable man' in (b). Nevertheless, psychiatrists do give evidence as to whether they think that the defendant was mentally responsible. The judge may withdraw this issue from the jury if the evidence does not disclose that the accused's mental responsibility was substantially impaired. What the jury is to consider is whether because of the mental illness the accused's capacity to control his behaviour was reduced ('substantially impaired') and, if so, did that reduced capacity lessen his moral blameworthiness for his acts?

Two other points of interpretation must be mentioned. The abnormality must arise from one of the causes listed in parenthesis in s 2(1). The question whether the abnormality of mind arose from one of the causes stated in s 2(1) is for the doctors: *Byrne*, above. Bad temper and jealousy (but see *Miller*, above) are excluded. If battered woman syndrome arises from abuse, the cause may fall within s 2(1). The Court of Appeal held in *Hobson* [1998] 1 Cr App R 31 that the syndrome could give rise to the defence of diminished responsibility. Presumably the syndrome has to come from 'inherent causes' or 'injury'. The Court of Appeal held in **Sanderson**, above, that 'induced by disease or injury' covered 'organic or physical injury or disease of the body including the brain' and that 'any inherent causes' covered 'functional mental illness'. Paranoid psychosis fell within 'inherent cause'. A 'disease' covered some if not all of the diseases of the mind which fell within the definition of insanity. Psychopaths remain a problem. They may fall within 'inherent causes' or perhaps 'arrested development' because their moral sense is not as developed as in normal people. The court held in **Sanderson** that the judge should refer only to the specified cause or causes which arise on the facts. Secondly, the judge should direct the jurors on the issue of the substantiality of the impairment on the basis either (a) that they are to approach the term 'substantial' in a common-sense way or (b) that the word means 'more than some trivial degree of impairment which does not make any appreciable difference to a person's ability to control himself, but it means less than total impairment'. This choice of expressions was approved in **Egan** (1992) 95 Cr App R 278 (CA). However, the Court of Appeal in **Mitchell** [1995] Crim LR 506 held that a direction on how substantial 'substantial' was need not be given.

The accused will have this defence when the words of the sub-section are fulfilled. There is, e.g., no need to prove that the accused was totally unable to resist his impulses, provided that the impulse was not a minor one: **Simcox** [1964] Crim LR 402 and **Lloyd** [1967] 1 QB 175. Furthermore, it does not matter that the killing was premeditated if the provisions of s 2(1) are fulfilled: **Matheson** [1958] 2 All ER 87. If all the elements of the defence are satisfied, the accused has a defence. It does not matter that the mental abnormality did not cause him to kill.

Points to note

(a) Diminished responsibility is only a defence to murder or being an accessory to murder. It acts as a defence even when there is evidence of planning: **Matheson** (above). It gets round the mandatory sentence by giving the judge discretion as to sentence. The effect, of course, is that irresistible impulse is no defence to other charges such as theft. Though there is a discretion it is not extraordinary for a judge to sentence the accused to life imprisonment when he succeeds in his plea, as occurred in **Byrne**, above. It should be recalled that even after the Criminal Procedure (Insanity and Unfitness to Plead) Act 1991, commitment is mandatory for insanity in a murder case and that diminished responsibility is a defence (only) to murder; therefore, an accused is more likely to rely on diminished responsibility than insanity when murder is charged.

(b) Diminished responsibility is not a complete defence but only a partial one. It reduces murder to manslaughter. A person may be sentenced to life imprisonment for manslaughter, and just as for murder he must receive that sentence. Accordingly for some defendants the effect of succeeding on this defence is nil, as occurred in **Gittens** [1984] QB 698. Some 30 per cent of those successful on this defence receive imprisonment. The court may make a hospital order under s 37 of the Mental Health Act 1983.

(c) If the accused seeks to prove that he is insane, the prosecution may put forward evidence that his defence is one of diminished responsibility. In that event the prosecution have to prove diminished responsibility beyond reasonable doubt.

(d) A judge may, not must, accept a plea of diminished responsibility where medical evidence is unchallenged: **Cox** [1968] 1 All ER 386. Pleas should not be accepted without clear evidence of an abnormality of mind: **Vinagre**, above. S. Dell (above) found that in only 13 per cent of her sample did the doctors disagree, but that if they did, the defence was likely to fail. The effect of *Cox* is to avoid a trial for murder, perhaps saving the public from the details of particularly savage murders. However, this did not happen in the case of the Yorkshire Ripper. In most cases pleas of diminished responsibility are accepted.

(e) All the evidence relating to mental abnormality, not simply the medical evidence, must be looked at by the jury, at least if the medical evidence is disputed: *Walton v R* [1977] AC 788 (PC), *Kiszko* (1978) 68 Cr App R 62. As Lawton LJ put it in *Robinson* (1979) 1 Cr App R (S) 108: 'these cases are to be tried by judges and juries and not by psychiatrists.' The jury can reject the medical evidence if there is other evidence: *Byrne*, *Walton v R* and *Tandy*, all above. If there is only medical evidence, the jury must accept it: *Matheson*, above and *Sanders* (1991) 93 Cr App R 245 (CA), *obiter*, which also approved the previous sentence's statement of the law. Medical evidence normally consists of a history of mental breakdown such as a series of attempts at suicide. Evidence may be given of the nature of the killing and the accused's conduct before, at the time of, and after the *actus reus*. As in insanity any medical evidence will not take place until some time after the killing. Psychiatrists have to try to reconstruct the accused's state of mind at an earlier time. The fact that the accused has killed may, of course, affect his state of mind. In *Sanders* two psychiatrists gave evidence that the accused was suffering from an abnormality of mind, depression, and the prosecution accepted that he was. However, the Crown contended that the abnormality did not substantially impair his mental responsibility. He had made preparations as if he was about to commit suicide but he did not include his victim, his long-term mistress, among the beneficiaries and while he wrote letters to three or four people in anticipation of his death, he did not write to her. The jury evidently thought the killing premeditated. The court held that the will and the letters demonstrated that there was evidence other than that given by psychiatrists which the jury could use to reject the defence. It should be noted that doctors will be examining the accused after he has allegedly killed the victim and the killing may have had some effect on his mind, and they have to judge his state of mind at the time of the killing from their examination of him at a later point in time.

(f) Sometimes flimsy evidence is used to get the accused off a charge of murder, e.g. *Price* (1971) *The Times*, 22 December: a father killing his severely disabled son. This looks like a mercy killing. The law has no category, of 'not guilty by reason of mercy killing'. The accused was suffering from a dissociative state. It may have been that his mental condition was brought about by an external cause, the disabled boy. However, this cause would not fall within the defence. Therefore, the court had to concentrate on the dissociation, not the cause of the dissociation. Some people argue that some battered wives cases are also examples of flimsy evidence because the accused has, after all, killed, and killing is not permitted, and that counsel know that juries are likely to be sympathetic to abused women. Again the court has to concentrate on the mental state, say depression, not on the cause of that abnormality of mind, the beatings. Lawton LJ commented in *Vinagre*, above, thus: 'There was clear evidence of a killing by a jealous husband which, until modern times, no one would have thought was anything else but murder.'

(g) Where the defendant has taken alcohol or drugs, the jury must disregard them: *Gittens*, above (CA), which disapproved *Turnbull* (1977) 65 Cr App R 242. Therefore, the accused has to prove on the balance of probabilities that the murder resulted from an abnormality of mind and not from the intoxication. *Gittens*, which the House of Lords approved in *Dietschmann* [2003] 1 AC 1209, was applied in *Egan*, above. In that case the accused, who was described as bordering on the subnormal, killed an elderly widow after breaking into her home. He had been drinking heavily. The court in a reserved judgment held that intoxication was to be ignored by the jury when considering whether the abnormality substantially impaired the accused's mental responsibility and considering the cause of the abnormality. Such disregard may be difficult for the jury. One effect of the authorities is that the accused to have the defence has to prove that he would have had the defence, had he not been drunk! The late Professor Griew criticised this proposition thus. For the accused to have this defence, there is no need to demonstrate that the abnormality of mind caused the killing; s 2(1) provides a defence when the accused killed while suffering from an abnormal mind. There is no need, therefore, for a causal link, but the position is different when the accused is intoxicated. He has to prove that the killing was due to the abnormality of mind, not the intoxication. In *Dietschmann* the accused killed his victim while both very drunk and suffering from an adjustment disorder consequent on the death of his girlfriend. The prosecution case was that he would not have killed, had he been sober. He was convicted of murder and his appeal dismissed by the Court of Appeal. However, the Lords allowed his appeal. Lord Hutton provided a model direction which restates the law:

> drink cannot be taken into account as something which contributed to his mental abnormality and to any impairment of his mental responsibility . . . but you [the jury] may take the view that both [the accused's] mental abnormality and drink played a part in impairing his mental responsibility . . . and that he might not have killed if he had not taken drink. If you take that view, then the question . . . is: has [the accused] satisfied you that, despite the drink, his mental abnormality substantially impaired his mental responsibility for his fatal acts . . . ?

Cases to the contrary are to be overruled: *Hendy* [2006] EWCA Crim 819 and *Robson* [2006] EWCA Crim 2749. In *Fenton* (1975) 61 Cr App R 261, the Court of Appeal said that they did not know how self-induced intoxication could be an abnormality of mind. This proposition was approved in *Gittens*. However, in *Fenton* it was stated that a craving for drink may create an abnormal mind, the cause being inherent. A permanent injury to the brain caused by alcohol is an 'injury' within s 2(1): *Tandy*, above (CA), which was approved in *Egan*. A mother, an alcoholic, drank nine-tenths of a bottle of vodka and strangled her daughter. Were her judgment and emotional responses greatly impaired; alternatively was she chronically incapable of resisting the impulse to drink, i.e. was her drinking involuntary? She would not have a defence if drink merely made her less able to resist temptation. On the facts it was held that there was no abnormality of mind within s 2(1). For comment see J. Goodliffe 'R v *Tandy* and the concept of alcoholism as a disease' (1990) 53 MLR 809, pointing out that the accused killed during a blackout; therefore she had no *mens*, never mind a *mens rea*; yet she had no defence. The comment of N. Lacey *et al.*, *Reconstructing Criminal Law*, 3rd edn (Butterworths, 2003) 772, is instructive.

> It would be interesting to compare the legally constructed 'biographies' of Moloney [see under murder] and Tandy. The House of Lords was clearly able to identify with the mess which Moloney, a soldier, had got himself into while drunk. The Court of Appeal shows no understanding of the emotional trauma Tandy must have experienced when she discovered her husband had abused her daughter.

It has been suggested that the temporary effect of alcohol on the brain could be classified as an injury, but the court thought not in *Di Duca* (1959) 43 Cr App R 167. The Court of Appeal in *O'Connell* [1997] Crim LR 683 held that the temporary effects of a (prescribed) sleeping drug could not be described as an 'injury'. If they had been, the effects of alcohol would also have to be called an 'injury' within s 2(1).

Alcohol dependence syndrome was seemingly accepted *obiter* in *Inseal* [1993] Crim LR 35 as a cause which can damage the brain, whether or not the accused had been drinking at the time of the killing. If he has been drinking and the syndrome makes the drinking involuntary, then provided that damage to the brain has resulted, the defence is available. *Dietschmann* above confirms that where alcohol does damage the brain, there is an abnormality of mind.

Gittens may be generalised thus: if there are two or more causes of the abnormality of mind, those which do not come within the terms in brackets in s 2(1) are to be disregarded. There is a Judicial Studies Board specimen direction which should be given when the accused raises the defence of diminished responsibility and was allegedly drunk at the time: *Roberts*, unreported, 27 January 2005 (CA). If, however, there are two or more causes which do fit within s 2(1), there is no need for the accused to prove that any one of the causes by itself was an 'abnormality of mind'; it is sufficient that the causes together constituted an 'abnormality of mind': *Dietschmann*, above.

(h) The Royal Commission on Capital Punishment, the Report of which led to the creation of this defence (Cmd 8932, 1953), stated that there were degrees of insanity: sanity and insanity shaded into each other. Similarly, there was no clear line between responsibility and irresponsibility. The defence of diminished responsibility was introduced to bring the law into line with these perceptions.

(i) Current law falls short of the European Convention on Human Rights. First, where the accused is charged with murder, the court does not have an opportunity to determine whether the mental incapacity is of such a kind as to warrant mandatory commitment. Secondly, the law must not be too far out of line with medical opinion, but as we have seen the decision whether the defence applies is one for the jury, not the psychiatrists.

Comment

It is important to realise that a person having the defence of diminished responsibility is convicted of manslaughter and is often imprisoned. The percentage of those imprisoned rather than placed in an hospital has been increasing over the last 30 years. Some, perhaps one-seventh, receive life sentences. This result makes the public safe. It does not necessarily cure the accused's problems. Moreover, the original justification of the defence has gone. It started as a defence to murder when the penalty for that offence was death. Death is no longer the sentence for murder, mandatory life imprisonment is. The modern rationalisation is that diminished responsibility serves to mitigate the sole remaining fixed imprisonment penalty in English law by allowing the court to be flexible in sentencing. If murder at some time lost its mandatory punishment, there would be little or no need for this defence. The trouble with this argument is that if diminished responsibility were abolished, a mentally disabled defendant might not be able to come within the defence of insanity because of its narrowness, and he would be convicted of murder: yet, surely mentally ill defendants should not be convicted of murder. Alternatively, diminished responsibility could be extended to all offences. Why should a partly excused criminal have a defence if he killed but not if, for example, he stole or raped? The accused by definition is not fully responsible for his actions. Probably the main effect of this defence is to put persons into prison who before the Homicide Act would have been sent to a secure hospital. What has occurred is that diminished responsibility was meant to provide a defence to persons who were not legally insane. Instead it has been used for persons who before 1957 would have been classified as insane, as well as those 'on the borderline of insanity'.

E. Griew sums up the present position 'The future of diminished responsibility' [1988] Crim LR 75 at 87:

> Section 2 is . . . badly worded . . . The Courts, by dint of a relaxed approach to interpreta-tion and to expert evidence, have enlarged the ambit of the section . . . [Reform] could make it a less effective device for evading the mandatory life sentence than the present position has proved to be.

The position remains the same today. A reformed law might lead to the exclusion of the mercy-killing father in *Price* (above) from the defence with the result that he would be convicted of murder.

Recommendations for reform 1980–2000

The Fourteenth Report of the Criminal Law Revision Committee, *Offences Against the Person*, Cmnd 7844, 1980, recommended that this defence should be reformed under the lines put forward by the Butler Committee (Cmnd 6244, 1975), above.

(a) The defence will succeed where there is evidence that the accused was suffering from 'severe mental illness' and if 'the mental disorder was such as to be a substantial enough reason to reduce murder to manslaughter'. If the accused agreed, he would be tried for manslaughter straightaway, without needing to look at murder.

(b) The burden of proof should be on the prosecution, though the accused should have the onus of adducing evidence.

(c) The Butler Committee thought that 'the provision for diminished responsibility is needed only because the offence of murder carries a mandatory life sentence. Its extension to offences other than murder is not justified.' It would not be needed if there was no mandatory sentence for murder (which is what the Committee preferred).

The Law Commission's team in 1985 (Law Com. No. 143, *Codification of the Criminal Law: A Report to the Law Commission*) and itself in 1989 (Law Com. No. 177, *A Criminal Code for England and Wales*) proposed to enact these recommendations. The 1989 version of the draft Criminal Code, cl 56, states:

(1) A person who, but for this section, would be guilty of murder is not guilty of murder if at the time of the act, he is suffering from such mental abnormality as is substantial enough reason to reduce his offence to manslaughter.

(2) In this section 'mental abnormality' means mental illness, arrested or incomplete development of mind, psychopathic disorder and any other disorder or disability of mind, except intoxication.

Clause 56(1) makes explicit what is implicit in current law: the jury is asked whether or not the accused's mental abnormality should reduce murder to manslaughter. Whether the accused falls within cl 56(1) would be for the jury, who would no doubt listen to psychiatric evidence. There is the possibility of one jury saying that one accused fell within the definition of mental abnormality but a second one holding the contrary. The terms, however, do reflect medical language better than current law does. Unfortunately both epilepsy and diabetes still fall within the definition 'any other disorder or disability of mind'. Unlike present law the burden of proof would be on the prosecution, and the requirement that the abnormality arise from a specified cause would be abolished. The proposed defence would therefore be wider than the present one. However, in practice the difference may be minimal because the concept of 'inherent causes' in s 2(1) is a broad one. The phrase 'other disorder or disability' would also make this defence wider than the present definition. The definition seems wishy-washy: what is 'substantial enough'? And how wide is 'any other disorder . . . of mind'? Would it cover Othello's jealousy? Nevertheless, the terms of cl 56(2) are narrower than those recommended by the Butler Committee. The Law Commission also recommended in the draft Criminal Code, 1989, that diminished responsibility (as well as provocation and self-defence where the force was excessive) should apply to attempted murder, mitigating the offence to attempted manslaughter: cl 61. This recommendation was based on the proposal of the Criminal Law Revision Committee's Fourteenth Report, *Offences against the Person*, Cmnd 7844, 1980. No move has been made to implement any of these proposals.

The (Nathan) Committee of the House of Lords on *Murder and Life Imprisonment* 1989, recommended the abolition of the mandatory sentence for murder but wished to retain the defence of diminished responsibility in order to afford a defence to those suffering from mental abnormality.

Reform of diminished responsibility: the Law Commission's 2004 proposals

As well as reviewing provocation and excessive force in self-defence the Law Commission in its Report No. 290, *Partial Defences to Murder*, 2004, considered whether the current boundaries of the defence of diminished responsibility should be amended. The Commission agreed with the consultees to their Consultation Paper of the same name, No. 173, 2003, that the defence should continue to exist as long as the mandatory sentence for murder remained. If the definition of murder were to be changed and the mandatory sentence abolished, then how diminished responsibility would be formulated would be for discussion.

As things presently are, there was a division between those consultees who wished to keep the current defence and those who wished it to be abolished. Those who wished to retain it, and did so even if the mandatory sentence were abolished, thought that the defence was a matter of fair labelling: people with diminished responsibility should not be convicted of murder. Moreover, an unreformed insanity plea was no help to those who currently have the defence of diminished responsibility because of the narrowness of the *M'Naghten* rules; jurors should not be obliged to choose acquittal (perversely) when their sole other choice was murder; culpability was an issue for the jury, not one for the judge at the sentencing stage; diminished responsibility is sometimes the sole defence open to battered women who kill on current law; and 'the defence may enable a merciful but just disposition of certain types of cases where all parties consider it meets the justice of the case' (para. 5.22). Even those who supported the retention of the plea argued that the defence had defects, in particular that it pathologised or stigmatised some of those who fell within its terms, especially battered women who kill. Nevertheless, those groups did not attempt to reformulate the defence, at least in part because they did not want a medically approved definition, which would have led to the stigma of being labelled as 'suffering' from diminished responsibility.

There were those who argued in favour of abolition and their arguments may be summarised thus. First, it was illogical to treat diminished responsibility as a defence; since responsibility is diminished, the defence should not be a defence but a mitigating factor. A person who kills but who has an abnormality of mind is, in other words, still a killer. Secondly, the definition is irredeemably unreformable in its use of concepts. Thirdly, the application of the defence is highly contentious, covering for instance mercy-killings which do not fit the definition in s 2 of the Homicide Act 1957.

In light of the differences of opinion about the desirability of retaining the defence and, if it were retained, its reformulation, the Law Commission did not propose any changes to the defence, including the burden of proof, in advance of the comprehensive review of the law of murder. Nevertheless, and with some trepidation, the Commission did advance a formula which it at present preferred if diminished responsibility was to remain a defence to murder. That redefinition was stated in para. 5.97. It is worth stating in full.

> A person, who would otherwise be guilty of murder, is not guilty of murder, but of manslaughter if, at the time of the act or omission causing death,
> (1) that person's capacity to:
>   (a) understand events; or
>   (b) judge whether his actions were right or wrong; or
>   (c) control himself;
> was substantially impaired by an abnormality of mind arising from an underlying condition and
> (2) the abnormality was a significant cause of the defendant's conduct in carrying out or taking part in the killing.
> 'Underlying condition' means a pre-existing mental or psychological condition other than of a transitory kind.

The Law Commission was strongly of the opinion that contrary to the view of some academics provocation and diminished responsibility should not be amalgamated. Their decision was succinctly and clearly expressed thus: '. . . the two partial defences rest on entirely different moral bases and the fact that they may be run together on occasions is not a reason for merging them. The jury can understand the difference and apply them separately.'

The Law Commission's Report No. 306 *Murder, Manslaughter and Infanticide*

The Law Commission endorsed to a large extent its proposals in Report No. 290 on *Partial Defences to Murder* (2004) in its Report No. 306 of November 2006 entitled *Murder, Manslaughter and Infanticide*, which is based on its Consultation Paper No. 177 *A New Homicide Act for England and Wales?* (December 2005). However, it is this Report which recommended a three-tier approach to murder and manslaughter: first degree murder, second degree murder, and manslaughter. See Chapter 11 for details of the proposed rearrangement of murder and manslaughter according to the seriousness of the mental element of the accused. The question then arises: how does diminished responsibility fit into this new scheme? The Commission proposes that diminished responsibility should remain a defence to first degree murder (i.e. when the accused killed and intended to kill or when he or she killed and intended to cause serious injury but was aware that there was a risk of death). However, in relation to other offences, including second degree murder, diminished responsibility should not be a defence. (The proposed maximum sanction for this type of murder is life imprisonment; in other words, life imprisonment would not be mandatory, as it would remain for first degree murder.) In respect of all offences except first degree murder the judge would have discretion as to sentence.

The Commission proposed to retain diminished responsibility as a defence to first degree murder on 'labelling' grounds. 'The mitigating factor of an abnormality of mental functioning can be such that a killer acting under its influence does not deserve to be labelled a first degree murderer.' (para. 5.99) Examples are provided in para. 5.100, one of which is: 'A woman kills her husband having been physically and mentally abused by him over many years, to the point where she admits she has "lost touch with reality."'

The recommendation that first degree murder would become second degree murder when the accused successfully pleaded diminished responsibility has come in for criticism. One argument is that it should reduce first degree murder to manslaughter, the proposed third tier of fatal offences. The Commission opined that since provocation and diminished responsibility were often run together, it would be unacceptable for the two defences to result in different outcomes. Secondly, '. . . if diminished responsibility reduced first degree murder to manslaughter, it would have to be a partial defence to second degree murder as well. Otherwise, those who have killed with the fault element only for second degree murder would irrationally be labelled more harshly (because they could not plead diminished responsibility) than those who had killed with the fault element for first degree murder but successfully pleaded diminished responsibility.' (para. 5.88)

However, there remained the problem of the definition of the defence. The Commission proposed to update it in light of developments in psychiatry and its recommendation on the degrees of murder. In response to comments on the definition proposed in the 2004 Report discussed above the Commission has revamped its proposed definition. It should be noted that the burden of proof will continue to lie on the accused.

(a) A person who would otherwise be guilty of first degree murder is guilty of second degree murder if, at the time he or she played his or her part in the killing, his or her capacity to:
(1) understand the nature of his or her conduct; or
(2) form a rational judgement; or
(3) control himself or herself,
was substantially impaired by an abnormality of mental functioning arising from a recognised mental condition, developmental immaturity in a defendant under the age of eighteen, or a combination of both; and
(b) the abnormality, developmental immaturity, or the combination of both provides an explanation for the defendant's conduct in carrying out or taking part in the killing.

The phrase 'understand the nature of his or her conduct' in (1) replaces 'understand events' in the 2004 formulation so that the accused's lack of understanding of (e.g.) 'global political events' (footnote 84 on p. 102) would not provide a defence. The phrase in (2) replaces 'judge whether his or her actions were right or wrong' because a person who believes himself to be Napoleon should have the defence, even if he knew it was morally and legally wrong to kill. One effect of the proposals is that the definition is no longer tied to outdated causes of mental aberrations as the 1957 definition is: see the phrase in brackets in the Homicide Act s 2(1). The revised definition will also clarify the role of medical experts: they are to give their opinions of whether the accused is suffering from an abnormality of mental functioning which stems from a recognised medical condition, and whether that abnormality had an effect on the accused's capacities. The term 'recognised mental condition' will allow the defence to be restricted or be extended as medical science moves on.

The Commission provides examples of each of the three substantial impairments (1)–(3) above.

(1) 'understand the nature of his or her conduct': 'a boy aged 10 who has been left to play very violent video games for hours on end for much of his life, loses his temper and kills another child when the child attempts to take a game from him. When interviewed, he shows no real understanding that, when a person is killed they cannot simply be later revived, as happens in the games he has been continually playing';

(2) 'form a rational judgement': 'a woman suffering from post-traumatic stress disorder, consequent upon violent abuse suffered at her husband's hands, comes to believe that only burning her husband to death will rid the world of his sins';

(3) 'control himself or herself': 'a man says that sometimes the devil takes control of him, and implants in him a desire that must be acted on before the devil will go away'.

The Commission furthermore explores causation. In present law it seems that there must be some kind of causation: the abnormality of mind must substantially impair (i.e. cause the impairment of) the accused's mental responsibility. The Commission's preferred phrase is that the abnormality of mind or developmental immaturity or both must provide an explanation of the killing or for taking part in the killing. 'This ensures that there is an appropriate connection (that is, one that grounds a case for mitigation of the offence) between the abnormality of mental functioning or developmental immaturity and the killing. It leaves open the possibility, however, that other causes (like provocation) may be admitted to have been at work, without prejudicing a case for mitigation.' (para. 5.124)

With regard to developmental immaturity the Commission states: '. . . it is unrealistic and unfair to assume that *all* children aged 10 or over who kill must have had the kind of developed sense of judgement, control and understanding that makes a first degree murder conviction the right result. . . . Instead, our recommendation is that it should be for the jury to decide in the individual case whether D had such a sense of judgement, control, or understanding.' (para. 5.131) It will not matter what the cause of the immaturity is: it could be the child's environment or social factors or biology or some mixture. It should also be remembered that the burden of proving developmental immaturity will lie on the child as it will throughout the revised definition of diminished responsibility.

The revised definition will not affect insanity, which will continue as now.

Automatism

Introduction

Lawton CJ in **Quick**, above, called the defence of automatism, which seems to have originated in **Chetwynd** (1912) 76 JP 544, 'a quagmire of law seldom entered into nowadays save by those in desperate need of some kind of defence'. It is a narrow defence, made narrower by the rule that insane automatism is insanity, not automatism. A decision which determines that some mental aberration such as epilepsy and sleepwalking is insanity narrows the potential scope of automatism. It is a question of law whether the cause of

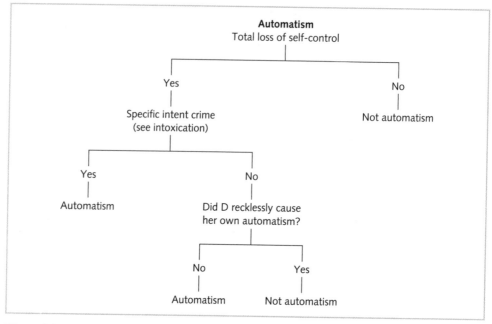

Figure 9.3 Automatism

the accused's mental condition is a disorder of the mind within the rules of insanity: **Sullivan**, above. A recent reminder of the law which distinguishes insanity and automatism is **Roach** [2001] EWCA Crim 2700. The Court of Appeal held that no matter what the doctors called the defendant's illness, the issue of whether the accused was suffering from insanity or automatism was a matter for the jury. The court said that 'the legal definition of automatism allows for the fact that, if external factors are operative upon an underlying condition which would not otherwise produce a state of automatism, then a defence of non-insane automatism should be left to the jury'. Here alcohol or drugs or both (external factors) had acted on the accused's 'mixed personality disorder' (a disease of the mind) to produce violence. The defence was one of automatism, not insanity. When allowed, it is a defence to all crimes, including strict offences. Therefore automatism cannot be simply a denial of *mens rea*, as some judges have said, for strict offences do not require *mens rea* in relation to one or more elements of their *actus reus*. Yet automatism is a defence to strict offences. Therefore, the defence is not one where the accused is saying just that he was not at fault (Fig. 9.3). Whether recklessly getting into a state of automatism is inconsistent with automatism is discussed below. It is sometimes said that automatism negates *actus reus*. If so, it should not matter how the accused came to be suffering from automatism, but the law is that he has no defence if he was at fault in getting into a state of automatism. It is suggested once again that *actus reus* and *mens rea* are sometimes but not always useful tools of analysis. The accused is really saying that what he did cannot be ascribed to him. He was not the author of the misdeed. Unlike insanity and diminished responsibility, the burden of proof is on the prosecution and the standard of proof is beyond reasonable doubt. Criticism has been directed at the outcome of a successful plea of automatism, total acquittal, because the public may be unprotected from a second attack. Lamer CJC in **Parks** (1993) 95 DLR (4th) 27 desired 'some minimally intrusive conditions which seek to assure the safety of the community', perhaps an order that the accused should see a sleep disorder specialist. Yet the accused was not found to have a mental disorder and how can the court make an order when the defendant has been acquitted? The fact that the outcome of a successful plea of automatism is an acquittal may have influenced the courts to keep the defence within narrow bounds.

The basic rule: complete loss of control

The law is not completely clear. Contrary to the view of Neill J in **Roberts v Ramsbottom** [1980] 1 All ER 7, the defence extends beyond complete unconsciousness. The Court of Appeal in **Quick** and **Isitt** [1978] Crim LR 159 referred to semi-conscious states falling within the definition. There is no clear line between consciousness and unconsciousness. The Court of Appeal in **Attorney-General's Reference (No. 2 of 1992)** [1994] QB 91, however, said that automatism denoted a total destruction of voluntary control. Impaired, reduced or partial control was insufficient. 'Driving without awareness', i.e. in a trance-like state, did not amount to a total loss of control. Therefore, the accused should have been found guilty of causing death by reckless driving when he drove his lorry 700 yards along the hard shoulder of a motorway before crashing into a stationary van, killing two people. The trance-like state could be stopped by stimuli such as flashing lights. This case has been criticised for holding that a person in such a state is criminally liable, but the decision seems correct. It is acceptable to punish those who have allowed themselves to get into a trance-like state on a motorway. **Charlson** would seem to be incorrect if this case is rightly decided for in **Charlson** the accused could not have hit his son with a mallet and defenestrated him without having some control over his bodily movements. **Broome v Perkins** (1987) 85 Cr App R 361 is to the same effect as **Attorney-General's Reference (No. 2 of 1992)**: there had to be a total loss of control. The Crown Court, however, held in **T** [1990] Crim LR 256 that a woman who had been raped was suffering from post-traumatic stress syndrome when she stabbed a victim during a robbery. She obviously did have some control over her movements but she acted as if in a 'dream', and accordingly had the defence. There have been suggestions by academics that the requirement of a total loss of consciousness is restricted to driving offences or offences of strict liability but the judiciary have not so held.

Which mental states give rise to automatism?

Non-insane automatism is a defence when the accused has not got control over his movements because of an external cause. His actions are involuntary. He is not guilty unless his movements were willed (though there may be problems with crimes of omissions, where the accused is guilty without bodily movements). A legally relevant act or omission occurs only when the accused's will has led to it. If there is muscular movement without volition, without will, the act is involuntary and is classified as automatism. It covers abnormal states of mind which are not insanity. It covers dissociations and psychological trauma if not prone to recur, according to the High Court of Australia in **Falconer** (1990) 65 ALJR 20, while Lord Diplock in **Sullivan** [1984] AC 156 spoke of 'concussion or the administration of an anaesthetic for therapeutic purposes'. For an Australian case involving a blow to the head see **Cooper v McKenna** [1960] Qd R 406. In **King** (1962) 35 DLR (2d) 386 a Canadian court held that delirium caused by an organism which originated outside the body was automatism. In **Hill v Baxter** [1958] 1 QB 277, the Divisional Court referred to confusions, delusions and strokes, while **Charlson** [1955] 1 All ER 859 was concerned with a brain tumour. In **Bell** [1984] 3 All ER 842, Goff LJ referred to a driver's being attacked by 'a swarm of bees or a malevolent passenger', his being 'affected by a sudden blinding pain' and his becoming 'suddenly unconscious by reason of a blackout'. It may cover hypnotism, according to **Quick and Paddison** [1973] QB 910. Because of the requirement of an external cause **Charlson** and some other cases seem incorrect. A brain tumour is a disease of the mind within the rules on insanity.

Lord Denning in **Bratty v Attorney-General for Northern Ireland** [1963] AC 386 mentioned spasms, reflex actions and convulsions. Some of these holdings may need revision in the light of **Sullivan**, above, and **Hennessy** [1989] 1 WLR 287. Sleepwalking was thought to give rise to automatism for many years: see **Bratty**, relying on Stephen J in **Tolson** (1889) 23 QBD 168; Toohey J did not question in **Falconer** that sleepwalking, like hypoglycaemia, amounted to automatism; and in **Lillienfield** (1985) *The Times*, 12 October, where a sleepwalker had stabbed a friend 20 times, a Crown Court judge held the defence to be automatism. In **Burgess**, above, the Court of Appeal held the defence to be insanity. Somnambulism was not an external factor such as a blow to the head, but an internal factor, which may result in violence. (See also under insanity.) The contrary authority of **Boshears** (1961) *The Times*, 8 February, was presumably overruled, as were other cases noted by Glanville Williams in *Criminal Law: The General Part*, 2nd edn (Stevens, 1961) 483. The court held further that 'external cause' did not cover the ordinary stresses and disappointments of everyday life such as unrequited love (unless the outburst reveals a previously hidden disease of the mind). Automatism is the defence where the accused is suffering traumatic stress after a rape because it was held that the cause, rape, was an external factor: **T**, above (Crown Court). Any normal person would have been severely affected by rape. **T** has been criticised on the grounds that the accused was conscious of what she was doing. She was capable of choosing not to take part in a robbery. The law in relation to post-traumatic stress syndrome is in a flux. In **White** [1995] Crim LR 393 the Court of Appeal held that the accused, a bouncer, who had earlier been stabbed, was not to be convicted of grievous bodily harm with intent when he stamped on the victim's head but of inflicting grievous bodily harm since because of his disorder he did not intend to commit grievous bodily harm. The court did not consider whether he should have been totally acquitted on account of automatism. If driving without awareness had given rise to a state of automatism in **Attorney-General's Reference (No. 2 of 1992)** the external cause would have been the motorway conditions. An irresistible impulse is not automatism: **Bratty**. The US Model Penal Code (Official Draft 1985), s 2.01(a), states that:

> The following are not voluntary acts . . . :
> (a) a reflex or convulsion;
> (b) a bodily movement during unconsciousness or sleep;
> (c) conduct during hypnosis or resulting from hypnotic suggestion;
> (d) a bodily movement that otherwise is not a product of the effort or determination of the actor, either conscious or habitual.

The Model Penal Code seeks to restate the best American criminal law. This definition is similar to the law in England and Wales.

It is not automatism where the accused's mind was not 'in top gear': **Isitt**, above, where the accused's act of driving was purposeful (see also below). He drove away after an accident. The Court of Appeal held that: 'because of panic or stress or alcohol, the appellant's mind was shut to the moral inhibitions which control the lives of most of us. But the fact that his moral inhibitions were not working properly . . . does not mean that the mind was not working at all.' If the automatism is caused by drunkenness, the defence is one of intoxication, and the rules on automatism do not apply. A Scottish case to that effect is *Finegan v Heywood* 2000 SCCR 460.

These different forms of behaviour giving rise to automatism show that it is difficult to find one basis for this defence. According to Gresson P in *Cottle* [1958] NZLR 999 in the Court of Appeal of New Zealand lack of consciousness is the essence. In *Bratty* Lord Kilmuir said that automatism is 'a defence because the mind does not go with what is being done'. It is also difficult to fit automatism into the category of 'defence'. Sometimes the accused is treated as if he did not commit the *actus reus* because his act was not voluntary or was not willed; alternatively, he did not possess the *mens rea* for the offence because his mind was blank. Whichever approach is adopted, there is no offence because the prosecution has failed to prove an element of the offence. Accordingly automatism is not a defence in the sense that the accused did the *actus reus* and had the *mens rea* but is excused or acted justifiably. There is doubt whether automatism fits into the traditional *actus reus*/*mens rea* dichotomy. It may be that, before the prosecution reach the stage of *actus reus* and *mens rea*, they have to show that the accused acted voluntarily. The accused does not act voluntarily if he injures someone as a result of a muscular spasm. Therefore, he is not guilty and the stage of *actus reus* and *mens rea* is not reached. A Scottish case to that effect is *Finegan v Heywood*, above. If this is so one must be careful in distinguishing involuntary from voluntary acts. As Lord Denning noted in *Bratty* on this approach an act is not involuntary simply because the actor could not resist the impulse or did not intend the consequences. However, to get the accused within the definition of automatism, the definition of involuntary behaviour must be stretched to accommodate the facts of *Charlson*. If the accused picks up a child, beats him and throws him through the window, the facts hardly present a picture of ordinary-language involuntarism; his conduct looked purposeful. In this context *Charlson* should be compared with *Broome v Perkins* (1987) 85 Cr App R 361. The accused drove home very erratically from his workplace. He collided with at least one other car and did not appear to have all his faculties. He said that he could recall only the start of his journey and his wife giving him a Mars Bar to counteract his hypoglycaemia. There was evidence that people in such states could drive along familiar roads without being conscious of having done so. He was charged with careless driving. The Divisional Court allowed the prosecution's appeal by way of case stated. The defendant was not entitled to the defence of automatism because his actions were voluntary. His mind was in control of his movements, enabling him to steer his vehicle along the roads. He had driven for six miles and had avoided crashing into lorries. This decision throws doubt on *Charlson*, where the father hit his son over the head and threw him out of the window. Surely he ought to be guilty when the accused in *Broome v Perkins* was. In both cases the acts were 'purposeful' as the Divisional Court put it. The verdict in *Charlson* might be supported, not by saying that the accused acted automatically, but that he had no *mens rea*. The alternative view is to hold that the true defence in *Charlson* was insanity. *Broome v Perkins* has been criticised as punishing someone who did his best. He was held to a very strict standard especially when another fact is added. He went to the police to tell them that he thought he had had an accident. Should we penalise such responsible behaviour?

Special rules in automatism

At least when the offence is one of strict liability or negligence and can be interpreted as occurring over a period of time, the accused will not be acquitted when the automatism is caused by his fault, such as occurred in *Kay v Butterworth* (1945) 173 LT 191 where the accused had fallen asleep. The accused was convicted of careless driving, a crime of negligence, for not stopping his car before he fell asleep. His fault constituted the carelessness necessary for the offence. The doctrine by which the accused was convicted is sometimes known as 'prior fault'. This doctrine is inconsistent with the rules on contemporaneity of *actus reus* and *mens rea* discussed in Chapter 3. It may be that the Divisional Court found that the accused had also fallen asleep at the wheel in **Hill v Baxter**, cited above. This rule applies even though the automatic state was induced by hypoglycaemia (see below) induced by the defendant's negligent failure to counteract the deficiency of sugar, as occurred in **Marison** [1996] Crim LR 909 (CA). The accused knew that he was liable to hypoglycaemic episodes. He had an attack; his car crashed into an oncoming vehicle, and the driver was killed. He did not have a defence of automatism because he knew that his driving was dangerous when he was undergoing a diabetic attack. This rule is sometimes phrased that the accused has no defence if he was reckless in getting into the state of automatism. Driving for many hours without a break would be the epitome of this rule. If a defendant 'drives without awareness', i.e. as if in a trance because he has not taken a rest, no defence is afforded him. **Marison** was distinguished in **G** [2006] EWCA Crim 3276, where the accused was charged with causing death by dangerous driving. She was suffering from hypoglycaemia at the time of the accident and was not at fault for getting into such a state.

Self-induced automatism, it used to be said, was no defence unless the accused's act was 'proper': **Quick and Paddison**, above. The term was undefined but it suggested that the defendant was not at fault. Possibly he was at fault, however, because he failed to prevent his diabetic coma, perhaps knowing what happened if he did not eat food. In **Quick**, the cause of automatism was the drug, insulin, prescribed by a doctor. It might be argued, however, that this rule should not exist. If this defence negatives *mens rea*, how can that be revived by fault? It may be that the case is inconsistent with previous authorities. In **Bailey** [1983] 2 All ER 503, the Court of Appeal cast grave doubt on this exception. See below for a full explanation of the relationship between **Quick** and **Bailey**.

Another rule is that according to Lord Morris in **Bratty**, 'It is not every facile mouthing of some easy phrase of excuse that can amount to an explanation.' It is not enough to say 'I had a blackout'. Voluntary conduct is assumed: the accused has therefore to bring forward some evidence of involuntary behaviour. The accused must show the nature of the incapability such as psychomotor epilepsy (**Bratty**) or abnormal consciousness (**Hill v Baxter**, above). Since the accused in the latter case could not point to medical evidence which would have founded his defence, the court directed the justices to convict. The usual way to show automatism is to adduce medical evidence: **Moses v Winder** [1983] Crim LR 233. The burden of proof, however, remains on the prosecution: **Stripp** (1978) 69 Cr App R 318 and **Bratty**. The contrary *dictum* of Lord Goddard CJ in **Hill v Baxter** is incorrect.

Lord Justice-General Hope in the Scottish High Court of Justiciary case of **Ross v HM Advocate** 1991 SLT 564 said: 'The requirement that the external factor must not be self-induced, that it must be one which the accused was not bound to foresee, and that it must have resulted in a total alienation of reason amounting to a complete absence of self-control, provide adequate safeguards against abuse.' English judges would no doubt express similar sentiments.

Automatism and diabetes

One somewhat uncertain point about automatism is whether diabetes gives rise to this defence. The first major authority is **Quick**, above. The accused, a male nurse at a mental hospital, was charged with assault occasioning actual bodily harm to a paraplegic spastic patient. He led medical evidence to show that he was a diabetic. He had taken insulin but had not eaten properly. He had been hospitalised on several occasions because he had not eaten. He contended that at the time of the alleged assault he was suffering from hypoglycaemia (deficiency of sugar in the blood – the attack need not be caused by diabetes: fasting can lead to it) caused by taking insulin and not eating, making him not know what he was doing, and that this disorder gave him this defence. The trial judge, however, ruled that the disorder was a disease of the mind within the *M'Naghten* Rules. On appeal, the defence argued that a temporary and reversible condition was not a disease of the mind. The judgment was delivered by Lawton LJ. He criticised the definition of disease of the mind given by Lord Denning in *Bratty*: 'any mental disorder which has manifested itself in violence and is prone to recur'. If that definition were correct, the accused would have to be detained in a mental hospital. Lawton LJ said:

> Common sense is affronted by the prospect of a diabetic being sent to such a hospital when in most cases the disordered mental condition can be rectified quickly by pushing a lump of sugar . . . into the patient's mouth.

Against this argument from common sense (and the Court of Appeal was strongly of the view that whether mental aberration constituted a disease of the mind had to be approached 'in a common-sense way', a way which is contradicted by more recent authorities on epilepsy, hyperglycaemia and sleepwalking) is the law that a disease of the mind need not be incurable or permanent (see Devlin J in *Kemp* [1957] 1 QB 399, see above). However, the law went further. In *Hill v Baxter* Lord Goddard CJ did not equate unconsciousness due to a sudden injury with disease of the mind. Lawton LJ held:

> A malfunctioning of the mind of transitory effect, caused by the application to the body of some external factor, such as violence, drugs, including anaesthetics, alcohol and hypnotic influences cannot fairly be said to be due to disease . . . A self-induced incapacity will not excuse . . . nor will one which could have been reasonably foreseen as a result of either doing or omitting to do something, as for example, taking alcohol against medical advice after using certain prescribed drugs, or failing to have regular meals whilst taking insulin.

In *Quick* there was held to be an external factor. The malfunction was caused not by diabetes, but by his use of insulin. Therefore, the accused should have had his defence of automatism put to the jury. The defence was not insanity but automatism. In medical terms, however, the cause of hypoglycaemic comas may be internal when the pancreas produces too much insulin. Moreover, the reason for the accused's taking insulin is an internal one for diabetes is an internal matter.

Quick was explained in *Bailey*. The accused, while suffering a hypoglycaemic episode, hit his girlfriend's lover with an iron bar. The Court of Appeal said *obiter* that even though his mental failure was due to his own act, i.e. was self-induced, in the sense that he could have avoided blacking out by having a meal:

(a) Self-induced automatism exculpated the accused from a crime of specific intent. Therefore, the accused could not be convicted of wounding with intent. This rule is the same as that in intoxication. The jury decides whether the defendant was acting as an automaton.

(b) In crimes of basic intent the rule relating to self-induced incapacity was a rule of drunkenness as a defence, not of automatism. Therefore, it does not apply to insulin. The jury is asked whether the accused was reckless and therefore had the mental element for a crime of recklessness.

The rule in **Quick** that the accused could have no defence where he was at fault was incorrect. However, the court said that the accused could not have this defence if he was subjectively reckless. Whether he was reckless or not was a question for the jury (cf. drunkenness). The jury has to investigate whether the accused himself knew that having no meal meant that he would act dangerously. Some diabetics, including the accused in **Quick**, apparently do not know the effect of their illness. It is suggested that in the years since **Quick** the effects of insulin have become more widely known and fewer people will nowadays be able to rely on their lack of knowledge than 35 years ago. Perhaps **Quick** would be decided differently nowadays: did he know of the consequences of failing to take insulin? From the wording of the judgment the test is subjective but in **Quick** Lawton LJ said that incapacity 'which could have been *reasonably* foreseen' (emphasis supplied) did not excuse, an objective formula. In **Hardie** [1984] 3 All ER 848 the Court of Appeal said that the correct direction on recklessness was not clear and it unfortunately did not rule one way or another. The reason for the distinction between the law on intoxication and automatism is hard to understand. Why should an intoxicated person have no defence to a basic intent offence, but an automaton in some circumstances have one? The court in **Bailey** emphasised that diabetes was not a disease of the mind. It was not a basis for insanity. As we have seen, the House of Lords in **Sullivan** held that epilepsy can be a disease of the mind. Accordingly, epileptics, or some of them at least, cannot rely on this defence. **Sullivan** approved the 'external factor' rule laid down in **Quick**.

The outcome in **Bailey** is open to the criticism that in reality the risk of dangerous behaviour if a diabetic does not take sufficient food after an insulin dose may be common knowledge. It certainly would be if the risk is published on the packet in which the drug comes. As an empirical matter, however, the answer is not clear. In fact the accused's appeal was dismissed because insufficient evidence had been adduced that he was in a state of automatism.

A case, one on hyperglycaemia (an excess of sugar in the blood) which leads to confusion and then a coma, is **Hennessy**, above. The Court of Appeal also approved the external/internal dichotomy. The accused was charged with driving while disqualified and taking a vehicle without consent. He was a diabetic, who had not taken food or insulin as prescribed. The court agreed with the trial judge that the true defence was insanity. **Hennessy** is one of several authorities which over the last 40 years have been extending the law of insanity and thereby reducing the law of automatism. Lord Lane CJ said: 'Stress, anxiety and depression can no doubt be the result of external factors, but they are not . . . external factors of the kind capable in law of causing or contributing to a state of automatism . . . They lack the feature of novelty or accident.' They were not like an anaesthetic or a blow to the head. Therefore, on the facts they were not automatism. Similarly, marital problems were not external factors. As N. J. Reville commented ([1989] LSG 19):

> [t]he implications of the external/internal factors distinction are disturbing, because it creates arbitrary rules. Should a diabetic, such as Mr. Hennessy, suffer a hyperglycaemic episode merely because he failed to eat enough, then any injury that he inflicts will result in an insanity verdict because his mental condition is not caused by an external factor. On the other hand, if the diabetic produced his state of automatism by taking insulin (and thereafter failing to eat), he would be regarded as being in a state of non-insane automatism.

One distinction between the two forms is that hyperglycaemia can come on slowly, whereas hypoglycaemia may come on quickly, but the two states are similar in effect: disorientation followed by loss of consciousness and death. It is strange therefore that one form leads to the stigma of being labelled insane whereas the other leads to a complete acquittal.

Certainly, the external/internal division does not necessarily differentiate between those who ought to be acquitted and those who ought to be treated or imprisoned. Yet the distinction between hypoglycaemia and hyperglycaemia was confirmed in *Bingham* [1991] Crim LR 433 (CA). The accused said that because of hypoglycaemia he was unaware of what he was doing, taking sandwiches and cola from a shop. The defence of automatism was available.

Summarising, taking too much insulin is an external factor. Automatism is a possible defence. Taking no insulin is an internal factor, which means that automatism is not available. Not enough sugar (hypoglycaemia) is automatism; hyperglycaemia (too much) is insanity, yet both involve the blood/sugar level and the difference in outcome is tremendous. In insanity the accused may be sent to a secure hospital even after the 1991 Act; in automatism the verdict is acquittal. The law should distinguish between dangerous persons and others: it does not.

The law in Australia is different. An accused suffering from an 'underlying mental infirmity' is insane but a temporary mental infirmity is automatism: see *Falconer*, above. One effect is that the defendant in *Hennessy* would be acquitted because of automatism if the Australian rule was imported into England.

Insanity and automatism

The previous section has shown the difficulty of distinguishing these defences in the context of automatism. *Quick* illustrates the problem. The accused's condition was due to the injection of insulin. The malfunction of the mind was held to be an external factor, not a disease. However, a high blood/sugar level, hyperglycaemia, is a disease and the *M'Naghten* Rules apply. In *Quick* the Court of Appeal said that a blow to the head was an external factor and therefore the defence was automatism. However, if the blow caused brain damage, then the defence is one of insanity provided that there is no other external blow. In *T*, above, if traumatic stress after a disease had been held to be a disease of the mind, the outcome was insanity quite possibly; if it was an illness caused by an external factor, the defence was automatism. Insane automatism is a rare defence in terms of successful pleas.

The basic distinction is that automatism stems from a 'temporary loss of consciousness arising accidentally', as Devlin J put it in *Hill v Baxter*, while insanity is founded on mental disease. In *Falconer*, above, where the High Court of Australia rejected the internal/external distinction, automatism was said to come from 'a transient non-recurrent mental malfunction caused by external forces which produces an incapacity' to control actions, whereas insanity was based on 'an underlying mental infirmity'. If the alleged automatism is a disease of the mind the plea really is one of insanity, and the burden of proof is on the accused, whereas if the automatism is of the non-insane variety the onus is on the prosecution to disprove beyond reasonable doubt that the accused has this defence. Therefore, the wider is 'disease of the mind', the narrower is automatism. It is arguable that if the accused's mental disorder is not likely to recur, there is little point in putting him into a secure hospital.

Even if a jury rejects evidence of insanity, they are entitled to consider automatism: *Burns* (1973) 58 Cr App R 364 (DC). As *Burns* also held, the jury must be directed separately on the differing burdens of proof. The cases stress that the burden in automatism is on the prosecution: *Budd* [1962] Crim LR 49 and *Bratty*, above.

One practical point remains. Counsel has the duty of choosing between advising the accused (a) to plead guilty and possibly get a light sentence or (b) plead automatism and so open the route to insanity. For example, in **Sullivan**, above, because the accused raised the plea of automatism, the prosecution could adduce evidence of insanity (which they had to prove beyond reasonable doubt).

The Criminal Procedure (Insanity and Unfitness to Plead) Act 1991, which was not in force at the time of **Sullivan** and **Hennessy**, means that commitment is not mandatory except in murder cases and the plea of insanity in theory ought to become more popular than before.

Reform

The Law Commission in its Report No. 177, *A Criminal Code for England and Wales*, 1989, cl 33(1), proposes to enact a large part of the Butler Committee on Mentally Abnormal Offenders, above:

A person is not guilty of an offence if –
(a) he acts in a state of automatism, that is, his act
    (i) is a spasm or convulsion; or
    (ii) occurs while he is in a condition (whether of sleep, unconsciousness, impaired consciousness or otherwise) depriving him of effective control of the act; and
(b) the act or condition is the result neither of anything done or omitted with the fault required for the offence nor of voluntary intoxication.

This proposal has been criticised for failing to define what 'effective control' is. Still excluded from the defence are epileptics and diabetics, though sleepwalkers would be included, reversing **Burgess**, above.

However, under cl 34 a defendant who was in a state of automatism (not resulting only from intoxication) which is a feature of a disorder, whether organic or functional and whether continuing or recurring, that may cause a similar state on another occasion would be subject to a mental disorder verdict, and by cl 39 the court would have wide powers of sentence. The present law of automatism has been criticised for permitting persons who ought to be treated to roam the streets.

The effect of cl 33(1) could be to get rid of the present internal/external debate: there would also be no need to speak of will, voluntary behaviour or volition. Since cl 33(1)(a) speaks of deprivation of 'effective control', **Broome v Perkins** and **Attorney-General's Reference (No. 2 of 1992)**, above, would presumably be reversed. However, phrases such as 'impaired consciousness' and 'effective control' could be read widely or narrowly, and outcomes may be different on the same facts, because what is 'effective' is a question of degree. The 1985 draft Criminal Code required that the accused was totally deprived of control of his movements. In criticism of that draft it may be said that to deprive defendants of this defence when they are not totally deprived of control seems severe. Certainly on this draft **Broome v Perkins** would have survived. Sleepwalking would again be part of automatism. Note also that sub-cl (b) takes away much of what is given in sub-cl (a). Sub-clause (b) also means that the principle of contemporaneity does not apply when cl 33(1) does.

Tabular summary of the defences

Table 9.1 gives a brief comparison of insanity, diminished responsibility and automatism.

Table 9.1 Insanity, diminished responsibility, automatism: a brief comparison

	Insanity	Diminished responsibility	Automatism
Defence to	All offences	Murder	All offences
Cause	Must be internal	Internal or external but must be listed in s 2(1), Homicide Act 1957	Must be external
Definition requires	Disease of the mind	Abnormality of mind	Loss of consciousness
Burden of proof	On the accused	On the accused	On the prosecution
Standard of proof	Balance of probabilities	Balance of probabilities	Beyond reasonable doubt
Outcome if successful plea	Not guilty by reason of insanity	(Voluntary) manslaughter	Acquittal

Loss of control over a car

In *Spurge* [1961] 2 QB 205 the court held that a sudden and total loss of control over a car is a defence, provided that the accused did not know nor should he have known of the defect. Similarly in *Burns* v *Bidder* [1967] 2 QB 227 the accused was not guilty of failing to accord precedence to a pedestrian at a crossing when the brakes failed. The analogy with automatism is close and indeed the court used the hackneyed automatism example of a driver being attacked by a swarm of bees when exculpating the driver. Similarly, in *Bell*, above, Goff LJ mentioned an attack by a swarm of bees and loss of control caused, e.g., by a blowout or a brake failure. The position may be different if a pedestrian jumps out. According to *Neal* v *Reynolds* [1966] Crim LR 393 the accused is guilty, but that case may be wrong. The courts have not been consistent in their use of terminology. If an accused has a defence of automatism because he is, e.g., attacked by a swarm of bees, the courts might say that the accused is not driving and is therefore not guilty of any offence involving the *actus reus* of driving. The act was involuntary; accordingly, there was no act. However, the court might say in different circumstances that the accused's act was voluntary even though he did not know of the circumstances of the activity. If an accused is driving with above the limit of alcohol in his blood because his drinks have been spiked, the court held in *Shippam* [1971] Crim LR 434 that he was guilty, under what is now s 5 of the Road Traffic Act 1988, because his driving was voluntary. (See the section on intoxication for the law on involuntary intoxication.) The point is this: be careful how the courts use the terms 'voluntary' and 'involuntary'. The terminology is inconsistent.

Summary

This chapter's coverage is summarised by its title: 'defences of mental disorder'. The first defence considered here is unfitness to plead. This occurs when the accused is insane at the time of the trial. The second defence, insanity, is when the accused is mentally fit to stand trial but alleges that she was insane at the time of the *actus reus* of the offence. The burden of proving this defence exceptionally lies on the accused. She must prove on the balance of probabilities that she (i) was labouring under such a defect of reason (ii) from disease of the mind (iii) that she either (a) did not know the nature and quality of the act or (b) that she did not know that what she was doing was [legally] wrong. The word 'legally' is in brackets because it is not sufficient to have this defence that the accused did not know that what she was doing was morally wrong: it will be a rare individual who does not know that killing is legally wrong. The law is based on the **M'Naghten** Rules of 1843. The consequences of the rules are worked out e.g. epileptics, sleepwalkers and some diabetics may be classified in law as being insane, no matter what the doctors say, while other diabetics may have the defence of automatism. Despite insanity's being a defence the accused who is found by the jury to be insane may appeal against that verdict. Indeed, particularly since the institution of the defence of diminished responsibility pleas of insanity are rare.

Diminished responsibility is, unlike insanity which applies to all offences, a defence only to murder, but like insanity the burden of proof is on the accused. Like insanity there are three hurdles for the accused to surmount. She must prove that at the time of the killing she was (i) suffering from an abnormality of mind (ii) which arose from one the causes specified in s 2(1) of the Homicide Act 1957 (iii) and which substantially impaired her mental responsibility for the crime. Like insanity the three issues are all questions of fact for the jury.

The third defence involving the accused's mental condition is automatism. Automatism is the defence where the accused's mind is not in control of her movements. There is debate about whether the accused must totally have lost control but modern authority is to that effect. Here the burden of proof is on the prosecution: and the prosecution must disprove the defence beyond reasonable doubt.

- Unfitness to plead: This defence is open to an accused who at the time of the trial cannot understand the trial process to make a proper defence. The issue of fitness to plead is for the jury. Except for murder the Criminal Procedure (Insanity and Unfitness to Plead) Act 1991 as amended provides a range of orders.

- Insanity: This common law defence affords a defence to persons who are 'insane' at the time of the offence but are fit to plead at the time of the trial. The burden of proof lies on the accused and the standard of proof is on the balance of probabilities (see Chapter 1). He or she must prove:
  1   he or she was suffering from a 'disease of the mind'
  2   which caused a defect of reason and EITHER
  3(a) which was such that the accused did not know the nature and quality of the act OR
  3(b) which was such that the accused did not know that what he was doing was legally wrong (even if he or she knew that he or she had acted in a morally wrong way).

Trenchant criticism of the rules on insanity has been made for many years, particularly of 'disease of the mind', a concept which covers epilepsy, sleepwalking and hypoglycaemia.

The jury decides whether a person is insane or not, but two medical practitioners must testify as to the accused's mental state. The same orders after a finding of insanity as are made after a finding of unfitness to plead may be made except in respect of murder when only one order is possible: Criminal Procedure (Insanity and Unfitness to Plead) Act 1991.

Despite insanity's being a defence the accused may appeal against the verdict of 'not guilty by reason of insanity'.

■ Diminished responsibility: Section 2(1) of the Homicide Act 1957 provides a defence to an accused who proves on the balance of probabilities that he or she is suffering from 'such abnormality of mind (whether arising from a condition of arrested or retarded development of mind or any inherent causes or induced by disease or injury) as substantially affected his mental responsibility for his acts or omissions in doing or being a party to the killing.' The offence, as may be obvious, is available only to those who kill or are accessories to a killing. The defence consists therefore of three elements:

1 abnormality of mind
2 a cause which is one of those found in the brackets of s 2(1) and
3 substantial impairment of mental responsibility.

These are not easy terms to understand (even though each issue is for the jury) but the purpose of s 2(1) was that of saving mentally disturbed killers from the death sentence on a broader basis than insanity already provided. There is empirical evidence to suggest that this defence is used both mercifully to defendants and as a substitute in murder cases for the defence of insanity.

■ Automatism: Automatism, a defence to all crimes, is based on either unconscious (as may be caused by diabetes) or reflex bodily actions or the external application of something e.g. force to the accused which causes him or her completely to lose control over bodily movements, to act involuntarily. If the accused felt himself or herself moving into a state of unconsciousness, there is no defence if he or she was at fault. Where the automatism was caused by insanity, the defence is one of insanity, not automatism. The burden of proving automatism lies on the prosecution, which must disprove it beyond reasonable doubt.

References

Reports

Criminal Law Revision Committee 11th Report, *Evidence (General)*, Cmnd 4991 (1972)

Criminal Law Revision Committee 14th Report, *Offences against the Person*, Cmnd 7844 (1980)

Law Commission Consultation Paper no. 173, *Partial Defences to Murder* (2003)

Law Commission Consultation Paper no. 177, *A new Homicide Act for England & Wales* (2005)

Law Commission Report no. 143, *Criminal Law: Codification of the Criminal Law – A Report to the Law Commission* (1985)

Law Commission Report no. 177, *A Criminal Code for England & Wales* (1989)

Law Commission Report no. 290, *Partial Defences to Murder* (2004)

Law Commission Report no. 306, *Murder, Manslaughter and Infanticide* (2006)

Model Penal Code, *Official Draft* (1985)

Report of the Committee on Mentally Abnormal Offenders (Butler) Cmnd 6244 (1975)

Books

Boland, F. *Anglo-American Insanity Defence Reform* (Dartmouth, 1999)

Clarkson, C. M. V. *Understanding Criminal Law* 1st edn (Fontana, 1987)

Clavkson, C. M. V. *Understanding Criminal Law* 4th edn (Thomson, 2005)

Dell, S. *Murder into Manslaughter* (Oxford University Press, 1984)

Lacey, N., Wells, C. and Quick, O. *Reconstructing Criminal Law* 3rd edn (Butterworths, 2003)

Mackay, R. D. *Mental Condition Defences in the Criminal Law* (Clarendon, 1995)

Journals

Ashworth, A. Comment on *H* Crim [2003] LR 818

Goodliffe, J. '*R* v *Tandy* and the concept of alcoholism as a disease' (1990) 53 MLR 809

Griew, E. 'The future of diminished responsibility' [1988] Crim LR 75

Grubin, D. 'Unfit to plead in England & Wales 1976–88 – a survey' (1991) 158 BJ Psych 540

Grubin, D. 'What constitutes fitness to plead?' [1993] Crim LR 748

Mackay, R. D. 'Fact and fiction about the insanity defence' [1990] Crim LR 247

Mackay, R. D. 'The decline of disability in relation to the trial' [1991] Crim LR 87

Mackay, R. D. and Kearns, G. 'An upturn in unfitness to plead?' [2000] Crim LR 532

Reville, N. 'Automatism and diabetes' [1989] 86 LSG 19

Further reading

Boland, F. *Anglo-American Insanity Defence Reform: The War Between Law and Medicine* (Ashgate, 1999)

Bynoe, I. 'Unfitness to plead' [1991] SJ 984

Dell, S. 'Wanted: an insanity defence that can be used' [1983] Crim LR 431

Duff, R. A. 'Fitness to plead and fair trials' [1994] Crim LR 419

Griew, E. 'Let's implement Butler on mental disorder and crime' [1984] CLP 47

Griew, E. 'Reducing murder to manslaughter: whose job?' (1986) 12 *Journal of Medical Ethics* 18

Griew, E. 'The future of diminished responsibility' [1988] Crim LR 75

Grubin, D. R. 'What constitutes unfitness to plead?' [1993] Crim LR 748

Grubin, D. R. 'Fitness to plead and fair trials – (2) A reply' [1994] Crim LR 423

Jones, T. H. 'Insanity, automatism and the burden of proof on the accused' (1995) 111 LQR 475

Loughnan, A. '"Manifest madness": towards a new understanding of the insanity defence' (2007) 70 MLR 379

Mackay, R. D. 'Fact and fiction about the insanity defence' [1990] Crim LR 247

Mackay, R. D. 'The automatism defence' (1983) 34 NILQ 81

Mackay, R. D. 'The abnormality of mind factor in diminished responsibility' [1999] Crim LR 117. (This author has written extensively in legal and medical journals in the UK and abroad and any article by him is worth reading. His book, *Mental Condition Defences in the Criminal Law* (Clarendon, 1995) is the main recent English work.)

Mackay, R. D. and Kearns, G. 'The continued underuse of unfitness to plead and the insanity defence' [1999] Crim LR 714

Mackay, R. D. and Mitchell, B. J. 'Sleepwalking, automatism and insanity' [2006] Crim LR 901

Mackay, R. D. Mitchell, B. J. and Howe, L. 'Yet more facts about the insanity defence' [2006] Crim LR 399

Mackay, R. D., Mitchell, B. J. and Howe, L. 'A continued upturn in unfitness to plead – more disability in relation to the trial under the 1991 Act' [2007] Crim LR 530

Ridgway, P. 'Sleep walking – insanity or automatism' (1996) 3 E LAW – *Murdoch University Electronic Journal of Law*

Virgo, G. 'Sanitising insanity – sleepwalking and statutory reform' (1991) 50(3) CLJ 386

Ward, T. 'Magistrates, insanity and the common law' [1997] Crim LR 790

Wells, C. 'Whither insanity?' [1983] Crim LR 787

Wilson, W. *et al.* 'Violence, sleepwalking and the criminal law (2): the legal aspects' [2005] Crim LR 614

Wootton, B. 'Diminished responsibility – a layman's view' (1960) 76 LQR 224

Yannoulidis, S. Y. 'Mental illness, rationality and criminal responsibility' [2003] Syd LR 10

For a Scottish view, see the Scottish Law Commission, *Discussion Paper on Insanity and Diminished Responsibility*, no. 122, 2003.

For an American approach, see R. F. Schopp, *Automatism, Insanity and the Psychology of Criminal Responsibility* (Cambridge University Press, 1991). The author provides a useful critique of English law.

Visit **www.mylawchamber.co.uk/jefferson** to access exam-style questions with answer guidance, multiple choice quizzes, live weblinks, an online glossary, and regular updates to the law.

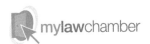

Use **Case Navigator** to read in full some of the key cases referenced in this chapter:

R v *Hennessy* [1989] 2 All ER 9
R v *Quick* [1973] 3 All ER 347

10

Inchoate offences

English law intervenes to punish persons who have not (yet) committed an offence. The crimes which penalise conduct before the commission of the (full or substantive) crime are called inchoate offences. Having these changes available is to deter offending in this category. The exception to this rule is conspiracy to defraud: the result to be achieved need not be a crime. Conspiracy to defraud cannot be described as a true inchoate offence. Unlike secondary offences, the full crime need not have taken place before the accused is guilty of an inchoate offence. If the principal offence is committed, the accused may also be liable as a secondary party. Inchoate offences are criminal only in relation to the full offence, i.e. one is not guilty of attempt but, e.g., of attempted murder.

There are three inchoate offences: incitement, conspiracy and attempt. This chapter deals with these offences. There are also specific offences. For example, there is an offence of inciting a person to commit murder contrary to s 4 of the Offences Against the Person Act 1861 (see below). Some other offences partake of the nature of inchoate offences. Two examples suffice: s 3 of the Criminal Damage Act 1971 deals with possessing anything with intent to damage property; s 1 of the Prevention of Crime Act 1953 penalises the carrying of offensive weapons. In neither crime need the accused have harmed any property or person. When assault was seen as attempted battery (which it no longer is), it was an inchoate offence. One form of burglary, entry into a building as a trespasser with intent to commit criminal damage, steal or commit grievous bodily harm is also an inchoate offence. The offences are discussed in the order incitement, conspiracy and attempt because generally speaking that sequence shows the movement towards the completion of the principal offence. For example, the crime of conspiracy is committed at an earlier stage than attempt and accordingly the police can intervene at an earlier time. It is also the sequence in the draft Criminal Code, Law Com. Report No. 177, 1989, *A Criminal Code for England and Wales*.

Encouraging, assisting & the former offence of incitement

Introduction

The Serious Crimes Act 2007, which came into force just before publication of this edition, makes the common law offence of inciting crimes (incitement) into a statutory one. The explanation of the common law offence is retained here because it will continue to exist until the new definition takes effect and because a comparison can be made between the common law and statutory definitions.

Part 2 of the 2007 statute repeals the common law offence of incitement (s 59) and creates the crimes of encouraging and assisting, which like the offence of incitement they replace, are inchoate offences (s 49(1)). It should be noted that 'encouraging or assisting' are to be read as covering situations where the accused put pressure on another to commit an offence (s 65(2)), a strange partial definition of 'encouraging or assisting' but one fully in line with the common law offence of incitement. Section 44(1) creates the crime of 'intentionally encouraging or assisting an offence'. It reads:

A person commits an offence if –
(a) he does an act capable of encouraging or assisting the commission of an offence; and
(b) he intends to encourage or assist its commission.

Section 44(2) makes the perhaps obvious point that:

. . . he is not to be taken to have intended to encourage or assist the commission of an offence merely because such encouragement or assistance was a foreseeable consequence of his act.

Section 45 creates a second offence, that of 'encouraging or assisting an offence believing that it will be committed'. Section 45(1) provides: 'A person commits an offence if –
(a) he does an act capable of encouraging or assisting the commission of an offence; and
(b) he believes –
    (i) that the offence will be committed; and
    (ii) that his act will encourage or assist its commission.

Section 46 deals with what are sometimes called 'laundry list' instances of encouraging or assisting, i.e. where the accused believes that one or more offences may be committed but is unsure as to which on will in fact be committed. On these facts the person who encourages or assists is guilty when he does an act capable of assisting or encouraging and he believes that 'his act will encourage or assist the commission of one or more' of the potential offences.

'Encouraging or assisting' also covers the following situation (s 66): 'If a person (D1) arranges for a person (D2) to do an act that is capable of encouraging or assisting the commission of an offence, and D2 does the act, D1 is also to be treated . . . as having done it.'

There is a partial definition of 'intends' in s 44(1)(b): '. . . it is sufficient to prove that he intended to encourage or assist the doing of an act which would amount to the commission of that offence.' The definition of 'believes' in s 45(1)(b) is found partly in s 47(3):

. . . it is sufficient to prove that he believed –
(a) that an act would be done which would amount to the commission of that offence; and
(b) that his act would encourage or assist the doing of that act.

There is a further explanation of the mental element in s 47(5):

In proving for the purposes of this section whether an act is one which, if done, would amount to the commission of an offence –
(a) if the offence is one requiring proof of fault, it must be proved that –
    (i) D [the accused] believed that, were the act to be done, it would be done with that fault;
    (ii) D was reckless as to whether or not it would be done with that fault; or
    (iii) D's state of mind was such that, were he to do it, it would be done with that fault.

(b) if the offence is one requiring proof of particular circumstances or consequences (or both), it must be proved that –
   (i) D believed that, were the act to be done, it would be done in those circumstances or with those consequences; or
   (ii) D was reckless as to whether or not it would be done in those circumstances or with those consequences.

For the avoidance of doubt, s 47(8) provides that an 'act' includes an omission and the continuation of an act.

Section 49 provides in part that a person may commit more than one offence under ss 44–46 on the same facts.

There is a special defence to these offences found in s 50, the defence of acting reasonably. It is a defence for the accused to prove (ss (2)) 'that he believed certain circumstances to exist; that his belief was reasonable; and that it was reasonable for him to act as he did in the circumstances as he believed them to be'. Subsection (3) goes on to provide:

> Factors to be considered in determining whether it was reasonable for a person to act as he did include –
> (a) the seriousness of the anticipated offence . . . ;
> (b) any purpose for which he claims to have been acting;
> (c) any authority by which he claims to have been acting.

Section 51 exempts protected persons from conviction for these offences. A protected person is one who is protected by a 'protective offence', which is one which exists 'for the protection of a particular category of persons' (s 51(2)).

The law superseded by the Serious Crimes Act is retained for comparison. That said it is a common law offence to solicit or invite a person to commit a crime, even if that solicitation has no effect: *Higgins* (1801) 102 ER 269, affirmed in *Whitehouse* [1977] QB 868 (CA). The person incited need not be induced to act criminally. The crime is complete when the accused solicits. For example, in *Higgins*, the accused solicited a servant to steal his master's property. He was guilty whether or not the servant acted on the suggestion. It may be fortuitous that the crime incited is not completed. The accused must show by his words or acts that he is disposed to having a crime committed. It is punishable with imprisonment or a fine at the judge's discretion when the case is tried on indictment even though the principal offence's maximum is substantially less. Potentially therefore the inciter of an assault is liable to life imprisonment but the principal offender's maximum sentence is only six months' imprisonment. Incitement to commit a summary offence is punishable to the same extent as the completed crime (Magistrates' Courts Act 1980, s 45(3)). Incitement to commit an either way offence if tried summarily has the same rule (s 32(1)(b)). Therefore, the accused may be punished more severely for inciting the offence than is the person who committed it, especially when trial is in the Crown Court. The inciter may have demonstrated that he can plan an offence whereas the incitee may simply have been told what to do.

Actus reus

There must be persuasion or encouragement: *Race Relations Board* v *Applin* [1973] QB 815 (CA), a case dealing with the crime of incitement to racial hatred, *Hendrickson* [1977] Crim LR 356 (CA), *James* (1985) 82 Cr App R 226 (CA) and *Marlow* [1997] Crim LR 197 (CA). In *Marlow* the accused published a book on how to grow marijuana and he advertised it in magazines. He was guilty of inciting others to cultivate a controlled drug even though the others would have cultivated the cannabis in any case and even though the same information was available elsewhere. It was also irrelevant that the acts of incitement were public ones. The court said in respect of the definition of incitement that 'encourage' 'represents as well as any modern word can the concept involved'. In *James* the defendants were not guilty of conspiracy to incite others to abstract electricity. Their intent was to sell machines which reversed meters but they did not persuade the buyer to use them, as charged. He would sell them to others. The Court of Appeal in *Fitzmaurice* [1983] QB 1083 spoke of 'suggestion, proposal or request'. In *Goldman* [2001] Crim LR 822 it was held that the accused suggested to, proposed to, induced or persuaded a company when he wrote to them requesting pornographic videos in response to their advertisement. As in *Marlow*, it was immaterial that the principal would have committed the crime of possessing pornographic videos without any encouragement from the accused. It was also immaterial that it is the person incited who invited the accused to encourage him, the person invited, to commit an offence. In criticism of *Goldman* it may be said that the accused did not persuade or encourage the child pornographers to do anything. They were willing sellers, he a willing buyer. Threats and pressure can be incitement: *Invicta Plastics Ltd* v *Clare* [1976] Crim LR 131 (DC) and *James*. The persuasion need not be oral. In *Invicta Plastics* the company advertised for sale an instrument useful in evading police speed traps. They were guilty of inciting an offence. The Divisional Court held that unlike in *James* the defendants were attempting to persuade motorists to break the law. In *James*, however, the selling of so-called 'black boxes', the sole purpose of which was to abstract electricity illegally, did not constitute incitement. The court held that there was no persuading or encouraging others to break the law when one facilitated their doing so. The incitement may be to the world in general as in *Most* (1881) 7 QBD 244, where the accused wrote an article in a newspaper advocating assassination. The incitement must come to the attention of the incitee but need not take effect: *Krause* (1902) 18 TLR 238. The incitement need not have any effect. The accused is guilty even though the person incited did not commit the crime. If the accused is the victim of the crime he cannot be guilty of inciting that offence, provided that the offence is one designed for his protection: *Tyrrell* [1894] 1 QB 710. The rule is the same in conspiracy (see below).

One outcome of the law as stated so far is (subject to *Goldman*) this. If the accused persuaded another orally to commit a crime, this is incitement. If, however, he sells her a gun knowing that she will shoot someone, he is not guilty of incitement because there is no persuasion or encouragement, and if the other does not, for example, kill that third party, there is no secondary liability either.

A very interesting recent case is *O'Shea* [2004] Crim LR 896 (CA) (also called *O'Shea* v *Coventry Magistrates' Court*). The accused, who had registered with and accessed child pornography on a US website, was guilty of inciting the US business to distribute indecent photographs (the substantive offence could be one of several including possession of an indecent photograph of a child contrary to s 160 of the Criminal Justice Act 1988). The court did not discuss whether a corporation could be incited. It is uncertain whether any human being was incited. The website was already in operation before the accused subscribed and surely one cannot incite a machine to commit an offence? *O'Shea* is a weak authority.

Mens rea

The *mens rea*, in part, is knowledge of or wilful blindness to the full offence's circumstances and intention as to the consequences. Accordingly, to be guilty of incitement to murder, the accused must intend that the victim be killed: intent to cause grievous bodily harm is insufficient. The accused is guilty if he does the *actus reus* of incitement with the intention that the principal offender should commit the offence. There is no need to show that the accused had the fault elements of the full offence. **Shaw** [1994] Crim LR 365 (CA) is incorrect insofar as it holds that the accused must have the *mens rea* of the full crime. It is hard to see why the inciter of theft must just as much intend to deprive permanently and be dishonest as the thief himself. Perhaps the issue did not cross the minds of the judges. Certainly incitement is complete, no matter whether the person incited intended to commit the offence: the state of mind of the incitee is irrelevant. See also the next section of this book. **Shaw** also suggests that the accused is not guilty if he does what would otherwise be an act of incitement in order to demonstrate failure of security at his employer's premises. His motive meant that he was not guilty. This ruling is incorrect in the light of general law that motive is irrelevant especially that of conspiracy noted below: see the discussion of **Yip Chiu-Cheung v R** [1995] 1 AC 111. Since the accused in **Shaw** persuaded his colleagues to commit theft, he should have been found guilty of incitement, no matter how good his motive was.

Statutory offences of incitement

The Offences Against the Person Act 1861, s 4 (as amended by the Criminal Law Act 1977) created the crime of incitement to murder. The accused is guilty if he acts to 'solicit, encourage, persuade or endeavour to persuade or . . . propose to any person to murder any other person'. The offence, which was at issue in **Most** and **Krause**, adds nothing to the common law offence of incitement in terms of substantive law. Section 4 includes inciting foreign nationals in England and Wales to commit murder abroad: **Abu Hamza** [2006] EWCA Crim 2918. It was not restricted to the solicitation of British subjects to commit murder. Parliament has created other incitement offences in, for example, the Sexual Offences Act 2003 (there are several such offences in the statute), the Incitement to Mutiny Act 1797 and the Incitement to Disaffection Act 1934.

The relationship between incitement and the full offence

(a) It is immaterial that the full offence is not committed. Where the crime does take place, the accused can be charged as inciter or secondary party or both. If the incitee gives way to the encouragement, conspiracy may take place. If the crime does not take place, the accused cannot be guilty of counselling but may be guilty of incitement.

(b) If the full crime is impossible to commit, **Fitzmaurice**, above, said that the accused was not guilty unless the means suggested were inadequate. (On the facts robbery of a woman believed to be carrying cash from a factory to a bank was a possible crime, even though the woman did not exist, because women do carry money from factories to banks.) The Court of Appeal did not, however, overrule the decision of the Court of Criminal Appeal in **McDonough** (1962) 47 Cr App R 37 in which it was held that the accused was guilty of inciting another to receive stolen lamb carcases even though there were no carcases at the relevant time. In **Fitzmaurice** the court said that **McDonough** was correct because there might have been at some time in the future. The Divisional Court in **DPP v Armstrong** [2000] Crim LR 379 held that the accused was guilty of inciting the offence of distributing indecent photographs of children when he asked a person to supply him with pornography involving girls 'not younger than say 12 years'. Unknown to the accused the other person was a police officer charged with catching paedophiles. He would not have supplied pornography.

The court held that the crime was not impossible because the officer could have access to a stock of pornography. The same rules as incitement apply to those conspiracies which remain crimes at common law. However, in relation to attempt and statutory conspiracies impossibility is not a defence. Therefore, if the accused solicits the 'full offender' to commit rape but the woman is dead, there is no offence of incitement. The defence of legal impossibility does apply, i.e. the accused is not guilty if he invites the principal to do something which is not a crime.

The full offence must be a crime: **Whitehouse**, above. A girl is exempt from the crime of committing incest with her father, though the father is guilty of the principal offence if incest is committed. Therefore, an accused, the father, was not guilty of inciting her to commit incest. While the principle remains and was applied in **Pickford** [1995] 1 Cr App R 420 (CA), the facts of **Whitehouse** now give rise to an offence. Under the Criminal Law Act 1977, s 54, it is an offence for a male to incite a girl under 16 to have sexual intercourse with him when he knows her to be his daughter, grand-daughter, sister or half-sister. This crime, however, is so worded that there is no offence for the male to incite the girl to have incestuous sex with someone else. The position would be different if the inciter applied duress to the alleged principal. It is thought that the inciter is guilty. The argument is that in duress the accused does have the *actus reus* and *mens rea* of the offence but the threat provides him with a defence. (Note that s 54 creates a principal offence of incitement: the accused could therefore incite someone to commit this offence. In theory A could incite B to incite C to commit the offence of inciting incestuous intercourse.) For the current criminal law on incest see the Sexual Offences Act 2003. In **Pickford** the accused was charged with inciting his stepson to commit incest with his mother, the accused's wife. At that time boys under 14 were irrebuttably presumed to be incapable of committing a crime involving sexual intercourse. (This presumption was abolished in 1993.) The stepson was 13. The accused was convicted at first instance. He contended that he had been found guilty of a crime unknown to law, inciting a boy under 14 to commit incest with his mother, because the boy could not in law have sexual intercourse with his mother at that time and incitement to commit a non-crime is not an offence. The court ruled that the presumption was to protect boys, not adults. It applied only to crimes committed by boys, not ones against them. A woman could commit incest with her son. Therefore, another person could incite her to commit incest. The accused was guilty of that offence, though not of inciting the boy to commit incest, which then was not a crime. The latest case is **C** (also called **Claydon**) [2006] 1 Cr App R 20. The Court of Appeal held, in relation to a charge of inciting a boy aged 13 to commit the offence of buggery before the Sexual Offences Act 1993 changed the law to permit boys of 12 and 13 to be charged with offences involving sexual intercourse, that since there was no substantive crime, there could be no offence of incitement to commit something which was not a crime at that time.

While it is true to say that the activity incited must be a crime, there is no need for it to be a crime at the time of the incitement. For example, an accused can be guilty of inciting another to handle stolen goods, even though at that moment the goods have not yet been stolen. This law should be distinguished from that governing impossibility. If the goods that the accused was persuading another to handle never existed, there is no crime of incitement (see (b) above).

The accused is not guilty of incitement if he believes that the principal does not have the *mens rea* for the principal offence, or if he knows that the alleged principal does not in fact have the mental element to fulfil the latter requirement. The main authority remains the much-criticised decision in *Curr* [1968] 2 QB 944 (CA). It was not shown that the alleged incitees had the *mens rea* for the offences, and the accused was not guilty of inciting them to commit those offences. The court did not discuss the *mens rea* of the *inciter* as it should have done. Card, Cross and Jones, *Criminal Law*, 14th edn (Butterworths, 1998) 528 (not in 17th edn, OUP, 2006) wrote: 'It is difficult to see why the mental element of the person incited should be relevant to liability for incitement since liability for that offence does not depend on the incited offence being committed or even intended by the person incited' (echoing the words of the 1985 Code team *Codification of the Criminal Law: A Report to the Law Commission* (Law Com. Consultation Paper, No. 143)). If the accused believes that the persons whom he has persuaded do not have the *mens rea* of the full offence, they will be innocent agents and he will be the principal offender if the full offence is committed. In this way the accused in *Curr* would have been guilty of a crime. *Curr* was distinguished in *DPP v Armstrong* [2000] Crim LR 379. The Divisional Court, which of course is bound by Court of Appeal decisions, held that the accused was guilty of incitement when he asked the incitee, an undercover police officer, to supply child pornography. Had the incitee done as requested, he would have committed a crime. It was said that the offence in *Curr* required the incitees to know that they were not entitled to collect welfare benefits. *Curr* was not overruled, only distinguished in *Armstrong*. However, in *C*, above, the Court of Appeal finally said *obiter* that *Curr* was wrong.

The law in this section demonstrates that incitement is a crime separate from the principal offence. It has different *actus reus* and *mens rea*. For this reason *Curr* and *Shaw* discussed above are wrong. As the court said in *DPP v Armstrong*, there is no parity of *mens rea* between the incitement and the crime incited.

Incitement and participation

There is no offence to incite one person to procure another to commit an offence: *Bodin* [1979] Crim LR 176 (Crown Court). The person incited must commit a crime as the principal offender, not as the secondary participant. The outcome may be accounted strange. If the accused persuades another to kill, that is incitement to murder; but if he persuades another party, a member of a terrorist organisation, to distribute arms to others to kill members of the security forces, that is not incitement to murder. A charge of inciting to incite a crime may be successful on these facts: see the next section. Although *Bodin* was mentioned without criticism by the Court of Appeal in *Sirat* (1985) 83 Cr App R 41, it is suggested that it was incorrectly decided. Surely there should be an offence of inciting another to procure, for example, others to commit murder. It is thought that there is no offence of incitement to counsel or aid and abet. This rule is retained by the draft Criminal Code, 1989, cl 47(5). The principle is that a person is guilty of a secondary offence only when the principal offence is committed. If none is, the accessory is not liable. However, the rule in incitement is that the act to be done by the person incited is a crime. A person can, however, be a secondary party to incitement and cl 47(5)(a) retains this rule. If the full offence has been committed, the inciter is also liable as accessory.

Incitement and other inchoate crimes

This section of text is devoted to what are sometimes known as double inchoate offences. The issue is partly which of the possible six crimes exist and partly whether the law *should* criminalise activity before the incitement, conspiracy or attempt.

(a) Incitement to conspire was abolished by the Criminal Law Act 1977, s 5(7). The draft Criminal Code, cl 47(5)(b), will, however, restore this offence if the draft becomes law. There would seem to be little point in charging incitement to attempt, because the accused will usually commit the full offence. The draft Criminal Code, cl 47(5)(b), expressly states that there is an offence of incitement to attempt. The Law Commission, *A Criminal Code for England and Wales*, Law Com. No. 177, 1989, 239, was persuaded that there should be this crime in the interests of consistency with incitement to incite and the revived crime of incitement to conspire and that the crime would fill the gap seen by Smith and Hogan, (D. Ormerod, ed.) *Criminal Law*, 12th edn (OUP, 2008) 444 'D gives E a substance which he knows to be harmless, telling E that it is poison and urging him to administer it to P. If E does as requested he will be guilty of an attempt to murder. D could scarcely be said to have incited murder but it is arguable that he should be liable for inciting an attempt to murder' (footnote omitted). The accused therefore is guilty of incitement to attempt if he knows that the principal offender cannot go beyond attempting to commit the full offence. For example, it is impossible to commit the offence through the means suggested. There is no reason in theory why the accused cannot be guilty of inciting one person to incite another to commit a crime, as the Court of Appeal has held in *Sirat*, above, and *Evans* [1986] Crim LR 470. If, however, the second incitement would lead to conspiracy, it may be that the courts would not allow the charge of inciting incitement because it would be an evasion of the abolition of incitement to conspire. The law is convoluted. The draft Criminal Code would put incitement to incite on a statutory footing.

(b) There is a crime of attempting to incite: *ex parte Amos* [1973] Crim LR 437 (DC). An example is where an inciting letter fails to reach the principal: *Bankes* (1873) 12 Cox CC 393 and *Ransford* (1874) 13 Cox CC 9. More up to date would be a failed attempt to leave a voicemail message or to send an e-mail. There may be a crime of conspiracy to incite: *James*, above.

(c) One spouse can be found guilty of inciting the other to commit an offence, though they cannot be found guilty of conspiracy if only the two of them joined the agreement.

It may be inquired whether incitement serves any purpose when there are two other inchoate offences and the law on complicity. The answer may be that incitement deters persons from getting others to commit crimes, and it allows the police to intervene before the offence is committed in the same way as do attempt and conspiracy.

Reform

Besides the matters mentioned in the text, the draft Criminal Code would reverse *Fitzmaurice* on impossibility. This recommendation in cl 50 was consistent with the Law Commission's Report No. 102, 1980, on *Attempt, and Impossibility in Relation to Attempt, Conspiracy and Incitement*. In that Report the Law Commission stated that incitement would have the same rules on impossibility as attempt and (statutory) conspiracy do after the Criminal Attempts Act 1981, i.e. impossibility is no defence. The Court of Appeal thwarted that expectation and now incitement is definitely to be brought into line with the other inchoate offences.

The elements of the offence were stated in cl 47(1):

A person is guilty of incitement to commit an offence or offences if –
(a) he incited another to do or cause to be done an act or acts which, if done, will involve the commission of the offence or offences by the other; and

(b) he intends or believes that the other, if he acts as incited, shall or will do so with the fault required for the offence or offences.

This proposed definition was said in **DPP v Armstrong**, above, to be an accurate statement of current law. The term 'incites' was retained in preference to 'encourages' as proposed by the drafters of the 1985 version of the Criminal Code (Law Com. No. 143) because the person incited need not be in fact encouraged. A person is guilty of incitement even though the principal party has already made up his mind to commit the offence and so does not need encouragement. **Curr** would be reversed by sub-cl (1)(b). The identity of the incitee need not be known (sub-cl (4)).

The rule about the statutorily protected intended victim found in **Whitehouse** and **Tyrrell** was retained (cl 47(3)), as was the reversal of the actual outcome in **Whitehouse** (cl 103(3)). Incitement of children under 16 to gross indecency (since repealed) would be made criminal by cll 114–115 on the recommendation of the Criminal Law Revision Committee's Fifteenth Report, *Sexual Offences*, Cmnd 9213, 1984, paras 7.12 and 7.23. The rule in **Most** was preserved ('offence or offences' in cl 47(1)).

Clause 47(1)(b) would effect a change in the law, which is discussed on pp. 237–8 of the Report.

> It should . . . be sufficient if the inciter believes that the person incited, if he acts at all, will do so with the fault required. For example, if D seeks to persuade E to have sexual intercourse with Mrs D, D believing that E knows that Mrs D does not consent to it, there seems to be a clear case of incitement to rape. It should not be necessary to prove that it was D's intention that E should have such knowledge. Whenever the fault required for a substantive offence includes knowledge of or recklessness as to circumstances (such as the absence of consent), it is likely to be more appropriate . . . to refer to the inciter's belief that such knowledge or recklessness exists rather than to his intention that it should.

Incitement to commit summary offences would be to be prosecuted only with the consent of the DPP.

The Law Commission in its Consultation Paper No. 131, *Assisting and Encouraging Crime*, 1993, proposed the abolition of incitement and its replacement by a new offence of encouraging crime. This development is discussed at the end of Chapter 5.

It took 13 years for the Law Commission to publish its Report No. 300 on *Inchoate Liability for Assisting and Encouraging Crime*, 2006. The Commission proposed to abolish incitement and replace it with two new inchoate offences of intentionally encouraging or assisting a criminal act and encouraging or assisting criminal acts believing that one or more of them will be done. The wording of both is contained in a draft bill. There will be two defences specific to these offences: that of acting to prevent the commission of an offence, which will be a defence to both offences, and that of acting reasonably, which will be a defence only to the second offence. The defence available to the victim (see **Tyrrell** above) will continue to apply. The *mens rea* of intent in the first offence is restricted to direct intent (purpose) and foreseeability is not sufficient. The Report aims to get rid of this issue:

> At common law if D [the accused] *encourages* P [the principal offender] to commit an offence that subsequently P does not commit or attempt to commit, D may nevertheless be criminally liable. By contrast, if D *assists* P to commit an offence, D incurs no criminal liability at common law if subsequently P, for whatever reason, does not commit or attempt to commit the offence (para. 1.3).

Both will be liable if the provisions of the Report become law. See the Introduction for the offences of 'encouraging or assisting', which came into force just before publication of this edition.

Conspiracy

Introduction

Lord Diplock in **DPP v Bhagwan** [1972] AC 60 (HL) said that common law **conspiracy** was 'the least systematic, the most irrational branch of English penal law'. Common law conspiracy has been largely abolished by s 5(1) of the Criminal Law Act 1977. The offence is now to a great extent a statutory one. When the full offence is committed conspiracy can still be charged, and will be if the charge is needed to give the full flavour of the criminal behaviour. The result is to make proceedings complex. However, the prosecution will not be allowed to proceed with both charges if the conspiracy count is prejudicial to the accused.

For those offences which remain common law conspiracies the famous definition in **Mulcahy v R** (1868) LR 3 HL 306 remains the touchstone: 'an agreement by two or more to do an unlawful act or do a lawful act in an unlawful way'. Statutory conspiracy is defined in s 1(1) of the 1977 Act, a new s 1(1) being substituted by the Criminal Attempts Act 1981, s 5(1).

> Subject to the following provisions of this Part of this Act, if a person agrees with any other person or persons that a course of conduct shall be pursued which if the agreement is carried out in accordance with their intentions, either –
>
> (a) will necessarily amount to or involve the commission of any offence or offences by one or more of the parties to the agreement, or
>
> (b) would do so but for the existence of facts which render the commission of the offence or offences impossible,
>
> he is guilty of conspiracy to commit the offence or offences in question.

The effect of the 1981 amendment was to bring the law on impossibility in statutory conspiracy into line with impossibility in attempt (which see later in this chapter). However, for conspiracies which remain ones at common law the pre-1981 law applies and impossibility is a defence in certain circumstances.

An example of s 1(1) is **Mulligan** [1990] STC 220 (CA). There is a common law offence of cheating the public revenue. If two persons commit this crime together, there is a conspiracy. In **Drew** [2000] 1 Cr App R 91 (CA) it was held that an accused is guilty of conspiracy even when he is the intended victim of the conspiracy, as when he is to be supplied with drugs. For exceptional cases relating to 'victims', see below. Section 1(1) has been interpreted in the following ways. In s 1(1) the 'other person' need not be identified: **Phillips** (1987) 86 Cr App R 18. A difficult authority on s 1(1) is **Anderson** [1986] AC 27 (HL). The accused, a person on remand in custody, was charged with conspiracy to effect a prisoner's escape. He contended that he never intended to go through with the plan; that is, he had no *mens rea*. The House of Lords dismissed his appeal. He had agreed with other persons that a course of conduct would be pursued which, when carried out 'in accordance with their intentions' – i.e. the others' intentions – would necessarily amount to or involve the commission of a crime. It was held that the accused had to play some part in the agreed course of conduct. The accused did not intend to let the prisoner escape but that was held to be irrelevant because it did not have to be proved that the individual accused intended that the agreement should be carried out. This reasoning leads to a problem if there is only one other person in the agreement. In that event the agreement will not be carried out in accordance with *their* intentions but only in accordance with one of their intentions. To say the least, the interpretation of s 1(1) is strained and *Anderson* is contrary to the intention of Parliament. On the wording at least two of the accused have to have the *mens rea*. The accused could have been convicted of being a secondary party, an aider and abettor, to the conspiracy.

In the much-criticised authority of *Yip Chiu-Cheung v R* [1995] 1 AC 111 (PC) a US drugs enforcement officer agreed to act as a courier of heroin from Hong Kong to Australia for the accused. The accused was arrested in Hong Kong and charged with conspiring with the officer to traffic in heroin. He contended that the officer could not be a conspirator because he did not have the *mens rea* for that offence; therefore, there was no conspiracy to which he could be a party for a conspiracy requires two participants. It was held that on the facts the officer did intend to commit the crime of trafficking in drugs: he did have the *actus reus* and *mens rea* for conspiracy. He too could be convicted of conspiracy. His motive and courage did not exculpate him. It was immaterial that he did not expect to be prosecuted: 'the fact that . . . the authorities would not prosecute the undercover agent does not mean that he did not commit the crime . . .'. The position would have been different if he did not intend to commit the crime. He would have no *mens rea* and there would be no conspiracy: *Anderson*, above. The *ratio* of *Yip Chiu-Cheung* is contrary to *Anderson* in that it requires two parties to intend and agree to commit an unlawful act.

The Law Commission's draft Criminal Code, *A Criminal Code for England and Wales*, Law Com. No. 177, 1989 rejected *Anderson* and preferred the plain meaning of the 1977 statute, which was based on the Law Commission's Report, *Conspiracy and Criminal Law Reform*, Law Com. No. 76, 1976. One recommendation was: 'Both must intend that any consequence in the definition of the offence will result.' Certainly the House of Lords ruling is contrary to the wishes of Parliament. The Court of Appeal in *Edwards* [1991] Crim LR 45 did not follow *Anderson* though they may not have realised what they were doing. The accused agreed to supply amphetamines but he may have intended to supply a drug called ephedrine. Since it was uncertain that he intended to supply amphetamines, he was not guilty of conspiracy to supply that type of controlled drug. In any case the decision in *Anderson* does not apply to the common law offence of conspiracy to defraud, for *Anderson* is based on the interpretation of the statute.

There is support in *Hollinshead* reported in [1985] AC 975 (CA) for the proposition that the phrase 'the commission of any offence . . . by one or more of the parties' should be read as requiring the involvement of one (or more) of them as the principal. Accordingly, if two secondary parties agree to assist the principal in killing the victim, they are not guilty of conspiracy to murder if the principal was not party to the agreement. (Presumably they could be convicted of conspiracy to incite the principal.) The Court of Appeal's judgment may be summarised as being that there is no statutory conspiracy to be a secondary party to an offence. One cannot therefore conspire to aid a murderer. One must conspire to commit the full offence, murder, as a principal. On appeal the House of Lords did not discuss the issue and did not approve or disapprove the Court of Appeal's decision. The ordinary meaning of the words in the statutory definition gives support to the Court of Appeal's proposition of law. If correct, when two parties agree to help a third party who is not part of the agreement between the first two, they are not guilty of conspiracy to commit whatever offence the third party committed. The Court of Appeal in *Kenning* [2008] EWCA Crim 1534 said that whether the reasoning of the same court in *Hollinshead* was binding was a matter of debate but that there was no crime of conspiracy to be a secondary party to a principal offence. This ruling is in line with s 1(4)(b) of the Criminal Attempts Act 1981, which states that there is no offence of attempting to be a secondary party.

Hollinshead applies only to statutory conspiracies and not to common law ones such as conspiracy to defraud.

Section 1(1) of the 1977 Act defines the *actus reus* of conspiracy. One might have expected s 1(2) to define the *mens rea*, but it seems to apply only when the crime agreed on is a strict offence:

> Where liability for any offence may be incurred without knowledge on the part of the person committing it of any particular fact or circumstance necessary for the commission of the offence, a person shall nevertheless not be guilty of conspiracy to commit that offence by virtue of subsection (1) above unless he and at least one other party to the agreement intend or know that fact or circumstance shall or will exist at the time when the conduct constituting the offence is to take place.

However, as we shall see in the discussion of the *mens rea* of statutory conspiracy, this provision is read as applying whatever the *mens rea* of the crime to be committed and not just to strict offences.

An agreement to commit a summary offence is a conspiracy but cannot be charged without the consent of the Crown Prosecution Service (s 4(1) of the 1977 Act and the Prosecution of Offences Act 1985, s 1(7)). In attempt, however, there is no offence of attempting to commit a summary offence.

Actus reus

General

One element of the *actus reus* is an agreement, which is manifested in some way such as by words, action or writing. Agreement, which to lawyers is often seen as a meeting of the minds, is without an external manifestation a mental state, and English law does not penalise people for entertaining wicked thoughts. Nevertheless, 'agreement' is a low threshold for a crime: compare the offence of attempt where an act more than merely preparatory to the commission of the offence is needed. The agreement must be communicated to the other party: *Scott* (1979) 68 Cr App R 164. It must have reached a definite conclusion and the parties must be beyond the stage of considering the possibility of committing a crime: *King* [1966] Crim LR 280. In *O'Brien* (1974) 59 Cr App R 222 (CA) the accused had talked about effecting the escape of three Irish nationalist prisoners from Winson Green Prison, Birmingham, but he had not reached the stage of agreement. Therefore, there was at that stage no conspiracy to effect an escape. In *Barnard* (1979) 70 Cr App R 28 the accused was talking with others about stealing from a jeweller's. The others had decided to rob the jeweller and were guilty of conspiracy to rob. He found out that the jeweller took the best pieces home at night. He decided to proceed no further because his way of stealing was to come through the ceiling at night. The others robbed the jeweller in the daytime. The accused was not guilty of conspiracy to rob. He had not agreed to join in that offence.

The parties need not have met previously provided that they acted in pursuance of a common purpose which was notified to at least one other party to the conspiracy: *Meyrick* (1929) 21 Cr App R 94 (CCA). This case has come in for criticism because it was not proved that each of the parties, night-club owners, knew that the other was paying a bribe to the same constable so that the police would turn a blind eye to breaches of the licensing laws, and it was suggested in *Griffiths* (1968) 49 Cr App R 279 that each knew what the other was doing because the premises were close, but that last fact does not explain why the court could say that there was an agreement. If there is no agreement and the parties are still negotiating, the situation looks like an attempted conspiracy, but there is no such offence: Criminal Law Act 1977, s 5(7). There is no need for the accused to play an active part in the conspiracy: *Siracusa* (1990) 90 Cr App R 340 (CA), not agreeing with the House of Lords in *Anderson* that the accused was guilty only if the accused played an active part in furthering the crime. *Siracusa* is an important authority, one assumed to represent the law, but *Hollinshead* is unfortunately a decision of the House of Lords. Since the focus is on the agreement, it does not matter that the parties have done something different from what they agreed. As Woolf LJ put it in *Bolton* (1992) 94 Cr App R 74 (CA): '. . . it is what was agreed to be done and not what was in fact done which is all important.' On the facts of the case it was irrelevant that mortgage fraudsters expected to be paid by cheque but the money was actually transferred electronically.

Sometimes the courts have used the analogy of contract to determine whether an agreement existed. In *Walker* [1962] Crim LR 458 (CCA), there was no conspiracy where there were negotiations, not an agreement, to steal wages. It should be noted that the analogy with contract is inexact. There is less certainty needed for an agreement in conspiracy than for a contract. Unlike in contract no consideration need have passed. Conspiracies are not, unlike contracts, enforceable in the courts. In the *Highwayman's Case* (1725), some persons had robbed stagecoaches. One person had taken all the loot. Another tried to sue for his share. He was hanged!

Once there is agreement that is sufficient. The conspiracy need not be put into effect. Since conspiracy is a continuing offence, the defendants are guilty even though they were not all parties to the same agreement at the same time. Provided that all the other elements exist, the conspiracy is complete at the time of the making of the agreement. If, e.g., two friends agree to steal a car on the next day, they are guilty, even though before that day one of them wins a car and they decide not to go ahead with their plan. Under the statute the agreement must necessarily amount to or involve the commission of a crime, if carried out. Donaldson LJ, as he then was, gave this example in *Reed* [1982] Crim LR 819 (CA): 'A and B agree to drive from London to Edinburgh in a time which can be achieved without breaking the speed limit, but only if the traffic which they encounter is exceptionally light . . . Accordingly the agreement does not constitute . . . conspiracy.' This passage was approved in *Jackson* [1985] Crim LR 442 (CA). In that case A, B and C agreed that C would be shot in the leg if he was convicted of the offence for which he was being tried in order that the court would feel sympathetic towards him and give him a light sentence. They were guilty of conspiracy to pervert the course of justice. Therefore, a conditional agreement ('We will shoot you if you are convicted') is a conspiracy. The men were guilty even though the trial was continuing. The person on trial might have been acquitted of burglary but the execution of the agreement would still be necessary in s 1(1) terms, for 'necessarily' does not mean 'inevitably' but 'if the agreement is carried out in accordance with the plan, an offence would take place'. In *Reed*, A and B agreed that A would visit persons who wished to commit suicide and either help or discourage them, depending on what he thought was the better approach. He was guilty of conspiring to abet suicide. Similarly, an agreement to make bombs during the IRA ceasefire in the early 1990s to be used after the ceasefire, if it ended, was a conspiracy to cause explosions. After all, the IRA did break that ceasefire by exploding the Canary Wharf bomb. In *Jackson* and *Reed* the objects of the agreements were unlawful whereas in the London–Edinburgh example the breaking of the speed limit was incidental to the agreement. The line may be hard to draw. An agreement to rob a bank when it is safe to do so is a conspiracy (*Reed*, *obiter*). There is no need that the full offence will necessarily be committed: the point is that the defendants must so intend (*mens rea*).

Under the statute the term 'course of conduct' limits what the defendants can be convicted of conspiring to do. The facts of *Siracusa*, above, illustrate this proposition. O'Connor LJ said: 'If the prosecution charge a conspiracy to contravene s 170(2) of the Customs and Excise Management Act 1979 by the importation of heroin, then the prosecution must prove that the agreed course of conduct was the importation of heroin. This is because the essence of the crime of conspiracy is the agreement and, in simple terms, you do not prove an agreement to import heroin by proving an agreement to import cannabis.' Therefore the defendants cannot in this way be guilty of conspiracy though they would be guilty of the full offence of importing heroin when they believed that the substance was cannabis. To clarify the point O'Connor LJ added that the accused would not be guilty of a conspiracy to murder unless they intended to kill, yet they are guilty of murder itself if they intended only grievous bodily harm. (The law on this point in conspiracy is the same as that for attempt.)

The requirement of two parties

Conspiracy is based on agreement. It does not matter that the accused does not know the identity of his partner or partners, and he need not be in contact with all of them. One person cannot conspire with himself. In *McDonnell* [1966] 1 QB 233 it was held that a person was not guilty of conspiracy when he was the sole director of a company, the other alleged party to the agreement, even though in law companies have separate legal personalities from the directors. This issue of liability for conspiring with a company with which one is identified is unaffected by the 1977 Act.

Spouses also cause difficulty. In *Mawji* v *R* [1957] AC 126, the Privy Council said, without the point being argued, that a husband could not conspire with his wife because she was assumed not to have a will independent from that of her husband. Oliver J accepted this *obiter dictum* as being the law in *Midland Bank Trust Co Ltd* v *Green (No. 3)* [1979] Ch 496, a civil law decision. It is uncertain whether the rule applies to actually or potentially polygamous marriages. The rule is preserved for statutory conspiracies in s 2(2)(a) of the Criminal Law Act 1977. The Law Commission's Report, *Conspiracy and Criminal Law Reform*, Law Com. No. 76, 1976, on which the Act was based, recommended that the rule should be preserved in order to maintain the stability of marriage and in accordance with the then policy of keeping the law out of marriage. If there is a third party, all become guilty of conspiracy. The wife is therefore guilty if she makes an agreement with her husband, knowing that he is conspiring with others: *Chrastny* [1991] 1 WLR 1381. There is no need to show that she herself came to an agreement with the third party. If the parties married after the agreement, they are liable. It should be noted that this rule is applicable only to conspiracy and not to incitement or secondary participation. It is also of course not applicable to all principal offences such as murder and theft which the husband and wife have agreed upon. No doubt it will be abrogated at some time in the future just as the husband's immunity in rape was in the early 1990s. There seems nowadays to be no good reason for keeping it. The fact that the accused is married has no bearing on the wrongfulness of criminal behaviour towards a victim.

An accused is not guilty of conspiracy if the sole other party is below the age of criminal responsibility: s 2(2)(b) of the 1977 Act. By s 2(3) a child is under the age of criminal responsibility when, by reason of the Children and Young Persons Act 1933, s 50, he cannot be guilty of any offence. The reference to the nonliability of the child means that s 2(2)(b) applies only to children under 10. A child aged 10–14 is guilty of conspiracy in the normal way. Section 2(2) provides for exemptions from the general principle of liability where there are two parties and if Parliament wished to exempt parties not expressly mentioned it should have said so. The statute says nothing about agreements with mentally deranged persons (who cannot form the intent necessary for conspiracy) but whether the same rule should apply as for infants under 10 is moot. Section 2 applies only to statutory conspiracies. It is suggested that the same rules apply at common law.

Section 2(2) goes on to provide that the accused cannot be convicted of conspiracy with the intended victim of the offence. Therefore if the accused elopes with a girl under 16, she is the intended victim. By s 2(2) the accused is not liable for conspiracy – perhaps he should be. The intended victim also is not guilty (s 2(1)). If two defendants agree with the under-age girl to have sexual intercourse with her they are guilty of conspiracy; the girl is not because of s 2(1). The 1977 Act gives no definition of 'intended victim'. It may be that the term is restricted to members of a class protected by Parliament such as girls under 16 in relation to unlawful sexual intercourse. If so, the law would be consistent with incitement and accomplice liability: see *Tyrrell*, above. On this approach the intended victim who is not a member of a specially protected class would be guilty, as would be the co-conspirator. A suggested illustration is where one party agrees with another that the latter will inflict harm on him or her in pursuance of sexual pleasure. Both would be guilty despite one being in ordinary language the intended victim. An accused to whom drugs are supplied is not a 'victim' within s 2 and can therefore be guilty of conspiracy.

There is no common law authority on infants and victims. For those agreements which remain conspiracies at common law (see later) the accused may be guilty. An example would be conspiring to defraud an infant or victim. It is, however, hard to envisage a victim agreeing to be defrauded. It has been suggested that the term 'intended victim' covers only a person who cannot perpetrate the full offence or be convicted as an accessory. On this approach a person aged 15 should be convicted of conspiring to commit homosexual offences even if he is the victim of the offence because he can be guilty of the full offence.

If one of the defendants does not fall within one of these exceptions, he is guilty of conspiracy even though he cannot commit the offence agreed upon. The crime of rape provides the best illustration. If a woman agrees with a man that he will rape a third party, she is guilty of conspiracy to rape despite her not being able to commit rape as a principal offender.

Immunity and acquittal of the other offender

May a person be convicted of conspiracy when the other is acquitted or immune from prosecution?

(a) *Immunity.* In *Duguid* (1906) 21 Cox CC 200, the accused agreed with a woman to remove the woman's child from the custody of the lawful guardian, contrary to s 56 of the Offences Against the Person Act 1861 (now repealed). By that section the mother is immune from prosecution. It was held that the accused could be found guilty of conspiracy. The Court for Crown Cases Reserved did not investigate the liability of the mother for conspiracy. It may be that she is liable, for in *Whitchurch* (1890) 24 QBD 420 a person was found guilty of conspiring to commit an offence which she could not have been convicted of as the principal. A woman who is not pregnant cannot be convicted of procuring her own abortion, but she is guilty of the conspiracy (though she is apparently never prosecuted nowadays), while in *Burns* (1984) 79 Cr App R 175 a father was found guilty of conspiring to steal his own child when he could not have been found guilty as the principal offender. (The exemption has since been abrogated.) The rule is not affected by s 2(2) of the 1977 Act. Contrary to the recommendation of the Law Commission, Parliament refused to overturn **Whitchurch**, and since the Act there is also **Burns**. The Court of Appeal looked at the purpose of the statute to see whether the exemption from the principal offence should apply to the conspiracy to commit that offence. Certainly on the facts of **Burns**, where the father and a 'posse of men' broke into his former wife's home to snatch the child, the husband would seem to have been justifiably convicted.

(b) *Acquittal*. Where one of two conspirators is acquitted, the old view was that, if both were tried together, the other could not be found guilty of conspiracy. However, the House of Lords held differently in **DPP v Shannon** [1975] AC 717. Two Law Lords said that the acquittal of one was not a bar to the conviction of the other (Viscount Dilhorne and Lord Simon); Lords Reid and Morris said that the traditional rule should apply; the casting vote was held by Lord Salmon who said that the orthodox rule should apply except in special circumstances. The common law therefore was confused. If the two accused were tried separately, the acquittal of one was not a bar to the conviction of another. (There might for instance have been a confession from one party but not from another, and the prosecution could not prove the case.)

In relation to statutory conspiracies, the 1977 Act, s 5(8), states:

> The fact that the person or persons who, so far as appears from the indictment on which any person has been convicted of conspiracy, were the only other parties to the agreement on which his conviction was based have been acquitted of conspiracy by reference to that agreement (whether after being tried with the person convicted or separately) shall not be a ground for quashing his conviction unless under all the circumstances of the case his conviction is inconsistent with the acquittal of the other person or persons in question.

The next sub-section, s 5(9), abolishes inconsistent 'law or practice'. While not so stating expressly, s 5(9) abolishes the common law on this topic. Therefore, s 5(8) applies to both statutory and common law conspiracies.

According to **Merrick** (1980) 71 Cr App R 130 (CA), **Longman** (1980) 72 Cr App R 121 (DC) and **Roberts** (1983) 78 Cr App R 41 (DC), a judge may tell the jury to acquit both if to convict one and let the other go would be inconsistent. If the evidence is the same against each member, the judge should direct the jury to convict all or acquit all. If the evidence is substantially stronger against one accused than against the other, the judge should instruct the jury to consider each party separately. The result may be that the jury accepts that the first accused conspires with the second accused but that the second did not conspire with the first!

Unlawful object of the conspiracy

Section 1(1) of the 1977 Act, as substituted by the Criminal Attempts Act 1981, s 5(1), quoted above, begins: 'Subject to the following provisions . . .'. That is a reference to s 5 of the 1977 Act which states that certain conspiracies remain crimes at common law. By s 5(2) an agreement to defraud is a common law crime. By s 5(3) conspiracies to corrupt public morals and outrage public decency remain common law offences if they would not necessarily amount to or result in a crime when performed by one person. If when done by one the behaviour does constitute a crime, the offence must be charged as a statutory conspiracy. For discussion see below. Unlike statutory conspiracies impossibility in some forms is a defence in common law conspiracies.

Conspiracy to defraud

This offence, which is unhelpfully defined as an agreement to practise a fraud on someone, is useful in financial and economic affairs. An agreement to occasion loss by dishonest means is a conspiracy to defraud. For a recent illustration, see **Norris v The Government of the United States of America** [2007] EWHC 71 (Admin), which involved a cartel with dishonest agreement to fix prices by representatives of companies. 'Dishonest' is of the normal **Ghosh** [1982] QB 1053 definition: see Chapter 15. A second form of this type of conspiracy is an agreement to persuade by dishonest means a person to act contrary to his or her duty. The former variety is very wide and has been criticised on this basis. For example, it is not theft to deprive the victim of an article temporarily. However, if two persons agree to do so, there is the offence of conspiracy to defraud. Similarly it is not the crime of theft if a person makes a secret profit from another's property (**Attorney-General's Reference (No. 1 of 1985)** [1986] QB 491 (CA) though the latest Privy Council authority (**Attorney-General of Hong Kong v Reid** [1994] 1 AC 324) is *contra*, see the discussion of 'Belonging to another' in Chapter 15), but it is a conspiracy to defraud if two persons agree to do so. The principal criticism of this offence is precisely that it makes unlawful something done by two which would have been lawful if done by one. A second criticism is that the offence is of uncertain width. The advantages to the prosecution are the reverse of these criticisms, and there is support for the view that a charge of conspiracy to defraud can reflect the overall criminality of the defendants' misconduct. Interrelated acts can be linked in one charge. The Criminal Justice Act 1987, s 12(1), provides that this common law offence and the statutory conspiracy offence are not mutually exclusive. An agreement to commit a fraud can be both. The effect is that only conspiracies to defraud which do not involve the commission of an offence need to be charged as conspiracy at common law. By s 12(3) the maximum sentence is 10 years' imprisonment. (It should be noted that the law is different with regard to conspiracies to corrupt public morals and outrage public decency. If there are substantive offences of corrupting public morals and outraging public decency, charges of conspiracies to commit them must be brought under the 1977 Act.)

Until recently the definition of this offence given by Lord Diplock in **Scott v MPC** [1975] AC 819 (HL) was considered to be correct: one in which the defendants either intend to cause (or are reckless as to causing) economic loss to another (or injure a proprietary interest) or to induce another to act dishonestly contrary to his public duty. The latter half of this definition comes from **Welham v DPP** [1961] AC 103 (HL) and was used in **Moses** [1991] Crim LR 617 (CA). There was a conspiracy when the parties agreed to facilitate the obtaining of work permits by immigrants who were prohibited from working by a stamp in their passport by deceiving the National Insurance Department into believing that the passports did not carry the stamp. The members of the department had acted contrary to their public duty. There was no need for the victim, the Crown, to suffer loss. Lord Denning in **Welham** rejected the contention that an intent to cause economic loss was required. The intent to defraud meant the intent to practise a fraud or to act to someone's prejudice. In this form of conspiracy to defraud there never existed a need to prove an intent to cause economic loss. It remains uncertain whether the public duty sub-head is indeed restricted to officials performing such obligations, but as stated in the next paragraph this type of conspiracy to defraud is now seen as merely an illustration of the general principle.

In the former part of the definition there must be depriving by dishonesty and it was thought there had to be an intention to cause or recklessness as to causing economic loss:

Scott, above, *Attorney-General's Reference (No. 1 of 1982)* [1983] QB 751 (CA) and *Wai Yu-Tsang v R* [1992] 1 AC 269 (PC). Viscount Dilhorne in *Scott* defined this version of the offence as 'an agreement by two or more by dishonesty to deprive a person of something which is his or to which he is or would be or might be entitled and an agreement by two or more by dishonesty to injure some proprietary right'. In *Attorney-General's Reference (No. 1 of 1982)*, the accused agreed to sell in the Lebanon whisky which was to be falsely labelled as made by a well-known firm. The court held that the true object of the conspiracy was to defraud the purchasers. There was no conspiracy to defraud in relation to the firm because their loss would have been incidental to the main object of the agreement. The case seems inconsistent with *Scott* where the principal object was to gain money for the defendants, yet they were guilty of conspiracy to defraud the copyright owners. Moreover, in most conspiracies to defraud the true object is to gain money, yet the agreement is still a conspiracy to defraud. The House of Lords in *Scott* did not distinguish between the true object of the agreement and the incidental effects. An oblique intention is sufficient as in *Scott*, *Hollinshead* and *Cooke* [1986] AC 909, where rail stewards were guilty of conspiring to defraud British Rail when their object was to make money for themselves. *Allsop* (1976) 63 Cr App R 29 (CA) held that recklessness was sufficient. Accordingly, the accused is guilty if he thought he could make good securities he had taken by striking a good deal on a different matter. The Privy Council in *Wai Yu-Tsang v R* said that the defendants were guilty if they realised that they had agreed to bring about a state of affairs which would or might deceive the victim into acting or failing to act in such a way that he would suffer economic loss or his economic interests would be imperilled. *Allsop* is to the same effect. Lord Diplock's division in *Scott* was incorrect. The public duty form of the offence was not a distinct category but merely an illustration of the general law. In neither type was economic loss necessary: it was sufficient that the defendants deprived the accused of something, actual or prospective, dishonestly. In *Adams v R* [1995] 1 WLR 52 the Privy Council emphasised this criterion: 'there must exist some right or interest in the victim which is capable of being prejudiced whether by actual loss or by being put at risk'. Therefore, the accused is not guilty when he makes it more difficult for the victim to find out whether he had an interest in a sum of money. On the facts of the case the Judicial Committee held that a dishonest agreement by directors to impede a company in the exercise of its right to recover secret profits made by them constituted a conspiracy to defraud. The accused himself had taken part in setting up a structure of overseas companies through which he had dishonestly concealed information, namely secret profits, in relation to which he had been under a legal duty to disclose to the company of which he was a director. Accordingly the company had a right or interest which could be prejudiced. Dishonesty must be proved. It bears the same definition as in theft (see Chapter 15). *Adams v R* was followed by the Court of Appeal in *Fussell* [1997] Crim LR 812. The fact that the conspirators did not wish to harm the victim was irrelevant: *Wai Yu-Tsang v R*. The fact that the fraudsters did not desire to cause loss was motive, as *Allsop* had also held. In *Wai Yu-Tsang v R* the defendant's desire, to stop a run on the bank, was a good one but irrelevant. It could be said that his true object was to stop the run on the bank, yet he was guilty. This authority is inconsistent with *Attorney-General's Reference (No. 1 of 1982)*, above, which should be taken to be overruled.

 Scott v MPC [1975] AC 819, discussed above, exemplifies the non-public duty part of the definition. There was an agreement to bribe cinema employees to make films available to be copied in breach of copyright. The House of Lords held this agreement to be a conspiracy to defraud. There was no need for deception. In *Hollinshead*, above, an agreement to make black boxes for others to get free electricity was a conspiracy to defraud. The conduct would probably amount to a fraud or some other offence against property by a third party who bought the equipment. Where the fraud agreed on amounts to a crime there is also a conspiracy under the 1977 Act. The Act states that a person is guilty of conspiracy under the Act only if at least one of the parties intends to perpetrate the offence. **Hollinshead**, as we have seen, holds differently for conspiracy to defraud. The parties themselves need not carry out the fraud. An agreement to have the fraud committed by others is sufficient. In **Dearlove** (1989) 88 Cr App R 280, the dishonest purchase of goods (Oxo cubes) at the lower export price intending to sell them at a higher price on the domestic market amounted to obtaining property by deception, an offence since abolished but now incorporated within that of fraud contrary to the Fraud Act 2006.

The Law Commission published its Working Paper on *Conspiracy to Defraud* (No. 104) as long ago as 1988. It listed four options: (a) do nothing; (b) put the law into a statute; (c) abolish the law and adjust offences to cover the gaps; (d) abolish present law and put into its place a wide fraud crime. Contrary to (a) are the policy arguments that judges should not make law and that Parliament is a better body than the courts to change the law. Contrary to (b) is the principle in the 1977 Act that agreements should not be conspiracies if they would not amount to a crime when carried out by one person. Contrary to (c) is the difficulty in seeing all the gaps. Contrary to (d) is the principle that the law should be clearly stated and not vague in its width. The Law Commission proposed a wide offence of dishonestly causing another to suffer economic prejudice or a risk of prejudice, or dishonestly making a gain for himself or another. The Law Commission published its Report No. 228, *Criminal Law: Conspiracy to Defraud*, 1994. At para 1.17 it averred that it wished 'to reduce the length and complexity of trials by simplifying the law, while always ensuring that the defendant is fully protected'. It summarised its conclusion in para 1.20: 'for practical reasons conspiracy to defraud performs a useful role in the present law of dishonesty, and we have concluded that it should remain intact pending our comprehensive review of the law. We have resolved that it would be inappropriate, at a time when we are about to re-examine the whole scheme of dishonesty offences, to make piecemeal recommendations for reform of other aspects of the law of dishonesty.' Defendants can be convicted of a crime appropriate to their conduct.

The Law Commission criticised the uncertainty surrounding the width of the offence and the fact that a conspiracy to defraud is lawful if done by one person. However, it referred to undesirable gaps in the law which would open up if the crime were abolished, such as a conspiracy to acquire confidential information and one to evade liability or to delay payment without intending to make permanent default. These lacunae were adjudged so substantial that the offence could not be abolished without replacement. An illustration from the case law after the publication of the Report is **Preddy** [1996] AC 815 (HL). A mortgage fraudster could not be convicted of the now repealed offence of obtaining property by deception, but had there been two of them acting in concert, they could have been convicted of conspiracy to defraud.

The Law Commission returned to the issue in its Report No. 276, *Fraud*, 2002. The Home Office issued a Consultation Paper *Fraud Law Reform* in 2004. The government in *Fraud Law Reform* (2005) rejected the abolition of the offence pending the settling in of the Fraud Act 2006. It stated that it was unclear whether the new offences in the 2006 statute would cover all the gaps in the law which conspiracy to defraud currently fills (para. 4). It does not cover the facts of **Scott v MPC**, above, because in that case there was no false representation.

A contention that conspiracy to defraud was contrary to Article 7 of the ECHR was rejected at the Divisional Court in **Norris**, above. The court agreed that conspiracy to defraud 'has long contained the clarity and precision required by the Convention and the common law, namely proof that two or more conspirators intended dishonestly to defraud another or others as explained in **Welham, Scott** and **Wai Yu-Tsang.**'

Conspiracy to corrupt public morals and outrage public decency

In **Shaw v DPP** [1962] AC 220, the defendants published *The Ladies' Directory*, a 28-page book advertising prostitutes' names, telephone numbers, addresses and services. The House of Lords held, Lord Reid dissenting, that there was an offence at common law of conspiracy to corrupt public morals. No proof was needed that anyone was in fact corrupted. It was for the jury to say whether on the facts the crime was committed, which leads to uncertainty in the law. There was no need for a conspiracy charge because the defendants could have been convicted of publishing an obscene article, a crime under s 2(4) of the Obscene Publications Act 1959. Since Parliament had spoken so recently on the topic it seems strange that the House of Lords should create a novel crime.

There was a retreat from **Shaw** in **Knuller (Publishing, Printing and Promotions) Ltd v DPP** [1973] AC 435. Two Law Lords, Morris and Kilbrandon, thought that **Shaw** was correctly decided. Two Lords, Reid and Morris, thought it was wrong. Lord Simon was unwilling to overrule **Shaw**. Therefore, **Shaw** remains part of the law. However, the test for corrupting public morals was changed from that in **Shaw**, leading astray, to corrupting public morals.

Lords Simon and Kilbrandon and probably Morris thought in **Knuller** that there was an offence of conspiracy to outrage public decency. If there is an offence when committed by one person and **Gibson** [1990] 2 QB 619 (CA) held that there was a substantive crime of outraging public decency, as did, among other cases, **Rowley** [1991] 1 WLR 1020 (CA) *obiter*, the charge is conspiracy contrary to s 1 of the 1977 Act. Therefore, the former common law offence of conspiracy to outrage public decency is now a statutory offence in accordance with s 5(3). An offence of conspiring to outrage *public* decency cannot take place in a private home. To 'outrage' means to disgust. No one actually needs to be outraged; it is sufficient that an ordinary person would be likely to be outraged if he saw the conduct. It is difficult to see which types of behaviour would be a conspiracy to outrage public decency if done by two people but not the crime of outraging public decency if done by one person. If conspiracy to corrupt public morals would amount to a crime when done by one person, the conspiracy is statutory, not common law: s 5(3)(b). There is doubt whether there is an offence of corrupting public morals. The Court of Criminal Appeal in **Shaw** thought that there was but the House of Lords considered only conspiracy and not whether a substantive offence existed.

Like conspiracy to defraud in s 5(2), the retention of the conspiracy in s 5(3) was meant to be temporary only, pending reform of the law on obscenity. The government had the opportunity to abolish these crimes when it enacted the 1977 statute but it postponed changes until the Committee on Obscenity and Film Censorship chaired by Bernard Williams had reported, but when it did in 1979 the law remained unchanged. In relation to these common law conspiracies impossibility is a defence unless the means to be used were inadequate to effectuate the plan, in which case the accused are guilty. The obvious tip to prosecutors is that where the facts give rise both to common law and statutory conspiracy the latter should be charged for impossibility has been abolished in respect of it. What may be called subsequent impossibility is no defence because conspiracy is complete on agreement. If the parties agree on 1 May to steal a gem on 1 July but another group steals it on 1 June, the original parties are guilty of conspiracy.

The draft Criminal Code did not affect these two types of agreement (the Code was drafted before **Gibson**) and conspiracy to defraud. Because the law is not clear, it is not always clear in advance of trial whether a certain form of behaviour is one of these common law conspiracies. It is unsatisfactory that people do not know whether their acts are illegal and it is costly and inefficient to find out by instigating prosecutions.

Conspiracy to trespass contrary to the 1977 Act

There was a crime at common law of conspiracy to trespass, provided that the execution of the agreement would invade the public domain or would inflict more than nominal damage. This type of conspiracy was abolished by the Criminal Law Act 1977. Sections 6–10 of that Act created five new offences of criminal trespass. An agreement by two or more persons to do any of these offences will be a statutory conspiracy. These crimes are:

(a) using violence to secure entry unless one is the displaced residential occupier or a person acting on his behalf (s 6(1)); there is a defence of lawful authority so that a police constable may use violence to secure entry in pursuance of a power granted by statute;

(b) remaining on premises, having entered as a trespasser and having been requested to leave by the displaced residential occupier or the protected intending occupier (s 7(1), as amended);

(c) trespassing while having with one a weapon of offence without lawful authority or reasonable excuse (s 8(1));

(d) trespassing on premises of diplomatic missions, or consular premises or private residences of diplomats. There is a list of the types of protected premises, s 9(2), which was amended by the Diplomatic and Consular Premises Act 1987 (s 9(1));

(e) obstructing a court officer who is executing a judgment for possession of any premises (s 10(1)).

There is also an offence of aggravated trespass in the Criminal Justice and Public Order Act 1994 aimed at hunt saboteurs.

Overseas conspiracies

The courts have treated the *actus reus* of conspiracy as a continuing matter. The principal authority is **DPP v Doot** [1973] AC 807 (HL). None of the five defendants was British, and the agreement to break UK drugs laws by importing cannabis was made outside the UK. Their Lordships held that conspiracy, being a continuing offence, was not complete at the moment the agreement was made. When one of the defendants arrived in England, he and his friends could be charged with conspiracy, even though originally English courts had no jurisdiction to try the offence. Viscount Dilhorne said: 'A conspiracy does not end with the making of the agreement. It will continue so long as there are two or more parties to it intending to carry out the design.' **Doot** involved conspiracy before the 1977 Act. That Act did not deal with the issue, but it is considered that the law remains the same.

In **Doot** there was an act in England. What if there was no such act? Lord Salmon in **Doot** considered that there was a conspiracy, as did Lord Diplock in **DPP v Stonehouse** [1978] AC 55 (HL), though Lord Keith spoke to the contrary. The position was in doubt until *Liangsiriprasert* v *Government of the USA* [1991] 1 AC 255 (PC), on appeal from Hong Kong, where the law on this point is the same as in England. Lord Griffiths said:

> Why should an overt act be necessary to found jurisdiction? In the case of conspiracy in England the crime is complete once the agreement is made and no further overt act need be proved as an ingredient of the crime. The only purpose of looking for an overt act in England in the case of a conspiracy entered into abroad can be to establish the link between the conspiracy and England or possibly to show the conspiracy is continuing. But, if this can be established by other evidence, for example the taping of conversations between the conspirators showing a firm agreement to commit the crime at some future date, it defeats the preventative purpose of the crime of conspiracy to have to wait until some overt act is performed in pursuance of the conspiracy.

Inchoate offences were aimed at frustrating the completion of crimes. 'If evidence is obtained that a terrorist cell operating abroad is planning a bombing campaign in London what sense can there be in the authorities . . . not acting until the cell comes to England to plant their bombs with the risk that the terrorists may slip through the net?' He continued:

> [t]heir Lordships can find nothing in precedent, comity or good sense that should inhibit the common law from regarding as justiciable in England inchoate crimes committed abroad which are intended to result in the commission of criminal offences in England. Accordingly a conspiracy entered into in Thailand with the intention of committing the criminal offence of trafficking in drugs in Hong Kong is justiciable in Hong Kong even if no overt act pursuant to the conspiracy has yet occurred in Hong Kong.

The result is in line with the recommendations of the Law Commission's *Report on Jurisdiction over Offences of Fraud and Dishonesty with a Foreign Element*, Law Com. No. 180, 1989, para 4.4. Defendants charged with a 'listed offence' would be triable in England and Wales if any part of the conspiracy took place there.

The Privy Council decision in *Liangsiriprasert* was followed by the Court of Appeal in *Sansom* [1991] 2 QB 130. The accused were charged with conspiring to evade the prohibition on the importation of a controlled drug, cannabis, into England. The agreement was made in Morocco, and no act pursuant to that agreement had been performed in England. Taylor LJ in a reserved judgment rejected the contention that *Liangsiriprasert* applied only to common law conspiracies. There was nothing in the 1977 Act which indicated that common law and statutory conspiracies were to be treated differently in relation to this point. It would be 'absurd' if *Liangsiriprasert* applied only to conspiracies to defraud, and the Privy Council would have restricted their opinions to the common law, if their advice had been only concerned with the common law. On the facts, moreover, there was an overt act in England, the hire of a fishing vessel to import the drugs from Morocco. Therefore, *Sansom* is like *DPP* v *Doot*. Although the endorsement of *Liangsiriprasert* is *obiter*, there is no doubt that it represents the law.

It should be noted that by s 1(4) of the 1977 Act an agreement for conduct to take place outside England and Wales is not a conspiracy unless the crime would constitute an offence triable in England and Wales. Therefore, an agreement to break foreign criminal law is not a conspiracy indictable in England and Wales unless it would amount to an offence if done in England and Wales. If there is an agreement made in England to commit abroad what would be an offence of conspiracy to defraud if committed in England, English courts have no jurisdiction: *Attorney-General's Reference (No. 1 of 1982)* [1983] QB 751 (CA). Exceptionally a conspiracy to murder is triable in England and

Wales even though it would not otherwise 'be so triable if committed in accordance with the intentions of the parties to the agreement'.

By virtue of the Criminal Justice Act 1993, which came into force in 1999 (and see the Criminal Justice (Terrorism and Conspiracy) Act 1998), a conspiracy to commit a 'group A' offence in England or abroad is triable in England whether the accused became a party to the conspiracy in England or abroad and whether 'any act or omission or other event in relation to the conspiracy occurred in England . . .' or not. This provision confirms **Liangsiriprasert** and **Sansom**, which, however, are not confined to listed offences. A 'group A' offence is one of those listed in the 1993 Act as amended. The list includes theft, fraud contrary to the Fraud Act 2006, blackmail, handling and evading liability by deception. The Act also inserts a new s 1A into the Criminal Law Act 1977. In relation to conspiracies to commit a 'group A' offence, whether or not the offence if committed would be an offence triable in England, the accused is now triable in England if he did 'anything' in England in relation to the agreement before its formation, or became a party to it in England, or did or omitted to do 'anything' in England in pursuance of it. Another provision deals with conspiracies where no element required to be proved for the commission of the offence occurred in England. An example is if the accused in England conspired with another in France to steal the *Mona Lisa* from the Louvre in Paris. Both defendants may be tried in England, even though the group A offence itself cannot be tried in England. The provisions apply also where the accused abroad has duped an innocent agent in England to start a conspiracy to purloin the *Mona Lisa*. If, however, everything took place abroad, there is no conspiracy justiciable here. An example is a purely French operation to steal the painting. In this eventuality the English courts have no jurisdiction.

Mens rea in statutory conspiracies

The mental element in conspiracy is the intention to play a part in the agreed course of conduct: **Anderson**, above. Recent cases, particularly ones involving drugs, have re-emphasised that recklessness is insufficient: **Harmer** [2005] 2 Cr App R 23 (CA), **Ali** [2005] Crim LR 864 (CA), and in particular **Saik** [2007] 1 AC 18 (HL). The accused must also intend to carry out the agreement and have the *mens rea* required for the offence he intends to commit. For example, in a conspiracy to steal the defendants must intend permanently to deprive and be dishonest. In conspiracy to murder the defendant must intend to kill; an intention to cause grievous bodily harm is insufficient: **Siracusa**, above. In a conspiracy to import heroin, there must be an agreement to import heroin, not just any drug. The reason is that according to s 1(1) the agreed course of conduct must necessarily amount to a crime if carried out, and an agreement to commit grievous bodily harm will not necessarily result in the death of their victim when carried out. A person is guilty even though he intended to take part in only a portion of the unlawful conduct. He must know that at least one of the conspirators intends to commit the full offence, but it need not be shown that he intended to carry it out, no matter that s 1 of the Criminal Law Act 1977 states 'in accordance with *their* intentions' (emphasis added). In **Anderson**, the facts of which are given above, the accused was held to be guilty. If he was guilty despite his not intending the agreed plan to be carried out, all of the other conspirators should also be guilty, even if those too did not intend the agreement to be carried out! The *ratio* of **Anderson** is inconsistent with s 1(1). Section 1(1) states when paraphrased that a person is guilty of conspiracy only when two or more of the defendants intended to carry out their agreement. This part of **Anderson** survives the clarification which another part of **Anderson** received in **Siracusa**, which is discussed below.

The House of Lords in *Churchill v Walton* [1967] 2 AC 224 (HL) held at common law that in relation to strict offences the accused is guilty only if he knows of the circumstances. Accordingly, an agreement to commit a strict offence requires *mens rea*. In relation to statutory conspiracies s 1(2) of the 1977 Act adopts the same position. The same applies where the *mens rea* of the substantive offence is satisfied by something less than knowledge. The principal authority is *Saik*, above. Suspicion was the relevant mental element but it was not for the crime of conspiring to commit that offence. Lord Nicholls said that 'know' meant true belief; suspicion did not constitute knowledge. Section 1(2) applies to all offences where at issue is the existence of a fact or circumstance. It is not restrictive to strict offences.

> Where liability for any offence may be incurred without knowledge on the part of the person committing it of any particular fact or circumstance necessary for the commission of the offence, a person shall nevertheless be guilty of conspiracy to commit that offence . . . unless he and at least one other party to the agreement intend or know that that fact or circumstance will exist at the time when the conduct constituting the offence is to take place.

It is suggested that s 1(2) is at base inconsistent with *Anderson*. If intention as to circumstances is required (s 1(2)) then, contrary to *Anderson*, intention as to consequence ought also to be required. The contrary view is that while intent as to circumstances is needed, recklessness as to consequences suffices. If so, two men who agree to rape, being reckless as to consent, are guilty of conspiracy to rape. It should also be pointed out that one cannot 'know' that something 'will exist' in the future. What is meant is that the accused must believe that a fact or circumstance will exist.

In *Anderson* Lord Bridge said that the accused had the mental element 'if, and only if . . . the accused, when he entered into the agreement intended to play some part in the agreed course of conduct in furtherance of the criminal purpose which the agreed course of conduct was intended to achieve'. On this view the defendant would not be guilty of conspiracy if he incites the principal to kill the third party but intended doing nothing else. (What about IRA 'Godfathers'? Can one see the House of Lords letting them go?) To state the proposition is to see how silly it is. This view was confirmed by the Court of Appeal in *Siracusa*, above. Contrary to what Lord Bridge said, there is no rule of law that the accused had to intend to play an active part in the agreed course of conduct. It was sufficient that the accused intended to continue to agree that the criminal behaviour of the other parties should continue. It must also be said that Lord Bridge's *dictum* is inconsistent with the thrust of his speech that intention is irrelevant and the *dictum* is inconsistent with his efforts to secure the acquittal of the law-abiding citizen who joins the conspiracy to entrap the co-conspirators. He is now liable if he does intend to play some part in the execution of the agreement. The House of Lords could have found the defendant guilty of being an accessory to the conspiracy to effect the escape.

In *Allsop*, above, a *dictum* of Lord Diplock in *Hyam v DPP* [1975] AC 55 (HL) that intention includes knowledge of the likelihood of consequences occurring was applied to conspiracy to defraud. The 1977 Act requires intent, and if *Allsop* is correct it is restricted to common law offences. It has, however, been argued that, as in attempt, recklessness as to circumstances should be enough. If two men agree to have sexual intercourse with a woman and believe that she may consent, under present law they are not guilty of conspiring to rape. If s 1(2) is applied not just to strict offences but generally, they do not 'intend or know that that fact or circumstance [lack of consent] will exist at the time when the conduct constituting the offence is to take place'. The accused is guilty of conspiracy only if he knew she did not consent. Recklessness as to the existence of circumstances, lack of consent, is not sufficient *mens rea* for statutory conspiracies, though it suffices for the full offence of rape. It also suffices for the crime of attempted rape (see below). The issue was discussed in **Mir** (1994) *The Independent*, 23 May (CA). Applying s 1(2) generally the court held that an accused is guilty of conspiracy only when he knows that a circumstance exists or intends that a consequence shall ensue. Recklessness is insufficient. Therefore, defendants are not guilty of conspiring to commit aggravated criminal damage if they are reckless as to a serious risk to life. This ruling should be contrasted with the law in attempt where recklessness as to endangering life is sufficient *mens rea*. The court in **Mir** made no effort to reconcile its ruling with the law of attempt. The decision is inconsistent with the rule that the accused must have the *mens rea* of the full offence. Recklessness as to danger to life is one of the fault elements for aggravated criminal damage. Yet the Court of Appeal held that the accused was guilty only if he intended to endanger life.

General comments on conspiracy

Under present law there remains the difficulty that three types of conspiracies remain common law offences. Two of them, corrupting public morals and outraging public decency, are vague. These offences continue to exist, it is thought, because prosecutions are rarely brought. If more prosecutions were brought, liberal thinkers would have a field day criticising the potential width of those offences. The width of conspiracy to defraud is also uncertain. It is wider than conspiracies to commit fraud offences (**Scott v MPC**, above) but is an agreement to damage property or to handle stolen goods a conspiracy to defraud? That is not to say that conspiracies under statute are perfect. If the width of the crime to be committed is uncertain, so is the conspiracy to commit it.

At common law and under the statute there is no maximum fine which a court may impose. In the common law conspiracies to corrupt public morals and outrage public decency there is no maximum sentence of imprisonment. By s 12 of the Criminal Justice Act 1987 the maximum sentence for conspiracy to defraud is 10 years. The maximum for statutory conspiracies is the maximum for the offence. If the offence is one triable either way, the maximum is that for trial on indictment. Conspiracy is an indictable offence even though the crime agreed on is only summary. There are special rules of evidence for conspiracy cases, by which prejudicial evidence against a conspirator may be adduced which would be forbidden for all other offences.

Ian Dennis in 'The rationale of criminal conspiracy' (1977) 93 LQR 39 gave five reasons for having a law of criminal conspiracy: (a) It is evidence of criminal intent, just as a 'more than merely preparatory' act is an attempt. (b) It allows intervention to prevent persons committing offences. Unless prevented, a conspiracy may lead to many organised crimes, not just one. (c) It gets the organisers of crimes before the courts. The Godfathers of crime, who do not soil their hands with carrying out crimes such as terrorism and robbery, can be caught by this offence. (d) Conspiracies constitute injurious combinations and persons joining such agreements ought to be punished. (e) The law provides a means of stopping partnerships in crime. It is possible that two persons egging each other on are more likely to commit an offence than one person by himself. The fact that two people are involved increases the dangerousness of their behaviour. A terrorist gang is more difficult to stop than one terrorist. (Incitement can be seen in a similar light.) In law a conspiracy applies even though the parties have not reached the stage of an attempt. The same activity may be a conspiracy if done by two persons, but not an attempt if done by one: the crime prevention rationale seems to apply much more strongly to conspiracy than to attempt. Indeed, in **Board of Trade v Owen** [1957] AC 602 (HL), Lord Tucker saw this as the rationale of conspiracy. 'The whole object of making such agreements punishable is to prevent the commission of the substantive offence before it has even reached the stage of an attempt.' It may be argued why the law applies more against two or more persons (who are guilty of conspiracy) than against one person (who is not guilty either of conspiracy or attempt). G. Fletcher, *Rethinking Criminal Law* (Little, Brown & Co, 1978) 133, thought that: '[T]he phenomenon of people forming criminal bands might be regarded as sufficiently unnerving to be prohibited for its own sake.' Nevertheless, one person can create just as much harm as two, and one gorilla-sized person may create as much alarm as two persons of restricted growth.

Reform

The draft Criminal Code, Law Com. No. 177, 1989, cl 48, provides:

> (1) A person is guilty of conspiracy . . . if –
>   (a) he agrees with another or others that an act or acts shall be done which, if done, will involve the commission of the offence or offences by one or more of the parties to the agreement; and
>   (b) he and at least one other party to the agreement intend that the offence or offences shall be committed.

The *ratio* in **Anderson** [1986] AC 27 is overruled and the *dictum* of Lord Bridge is not to be enacted.

> (2) For the purpose of sub-[clause] (1) an intention that an offence shall be committed is an intention with respect to all the elements of the offence (other than fault elements), except that recklessness with respect to a circumstance suffices where it suffices for the offence itself.

As in attempt, recklessness as to circumstances, e.g. consent in rape, is to be sufficient.

The draft omits the word 'necessarily' found in s 1(1). The issue of conditional intention is left to the general law and no longer would depend, as *Jackson* [1985] Crim LR 442 had held, on whether the agreement necessarily amounts to an offence if carried out in accordance with the defendants' intentions.

The exemption of intended victims as conspirators themselves is preserved by cl 48(4). However, the class exempted must be 'protected persons'. That is, those who are intended victims *and* are the subject of Parliament's intention to protect them. By sub-cl (8) a person is guilty of conspiracy although:

> (a) no other party has been or is charged with such conspiracy;
> (b) the identity of any other party to the agreement is unknown;
> (c) any other party appearing from the indictment to have been a party to the agreement has been or is acquitted of such conspiracy, unless in all the circumstances his conviction is inconsistent with the acquittal of the other; or
> (d) the only other party to the agreement cannot be convicted of such conspiracy (for example, because he was acting under duress by threats . . . , or he was a child under ten years of age . . . , or he is immune from prosecution).

These sub-clauses largely restate current law.

The present exceptions where the accused agreed with the spouse, a child under the age of criminal responsibility and the intended victim are to be abrogated. Whether the accused is to be liable will depend on the general law. If there is now any difference between the law relating to conspiracy with children and conspiracy with mentally disordered adults, the draft Criminal Code would remove it. The Law Commission thought that the social policy behind the marital exemption which existed earlier, that the criminal law should not disturb the confidential relationship of marriage, had disappeared. Moreover, since one spouse can be an accessory to the other's principal offence, it was nonsensical that they could not be liable for conspiracy.

Clause 48(7) clarifies the law. There is to be no crime of conspiracy to be a secondary party to the commission of a crime by a person not party to the agreement, but there are offences of being an accessory to conspiracy by others and of conspiracy to incite. The first (non-liability) proposition restates the Court of Appeal decision in **Hollinshead** [1985] AC 975, above.

Conspiracy to defraud is not affected by the draft Criminal Code or by the Fraud Act 2006.

The Law Commission issued its Consultation Paper No. 183, *Conspiracy and Attempts*, in 2007. In it it made the following proposals. First, and contrary to the current law in *Saik*, above, it was recommended that recklessness should suffice as to any circumstance element in the substantive offence. Secondly, and widening the law found in s 1(2), if knowledge or belief suffices for the full offence, it should also suffice for the conspiracy to commit that offence; s 1(2) demands that knowledge alone suffices at present. Thirdly, two parts of the law in **Anderson** – that the accused to be guilty of conspiracy must intend 'to play some part in the agreed course of conduct' and that conspiracy does not require that the accused intends that the agreement is to be carried through to completion – are to be abolished. Paragraph 1.39 expresses the Commission's concerns:

> First, there is no reason, in terms of statutory language or policy, for insisting that D must intend to play some part in implementing the agreement. If D1 and D2 agree to murder V, D1 ought to be convicted of conspiracy to murder even if it was not his or her intention to play any party in V's murder. Secondly, an agreement to commit an offence implies an intention that it should be committed, as section 1(1) of the 1977 Act seems to make clear. The idea of a conspiracy that the conspirators agree to take part in but which none intends to see carried out is very unsatisfactory.

Thirdly, the spousal immunity is recommended for abolition. Fourthly, the law that exempts both parties when a non-victim and his victim agree to commit a crime will be abolished with the result that the non-victim is to be liable for conspiracy; however, a defence will be given to the victim. The obvious example is when a man of mature years persuades an underage person to have sexual intercourse with him. Currently, both the man, the 'non-victim', and the other party, the victim, whose interests are protected by the law of sexual offences (now s 9 of the Sexual Offences Act 2003), have a defence. The proposal is that only the victim should have a defence. Fifthly, however, the law on conspiracy with a child under 10 is preserved, a recommendation with is hard to square with the previous one, especially when it is recalled that current law protects an adult who targets a vulnerable young child to enter into what would otherwise be a conspiracy. The Commission's argument (para. 1.47) is that when an adult agrees with a child to commit an offence, 'there can be no meeting of "criminal" minds of a kind at the heart of any criminal conspiracy'. It then notes that the adult should unless excluded be guilty of the crimes of attempt or criminal preparation, as it proposes in the same Consultation Paper (see later in this chapter). Sixthly, and in line with the Serious Crime Act 2007 in respect of assisting or encouraging crime (see earlier in this chapter), there should be a defence of acting reasonably. This defence would reverse the law in **Yip Chiu-Cheung**, above, so that for example an undercover officer would not be guilty of conspiracy. Finally, at present conspiracies to commit summary offences are, like other conspiracies, triable only on indictment; and the Director of Public Prosecutions' consent is required. The proposal is that such conspiracies should be triable summarily; one result is that the consent of the DPP would no longer be needed.

Attempt

Introduction

Attempt originated in the Star Chamber in the early seventeenth century. Its purpose was to criminalise conduct before the full offence had taken place. Attempt is a crime under statute, the Criminal Attempts Act 1981. Section 6(1) abolished attempt at common law. It is punishable in general to the same extent as the complete or full offence: s 4(1). A person may be convicted of an attempt even though he is guilty of the full offence: **Webley v Buxton** [1977] QB 481 (DC) in relation to summary trials and s 6(4) of the Criminal Law Act 1967 in relation to trials on indictment. Where there are two counts in the indictment, attempt and the full offence, the accused may be convicted of the full offence but found not guilty of the attempt. One way of explaining this rule is to say that the attempt is merged with the full offence when the attempt is successful. However, a person convicted on one indictment of attempt cannot later be charged with the full offence: **Velasquez** [1996] 1 Cr App R 155.

Attempt is a crime where principles of criminal law collide. First, people who are dangerous should be restrained. A person who shoots and misses is just as culpable as one who shoots and hits. His actions demonstrate a criminal intent. The law should prevent future misconduct as well as punish past misbehaviour. Both are dangerous. Moreover, the line between success and failure may be slight. In both eventualities the accused must be deterred. Secondly, people should not be penalised for simply thinking about committing crimes. Balancing these principles leaves the police in an invidious position. They have to hold back until the moment when the accused is well on his way towards committing the offence, even though it is certain that a crime will be performed. The Law Commission Report No. 102, 1980, on *Attempt, and Impossibility in Relation to Attempt, Conspiracy and Incitement*, see above, said that the rationale of the offence was to stop persons from committing the full offence. The law adopts the view that attempt is an offence where the accused both has the intent of carrying out the full offence and he has put that intention partly into effect: in the words of the Act he must have done a 'more than merely preparatory' act. Both firmness of purpose and antisocial behaviour are looked at.

Each time a new indictable offence is created the crime of attempting to commit that offence is automatically created. Since, however, there is no offence of attempting to commit a summary offence, changing the category of an offence to make it summary means that the attempt is abolished unless Parliament expressly provides for the attempt. Accordingly because of ss 39 and 37 respectively of the Criminal Justice Act 1988 there are no longer crimes of attempting to assault or to take a vehicle without consent. Perhaps there should be. This law is laid down in s 1(4) of the 1981 Act, which also provides that one cannot attempt to aid, abet, counsel or procure a crime. One can, however, be a secondary party to attempting to commit an offence: **Dunnington** [1984] QB

472 (CA). Section 1(4) further states that one cannot attempt to conspire, assist offenders, or conceal information about arrestable offences. (Attempt to conspire is at least covered by the crime of incitement.) The draft Criminal Code, Law Com. No. 177, 1989, will reverse non-liability for attempt to conspire but preserve it for the other two offences.

It may be that one cannot be convicted of at least some forms of attempted manslaughter. The Criminal Attempts Act 1981, s 1(1), provides that the *mens rea* of attempt is intent. The test of gross negligence manslaughter is that the accused fell short, grossly, of a certain standard of care and thereby killed the victim; he does not have to intend a certain consequence. How can one intend to be grossly negligent? This argument does not, however, hold true of voluntary manslaughter. If a person attempts to kill and would have had the defence of provocation or diminished responsibility if he had killed, surely he may be convicted of attempted manslaughter if the victim does not die. In *Bruzas* [1972] Crim LR 367 the Crown Court did not accept the existence of such a crime. If the draft Criminal Code were enacted, cl 61 would permit the charge in relation to diminished responsibility and provocation. It is thought that one cannot attempt to attempt the full offence. If it were a crime, the accused would be guilty before he had reached the stage of a more than merely preparatory act, which the 1981 Act requires.

Where Parliament changes the law relating to the substantive offence, the width of the attempt to commit that offence may be affected. A good illustration is the new crime of fraud contrary to the Fraud Act 2006. If the accused sent an email to a person who unbeknown to him was dead, begging for money, there would before the 2006 Act have been the offence of attempting to obtain property (money) by deception. Here, amending the substantive law has changed the offence from one of attempt (attempted deception) to one of the full offence (fraud, not merely attempted fraud). See also the former defence of impossibility discussed below.

Criminal Attempts Act 1981

Parliament substantially implemented the recommendations of the Law Commission in the 1981 Act, the main difference being that there is no crime of attempting to commit a summary offence unless Parliament says differently. The principal provisions of the Act are:

(a) the definition of the *mens rea*;

(b) the establishment of a new test of the *actus reus*;

(c) the abolition of the defence of impossibility, reversing *Haughton v Smith* [1975] AC 476 (HL);

(d) the abolition of 'sus' (see below) and the creation of an offence of interference with vehicles;

(e) the abolition of the offence of procuring materials for crime, though other preparatory offences continue to exist, such as those found in s 25 of the Theft Act 1968 (see Chapter 17) and s 3 of the Criminal Damage Act 1971 (see Chapter 18).

The Act was meant to remedy several defects in the law and to codify the law in preparation for the general codification of criminal law.

The definition of the *mens rea*

Section 1(1) of the Criminal Attempts Act 1981 provides that the mental element for attempt is 'intent'. There is no definition of this term in the Act. The government rejected a clause stating that recklessness as to circumstances sufficed if it sufficed for the full offence. In view of the legislative history one might have expected that intent meant intent with regard to *every* element of the *actus reus*. In **Mohan** [1976] QB 1 the Court of Appeal had defined intent in attempt as 'a decision to bring about . . . the commission of the offence . . . no matter whether the accused desired that consequence or not'. The second part was meant to cover oblique intent, such as putting a bomb on a plane to claim the insurance on freight without desiring the death of the passengers and crew according to Stuart-Smith J in **Pearman** (1985) 80 Cr App R 259. Therefore, the accused is guilty when his intention cannot be achieved without the occurring of another consequence first. It will, using an example from **Pearman**, not be difficult to find that the accused intended to injure a constable if he drove straight at him. Section 6 of the 1981 Act abolished the common law of attempt but s 1(1) still requires 'intent' and in **Pearman** the Court of Appeal said that the definition in **Mohan** applied to the Act. No case has as yet discussed the effect of **Woollin** [1999] AC 82 (HL) on attempt. See Chapter 3 for an exposition of the general law of intent. **Woollin** was expressly restricted by the Lords to murder. If it applies generally throughout the criminal law, foresight of a consequence as virtually certain *is only evidence of* intent. However, attempt may be restricted to direct intent: how can one attempt something without having the achievement of that result as one's purpose?

See Chapter 3 for an explanation of intent.

The requirement of intent continues to apply as to the consequences of conduct. The accused is not guilty of attempting to cause grievous bodily harm by driving so recklessly that he foresaw harm as likely. On usual principles the higher degree of foresight the more likely it is that the accused intended the result. However, in relation to circumstances the requirement of intent has been watered down. In **Pigg** [1982] 1 WLR 762, a case decided on the common law, the Court of Appeal, seemingly without reflecting on the matter, held that recklessness as to circumstances was sufficient if it sufficed for the substantive offence. Recklessness as to the woman's consent in rape was therefore sufficient for attempted rape. (The law of rape was subsequently amended by the Sexual Offences Act 2003 but the principle stands.) In **Breckenridge** (1984) 79 Cr App R 244, the court had 'no criticism' of the trial judge's ruling that recklessness as to consent was sufficient for rape. In **Millard** [1987] Crim LR 393, the Court of Appeal saw the problem about attempted rape but did not resolve it. It did state that it was wrong to say that attempted criminal damage could be committed recklessly. In **O'Toole** [1987] Crim LR 759, the Court of Appeal confirmed that recklessness as to criminal damage was insufficient for attempting to damage property by fire being reckless as to whether life was endangered. He had tried to set fire to a pub in which there was a barmaid. The courts appeared to be drawing a line between consequences (recklessness insufficient) and circumstances (recklessness sufficient), though s 1(1) of the Act is not so phrased; it speaks only of 'intent'. The principal authority is now **Khan** [1990] 1 WLR 815 (CA). The defendants tried but failed to have sexual intercourse with a 16-year-old girl, whom they had met at a daytime disco. Russell LJ argued thus. The then *mens rea* in rape, the full offence, was the intention to have sexual intercourse with a woman, knowing that she was not consenting or being reckless whether she consented. (Nowadays men as well as women can be raped.) The same applied to attempted rape. The difference between rape and attempted rape lay in the *actus reus*: in attempt, the sexual intercourse had not taken place. The difference therefore related to a physical matter, but the state of mind was the same. 'The words "with intent to commit an offence" . . . in s 1 of the Act of 1981 mean when applied to rape, "with intent to have sexual intercourse with a woman in circumstances where she does not consent" and the defendant knows or could not care less about her absence of consent. The only "intent" . . . of the rapist is to have sexual intercourse.' Therefore, the accused is guilty of attempted rape, even though he does not know that the victim was not consenting. He is guilty of attempted rape if he is reckless as to consent. Yet, according to *Millard*, one is not guilty of attempted criminal damage if one is reckless as to who owns the damaged property. Ownership, a circumstance, is not an element to which one can be reckless. The distinction between being reckless as to ownership (not guilty) and being reckless as to consent (guilty) is not easily acceptable.

Khan stated that recklessness as to circumstances (such as consent in rape) is sufficient to convict of the attempt but intent as to consequences (the intention to have sexual intercourse in rape) is needed. The rule still stands that intention as to consequences is necessary for the attempt even if recklessness as to consequences is sufficient for the full offence. *Khan* presumably applies to all 'circumstances' crimes, though it is in fact an authority on attempting to commit the crime of rape as defined in a since repealed statute. Presumably the law applies to attempts to commit strict offences.

The width of *Khan* is uncertain. The Court of Appeal said: 'our reasoning cannot apply to all offences and all attempts. Where for example, as in . . . reckless arson, no state of mind other than recklessness is involved in the offence, there can be no attempt to commit it.' In the first draft Criminal Code, Law Com. No. 143, 1985, the academic drafters thought that the distinction between circumstances and conduct was not workable and, indeed, used rape as their example. On consultation their formulation of the mental element in attempted rape was criticised as being too narrow. The present draft Criminal Code, Law Com. No. 177, 1989, which predated *Khan*, is consistent with the ruling, despite the fact that the draft Criminal Code team and the Law Commission itself in Report No. 102 on *Attempt*, 1980, para 2.18, on which the Act was based, had previously rejected it. Indeed, if the Court of Appeal in *Khan* had looked at the Report (and under current law expressed in *Pepper* v *Hart* [1993] AC 593 it was entitled to do so), it would have discovered that it was wrong. Clause 49(2) of the 1989 version stipulates that for all attempts:

> An intention to commit an offence is an intention with respect to all the elements of the offence other than fault elements, except that recklessness with respect to circumstances suffices where it suffices for the offence itself.

The Law Commission did not define the line between circumstances and consequences, which was to be left for the courts. The Law Commission opined that in rape (as it was then defined) the distinction was easy in that absence of the victim's consent was a circumstance. But what about the former requirement that the victim was a woman? It looks like a circumstance but the Court of Appeal in *Millard* said that it was a consequence. It is thought that judges may require guidance if the draft Criminal Code is enacted.

In relation to the other inchoate offences *Khan* does not apply to statutory conspiracies because s 1(2) of the Criminal Law Act 1977 requires intention or knowledge of 'the fact or circumstance'. *Khan* may apply to common law conspiracies. Under the draft Criminal Code, conspiracy would be brought into line with attempt: cl 48(2) does for conspiring what cl 49(2) does for attempt. Presumably *Khan* applies to incitement.

Graham Virgo wrote in 'Reckless attempts – rape and circumstance' [1990] CLJ 390 that *Khan* is 'justifiable because "intention" cannot relate to circumstances; whether a woman is consenting or not cannot be intended, but can be known or believed. No provision for circumstances was made in the Criminal Attempts Act 1981, so allowing the Court of Appeal's interpretation here.' On the other hand, the statute does say 'intent' not 'intent as to consequences and recklessness as to circumstances'. Certainly

Parliament could have expressed itself more clearly but it did not do so. Furthermore, the term 'attempt' may imply intent: how can the accused attempt to do something unless one does intend it? Such was the view of Edmund-Davies LJ, as he then was, in **Easom** [1971] 2 QB 315 (CA). One might even argue that, accepting the circumstances/consequences split, the consequences in rape could be defined as sexual intercourse with a woman who does not consent. All the elements are consequences; therefore, intent is required throughout: therefore, recklessness as to consent is insufficient, and **Khan** is wrong. Whatever is said about statutory construction it would have been strange in principle to convict a person who had just achieved penetration, being reckless as to the victim's consent, and not convicting the accused of attempted rape in a similar situation where he was stopped just before penetration. For a criticism of the circumstance/consequence dichotomy and a proposed solution, see Glanville Williams 'Intents in the alternative' [1991] CLJ 120.

Khan was approved in **Attorney-General's Reference (No. 3 of 1992)** [1994] 2 All ER 121 (CA). Schiemann J speaking for the court said in a reserved judgment that **Khan** was in accord with policy and common sense and did no violence to the words of the statute. **Khan** was not restricted to rape. He extended **Khan** from recklessness as to circumstances to recklessness as to endangering life in aggravated criminal damage. This element, it is suggested, is neither consequence nor circumstance but a further part of the mental element. Accordingly the mental element in the offence of attempted aggravated criminal damage is, at its lowest, intending to cause criminal damage, being reckless as to whether life would be endangered by the damage, a state of mind which on the facts of the case covered throwing a petrol bomb at the complainant's property but missing, being reckless as to endangering life. In the present case damage was missing, in **Khan** sexual intercourse had not taken place. With regard to that missing element intent was needed, but with regard to the other constituents of the attempt the same state of mind which sufficed for the substantive crime sufficed for the attempt. On the facts of the case what was missing was damage. Therefore, to be guilty of the attempt the accused had to intend to cause damage. However, the element of endangering life existed. Therefore, it was sufficient that the accused was reckless as to this element. Accordingly the *mens rea* for the attempt was intending to cause criminal damage, being reckless as to whether life would be endangered. If the accused does not intend to cause criminal damage he is not guilty of the attempt even though he is reckless as to endangering life. In criticism of this *dictum* may be instanced the crime of attempted sexual intercourse with a girl under 16. Surely the accused is not guilty of this offence if the accused believes the victim to be over 16. The full crime is strict as to the age of the girl. It cannot be that the attempt is also strict. If it were, one might have expected the courts (and Parliament) to have said so in their analysis of attempt. Nevertheless, the missing-element point would make the accused guilty of the attempt. Another problem with current law is this: for the crime of attempted criminal damage it must be proved in the basic offence that the accused intended to damage property belonging to another; in attempted rape the prosecution must prove that the accused intended to have sexual intercourse but it is sufficient that the accused was reckless as to the victim's consent. It seems strange that 'belonging to another' is central to the crime of attempted (basic) criminal damage but 'without the consent of the victim' is not central to the crime of attempted rape, especially when both elements constitute circumstances of the crime. This proposition is preferred by Professor P. Dobson in his commentary on the **Reference** case (1994) 11 Student LR 17 thus: 'ask "if the accused had succeeded in carrying out his intention, would the full offence have been committed?" If the answer is yes, then the accused had sufficient *mens rea* for the attempt.'

One issue which was not discussed in ***Attorney-General's Reference (No. 3 of 1992)*** was whether the type of recklessness mentioned was subjective or objective. From the phrasing of the judgment objective recklessness was presumably meant. The court said that once the Crown had proved the intent to cause criminal damage, the sole other mental element is the remaining state of mind required for the offence of aggravated arson, i.e. objective recklessness. The result was that an accused is guilty of attempted aggravated criminal damage if he sets light to a house, intending to do so, and does not realise that anyone is in the house, provided that there was an obvious and serious risk of endangering the life of any person who was in fact in the house. The court did not seem to have considered this issue. In any case the abolition of ***Caldwell*** recklessness in criminal damage in ***G*** [2004] 1 AC 1034 now means that subjective recklessness is the appropriate test. It should be noted that the definition of intention in ***Khan*** and ***Attorney-General's Reference (No. 3 of 1992)*** is restricted to attempt and does not extend throughout criminal law. For the definition of intent elsewhere, see Chapter 3.

Two further matters relating to intent in s 1(1)

In attempted murder the accused must intend to kill. It is not sufficient if he intended only to cause grievous bodily harm. Therefore, the more serious crime, murder, has a wider mental element than the lesser, attempted murder. In ***Whybrow*** (1951) 35 Cr App R 141, the accused wired up the bath in an attempt to kill his wife. In ***Walker and Hayles***, above, the victim was dropped by the accused from a third-floor window. In both cases the Court of Criminal Appeal and the Court of Appeal respectively held that intention to commit grievous bodily harm was insufficient.

The case of ***Walker and Hayles***, which was discussed in Chapter 3, demonstrates how simple questions can become difficult. When the accused did what they did, did they intend to kill? The trial judge might have directed the jury that the accused were guilty if they intended to kill; in the event of any difficulty the jury might have been instructed in accordance with ***Mohan*** that the accused were guilty if they had made up their minds to kill or decided to kill. The case was one of direct intent or nothing. There was no oblique intent problem. The judge, however, directed the jury in terms of foreseeing death as a high probability. The Court of Appeal preferred the term 'virtual certainty' to a high probability of death but did not quash the conviction on the basis that a high probability of death was sufficient. On the facts the probability or certainty of death was in truth irrelevant if the accused did (directly) intend to kill. It is only when there is doubt about what the accused did intend to do that one need look at virtual certainties or high degrees of probability as matters of evidence. In those circumstances the jury could infer intention to kill from the accused's foresight of death as a virtually certain consequence.

Section 1(3) and intent

Section 1(3) of the 1981 Act provides:

> In any case where –
> (a) apart from this subsection a person's intention would not be regarded as having amounted to an intent to commit an offence; but
> (b) if the facts of the case had been as he believed them to be his intention would be so regarded,
> then, for the purposes of subsection (1) above, he shall be regarded as having had an intent to commit that offence.

What s 1(3) seems to means is this. The common law rule as to impossibility in attempt was laid down by the House of Lords in **Haughton v Smith**, above. That case decided, *inter alia*, that the accused was not guilty of an attempt if he had done everything he wished to do but contrary to his belief his actions did not amount to a crime. In the case itself the accused had done all he intended to do in relation to the property, but he did not know that in law the goods were no longer stolen. Contrary to his belief what he did did not constitute the offence of handling stolen goods. By s 1(3) the accused is deemed to have the necessary intent for handling stolen goods on the facts as he believed to exist. He intended to handle goods which were stolen; he believed he was handling goods which were stolen; applying s 1(3) the *mens rea* of attempted handling is satisfied.

The establishment of a new test for the *actus reus*

The *actus reus* is defined in s 1(1) of the 1981 Act as doing 'an act which is more than merely preparatory to the commission of the offence'. There is no such requirement in conspiracy. 'An act' is wide. It need not be a dangerous act. It is the *mens rea* which converts the act into a crime. I may be driving my car towards you. Only if the jurors know that I intend to run you down can they convict me of an offence. By s 4(3) the question whether the accused committed an attempt is for the jury, provided that there is sufficient evidence in law to support that finding: that is, the judge can rule that the act may be an attempt but it is for the jury to determine that it was so. The judge cannot instruct the jury that a situation amounts to a more than merely preparatory act. However, he or she may tell the jury that there is no evidence that what the accused has done amounts to a more than merely preparatory act, and the issue can be withdrawn from the jury: **Campbell** (1991) 93 Cr App R 350. On the facts the accused was not guilty of attempted robbery even though he had reconnoitred a sub-post office he had intended to rob and he had an imitation gun (and he was convicted of possessing an imitation firearm) and a threatening note. He was arrested near to the office door. He said he was going back to his motorcycle, having decided not to rob. Presumably he would not on this approach have been guilty until he had crossed the threshold of the sub-post office – not a helpful decision in the prevention of crime. If the facts had been left to the jury a conviction may well have been secured, and presumably he could have been convicted of a different attempted crime, attempted burglary, for he had performed a more than merely preparatory act on his way towards entering the building as a trespasser with intent to steal. The Court of Appeal said that cases had to be decided on a case-by-case approach, which is not a help to juries. A contrasting case is **Griffin** [1993] Crim LR 515. A mother was guilty of attempting to abduct her children and take them out of the UK when she had bought ferry tickets for Ireland and told her children's teacher that she was taking them to the dentist's. She had not yet taken charge of the children, never mind set off for the port. She was found guilty, despite the fact that she was nowhere near removing them from the jurisdiction.

The rationale behind cases such as **Campbell** is that the accused is not guilty until he has gone through the psychological barrier on the way towards committing the offence. The accused is within striking distance of committing the offence. It is not sufficient that the accused merely thought about committing the offence. The line at present is between preparatory activities and others.

In **Qadir**, unreported, 25 July 1997, the Court of Appeal said, as it has done before, that *actus reus* of attempt as laid down in the Act seeks to steer 'a midway course . . . [t]he attempt begins at the moment when the defendant embarks on the crime proper, as opposed to taking steps rightly regarded as merely preparatory'. Potter LJ continued: 'Whether or not an act crosses the threshold between preparation and embarkation on the commission of the crime will always depend on an examination of the scope or substance of the crime aimed at.' He gave several examples: 'in a case of [killing], wounding or causing [sic] actual bodily harm, it would be likely that any act leading up to the commission . . . of the crime but substantially anterior to it in time will be an act merely preparatory. In a case of deception . . . , since the *actus reus* of the crime itself may take place over an extended period of time, the moment of embarkation upon it may be quite remote in time from the point of its anticipated successful outcome.'

Present law does little to encourage the prevention of crime, for preparations to commit offences are not attempts, though there is the possibility that other crimes may have been committed (including conspiracy if there were two or more parties). In **Sidaway**, unreported, 11 June 1993, the Court of Appeal held that making an imitation bomb and taking it to London *en route* for Ramsgate did not amount to attempting to commit a bomb hoax in Ramsgate. In **Gullefer** [1990] 3 All ER 882, the accused backed a greyhound which was going to lose. He jumped onto the track trying to distract the dogs so that the stewards would call 'no race' and bookmakers would return stake money. He failed. The Court of Appeal held that he was not guilty of attempt. There was no evidence to go to the jury. His acts were preparatory. The position would have been different if the stewards had called 'no race'. In that eventuality there would have been evidence for the jury. The jury might have, however, held that the accused was guilty only when he had presented his betting slip, or perhaps when he joined the queue. The court said that the accused was guilty only when he had embarked on the 'crime proper'. On the facts juries might have different views as to when the accused did that. After all, he did not have to do anything more. It was for the stewards to declare the race void. The Court of Appeal in **Tosti** [1997] Crim LR 746 held that the two defendants were guilty of attempted burglary of a barn when they had brought oxyacetelene equipment to the scene, hidden it in a hedge and examined the padlock because they were 'evidentially the first steps in the commission of the offence', and not merely preparatory steps. **Gullefer** was applied in **Attorney-General's Reference (No. 1 of 1992)** [1993] 1 WLR 274 (CA). The accused was guilty of attempted rape when he had embarked on committing rape itself. 'The evidence of the young woman's distress, of the state of her clothing, and the position in which she was seen, together with the respondent's acts of dragging her up the steps, lowering his trousers and interfering with her private parts . . . left it open to a jury to conclude that the respondent had the necessary intent and had done acts which were more than merely preparatory.' There was no need to show that he had tried to penetrate the vagina. However, since rape requires penetration and the accused's penis was flaccid, it is perhaps strange that he was convicted of attempted rape. This case does not seem distinguishable from **Campbell**, yet there the accused was acquitted. Similarly in **Patnaik**, unreported, 5 November 2000 (CA), the accused had threatened the victim, attempted to kiss her and straddled her, but had not removed any of her or his own clothing and he had not touched her intimately. It was held that there was sufficient evidence of attempted rape to be left to the jury. In criticism it may be questioned whether the accused had embarked on the crime of rape. He had completed several offences of the then existing crime of indecent assault but the facts are far from as convincing as **Attorney-General's Reference (No. 1 of 1992)**. **Dagnall** [2003] EWCA Crim 2441 is similar as far as can be seen from the facts given. The accused had followed the victim, put his arms around her, told her that he wanted sexual intercourse, said that no-one would hear her if he took her onto a dark road, pulled her backwards by her hair, put her into an arm-lock, covered her mouth and dragged her to a bus stop. The court rejected his argument that because he had not touched her in a sexual way, his actions were no more than merely preparatory.

Under present law intervention seems in many cases to come too late in the interests of crime prevention. For example, 'casing the joint', as in *Campbell*, is too early in the train of events leading to the crime and the judge withdraws the issue from the jury. In *Geddes* [1996] Crim LR 894 the accused intended to kidnap a boy from a school. He ran away when he was discovered in the boys' toilets in which, of course, he was a trespasser. In his rucksack were a large knife, masking tape and rope. The Court of Appeal held ('with the gravest unease') that he was still at the preparation stage and therefore not guilty of attempted false imprisonment. Presumably he would have been guilty if he had made contact with the boy. The court felt uneasy about its decision, but no doubt parents feel much more uneasy. The decision does not encourage the inhibition of the conduct of dangerous people. The reader may also think that the accused was deserving of punishment. (Since the case Parliament has created the offence of trespass with intent to commit a sexual offence while on any premises where he is a trespasser, contrary to s 63 of the Sexual Offences Act 2003, and the accused would be guilty of this offence.) Similar is *Nash* [1999] Crim LR 308 (CA). The accused appealed against a conviction of attempting to procure an act of gross indecency. He had written three letters addressed to 'paper boy'. The first two contained invitations to indulge in mutual masturbation or oral sex or both. The third offered work with a security company. In respect of the third letter it was held that the accused had not gone beyond the stage of mere preparation. *Geddes* was approved. The most recent case is *Bowles & Bowles* [2004] EWCA Crim 1608. The two accused had set out on a plan to get hold of an old woman's money on her death. They had already received large sums from her. They drafted her last will and testament, which named them as beneficiaries. The unexecuted will was then put into the victim's bedside drawer and left for several months. The court held that they were not guilty of attempting to make a false instrument, the will, because they had performed only preparatory acts.

Glanville Williams 'Wrong turnings on the law of attempt' [1991] Crim LR 416 wished the law to be that a judge would rule when preparation became an attempt. 'What the judges have lost is their power to protect the public by telling the jury firmly that the defendant's act, if proved, . . . did amount to an attempt' (at 425). There is nothing to prevent two juries reaching different conclusions on the same facts. This means that juries may reach their verdicts by taking into account non-legal matters. Even the judges are inconsistent, as this section has showed, as to when the accused moves to a 'more than merely preparatory' stage.

May judges refer to common law authorities?

At law the judges had several tests to which they could refer.

(a) The last act test inquired whether the defendant did the last act dependent on him. A modern phrasing of that test was to ask whether the accused had 'crossed the Rubicon and burnt his boats', as Lord Diplock put it in *DPP v Stonehouse* [1978] AC 55 (HL). This test was not always adopted at common law. In *White* [1910] 2 KB 124, the accused was guilty of attempted murder despite the fact that he needed to put more doses of potassium cyanide into his mother's drink before he killed her. This last act test was approved in *Widdowson* (1985) 82 Cr App R 314 (CA) after the Act but rejected in *Gullefer*.

(b) The any-act-carrying-the-*mens-rea*-into-effect test was laid down in ***Gurmit Singh*** [1966] 2 QB 53 but overruled by s 6(1) of the 1981 Act: see below.

(c) The equivocality test, laid down in cases such as ***Davey v Lee*** [1968] 1 QB 366, asked whether the accused's conduct had any purpose other than the commission of the full offence.

(d) The test most often used was the proximity test. Parke B in ***Eagleton*** (1855) [1843–60] All ER Rep 363 said that: 'Acts remotely leading towards the commission of the full offence are not to be considered as attempts to commit it, but acts immediately connected with it are.' Three Law Lords approved the ***Eagleton*** test in ***Stonehouse***. This test did, however, give rise to cases such as ***Robinson*** [1915] 2 KB 342, in which the accused was not guilty of attempting to obtain money from his insurance company when he faked a robbery at his jeweller's shop because he had not sent in the claim form. The argument was that the accused (as also in ***Gullefer***) was not yet engaged in the business of fraud. He had prepared the way but not reached the stage where deceit could be practised. Yet in both ***Robinson*** and ***Gullefer*** the accused did not have himself to do very much else. In ***Gullefer*** the only act for him to do was to collect his stake. The Law Commission's Report No. 102, 1980, on which the Criminal Attempts Act 1981 was based, wished to consign this case to the dustbin of history (paras 2.30, 2.42 and 2.48) but the same result could be reached on analogy with ***Gullefer*** and ***Campbell*** after the 1981 Act. Any resurgence of the proximity test would be contrary to the wishes of the Law Commission, the words of the statute and, it is suggested, common sense.

In ***Ilyas*** (1983) 78 Cr App R 17 (CA), a case decided at common law but after the enactment of the statute, the court used the statute's terminology. It said that it was acceptable under the new law to look at the old cases. In ***Boyle*** (1987) 84 Cr App R 270, the Court of Appeal held similarly in a case on the 1981 Act. The same occurred in ***Widdowson***, above. In these cases it did not matter which of the two main pre-Act tests, last act or proximity, were used because the facts satisfied both tests. Later cases have taken a different view. In ***Gullefer***, however, the court determined that the 1981 Act did not enact previous law. The draughtsmen could have done that but did not. Instead a middle course was steered. That midway course was the natural meaning of s 1(1). In ***Jones*** [1990] 1 WLR 1057 the Court of Appeal in a reserved judgment held that the Act did not incorporate any of the common law tests and judges should not refer to the previous law. It is the words in the Act which count. Taylor LJ said that the accused's 'actions in obtaining the gun, in shortening it, in loading it, in putting on his disguise, and in going into the school could only be regarded as preparatory acts. But . . . once he had got into the car, taken out the loaded gun and pointed it at the victim with the intention of killing him, there was sufficient evidence for the consideration of the jury on the charge of attempted murder.' There was no need to wait until the accused had done the last act. There was evidence of a more than merely preparatory act even though the safety catch was on. There was no need to wait until the accused had released the catch, put his finger on the trigger, and started to squeeze it. The prosecution had to prove only that the accused's actions were 'more than merely preparatory' and those words bore their ordinary meaning. In ***Campbell*** the court held that the judge should not refer to the common law but direct the jury in terms of the 1981 Act.

Despite these strong authorities the Court of Appeal in ***Rowley*** above referred to ***Ransford*** (1874) 13 Cox CC 9, referred to under incitement, when asking whether notes passed to boys to lure them away for immoral purposes constituted the offence of attempting to incite a child under 14 to commit gross indecency. The notes were passed to set up meetings. They contained no express sexual invitation. The court ruled that they constituted preparation, not more than merely preparatory acts. Yet the question remains: what else did he have to do to be guilty? If he had actually met the boys and made lewd suggestions, he would have been guilty of incitement. Presumably attempted incitement occurs when he meets them but before making any proposition.

In at least one way the new law is better for students than the old. There is only one test of the *actus reus*, not several. The form of words is bound to lead to uncertainty, with juries disagreeing whether a more than merely preparatory act has been performed. Whatever happens juries without express provision will come to inconsistent verdicts as to at which point, to use an old example, an accused is guilty when he approaches a haystack intending to set light to it.

Three other points of interpretation

(a) It is cumbersome to speak of a 'more than merely preparatory' act. Unfortunately, to escape from the old law of proximity a different term had to be picked. Now that the courts have eschewed reference to the old law 'proximate' could be reinstated as an adjective which encapsulates the law.

(b) The adverb 'merely' seems to add nothing to 'more than preparatory'. It could mean that only 'merely preparatory' acts are not attempts, whereas 'preparatory' ones are, but such interpretation is inconsistent with the cases. What it seems to mean is that people such as the accused in **Robinson** would now be guilty: they went beyond mere preparation. Therefore, some preparatory acts are attempts.

(c) Section 1(1) refers to 'acts'. Does the term cover omissions? There is a division among commentators, and there is no case law. The government meant 'act' to cover omissions so that it would, e.g., be a crime for a parent to fail to give food to her child but the infant is saved before death. An amendment that crimes of omission could not be attempted was defeated. However, if a statute says the accused is guilty if he does an 'act', an omission does not suffice (unless the omission can also be interpreted as an act). The Act could have been better drafted. If 'act' does include omissions, it may well be difficult to say when the accused commits a 'more than merely preparatory' omission. When, for example, does a father commit a more than merely preparatory omission when he is starving his daughter to death? (See below for the draft Criminal Code's solution.)

An alternative to 'more than merely preparatory'

The Law Commission's Working Party published a Paper, No. 50, *Codification of the Criminal Law: General Principles, Parties, Complicity and Liability for the Acts of Another*, 1973 which recommended the 'substantial step' test as adopted in the US Model Penal Code, 1962, s 5.01. The Model Penal Code in para (2) had a list of illustrations:

> The following, if strongly corroborative of the actor's criminal purpose, shall not be held insufficient as a matter of law:
> (a) lying in wait, searching for or following the contemplated victim . . . ;
> (b) enticing or seeking to entice the contemplated victim of the crime to go to the place contemplated for its commission;
> (c) reconnoitring the place contemplated for the commission of the crime;

(d) unlawful entry of a structure, vehicle or enclosure in which it is contemplated that the crime will be committed;

(e) possession of materials to be employed in the commission of the crime which are specially designed for such unlawful use or which can serve no lawful purpose of the actor under the circumstances;

(f) possession, collection or fabrication of materials to be employed in the commission of the offence, at or near the place contemplated for its commission, where such possession, collection or fabrication serves no lawful purpose in the circumstances;

(g) soliciting an innocent agent to engage in conduct constituting an element of the crime.

The commentary found in the Proposed Official Draft 1985 stated that in each of these instances the accused had broken the psychological barrier and would be unlikely to desist. The US National Commission on Federal Criminal Laws, Final Report upon *A Proposed New Federal Criminal Code*, 1971, omitted these illustrations but only because the list could be extended.

One reason for the rejection of the substantial step test by the Law Commission in its Report No. 102, 1980, was that it was imprecise. After two decades it can be said that the 1981 Act's 'more than merely preparatory' test is just as imprecise, if not more so. The Court of Appeal recognised the difficulty in **Geddes** (above): 'There is no rule of thumb test. There must always be an exercise of judgment based on the particular facts of the case.' As A. Ashworth wrote: 'If the protection of individual rights and the confining of police discretion are regarded as important goals, does not its imprecision count against the test?' ('Criminal attempts and the role of resulting harm under the Code and in the common law' (1988) 19 Rutgers LJ 725 at 752). He was in favour of the list of authoritative examples as in the Model Penal Code, for without them the law is unsettled. Since there is no doubt that if two or more persons agreed to do one of the acts mentioned in the list, they would be guilty of conspiracy, surely if done by one person, a crime – attempt – should be committed.

The abolition of the defence of impossibility

Haughton v Smith [1975] AC 476 and **DPP v Nock** [1978] AC 979 were taken to have laid down a rule that a person was not guilty of attempt or conspiracy respectively where the facts were such that it was impossible to commit the full offence. For instance, if the accused put his hand into a pocket, having made up his mind to steal, he was not guilty of attempted theft if there was nothing in the pocket. Though this statement of law, which has been simplified for present purposes, had its defenders, most commentators thought it ludicrous, and the Law Commission and Parliament agreed. After all the accused had demonstrated an intent to break the law. The law is now stated in s 1(2) of the Criminal Attempts Act 1981:

> A person may be guilty of attempting to commit an offence to which this section applies even though the facts are such that the commission of the offence is impossible.

Section 1(2) states 'may be'. 'Is' was meant. The Court of Appeal in **Shivpuri** [1985] QB 1029 thought that 'may be' was used to emphasise the requirements of *actus reus* and *mens rea*. On the pickpocket facts, the accused is now guilty. In an illustration based on **Partington v Williams** (1975) 62 Cr App R 225, the accused is guilty if he tried to take money from a wallet in a drawer but there was no money there. In an example based on **Farrance** [1978] RTR 225, the accused is guilty where he attempts to take a car but it is impossible to drive away because the clutch has burnt out.

The House of Lords applied s 1(2) in *Shivpuri* [1987] AC 1. The accused was charged with attempting to be knowingly concerned in dealing with a controlled drug, heroin. He was found carrying a package containing a powdered substance and more was found in his flat. He thought the substance was heroin, but in fact it was not. The House of Lords dismissed his appeal. Lord Bridge said that the accused had intended to commit the offence and he had performed a more than merely preparatory act. Though he could not have committed the full offence, s 1(2) deems him to be guilty. The House of Lords stated that the accused should also have been guilty in *Anderton v Ryan* [1985] AC 560 (HL) for attempting to handle a video which he believed to have been stolen. The law is plainly stated in s 1(2). To argue differently is to go against the words of the statute, which represent the intention of Parliament. One can nowadays be guilty of attempting to steal property which one already owns. Whether one should be guilty is a matter of policy, and should not be left to the discretion of the prosecution.

Cases since *Shivpuri* on impossible attempts have been rare but an example is *Brown*, unreported, 2 March 2004. The accused was convicted of attempting to pervert the course of justice when he made allegations of sexual and physical abuse by a person who was dead at the time to which the allegations related.

The law has, however, not always been applied. In *Galvin* (1987) 88 Cr App R 85 (CA), the accused was charged under s 2(2) of the Official Secrets Act 1911, since repealed, with unlawfully receiving a government document. The court held that his conviction should be quashed because the government had disclosed the document so widely that the accused believed that he could use it. Perhaps he should have been convicted of attempting to receive the document unlawfully, which is what he believed was happening. Perhaps the accused in *DPP v Huskinson* [1988] Crim LR 620 should have been convicted of attempt too. He was given money by the Housing Services Department. He thought he was under a legal duty to use that money to pay off his rent arrears; in fact he was not. In those circumstances he could not be convicted of theft, which by s 5(3) of the Theft Act 1968 requires a legal obligation to exist in such circumstances (see Chapter 15). Perhaps *Shivpuri* does not apply to mistakes of law, which was the issue in *Huskinson*. He thought mistakenly he was breaking the law: he did not understand the legal nature of the money he was given. In *Shivpuri* there was a mistake of fact, the nature of the substance, and in *Anderton v Ryan* the mistake was as to the nature of the goods: were they stolen or were they not? The answer to *Huskinson* in terms of statutory interpretation is whether 'facts' in s 1(2) can cover a mistake of civil law – it may do. This construction would also cover this example. The accused agrees to buy a car and takes possession. He believes that he does not become the owner until he had paid for it. In fact by the Sale of Goods Act 1979, s 18, he does become owner. If he kicks in the boot, he is guilty of attempted criminal damage if 'facts' include mistakes of civil law. (Under the pre-Act law he would not have been guilty.)

Many cases will not give rise to problems. If the accused fires a gun at a pillow intending to kill someone, he is guilty of attempted murder. If the accused puts potassium cyanide into his mother's drink, intending to kill her, but the dose is too weak, he is guilty of attempted murder. If the accused tries to open a safe with the wrong tools, intending to steal, he is guilty of attempted theft. A slightly more difficult case is the well-known example of the accused who takes an umbrella from a London club, believing he has stolen it from another member. In fact it belongs to him. Because it does not belong to another, he is not guilty of theft. He is, however, guilty of attempting theft. It does not matter that the property in fact belongs to him. Leaving the solution to the discretion not to prosecute seems weak, but the law is clear.

The exceptional case of the imaginary crime

In *Taaffe* [1984] AC 539 (HL), the accused believed he was importing foreign currency into the UK in breach of the law. There is no such law. The accused was not guilty despite his state of mind. He could not be convicted of attempting to commit an imaginary offence. If someone does an act which he believes to be illegal but which is not, he is not guilty of attempt. Therefore, in this area there still is a law of impossible attempts.

A couple of illustrations make the point. If the accused believes adultery to be an offence, he is not guilty of attempted adultery when he has an affair with a married woman. Adultery is no offence. Therefore, attempted adultery is no offence. If the accused mistakenly believes that he is guilty of having sexual intercourse with a consenting girl of 17, he is not guilty, because there is no such crime. The position is different when the accused has sexual intercourse with a girl of 17, thinking her to be 15. There is a crime of sexual intercourse with a girl under 16. The crime is not imaginary, and the accused will be convicted of the attempt.

Christopher Ryan, *Criminal Law*, 4th edn (Blackstone, 1995) 143, commented:

> What distinguishes Mr Taaffe (who was not found guilty) from Mr Shivpuri (who was)? Both are morally reprehensible, both think they are engaged in committing a crime . . . If social danger is to be the governing factor then surely each of these men has evidenced that he is a danger, that he is prepared to break laws (or what he perceives to be laws) although it is impossible for either actually to do so.

Abolition of 'sus' and the creation of the offence of interference with vehicles

Section 9 of the Criminal Attempts Act 1981 repealed s 4 of the Vagrancy Act 1824, as amended, which contained the offence which came to be known as 'sus', suspected person loitering with intent to commit an arrestable offence. This crime had acquired a bad reputation because it was alleged that the police had used it selectively. In place of 'sus' there was instituted the crime of interference with vehicles in s 9. Besides being narrower and therefore more acceptable than 'sus', it got rid of a troublesome difficulty in the law. If a person was seen tampering with a car door, with which offence was he charged? Attempted theft of the car contrary to s 1 of the Theft Act 1968 would fail if he pleaded that he was going to joy-ride under s 12 of that Act; the same problems arose with the crimes vice versa; or the accused might contend that he wanted to steal the contents, not the car itself. Section 9 of the 1981 Act remedies this difficulty:

> (1) A person is guilty of the offence of vehicle interference if he interferes with a motor vehicle or trailer or with anything carried in or on the motor vehicle or trailer with the intention that an offence specified in sub-section (2) below shall be committed by himself or some other person.
>
> (2) The offences mentioned in sub-section (1) above are –
>   (a) theft of the motor vehicle or trailer or part of it;
>   (b) theft of anything carried in or on the motor vehicle or trailer; and
>   (c) an offence under s 12 of the Theft Act 1968 (taking and driving away without consent): and, if it is shown that a person accused of an offence under this section intended that one of these offences should be committed, it is immaterial that it cannot be shown which it was.

A 'motor vehicle' is defined as a mechanically propelled vehicle intended or adapted for use on roads. This definition is narrower than that of 'conveyance' in the offence of taking without consent.

Points of interpretation

(a) One act of interference is enough. The accused need not be a suspected person.

(b) One of the intents specified in s 9 must be proved. There is no offence under this section if, e.g., the accused intends to commit criminal damage.

(c) 'Interference' seems to require some kind of meddling. Touching a vehicle or leaning against it may not suffice. In **Reynolds v Metropolitan Police** [1982] Crim LR 831, a judge in the Crown Court thought *obiter* that opening the door or applying pressure to the handle would amount to interference. Opening a door would not normally be called an interference but it is for the purposes of this offence.

(d) The long title of the Act speaks of 'unauthorised interference with vehicles'. Moving a car to create a space may be an authorised interference. However, s 9 does not speak of 'unauthorised interference', but only of 'interference', though the intention specified in sub-s (2) must be proved.

(e) The intents in sub-s (2) refer to Theft Act offences. The accused has a defence to s 9(1) if he has a defence under that statute. Belief in the owner's consent is a defence to taking a conveyance without consent. The accused has a defence to s 9(1) if he interferes but believes that the owner would have consented, had he or she known about it.

(f) This offence is a summary one. By s 1(4) of the Criminal Attempts Act 1981 there is no offence of attempting to commit summary offences. Therefore, there is no such crime as attempting to interfere with vehicles.

The abolition of the common law offence of preparation

Section 6 of the 1981 Act abolished the offence of procuring materials to commit a crime. It could be that there still exists at law a more general offence of preparing where the stage of a 'more than merely preparatory' act has not been reached. It is thought, however, that no such offence exists.

Withdrawal

In all three offences there is no defence of withdrawal. Lord Hailsham said so in relation to attempt in **Haughton v Smith**, above. Wright J in **Toothill** [1998] Crim LR 876 (CA) called it 'trite law' that withdrawal was no defence to attempts. Repentance can be taken into account in sentencing, and the Crown Prosecution Service may decline to prosecute. It could be argued that such a defence would accord with the policy of the law which is to encourage people to desist from offending. That argument is weakened where the reason for not committing the full offence is the presence of the police! In other words, if a defence were afforded, it should be restricted to the voluntary abandonment of purpose.

Reform

The draft Criminal Code, Law Com. No. 177, 1989, would if enacted restate s 1(1) of the Criminal Attempts Act 1981 (cl 49(1)) with the addition that **Khan**, above, would be enacted (cl 49(2)); that is, that recklessness as to circumstances would suffice for the attempt if it sufficed for the full crime. Since the draft Criminal Code's terms do not include **Caldwell** recklessness, only **Cunningham** recklessness would suffice. As in present law only attempts to commit indictable offences would be sufficient (cl 49(1)). The problem whether 'act' in the 1981 statute includes omission (the government assumed that at least some omissions were sufficient to found liability) is dealt with in cl 49(3). 'Act' in this section includes an omission only where the offence intended is capable of being committed by an omission. The example given by the Law Commission (Law Com. No. 177, 1989, 168–169) is this:

> D has custody of P, her mentally handicapped child by her divorced husband. E moves in to live with D and P. The police visit the home some weeks later and find P emaciated and very ill. D and E confess that, hoping P would die, they agreed not to feed P or to call medical attention when P fell ill. Murder is an offence capable of being committed by an omission; therefore an attempt to commit murder by omission is within the scope of the section. D would have a duty to feed and obtain medical care for her child; if her failure to discharge this duty was more than merely preparatory to the causing of death she would be guilty. E would also be guilty, either as a principal if he owed a similar duty himself or as an accessory to D's offence.

Clause 49(4) restates s 4(3) of the 1981 Act about the roles of judge and jury. Attempt to conspire becomes an offence again (as does incitement to conspire). Clause 49(5) restates s 1(4)(c) of the Act. Clause 49(6) is in part the same as s 1(4)(b) but is clearer and enacts *Dunnington* [1984] QB 472, above. The Law Commission stated (at 245) that '[a] charge of attempt to attempt would of course be inept'. Accordingly one cannot attempt to be a secondary party but one can be a secondary party to an attempt. The crime of attempt to conspire, which was abolished in 1981, would be resurrected. Impossibility is no defence to all inchoate offences (cl 50). The difficult language in s 1(2) and (3) would be simplified. Jurisdiction is dealt with in cl 52.

The latest set of proposals from the Law Commission is found in Consultation Paper No. 183, 2007, *Conspiracy and Attempts*. In respect of attempts the Commission proposes to abolish the current offence found in s 1(1) of the Criminal Attempts Act 1981 and to replace it with two offences, one of 'attempt', which would be restricted to the accused's last acts, and 'criminal preparation', which would cover behaviour which was part of the execution of his plan: the accused was still only preparing to commit the substantive offence but had proceeded beyond the stage of mere preparation. The mental element for both offences would be intent to commit the full offence and with regard to consequences (if any) but recklessness as to circumstances. The aim is not to extend liability but to clarify the law.

The proposals may be encapsulated thus. First, in respect of the actus reus, the Commission was concerned that the courts had struggled to draw the line between 'merely preparatory' and 'more than merely preparatory' conduct and instanced *Geddes*, above, as an example of where the courts had gone wrong. The Commission puts the result down to the wording of s 1(1) in that 'attempt' seems to imply 'trying' – the accused is not to be convicted unless the attempt is 'complete or all-but complete' (para. 1.77). Having two offences would get round the problem of definition found in cases such as *Geddes*. There should be a list of examples in the forthcoming Report which would fall within the proposed offence of criminal preparation but these would not appear in the legislation: see para. 12.39 for the illustrations and para. 16.40 for the proposal not to include the list in the legislation, though the Commission was open to persuasion (para. 16.47) as to whether the legislation should include a list of examples. Secondly, it should be made clear that if the substantive offence may be committed by an omission, so can the attempt to omit that offence. Thirdly, in respect of the fault element there should be intent (defined as in *Woollin* [1999] 1 AC 82) as to conduct and consequences but (subjective) recklessness as to circumstances. Similar fault elements are proposed for conspiracy. Fourthly, under the Criminal Attempts Act 1981, s 4(3), see above, the judge has to rule whether the accused did commit a 'more than merely preparatory' act but then the jury has to be instructed to answer the same question! The Commission proposes to revise the law so that the judge in the normal fashion rules whether the accused's behaviour could in law constitute an attempt but the jury holds whether or not that conduct did in fact constitute an attempt. Fifthly, the rule that there is no offence of attempting to commit a summary offence is seen as an 'anomaly' (para. 1.87) to be abrogated. This proposal would apply not just to the proposed attempt crime but also the proposed offence of criminal preparation. Sixthly, in relation of crimes of double inchoateness (e.g. attempting to conspire and conspiring to attempt) the Commission recommends the reversal of s 1(4)(a) of the 1981 Act: there should be a crime of attempting or criminally preparing to commit a statutory conspiracy. However, since the law would catch activities 'very remote' (para. 1.98) from the commission of offences, the Commission is open to consultees' proposing a defence of 'acting reasonably'.

Summary

This chapter on inchoate offences forms the last of those which deal with general topics. The remainder of the book considers specific offences such as murder, theft and rape. 'Inchoate' offences mean ones where the alleged principal offender has not yet committed the full offence such as murder (cf. secondary participation, where the full offence has been committed). Anglo-Welsh law has three such offences: incitement, conspiracy and attempt. Incitement, a common law offence, consists of the accused's persuading or encouraging the principal offender to commit a crime (it will become a statutory offence on the coming into force of the Serious Crime Act 2007); conspiracy, which has two forms, statutory (contrary to the Criminal Law Act 1977) and common law, exists where two or more offenders agree to commit conduct which constitutes an offence; attempt, a crime contrary to the Criminal Attempts Act 1981, occurs where the accused has embarked on behaviour which will lead to the principal offence being committed – the law demands that the defendant has committed a 'more than merely preparatory' act. All three offences have difficult issues attached to them. What is the mental element in incitement? What is the *actus reus* in conspiracy? Why does conspiracy to defraud continue to exist at common law? When can it be said that the accused has performed a 'more than merely preparatory act'? A problem which underlies the law of all three offences is whether the accused may be guilty of one of them when the crime is one which it is impossible to accomplish. A policy issue, again underlying all three offences, is: should the accused be convicted when the principal offence has not been committed? The proposals for reform are discussed after each inchoate offence.

- Incitement: this is a common law crime which is concerned with soliciting or encouraging people to commit offences. The mental element remains, even after recent cases, controversial but the position being moved towards is that the *mens rea* consists of the intention to produce the consequences (e.g. intention that the principal offender will kill) and knowledge of the circumstances. Impossibility is a defence, perhaps surprisingly in light of legislative changes to attempt and statutory conspiracy. It should also be noted that there must be a crime incited: inciting a 'non-crime' is not the offence of incitement. The offence of incitement will be abolished and replaced by a new offence on the coming into force of the Serious Crime Act 2007.

- Conspiracy: almost all conspiracies are statutory ones contrary to s 1(1) of the Criminal Law Act 1977 as amended. The principal exception is conspiracy to defraud. Impossibility is not a defence to statutory conspiracy, but is to the common law variety. The *actus reus* is an agreement to commit an offence and the *mens rea* is the intent to play a part in the prohibited conduct (according to the HL in **Anderson** [1986] AC 27), intention to carry out the crime and the mental element specified in the crime agreed on. The need for two parties has led to non-liability for conspiracy where the accused has reached an agreement to commit an offence with the company he or she controls, with a spouse and with a person such as a child or one who is insane.

- Attempt: the law is laid down in the Criminal Attempts Act 1981. The *actus reus* is a more than merely preparatory act; the *mens rea* is the intent to commit the full offence. There is no crime of attempting to commit a summary offence unless Parliament has stated otherwise. Impossibility is not a defence.

References

Reports

Criminal Law Revision Committee 15th Report, *Sexual Offences*, Cmnd 9213 (1984)

Home Office Consultation Paper, *Fraud Law Reform* (2005)

Law Commission Consultation Paper no. 131, *Assisting and Encouraging Crime* (1993)

Law Commission Report no. 76, *Conspiracy and Criminal Law Reform* (1976)

Law Commission Report no. 102, *Attempt, and Impossibility in Relation to Attempt, Conspiracy and Incitement* (1980)

Law Commission Report no. 143, *Criminal Law: Codification of the Criminal Law – A Report to the Law Commission* (1985)

Law Commission Report no. 177, *A Criminal Code for England & Wales* (1989)

Law Commission Report no. 180, *Jurisdiction over Offences of Fraud and Dishonesty with a Foreign Element* (1989)

Law Commission Report no. 228, *Criminal Law: Conspiracy to Defraud* (1994)

Law Commission Report no. 276, *Fraud* (2002)

Law Commission Report no. 300, *Inchoate Liability for Assisting and Encouraging Crime* (2006)

Law Commission Working Paper no. 50, *Codification of the Criminal Law: General Principles, Complicity, and Liability for the Acts of Another* (1973)

Law Commission Working Paper no. 104, *Conspiracy to Defraud* (1988)

Model Penal Code (1962)

National Commission on Federal Criminal Laws *A Proposed New Federal Criminal Code* (1971)

Books

Card, R., Cross, P. and Jones, P. A. *Criminal Law* 14th edn (Butterworths, 1998, and (17th edn), Oxford University Press, 2006)

Fletcher, G. *Rethinking Criminal Law* (Little, Brown & Co., 1978)

Ryan, C. *Criminal Law* 4th edn (Blackstone, 1995)

Smith, J. C. and Hogan, B. *Criminal Law* (ed. D. Ormerod) 11th edn (Oxford University Press, 2005)

Journals

Ashworth, A. 'Criminal attempts and the role of resulting harm under the Code and in the common law' (1988) 19 Rutgers LJ 725

Virgo, G. 'Reckless attempts – rape and circumstance' [1990] CLJ 390

Williams, G. 'Intents in the alternative' [1991] CLJ 120

Williams, G. 'Wrong turnings on the law of attempt' [1991] Crim LR 416

Further reading

Dennis, I. 'The rationale of criminal conspiracy' (1977) 93 LQR 39

Duff, R. A. 'The circumstances of an attempt' [1991] CLJ 100

Duff, R. A. 'Attempts and the problem of the missing circumstance' (1991) 42 NILQ 87

Duff, R. A. 'Recklessness in attempts (again)' (1995) 15 OJLS 309. See also R. A. Duff, *Criminal Attempts* (OUP, 1996).

Husak, D. 'The nature and justifiability of nonconsummate offenses' (1995) 37 Ariz LR 151

Johnson, P. E. 'The unnecessary crime of complicity' (1973) 61 Col LR 1137

Katyal, N. K. 'Complicity theory' (2003) 112 Yale LJ 1307

Robbins, I. P. 'Double inchoate crimes' (1989) 26 Harv JL 1

Rogers, J. 'The codification of attempts and the case for "preparation"' [2008] Crim LR 937

Smith, J. C. 'Conspiracy to defraud: Some comments on the Law Commission's Report' [1995] Crim LR 209

Smith, K. J. M. 'Proximity in attempt: Lord Lane's "midway course"' [1991] Crim LR 576

Stannard, J. 'Making up for the missing element: a sideways look at attempts' (1987) 7 LS 194

Sullivan, G. R. 'Inchoate liability for assisting and encouraging crime' – the Law Commission Report Crim [2006] LR 1047

Virgo, G. 'Laundering conspiracy' [2006] CLJ 482

Williams, G. 'Intents in the alternative' [1991] CLJ 120

Williams, G. 'Wrong turnings on the law of attempt' [1991] Crim LR 416

For conspiracy to defraud, see A. T. H. Smith, *Property Offences* (Sweet & Maxwell, 1994), ch. 19.

For a recent Irish view, see Law Reform Commission (2008) Consultation Paper No. 48, *Inchoate Offences*.

Visit **www.mylawchamber.co.uk/jefferson** to access exam-style questions with answer guidance, multiple choice quizzes, live weblinks, an online glossary, and regular updates to the law.

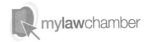 mylawchamber

Use **Case Navigator** to read in full some of the key cases referenced in this chapter:

R v *Cunningham* [1957] 2 All ER 412
R v *G* [2003] 4 All ER 765
R v *White* [1910] 2 KB 124
R v *Woollin* [1998] 4 All ER 103

Part 3

Particular offences

11

Murder

If the accused kills someone who has been born alive, one or more of the following crimes may occur: murder, manslaughter, causing death by dangerous driving, infanticide or genocide. These offences are generally called 'homicide', but that word is not a term of art in English law. People are charged with murder, not with homicide. A killing may not always constitute a crime, and one must be careful that not too much is swept up into manslaughter, especially the gross negligence form, discussed later. Murder and manslaughter are distinguished by a difference in the state of mind of the accused at the time of killing (Fig. 11.1). In both offences he has caused someone's death. Murder is a more serious crime than manslaughter because to be guilty of it he must have intended to kill or commit grievous bodily harm, whereas a lesser (which means 'less blameworthy') state of mind suffices for manslaughter. The difference resides in morality: the murderer is more morally culpable than a person guilty of manslaughter.

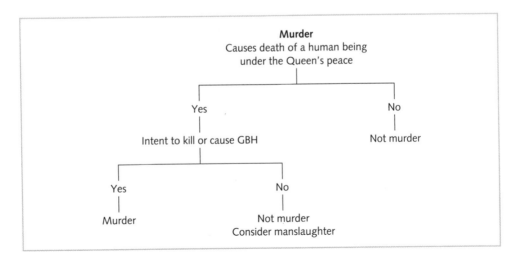

Figure 11.1 Murder

General introduction

Most murders arise out of quarrels, jealousy, arguments over money and robbery. Many murders are committed against persons from the accused's family or friends and the killing often takes place in the home of the victim or killer. Indeed, the age category into which more victims fall than any other is being aged under one: C. Flood-Page and J. Turner (eds), *Crime in England and Wales 2001/2002*, Home Office, 2003. Most are committed by men, but victims are more or less evenly divided among males and females. In 2001–02 46 per cent of female victims of homicide were killed by their former partner. See the Home Office's *Criminal Statistics*, published annually. However, vastly more men than women are killed; 73 per cent of victims in 2001–02 were males. See Flood-Page and Turner, above, at p. 3. In 1987 there were 687 deaths from murder, manslaughter and infanticide. In 1990, 116 people were convicted of manslaughter, 107 of the types of manslaughter discussed in Chapter 12 and three of infanticide. In 1992 of 5.6 million crimes notified to the police, 689 were for murder, manslaughter and infanticide. The number of homicides per annum did not vary much throughout the 1990s, being around 600 per year. In 1999–2000 there were 761. The figures for 2002–03 were 1,048 homicides, an increase of 18 per cent on the previous year, but including 172 killings by Dr Harold Shipman.

There were 859 homicides in 2004–05. The risk to the general population in 2001 was 15 per million, rising to 82 per million for children under one: see the Home Office's annual *Criminal Statistics*. Overseas readers, especially those in US cities, may wish to compare this level with that in their home towns.

The definition of murder

Parliament has not defined murder. There have been several calls for placing murder on a statutory footing. For example, the (Nathan) *Report of the Select Committee of the House of Lords on Murder and Life Imprisonment* (HL Paper 78–1) made such a call in 1989. Despite such calls, the definition is left to the common law. The task is left for judges, who mostly adopt and adapt the definition of Chief Justice Coke from the early seventeenth century (3 Co Inst 47):

> Murder is when a man of sound memory and of the age of discretion unlawfully killeth . . . any reasonable creature *in rerum natura* under the King's peace, with malice aforethought, either expressed by the party or implied by law, so as the party wounded or hurt etc., die of the wound or hurt etc. . . . .

(a) The phrase 'any reasonable creature' means a human being. It is thought that persons born without heads are protected.

(b) '*In rerum natura*' is translated as 'in being'. Accordingly one cannot murder an unborn person, even if that foetus could have survived had it been born naturally; one can murder only a child who is born alive and fully extruded from the mother, though the law, being based on nineteenth-century cases, is not pellucid. Apparently there is no need for the child to breathe, and the umbilical cord need not be cut or the afterbirth expelled. The principal English authorities are pre-Victorian and may require reconsideration in the light of modern science. Nevertheless, they were followed by the New South Wales Court of Criminal Appeal in *Iby* [2005] NSWCCA

178. The accused drove a stolen car at excessive speed and collided head-on with a woman who was 38 weeks pregnant. An emergency caesarean was performed and the baby had a heartbeat and was put on the ventilator but he had no (or little) electrical activity in the brain and by two hours after birth there was no heartbeat, the court held that the baby had been born alive and therefore could be the subject of a manslaughter charge. Though there was no one definition of being 'born alive'. The child had an existence independent of its mother, both as to breathing and as to heartbeat, and it was irrelevant that the heartbeat had been sustained mechanically. The case examines and applies the English authorities.

The Infant Life (Preservation) Act 1929 created the offence of child destruction to deal with killing before the definition of murder could be satisfied. It is an offence wilfully to cause the death of a child who is capable of being born alive at any time before he obtains an independent existence. It is a defence to prove that the act was done in good faith for the preservation of the mother's life. The Fourteenth Report of the Criminal Law Revision Committee, *Offences Against The Person*, Cmnd 7844, 1980, adopted the test that 'the victim should have been born and have an existence independent of its mother' (para 35). Before that the 1929 Act would apply; after that the law of homicide would.

In *Attorney-General's Reference (No. 3 of 1994)* [1998] AC 245 the accused was charged with the murder of a child. While the child was a foetus, the accused had stabbed the mother in the abdomen. He knew that the woman was pregnant. The child was born prematurely because of the injury and died six months after birth. The trial judge ruled that there was no *actus reus* for murder (or manslaughter) because a foetus was not a live person protected by the law of murder, and that there was no *mens rea* towards the foetus: the defendant intended to wound the mother, and malice towards her could not be transferred to the foetus because it was not a live person protected by the homicide law. Therefore, according to the trial judge, there was no crime. The Court of Appeal disagreed and would have convicted of murder. The House of Lords in turn disagreed with the Court of Appeal and would have found the accused guilty of manslaughter. Lord Mustill said that the Court of Appeal was wrong to hold that a foetus is part of the mother and therefore that an intent to injure the mother is an intent to injure the foetus. 'The mother and the foetus were two distinct organisms living symbiotically, not a single organism with two aspects.' Moreover, a foetus does not share human personality with its mother: it is an organism in and of itself, not part of the mother. Accordingly, when the accused acts without intent to injure the foetus, the intent to injure the mother seriously cannot be transferred from the mother to the foetus, and then from the foetus to the child, who is born alive but later dies as a result of the attack on the mother. Therefore, the accused could not be guilty of murder. He was, however, guilty of constructive manslaughter (see Chapter 12), because for that crime the unlawful and dangerous act can be a risk to anyone including a woman carrying a foetus, and that law applies whether or not the accused knew that she was pregnant.

See Figure 12.3 in Chapter 12 for a diagram illustrating constructive (unlawful act) manslaughter.

There are difficulties integrating the offences of child destruction (and procuring a miscarriage contrary to s 58 of the Offences Against the Person Act 1861) with murder and manslaughter. If, as in the *Reference* case, the accused tries to kill the foetus, the child is born but then dies from its injuries, he may be guilty of murder or manslaughter. However, if the foetus is killed in the womb, murder and manslaughter are not applicable and the charge is one of child destruction (or procuring a miscarriage).

A conjoined twin is a human being even though he has 'a useless brain, a useless heart and useless lungs': *Re A* [2001] Fam 147 (CA).

A human clone would presumably be a creature *in rerum natura*.

(c) 'Under the King's peace' exempts from liability those who kill active enemy aliens in time of war; it remains murder, however, to kill prisoners of war. It may well be that killing rebels against the Crown is also not murder.

(d) Malice aforethought is the mental element in murder and is dealt with separately below.

(e) For both murder and manslaughter it was until recently a rule of English law (though not of Scotland, of European Union member states, or of some parts of the Commonwealth) that the death must occur within a year and a day, even though it could otherwise be said that the accused caused the victim's death. This rule was abrogated by the Law Reform (Year and a Day Rule) Act 1996. For discussion see below.

(f) Murder or manslaughter by a citizen of the UK or colonies is triable in England and Wales, even if the crime was committed outside England, and a killing by a non-British citizen on a British ship or aircraft is triable in England. One effect of this rule should be noted. Because of it, the rule about killing persons not under the Queen's peace is needed; otherwise UK citizens who killed enemy aliens in battle abroad would be guilty of murder in England and Wales.

(g) Coke's definition has the term 'unlawfully' in it. For that reason the law of murder demonstrates that the sanctity of life is not always upheld and the following are not murder:

   (i) execution carried out by the person whose duty it is and in the manner appointed;

   (ii) killing by an officer of justice in the execution of his duty to arrest, search or seize property, provided that the force was necessary to protect himself and execute his duty; a private person helping such an officer will also not be guilty;

   (iii) killing by a citizen effecting a lawful arrest and using reasonable force;

   (iv) killing by a person using force to prevent a crime;

   (v) killing by a person using reasonable force to prevent trespass to land or goods (this is questionable because in the modern era it is difficult to justify or excuse the killing of a human being in order to preserve property.);

   (vi) killing as a result of lawful chastisement;

   (vii) killing as a result of a lawful operation.

(h) The width of the definition should be noted. It covers, for example, both terrorists who set out to kill as many people as possible and mercy-killers. Mercy-killers are murderers, but those who drive recklessly and cause a crash in which many people die are not: reasonable people may disagree as to who is more blameworthy.

The sentence for murder

... the gradations of culpability in the crime of murder are almost as infinite as the variations in the human psyche itself. (Keane CJ 'Murder – the mental element' (2002) 53 NILQ 1, 8)

The sentence for murder must be life imprisonment. In 1995 there were 238 convictions for murder, the highest total ever. Figures show that the average time served for those released in 1992 was 12.5 years, a substantial increase on 1988 when it was 10.1 years. These are averages. The actual time spent in prison varies tremendously. The case of **Cocker** [1989] Crim LR 740 is discussed below under provocation. The accused was convicted of murder of his terminally ill wife. He served four years. The Moors murderers served over 30 years in prison before Myra Hindley died in November 2002.

The House of Lords in **Lichniak** [2003] 1 AC 903 held that the indeterminate life sentence was not contrary to Article 3 (inhuman or degrading treatment) or Article 5 (right to liberty) of the European Convention on Human Rights.

In a parliamentary debate on the subject, on 25 June 1991, the House of Commons overturned a House of Lords majority in favour of giving the judges discretion as to sentence. The then Home Secretary supported the life sentence on the ground that the seriousness of murder had to be marked out, while gradations in the type of killing could be dealt with by varying the amount of time actually spent in prison serving the mandatory life sentence: a mercy-killer would serve less than a sadistic murderer. The Opposition thought that the sentence should be determined by the judge, not by the Executive, which after all is what happens in other offences; the judge has seen the demeanour of the accused during the trial but the Executive has not; and sentences should not be determined and given behind closed doors. Giving judges discretion would also alleviate one problem: duress is not a defence to murder, but if a life sentence was no longer compulsory, duress could be taken into account in the sentence. Similarly, the battered spouse whose reaction is not quick enough for provocation could have a determinate sentence. Moreover, the difference between murder and another offence may depend on fortuitous circumstances such as a doctor being at hand; and in respect of attempted murder only an intent to kill will suffice, yet in murder itself the mental element also covers an intent to commit grievous bodily harm; in terms of *mens rea* attempted murder can be more serious than murder, but only the latter crime attracts a mandatory sentence. As Lord Hailsham, the former Lord Chancellor, put it in **Howe** [1987] AC 417 in the House of Lords:

> [m]urder . . . , though often described as one of the [crimes of] utmost heinousness, is not in fact necessarily so, but consists in a whole bundle of offences of vastly differing degrees of culpability, ranging from brutal, cynical and repeated offences like the so-called Moors murders to the almost venial, if objectively immoral, 'mercy killing' of a beloved partner.

A survey of public attitudes about the mandatory life sentence was conducted by Professor Barry Mitchell and published by the Law Commission as part of its Report No. 290, *Partial Defences to Murder*, 2004. Paragraph 2.35 states: 'The notion that all murders, as the law is presently framed, represent instances of a uniquely heinous offence for which a single uniquely severe penalty is justified does not reflect the views of a cross-section of the public when asked to reflect on particular cases.' This survey of public opinion is reflected in the views of consultees on the Consultation Paper, also called *Partial Defences to Murder*, No. 173, 2003. However, some groups such as Support after Murder and Manslaughter support the mandatory sentence.

The Nathan Report, *Report of the Select Committee of the House of Lords on Murder and Life Imprisonment*, 1989, recommended that the mandatory life sentence for murder should be abolished. The judge should have a discretion in order that he can take into account the many forms of murder. The government rejected this proposal. An amendment to a Bill which would have made the sentence discretionary failed in 1991. No change is likely for the next few years, despite the Human Rights Act 1998. The then Home Secretary said that arguments of deterrence and retribution supported the mandatory sentence and by murdering the accused had forfeited his liberty to the state and it should therefore be the state which decided on release. The current government said in 1997 that it would not abolish the mandatory sentence. However, in a leaked memo reported in *The Guardian*, 11 July 2000, the Prime Minister is reported as suggesting that a senior judge should report on whether the life sentence should remain mandatory in the light of the conviction for murder of Tony Martin who shot a teenage burglar dead at his isolated farm. However, nothing was done. Pressure for reform has been expressed elsewhere and Lord Mustill said in *Powell*; *English* [1998] AC 147 that England and Wales 'need a new law of homicide, or a new law of punishment for homicide, or preferably both'. Since the judges could not alter the law, he called for parliamentary intervention, but noted that a change in the law may not be popular. However, one straw in the wind was a prematurely released Home Office press release in 2004 which said that a revised law of murder had to be 'clear, comprehensive and fair', and surely it is not fair to sentence terrorists and mercy-killers to the same length of imprisonment.

The death sentence for murder was completely abolished in 1965. In 1998 the United Kingdom ratified the Sixth Protocol to the European Convention, by which execution in peacetime is prohibited and the Crime and Disorder Act 1998 abolished the death penalty for piracy and treason. The only way of restoring the death penalty would be to revise the Human Rights Act 1998.

Death

There is no accepted definition of death in homicide cases: is it when the heart and breathing stop or is it brain-death? Certainly people whose heart has stopped and whose breathing has ceased have been revived. Probably, if the judges had to choose, they would select brain-death. This definition means that the brain stem has ceased to function with the result that reflex actions, in particular circulation of the blood and breathing, have ceased to function. If so, an accused who decapitated a brain-dead person would not be guilty of murder, even though the victim is 'breathing' by means of a ventilator. Three Law Lords accepted this definition (apparently) *obiter* in *Airedale NHS Trust v Bland* [1993] AC 789 and there is authority from a lower court to the same effect: *Re A (a Minor)* [1992] 3 Med LR 303. A person in a persistent vegetative state is not brain-dead. Presumably therefore someone in a deep coma is also not dead. One who is not brain-dead but who is on a ventilator can be the subject of homicide, as *Malcherek* [1981] 2 All ER 422 (CA) demonstrates. The Criminal Law Revision Committee in its Fourteenth Report, *Offences Against the Person*, Cmnd 7844, 1980, recommended that there should not be a statutory definition of death because it might become out of date through improvements in medical technology.

For causation, see Chapter 2.

For an explanation of causation, see Chapter 2. This is illustrated in Figure 2.1 on p 52.

Abolition of the Year-and-a-Day Rule

The Law Commission in 1995 recommended the abolition of the year-and-a-day rule, which was arbitrary in its effect (Report No. 230, *The Year and a Day Rule in Homicide*). A Bill was attached to the Report, and it was enacted as the Law Reform (Year and a Day Rule) Act 1996. The Act applies to cases where the act or omission causing death occurred on or after 17 June 1996. The year-and-a-day rule came increasingly under attack both for not being in accord with modern medical science and for reducing the nature of the crime in a fortuitous way. If the victim died within a year, the crime was one of the homicide offences. If he died a year and two days after the attack, it was not, yet the survival for slightly longer in the second instance than the first may be dependent on factors such as the use of a ventilator, outside the control both of victim and accused. The Law Commission opined (at para 3.19) that 'it is wrong that a defendant should be charged with an offence which does not properly reflect the consequences of his conduct merely because his victim happens to survive for more than 366 days'. Sentences lower than would otherwise be the case are imposed. The law also meant that offenders were incorrectly labelled and sentenced. The Law Commission received a petition requesting abolition of the rule and noted a case from Darlington: the attacker could be convicted only of inflicting grievous bodily harm and was sentenced to two years' imprisonment.

Another problem was that the rule permitted the accused to escape liability where he had infected the victim with a long-term illness such as AIDS. Furthermore, if the victim of what would otherwise be manslaughter by gross negligence survived for longer than a year and a day, the accused could not be found guilty of any crime because there is no non-fatal gross negligence offence. Various Australian states such as Victoria have abolished the rule: Crimes (Year-and-a-Day Rule) Act 1991, s 3. The sole Australian state to preserve the rule is Queensland, but the Criminal Code Review Committee recommended its abolition.

The argument that the rule prevented prosecutions long after the attack is ill-founded. Persons are prosecuted many years after they have killed, an obvious instance being Frederick West, the Gloucester builder. If there is no time limit for homicide in this sense, why should there have been one in relation to the gap between the attack and the killing? It might be argued that a person who is convicted for a non-fatal offence should not be retried for a fatal offence on the ground of double jeopardy, but the situation does occur when the victim dies before a year and a day. The fact that the death happened after that period does not affect the issue. The judge may stop the trial if there is an abuse of process, which there might be if the trial is many years after the events giving rise to the offence.

In light of these criticisms, the Law Reform (Year and a Day Rule) Act 1996 abolished the rule for all offences. The Attorney-General's consent (which will be refused if the prosecution is oppressive) is required when the death occurred more than three years after the injury or when the accused had been convicted of another offence in connection with the injury. The offence will normally be a non-fatal offence but could, for example, be burglary. The Law Commission in Report No. 230 proposed that the first exception, which relates to death more than three years after the injury, is to protect the accused in situations where his memory may not be reliable or where evidence has disappeared but this exception does not apply to other offences where memory may have become defective or evidence may have disappeared.

Malice aforethought

In human affairs we are always concerned with probabilities rather than certainties. The difference between intention and recklessness is the difference between a virtual (or moral) certainty and a high probability (Lord Edmund-Davies in **MPC v Caldwell** [1982] AC 341 at 359).

The mental element in murder is:

(a) the intention to kill;

(b) the intention to cause grievous bodily harm.

The House of Lords in **Cunningham** [1982] AC 566 settled a dispute as to whether the second form was indeed an alternative mental element. To say that intent is the fault element for murder is, therefore, only partly true, for an intent to frighten, say, is insufficient. In respect of both intention and recklessness, the harm required for the offence to be consummated must be stated. One can extend the formulation of the mental element, also known as malice aforethought, in this way: the accused must intend to kill, or cause grievous bodily harm to, a human being, knowing or perhaps only foreseeing that the victim is under the Queen's Peace. As is general in criminal law, motive is no defence, but there may be a defence such as provocation. Malice aforethought is a legal term of art. It is not necessary that the accused acted spitefully or gave much thought to the killing. Intention does not require a plan. A fleeting state of mind suffices.

That these two forms of *mens rea* were the sole ones was affirmed by the House of Lords in **Moloney**.

Moloney [1985] AC 905

The accused and victim had been celebrating the ruby wedding anniversary of the accused's grandparents. The victim was the accused's stepfather. They had both been drinking heavily. The victim claimed that, even with his crippled arm, he could outload, outdraw and outshoot the accused. They put the claim to the test. Unfortunately for the victim the accused won, and blew off the victim's head with a twelve-bore shotgun. The accused said that he had no idea that by shooting the gun, he would injure his stepfather. He was convicted of murder. The House of Lords allowed his appeal but substituted a conviction for manslaughter (on the grounds of gross negligence or recklessness) for there was no doubt in the mind of Lord Bridge that the accused acted with 'a high degree of recklessness'. The case was remitted for sentence to the Court of Appeal, and an immediate release was ordered.

Morally conduct committed intentionally should be punished more severely than recklessly committed behaviour. For this reason a sharp line should be drawn between intention and recklessness.

The European Convention on Human Rights, Article 2(1), protects persons from being intentionally deprived of life. Brooke and Walker LJJ in **Re A** [2001] Fam 147, a civil case concerning surgical separation of conjoined twins, said that doctors did not kill 'intentionally' when they knew that the separation would cause the death of one of the twins within minutes, because they acted to save the life of the other twin, her life before separation being shortened by her twin. 'Intentionally' therefore covers only 'direct intent' (see Chapter 3), not oblique intent.

See Chapter 3 for a definition of intent.

 ## The intention to cause grievous bodily harm

As stated above, the present law holds that this head of malice aforethought exists, and the House of Lords said in **Moloney** and **Attorney-General's Reference (No. 3 of 1994)** that any amendment was for Parliament. The law was laid down in **Cunningham** [1982] AC 566, see 'Malice aforethought' above, where the accused hit his victim, who was lying defenceless on the floor, over the head with a chair. He argued that he had only 'implied malice', that is he only intended to cause grievous bodily harm, and that the head of malice aforethought no longer existed. Lord Hailsham said:

(a) The Homicide Act 1957 did not abolish implied malice. Two cases to that effect, *Vickers* [1957] 2 QB 664 and *Hyam v DPP* [1975] AC 55 were approved.

(b) The test for proving intent is subjective, as the Criminal Justice Act 1967, s 8, laid down. On this point also *Hyam* was approved.

(c) 'Grievous bodily harm' meant 'really serious bodily harm', as the House of Lords had held in *DPP v Smith* [1961] AC 290, above, and the Court of Criminal Appeal had determined in *Metharam* [1961] 3 All ER 200 (though the modern approach is to drop 'really' where there is no doubt that the injury was serious (see *Janjua* [1999] 1 Cr App R 91 where it was said that 'really' might be required in some cases but normally it was not and it was definitely not required when the accused had used a 5$\frac{1}{2}$ inch sharp knife with which the victim had been killed); *Saunders* [1985] Crim LR 230 (CA) where the victim suffered a broken nose and cuts).

(d) *Vickers* as endorsed by *Smith* was correct as to the definition of grievous bodily harm. It did not mean endangering life as the dissentients had stated in *Hyam*. Moreover, the test of intent to cause serious harm was not too difficult for a jury, and changing it to intent to endanger life would not facilitate the jury's task.

The House of Lords refused to use their *Practice Statement* on precedent to overrule *Smith* on this point, for (a) their power to overrule their previous cases must be used sparingly, especially in the criminal law; (b) to rule otherwise would mean that some people including Vickers had been wrongfully hanged; (c) such a change is too great for the judges and should be left for Parliament. Accordingly, murder remains what might be called a crime of 'half *mens rea*': the defendant's *actus reus* is killing, but his *mens rea* need not be that. He is guilty if he intended to commit grievous bodily harm. For example, in *Middleton*, unreported, 11 March 1999, the defendants attacked their victim with their fists and feet. The Court of Appeal held that the jury were entitled to find that they intended (at least) serious harm.

The arguments in favour of the rule are that whether death results when the accused intended to commit grievous bodily harm may depend on chance (such as proximity of an accident and emergency unit) and that there is insufficient moral distinction between one who intends to kill and one who intends to cause grievous bodily harm. Lord Edmund-Davies said that the result of causing serious harm was so unpredictable that the person who inflicted it deserved to be called a murderer if the victim died because he had acted 'wickedly'. The minority in *Cunningham* strongly criticised this result. Lord Edmund-Davies thought it 'strange that a person can be convicted of murder if death results from, say, his intentional breaking of another's arm, an action which . . . would in most cases be unlikely to kill'. There is also the argument contrary to the one noted above, that there is a moral difference between the two forms of intent. Lord Mustill in *Attorney-General's Reference (No. 3 of 1994)* [1998] AC 245 criticised the fact that intent to cause grievous bodily harm was part of malice aforethought. The Law Commission in one of its first reports, *Imputed Criminal Intent (DPP v Smith)*, No. 10, 1967, argued in favour of changing current law.

(a) Murder is commonly understood to mean the intentional killing of another human being; and, unless there are strong reasons which justify a contrary course, it is generally desirable that legal terms should correspond with their popular meaning.

(b) To limit intent in murder to the intent to kill is not to disregard the very serious nature of causing death by the infliction of grievous bodily harm, but . . . if such an offence were to be treated as manslaughter only, it could nevertheless be punished by a maximum penalty as severe as the penalty prescribed for murder . . .

(d) . . . [A] man should not be regarded as a murderer if he does not *know* that the bodily harm which he intends to inflict is likely to kill.

The proposed reform dealt with in the previous section would not abolish this head of *mens rea*, but narrow it slightly.

It may be noted that this head of *mens rea* may not always be correctly applied. Barry Mitchell found a case where the accused had gagged a victim, who died. The accused was convicted of murder, but doubt must remain whether the defendant did intend to cause serious harm. The intent seems to have been to incapacitate: 'Distinguishing between murder and manslaughter' [1991] NLJ 935. Accordingly, even if the law were tightly defined, the jurors might let their feelings lead to the conviction of the 'bad' person and acquit the 'good'. The same point can be made in relation to provocation and the prosecution of terrorists for murder.

One point of interest is that when Parliament overrode **DPP v Smith** in relation to the presumption that a person intends the natural consequences of his conduct so that he is no longer taken to have the intention to commit murder when he killed someone, it was given the opportunity to abolish another part of **DPP v Smith**, namely that implied malice had survived the enactment of the Homicide Act 1957. The Law Commission Report *Imputed Criminal Intent (**DPP v Smith**)*, 1967, was partly enacted in the Criminal Justice Act 1967, s 8. Another part was not. The Commission recommended (para 18): 'So long as a distinction between murder and manslaughter is to be maintained, there must be a defensible criterion for distinguishing between them. In our view the essential element in murder should be willingness to kill, thereby evincing a total lack of respect for human life.' But Parliament's rejection of the proposal shows that it did not wish to remove the intent to commit grievous bodily harm from malice aforethought.

The Fourteenth Report of the Criminal Law Revision Committee, *Offences Against the Person*, Cmnd 7844, 1980, para 31, supported the Law Commission's 1967 proposal, as did the draft Criminal Code, Law Com. Report No. 177, 1989. Clause 54(1) is quoted above.

Retaining the offence of murder

Lord Kilbrandon in **Hyam v DPP** [1975] AC 55 was the main proponent of the view that murder and manslaughter should be amalgamated to form a crime of unlawful homicide in respect of which the judge would have a discretion as to sentencing. Only on the most heinous facts would the accused receive life imprisonment. This reform would receive the support of those involved in or supporting euthanasia. The defences of provocation, diminished responsibility and killing in pursuance of a suicide pact, which reduce murder to manslaughter, could be abolished. The argument against is that there should be marked a category for those particularly serious killers, and the crime of murder, perhaps with the deletion of the intent to cause grievous bodily harm, reflects that moral distinction. This principle is sometimes known as 'fair labelling'. Murder is a well-established term with moral connotations, and the public accepts that murderers should be distinguished from those who are guilty of less blameworthy homicides. There is a vast difference between the contract-killer and a person who kills through gross negligence. The former deserves to be called a murderer and be stigmatised, whereas the latter does not. Decisions on issues such as whether the killing was grave or not should be for juries, not for judges.

Murder, manslaughter and infanticide

The Law Commission Report *Murder, Manslaughter and Infanticide* No. 306 of November 2006 is a follow-up to the Consultation Paper (CP) No. 177, *A New Homicide Act for England and Wales?* December 2005. For a summary of this Paper, see the website attached to the seventh edition of this book.

'The law governing homicide . . . is a rickety structure set upon shaky foundations . . .' (para 1.8). Therefore, '. . . for the first time, the general law of homicide [must be] rationalised through legislation. Offences and defences specific to murder must take their place within a readily comprehensible and fair legal structure.' (para. 1.10) 'Although twentieth century legislation on murder brought many valuable reforms, the definitions of murder and the partial defences remain misleading, out-of-date, unfit for purpose, or all of these.' (para 1.70) There should be a new Homicide Act, replacing the 1957 version, with 'clear and comprehensive definitions of the homicide offences and the partial defences.' (para 1.63)

The main difficulties with the current definition of murder

The following are the major problems.

1 The 'serious harm' rule in murder.

   Example: 'D intentionally punches V in the face. The punch breaks V's nose and causes V to fall to the ground. In falling, V hits his or her head on the kerb causing a massive and fatal brain haemorrhage.'

   Parliament in passing the Homicide Act 1957 did not expect that the courts would construe malice aforethought so widely: see *Vickers* (1957) CCA.

   Recommendation: where D intends serious harm and was aware that the conduct posed a serious risk of death, that should be top-tier (first degree) homicide; however, where D intends serious harm but was not aware of a serious risk of death, that would be second tier homicide.

2 'The law is too generous in treating all those who realise that their conduct poses a risk of causing death but press on regardless as guilty only of manslaughter.' These killers should be guilty of top-tier homicide.

The first problem stems from murder being too wide, the second from murder being too narrow.

The principal recommendations

The outcome is a three-tier structure with the terms 'murder' and 'manslaughter' preserved. This structure is 'clearer and more intelligible, as well as being morally more defensible.' (para 2.4)

1 'first degree murder':
   (a) intentional killing e.g. contract killers: there is an intention to kill;
   (b) killing through an intention to do serious injury with an awareness of a serious risk of causing death.
   There would be a mandatory life sentence.

   This proposal differs from that in the CP where first degree murder was restricted to intentional killing. The recommendation is based on morality: some reckless killings are as heinous as intentional killings (para 2.60).

2 'second degree murder'
   (a) killing through an intention to cause serious injury (even without an awareness of a serious risk of causing death);
   (b) killing where D was aware of a serious risk of causing death coupled with an intent to cause some injury, or fear of injury or a risk of injury (this would cover the terrorist who gave insufficient warning of a bomb);
   (c) provocation;
   (d) diminished responsibility;
   (e) suicide pact.
   The concept of second degree murder would be new to Anglo-Welsh law. There would not be a mandatory life sentence for this second rank of murder: the maximum sentence would be life imprisonment. However, it must be noted that second degree murder is still 'murder' with the result for example that a successful plea of provocation would lead to a verdict of murder, admittedly in the second degree, and not as now manslaughter. In this respect second degree murder covers some who now are murderers, some who are guilty of manslaughter and some who have a successful partial defence to manslaughter. The current partial defences to murder would not lead to a verdict of manslaughter because D did kill intending to kill: such killers fall within the label of first degree murderers except for the defence (para 2.156).

   The term 'injury' would replace 'bodily harm' to ensure that psychiatric harm is covered. However, there would be no definition of 'serious' injury (para 2.94) and whether injury is serious or not would be left to the jury.

   The term 'reckless indifference' used in the CP would be replaced by (b) above.

   It should be noted that to be guilty of second degree murder, an accused who kills being aware that his or her conduct involved a serious risk of death would also have to intend to cause injury, fear of injury or risk of injury. Without that intent, D would be guilty of manslaughter. For example, an electrician who believes that she can cut corners may be aware of the risk of death but would not be guilty of second degree murder but of manslaughter because she did not intend injury or fear of injury or the risk of injury (para 2.110).

   It should be added that provocation, diminished responsibility and suicide pacts will not provide defences to second degree murder. They are to be taken into account in the sentence.

3 'manslaughter'
   (a) death caused by a criminal act intended to cause injury;
   (b) death when D was aware that the criminal act involved a serious risk of causing injury;
   (c) death where D was grossly negligent as to causing death.
   The remit of the Law Commission did not allow it to make recommendations as to manslaughter but (a) and (b) are very similar to the Government's proposals for

replacing unlawful act (or constructive) manslaughter found in the Home Office's *Reforming the Law on Involuntary Manslaughter: The Government's Proposals* (2000).

In this way there would be a 'ladder' (para 1.64) of offences.

The specific defences to murder

See Chapter 9 for more on diminished responsibility and Chapter 12 for more on provocation.

Problems with provocation and diminished responsibility are dealt with in Chapters 12 and 9 respectively. However, for the moment it is sufficient to say that the Law Commission wishes to expand the defence of provocation: for example, at present there is the restriction of sudden loss of self-control; therefore, those who kill fearing serious violence in the future have no defence. In respect of diminished responsibility, this defence, created in 1957, is based on outmoded psychiatry and should be modernised.

Additional proposal

There should be a defence of excessive self-defence when D overreacts to a threat of serious violence from an aggressor. This recommendation is dealt with in Chapter 8.

Summary

The chapters from here until the end deal with specific offences. This one is on murder, which is defined as the unlawful killing of a human being with malice aforethought. 'Unlawful' is in the definition to remind the reader that killings may be lawful as when the accused used reasonable force in self-defence or where the killing was of the enemy in wartime in the heat of battle. 'Malice aforethought' does not mean that the accused must act spitefully or with premeditation. All the phrase means is that she acted either with the intent to kill or with the intent to commit grievous bodily harm. Intent is defined in Chapter 3. Whether a person has been born or is dead is discussed because only a live human being may be murdered. The former restriction that the victim must have died within a year and a day of the accused's act is noted. The sentence for murder, the mandatory life sentence, is considered. The width of murder, particularly the fact that it may be committed when the accused intended only grievous bodily harm, is debated. Again, reference is made to possible reform, including the recommendations of the Law Commission.

- Murder: Murder is the unlawful killing of a human being under the Queen's peace with malice aforethought. 'Malice aforethought' is simply the *mens rea* of murder and comprises the intent to kill and the intent to cause grievous bodily harm (GBH). Intention is considered in Chapter 3. Death means the non-functioning of the brainstem; GBH means (really) serious bodily harm.

References

Reports

Criminal Law Revision Committee 14th Report, *Offences against the Person*, Cmnd 7844 (1980)

Home Office *Reforming the Law on Involuntary Manslaughter: The Government's Proposals* (2000)

Law Commission Consultation Paper no. 173, *Partial Defences to Murder* (2003)

Law Commission Consultation Paper no. 177, *A new Homicide Act for England & Wales?* (2005)

Law Commission Report no. 10, *Imputed Criminal Intent (DPP v Smith)* (1967)

Law Commission Report no. 177, *A Criminal Code for England & Wales* (1989)

Law Commission Report no. 230, *The Year and a Day Rule in Homicide* (1995)

Law Commission Report no. 290, *Partial Defences to Murder* (2004)

Law Commission Report no. 306, *Murder, Manslaughter and Infanticide* (2006)

Report of the Select Committee of the House of Lords on Murder and Life Imprisonment (Nathan) (1989) HL Paper 78-1

Journals

Keane, C. J. 'Murder – the mental element' (2002) 53 NILQ 1

Further reading

Ashworth, A. 'Principles, pragmatism and the Law Commission's recommendations on homicide law reform' [2007] Crim LR 333

Justice Response to Law Commission Consultation Paper No. 177, *A New Homicide Act for England and Wales?* (2006) (written by Sally Ireland)

Mitchell, B. 'Further evidence of the relationship between legal and public opinion on the homicide law' [2000] Crim LR 814

Mitchell, B. 'Distinguishing between murder and manslaughter in practice' (2007) 71 JCL 318

Rogers, J. 'The homicide ladder' (2007) 157 NLJ 48

Smith, J. C. 'A note on intention' [1990] Crim LR 85

Tadros, V. 'The homicide ladder' (2006) 69 MLR 601

Taylor, R. 'The nature of "partial defences" and the coherence of (second degree) murder' [2007] Crim LR 345

Tur, R. H. S. 'The doctor's defence and professional ethics' (2002) 13 *King's College Law Journal* 75

For an Irish approach, see *Homicide: Murder and Involuntary Manslaughter*, Law Reform Commission Report No. 87, 2008.

Visit **www.mylawchamber.co.uk/jefferson** to access exam-style questions with answer guidance, multiple choice quizzes, live weblinks, an online glossary, and regular updates to the law.

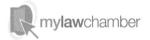

12

Manslaughter

Introduction

Manslaughter is not defined in a statute. In *Church* [1966] 1 QB 59 (CCA), Edmund Davies J was driven to say that 'there has never been a complete and satisfactory definition of manslaughter'. It acts as a sort of catch-all offence where the accused has caused death but did not have malice aforethought or has a defence to murder. Since 'murder' is a strong term and some killings are not seen to be as heinous as the archetypal murder case, the retention of a second form of criminal killing is probably a good idea. One difficulty, however, is that this offence covers a wide range of situations from killings just short of murder to carelessly causing death (Fig. 12.1). In some instances death is caused fortuitously. It is unfair to use the same label for those who kill accidentally and those whose conduct is just short of murder. The *actus reus*, death, is very serious, but the accused is guilty though his *mens rea* is substantially less than intending or foreseeing death. There is therefore no gradation in the types of manslaughter, though there is in the sentence. The maximum is life imprisonment, but the average in the 1980s was four and a half years. The average crept up in the 1990s and is now about six years. The law is not easy to state and is obscure in places.

The old classification of manslaughter was into **voluntary** and **involuntary**, the former being when the accused had the *mens rea* for murder but there is some mitigating factor, which could be provocation, diminished responsibility or killing in pursuance of a suicide pact. Involuntary manslaughter is unlawful homicide without malice aforethought.

Types of manslaughter	
Voluntary	*Involuntary*
(all Homicide Act 1957)	(all common law)
Diminished responsibility (s 2)	Constructive (or unlawful acts)
Provocation (s 3)	Gross negligence
Killing in pursuance of a	(Subjectively) reckless
suicide pact (s 4)	

Figure 12.1 Types of manslaughter

The accused has acted unlawfully and the consequence is that someone has died. He is guilty even though he did not foresee that his activity might cause death or even serious bodily harm. A person does not need to be acting involuntarily (see Chapter 2) to be guilty of this form of manslaughter. As can be seen, there is a conceptual difference between voluntary manslaughter (the accused had malice aforethought) and involuntary manslaughter (the accused did not have malice aforethought). A person cannot be charged with voluntary manslaughter. The charge is one of murder, but if one of the three mitigations applies, the verdict is (voluntary) manslaughter.

The order in this chapter is that voluntary manslaughter is treated before involuntary manslaughter because the former, but not the latter, requires the *mens rea* of murder, the subject of the previous chapter. A modern categorisation is this:

(a) killing by gross negligence, including omission to act;

(b) killing by an unlawful act, also called constructive manslaughter;

(c) killing by (subjective) recklessness;

(d) killing where there is provocation (see later in this chapter), diminished responsibility (see Chapter 9), or a suicide pact (see below).

'Involuntary' therefore bears a meaning different from elsewhere in criminal law: for example, in mental condition defences the act of the accused may be involuntary because he suffers from a disease of the mind or an abnormality of mind; in duress the accused may act involuntarily because of pressure placed on him (e.g. 'Kneecap her or I will kill you.')

Because these forms of manslaughter have very different requirements, it may be a good idea to think of each of them as separate offences. The Court of Appeal, as noted below, twice in 1993 called for reform of involuntary manslaughter, and a head of steam is developing in favour of radical change, two aspects of which are the reform of provocation and the proposed abolition of constructive manslaughter. For proposals for reform of involuntary manslaughter see the end of this chapter.

It seems very likely but it is not yet quite clear that there is a defence of (subjectively) reckless manslaughter. This is, as it were, a companion offence to murder. It occurs where the accused foresees (subjectively) that death or serious injury may occur as a highly probable consequence. It would seem that facts falling within subjectively reckless manslaughter also always fall within unlawful act manslaughter. The Court of Appeal in *Lidar* [1999] 11 November, unreported, seems to confirm this crime's existence. See below for further discussion.

Provocation

Introduction

The Homicide Act 1957, s 3, gives a partial definition of the defence of provocation:

> [W]here on a charge of murder there is evidence on which the jury can find that the person charged was provoked (whether by things done or by things said or by both together) to lose his self-control, the question whether the provocation was enough to make a reasonable man do as he did shall be left to be determined by the jury; and in determining that question the jury shall take into account everything both done and said according to the effect which, in their opinion, it would have had on a reasonable man.

The Court of Appeal stated in **Davies** [1975] QB 691 that s 3 constituted a new test and the words were to be given their ordinary meaning. However, the section does not state the whole of the law. It does not say, for example, what amounts to provocation and what the effect of a successful plea is. Therefore, to understand this defence the common law and the changes wrought by the Act must be considered.

Before reaching those answers, it is worthwhile stressing some points.

(a) The opening words of s 3 are 'where on a charge of murder . . .'. The accused must, subject to what is said in the next paragraph, have performed the *actus reus* of murder and have had malice aforethought. If there is no such intent, the defence is otiose. Provocation is a defence only to murder. It is not even a defence to attempted murder: **Bruzas** [1972] Crim LR 367 (Crown Court). The High Court of Australia in **McGhee** (1995) 69 ALJR 650 ruled to similar effect in relation to the Tasmanian Criminal Code on the ground that provocation was 'a peculiar doctrine founded historically in the need to ameliorate what was the automatic and drastic consequence of a conviction for murder' (to use the words of Hampel J in **Farrar** [1992] 1 VR 207). The court noted that 'the accused must have caused death with the intention of killing or inflicting grievous bodily harm . . . it is only then that provocation may operate . . .'. In other words, the accused must have the *actus reus* and *mens rea* of murder before the defence can apply. The reader may wish to compare provocation's application with that of duress which is not a defence to murder, and with mercy-killing, which again does not exculpate the accused. The reader is invited to think why provocation is, but duress is not, a defence to murder. Despite provocation not affording a defence to charges other than murder, it is relevant to other offences in that if, as a result of provocation, the accused did not foresee the consequences of his actions, he is alleging that he did not have *mens rea*. Because provocation is a defence only to murder, it is known as a 'special defence'. The term for a defence which applies to all or most offences is 'general defence'. In crimes other than murder provocation is taken into account in the sentence.

The Court of Appeal accepted in **Marks** [1998] Crim LR 676 that provocation was a defence to a charge of being an accessory to murder. The accused, the principal offender and the victim were drug dealers who had fallen out. On the assumed facts the accused had told the perpetrator to kill the victim. On the facts there was no loss of self-control and it had not been shown that the victim had said or done anything which led to a loss of control.

(b) The effect of a successful plea is to reduce murder to manslaughter. Formerly, the effect of success would be to avoid capital punishment. Nowadays, it is to give the judge discretion as to sentence. Nevertheless, the outcome in murder and in murder reduced to manslaughter by provocation may be the same. For example, in **Whitfield** (1976) 63 Cr App R 39 a conviction for murder was quashed, but the life sentence was maintained.

Like diminished responsibility and suicide pacts, which also had their origin in the 1957 Homicide Act, manslaughter by provocation is classified as 'voluntary manslaughter'. That term means that the accused may well have had malice aforethought, but there exists a mitigating element which reduces murder to manslaughter.

(c) It is thought that some 45 per cent of all homicide killings are committed by persons in a temper. Provocation is therefore potentially an important matter.

(d) To gain this defence the accused must have killed because he was provoked. It is not sufficient that some provocation existed.

(e) Section 3 is traditionally divided into two 'limbs' for the purposes of exposition. The first limb is whether the accused was in fact provoked; the second limb is whether a reasonable person would have been provoked. This approach is dealt with below. The first limb by itself would exculpate those who killed in a temper: this outcome was felt to be unacceptable. The second limb by itself would exculpate killers who were so phlegmatic that they kept their self-control when ordinary people would have lost theirs: again such an outome was not acceptable. It is, however, worth mentioning *Clarke* [1991] Crim LR 383, where the Court of Appeal determined that provocation covers the whole course of conduct, not just the act which caused death. In this case the accused head-butted the victim, his former cohabitee, and strangled her. He then electrocuted her by putting live wires into her mouth. She could have been dead before the electrocution. (If she was not dead, the electrocution would have killed her.) The court refused his application for leave to appeal. The whole sequence had to be looked at to see whether the accused had lost his self-control. The deed of electrocution formed part of the circumstances. The electrocution followed very soon after the strangulation and it would have been artificial to ask of the jury to consider only the acts which they decided actually caused death. Provided that the conduct causing the death was part of one continuing assault, the jury should look at everything the accused had done in considering whether a reasonable man would have acted in the same way. In other words, the phrase 'do as he did' is not limited to the act which caused death: might a reasonable person have killed? If so, might a reasonable person have killed in the way in which the accused did? It is suggested that the court was incorrect. 'Do as he did' means 'do the act which caused death'. Therefore, any conduct after the victim's death is irrelevant (such as putting the electrical wires into the victim's mouth), including the fact that very shortly after the killing the accused retained his self-composure. *Clarke*, however, is inconsistent with the requirement that there was a loss of self-control at the moment of provocation. Surely the whole course of conduct cannot be taken into account if the accused has at some time recovered his self-control and then killed. On the facts the electrocution was simply a way of attempting to hide how the victim's death was caused. If the accused has not in fact been provoked, he will not have this defence, even if a reasonable person would have lost control.

(f) Provocation is a defence only to murder. Therefore, before the accused may rely on this defence, he must have intended to kill or commit serious bodily harm. If he did not so intend, he is anyway not guilty of murder. Therefore, provocation does not destroy intent: rather it is a defence separate from malice aforethought. Similarly, it is thought that the accused is acting voluntarily when he is provoked. Nevertheless, at times he may be in such a rage that he is not conscious of his actions. If so, logically provocation should be a complete defence and a defence to all offences.

(g) The judicial foundation of the defence was succinctly stated by Viscount Simon in *Holmes v DPP* [1946] AC 588: '. . . the law has to reconcile respect for the sanctity of human life with recognition of the effect of provocation on human frailty'. It may seem strange that the jury may use the defence of provocation to find an accused not guilty of murder, but cannot use the defence of duress to do the same. Why is an angry person able to avoid liability when a coerced person is not? Lord Hoffmann in *Smith* [2001] 1 AC 146 (HL) astutely noticed that the emotions which gave rise to provocation were not restricted to anger but included quite possibly 'fear and despair'. A battered woman who killed her sleeping or drunk partner may have lost control not because of anger but because she lived in fear of being abused and had no means of leaving her partner, perhaps because of a lack of money or accommodation.

(h) Although provocation is called a defence, the burden of proof remains on the prosecution. Authorities from the Privy Council include *Lee Chun Chuen v R* [1963] AC 220 and *Rolle v R* [1965] 1 WLR 1341.

(i) Section 3 is restricted by its wording to things said or done; therefore, circumstances cannot constitute provocation. If a rockfall knocks the victim off a mountainside and the accused cuts the rope attaching him to the victim, who falls to her death, he does not have a defence of provocation.

The Court of Appeal of New Zealand said in *Campbell* [1997] 1 NZLR 16 that provocation was 'a notoriously difficult aspect of criminal law'. The truth or otherwise of this statement will be demonstrated in the following pages.

Which activities constitute provocation?

As stated above, the Homicide Act 1957 does not fully explicate the definition of provocation. The best-known definition before the statute was that of Devlin J in the Court of Criminal Appeal in *Duffy* [1949] 1 All ER 932:

> [p]rovocation is some act or series of acts (done by the dead man to the accused) which would cause in any reasonable person, and actually causes in the accused, a sudden and temporary loss of self-control, rendering the accused so subject to passion as to make him or her for the moment not master of his mind. [The words in round brackets have been put into parenthesis because the law has since changed.]

The phrase 'a sudden and temporary loss of self-control', which also appears in *Holmes v DPP*, above, constitutes the governing principle of the first, the subjective, limb of the defence. It is suggested that if 'temporary' means anything, it means that the accused has the defence of insanity if he has permanently lost self-control. If one compares *Duffy* with s 3, one difference is obvious. The law before 1957 took into account only acts, though there was some authority that words alone could constitute provocation in exceptional circumstances. As we shall see, the Act also altered the role of judge and jury. On one interpretation the 1957 Act made no other changes to the common law. This construction is to the effect that the Act places the question 'whether the provocation was enough to make a reasonable man do as he did' before the jury, but does not change the definition of provocation except that nowadays the jury can take into account words as well as deeds. On this approach the pre-1957 rules on provocation remain. For example, *Duffy* asks for an act 'done by the dead person to the accused'. Accordingly, acts done by the deceased to someone other than the accused, and also done by someone other than the victim, do not amount to provocation. The alternative approach is to state that s 3 redefines provocation: the jury are to take everything into account with the result that, for instance, there is no restriction that the provocation did not come from the victim or was not directed at the accused. There is certainly support for the first, narrow, approach both from early cases interpreting the Act, especially the Privy Council decision in *Phillips v R* [1969] 2 AC 130, and from the parliamentary debates (see below). However, since the 1970s the courts have adopted the view that s 3 marks a fresh start in the law and that the section abolished the earlier law. Nevertheless, the revised definition in *Duffy* still stands. There must be a sudden and temporary loss of self-control, e.g. *Ahluwalia* [1992] 4 All ER 889 (CA). The test is subjective. The jury looks at this specific accused. At this stage drunkenness and irascibility are relevant. What the subjective test ensures is that an accused does not have this defence if he has not lost self-control even though a reasonable man, an ordinary person in current parlance, would have lost it.

This development may be seen by examining the previous limitations on which matters could not amount to provocation. These rules of law have either been abolished or have been eroded into factors which the jury may consider in determining whether s 3 is satisfied.

(a) In *Holmes v DPP* [1946] AC 588 the House of Lords held that 'in no case could words alone, save in circumstances of a most extreme and exceptional character', amount to provocation. What those exceptional circumstances were the House of Lords did not vouchsafe. Section 3 definitely changes the law stated in *Holmes*: words alone now suffice.

(b) If the accused found his wife having sexual intercourse with another man (*in flagrante delicto*), there was provocation. Catching one's common law wife (i.e. long-term mistress) (*Greening* [1913] 3 KB 846) or fiancé (*Palmer* [1913] 2 KB 29) *in flagrante* was insufficient. There was no authority whether it was provocation where the wife caught her husband *in flagrante*. Despite the fact that as recently as 1964 Hollis in *The Homicide Act*, mentioned by J. K. Webster, 'Some provoking aspects of voluntary manslaughter law' in (1981) 10 *Anglo-American Law Review* 159 at 175, n 15, thought that killing a wife *in flagrante* was manslaughter but killing a mistress in such circumstances was murder, even before 1957 the rule seemed to have evaporated, for in *Larkin* [1943] KB 174 and *Gauthier* (1943) 29 Cr App R 113 the courts did not take into account that the deceased women were mistresses. After the 1957 Act it is universally thought that the common law rules in this area have disappeared, though it has to be said that there is nothing in the Act which expressly says so. The legal argument to the effect that these rules have been abolished must rely on the phrase 'everything . . . done', which can cover catching one's spouse, lover or fiancé(e) in bed with someone else.

(c) It was sometimes said pre-1957 that provocation had to derive from the deceased, e.g. *Simpson* (1915) 84 LJKB 1893. Devlin J also said so in *Duffy*. It may be that this rule was not truly a common law proposition. Certainly on the facts of *Duffy* the point did not arise, and R. S. O'Regan, 'Indirect provocation and misdirected retaliation' [1968] Crim LR 319 argued that the statement in *Duffy* was incorrect insofar as it purported to state the law before 1957. *Davies*, above, decided that at least after the Act it was a misdirection to instruct the jury to investigate only the words and acts of the deceased. She had been having an affair with a man and was killed by her husband. The acts and words of her lover had to be taken into account when assessing whether the husband was provoked.

The concomitant rule was that the acts of provocation had to be directed at the accused. There were two exceptions, although they could also be seen as acts directed at the accused: adultery with the accused's wife and sodomy with the accused's son. This rule also disappeared after the Act, perhaps because there is no restriction against whom the words or acts were directed in the statute: for a case see *Pearson* [1992] Crim LR 193, discussed below.

(d) At common law provocation did not apply where there was a cooling-off time: *Hayward* (1833) 172 ER 1188. In *Duffy*, above, the accused had an argument with her husband. She got a hammer and hatchet, went upstairs, and killed him. It was held that she did not have this defence because there had been a cooling-off time. After the 1957 Act it seems that this rule has vanished and the fact that the accused has had time to calm down is one element in the equation whether the accused was labouring under the provocation at the time of the killing. In *Ibrams* (1982) 74 Cr App R 155, where the Court of Appeal also approved *Duffy*, there was a gap of five days between the last act of provocation and the killing. The victim had been lured to his death by his wife, whom he had bullied. He was killed by the accused, whom he had bullied over a long period. Accordingly, the trial judge had been correct, the Court of Appeal ruled, to hold that there was no evidence of a loss of self-control. Therefore, provocation was ruled out. The facts, however, look like those of a killing in revenge. The defendant had planned the killing. Perhaps the true defence on the facts should have been self-defence/prevention of crime. Whether the accused had regained control is judged by reference to the accused, not by reference to the ordinary or responsible person: *Masciantonio v R* (1995) 69 ALJR 598 (HCA).

Provocation normally occurs on impulse, in hot blood. Section 3 speaks of the loss of self-control, a point sometimes forgotten. A recent restatement of this principle occurred in the speech of Lord Steyn in *Smith* [2001] 1 AC 146: 'One essential element for the availability of a plea of provocation has always been that the act be done in the heat of passion fired by the provocation before reason has returned.' As Devlin J put it in *Duffy*, 'the further removed an incident is from the crime, the less it counts'. He added that 'the conscious formulation of a desire for revenge . . . would negative a sudden temporary loss of self-control, which is of the essence of provocation'. Since the issues of provocation are for the jury (see below), it may happen that jurors may find that the accused was provoked despite 'the desire for revenge, . . . a lapse of time, . . . planning', because the judge is not entitled to withdraw the subjective question from the jury where there is any evidence that the defendant was provoked: *Baillie* [1995] 2 Cr App R 31 (CA), a case which incurred the wrath of the Law Commission in its Report No. 290, *Partial Defences to Murder*, 2004. The fact that the accused got a gun from the attic, picked up a cut-throat razor and drove a car for two miles (and filled it with petrol) shows that the law does not demand an instantaneous reaction. Continuing rage demonstrates that self-control has not been regained but where there is a cooling down, there is no loss of self-control as s 3 demands. Whether the accused has calmed down is a matter for the jury using its common sense.

This aspect of manslaughter has been to the fore in cases such as *Ibrams* where the wife killed her husband who had been battering her. In *Ahluwalia*, above, the accused's husband had beaten and burnt her. She had taken paraffin and a taper upstairs, and set her sleeping husband alight, killing him. Since there had been a cooling-off time, murder was not reduced to manslaughter on the grounds of provocation. The Court of Appeal approved *Duffy*. The enactment of s 3 had not affected the requirement of a sudden and temporary loss of self-control. The longer the delay between the provocation and the killing and the stronger the evidence of premeditation, the less likelihood there was of the defence's success. It should be noted that the court did not decide that a lapse of time was an absolute bar to the defence. If there is a sudden and temporary loss of self-control at the time of the killing, it does not matter that the outburst was the outcome of a 'slow-burn' reaction rather than an immediate loss of self-control. Accordingly, 'sudden' in the *Duffy* formula does not mean 'immediate in response to what the victim said or did'. Similar is *Thornton* [1992] 1 All ER 306. The Court of Appeal ruled that the accused must be deprived of self-control 'at the moment the fatal blow was struck', as Beldam LJ put it. The accused, who disclaimed that she had lost her self-control, had told a friend that she was going to kill her husband, and she had sharpened the knife. Such deliberation was inconsistent with provocation. Accordingly she did not have the defence. The court refused to certify that a point of law of general public importance was involved. Short of the House of Lords, the law is clear and it was applied by the Court of Appeal in *Richens* [1993] 4 All ER 877. The ruling in *Thornton* that there had to be a loss of self-control at the time when the blow was struck, not necessarily at the time of the provocation, should be contrasted with *Ibrams*, above, where the Court of Appeal ruled that the loss of control had to happen immediately after the last act or words of provocation. *Thornton* states current law.

There is no doubt that these decisions have come under attack. The basis of the criticism is that they distinguish between men and women. Women are more likely to kill their spouses as a result of planning (the jargon phrase is 'slow burn') than men, who tend to kill in the heat of the moment. On this approach men get the defence, but women do not. Yet a woman may feel powerless against a strong husband and may not be able to act on the spur of the moment. She may have to wait to strike when he is drunk or asleep. Furthermore, the use of the battered woman syndrome switches the emphasis of the defence from provocation by the victim to the accused's mental condition and can lead to diminished responsibility, a defence at times akin to insanity, rather than provocation. Such occurred in *Ahluwalia.* The accused's depression constituted an 'abnormality of mind' within the law of diminished responsibility. A woman may well not wish to be classified as having a defence of diminished responsibility through her mental disorder. The trial judge in *Thornton* thought that the accused should have sought alternatives, such as walking out on her husband. The criticism is this: where is she to walk to, especially when she has children or is economically dependent on her husband?

It is interesting to note that while the law is laid down in *Thornton*, B. Mitchell in his survey of homicide [1991] NLJ 935 found a couple of cases where the defence succeeded despite cooling off. The jury seems to have taken a moral, not a legal, attitude to the facts. If *Ibrams* is correct in stating that cooling off is a factor and not a nullification of the defence in itself, that factor could be overwhelmed by other factors. Moreover, in *Pearson*, above, there was said to be evidence of provocation even though two brothers had armed themselves and had jointly set off to kill their abusive father, who was sleeping at the time. There was no sudden loss of self-control, no final straw. There are other similar cases, both reported and unreported. Sympathy for the accused should not obscure the law that in the words of s 3 'the person charged' must have been 'provoked . . . to lose his self-control'. If the accused retains self-control, there is no provocation. It is arguable that some judges do not wish to see this requirement in the law. Furthermore it may sometimes happen that the accused may let matters fester, but the test in *Duffy* is based on the assumption that temper will cool down over time. The law at present (and certainly there have been jury findings of provocation when there was a substantial time between the provocation and the killing) was summarised by Lord Taylor CJ in *Ahluwalia*: 'The subjective element . . . would not as a matter of law be negatived simply because of the delayed reaction . . . , provided that there was at the time of the killing a "sudden and temporary loss of self-control" caused by the alleged provocation. However, the longer the delay and the stronger the evidence of deliberation . . . , the more likely it will be that the prosecution will negative provocation.' For criticism of

Pearson, see the case comment of J. C. Smith [1992] Crim LR 194, who suggests that it 'is perhaps one of the consequences of the mandatory penalty for murder that defences will be artificially extended so as to untie the judge's hands in hard cases'.

The rationale behind the *Duffy* test was stated by McHugh J in *Masciantonio v R*: 'The concept of suddenness negatived any question of premeditation. The concept of temporariness ensured that an intentional killing would be excused as manslaughter only when it was committed while the killer's capacity for self-control had been overwhelmed by the desire for retribution that often arises when an interest or relationship that a person values is harmed or threatened by the conduct of another person.' A full account of US law on women (though the defence is not limited to women; it has been applied to male homosexuals) who kill is C. K. Gillespie, *Justifiable Homicide* (Ohio State UP, 1989). From a battered person's point of view, a better defence is self-defence. If an accused successfully pleads this defence, he is totally acquitted. It is possible that English juries may accept quite thin evidence of self-defence and acquit the battered person. For a Scottish case involving a battered girlfriend see *HM Advocate v McNab*, unreported, 30 August 1995 (High Court). The distinction between the two defences was summarised by Hampel J in *Farrar*, above, thus: 'Self-defence . . . is a complete defence because in appropriate circumstances it justifies extreme violence and even a killing which would otherwise amount to murder. Provocation, on the other hand, excuses a person from incurring the consequences of a conviction for murder but does not justify a killing which would otherwise amount to murder.'

(e) Before 1957 the law was that the response had to be proportionate to the provocation. In *Mancini v DPP* [1942] AC 1 the House of Lords held that 'the mode of resentment must bear a reasonable relationship to the provocation', and in *Duffy*, above, Devlin J said that 'fists might be answered with fists but not with a deadly weapon'. The rule was criticised on the grounds that a provoked person has so lost his self-control that he has killed. To say that he overreacted was inappropriate because to say that he had lost his self-control but had acted proportionately were not necessarily consistent statements. One problem of interpretation of s 3 is the width of the phrase 'does as he did'. It could mean that this reasonable retaliation rule survived (the provocation must be 'enough to make a reasonable man do as he did', words which seemingly state a rule) or it could mean that the rule had not survived the treatment of s 3. Since 1957 the Privy Council has advised that judges should not stick close to the *Mancini* formula and the Court of Appeal in *Brown* [1972] 2 QB 229 considered that this reasonableness of the retaliation was a factor to be weighed in determining whether a reasonable person would have been provoked. The High Court of Australia held similarly in *Masciantonio v R*, above. This interpretation, in the view of the author, does violence to the words of the statute. Lord Goff in *Morhall* [1996] 1 AC 90 (HL) stated that the term 'reasonable man' in s 3 should not be used because a jury might be misled into thinking that the accused had to have the power of self-control of a reasonable person, whereas the true inquiry of s 3 was whether he had the self-control of an 'ordinary person'. Such a person can presumably act unreasonably, i.e. disproportionately. The relationship between the gravity of the provocation and the retaliation is judged by current social standards.

(f) There is no need to prove that the defendant so lost his self-control that he did not know what he was doing. The correct direction is to ask whether or not the accused so suddenly and temporarily lost his self-control that he could not stop himself doing as he did: *Richens*, above. The accused need not be insane within the criminal law definition of insanity. Accordingly, an accused can have the defence even though he is acting purposely. Devlin J said in *Duffy* provocation arose when the accused was 'for the moment not master of his mind', demonstrating that a complete lack of self-control was not a necessary precondition. Other metaphors such as 'in the heat of passion' and 'in hot blood' are also used. In *Richens* the accused stabbed the victim to death when the latter told him that he had had sexual intercourse with his girlfriend. She had complained of rape. The accused became enraged when the victim said that she had wanted and enjoyed the intercourse and that it was the first time that she had had sex with a real man. Applying the *dictum* in *Duffy*, he did lose his self-control. In sum, an accused need not be acting as an automaton but a mere loss of temper does not suffice. After all the accused only needs the defence of provocation if he has the *mens rea* for murder. If he does not possess it, as when he does not know what he is doing, he has no need of the defence for even without it he is not guilty of murder. An example of loss of self-control is when the accused has inflicted numerous wounds on the victim.

This shift from rule to factor does not mean that the judge may disregard the relevant elements in summing up: *Jones* [1987] Crim LR 701. The Court of Appeal held that the trial judge should have dealt with the serious nature of the provocation: an attack with a pick-axe handle. The accused had received injuries before he had taken over the handle and struck the fatal blow.

Four other points which are not dependent on the Homicide Act 1957 are these:

(a) An honest, but mistaken, belief in the existence of facts which, had they existed, would have provoked a reasonable person will give a defence: *Brown* (1776) 168 ER 177. The accused killed the victim whom he wrongly supposed to be part of a mob. He had a defence, because he would have done if the facts as he believed them to be had truly existed. On analogy with self-defence, the mistake need not be a reasonable one. Even if the mistake affected an accused who was drunk, he has a defence: *Letenock* (1917) 12 Cr App R 221 (CCA). Because he was drunk, the accused believed he was about to be attacked. In fact he was not. The court quashed the conviction for murder. A reasonable person in the position of the accused, thinking as the accused did, might have reacted in the same way. It is suggested that *Letenock* may not survive challenge. In the context of self-defence a drunken mistake is no defence (*O'Grady* [1987] QB 995 (CA)). To have different rules is indefensible. An alternative approach is to say that *O'Grady* is wrong and that honest mistakes, even those brought about by intoxication, should give a defence. See below for the different rule applying to the attributes of the reasonable person who is not intoxicated.

See p 337 in Chapter 8 for more on drunken mistake.

(b) Cruel conduct over a period of time may amount to provocation: the case of the *Maw* sisters, unreported, 1980, where the sisters had killed their bullying father. Accordingly, cumulative provocation can provide a defence, and the last straw can break the camel's back, i.e. the last act of provocation can be a small one. 'Boiling point can be just as effectively reached by a continuing low fire as by some momentarily fierce flame': *Stone* [1965] NSWLR 898 *per* Herron CJ. For example, the fact that a husband has been beating his wife over a long period can be taken into account to explain why she killed him after what would otherwise be a trivial row. In *Thornton (No. 2)* [1996] 1 WLR 1174 (CA) Lord Taylor CJ said that battered woman syndrome could explain why a minor incident could lead to the killing. (See below for how the syndrome relates to the objective reasonable person test.) It is surprising that in recent cases the Court of Appeal has had to emphasise that cumulative provocation is part of the law (but the killing must still be in hot blood). As long as the loss of self-control was sudden it does not matter that the provocation itself was not sudden.

(c) The acts or words of provocation need not be unlawful. In **Doughty** (1986) 83 Cr App R 319 the Court of Appeal held that provocation can be effected by the crying of a baby. The Act's terms were not restricted to wrongful acts or words. Interestingly, Minnesota law expressly provides that: 'the crying of a baby does not constitute provocation' (Code s 609.20(1), 2006). There was no need for an assault such as by a threat. It is suggested that **Doughty** is wrong. It is arguable that a baby who cries is a natural event like a thunderstorm and natural events do not give rise to provocation; and the fact that the killer became angry does not mean that he has necessarily been provoked.

Since the question of what suffices for provocation is one for the jury, two juries might come to different conclusions on the same facts. In the unreported first instance decision in **Corlett**, *The Lawyer*, 29 August 1995, moving a mustard pot constituted the provoking act. What about a constable making a lawful arrest? This is a lawful act. Surely the law is not that an accused passes the subjective test if he kills the constable? Furthermore, there is nothing in s 3 to restrict the provoking act to one which comes from a human. Can a provoking act come from nature? The usual answer is that circumstances such as one's house being set on fire by lightning cannot constitute provocation. However, the crying of a baby is perhaps more akin to natural circumstances than to 'human' acts or words. **Doughty** brings to the fore one of the most morally difficult issues in criminal law. It seems strange that an accused potentially has a defence when he kills his crying baby, but not when he kills his terminally ill aged parent who is in great pain. It must be emphasised that **Doughty** is authority on the first, subjective test for provocation. The court held that the issue of provocation had to be left to the jury: it did not decide whether the accused's reaction was reasonable, the second test.

(d) An issue not often raised before 1957 is that of self-induced provocation. Self-induced provocation is where the accused has acted or spoken in such a way that the predictable outcome of his behaviour is that his deeds or words will provoke the victim into attacking him physically or verbally and the accused kills him. In **Johnson** (1989) 89 Cr App R 148 it was held that s 3 covers such conduct because it stipulates that everything both done and said has to be considered. It contemplates a situation where the accused had started the trouble and caused the victim to provoke him. In **Johnson** there was a fight in a nightclub. The victim pinned the accused against a wall. The accused retaliated by stabbing the victim with a flick-knife. (Note that a successful defence of self-defence on these facts would lead to complete acquittal.) In **Edwards v R** [1973] AC 648 the Privy Council had said that self-induced provocation could not be relied on where the reaction was predictable but could be where the reaction went to extreme lengths. This was inconsistent with s 3, which requires *any* evidence to be left to the jury: the source of the events leading to the killing is not relevant. On the facts the reaction of the victim to blackmail had been extreme in relation to the blackmail. If, however, that had not been so, the judge should not leave the issue to the jury. Watkins LJ in **Johnson** thought that this proposition as to extreme lengths of the hostile reaction was restricted to the facts of the case. (This is equivalent to saying: 'It is wrong and, if I could, I'd overrule it!') What the victim did in *Johnson* was probably unpredictable, so the cases can be reconciled. Section 3 left all issues to the jury, who had to take 'everything' into account. 'Everything' includes even the unpredictable result of the accused's behaviour. The judge, therefore, cannot withdraw the issue of provocation from the jury on the basis that it was self-induced. The position would appear now to be this: even a self-induced arrest can be a provoking act and this proposition is true even when the arrest was lawful: see *Doughty*, above. One point which was not discussed in *Johnson* is the situation where the accused sets out deliberately to induce the victim to provoke him. Such was not the situation in *Johnson*. While there is no decided case, it may be that this accused's original fault – the decision to induce the other to provoke him – negates the later provocation. This explanation, however, runs up against the terms of s 3. One argument against the law in *Johnson* is that the accused, if successful in his plea of provocation, has his crime reduced to manslaughter. Why should he again be able to slough off responsibility for causing the situation in which the provocation arose? The contrary view is that the provocation 'trumps' the fault of the accused in getting into the situation in which the provocation arose.

See pp 305–6 in Chapter 8 for more on self-induced intoxication.

The reader is invited to compare the defence of self-induced provocation with the lack of a defence of **duress** when the accused had joined a terrorist gang, and the narrowness of the defence of self-induced intoxication.

Who is the reasonable person in the Homicide Act?

(a) The 1957 Act and the reasonable man

The Homicide Act 1957, s 3, lays down a two-stage test for provocation: Was the accused provoked? If so, might a reasonable (or in modern parlance 'ordinary') person have been provoked and acted as the accused did? This second stage is often known as the 'objective' test, just as the first stage is known as the 'subjective' test. The statute speaks of a 'reasonable man'. To the question 'who is the reasonable man in s 3?' one might have expected a purely hypothetical, abstract reasonable man, and the law started with that concept. However, the position was vastly changed by *Smith* [2001] 1 AC 146. The accused was no longer to be assessed against the standards of the 'reasonable man', as s 3 demands; rather and subject to some exceptions the question was: did this person fall short of the standard expected *of him*? Despite some statements to the contrary the position was that just about every characteristic of the accused was attributable to the reasonable person in s 3 after *Smith*, above. In the words of Andrew Ashworth in his case-note on *Weller* [2003] Crim LR 725 there was an 'evaluative free for all'. How far the law moved in some fifty years! The law is now that stated in *Attorney-General for Jersey v Holley* [2005] 2 AC 580 (PC).

(b) What might a reasonable man or woman have done?

The judge should direct the jury that the relevant question at this point is whether a reasonable person might or could have killed, not whether she would have killed: *Stewart* [1995] 4 All ER 999 (CA). Section 3 speaks of a 'reasonable man'; if the accused is a woman, the term 'reasonable woman' is used: see below for details. Despite the section's reference to a reasonable man, modern cases (in particular, *Smith*, above, *per* Lords Hoffmann and Clyde) tend to judge the accused against the standard of an ordinary person, though the use of the term 'reasonable man' in a jury instruction is not a misdirection: *Jenkins*, unreported, 14 February 2002 (CA). This rewording is the result of antipodean authorities. For example, s 169(2)(a) of the Crimes Act 1961 talks of 'a person having the power of self-control of an ordinary person . . .'. Australian courts, like English ones, ask whether the reasonable person *could* have lost self-control to the extent that the accused did: *Stingel* v *R* (1990) 171 CLR 312 (HCA). This section is concerned with the second stage of the test in s 3.

While one might think that a reasonable person would never kill, Parliament by laying down the stages has assumed to the contrary. By replacing the 'reasonable man' with the concept of the 'ordinary person', the courts have ensured that juries are less concerned with the issue of whether a reasonable man might have killed and more concerned with whether the accused did act like an ordinary, average person might have reacted. What, however, Parliament did not do was to state clearly the attributes of the reasonable man. For example, could a reasonable woman be a 'reasonable man' within the Act? Such a proposition looks absurd nowadays, but was not before 1957. It was in line with the pre-1957 law of *Bedder* v *DPP* [1954] 2 All ER 801, which would have ruled matters not to be provocation which would not have provoked a reasonable man but would have provoked a reasonable woman. The law remains controversial and continues to develop. Certainly not all of the accused's characteristics or history can be taken into account. If they could, there would not be a second stage of reasonableness. Without this second stage any insult which had led to a sudden and temporary loss of self-control would constitute provocation and the accused would be guilty only of manslaughter and not of murder. Present law promotes both the policy of encouraging self-restraint and the policy of non-violence.

(c) The objective nature of the responsible person

Section 3 relates that 'the question of whether the provocation was enough to make a reasonable man do as he did' is for the jury. The more obvious of the possible interpretations of that phrase is to ask whether the totally objective reasonable person would have acted in such a way. The less obvious construction is to ask whether a reasonable person imbued with the relevant characteristics would have done as the accused did. The former interpretation controlled throughout most of this century. In *Lesbini* [1914] 3 KB 1116 the accused killed a girl who had called him a racially pejorative name. He was mentally unbalanced, indeed, so much so that one of his defences was insanity. That defence failed, and so did provocation because, the Court of Criminal Appeal held, the provoking behaviour had to be such as would affect the mind of a reasonable man, not the mind of a mentally defective person. (The defence would have failed anyway at that time, because it was based on words alone.) The apotheosis of the purely objective test was *Bedder*, above. The accused, a sexually impotent youth of 18, failed to have intercourse with a prostitute. She mocked him. He tried to stop her leaving. She slapped and punched him, and kicked him in a painful place. He killed her. The House of Lords held that the jury was to be told to consider whether a reasonable man would have reacted to the provocation, not whether an impotent 18-year-old would have reacted, despite the fact that a reasonable man is not an impotent 18-year-old.

(d) *Camplin*

Accordingly, at the time of the 1957 statute there was the highest authority that no account should be taken of the accused's characteristics, such as religion, race, age or sexual potency. The consequence was that in cases such as *Bedder* the accused was guilty of murder, an outcome which many would consider to be unjust. Debates in both the

House of Commons and the House of Lords demonstrated no desire to change the law. Cases after the Act rejected the view that it changed the law. In **Williams** [1968] Crim LR 678 and **Ives** [1969] 3 All ER 470, the Court of Appeal unsurprisingly rejected the contention that the reasonable man test had been affected by s 8 of the Criminal Justice Act 1967, which is a section governing evidence, not substantive criminal law. On the face of it the 1957 Act with its 'reasonable man' did not change the law. However, in **Camplin** [1978] AC 705 the House of Lords decided that **Bedder** was no longer to be followed. The accused, aged 15, went to the house of a male in his fifties. The latter forcibly buggered him. The man laughed at him and the accused hit him over the head with a chapatti pan. The trial judge instructed the jury in terms of **Bedder**. The Court of Appeal distinguished it as dealing with abnormality whereas the accused's age was something normal. The Lords went further and departed from **Bedder**.

It is important to understand how the House of Lords did this. In reviewing the history of the law of provocation, Lord Diplock noted that the reasonableness of reactions depends on social circumstances. In the seventeenth century pulling a man's nose made a reasonable man react with a sword; the same did not apply now. In a significant passage he said that the 1957 Act 'abolished all previous rules as to what could or could not amount to provocation'. He emphasised that, since words alone could now constitute provocation, the context for applying **Bedder** had been altered by the statute: the gravity of verbal provocation might well depend on the particular characteristics or circumstances of the person to whom a taunt or insult was addressed. Accordingly, those characteristics could now be taken into account in determining whether a reasonable person would have reacted as the accused did. One had to compare the accused's behaviour to the reaction of a reasonable person imbued with the relevant traits of the defendant, but only traits which affect the gravity of the provocation could be considered. For example, to call a woman a 'whore' might be expected to raise a reaction, but to call a man the same might not.

As a result **Bedder**, like **Holmes** and it appears **Mancini**, should be discarded, despite the fact that as a matter of legislative intent Parliament in 1957 did not wish to alter **Bedder** and, had it wished to have done so, it could and would have used different words to make the meaning plain. There is quite simply no mandate in s 3 for **Camplin** or indeed for later cases which have said that certain characteristics are or are not proper ones to be left to the jury.

Lord Diplock in **Camplin** laid down the rule: that the reasonable man in the statute is a person having the power of self-control to be expected of an ordinary person of the age and sex of the accused, but otherwise sharing such of his characteristics as the jury thought would affect the gravity of the provocation to him. Therefore, a young man is to be judged against the standards of reasonable (or ordinary) young men because age is a characteristic of being an ordinary person. As Lord Diplock put it, 'to require old heads on young shoulders is inconsistent with the law's compassion of human infirmity'. The provocation need not be directed at the accused's age or sex. The judge should refer only to age and sex if there are no other relevant characteristics. These characteristics were relevant both to the reasonable person standard and to the gravity of the provocation. Other matters were thought to be relevant only to the gravity of the provocation. The term 'characteristics' is something of a misnomer because circumstances in which the accused was placed and his history can be considered. Lord Diplock spoke of 'the particular characteristics or circumstances' and Lord Simon referred to 'the entire factual situation'. For example, the accused may be peculiarly sensitive to a homosexual advance because of his family history: **Green v R** (1997) 72 ALJR 19 (HCA). The relationship between the accused and the victim is not a characteristic: *Horrex* [1999] Crim LR 500 (CA). However, as the transcript shows, that emotional relationship was part of the circumstances, which could be taken into account. Having attached the relevant traits to the hypothetical reasonable person, the question then is: might this reasonable person have reacted as the accused did? For example, on the facts of *Raney* (1942) 29 Cr App R 14, how would a one-legged person have reacted? (In fact *Raney* was one of those pre-*Bedder* cases which applied the post-*Camplin* law, i.e. the same question was asked there and then as could be asked nowadays.) The jurors answer such questions 'drawing on their experiences of how ordinary human beings behave in real life', as Lord Diplock put it in *Camplin*. In *Burke* [1987] Crim LR 336 the Court of Appeal decided that the exact words of Lord Diplock need not be used. It is enough that the substance is given.

(e) *Smith*

For 30 years there has been debate as to which characteristics may be taken into account when assessing how an ordinary person might have reacted to the provoking act or insult. The structure of the law in the last years of the twentieth century seemed to be that some characteristics could never be taken into account. Examples of these included intoxication, whether by alcohol or drugs, excitability and pugnacity. The exclusion was largely on the basis that to imbue the reasonable person with these traits would undermine the concept of rationality. Lord Goff in *Morhall* [1996] AC 90 (HL) excluded intoxication from the list of permitted characteristics because the policy of the law was that intoxication was no defence to crime. There is no 'reasonable drunkard' or 'reasonable glue-sniffer' test. Potter LJ in *Rowland* [2003] EWCA Crim 3636 said that even after *Smith* [2001] 1 AC 146, discussed below, drunkenness is not a characteristic with which the ordinary person is imbued. However, it can be said that intoxication reduces self-control: a drunk or drugged person is more likely to react to provocation than is a sober one. Two characteristics seemed to be always relevant, youth and sex. Lord Diplock in *Camplin* had mentioned 'age', but 'age' was to be read in its context, which concerned a 15-year-old boy. Such a person could not be expected to react in the same way as a middle-aged person. However, once the accused was out of youth, age became irrelevant. The reasonable person standard admitted no characteristic of 'age' once adolescence was passed. (No case discussed old age, but presumably that could be considered on the ground that elderly people might in the circumstances have to act with more force to provoking acts or words than a reasonable but not old person might have reacted. Ordinary people become old; therefore, age was a characteristic.) 'Sex' was included, it is thought, not because one gender has a lower threshold of anger than another but because a woman might react differently from a man even though both were taunted by the same words. Sex could also be seen as an 'ordinary' characteristic. Just as people are at some time young, so they belong to one sex. It was the third category which caused particular difficulty. This class particularly concerned 'mental' characteristics. Could such character traits be taken into account at all stages, i.e. at the stage both of judging the self-control a reasonable person might have and of judging the seriousness of the provocation, or were they relevant only to the latter issue? For instance, was the reasonable man in the 1957 Act an attention-seeking ordinary person or was the mental characteristic of being attention-seeking to be disregarded? *Camplin* seemed to say that only 'ordinary' characteristics could be considered when dealing with the degree of self-control expected of the ordinary person.

The issue divided the Court of Appeal and the Privy Council in the late 1990s but was temporarily resolved by the 3:2 decision of the House of Lords in *Smith* [2001] 1 AC 146.

The accused killed his friend while severely depressed. The trial judge rejected the contention that the jury had to judge his reaction against that of an ordinary severely depressed person. The standard of control of the ordinary person was not affected by such a state of mind. The Court of Appeal allowed the appeal in accordance with its previous determinations. The House of Lords by a majority agreed. Depression affecting either or both of the accused's level of self-control and the gravity of the provocation to him could be taken into account by the jury. Previous law excluding depression was incorrect, as was evident from *Smith* itself but expressly said in *Farnell* [2003] EWHC 835 (Admin). As Mitchell J put it: 'the decision of the House of Lords in *Smith* puts beyond doubt the relevance of the depressive illness to the issue of provocation in this case – regardless of the issue of diminished responsibility.' It must be borne in mind that as a result of *Holley* discussed below, the law has reverted to its *Camplin* position and mental conditions such as depression are no longer relevant to the standard of self-control to be expected of a reasonable person. However, *Holley* cannot be understood without discussion of *Smith*.

The principal speech was delivered by Lord Hoffmann. He rejected the dichotomy which Professor Andrew Ashworth had stated in 'The doctrine of provocation' [1976] CLJ 292: 'the proper distinction is that individual characteristics which bear on the gravity of the provocation should be taken into account, whereas individual particularities bearing on the accused's level of self-control are not'. If one takes the facts of *Morhall* as illustrative, the accused's glue-sniffing was a characteristic; he was taunted about that; therefore, the provocation was more serious to him than to others. However, that characteristic was not to be taken into account when considering the accused's power of self-control. It was this distinction which Lord Hoffmann got rid of in *Smith*. Furthermore, if the provocation had not been directed at his glue-sniffing, the fact that he sniffed glue could not be taken into account even when the jury was considering the gravity of the provocation. Lord Hoffmann said that Lord Diplock's references to age and sex in *Camplin* were merely illustrations of the characteristics which were relevant in provocation cases: they were relevant in *Camplin* itself but were not conclusive of the traits which were to be attributed to the ordinary person. What was material depended on the facts of the case. He added that: 'it would not be consistent with s 3 for the judge to tell the jury that they should ignore any factor or characteristic of the accused in deciding whether the objective element of provocation had been satisfied. That would be to trespass on their province.' He opined that the distinction sought to be drawn by Ashworth was confusing to juries and he rejected the view that mental characteristics fell solely within s 2 of the Homicide Act 1957, which dealt with diminished responsibility, for not all such traits constituted mental abnormalities. The law remained that some characteristics still could not be attributed to the reasonable person, the usual illustrations being intoxication, pugnacity and excitability. (Smith himself suffered from 'violent rages', which Lord Hoffmann excluded, yet he had a defence.) To those Lord Hoffmann added jealousy and obsession. Unfortunately those two traits were given only as examples of excluded characteristics, and in *Weller* [2004] 1 Cr App R 1 the court said that jealousy and possessiveness could be attributed to the reasonable man. The accused strangled his girlfriend during an argument as to her behaviour with other men. He was extraordinarily jealous and possessive. The trial judge refused to direct the jury specifically on these personal attributes. The Court of Appeal, dismissing the appeal, held that while the trial judge should have directed the jury as to the characteristics, she had not excluded them and she was right not to have done so. Moreover, her direction that the jury has to consider 'all the circumstances' and the jurors had to apply the standard of 'what society expects of a man like this in his position' did permit them to take into account the accused's characteristics. Paul Dobson commented in his summary of this case (2004) 42 *Student Law Review* 20: 'If a jury decides for itself to give [the characteristic such as jealousy] no weight, that is absolutely fine. In any case, no-one will know that that is what they did! Indeed, they might decide that his jealousy is a factor rendering his actions less excusable. Again that is fine and again no-one will know.' Therefore, the law still remains unclear as to which characteristics can be taken into account. This issue is developed below. Lord Hoffmann noted that both permanent and temporary characteristics could be taken into consideration, as Lord Goff had previously said in **Morhall**. Lord Hoffmann considered that there was no one right way of instructing juries and he did not wish judges to refer to 'monsters like the reasonable obsessive, the reasonable depressive alcoholic and even the reasonable glue sniffer'. Such attributions were 'highly artificial'. Instead juries should be instructed as to whether 'there was some characteristic of the accused, whether temporary or permanent, which affected the degree of control which society could reasonably have expected of him and which it would be unjust not to take into account'. This was a strange interpretation of s 3, which speaks of the 'reasonable man'.

It should be noted that the fact that the accused was young and so on was not in itself a defence. As Lord Slynn put it in **Smith**, 'The jury must ask whether he has exercised the degree of self-control to be expected of someone in his situation'. Therefore, a response which is unreasonable by the standards of a young person and so on does not provide a defence.

There was a fiery dissenting speech by Lord Hobhouse. He argued that it was the judges' task to provide the jury with help as to the objective criterion in the test for provocation. If all the accused's characteristics could be attributed to the reasonable person, 'the reasonable man becomes "reincarnated" in the defendant'. In other words, the objective test becomes a subjective test. He thought that unreasonable characteristics should not be attributed to the reasonable person: to do so was 'artificial and self-contradictory'. And he stated that the defence of diminished responsibility was available for abnormalities of mind; therefore, mental characteristics fell within s 2, not s 3. This important dissent can be seen as the basis for **Holley**.

Five comments may be made. First, the objective test virtually disappeared. The question was, subject to exceptions such as intoxication and pugnacity, whether the accused exercised the degree of self-control which could reasonably be expected of him. The test which the 1957 Act seemed to lay down, whether the accused exercised the degree of self-control to be expected of a reasonable man, has gone. Even the exceptions do not constitute one group. Lord Hoffmann said that they were 'defects of character', not excuses. The glue-sniffing in **Morhall** could perhaps be both a defect in character (I did not have the strength of mind to resist) or an excuse (I should not be guilty of murder because I did not intend to kill or commit GBH since I was a glue-sniffer or because I did not have a free choice whether to kill or commit GBH). Secondly, since the reasonable man (or in modern guise, ordinary person) test was reduced in importance, the weight which the subjective test had to bear correspondingly increased. Thirdly, **Luc Thiet Thuan v R** [1997] AC 131, see below, remains binding in those countries which have the Privy Council as their final court of appeal. Fourthly, provocation has been criticised in the past for male bias, but there is a *dictum* of Lord Hoffmann that 'male possessiveness and jealousy should not today be an acceptable reason for loss of self-control leading to homicide . . .'. This *dictum* seems inspired by anti-male sentiment and is inconsistent with authorities stretching back several centuries. **Dryden** [1995] 4 All ER 987 is noted in the next paragraph. The accused, a male, was obsessed about planning permission. This characteristic was taken into account, and **Dryden** was approved by Lord Clyde in **Smith**, yet Lord Hoffmann said that male obsessiveness was not a relevant trait. Finally, Lord Hobhouse's dissenting speech made several strong points. Sections 2 and 3 should be read together: s 2 covers those with abnormalities of mind; the rest fall within s 3; therefore, those who have mental problems do not fall within the defence of provocation. It can hardly be expected that the same mental state would fall within both defences. In diminished responsibility the accused would have to prove on the balance of probabilities that he was suffering from it, whereas in provocation the prosecution would have to prove beyond reasonable doubt that he did not! When both defences are raised on the same facts, jurors may be mightily confused. Lord Slynn, however, disagreed about any overlap. Diminished responsibility arose from an internal cause, 'abnormality of mind', whereas provocation came from an external cause, 'something said or done'. Except for age and sex Lord Diplock in **Camplin** was speaking about reaction to provocation, not of the standard to be expected of a reasonable person. The distinction between provocation and diminished responsibility came to the fore in **Holley**, discussed below.

The Court of Appeal was faced in several cases with applying **Smith**. In **Rowland**, above, the Court was faced with facts which occurred before **Smith**. The accused had killed his wife during an argument. He was distressed at the break-up of their marriage. He was convicted of murder. The Court of Appeal, after **Smith**, permitted him to adduce evidence as to his depression. Such evidence was inadmissible on the pre-**Smith** law. The court held that the jury should have been permitted to hear the evidence. In relation to the subjective test depression may have reduced his threshold for losing self-control, and in relation to the objective test depression was a characteristic which affected the gravity of the provocation. Another important post-**Smith** authority was **Weller** [2004] 1 Cr App R 1 (CA), which is noted above. A third case of the post-**Smith** era was **Miah** [2003] EWCA Crim 3713. The trial judge did not specifically draw to the jury's attention the facts that the accused was short, young and a man. The Court of Appeal held that there was no duty on the judge to point out each attribute to the jury. The court said: 'It is clear from **Smith**, in particular Lord Hoffmann's speech, that provided a judge states that these are matters for the jury to decide then it is for a judge to consider precisely how he puts the matter to the jury.' Mantell LJ, in **Weller**, said: 'The judge should not tell the jury that they should, as a matter of law, ignore any aspect . . . This approach has the considerable advantage that it is unnecessary to determine whether . . . a "characteristic" is an eligible characteristic. . . .' Nevertheless, some characteristics remain ineligible: see (g) below.

(f) Holley

The Privy Council delivered its advice in **Holley v Attorney General for Jersey** [2005] 2 AC 580 as to whether **Smith** above was correct. By a majority of six to three insofar as it could consistently with the doctrine of precedent it rejected **Smith**, the leading modern House of Lords decision on provocation. The first limb (was there a sudden and temporary loss of self-control?) was unaffected. While the advice of the Privy Council is not binding on courts in England and Wales there are several grounds for saying that **Holley** is now the leading authority on provocation's second, objective, limb: all of the members of the Judicial Committee on this occasion were members of the House of Lords; the Jersey statute is phrased in exactly the same terms as s 3 of the Homicide Act 1957; and most important, all of the advice of the majority and minority was devoted to discussing **Smith**. There were no reflections on Jersey law. To quote Lord Nicholls, who delivered the advice of the six Law Lords in the majority:

Jersey law on this subject is the same as English law. In July 2000 the House of Lords considered the ingredients of this defence in the **Morgan Smith** case. . . . The decision of the House in that case is in direct conflict with the decision of their Lordships' Board in **Luc Thiet Thuan v The Queen** [1997] AC 131. And the reasoning of the majority in the **Morgan Smith** case is not easy to reconcile with the reasoning of the House of Lords in **R v Camplin** [1978] AC 705 or **R v Morhall** [1996] AC 90. This appeal, being heard by an enlarged Board of nine members, is concerned to resolve this conflict and clarify definitively the present state of English law, and hence Jersey law, on this important subject.

This quote proves that the heart of the matter was the standing of **Smith** in England and Wales.

The accused was a chronic alcoholic who had killed his girlfriend with an axe while inebriated. He was convicted of murder but the Court of Appeal of Jersey substituted a conviction of manslaughter on the ground of provocation. The appeal directly raised the status of the rule in **Smith**. Lord Nicholls said that the objective test in provocation had two subtests: how grave was the provocation? And was the provocation 'enough to make a reasonable man do as he [the accused] did . . .'? The Law Lord took the modern approach (see the text of this book) to the definition of the reasonable man. That is, because it is difficult to see a reasonable man ever killing, what the term meant was 'an ordinary person, that is, a person of ordinary control'. Therefore, since a person of ordinary control might kill, s 3 could be satisfied when a reasonable person killed. What kind of man was a reasonable or ordinary person? The answer came from Lord Diplock's celebrated definition in **Camplin**: 'It means an ordinary person of either sex, not exceptionally excitable or pugnacious, but possessed of such powers of self-control as everyone is entitled to expect that his fellow citizens will exercise in society as it is today.' Here we see Lord Diplock holding that a 'reasonable man' in s 3 includes a reasonable woman (for example, a reasonable woman might react differently from a reasonable man when taunted as being a 'whore'); that certain characteristics are excluded, two being mentioned, excitability and pugnacity, but also including intoxication whether by alcohol or by drugs; that the level of self-control may differ over time; and that the test is an objective one. Of course the whole law as to the second limb cannot be summed up in one sentence and Lord Diplock was alert to this possible criticism. The case itself involved a 15-year-old boy and the definition of a 'reasonable man' was to be extended to a boy of 15: how might an ordinary boy of 15, not exceptionally excitable or pugnacious, have reacted to being forcibly buggered? The reason for this exception to the level of self-control to be expected of people living in a modern society was that old heads cannot be expected on young shoulders. If none of these included or excluded characteristics was relevant, the judge should not direct the jury as to them. For instance, if the accused was a man of say 45, the instruction should be 'how might a reasonable man have reacted?', not 'how might a reasonable man of 45 have reacted'? The same applies to intoxication, excitability and pugnacity. For example, if the accused was not intoxicated, there is no need to refer to intoxication.

Lord Diplock was also alert to another possibility. Gender, age, excitability, pugnacity and to a lesser degree intoxication could be described as characteristics. How might a reasonable person with these characteristics (age, sex) but excluding those characteristics (excitability, pugnacity, intoxication) have reacted? However, if one was tempted to go down the line of saying that there were certain included and certain excluded characteristics to be attributed to the 'reasonable man' in s 3, then what about circumstances? These could be taken into account at the stage of assessing the gravity of the provoking act or words. In Lord Diplock's words, the gravity of the provocation could depend on 'the particular characteristics or circumstances of' the accused. '. . . [T]he reasonable man . . . is a person having the power of self-control to be expected of an ordinary person of the sex and age of the accused, but in other respects sharing such of the accused's characteristics as they [the jurors] think would affect the gravity of the provocation to him . . .'.

An example of the application of post-*Camplin* law was given by Lord Nicholls: '. . . if a homosexual man is taunted for his homosexuality, it is for the jury to consider whether a homosexual man having ordinary powers of self-control might, in comparable circumstances, be provoked to lose his self-control and react to the provocation as the defendant did.' *Morhall* above demonstrates exactly this proposition of law. The accused's glue sniffing was to be taken into account in determining the question of the gravity of the provocation. Lord Goff in *Morhall* gave the example of a rapist taunted by the victim as to the rape; the history of the accused, here the fact that he was a rapist, was to be taken into account when assessing the gravity of the provoking words spoken by the victim. Therefore, as was made obvious in *Morhall*, 'bad' characteristics and history are to be considered by the jury when judging the gravity of the provocation. Lord Nicholls deftly pointed out the real problem for the 'reasonable glue sniffer' in the law of provocation: '. . . assessing the conduct of a glue-sniffing defendant against the standard of a glue-sniffing man having ordinary powers of self-control may mean that the defendant is assessed against a standard he cannot attain. He may be exceptionally excitable or pugnacious. But this is so with every defendant who seeks to rely upon provocation . . . [T]he statutory reference to a "reasonable man" . . . is of general application. Inherent in the use of this prescribed standard as a uniform standard applicable to all defendants is the possibility that an individual defendant may be temperamentally unable to achieve this standard.'

The effect is, to use the 'homosexual' illustration, that if the accused is taunted as to being a homosexual, the gravity of the taunt is judged by looking at the effect of the taunt on the reasonable accused who is a homosexual; however, the s 3 test of 'whether the provocation was enough to make a reasonable man do as he did' is assessed by looking at the standard of the reasonable man. 'The statutory reasonable man has the power of self-control to be expected of an ordinary person of like age and sex. In other respects, that is, in respects other than power of self-control, the reasonable man shares such of the accused's characteristics as the jury think would affect the gravity of the provocation to the defendant.' This is Lord Nicholls' summary of the post-*Camplin* law on the second limb of the defence of provocation. This is very much the view of Andrew Ashworth in 'The doctrine of provocation' [1976] CLJ 292, 300:

> The proper distinction . . . is that individual peculiarities which bear on the gravity of the provocation should be taken into account, whereas individual peculiarities bearing on the accused's level of self-control should not.

How then does this view of provocation fit in with diminished responsibility? Lord Nicholls stated:

> . . . when adopting the 'reasonable man' standard in section 3 of the Homicide Act 1957 Parliament recognised that, standing alone, this provision might work harshly on defendants suffering from mental abnormality. Accordingly, cheek by jowl with section 3 Parliament introduced into English law the partial defence of diminished responsibility. . . . This provision . . . is apt to embrace some cases where it is inappropriate to apply the standard of control of an ordinary person. . . . Section 2 represents the legislature's view on how cases of mental abnormality are to be accommodated in the law of homicide. *Raven*

[1982] Crim LR 51 appears to be an instance of a case where this defence would have been relevant . . . Similarly in *Ahluwalia*, where a defence of provocation failed, the Court of Appeal ordered a retrial on the issue of diminished responsibility.

Section 3 is therefore to be read in light of the fact that s 2 is appropriate for instances of defendants suffering from mental abnormality. 'Section 3 should not be distorted to accommodate the types of case for which section 2 was specifically enacted.'

The use by Lord Nicholls of the defence of diminished responsibility, as a defence specifically enacted to benefit those defendants suffering from a mental abnormality who could not comply with the ordinary powers of self-control expected of an ordinary person, effectively ended the contest between the view that mental abnormality could not (*Luc*) or could (*Smith*) be taken into account when assessing the power of self-control to be expected of an ordinary person. Nevertheless, Lord Nicholls went on to discuss the issue. The majority view in *Smith* was that the accused had to be judged against the standard of someone 'in his situation' (per Lord Slynn); a mentally infirm defendant therefore was not to be assessed against an unvarying standard. Lord Nicholls rejected the view of the majority in *Smith* as usurping the function of Parliament. Their ruling was an impermissible development of the law laid down by Parliament in 1957. 'Whether the provocative act or words and the defendant's response met the "ordinary person" standard prescribed by the statute is the question the jury must consider, not the altogether looser question of whether, having regard to all the circumstances, the jury consider the loss of self-control was sufficiently excusable.' Therefore, the view of the majority in *Smith* was wrong.

Lord Nicholls added four more 'ancillary points':

(1) 'If the defendant is taunted on account of his intoxication, that may be a relevant matter for the jury to take into account when assessing the gravity of the taunt to the defendant. But the defendant's intoxicated state is not a matter to be taken into account by the jury when considering whether the defendant exercised ordinary self-control. The position is the same, so far as provocation is concerned, if the defendant's addiction to alcohol has reached the stage that he is suffering from the disease of alcoholism.'

(2) Where a woman suffers from a personality disorder, postnatal depression or battered woman syndrome, the law is this. 'The jury will decide . . . whether in their opinion, having regard to the actual provocation and their view of its gravity for the defendant, a woman of her age having ordinary power of self-control might have done what the defendant did. More importantly, . . . the defendant will in principle have available to her the defence of diminished responsibility.'

For more on diminished responsibility, see pp 367–79 in Chapter 9.

(3) '. . . in recent years much play has been made of the "mental gymnastics" required of the jurors in having regard to a defendant's "characteristics" for one purpose of the law of provocation but not another. Their Lordships consider that any difficulties in this regard have been exaggerated. The question is largely one of presentation.' In particular, the majority considered that any reference to 'characteristics' should be eschewed.

(4) 'In expressing their conclusion . . . their Lordships are not to be taken as accepting that the present state of the law is satisfactory. It is not. The widely held view is that the law relating to provocation is flawed to an extent beyond reform by the courts: see the Law Commission report *Partial Defences to Murder*, Law Com. No. 290, 2004, para. 2.10. But the law on provocation cannot be reformed in isolation from a review

of the law of homicide as a whole. In October 2004 the Home Secretary announced the government's intention to review the law of murder. Given the importance of this area of the criminal law it is imperative that a review . . . should be undertaken as soon as possible.'

[This review has been undertaken and the Commission's Report No. 306 of November 2006, *Murder, Manslaughter and Infanticide*, is discussed at various pages in the text.]

Applying the law to the facts of the present case, their Lordships held that 'evidence that the defendant was suffering from chronic alcoholism was not a matter to be taken into account by the jury when considering whether in their opinion, having regard to the actual provocation and their view of its gravity, a person having ordinary powers of self-control would have done what the defendant did.' Two comments on this ruling may be made at this stage. First, the application of the law to the facts demonstrates that a judge can instruct the jury without using the concept of 'characteristic'. The second is that right at the end, Homer has nodded. The final part of the sentence ought to have been expressed as '*might* have done what the defendant did', not '*would* have done'. In any case the appeal was dismissed by the majority in **Holley**.

The advice of two members of the dissenting minority, Lords Bingham and Hoffmann, started from the basis that the defence was 'a humane concession to human infirmity'. Therefore, provocation's boundaries should be set consonantly with its rationale. Moreover, another policy was to reduce violence. 'The public policy underlying adoption of the reasonable man test in the common law doctrine of provocation was to reduce the incidence of fatal violence by preventing a person relying upon his exceptional pugnacity or excitability as an excuse for loss of self-control . . .' The changes made by Parliament in 1957 were two: the permitting of words to be taken into account and the placing of the decision whether the defendant killed under provocation, having regard to the objective standard of the reasonable man, into the jury's hands. With regard to the latter amendment to the common law, their Lordships instanced **Bedder** v **DPP** above: 'a trial jury could no longer be directed that the reasonable (or ordinary or average) man should not be treated as a sexually impotent man . . .' With respect to the argument of the majority that **Camplin** was restricted to the extension of the 'ordinary person' to an 'ordinary person sharing the accused's age and gender' the dissentients said that if that were so, the speeches in **Camplin** 'would have been shorter, simpler and to different effect.' Their Lordships had in that case reminded themselves of the 'concession to human frailty' rationale of the defence; they had accepted that the law laid down in **Bedder** was wrong after 1957; they had rejected 'the notion that the objective comparison should be made with an abstract, hypothetical, reasonable man'; and the reference to age was merely an illustration that like should be treated alike. This view of **Camplin** was taken shortly afterwards by the highly experienced Lord Lane CJ in **Newell** (1980) 71 Cr App R 331. His judgment was to the effect that 'the defendant should be presumed to possess in general the power of self-control of the ordinary man, save insofar as his power of self-control was weakened because of some particular characteristic possessed by him, such characteristics potentially including not only physical qualities but also mental qualities and such indeterminate attributes as colour, race and creed, the question being whether such characteristic or attribute distinguished the defendant from the ordinary member of the community.' On this basis the *ratio* or *dicta* in the following cases was or were correct:

Raven above: mental age;

Ahluwalia [1992] 4 All ER 889: 'mental state or personality';

Dryden [1995] 4 All ER 987: 'features of character or personality';

Humphreys [1995] 4 All ER 1008: 'seriously abnormal characteristics';

Morhall above: habitual glue-sniffing;

Thornton (No. 2) [1996] 1 WLR 1174: 'her personality disorder and the effect of the deceased's abuse over a period upon her mental make-up'.

In their Lordships' opinion these authorities were true to the spirit of *Camplin*. 'The effect of these decisions was not to abrogate the important safeguard provided by the objective comparison, and there is nothing in these cases to suggest that short temper or undue pugnacity or excitability could begin to excuse the deliberate taking of a human life. The cases do, however, make clear that the objective comparison is a matter for the opinion of the jury, as Parliament had enacted, with such properly expressed judicial guidance as might be appropriate in the particular case. And they make clear, as *Camplin* had done, that the question is not whether the defendant showed such self-control as would reasonably be expected of a person having such of his attributes as the jury thought relevant in the factual situation in which the defendant actually found himself at the relevant time.' Accordingly, *Luc* was incorrectly decided.

In summary, for the minority, as Mantell LJ put it in *Weller*:

> . . . the question whether the defendant should reasonably have controlled himself is to be answered by the jury taking all matters into account. That includes matters relating to the defendant, the kind of man he is and his mental state, as well as the circumstances in which the death occurred. . . . This approach has the considerable advantage that it is unnecessary to determine whether what has been called a 'characteristic' of the accused is an eligible characteristic for the purposes of the second element in provocation.

Applying the law to the facts, the jury according to the minority should have been directed to take into account the accused's chronic alcoholism. He should have had a defence of provocation.

The third member of the dissenting threesome was Lord Carswell. He agreed with the other two and added that the distinction between the gravity of the provocation and the level of self-control 'cannot readily be made comprehensible to a jury by the directions fashioned by a judge with the greatest care and clarity.' The dichotomy accepted by the majority was 'illogical, inexplicable and unjust'. He accepted that the law was as stated by Lord Nicholls in *Smith*:

> The general principle is that the same standards of behaviour are expected of everyone, regardless of their individual psychological make-up. In most cases, nothing more will need to be said. But the jury should in an appropriate case be told . . . that this is a principle and not a rigid rule. It may sometimes have to yield to a more important principle, which is to do justice in the particular case. So the jury may think that there was some characteristic of the accused, whether temporary or permanent, which affected the degree of control which society could reasonably have expected of him and which it would be unjust not to take into account.

On the facts of this case, the accused's chronic alcoholism should have been taken into account.

All three dissentients agreed with the majority that homicide law in the words of Lord Carswell 'needs comprehensive and fundamental reform. It is a patchwork of rules which makes coherent direction of juries unnecessarily difficult and reflects no credit on our legal system.' The Law Commission's 2006 Report has been mentioned above and is discussed below.

(g) Relevant and irrelevant characteristics

Lord Simon in *Camplin* said that the reasonable person was not unusually excitable, pugnacious or ill-tempered. It did not matter whether the excitability arose out of the 'cultural environment or ethnic origin' or whether the characteristic was idiosyncratic to the accused. These character traits are inconsistent with what Lord Diplock in *Camplin* called the 'powers of self-control as everyone is entitled to expect that his fellow citizens will exercise in society as it is today'. In an old case, *Kirkham* (1837) 8 C&P 115, Coleridge J in his address to the jury said: 'Though the law condescends to human frailty, it will not indulge to human ferocity. It considers man to be a rational being, and requires that he should exercise a reasonable control over his passions.' Presumably he is sane.

Before *Camplin* it was accepted that he was not drunk, at least if the intoxication was not self-induced: *McCarthy* [1954] 2 QB 105 and *Wardrope* [1960] Crim LR 770. Both Canada and New Zealand have authorities which hold that drink can affect whether the accused was in fact provoked, i.e. the first limb: *Squire* (1975) 31 CRNS 214 and *Barton* [1977] 1 NZLR 295. There is old English authority to like effect: *Thomas* (1837) 173 ER 356, but the law seems settled that drink has no effect on the standard of reasonableness. Intoxication can be seen as the reason why the accused is unusually excitable, pugnacious or ill-tempered, and Lord Goddard CJ explained the law in this way in *McCarthy*. The modern explanation is that intoxication is in general no defence to a crime: *Morhall*, above, and *Rowland* above. Furthermore, it is inconsistent with the idea of a person of ordinary or reasonable self-control. The previous explanation was that intoxication was a temporary characteristic and such a trait was not one of those which could be attributed to the reasonable person. However, self-induced glue-sniffing may be a characteristic of a reasonable person: *Morhall*. The House of Lords moved away from the law as stated in *Newell* (1980) 71 Cr App R 331 that the characteristic had to be sufficiently permanent and it appears that permanence is no longer a requirement. Since eczema is a temporary matter, the temporary nature of the characteristic does not exclude its being taken into account.

The House of Lords in *Morhall* also stated that undue emphasis should not be placed on the need for the accused to have a particular *characteristic*. The accused's entire circumstances, such as his history, his generosity and his success in business, are relevant. *Morhall*, above, *Dryden* [1995] 4 All ER 987 (CA) and *Humphreys* [1995] 4 All ER 1008 (CA) exemplify the proposition that the jury must consider almost all characteristics, such as an obsessional and eccentric nature as in *Dryden* and an attention-seeking personality coupled with immaturity in *Humphreys* (but not the accused's 'explosiveness'). Physical matters which affect the brain causing 'reduced impulse control' must be considered: *Horsman* [2001] EWCA 3040. While not overruled, the attention-seeking trait in *Humphreys* seemed inconsistent with *Smith*. Glue-sniffing, having an obsessional personality and possessing an attention-seeking complex respectively were traits which distinguished the defendants from ordinary people. As Susan Edwards put it, 'The erosion of the objective test in provocation' (2001) 23 JSWFL 227, 237: 'Leaving the question to the jury's subjectivism may produce a reasonable man who is racist, sexist, and ethnocentric.' The problem which results was well addressed by Lord Lane CJ in *Dryden*: 'If one adds all the characteristics of the appellant to the notional reasonable man, there is a danger that the reasonable man becomes reincarnated as the appellant.' Subject to exceptions such as pugnacity and intoxication the law arrived at this position as a result of *Smith*.

It should be noted that even though the relevant characteristic is imputed to the reasonable person, the defence fails if a reasonable person would have acted differently from the accused. For example, in *Dryden* 'the jury would inevitably have rejected the suggestion that to go in, deliberately put on the holster, come out with a loaded gun and fire it to kill, was something which someone with the self-control of a reasonable man would have done' (*per* Lord Taylor CJ). Lord Taylor CJ in *Thornton (No. 2)*, above, held that where battered woman syndrome had affected the accused's personality it became a relevant characteristic.

Potter LJ in *Rowland*, above, said: '. . . there may be difficult borderline cases, particularly as between mere bad temper or excitability on the one hand and identifiable mental conditions and personality traits on the other'. In such instances the judge should be careful in directing the jury.

If the characteristic is one which is permissible to take into account, the law presumably excludes from the defence of provocation those subjected to what might be called 'untrue name-calling'. Take, for instance, a non-paedophile who is called a child molester. He cannot rely on the taunt because it is not addressed to any characteristic he possesses, yet it may well be that he deserves a defence.

The first case to apply *Camplin* was *Newell* (1980) 71 Cr App R 331. The accused, a chronic alcoholic for 10 years, had been deserted by his woman, and he attempted to commit suicide. His feelings of depression continued. A few days later he was drinking again as well as taking drugs. A friend spoke disparagingly about his former mistress and made a homosexual suggestion. The accused responded by picking up a heavy ashtray and striking him more than 20 times around the head, thereby killing him. The Court of Appeal held, first, that while applying the reasonable man test, the jurors should be guided by their own individual and collective reaction to the suggestion that the reasonable person could not have reacted in a certain way; secondly, characteristics which were to be considered under *Camplin* had to have a sufficient degree of permanence so as to be regarded as part of the accused's personality, e.g. 'mental qualities', sex, religion, and ethnicity and on the facts the accused's alcoholism. In the words of the court the characteristic had to make the accused 'a different person from the ordinary run of mankind'. The fact that the accused was drunk, drugged and depressed were insufficient. This *dictum* must now be incorrect in the light of *Morhall* where emphasis was placed on the fact that the reasonable person was an ordinary one and therefore was not different from the ordinary run of mankind. Glue-sniffing in *Morhall* was a characteristic which could be taken into account when determining the effect the taunt might have on an ordinary reasonable person for the provocation would affect a solvent abuser more than it would a non-glue-sniffer. The taunt was aimed at the characteristic of glue-sniffing. Battered woman syndrome may fit into the first class. Something transitory such as a temporary suicidal disposition and exhaustion brought about by drugs and alcohol of short duration was irrelevant, according to *Newell*. Last, there had to be a causal link between the particular characteristic and the nature of the provocation. There was none such in *Newell* on the facts. Alcoholism was a possible characteristic but the provocation from the victim was not directed at it. In *Morhall* the House of Lords clarified the law and there is now no doubt that an addiction, such as one to alcohol, can be a relevant characteristic.

The requirement that the provocation must be directed at the relevant characteristic of the accused has been criticised on the ground that it complicates the application of the reasonable person test, but the principle is sound: to say that the accused in *Raney*, above, was 'legless' might be provoking but the fact that he had one leg is irrelevant if he is taunted as to the colour of his skin. The court did not say that chronic alcoholism could or could not be a characteristic. The fact was that that illness had nothing to do with the words by which he was provoked. The court refused leave to appeal. The law has moved on.

Temporary physical and mental states such as impotence can be taken into account. Lord Goff in *Morhall* expressly said 'some physical conditions (such as eczema) may be transitory in nature and yet can surely be taken into account in the subject of taunts'. The depression in *Smith* itself was of a temporary nature. Accordingly *Newell* is no longer correct on this issue.

In *Camplin* itself Lord Simon suggested that a female accused's suffering from PMT, being pregnant or undergoing the menopause were features with which the reasonable person might be endowed. These are not extraordinary features, nor are they peculiar to a particular accused. The Court of Appeal in *Ahluwalia*, above, declined to consider the appellant's contention that she had a characteristic of 'learned helplessness' which was part of the battered woman syndrome because no evidence to support it had been led. The position might have been different if such evidence had been adduced. Her heightened sensitivity to the victim's behaviour brought about by the syndrome would have been a characteristic within *Camplin* and the battering would have been part of the context. Lord Taylor CJ applied the words of North J in the New Zealand case of *McGregor* [1962] NZLR 1069 as the Court of Appeal had earlier done in *Newell*. Although the accused had been severely maltreated by her husband there was no evidence that she was 'marked off or distinguished from the ordinary [woman] of the community'. Accordingly, her plea failed. Nevertheless, the court did not totally rule out a situation in which a defendant could rely on the battered woman syndrome. The accused's successful plea of diminished responsibility is difficult to square with the principal plea, provocation. The latter defence in her case was partly based on her contention that her response to the victim's behaviour was reasonable, whereas diminished responsibility is not grounded on reasonableness. (Indeed in the USA the syndrome has been used by battered children and homosexual lovers. In England evidence of 'battered husbands' syndrome' was led in *Irons* (1995) 16 Cr App R (S) 46.) A difficulty with the syndrome is that not all battered women suffer from it with the result that those who do not fall within the proposed definition cannot rely on it, though it must be said that the definition is only a working one and that it is a nature of syndromes (such as post-traumatic stress disorder) that not all potential sufferers do in fact suffer from them. The US definition may not become the English one. One criticism of the syndrome from the English law viewpoint was that it may be difficult to envisage the dead male directing his onslaught at this characteristic but after *Camplin*, *Morhall* and *Smith* this issue is less relevant than before.

It is suggested that the rule should be whether the characteristic excused the accused's fatal response. The defendant's control over her reactions may be reduced in comparison with those of a reasonable person through the syndrome. Supporters of abused women argue that battered woman syndrome turns such women into abnormal people, it medicalises them. In *Humphreys*, the accused, who had a history of slashing her wrists to gain attention, killed the victim with whom she was cohabiting. He had said to his son and two friends: 'We'll be all right for a gang bang tonight', and he told her on the same evening when he arrived home to discover that she had again slashed her wrists that she had not made a very good job of her attempted suicide. She immediately stabbed him with a kitchen knife. The court held that her immaturity and attention-seeking traits were characteristics within *Camplin* and that the taunts were directed at these abnormal aspects of her personality.

Two contrasting cases to the above are **Roberts** [1990] Crim LR 123 and **Ali** [1989] Crim LR 736. In the former the Court of Appeal held that on the facts the reasonable man was 23 years old, suffering from a large degree of deafness, and having a consequent speech impairment. However, the fact that he reacted with irrational explosions of violence (which was part of his frustration at being a deaf-mute) was not a trait of the ordinary person because excitability was to be disregarded by the jury. Deaf-mutes did not necessarily react violently when taunted about their condition. In the latter case the victim seized the accused, aged 20, at a disco and punched him to the ground. The accused stabbed him to death. The Court of Appeal held, following **Newell**, that there was no causal nexus between the accused's age and the provocation. Therefore, his age was irrelevant. The question was therefore, on the facts, not how would a reasonable 20-year-old react but how would a reasonable person of, say, 35 react? His sex was also irrelevant. No reasonable jury could have considered that his age or sex affected his behaviour.

The authority of the English cases of **Newell**, **Dryden** and **Thornton (No. 2)** in relation to mental characteristics was undermined by the Privy Council advice in **Luc Thiet Thuan v R** [1997] AC 131. The trial judge did not refer to the fact that the appellant had brain damage which caused him to lack self-control. Lord Goff, delivering the opinion of the majority, referred to **Camplin** and said that an accused was imbued with the powers of self-control expected of a reasonable person of the same age and sex as he was. 'But it is an entirely different question whether the mental infirmity of the defendant which impairs his power of self-control should be taken into account; and indeed it is difficult to see how it can be consistent with a person having the power of self-control of an ordinary person.' Accordingly, 'there is no basis upon which mental infirmity on the part of the defendant which has the effect of reducing his powers of self-control below that to be expected of an ordinary person can, as such, be attributed to the ordinary person . . .'. However, applying **Camplin** and **Morhall**, 'mental infirmity of the defendant, if itself the subject of taunts by the deceased, may be taken into account as going to the gravity of the provocation as applied to the defendant'. The majority averred that to accept that the reasonable person's power of self-control was reduced by mental imbalance would mean that the law of diminished responsibility was to be incorporated into the law of provocation. Such a result was not intended by Parliament. Lord Goff accepted that provocation could be cumulative but expressed no opinion on the effect of cumulative provocation on the battered persons' syndrome. One point of authority is that although the case is a Privy Council one, there was only one Law Lord in the majority; the other Law Lord there formed the minority. It was not that there were four Law Lords in the majority as had sometimes been the case. English courts continue to apply the Court of Appeal authorities, which are binding on them, whereas the advice of the Privy Council is only of persuasive authority: **Campbell** [1997] 1 Cr App R 199 and **Parker** [1997] Crim LR 760 (a case where alcoholism had caused brain damage). The House of Lords in **Smith** [2001] 1 AC 146, as we have seen, rejected the reasoning behind **Luc Thiet Thuan**, above. In the words of Lord Hoffmann in **Smith**, the jury has to enquire whether 'the behaviour of the accused . . . measured up to the standard of self-control which ought reasonably to have been expected of him'. This subjectivised test ('of him') is not what Parliament intended. However, as we have also seen, the fortunes of **Luc** were restored by **Holley**.

(h) The ordinary person test

Lord Goff in **Morhall** said that the reasonable person test in provocation was not the same as that in tort. It was not concerned with reasonable foreseeability and reasonable care.

The function of the test is only to introduce, as a matter of policy, a standard of self-control which has to be complied with if provocation is to be established in law. . . . It would be entirely consistent with the law as stated in s 3 of the 1957 Act . . . to direct the jury simply by reference to a hypothetical person having the power of self-control to be expected of an *ordinary* person of the age and sex of the defendant but in other respects sharing such of the defendant's characteristics as they think would affect the gravity of the provocation to him . . .

Lord Goff in **Morhall** spoke of the ordinary person, rather than the reasonable man or reasonable person but in **Smith** the House of Lords, perhaps without noticing the point, reverted to 'reasonable man', which after all is what the statute says. The point which Lord Goff was making was that in s 3 the 'reasonable man' was not a paragon, an exemplary person, but an ordinary one who may be addicted to drugs.

Summary of the current law

The Judicial Studies Board issued a Specimen Direction on Provocation in 2003. It was an attempt to provide to trial judges a 'Court of Appeal – proof' instruction to juries after **Smith**. Paragraph (iv) reads in part:

It is . . . for you [the jury] to decide whether or not [the accused's] loss of self-control was sufficiently excusable to reduce the offence from murder to manslaughter. When deciding this, bear in mind that the law expects people to exercise control over their emotions. If a person has an unusually volatile, excitable or violent nature (or is drunk), he cannot rely on that as an excuse. Otherwise, however, it is entirely for you . . . to decide what are appropriate standards of behaviour, what degree of control society could reasonably have expected of [the accused], and what is the just outcome of the case. You should make allowances for human nature and the power of emotions.

After **Holley** the law has reverted to that as stated in **Camplin** and characteristics of the accused are relevant to the gravity of the taunt but not to the potential for loss of self-control. A revised specimen direction is awaited. However, still excluded are personality defects such as excitability, pugnacity, and 'explosiveness' (as in **Humphreys**) as well as intoxication. Indeed, there is some support of omitting reference to the reasonable person altogether.

The Court of Appeal confirmed in **James** [2006] 1 All ER 759 that **Holley** has overruled **Smith** despite **Holley** being the advice of the Privy Council and **Smith** being a decision of the Lords. The fact that **James** was composed of a five-person bench emphasises its authority. The fact also that the Privy Council in **Holley** comprised Law Lords is to the same effect. For the cases applying **Holley** see **Mohammed** [2005] EWCA Crim 1880, **Van Dongen** [2005] 2 Cr App R 632 (CA) and **Shickle** [2005] EWCA Crim 1881.

What are the functions of judge and jury?

Since the Homicide Act 1957 matters which were previously rules of law have become factors. For example, the accused may now have a defence of provocation even though his reaction was not proportionate to the attack. What was part of the judge's function has become an issue for the jury. As Lord Diplock said in **Camplin** [1978] AC 705:

Until the 1957 Act there was a condition precedent: the deceased's conduct had to be of a kind capable in law of constituting provocation. The House so held in **Mancini** . . . Section 3 . . . abolished all previous rules as to what could or could not amount to provocation.

Provocation may be lawful; it may be self-induced; there may be something of a cooling-off time, though recent cases such as **Thornton** seem to be remaking this factor into a rule of law; and so on. All that the judge on this approach has to do is to instruct the jury that the accused must have lost his self-control (which she had not, for instance, in **Thornton**) and that he is to be judged against the reasonable person imbued with the characteristics relevant under **Camplin** and its progeny. The argument against Lord Diplock's interpretation of s 3 is that in 1957 Parliament intended and did change the law in certain ways only. It did not amend the normal common law rule about leaving evidence to the jury.

These remaining matters need some analysis. The first 'limb' of provocation is whether the accused was in fact so provoked as to lose his self-control. May the judge withdraw this issue from the jury on the grounds that no reasonable jury could find that he had done so? The law seems to have been settled by **Whitfield** (1976) 63 Cr App R 39 and **Camplin** (above): if there is any evidence of provocation, it must be left to the jury, no matter how thin that evidence is and no matter whether the judge believes that no reasonable jury would have found that the accused had been provoked. Recently, however, there seems to have been a retreat from these propositions.

In the case of **Whitfield** the defendant killed his wife and sister-in-law after a quarrel. He said that his wife had told him that her child was not his, and that when he said he would kill himself, she said: 'see if I care'. His evidence was hard to follow. The Court of Appeal held that the trial judge was wrong to withdraw the issue on the basis that no jury could find that the accused had been provoked. In **Jones** [1987] Crim LR 701 and **Stewart** [1995] 4 All ER 999 the same court determined that there should be a full direction on the law if provocation was raised on the facts. A direction on provocation must be given, even if counsel objects: **Burgess** [1995] Crim LR 425 (CA). In **Rossiter** (1992) 95 Cr App R 326 the accused, a battered wife, killed her husband, stabbing him deeply twice and superficially 17 times. Though the defence had not been raised, the Court of Appeal quashed the conviction for murder and substituted one for manslaughter on the basis that the judge should have put the defence to the jury because there was clear evidence of it. She may have been attacked with a rolling-pin, half-strangled and attacked with a mitre block. In several cases such as **Johnson** (1989) 89 Cr App R 148 the Court of Appeal has approved **Cascoe** (1970) 54 Cr App R 401:

> Whether the issue is raised at the trial or not, if there is evidence which might lead the jury to find provocation, then it is the duty of the Court to leave that issue to the jury.

This principle governs even if, as was said in **Cascoe** itself, the evidence is 'very thin indeed'. Lord Diplock approved this principle in **Camplin**, as did the Court of Appeal in the second **Newell** case [1989] Crim LR 906. It seems, therefore, that even if the sole evidence is that of the accused, the issue of loss of self-control is for the jury. This rule applies even though as in **Newell** the accused has not attempted to raise provocation, where his defence is one of diminished responsibility as in **Cox** [1995] 2 Cr App R 513 (CA), where the accused's defence was that he was attempting to escape from the deceased and the death was an accident as in **Dhillon** [1997] 2 Cr App R 106 (CA) or as in **Sawyer** [1989] Crim LR 906 (CA) where the accused relied on self-defence. The defence may attempt not to adduce evidence of provocation, fearing that it will undermine the principal defence, but the judge must instruct the jury on provocation. Where there is evidence of provocation, it must be left to the jury, and this rule applies even when as in **Sawyer** and in **Stewart**, where the accused pleaded that the death of his wife was an accident, provocation is inconsistent with the defence on which the accused is seeking to rely. Even where the accused contends that he did not cause the death of the victim, provocation must be left to the jury, provided that there is evidence from which a reasonable jury might conclude that there has been provocation, even though the judge does not believe that no reasonable person would have responded as the accused did: *Cambridge* [1994] 2 All ER 760 (CA). On the facts the issue had to be left for the jury, despite a possible finding of provocation being inconsistent with the defence submission that the accused did not cause the victim's death. *Newell* goes further. Provocation must be left to the jury if there is evidence of it, even when the accused says he was not present at the scene of the killing. There is a duty on counsel to inform the judge of the need to direct the jury on provocation when there is evidence that the accused lost his self-control: *Cox*. A direction on provocation must be given if the facts give rise to it, even if both prosecution and defence counsel think one is unnecessary: *Dhillon*. A conviction will be quashed if, at first instance, the defence waives reliance on provocation where there is any evidence of it: *McDonald* [2004] EWCA Crim 401.

If, however, there is no evidence of provocation at all, the issue should be withdrawn from the jury: *Robinson* [1965] Crim LR 491 (CA) and *Dryden*, though in the view of the author there was at least a modicum of evidence in the latter case that the accused had lost self-control. The leading authority is *Cocker* [1989] Crim LR 740. The Court of Appeal held that the judge was right to withdraw the issue from the jury when the evidence was that the accused had deliberately smothered his wife. He had given in to his wife's entreaties to kill her because she was suffering from an incurable wasting disease. The mere fact that he had not acted as he did beforehand did not mean that he had lost his self-control on this occasion, rather he had lost his self-restraint. Lord Lane CJ said: 'This was almost . . . the very opposite of provocation. It was his giving way to her entreaties and acting . . . perfectly in self-control . . . , however terrible that act was in its meaning.' There have been similar cases such as *Gilbert* (1978) 66 Cr App R 237 (CA), but *Cocker* has come under criticism, partly because if the accused in *Cocker* was in control of his actions, why was not the accused in *Steane*, dealt with above under malice aforethought, not also in control and therefore guilty? Perhaps the true defence in *Cocker* was diminished responsibility. *Cocker* also demonstrates the subjective nature of the first limb. It does not matter that any reasonable person might have killed the wife as a result of her entreaties – the question is whether this accused, having suddenly and temporarily lost control, killed the victim. *Cocker* demonstrates one limitation on the jury's discretion. The other was elucidated by the House of Lords in *Acott* [1997] 1 WLR 306. The provocation must be something said or done (or both). If the loss of self-control cannot be attributed to one (or both) of these causes, the defence of provocation is irrelevant. Lord Steyn said that if there was 'insufficient material for a jury to find that it is a reasonable possibility that there was specific provoking conduct resulting in a loss of self-control, there is simply no issue of provocation to be considered by the jury'. An example is when the accused killed in a fit of temper and the outburst has no external causes. Lord Steyn instanced 'fear, panic, sheer bad temper or . . . a slow down of traffic due to snow'. *Acott* was applied in *Marks*, the facts of which are stated at the start of the section on provocation above. The victim had not done or said anything which caused the accused to lose his self-control. There has to be evidence that something was said or done. A more recent case is *Miao* [2003] EWCA Crim 3486. The accused admitted to killing his partner. He contended that she had accused him of having an affair and had hit him. He said that in order to stop her shouting, he had put his hand over her mouth and that when she bit his hand, he had put it on her throat. The trial judge found that evidence of provocation was minimal and the accused was convicted of murder. The

Court of Appeal applied *Acott* and upheld the trial judge's decision. While there was evidence of provoking conduct, there was no evidence that he had lost self-control. The court held, using the words of Lord Steyn in *Acott*, that 'a speculative possibility' of provocation was insufficient to leave the issue to the jury. It should be noted that where there is evidence of a loss of self-control due to things said or done, or both, the rule in *Whitfield* and *Camplin* applies with full force.

What about the second issue, whether a reasonable person would have been provoked? Before the Homicide Act 1957 the judge could rule that the evidence was not such as would provoke a reasonable person to react as the accused did. The 1957 Act specifically reversed the law: 'The question whether provocation was enough to make a reasonable man do as he did shall be left to be determined by the jury . . .' If confirmation is needed, the Privy Council in *Phillips v R* [1969] 2 AC 130 and the House of Lords in *Camplin* (above) ruled that such was the law. The Criminal Law Revision Committee, Fourteenth Report, *Offences Against the Person*, Cmnd 7844, 1980, recommended the abolition of the rule that the judge could not withdraw the issue from the jury on the ground that there was no evidence on which the jurors could hold that the provocation was enough to make a reasonable person do as the accused did.

The effect of the shift from law to fact, from withdrawal of the issue to leaving it to the jury, means that the role of the judge is narrow, narrower than in other areas of the law. It could be that because the jury cannot be controlled in the ways that it was under the pre-1957 law, there could be inconsistent verdicts. A one-sentence summary of this section would be: if there is any evidence of provocation, the defence must be left to the jury.

It is possible, though rare, for the Crown to accept that the accused had a defence of provocation: *Gopal* (1995) *The Independent*, 25 April (CCC).

Conclusion

The Homicide Act 1957, s 3, reversed earlier law by providing that provocation may consist of words. It also removed the power from the judge to rule that a reasonable person would not have been provoked. For some time after the Act it was uncertain if the fact whether the accused retaliated as a reasonable person might have done was a matter for the judge or for the jury. This reasonable relationship rule could have survived either because the statute said 'do as he did' or because provocation was left undefined in the statute, except that it included words. The argument ran that since provocation otherwise bore its common law meaning, that definition included this proportionality rule, and therefore the rule was preserved. This argument was supported by the interpretation of 'do as he did' as covering the whole sequence of events, i.e. 'kill in the way that he killed'. On this approach the rule might survive as a matter of law. The contrary argument is that s 3 permits the jury to determine on the evidence whether a reasonable person would have done as the accused did. The judge was to state the law but leave the conclusions to be drawn from the evidence to the jury. The Court of Appeal accepted in *Walker* [1969] 1 WLR 311 that the Act overruled *Mancini v DPP* [1942] AC 1 on this point and that opinion has come to be accepted. That such an opinion is not in line with what the Royal Commission on Capital Punishment, Cmd 8932, 1953, the Report of which formed the basis of the 1957 Act, proposed, or with what the MPs who debated the Homicide Bill thought they were doing, is well demonstrated by P. English 'What DID Section 3 do to the law of provocation?' [1970] Crim LR 249. He showed that

Parliament wished to change only the two matters mentioned at the start of this section. The Court of Appeal in *Thornton*, *Ahluwalia* and *Richens* rejected the argument that s 3 provided a self-contained definition of provocation. In *Ahluwalia* the court stated that: 's 3 of the Homicide Act 1957 did not provide a general or fresh definition of provocation which remains a common law and not a statutory defence'. On this approach the (partial) definition in *Duffy* remains good law.

Certainly Parliament did not intend to alter the law in the way that *Camplin* and *Smith* did. The Lords in *Camplin* stated that the 1957 Act undermined the test in *Bedder* (above) that the reasonable person was not imbued with the defendant's traits. Lord Diplock said:

> It would stultify much of the mitigation of the previous harshness of the common law in ruling out verbal provocation . . . if the jury could not take into consideration all those factors which in their opinion would affect the gravity of taunts and insults when applied to the person to whom they are addressed.

Holley restores the law as to the attributes to be attributed to the reasonable person to those laid down in *Camplin*.

Reform

Lord Hoffmann's speech in *Smith* is highly apposite: '. . . it is impossible to read even a selection of the extensive modern literature on provocation without coming to the conclusion that the concept has serious logical and moral flaws'. The main argument for keeping provocation as a defence to murder is that, morally, killings which are provoked are not as serious as ones which are not. Nevertheless, severe criticisms have been made of the defence and there have been several consequent proposals for reform.

(a) There have been calls for the abolition of the mandatory life sentence for murder, e.g. by Lord Lane CJ in 1991. If that proposal were ever adopted, there would be no need for a special defence of provocation, which would be a factor in sentencing as it is in crimes other than murder. Contrariwise, if murder is to continue to be regarded as the most heinous crime, its gravity marked by a mandatory sentence, provocation would remain a useful defence. Perhaps it could be extended to all 'heat of passion' killings. The US Model Penal Code, s 2.01(3)(b), exculpates an accused who kills under the influence of 'extreme mental or emotional disturbance for which there is reasonable explanation or excuse'.

(b) Sometimes the objective 'limb' of the defence has been criticised as not being necessary. The reasonable person is not pugnacious. If a pugnacious man kills, his pugnacity is not considered, yet that characteristic is the reason why he killed when another man would not have done so. Andrew Ashworth put the opposite view in 'The doctrine of provocation' (1976) 35 CLJ 292 at 319: the abolition of the reasonable man test would mean that every trivial affront which caused a loss of temper could be provocation. People prone to anger would otherwise escape responsibility. Murphy J, dissenting in *Moffa* v *R* (1977) 13 Aust LR 225, put the contrary view to that of Ashworth:

> [m]uch of the opposition to discarding the objective test is based on the assumption that this will undermine the social fabric and cheapen the value of human life. It is easily overlooked . . . that the defence is only to murder, and its success results in a conviction for manslaughter.

He added that:

> the more heterogeneous our society becomes, the more inappropriate the test is. Behaviour is influenced by age, sex, ethnic origin, climatic and other living conditions, biorhythms, education, occupation and, above all, individual differences. It is impossible to construct a reasonable or ordinary [person].

See also the Irish case of **The People** v **MacEoin** (1978) 112 ILTR 53 (CA). The objective test's rationale was pinpointed by Lord Goff in **Morhall**. 'The function of the test is only to introduce, as a matter of policy, a standard of self-control which had to be complied with if provocation is to be established in law.' Accordingly, if policy changes, this test could be modified or even abandoned.

(c) The Law Commission draft Criminal Code, Law Com. No. 177, 1989, cl 58, would put into statutory form the 1957 Act and subsequent cases.

> A person who, but for this section, would be guilty of murder is not guilty of murder if –
> (a) he acts when provoked (whether by things done or by things said or by both and whether by the deceased person or by another) to lose his self-control; and
> (b) the provocation is, in all the circumstances (including any of his personal characteristics that affect its gravity), sufficient ground for the loss of self-control.

Clause 55 provides that a defence of provocation results in a conviction for manslaughter. The comment (para 14.18) on cl 58 is not too helpful but it notes that the same types of characteristics may be of relevance to provocation as with regard to duress by threats or duress of circumstances. The student should be grateful! The clause would remove reference to the reasonable or ordinary person, but the jury would still have to use their moral sense: were the circumstances such that the accused does not deserve to be convicted of murder? This seems to be very much the position reached in **Smith**. It also removes the references to sudden loss of self-control and to 'doing as he did' (found in s 3), which is a survival of the era when the killing had to be proportionate to the provocation. Clause 58 is based on the recommendations of the Criminal Law Revision Committee, *Offences Against the Person* Cmnd 7844, 1980. The Committee commented (at 35): 'This formulation has some advantage over the present law in that it omits reference to the entirely notional "reasonable man", directing the jury's attention instead to what they themselves consider reasonable – which has always been the real question.'

(d) In 1993 the Home Affairs Committee called for review of the law of murder and manslaughter so as to widen the defence of provocation to cover more women who kill their partners than does the law at present. It has to be said that, in the view of the author, it will call for excellence in drafting to exculpate women who kill when suffering from battered woman syndrome but convict those who kill in revenge. It might be a good idea to provide money for more refuges for women than is given nowadays.

(e) The principal academic critic of provocation at the present time is Jeremy Horder. In his book *Provocation and Responsibility* (Clarendon, 1991) he contends that the defence should be abolished. He asks why the emotion of anger should be privileged above greed, lust and envy, which do not partially excuse the accused. He argues that the requirement of sudden retaliation in **Duffy**, above, fails to capture the reality of the lives of many women. These women kill, not because they have lost their self-control, but because they see no other way out of their predicament. (Compare the research at researchnews.osu.ed/archive/symmetry.htm by Zeynep Benderlioglu that on provocation women become more aggressive than men.) They do kill deliberately and therefore provocation is not available. Even, however, if the prerequisite of sudden killing were removed, provocation would still not be the appropriate defence because the killing was not in anger but out of despair. Horder believes that killing in such circumstances is not acceptable morally. Accordingly, both on the grounds that provocation is a sexually biased defence being consistent only with the masculine psyche and that it should not be available for deliberate killings (even by battered women), it should be abolished. The acknowledgement that the defence is sex-biased seems generally accepted by commentators (such as Celia Wells in A. Ashworth and B. Mitchell (eds) *Rethinking English Homicide Law*, OUP, 2000) and by law reform bodies such as the Australian Model Criminal Code Officers Committee's *Discussion Paper on Fatal Offences against the Person*, 1998.

(f) At present provocation is a defence only to murder. If a reasonable person in the position of the accused might have killed, why might he not have wounded or otherwise harmed someone? There does not seem to be a good reason for restricting this defence to one offence.

(g) As noted already, it is strange that provocation is a defence to those who give way to their emotions, but no defence to those who kill under duress or who perform a mercy-killing. Killings under provocations are intentional killings. Why should this form of intentional killing receive special treatment? Why single out hot-blooded killers? The Australian Committee mentioned in (e) wrote: 'Why is a conservative Turkish Muslim father partially excused when he stabs his daughter to death because she refuses to stop seeing her boyfriend?' It should be added that while anger remains the core emotion in provocation, the battered women's cases show that it now extends to despair and fear, as Lord Hoffmann noted in *Smith*.

(h) If provocation were to be widened to allow battered persons to rely on it, it would be difficult to permit them to rely on the defence while keeping those who kill in revenge out of the defence.

(i) Another difficulty occurs when provocation and diminished responsibility are, as they sometimes are, pleaded together. In the former the prosecution must disprove it beyond reasonable doubt but the burden is on the accused in diminished responsibility. It may be difficult for juries to understand this distinction.

Various Bills have been proposed to reduce the requirements of the defence. In the Homicide (Defence of Provocation) Bill 1992/3 a clause would have permitted the jury to take into account 'any conduct of the deceased, including domestic violence, violence to immediate family members, and the threat of such violence'. The outcome would be that the reaction would no longer need to be sudden. It is indeed difficult to see how a person who has been battered over a long period could react as an ordinary person might.

The Law Commission 2004 proposals on provocation

The Law Commission issued its Report Law Com. No. 290, *Partial Defences to Murder*, in 2004. Its remit was restricted to provocation and diminished responsibility and to the question whether or not excessive force should be a defence to murder in the same way that provocation and diminished responsibility are; that is, by reducing murder to manslaughter. The issues of diminished responsibility and excessive self-defence are dealt with elsewhere. In respect of provocation the Home Secretary invited the Commission to review the defence particularly in light of its impact on domestic violence cases and whether it should be merged with diminished responsibility or self-defence or both. The Commission has for several years wished to examine the law of murder as a whole but its reports are restricted by the terms of reference given to it by the Home Secretary.

The Report is a vastly different document in respect of provocation from its precursor Consultation Paper (No. 173) of the same name in 2003. That Paper expressed the opinion that provocation existed solely to prevent some killers being adjudged to be murderers and therefore subject to mandatory life imprisonment, and the Commission was strongly of the view that no reformulation of the defence would enhance current law. For these reasons and unlike other Consultation Papers in criminal law the Commission's Paper did not contain proposals for reform; instead it asked readers whether provocation should be abolished (whether or not the mandatory sentence for murder was retained). As the Commission states in para 1.8 of its Report, the response to its Paper took it 'somewhat by surprise'. There was a groundswell in favour of retention even if the mandatory sentence were abolished. In light of this groundswell the Commission decided not to abolish the defence but to retain it with (substantial) amendments.

It is worth setting out the summary of the recommendations in full.

> . . . the principles which should govern a reformed partial defence of provocation are:
> 1. unlawful homicide that would otherwise be murder should be manslaughter if:
>   a. the defendant acted in response to
>   i.   gross provocation (meaning words or conduct or a combination of words and conduct which caused the defendant to have a justifiable sense of being seriously wronged); or
>   ii. fear of serious violence towards the defendant or another; or
>   iii. a combination of i and ii [The Commission wrote a. and b. but it meant i and ii]; and
>   b. a person of the defendant's age and of ordinary temperament, i.e. ordinary tolerance and self-restraint, in the circumstances of the defendant might have reacted in the same or a similar way.
> 2. In deciding whether a person of ordinary temperament in the circumstances of the defendant might have acted in the same or a similar way, the court should take into account the defendant's age and all the circumstances of the defendant other than matters whose only relevance to the defendant's conduct is that they bear simply on his or her general capacity for self-control.
> 3. The partial defence shall not apply where
>   a. the provocation was incited by the defendant for the purpose of providing an excuse to use violence, or
>   b. the defendant acted in considered desire for revenge.
> 4. A person should not be treated as having acted in considered desire for revenge if he or she acted in fear of serious violence merely because he or she was also angry towards the deceased for the conduct which engendered that fear.

The Commission proposed that any overlap between provocation and duress (by threats) should be resolved thus.

> 5. The partial defence should not apply to a defendant who kills or takes part in the killing of another person under duress of threats by a third person.

This recommendation was made pending review of the law of murder.

The Commission also proposed to change the law relating to the functions of judge and jury.

> 6. A judge should not be required to leave the defence to the jury unless there is evidence on which a reasonable jury, properly directed, could conclude that it might apply.

The actual drafting of the revised defence was for Parliamentary counsel.

In sum the proposals at the same time widen and reduce the width of the current defence, and the final proposal would give the court the power to withdraw the issue from the jury, unlike at present, thereby bringing provocation into line with other defences.

The Commission expressed dissatisfaction with provocation as it exists at present. It identified the following defects: the difficulty of fitting 'slow burn' and delayed reaction into the first subjective limb of the defence, for example, a battered woman who kills her abuser while he or she is asleep or drunk; the effect of **Smith** on the second objective limb (now gone as a result of **Holley**); the difficulty in finding a 'truly coherent, logical or consistent' rationale for the defence (para 3.21). The arguments in favour of abolishing provocation are summarised in para 3.36:

> . . . a person who is sane and who kills another person unlawfully, with the intent required for murder, ought to be guilty of murder however great the provocation may have been. . . . Not only is it inappropriate that provocation should be singled out among other possible mitigating circumstances as providing a special partial defence, but there are great difficulties in trying to define what may amount to provocation and how serious it has to be in order to amount to a partial defence.

The arguments in favour of retaining it are aptly summarised in the following paragraph of the Report:

> Where the defendant's conduct was precipitated by really serious provocation, it is morally right that this should be reflected in the way society labels and sentences the defendant. . . . The existence of such a partial defence is justifiable in the law of murder, although there is no similar partial defence to non-fatal offences of violence, not only because the sentence for murder is fixed by law but also because of the unique gravity and stigma attached to murder. The real problem with provocation is not the underlying concept, but the way it has developed. It needs to be reshaped.

The Commission itself opines (para 3.63):

> . . . the moral blameworthiness of homicide may be significantly lessened when the defendant acts in response to gross provocation in the sense of words or conduct (or a combination) giving the defendant a justified sense of being severely wronged. . . . We do not suggest that these are the only circumstances which could significantly extenuate moral responsibility for homicide, but we do think that they fall into a distinct category. . . . An example is the genuine case of mercy killing, but that falls outside the terms of our present review.

Accordingly, the Law Commission proposed in line with the consultees' responses that the defence should be reformed by statute, and its preferred reformulation has been stated above.

One concept in that reformulation requires elucidation. 'Gross provocation' denotes that the defendant must have a 'justifiable sense of being seriously wronged' (para 3.68). By 'justifiable' the Commission means that the test is objective but the jury is to take into account the accused's circumstances and characteristics; therefore, the jury could reject traits as not being consonant with society in the twenty-first century. Gross provocation was not to be restricted to threats of or actual physical violence but would extend, for example, to words such as racial taunting.

The Commission was strongly of the view that the proposals should not differentiate between domestic and other killings and that they should be 'gender-neutral unless it is absolutely necessary to depart from that principle' (para 3.78).

The objective limb is preserved and reformulated as stated above. To repeat (para 3.109): 'The defence should only be available if a person of ordinary temperament, i.e. ordinary tolerance and self-restraint, in the circumstances of the defendant might have reacted in the same or a similar way.' Age would be relevant to the capacity for self-control. Overall, this is a significant change from the then existing law found in *Smith* and to a large degree restates the reasoning of the minority of their Lordships. Since the Commission proposes to abolish the subjective test as it presently exists, the stress that the reformulated objective limb will bear will be great.

Critique of the 2004 Proposals on Provocation

Some comments are necessary. First, because the Commission proposes to give the judge the ordinary power to withdraw issues from the jury in provocation cases, a member of a criminal gang will not be able to rely on the defence to kill members of rival gangs without being in imminent peril because no reasonable jury would so find. Secondly, the need for the objective limb is supported by Lord Hoffmann in *Smith*, where he said: 'A person who flies into a murderous rage when he is crossed, thwarted or disappointed in the vicissitudes of life should not be able to rely upon his anti-social propensity as even a partial excuse for killing.' Thirdly, people must exercise reasonable restraint and for this reason the excitable still would not fall within the revised defence. Fourthly, the test is not one whether or not the accused's reaction was reasonable but whether a person of ordinary temperament might have been driven to kill. Fifthly, the test is 'might', not 'would', just as in current law. Sixthly, while physical age is to be taken into consideration, mental age is not because to include mental age would complicate the law and would undermine the objective test. To quote the Law Commission (para 3.130): 'A person who is a psychopath or suffers from retarded development of mind may be eligible for a defence of diminished responsibility. We do not think that factors of that nature should be taken into account in adjusting the objective test for the purposes of provocation.'

As may be obvious, the defence will not be open to those who act out of 'considered revenge'. This concept is to replace the current subjective limb of provocation, that of the sudden and temporary loss of self-control. Furthermore, the defence would not be available when the accused himself or herself incited the gross provocation in order to have an excuse for using violence. In other words, this form of self-induced provocation would not fall within the amended defence.

The Law Commission agrees with Lord Hoffmann in *Smith* that:

> Male possessiveness and jealousy should not today be an acceptable reason for loss of self-control leading to homicide, whether inflicted upon the woman herself or her new lover. In Australia the judge [in *Stingel* (1990) 171 CLR 312] was able to give effect to this policy by withdrawing the issue from the jury. But section 3 prevents an English judge from doing so.

The Commission said (para 3.144): '. . . provocation should not be left to the jury in such a case because we do not see how any reasonable jury, properly directed, could conclude there had been gross provocation or that a person of ordinary tolerance and self-restraint might have acted in the same way as the defendant.' The adjustment to the functions of judge and jury would permit the judge to do so if the proposals were enacted.

Facts which in previous cases gave rise to the defence will no longer do so. The Commission instances *Baillie* ('considered revenge'), *Doughty* (the crying baby: no provocative conduct), and *Dryden* (similarly).

The Commission proposed neither to merge provocation and self-defence nor provocation and diminished responsibility. The burden of proof is to remain on the prosecution.

In conclusion, the Commission stated in para 3.152: 'Nobody pretends that this is an easy area of the law but we believe that this scheme would be workable and it would be a real improvement on the present law.'

The Law Commission, murder in the first and second degrees and provocation

In 2006 the Law Commission published its Report no. 306, *Murder, Manslaughter and Infanticide*, which is the follow-up to its Consultation Paper No. 177 *A New Homicide Act for England and Wales?* of 2005. The Report proposes a three-tier structure of murder and manslaughter which involves the reclassifying of the current law of murder and manslaughter into three categories. For example, where the accused intended to cause serious injury and foresaw a risk of death would be one of the states of mind required for first degree murder, but where the accused intended to cause serious injury but was not aware of the risk of death would become second degree murder. The scheme is outlined in Chapter 11 on Murder.

The Law Commission recently made proposals in its Report No. 290 *Partial Defences to Murder* 2004, which are explained in the previous section of this book. The Commission wishes to retain those recommendations. For example, it would be unjust that the boy in *Camplin* (above) who had been forcibly raped and laughed at should be sentenced to the mandatory life sentence for murder. However, the Commission did not place the defence within the proposed framework for homicide. Report No. 306 does just that. Provocation is to be retained as a defence but it will be restricted to first degree murder. Therefore, it will no longer be a defence in some instances where it is currently a defence: where there is second degree murder, provocation will not afford a defence. Provocation will still not remain a defence to other offences. With regard to those, provocation may be taken into account in the sentence. Similarly, with regard to second degree murder: the recommended maximum sentence for this kind of murder is life imprisonment; second degree murder unlike first degree murder will not attract the mandatory life sentence; therefore, a defence of provocation is not needed. In this way the defence of provocation will be narrowed. In other words, it will be more difficult to plead provocation successfully than it is now. It will also be narrowed because the judge will be given the power to withdraw weak cases from the jury in accordance with normal practice: a judge will no longer be required to leave the defence to the jury unless there is evidence on which a reasonable jury might find provocation. One advantage to the accused of this reversion to the normal rule (reversion because it seems that the current law was not intended by Parliament when it reformed provocation in s 3 of the Homicide Act 1957) is that he or she is no longer forced to rely on inconsistent defences where there is any possible evidence of provocation. For example, an accused may wish to rely on self-defence, where the outcome of a successful plea is an acquittal, but such a plea is in some respects inconsistent with a plea of provocation: in self-defence one may not have acted in hot blood whereas classically one must do so for a successful defence of provocation; yet if there is a scintilla of evidence of provocation, the judge must leave that issue to the jury. The present law is perhaps perverse when provocation is inconsistent with the defence, as occurs when the defendant's plea is one of alibi or 'no malice aforethought'. The Commission does, however, propose an interlocutory appeal against a judge's ruling that the defence should not be left to the jury (para 5.16). The provocation will have to be 'gross', and again some successful pleas under current law may fail at this hurdle.

The defence, however, will at the same time be widened. It will cover not just 'gross provocation' but also 'fear of serious injury'. 'It should be made possible in English law to plead provocation when the killing was in response to a fear of serious violence, if someone of an ordinary temperament but otherwise acting in circumstances facing the accused, might have reacted in the same or in a similar way.' (para 5.50) '. . . D should not be prejudiced because he or she overreacted in fear or panic, instead of overreacting due to an angry loss of self-control.' (para. 5.54) The requirement of loss of self-control, which the Law Commission call 'unnecessary and undesirable' (subheading before para. 5.17), is to be abrogated. Currently the law is unclear as to how immediate the accused's response must be and in the words of the Commission (at para 5.18): '. . . the requirement of loss of self-control has been widely criticised as privileging men's typical reactions over women's typical reactions. Women's reactions to provocation are less likely to involve a "loss of self-control", as such, and more likely to be comprised of a combination of anger, fear, frustration and a sense of desperation. This can make it difficult or impossible for women to satisfy the loss of self-control requirement, even where they otherwise deserve at least a partial defence.' The Commission adds: '. . . when a battered woman uses excessive force against her abusive partner only because she fears for her safety in any direct confrontation, it would be wrong to rule out her plea simply because there was no evidence of loss of self-control.' (para 5.29) Therefore, some battered partners will be afforded the defence in the future when they are not afforded it nowadays.

The Commission, however, rules out killings committed 'in considered desire for revenge'. Some battered persons may fall foul of this rule. The Commission singles out so-called 'honour killings' as ones falling within this exception to provocation. In most of these cases there will be a desire for revenge: 'The offender is seeking to make an example of the victim because she (and it normally will be a "she") has defied tradition, custom or parental wishes in her choice of boyfriend, spouse or life-style.' (para 5.25, footnote omitted) The Law Commission restates its views on the objective test and proposes to retain the definition previously proposed in their Report No. 290, *Partial Defences to Murder*, a recommendation very like current law found in **Holley** above and therefore completely different from that in **Smith** above.

Killing in pursuance of a suicide pact

Like provocation, this form of manslaughter is applied to someone who has malice aforethought. By s 4(1) of the Homicide Act 1957 if the accused kills in pursuance of a suicide agreement by two or more persons, the crime is manslaughter. Unlike the normal rule, the consent of the victim to being killed is significant. The burden of proof demonstrating this mitigating factor is on the accused: s 4(2). By s 4(3) a suicide pact is defined as:

A common agreement between two or more persons having for its object the death of all of them, whether or not each is to take his own life, but nothing shall be treated as done by him in pursuance of the pact unless it is done while he has the settled intention of dying in pursuance of the pact.

If each individual intends to take his or her own life, there is obviously no liability for murder or manslaughter.

Placing the burden of proof on the accused is not incompatible with Article 6(2) of the European Convention on Human Rights: *A-G's Reference (No. 1 of 2004)* [2004] I WLR 2111 (CA).

In its Report No. 304 *Murder, Manslaughter and Infanticide*, 2006, the Law Commission proposed to retain the defence pending reform of the law on mercy killings. This is a change from their previous recommendations that the defence should be abolished but that some killings in these circumstances would fall within a revised defence of diminished responsibility: Consultation Paper No. 177, *A New Homicide Act for England and Wales?*, 2005.

Subjectively reckless manslaughter

Before *Seymour* there was a type of manslaughter where the accused, being aware of the possibility of injury (i.e. subjectively reckless), killed someone. It is a pity that this type does not have a snappy title. *Pike* [1961] Crim LR 547 (CCA) illustrated this form. The accused gave his mistress carbon tetrachloride to increase sexual satisfaction. He had administered the fumes to a number of women over several years with no side-effects. However, on this occasion the victim died. It was held that the trial judge was correct to direct the jury that the accused was guilty of manslaughter if he was aware of the risk that some physical harm might occur. This test is less than that in manslaughter by gross negligence, which may require a risk as to life or safety (see the next section). It is suggested that this form of (subjectively) reckless manslaughter survives the abolition of (objectively) reckless manslaughter discussed next. In the Crown Court case of *Smith* [1979] Crim LR 547 the judge referred to a civil case where it had been said that 'to do a lawful act which is dangerous with reckless disregard whether or not it injures another is also manslaughter'. Griffiths J read 'reckless disregard' as meaning 'fully appreciating that there was a real risk to her health'. Both this formula and that in *Pike* are ones of 'subjective recklessness'.

The Court of Appeal in *Lidar*, unreported, 11 November 1999, where the accused drove off with the victim's foot caught in the wheel, the victim fell off and was run over and killed, said that manslaughter could be committed by consciously taking a risk of serious injury and that 'to some extent' this form of manslaughter survives the revival of gross negligence manslaughter. It is not absolutely certain whether the court considered subjectively reckless manslaughter to be a separate offence or whether it was part of gross negligence manslaughter. While the existence is admitted, it is uncertain whether the formulation is correct. Perhaps there must be a high probability of serious injury, as *Lidar* suggested, and not just foresight of a risk of serious harm as possibly occurring. At present it seems that facts giving rise to this form of manslaughter are treated as ones which fall within constructive and gross negligence manslaughter, which are easier to prove than subjectively reckless manslaughter. If constructive manslaughter were abolished, there would be a need for (subjectively) reckless manslaughter, and pressure would develop for an exact definition of its elements. The existence of this offence has simply not been discussed in the cases noted elsewhere in this section.

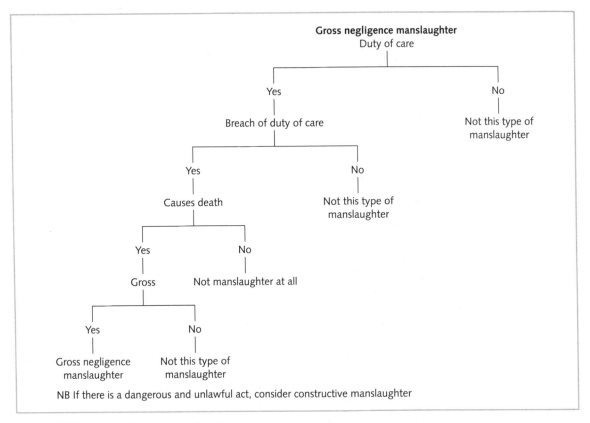

Figure 12.2 Gross negligence manslaughter

Killing by gross negligence

There is a form of manslaughter where the accused had killed the victim in a grossly negligent fashion (Fig. 12.2). Anybody may be convicted of the offence of **gross negligence**, though often the defendants occupy professional jobs. With the development of the form of recklessness found in *MPC v Caldwell* [1982] AC 341 (HL), which applied in this area (*Seymour* [1983] 2 AC 493 (HL)) there were authorities to the effect that manslaughter by gross negligence had been totally swallowed up by objectively reckless manslaughter: *Kong Cheuk Kwan v R* (1985) 82 Cr App R 18 (PC) and *Goodfellow* (1986) 83 Cr App R 23 (CA). The basic rule of liability for reckless manslaughter was stated in *Goodfellow*: has the accused acted in such a way as to create an obvious and serious risk of causing physical harm and, having recognised it, gone ahead, or not given any thought to that risk? The accused need not realise that he is putting someone at risk: *Seymour*. As a result of *Seymour*, an accused was guilty if he did not realise that there was an obvious risk of some personal injury to another.

In *Reid* [1992] 1 WLR 793 (HL) Lord Ackner used the illustration of a diver jumping off a springboard into a pool and colliding with a swimmer without having considered whether anyone might be harmed. If the swimmer died, the crime would be reckless manslaughter if the ordinary prudent bystander would consider that the risk was obvious and serious. If, however, the swimmer survived, the accused would not be guilty of any non-fatal offence because all of them are defined in terms of subjective recklessness. In modern post-*Caldwell* terms if an accused kills by gross negligence, he is killing in this type of manslaughter. If the victim survives (perhaps through the fortuitous intervention of a paramedic), the accused is not guilty of any non-fatal offence, because non-fatal offences cannot be committed by gross negligence, only intentionally or in a subjectively reckless manner.

Although the *Caldwell* formulation is no longer to be used, even though it was by the House of Lords as recently as 1992 in *Reid*, only by looking at history can one understand present law.

A risk of what?

Before the irruption of reckless manslaughter Fenton Atkinson LJ in *Stone and Dobinson* [1977] QB 354 rejected the view that the accused had to be grossly negligent as to the likelihood of death or serious injury. He said that gross negligence signified a high degree of negligence and 'indifference to an obvious risk to health and welfare [or] an appreciation of such risk coupled with a determination to run it'. After *Caldwell* Lord Roskill in *Seymour* spoke of a very high risk of death, but he said that in the context of manslaughter caused by a car ('motor manslaughter') in order to distinguish that offence from causing death by reckless driving, or at least such is the construction put on his words in *Kong Cheuk Kwan v R*, and Lord Roskill did uphold the trial judge's direction which included a reference to an obvious and serious risk of physical injury. There was no need for the recklessness to be gross. Both *Goodfellow* and *Kong Cheuk Kwan v R* demanded only a risk of physical injury. Therefore, it can be said that there need not be an obvious and serious risk of death or even serious injury in reckless manslaughter. *Stone and Dobinson*'s test of 'obvious risk to health or welfare' would broaden manslaughter perhaps unacceptably, and the position until 1993 was that accepted by the Privy Council and Court of Appeal. Manslaughter is a serious crime, for which the maximum sentence is life imprisonment; yet the requirement of only a risk as to some physical injury is not commensurate with the gravity of the offence.

In *Lawrence* [1982] AC 510, Lord Diplock said that there had to be an obvious and serious risk of some physical harm or substantial damage to property in relation to reckless driving and causing death by reckless driving. Omitting the reference to property this decision was extended to manslaughter involving cars in *Seymour* though the Crown wished to reserve the question whether a risk to property was sufficient: on the facts it was not relevant. In *Kong Cheuk Kwan v R*, Lord Roskill referred to a risk of causing damage but on the facts that was a relevant risk because a collision between two hydrofoils did create such a risk. It is not certain whether he realised that his reference to 'physical damage' was different from 'substantial damage to property' in *Caldwell*. In *Goodfellow* the Court of Appeal ruled that there should be no reference to the risk of damage to property. These cases illustrate that *Seymour* was not restricted to manslaughter through the use of a car. In *ex parte Jennings* [1983] 1 AC 624, the House of Lords decided that in both causing death by reckless driving and reckless manslaughter there had to be 'an obvious and serious risk of causing physical injury'. Since *Lawrence* had held that a risk of substantial damage to property was sufficient in causing death by reckless driving, the effect of *ex parte Jennings* was that the same was true of manslaughter. The point was not discussed in cases such as *Goodfellow*. Lord Roskill in *Seymour* simply stated that on the facts there was no need to refer to damage to property. He did not say that it was never relevant. If it was relevant, the law had been extended, for previous law required gross negligence as to life or safety and no reference was made to property.

Lord Goff in *Reid*, above, reformulated the test in *Caldwell* and *Lawrence* in relation to causing death by reckless driving. The law on recklessness in that offence, criminal damage, and subject to the 'property' point above reckless manslaughter was to the same effect. Reckless manslaughter was in the normal run of cases defined thus: did the accused create a serious risk of causing physical injury to some other person and either (a) did he recognise that there was some risk of that kind involved but nevertheless did he go on to take it or (b) did he not address his mind to the possibility of there being any such risk, the risk being obvious to the reasonable person? This reformulation changed the law (and reversed the second part of Lord Diplock's speech in *Caldwell*). In (a) the risk need not be obvious to the reasonable bystander. Lord Browne-Wilkinson supported Lord Goff's formula. Lords Ackner and Keith did not mention it and Lord Roskill agreed with all the speeches. Accordingly it could not be said that the law on 'obviousness' was settled. If the formula was correct, in (a) there had to be a serious risk but it need not be a risk obvious to the reasonable individual. In the words of the Court of Appeal in *Reid*, 'serious' meant 'to be taken seriously'. A risk which is one to be taken seriously is one which is dependent on the inverse proportionality between the harm which would occur if the risk of injury eventuated and the degree of probability of harm occurring. The greater the harm, the less the degree of occurrence is the test postulated. On the facts of the Zeebrugge ferry disaster case the chance of harm was thought to be small enough to be disregarded, but if the bow doors did take water in, the results would be disastrous. If the reasonable person would classify the risk as serious, then if the accused knew of the risk, he would be reckless on the reformulation in (a).

The survival of gross negligence manslaughter

While most of the cases which were decided under the heading of gross negligence would have been decided the same way under objectively reckless manslaughter, apart from cases such as *Lamb* [1967] 2 QB 981 where the accused was guilty of gross negligence manslaughter but would not have been guilty of objectively reckless manslaughter because he, mistakenly, thought about the risk and thought there was none, manslaughter by gross negligence does survive, despite Lord Roskill's statement in *Kong Cheuk Kwan* v *R* that the term was not to be used.

The term gross negligence was never clearly defined in the cases. The criminal law, however, did recognise that an accused could be guilty only if he acted in a grossly negligent fashion. Acting carelessly was insufficient. As was said in the classic authority, *Andrews* v *DPP* [1937] AC 576 (HL), 'simple lack of care as will constitute civil liability is insufficient'. The accused must break a duty he owed the victim, the victim must die, and the accused's carelessness must be gross, taking into account all the circumstances of the case. In *Bateman* [1925] All ER Rep 45, Lord Hewart said that a person was guilty only if he demonstrated 'such disregard for the life and safety of others as to amount to a crime against the State and conduct deserving of punishment', a circular definition (the judges have accepted that this is so) but one which gives a flavour of the topic. (He talked of the negligence being 'criminal', 'culpable', 'wicked', 'clear' and 'complete' as synonyms for 'gross'. None of these terms is of much help to a jury. Indeed, different juries may convict or acquit on the same facts, one finding the carelessness not gross, the other disagreeing.) This formula has also been criticised for leaving a question of law to the jury. See below for further criticism of juries and the grossness of the accused's behaviour.

In the Zeebrugge case, *Stanley*, unreported, 10 October 1990, Turner J at the Old Bailey said that gross negligence manslaughter no longer existed (if it had done at that time, quite possibly the jury would have convicted). Yet in *Ball* (1990) 90 Cr App R 378 the Court of Appeal did refer to negligence but the mention was *obiter*. It did not mention *Seymour*. It was as if *Kong Cheuk Kwan v R* and *Seymour* had never occurred. The former Lord Chief Justice said in *Goodfellow*, above, that the face of *Kong Cheuk Kwan* raised the issue whether the accused was 'guilty of recklessness (or gross negligence)'. Yet in *Kong Cheuk Kwan* the Privy Council made no reference to gross negligence. Accordingly, the cases were equivocal whether this form of manslaughter survived. Indeed the House of Lords purported to follow *Andrews* in *Seymour* but the two definitions were different.

 The Court of Appeal blew fresh life into manslaughter by gross negligence in *Prentice* [1994] QB 302, which on appeal to the House of Lords is known as **Adomako** [1995] 1 AC 171. The accused, an anaesthetist who had been working long hours, failed to notice that a tube carrying oxygen to a patient had become disconnected and the patient died. The case was joined with others in the Court of Appeal and all appeals were allowed there except for this accused's. The prosecution alleged that the appellant, who conceded that he had been negligent, had been grossly negligent for not noting the obvious signs of disconnection, e.g. the chest was not moving, the dials on the ventilator were not moving, the patient was turning blue, and the pulse and blood pressure were dropping. He had also failed to see that the alarm on the ventilator was not switched on. Only when the alarm on the machine monitoring blood pressure went off did he check that machine and only after the patient had had a heart attack and was undergoing resuscitation was the disconnection discovered. Lord Mackay stated that the law in *Bateman* and *Andrews*, above, was correct and 'satisfactory'. He approved the classic if circular definition of Lord Hewart CJ in *Bateman*: '. . . the facts must be such that, in the opinion of the jury, the negligence of the accused went beyond a mere matter of compensation between subjects'. He also approved the opinion of Lord Atkin in *Andrews* that '. . . a very high degree of negligence is required, and that the crime's mental element covers both an indifference to a risk and the situation where the accused appreciated the risk and intended to avoid it and yet [showed] such a high degree of negligence in the manner adopted to avoid the risk as would justify a conviction'. The jury has to assess whether 'the conduct of the defendant was so bad in all the circumstances as to amount . . . to a criminal act or omission'. Lord Mackay in a highly important passage summarised the offence thus:

> . . . [t]he ordinary principles of the law of negligence apply to ascertain whether or not the defendant has been in breach of a duty of care towards the victim who has died. If such a breach of duty is established the next question is whether that breach of duty caused the death of the victim. If so, the jury must go on to consider whether the breach of the duty caused the death of the victim. If so, the jury must go on to consider whether the breach of the duty should be characterised as gross negligence and therefore as a crime. This will depend on the seriousness of the breach of duty . . . in all the circumstances in which the defendant was placed. The jury will have to consider whether the extent to which the defendant's conduct departed from the proper standard of care incumbent upon him, involving as it must have done a risk of death . . . , was such that it should be judged criminal.

It will in the normal run of cases not be difficult to demonstrate that a duty of care existed. Surely all neighbours must take care not to endanger the lives of others. So, for example, a car driver owes a duty of care to his passengers during the journey. Doctors and other similar professionals owe such a duty, but the duty is not restricted to professional persons. It is uncertain how far one can take the tort analogy into criminal law, despite Lord Mackay's words quoted above. Kennedy LJ in *R* (*on the application of Lewin*) *v DPP* [2002] EWHC 1049 (Admin) (DC) spoke of applying the ordinary principles of negligence, but it is by no means certain that he was correct. The tortious duty of care is explicitly founded on public policy and serves the function of shifting financial loss from one person to another, but criminal law does not promote this aim.

There are differences too in relation to omissions. Surely the House of Lords did not intend to overrule *Stone and Dobinson*, which they would have done if the narrower tort law on omissions had replaced the quite possibly wider criminal liability for omissions. See Chapter 2 for examples of situations in which the criminal law imposes a duty to act. *Adomako* itself was a case on omissions. It cannot be stated for certain if this is the case; indeed, there may be areas of tort law on omissions which are broader than criminal law. Furthermore, if tort law is to be incorporated into gross negligence manslaughter, there may be instances where there is no duty of care in tort but there should be one in criminal law. Surely everyone is under a duty not to do anything which causes danger to the lives of others, even though no duty of care arises in tort law. If this is the law, the duty of care issue which occurs in the tort of negligence is irrelevant. The contrary argument is that the former Lord Chancellor was very definite that 'the ordinary principles of the law of negligence apply'. If so, changes in tort, such as whether a duty exists, will affect criminal law, an unexpected development. For more on the position in relation to omissions, see below. One other issue is problematical. If the accused did foresee the risk of death, why should it matter that in applying the law of negligence a reasonable person would not?

For an explanation of the law on omissions, see pp 70–79 in Chapter 2.

Cases from *Adomako* onwards exemplify situations where the accused owed a duty of care to his victim.

Adomako: doctor to patient;

Prentice, which was one of the cases joined with *Adomako* at the Court of Appeal stage: electrician to customer;

Litchfield [1998] Crim LR 507: captain of ship to sailors (for facts see below).

Adomako brings up an issue of who should be criminally liable. In this case the doctor was tired after working long hours, and it seems that his training had been deficient. Should not the National Health Service have been on trial? Prosecuting the anaesthetist will not *per se* improve the system.

The statement by Lord Mackay LC that 'the ordinary principles of the law of negligence' govern whether or not there has been a breach of the duty of care must, therefore, not be read as a definitive outline of the law. The Law Commission in its Consultation Paper No. 135, *Involuntary Manslaughter*, said that 'negligence' meant 'carelessness'; it did not mean duty/breach/damage as found in tort. In *Wacker* [2003] QB 1207 the accused drove a lorry from the Netherlands to the UK. At Dover 58 illegal immigrants were found dead in the back of the lorry. The accused had closed a vent and the victims suffocated. He argued that he was not guilty of manslaughter because *ex turpi causa non oritur actio* (that is, no legal action may be founded on an unlawful event). In other words, the joint unlawful conduct, the smuggling of immigrants, prevented any duty of care arising between claimants and defendants in tort. The Court of Appeal held that civil law and criminal law served different purposes. The fact that the civil law of compensation for wrongs was disapplied did not mean that the criminal law was also disapplied. Accordingly, the *ex turpi* doctrine was inapplicable to gross negligence manslaughter. Thus it is true to say, as the Law Commission did in its Report No. 237, *Involuntary Manslaughter*, that the concepts of tort law are best avoided. **Wacker** also illustrates the point that an accused can be grossly negligent even though the victims have consented to the activity.

 The law in **Caldwell**, **Lawrence** and **Seymour** no longer applied to involuntary manslaughter even before the expurgation on **Caldwell** from criminal law in **G** [2004] 1 AC 1034 (HL). The abolition of causing death by reckless driving in the Road Traffic Act 1991 was said to justify this approach. This *dictum* cannot be right, for the statute did not affect the common law of manslaughter. The Court of Appeal in **Prentice** had, as they were obliged to do by the doctrine of precedent, stated that **Seymour** still governed motor manslaughter. Lord Mackay said, however, that manslaughter by gross negligence now included motor manslaughter. If the exception had been retained the law would have been unnecessarily complex. 'For example, in **Kong Cheuk Kwan v R** it would give rise to unnecessary differences in the law applicable to those navigating vessels and the lookouts on the vessels.' It should be noted that **Andrews** itself is a case of motor manslaughter.

The term 'reckless' can still be used in manslaughter, but not in its **Caldwell** sense, which in any case has since been abolished throughout criminal law. There was, in Lord Mackay's view, no need to use it. The Court of Appeal used it in **Lidar**, above, applying the *dictum* of Lord Mackay. It would have been elegant if the use of the term 'recklessness' had been wiped out in this context.

Elaborate directions such as those laid down in **Prentice** were to be avoided because of the manifold circumstances in which this form of manslaughter applies. Professionals were to be judged against the standard of their 'reasonably competent' colleagues. On the facts the trial judge had given a correct instruction and the Court of Appeal had been right to dismiss the appeal, though their approach had been overelaborate. It is suggested that while elaborate directions are likely to confuse juries, there are two points which need elucidation, and enlightenment is not found in Lord Mackay's speech. First, which kind of risk must the accused have failed to notice? The Lord Chancellor approved specifically the **Bateman** test of 'life and safety' and he speaks of 'the risk of death' (that is a risk of death foreseeable by a reasonably prudent person) in a passing comment on the issue of grossness being supremely a jury question, and he did not specifically overrule the test in **Stone and Dobinson** [1977] QB 354 of 'injury to health and welfare' (indeed he said that this case defined gross negligence 'with complete accuracy') or Lord Taylor's test in **Prentice** of 'injury to health'. Perhaps **Stone** is impliedly overruled on this point. (The House of Lords expressly approved another part of **Stone and Dobinson**, the proposition that gross negligence covers indifference.) The fact that someone has died shows that there was a risk of death. The requirement must mean something other than this, otherwise it serves no purpose. In the light of the difficulty which this issue caused after **Seymour**, one might have hoped that it would have been addressed by the House of Lords. It is suggested that as in murder, the law is that risk of death or serious injury has to exist. In **Singh** [1999] Crim LR 582, the Court of Appeal held that only a risk of death sufficed, though the issue was not fully aired, and the Court of Appeal in **Lewin v Crown Prosecution Service** [2002] EWHC (Admin.) 1049 cited this passage approvingly (as did the Court of Appeal in **Yaqoob** [2005] EWCA Crim 1269), though later that year the same court in **Lidar**, above, spoke *obiter* of a risk of death or injury, where the accused had managed properties owned by his father and a gas fitter had grossly negligently installed a fire. If confirmation is needed that only a risk of death suffices, it is found in

Judge LJ's judgment in **Misra** [2005] 1 WLR 1. The Court of Appeal approved the statement in **Singh** that: 'The circumstances must be such that a reasonably prudent person would have foreseen a serious and obvious risk not merely of injury, even serious injury, but of death.' This passage was also approved by the same court in **Yaqoob**. The requirement of a risk of death or perhaps a risk of serious injury should be compared with the requirement of a risk of (only) injury in unlawful act manslaughter. Secondly, which type of level of risk is needed? Would a risk suffice or is a substantial risk needed? Lord Mackay's speech provides no assistance. Lord Taylor CJ mentioned in separate places an 'obvious' risk and a 'serious' risk. Perhaps he was under the influence of objective recklessness. It is a pity that further cases (and time and expense) will be needed to settle this point. Furthermore, since the House of Lords in **Adomako** got rid of the 'elaborate' directions of the Court of Appeal in **Prentice**, there is little law for the judge to direct the jury to consider.

Because the issue of grossness is one for the jury and the issue is one whether or not the accused's act of omission was 'bad', the criticism is easy to make that juries may be sympathetic to one accused and find him not guilty but unsympathetic to another and find him guilty. Moreover, how is a jury to assess whether what the accused did was so gross as to be deserving of punishment? There is a possibility of two juries holding one accused to be guilty and another not guilty, on exactly the same facts, and the Court of Appeal would be powerless to intervene. If they say that the negligence was not gross, there is no criminal liability though the defendant may be liable in tort.

The grossness of the conduct will vary with regard to the facts of each case. This point was adopted by a majority of the Supreme Court of Canada in **Creighton** (1993) 105 DLR (4th) 432. For example, a surgeon may justifiably run the risk of killing the patient if the operation is necessary to save life, whereas employers may not take a substantial risk with the lives of their workers in order to increase profits. Even a bad mistake need not be the result of gross negligence but the jury may be instructed to take into account the 'badness' of the accused's behaviour: ***R (on the application of Rowley) v DPP*** [2003] EWHC 693. Grossness is a question for the jury.

Litchfield [1998] Crim LR 507

The accused asserted that he was not guilty of gross negligence manslaughter when he both sailed his sailing ship too close to land and knew that the fuel in the engines was contaminated. He contended that **Adomako** required the jury to ask whether his behaviour was so bad that it demonstrated a lack of regard for the lives of others such that it amounted to a crime, but he was already guilty of a crime, one under the merchant shipping laws; therefore, **Adomako** was irrelevant. The Court of Appeal dismissed his appeal. **Adomako** applied generally and it was immaterial that the accused was also guilty of another offence. The accused's conduct was grossly negligent.

Litchfield also demonstrates that the accused has to be judged against the standards of a reasonably competent person undertaking the task he was performing, e.g. a reasonably competent driver, a reasonably competent doctor. In **Litchfield** the standard to be measured against was that of a reasonably competent sailor. **Litchfield** furthermore shows that the **Adomako** test applies whether the accused failed to act or did not, omission or commission.

The facts in **Litchfield** look like ones which could give rise to a charge of (subjectively) reckless manslaughter. The accused knowingly took the risk of death. He was advertent. **Adomako** by contrast is a case of carelessness: the accused did not know of any risk of death to his patient. He was inadvertent.

The Court of Appeal in *Attorney-General's Reference (No. 2 of 1999)* [2000] QB 796 stated: 'Although there may be cases where the defendant's state of mind is relevant to the jury's consideration when assessing the grossness and criminality of his conduct, evidence of his state of mind is not a prerequisite to a conviction for manslaughter by gross negligence.' The accused himself therefore need not foresee the risk of death. If, however, he did do so, that is evidence going towards proving that his behaviour was *grossly* negligent. The Divisional Court approved this passage in *DPP ex p Jones* [2000] IRLR 373. The test for negligence is an objective one. The Court of Appeal spoke to similar effect in *Misra*, above rejecting the application of the subjective test for recklessness found in *G* [2004] AC 1034.

Because the test for grossness is left to the jury there is a possibility that the offence contravenes Article 5, the right to liberty, and Article 7, the right not to be punished without law, of the European Convention on Human Rights. The Court of Appeal in *Misra*, above, a case where two doctors failed to diagnose a serious infection after a routine knee operation, held that the definition did not infringe Article 7. Judge LJ stated that a law achieved the standard laid down in that Article if it was sufficiently certain; it need not be absolutely certain in its scope. Moreover, Article 7 did not apply to situations where juries had to evaluate an accused's conduct. Furthermore, the jurors were not deciding an issue of law. All that was meant by saying that they had to determine whether the accused was 'criminal' was that his conduct or omission had to be grossly negligent as to the risk of death. There was no extra requirement of *criminal* negligence. The jury was simply applying the law to the facts, as it does for example with intent and dishonesty.

Examples involving medical facts help to show the distinction between carelessness and gross negligence. In *Akerele v R* [1943] AC 255 (PC), which approved the law in *Bateman*, a doctor's careless mixing of a powder with the result that five children died was not manslaughter. The fact that someone died is not by itself gross negligence, and one cannot multiply the carelessness by the five deaths to create gross negligence. Grossness was a question of degree for the jury, and it would be rare to find a professional person so negligent. A jury should look at the quality of the accused's behaviour, not at the quantity of it. In *Bateman* itself the accused took part of the victim's uterus away during childbirth and did not remove her to hospital for five days. She died. On appeal he was found not guilty because he was carrying out a normal procedure approved by the medical profession. It was merely that the procedure had gone wrong. *Bateman* emphasises that the accused's behaviour is to be judged against the current standards of the industry or profession. An error, even one with grave consequences, is not necessarily gross negligence. In *Long* (1830) 172 ER 756, a person who was not a doctor killed two patients by applying corrosive plasters to their chests. There was 'gross and improper rashness and want of caution'. He was convicted (but fined £250). Cases such as these demonstrate how far the assessment of whether the accused was grossly negligent is a question for the jury.

Recklessness as a synonym for gross negligence

One difficulty in knowing whether gross negligence manslaughter did survive is the use in older cases of recklessness as a synonym for gross negligence. The Court of Oyer and Terminer, Dublin, required 'gross negligence' or 'recklessly negligent conduct': *Elliott* (1889) 16 Cox CC 710. The accused was not guilty of manslaughter of 76 passengers when he separated a train on an incline, causing coaches to run backwards into another train. The court said in a phrase which academics today could still use: '. . . the degree of care to be expected from a person, the want of which would be gross negligence or less than that, must in the necessity of things . . . have some relation to the subject and the consequences . . . [T]here must be a certain moral quality carried into the act for which [the accused] is made criminally responsible.' In *Andrews v DPP* [1937] AC 576 Lord Atkin defined gross negligence as 'a very high degree of negligence' or recklessness. Gross negligence was thought to be more appropriate because it covered the situation where the accused appreciated the risk but was grossly negligent as to how he sought to avoid it whereas recklessness did not. Recklessness was therefore either a synonym for gross negligence or only one form of it. In *Cato* [1976] 1 WLR 110 gross negligence and reckless-ness were used synonymously. Even after *Seymour*, gross negligence and recklessness were used interchangeably. In *Sargent* (1990) *The Guardian*, 3 July, Boreham J at Leeds Crown Court is reported as saying: 'You were so negligent as to be reckless as to this woman's welfare', by pumping so much oxygen into her during an operation that she swelled up like a Michelin man. Note the reference to 'welfare', a low test which was below that required for reckless manslaughter. It is uncertain what is meant by 'welfare'. In the cases it is something separate from and less serious than recklessness as to injury. The obvious comment is that manslaughter, being a serious crime, should not be founded on gross negligence as to welfare. It would appear that when the Court of Appeal referred to 'health and welfare' in *Stone and Dobinson* it did not realise that it was departing from the *Andrews* test.

Summary of gross negligence manslaughter

In summary, gross negligence manslaughter is wider than objectively reckless manslaughter when it existed because, provided that the carelessness was gross, the lacuna case is covered. However, according to *Reid* [1992] 1 WLR 793 (HL) the accused was, it seems, guilty of reckless manslaughter if he did not advert to a risk which ought to have been taken seriously and someone died. Inadvertence is another way of saying 'negligence'. Accordingly (simple) carelessness fell within reckless, but not gross negli-gence, manslaughter. Another distinction is that in objectively reckless manslaughter recklessness as to physical injury was needed; in gross negligence the criterion has usu-ally been gross negligence as to death. Such tests are also low thresholds for such a seri-ous crime as manslaughter. The point about gross negligence has already been made but consider too the nature of the risk in reckless manslaughter. The accused did not need to be objectively reckless as to serious harm. *Caldwell* recklessness as to any physical harm sufficed. In another respect reckless manslaughter is narrower than the gross negligence variety for in it the accused must have caused the risk.

Manslaughter by omission

The general issue of omissions in the criminal law was discussed in Chapter 2, though is should be noted that in *Adomako* itself there was no reference to the general rule on omissions. Manslaughter by omission occurs where the accused, in breach of a duty imposed by law, fails to carry out an undertaking, whether contractual or otherwise, and the victim dies as a result: *Khan* [1998] Crim LR 830 (CA). The court ruled that the jury should be left four questions: '(1) Was there in the circumstances a duty of care owed by the defendants to the deceased . . . ? (2) Was there a breach of that duty? (3) Did the breach cause the death of the deceased? (4) Should the breach of duty be characterised as gross negligence . . . ?' The rule in gross negligence that the duty of care's existence is determined by the tort law of negligence is somewhat controversial but in respect of omissions the position is plain: if in respect of omissions there is a duty of care in tort, there is also a duty of care in criminal law.

It is suggested that the issue whether a duty of care exists is really a matter of law for the judge, not a matter of fact for the jury, and **Singh** [1999] Crim LR 582 (CA) so held. See also **Willoughby** [2005] 1 WLR 1880 where the Court of Appeal rejected a contention that the accused owed a duty to the victim of arson because he was the owner of the premises he had set alight. However, there was on the facts a duty because he had enlisted the victim's help in committing the arson. Controversially the court said that whether a duty existed was a matter for the jury: the general principle is that whether a duty exists is a decision for the judge but it is the jury's task to apply the law to the facts. In **Pittwood** (1902) 19 TLR 37, a level-crossing keeper failed to close a gate. A person crossing the line was killed. The court held that the keeper was guilty of gross negligence manslaughter, even though he did not owe the contractual duty to open and close the gate to the victim. (Other cases are given in Chapter 2.) If there is no legal duty to act, this form of manslaughter is not committed. In **Khan** the defendants supplied the victim with heroin. She snorted it and overdosed. They failed to summon medical assistance and she died. Drug dealers did not on the facts owe a duty to their customer. **Khan** makes plain that there is no separate category of manslaughter by omission, but it is one way in which gross negligence manslaughter is committed. (There is in fact a way of making the drug dealers in this case criminally liable: they created a dangerous situation and failed to rectify it.)

In *Sinclair* [1998] NLJ 1353 the Court of Appeal held that the accused was under a duty of care when he was a close friend of the victim, a drug addict, had previously supplied him with methadone, had helped to obtain the fatal dose, and had stayed with him until he died.

See the further discussion of omissions in Chapter 2.

Singh exemplifies this area of law. Tenants told the accused that gas fires in their flats were not working properly. The accused did not have an expert to check the fires. The victim died. It was held that the accused did owe a duty of care; that duty was broken by his not bringing in an expert; his negligence caused the victim's death.

The mental element is that laid down in **Adomako** (above). The test is objective pure and simple, which is objectionable from the viewpoint of subjectivists for such a serious crime.

It should be noted that an omission is not sufficient for unlawful act manslaughter. The lack of liability in unlawful act manslaughter for an omission which caused death has been criticised on the grounds that an omission, especially a deliberate one, is blameworthy, and it can cause death. Subjectively reckless manslaughter may be committed by omission.

The Law Commission's Report No. 227, *Legislating the Criminal Code: Involuntary Manslaughter*, 1996 does not affect the occasions when a duty of care arises. The Law Commission considered that the topic of omissions should be separately reviewed.

Unlawful act or constructive manslaughter

This type of manslaughter gets its name from the requirement that the victim must have died as a result of an unlawful criminal act and liability is **constructive** because the accused is guilty even though he did not foresee death. A similar doctrine in relation to murder was abolished in 1957. Both doctrines are harsh in the effect on the accused. They might however represent current opinion which focuses on results, death, and there is correspondingly a reduced emphasis on the accused's fault. In *Creighton*, above, McLachlin J endorsed this proposition. 'To tell people that if they embark on dangerous conduct which foreseeably may cause bodily harm which is neither trivial nor transient, and which in fact results in death, that they will not be held responsible for the death but only for aggravated assault, is less likely to deter such conduct than a message that they will be held responsible for the death . . . Given the finality of death and the absolute unacceptability of killing another human being, it is not amiss to preserve the test which promises the greatest measure of deterrence, provided the penal consequences of the offence are not disproportionate.'

The same act could be both this form of manslaughter and gross negligence manslaughter. In *Goodfellow* above, the accused set fire to a house so that he could be rehoused. Three died. The unlawful act was arson, and he was grossly negligent as to the risk of injury.

This type of manslaughter occurs when death is caused by an unlawful act intentionally or recklessly committed by the accused which reasonable persons would foresee as liable to cause some injury, though not necessarily serious injury: *Church* [1966] 1 QB 59, as approved in *DPP v Newbury* [1977] AC 500 (HL) and *Goodfellow*. Lord Hope in *Attorney-General's Reference (No. 3 of 1994)* [1998] AC 245 stated:

> The only questions which need to be addressed are (1) whether the act was done intentionally, (2) whether it was unlawful, (3) whether it was dangerous because it was likely to cause harm to somebody and (4) whether that unlawful and dangerous act caused the death.

A similar definition was laid down by the House of Lords in *Kennedy (No. 2)* [2008] 1 AC 269. Some of these phrases need lengthy exposition in the light of the unclear case law but some issues can be dealt with quickly. The fact that death ensues converts the crime from a lesser offence to manslaughter. The accused is guilty even though he personally foresaw no risk of injury. An example occurs when the accused punches the victim, who loses his balance, falls to the ground, bangs his head on a kerbstone and dies. If the victim had not died, the accused might have been guilty only of a battery. By mischance he is, however, guilty of manslaughter. This bad luck has converted a minor offence against the person into a major crime of homicide. Furthermore, not even the reasonable bystander need foresee serious injury, never mind death. 'Injury' covers shock causing physical injury, but not emotional disturbance: *Dawson* (1985) 81 Cr App R 150 (CA). It is only where a reasonable person might foresee physical harm resulting from an emotional disturbance that frightening someone to death amounts to this type of manslaughter.

A recent case gives a flavour of this offence.

R v A [2005] All ER (D) 38 (July)

The two 16-year-old defendants and the victim were celebrating finishing their exams. Some drink having been taken, the accused hoisted the victim over a railing and he fell into the river and drowned. The act of the defendants was dangerous within the definition used in this form of manslaughter and it had caused death. The defendants argued that what they did was horseplay and therefore since the victim had consented to the horseplay, there was no 'unlawful' act, here the crime of battery. The Court of Appeal held that the victim had not in fact consented. The accused were guilty of manslaughter.

The accused's unlawful act must of course cause the death of the victim. Where the accused hits the victim, it is only if that act caused her death that the accused is guilty. In *Carey* [2006] EWCA Crim 17 it was said that the accused's blow did not cause the death and therefore he could not be guilty of manslaughter. For a case comment see D. Ormerod 'Manslaughter: unlawful act – affray – dangerous act' [2006] Crim LR 843.

It was said at one time that the act had to be directed or aimed at the victim. In *Dalby* [1982] 1 WLR 425 (CA), the accused was found not guilty because the unlawful act, the supply of a dangerous drug, did not cause the victim's death. (Both the accused and the victim had injected themselves. There was no argument run that the victim's self-injection was an unlawful act.) *Obiter* the court said that the supply of the drug was not directed at the person of the accused. The drug, which was obtained on a prescription, was taken by the accused and the victim together, but each individual injected himself. The act of the accused was not aimed at the victim but at herself. This was a novel requirement and appeared inconsistent with the decision of the House of Lords in *Newbury*, where the defendants did not aim at the victim the stone which killed him. They aimed at the train. Nevertheless, the House of Lords refused leave to appeal in *Dalby*. A comparison case is *Cato*, above. The accused was guilty when he injected heroin into his friend. It could thus be said that the accused aimed the act at the victim. In *Dalby* the victim injected herself. In *Mitchell* [1983] QB 741 the Court of Appeal held that there was a *novus actus interveniens* in *Dalby*. The chain of causation had been broken. In this way the result in *Dalby* can be reconciled with earlier law. Even at the time when *Dalby* was taken to represent the law, it was not quite true to say that the act had to be directed at the victim, since the doctrine of transferred malice applies. In *Mitchell* the accused pushed a man who fell against an 89-year-old woman in a queue at a post office. She suffered a broken leg, developed thrombosis and died. The accused was guilty of manslaughter even though he did not direct his attack at the victim. The chain of causation had not been broken. It should be noted that the accused was guilty of manslaughter, even though he intended only a battery. In *Pagett* (1983) 76 Cr App R 279 (CA), where a girl was used as a shield by the accused (see Chapter 2), the court did not deal with the point that under *Dalby* the act had to be directed at the victim. The court said *obiter* that the accused would have been guilty even if the police had shot dead an innocent bystander, though the actual victim was innocent too. The point is that the accused did not direct his act at her. *Mitchell* followed *Pagett* and did not make any special rule for constructive manslaughter, but instead applied general rules on causation, and did not refer to *Dalby* or the principle there stated.

The Court of Appeal finally gave the 'aimed at' rule its quietus in *Goodfellow*. *Dalby* was held to have been decided in the way that it was because a direction was needed whether or not there was an intervening act, i.e. the words in *Dalby* did not mean what they said. The result in *Dalby* is preserved. The accused did not (now) cause the victim's death. On the facts of *Goodfellow* where the accused set fire to his dwelling, there was no break in the chain of causation which led to the death of his wife, son and son's girlfriend. He did not aim his arson at the victims. In *Ball*, above, the court mentioned the 'aimed at' doctrine but did not treat it as a separate element. It *obiter* referred to both the **Dalby** test and the **Goodfellow** test of no *novus actus interveniens*. This may signify a return to **Dalby**. The court instanced a pub landlord who sold alcohol to an under-age drinker. The alcohol contained poison but the landlord did not know it. If the drinker imbibed the poison, the landlord would not be guilty of this type of manslaughter because he did not direct the unlawful act, sale of alcohol to a person under age, at the victim. The law was clarified by the House of Lords in **Attorney-General's Reference (No. 3 of 1994)**, above, in which Lord Hope *per curiam* stated that the 'aimed at' rule was not a requirement of constructive manslaughter. **Goodfellow** is therefore correct. Unfortunately **Dalby** was not overruled.

The argument in favour of the 'aimed at' doctrine is that it is a limit on the very wide ambit of constructive manslaughter. If a person drops some chips on the floor, the victim happens to slip on them, falls to the ground banging her head and dies, he is guilty of manslaughter, a serious offence. A contrary argument is that since the harm need not be foreseen by the accused for him to be guilty of this type of manslaughter, why should the accused have to aim his act at the victim?

The elements of the offence

(a) This type of manslaughter is different from gross negligence manslaughter, as Fig. 12.3 illustrates. A lawful act which is performed carelessly does not automatically become an unlawful act for this purpose, even if a lawful act done carelessly amounts to an offence (e.g. careless driving): **Andrews v DPP**, above, where the crime was that of dangerous driving in that the accused knocked down and killed a pedestrian while

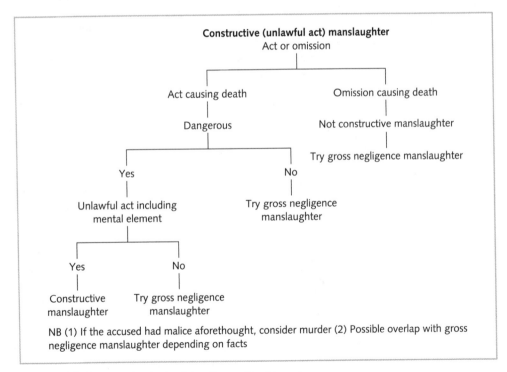

Figure 12.3 Constructive (unlawful act) manslaughter

overtaking. Therefore a person who kills while driving carelessly is not guilty of this form of manslaughter, but may be guilty of manslaughter by gross negligence. It should be said that the width of this exception is uncertain.

(b) The unlawful act need not be a violent act but it must be 'a dangerous act, that is, an act which is likely to injure another person': **Larkin** [1943] 1 All ER 217. Previous law did not require this element. The Court of Criminal Appeal held that brandishing a razor was an assault, a dangerous act. When a woman inadvertently fell against the razor, cut her throat and died, the person holding the razor was guilty of manslaughter. **Church** adopted a like definition. In some cases, as Lord Hope put it in **Attorney-General's Reference (No. 3 of 1994)**, 'dangerousness in this context is not a high standard' and in others the danger is obvious. In **Mahal** [1991] Crim LR 632 (CA), it was held that a jury could find that pushing someone through an open window 22 feet from the ground could lead to 'the risk of some harm'. In **Attorney-General's Reference (No. 3 of 1994)** the accused's attack on the child's mother was a dangerous act likely to injure her. The death of the child, therefore, was constructive manslaughter. A risk of danger to anyone, therefore, suffices. The attacker need not even know that the woman attacked was pregnant. There is no need to foresee death or serious harm. The element of dangerousness must be proved: **Scarlett** [1993] 4 All ER 629.

(c) There must be an act which must be unlawful: see Lord Hope in **Attorney-General's Reference (No. 3 of 1994)**, above. Both an *act* and an *unlawful* act are needed. An omission, even a deliberate one, which causes death, cannot be a wrongful act: **Lowe** [1973] QB 702 (CA), not following **Senior** [1899] 1 QB 283 (Court for Crown Cases Reserved). The fact that the accused was guilty of wilful neglect of his child who died as a result did not mean that he was guilty of this type of manslaughter. The court drew a line between an act which was likely to cause harm and an omission which was likely to do the same. But in both instances the accused caused the death of the child. Starving a child to death does not seem morally less reprehensible than beating it to death. In this context the drawing of a distinction between act and omission has been strongly criticised. It seems strange that murder can be committed by an omission (**Gibbins & Proctor** (1918) 13 Cr App R 134) but unlawful act manslaughter cannot. Both gross negligence and subjectively reckless manslaughter may be committed by omissions.

Normally the unlawful act, which must be a crime, is a non-fatal offence such as battery but it could, for example, be arson, as in **Goodfellow**, above. Other examples include attempted robbery in **Dawson**, above, and burglary in **Watson** [1989] 1 WLR 684 (CA). In **Andrews** [2003] Crim LR 477 the Court of Appeal held that if the underlying crime (here, supplying a prescription-only drug without a prescription) is one of strict liability, no *mens rea* as to that crime need be proved for the accused to be convicted of unlawful act manslaughter. However, **Andrews** is a weak case. The court did not discuss the issue, and if a careless act is not an unlawful act for this purpose (see (a) above), *a fortiori* a strict offence is not. **Andrews** is also contrary to the statement in **Lamb** that *mens rea* is 'an essential ingredient in manslaughter'. Furthermore, there in fact was a *mens rea* offence which could have formed the basis of the charge: s 23 of the Offences against the Person Act 1861, administering a noxious thing. An act which is a tort only and not a crime is not an unlawful act for the purposes of unlawful act manslaughter: **Franklin** (1883) 15 Cox CC 163, where the tort was one of trespass to goods when the accused threw a box from one of the piers in Brighton and it struck and killed a swimmer. (In **Franklin** there was a crime, larceny (nowadays theft), but that crime was not mentioned and it was not in itself dangerous.) Civil liability remains immaterial today: **Lamb**, above, *per* Sachs LJ. It seems strange to reduce the width of unlawful act manslaughter in **Franklin** because manslaughter is a serious crime, yet in **Andrews** to hold that no *mens rea* as to the underlying offence need be established, even though manslaughter is a serious crime.

Jennings [1990] Crim LR 588 (CA) confirmed the need for there to be a crime and for the unlawful act to be identified. Possessing a knife was not *per se* an unlawful act under the Prevention of Crime Act 1953, s 1. The accused's intention had to be considered to determine whether he wished to use it to inflict injury. Whether the accused had that intent had to be left to the jury. Without that state of mind there was no unlawful act manslaughter when the accused stabbed his brother who was trying to restrain him. There must, therefore, be a mental element in the 'unlawful act', though this proposition is not always stated in the cases. (See e.g. **Newbury**, where it is difficult to state what the unlawful act was: the House of Lords did not refer to this point, counsel having conceded that there was an unlawful act. One possible crime is endangering the safety of passengers conveyed by rail. Other possibilities include criminal damage and assault occasioning actual bodily harm. It is unclear whether a property offence can be an unlawful act.) See also **Lamb**, below, which clearly demonstrates the condition that there must be *mens rea* as to the unlawful act. The requirement of *mens rea* for unlawful act manslaughter may be easily satisfied. If the accused kills by fire, the unlawful act is arson as in **Goodfellow**. That offence can be committed by a person who was reckless. Therefore, he is guilty of manslaughter, even though he gave no thought to an obvious (and serious) risk of criminal damage. The *actus reus* and *mens rea* are totally out of step. A lawful act, such as a killing in self-defence, or a minor harm committed with the victim's consent, such as a tackle in a game of football, is not an unlawful act for this purpose. If, however, the force used was excessive, the act is a crime and unlawful for this purpose. **Jennings** demonstrates that the unlawful act need not in fact be an act but can be a state of affairs crime, in this case possessing an offensive weapon. If the crime is one of specific intent and the accused was intoxicated, he is not guilty of unlawful act manslaughter based on that offence: **O'Driscoll** (1977) 65 Cr App R 50 (CA). However, if there is a basic intent crime as a fall-back to the specific intent one, he is guilty because intoxication is no defence to such an offence.

In two cases the 'unlawful act' is hard if not impossible to find despite the requirement of an unlawful act. The courts suggested that the unlawful act need not be a recognised crime. It is sufficient that the accused acted voluntarily; in other words, there need be no *mens rea*. In **Cato**, above, the victim produced heroin and syringes and invited the accused to have a fix. Several times during the night they injected one another with heroin and water. In the morning the victim died. The accused's conviction for manslaughter was upheld. There was a crime, administering a noxious thing. Lord Widgery CJ went on, however, to say that injecting the victim irrespective of this crime was an unlawful act for the purposes of constructive manslaughter. Yet injecting someone with heroin at his request is not a crime. Lord Widgery CJ's suggestion was *obiter*, for as he noted there already was an offence, administering a noxious thing.

Other drug cases have caused difficulty. In **Dias** [2002] 2 Cr App R 96 where the accused prepared a needleful of heroin and passed it to the victim who injected himself with it, the Court of Appeal said that 'it is not easy to see on what basis the court [below] concluded that the act of self-injection was unlawful . . .'. The Crown in **Dias** found it 'difficult' to uphold that reasoning. There is no crime of injecting drugs; supplying drugs is the offence. Whether supplying drugs caused the death is a question of fact, which must be left to the jury. In **Dias** because the question of causation had not been considered at first instance the conviction was quashed but the court did not rule out the possibility that causation may be established on similar facts; however, the court recognised that the victims in such circumstances may have a choice, in which event causation will not be proven. A similar case to **Dias** is **Rogers** [2003] 1 WLR 1374 (CA). The accused applied a tourniquet to the arm of the victim, who then injected himself with heroin. The court said that while self-injection is not an unlawful act (indeed there is no offence of self-manslaughter), the application of the tourniquet and the self-injection were part of the same transaction: they could not be separated. Therefore, the accused caused in part the injection which in turn caused death. He had played a part in the mechanics of the victim's death. On these facts there was both causing death and an unlawful act. The court applied **Dias** and like other courts thought that **Kennedy** was incorrectly decided. The Court of Appeal in **Andrews** [2003] Crim LR 477 strongly agreed with **Dias** that there has to be an unlawful act. The victim's consent to the accused's injecting her with insulin in order to have a 'high' was irrelevant to the criminal charge that the accused administered a prescription-only medicine when he was not qualified to do so. The court in **Dias** suggested *obiter* that where the facts gave rise to a duty of care, there could be a conviction for manslaughter by gross negligence. It also added that where the victim was a child or mentally disturbed, the chain of causation may still be established. **Cato** must be incorrect, for as the court said in **Dias**: '. . . "unlawful" means that the act has to be a criminal offence.'

In the second troubling case, **Lipman** [1970] 1 QB 152, the defendant was also convicted of manslaughter (for facts see Chapter 8). In these cases the taking of drugs was not a crime. Possession is the offence but possession did not cause the death. The defendants in **Cato** and **Lipman** at the time of the victims' deaths were presumably unconscious and it is accordingly difficult to attribute to them any *mens rea*. Getting into a state as a result of which someone died may have been reckless in ordinary language but there was a gap in time, a lack of contemporaneity, between the getting into the state and the victim's death. The House of Lords refused leave to appeal in **Lipman**, and it was approved by the House of Lords in **DPP v Majewski** [1977] AC 433. The issue whether the act had to be unlawful was not addressed in **Newbury**, above, though as a minimum criminal damage existed, as did the more esoteric offence of endangering the safety of any person conveyed upon a railway, but Lord Hope did require it in **Attorney-General's Reference (No. 3 of 1994)**, quoted above. It is suggested that cases such as **Cato** are incorrect. Surely it cannot be the law that a person who commits the *actus reus* only of battery can be convicted of manslaughter, but not of battery itself? Moreover, if the act need not be criminal, the courts spent a long time in cases such as **Lamb** overruling the first instance judgment, considering whether an offence existed. The accused need not know that the act is unlawful: **Newbury**, **DPP v Daley** [1980] AC 237 (PC). However, his state of mind must be investigated to see whether he intended to commit an *actus reus*.

As we have seen, the unlawful act need not be an offence against the person. Stanley Yeo criticised this law in *Fault in Homicide* (Federation Press, 1997) 188:

'To convict a person of manslaughter on the basis of a property offence seems almost as objectionable as convicting her or him on account of a tort.'

A final point is this. As we have seen, the rule is that the unlawful act must be a crime. This means that mere psychological harm is by itself insufficient: *Dhaliwal* [2006] EWCA Crim 1139 (CA).

(d) Whether the unlawful act was a dangerous one is judged not by the accused's state of mind, but by a sober and reasonable person in the defendant's position. It is the act which has to be dangerous, not whether the accused believed it to be dangerous. The test is objective: *Church*, *Lipman*, *Newbury*, *Dawson* and *Ball*, above. In *Newbury*, two teenagers pushed part of a paving stone from the parapet of a railway bridge as a train was approaching. The stone passed through the window of the cab and killed a guard. The House of Lords held that the boys were guilty even though they did not realise that what they were doing might harm others. They were guilty if they did an act which was unlawful and which 'all sober and reasonable people' would recognise as being dangerous. Accordingly, whether the boys recognised that there was a risk or not was irrelevant (cf. the law of objective recklessness). In *Church* the accused did not know that there was a risk of harm to his victim when he threw her into the river, because he believed her to be dead. His mistaken belief was immaterial: reasonable people would have recognised that there was such a risk. As the next paragraph demonstrates, the test is not a purely objective one. In *Kennedy*, above, encouraging the victim to take heroin by injection would be recognised as creating the risk of some harm. That harm could be as little as the prick caused by a needle. In *Carey* [2006] EWCA Crim 17, the Court of Appeal said that despite the principle in *Church* being wide, it is 'clear and now well-established as part of our law . . . This principle must . . . be loyally applied and without reservation.'

The jury must place themselves in the accused's position with the accused's knowledge. In *Dawson* it was held that a reasonable person robbing a petrol station would not know of the attendant's bad heart. A sober and reasonable person would foresee that an attack by several persons, one of whom was clad in a balaclava, would cause fear through their pointing a replica gun at the attendant, banging a pick-axe handle on the counter and demanding money but he or she would not foresee physical harm resulting from the fear. Therefore, there was no dangerous act. However, the accused would be guilty if he became aware of the condition during the robbery. A contrasting case is *Watson*, above (CA): the jury were to take into account the burglar's knowledge of the victim's age and (frail) condition, which he had acquired after he had broken into her house. The accused was guilty even though his intent was only to steal. Theft or burglary is an unlawful act; on the facts it was a dangerous act because of the victim's physical state; and the victim died from a heart attack caused by the burglar. The reasonable person was fixed with the accused's knowledge acquired during the burglary.

If the accused had not become aware of the victim's frailty, the reasonable person in this context knows the facts which are obvious to a reasonable person, but not those facts which are not obvious. On the facts of *Watson*, however, the prosecution could not prove that the accused's acts caused the victim's death.

The reasonable person, while imbued with the knowledge the accused acquired throughout the crime, is not imbued with the mistaken beliefs he had. In *Ball*, above, the accused killed his neighbour with a shotgun. He said he thought the gun contained blanks. He had grabbed a handful of cartridges from his pocket, which as he knew contained both blank and live cartridges. The court held that it did not matter whether the accused thought about dangerousness. Whether the act was dangerous was to be judged by what the reasonable person would have appreciated. The reasonable person would have realised that he was inserting live cartridges because they were heavier than blanks: he would by definition not have made an unreasonable mistake. The accused's own 'intention, foresight or knowledge is irrelevant', said Lord Lane CJ. Therefore, the accused is not to be judged on the facts which he believed existed, but on the reasonable person's assessment of the facts. Accordingly, the reasonable person is imbued with the accused's knowledge, including expert knowledge, but not his mistaken beliefs. *Dawson* was distinguished as being an authority on the victim's vulnerability, whereas *Ball* was about the dangerousness of the accused's act. In a situation like *Ball* the jury is to look at all the facts, not just at the facts known to the accused. In actual fact *Ball* is similar to *Dawson* and there is no need to talk about mistake. The reasonable person with the accused's knowledge that his pocket contained both live and blank cartridges would have realised that what was done was dangerous.

In other areas of law, in particular provocation and duress, the reasonable person standard is modified by at least some of the accused's personal characteristics. No English case has discussed this eventuality in the context of manslaughter, but the possibility is there. The ruling as to the objective test is not affected by s 8 of the Criminal Justice Act 1967, which relates to proof: *Newbury*. Section 8 concerns the accused's intent or foresight: neither state of mind constitutes an element in the objective test of whether the accused's act was a dangerous one.

(e) The unlawful and dangerous act must cause the death of the victim. In *Carey*, above, the defendants punched the victim, who ran away. She died: she had a severely damaged heart which no one knew about. The harm to the victim caused by the defendant did not bring about her death.

Further examples of unlawful act manslaughter

Hayward (1908) 21 Cox CC 692: 'death from fright alone, caused by an illegal act, such as threats of violence, would be sufficient' (Ridley J).

Larkin, above: brandishing an open razor, intending to frighten the victim's man and inadvertently killing the victim.

Hall (1961) 45 Cr App R 366: producing a knife, intending to terrify his wife. *Larkin* was applied.

Mackie (1973) 57 Cr App R 453: using excessive violence on a child. This case was approved by the Privy Council in *DPP v Daley*, above. A similar case on chastisement is *Conner* (1835) 173 ER 194. (For more on the 'escape cases', see Chapter 2.)

Buck and Buck (1960) 44 Cr App R 213: illegal abortion.

Mahal, above: pushing the victim through an open window 22 feet above ground.

Where there is no unlawful act, there is no unlawful act manslaughter. In *Lamb*, above, the accused pulled the trigger of a gun and killed his best friend, but there was no assault because both did not expect a bullet to come out of the barrel. Sachs J said that *mens rea* was an essential part of this type of manslaughter. In *Jennings*, above, the accused had a sheathknife to protect himself from a person with whom he had been quarrelling. He was told by his brother that the person was looking for him. He got out his knife but stabbed to death his brother, who was attempting to restrain him. Since the possession of the knife was not in itself illegal, the jury should have been directed to look at the accused's intent. He might have had it with him to protect himself against 'an imminent and particular threat'. It was not sufficient that any bystander would on those facts have realised that some injury was inevitable.

Summary

Goodfellow sums up this area of law. The accused is guilty of unlawful act manslaughter if the responses to these questions are in the affirmative: '(1) was the act intentional? (2) was it unlawful? (3) was it an act which any reasonable person would realise was bound to subject some other human being to the risk of physical harm, albeit not necessarily serious harm? (4) was the act the cause of death?' (This summary may be too favourable to the accused. There is debate whether the unlawful act must be intentionally committed. For example, in *Scarlett*, above, the Court of Appeal assumed that a reckless battery was an unlawful act.) The Court of Appeal took a similar view in *Watson*, above, when it approved the trial judge's direction.

> Manslaughter is the offence committed when one person causes the death of another by an act which is unlawful and which is also dangerous, dangerous in the sense that it is an act which all sober and reasonable people would inevitably realise must subject the victim to the risk of some harm resulting whether the defendant realised that or not.

The same scenario can give rise to both gross negligence and unlawful act manslaughter, as the facts of *Goodfellow* demonstrate but need not. The differences are, first, that the former requires 'grossness' whereas the latter does not and, secondly, the former requires foresight of death whereas the latter requires only reasonable foreseeability of some harm however slight. For a case where the Court of Appeal said that on the facts the prosecution should have pursued unlawful act manslaughter and not gross negligence manslaughter, see *Willoughby* above. Since criminal damages had been proved, the prosecution had only one element of unlawful act manslaughter to prove: did the accused cause the victim's death?

Reform of manslaughter

The main criticism of unlawful act manslaughter is that it is a serious crime, yet a person is guilty of it if a reasonable person might foresee that some harm might occur: it is not necessary that some reasonable person might have foreseen death or GBH. Subjectivists are of course most unhappy that the accused is not being judged by what he foresaw but by what a reasonable person might have foreseen. Subjectivists also think that gross negligence manslaughter is unsupportable because again a jury does not consider what the accused intended or foresaw but uses the tort test of reasonable foreseeability.

The Law Commission's draft Criminal Code, Law Com. No. 177, 1989, proposed to abolish manslaughter by gross negligence. The Criminal Law Revision Committee had recommended the same in its Fourteenth Report, *Offences Against the Person*, Cmnd 7844, 1980. In cl 55 of the draft Criminal Code 'reckless' manslaughter is defined in accordance with cl 18(c) (see Chapter 3), which would restore the subjective meaning.

There have been two recent attempts to put manslaughter on a defensible statutory footing. The first was undertaken after the irruption of objective recklessness, the second after the resurrection of manslaughter by gross negligence.

By cl 55 of the draft Criminal Code, Law Com. No. 177, 1989:

A person is guilty of manslaughter if –

(a) he is not guilty of murder by reason only of the fact that a defence provided by s 56 (diminished responsibility), 58 (provocation) or 59 (use of excessive force) applies; or

(b) he is not guilty of murder by reason only of the fact that, because of voluntary intoxication, he is not aware that death may be caused or believes that an exemplary circumstance exists; or

(c) he causes the death of another –

(i) intending to cause serious personal harm; or

(ii) being reckless whether death or serious personal harm will be caused.

Since by definition in the draft Code 'recklessness' is given its subjective meaning, there is no place for *Caldwell* recklessness. Sub-clause (i) would move implied malice out of the law of murder into that of manslaughter, in cases where the accused knew that there would be a risk of death. Sub-clause (ii) does not state how high the probability of the harm's occurring is to be. It should be reformulated in a manner approximating to 'being reckless whether death or serious personal harm will be caused'.

Manslaughter would remain a catch-all offence. Because of the narrowing of one aspect of the fault element of murder (cl 54(1)(b)) to 'intending to cause serious personal harm and being aware that he may cause death', manslaughter is extended into part of the area currently covered by murder. Unlawful act manslaughter, as it now stands, is abolished. Suicide pact killings are retained (cl 62), not as manslaughter but as a separate offence, punishable with a maximum of seven years' imprisonment. This reform is in accordance with the recommendation of the Criminal Law Revision Committee.

It should be noted that contrary to present law, where the accused kills using excessive force in self-defence, he will be guilty of manslaughter (cl 59), not acquitted. Killing in pursuance of a suicide pact would become a separate offence, not manslaughter, with a maximum sentence of seven years' imprisonment.

If the 1989 reforms were adopted, the law would be clarified and the confusions which have arisen since the mid 1970s abolished. Indeed, the draft Criminal Code would also abolish the doctrine of constructive manslaughter, odious to subjectivists because a person is convicted for a result, death, which he did not intend and as to which he was not reckless.

The 1996 recommendations on involuntary manslaughter

Other reform proposals emanate from the Law Commission in its Report No. 237, *Legislating the Criminal Code: Involuntary Manslaughter*, 1996. There are four major recommendations in relation to the liability of natural persons. The Commission was concerned that the current law of manslaughter is too all-encompassing, ranging from a person who commits arson knowing that his family is in the burning house to a very careless electrician. It thought that juries may be reluctant to find incompetent doctors guilty of manslaughter, which has stigma attached to it. Two principal forms of unlawful killing, (a) and (d) below, are proposed.

(a) The crime should be reckless killing when the accused kills, being subjectively reckless as to death or serious injury. The risk must be one which in all the circumstances which he knows or believes to exist it is unreasonable for him to take. The Law Commission expressed some doubt about whether recklessness as to serious injury was sufficient *mens rea* for such a serious crime in its Consultation Paper No. 135,

Involuntary Manslaughter, 1994, which preceded the Report, but wished the law to be in line with murder; moreover, 'there is a very thin line between behaviour that risks serious injury and behaviour which risks death, because it is frequently a matter of chance, depending on such factors as the availability of medical treatment, whether serious injury leads to death' (para 4.19). The maximum sentence should be life imprisonment. This offence covers killings only a little short of murder (and pre-*Moloney* [1985] AC 905 such killings may have amounted to murder). Recklessness is defined as in the draft Criminal Code 1989 and the Law Commission Report No. 218, *Legislating the Criminal Code – Offences against the Person and General Principles*, 1993. As in that Report no definition is given of 'serious injury'.

(b) Unlawful act manslaughter should be abolished. The mishap that a person kills when he had the fault element for a crime less than causing serious injury is unfortunate, and the crime should not be manslaughter. The Law Commission has generally opposed constructive liability. In its opinion manslaughter is a crime about causing death when there is a significant risk of death or serious injury. Causing death by accident was not appropriately called manslaughter. Present law was also thought to be confused and uncertain. In its words, 'unlawful act manslaughter is ... unprincipled because it requires only that a foreseeable risk of causing some harm should have been inherent in the accused's conduct, whereas he is actually convicted of causing death'. This recommendation is consonant with the proposed abolition of constructive liability in ss 18 and 20 of the Offences Against the Person Act 1861: see Law Commission Report No. 218. The accused should be punished for what he did and thought – reckless injury or assault – not for the unexpected outcome of his act. The effect of the abolition of this form of manslaughter would not be that the accused would escape liability. He could be convicted of the types of manslaughter noted in (a) or (d) or of a non-fatal offence.

(c) The special category of motor manslaughter which received the sanction of the Court of Appeal in *Prentice* should be abolished on the basis that the law of manslaughter should apply generally, and not become divided into several crimes dependent on the accused's activity. There already is the offence of causing death by dangerous driving which since 1993 has been punishable by 10 years' imprisonment, and the new offence in (a) would cover the most heinous instances of killing through the use of a vehicle. Other fact situations would fall within (d).

(d) There should be an offence called killing by gross carelessness where the accused did not subjectively act recklessly as to death or serious injury. The Law Commission wished to avoid references to negligence and the duty of care, which are concepts of uncertain scope, as well as to recklessness and so formulated a new crime penalising the accused who has killed and reasonably ought to have been aware of a risk, which would have been obvious to a reasonable person in his position, that his act might result in death or in serious injury and whose conduct fell far below that which could reasonably have been demanded *of him* in preventing the occurrence of the risk (or in preventing the risk that had arisen from resulting in death). The bracketed phrase is where the liability of doctors will arise. The accused must also have been capable of appreciating that the risk of death or serious injury would have been obvious to a person in his position. As an alternative to the test of the accused's conduct falling far below what could reasonably be expected of him in the circumstances, the Law Commission proposed a test whereby the accused would be guilty if he intends to cause some injury or realises and unreasonably takes the risk that injury may be caused and the conduct causing the injury is an offence. If the risk was apparent to the accused, he will be guilty of reckless manslaughter, as defined in (a) above. The term 'of him' means that the accused will not be guilty if, e.g., he does his best to give assistance at a car crash, but means too that practice in the relevant field of activity could be investigated: the defendant may still be guilty even though he followed normal procedure in the sphere of action concerned. The Law Commission phrases liability for this possible offence as serious negligence and considers that the main application will be in relation to public services such as transport. While the Law Commission was of the view that the maximum sentence should be a determinate one of less than life imprisonment, it made no recommendation as to length. In Consultation Paper No. 134, *Involuntary Manslaughter*, which preceded the Report, the suggestion of the Law Commission was 10 years' imprisonment as the maximum. This offence would replace the crime of manslaughter by gross negligence. The Law Commission thought that an accused should be liable for a result he had not foreseen when the risk of harm was high and the failure to notice that risk was blameworthy. For recommendations as to corporate manslaughter, see Chapter 6.

(e) There is no proposal relating to omissions. The Law Commission recommended that the topic form the subject of another law reform project.

The Court of Appeal has twice called for an urgent and full review of the law of manslaughter: *Prentice* and *Scarlett* [1993] 4 All ER 629. The overruling of *Scarlett* does not affect this call for reform. The Law Commission's proposals are complex in that the jury would have to answer more questions than exist in present law.

The government's proposals

In its Consultation Paper, *Reforming the Law of Involuntary Manslaughter: The Government's Proposals*, 2000, the Home Office accepted most but not all of the recommendations of the Law Commission in its Report No. 237. In particular, it welcomed the new offences of (subjectively) reckless killing and killing by gross carelessness. However, it did not support the abolition of constructive manslaughter. On public consultation there was a strong response that constructive manslaughter in some form should be retained. In para 2.10 it stated: 'The Government is concerned that the Law Commission's approach would mean that behaviour which may be regarded as seriously culpable because it involves intentional or reckless criminal behaviour which results in death would no longer attract an appropriate charge. It might be viewed as unacceptable if the law permitted only a charge of assault where that assault had in fact resulted in death. The Government considers that there is an argument that anyone who embarks on a course of illegal violence has to accept the consequences of his act, even if the final consequences are unforeseeable.' Accordingly, another homicide offence was needed when the accused killed intending to injure or being reckless as to some injury and 'the conduct causing, or intended to cause, the injury constitutes an offence'. This crime would differ from constructive manslaughter because the objective test of dangerousness would be replaced by a subjective *mens rea* test. Excluded from this offence would be death caused by normally minor diseases which were fatal to susceptible persons (para 4.14). In respect of the transmission of fatal diseases, those who recklessly or by gross carelessness pass on a disease which results in death would be liable except where there is direct transmission from one person to another as by sexual contact. To this exception there is engrafted another exception: where a person owed a professional duty to the victim, he would be liable (para 4.12). The government has since announced that it does not intend to legislate on the basis of the Home Office's paper. Its focus currently is on corporate manslaughter. However, the Law Commission has returned to the fray, as is discussed in the next section of the book.

The Law Commission's 2006 proposals on involuntary manslaughter

The Law Commission in its Report No. 306 of November 2006 *Murder, Manslaughter and Infanticide* recommended a three-tier structure for fatal offences: first degree murder, second degree murder and manslaughter. The terms of reference did not permit it to examine involuntary manslaughter in depth, particularly as it had made proposals for reform in its 1996 Report, noted in the previous section of this book, and the Home Office had given the government's response, also noted there. What the Commission did do, however, was to redefine unlawful act manslaughter and gross negligence manslaughter. The former has come in for much criticism because (para 3.42): '. . . a person can be convicted of a very serious offence even though he or she was not aware that their criminal act posed a risk of any harm occurring. It suffices if a reasonable person would have been aware.' Nevertheless, the consultees to the Consultation Paper *A New Homicide Act for England and Wales?* 2005 supported the continued existence of both offences.

Unlawful act manslaughter would be defined as: killing another through a criminal act intended to cause injury or through a criminal act being aware that it involved a serious risk of causing injury. The Law Commission rejected a suggestion that there should be awareness of a risk of *serious* injury because that would overcomplicate the law: there should not be debate before the jury whether the injury was serious or not.

Gross negligence manslaughter differs somewhat from that found in the Home Office's 2000 proposals. First, there would be no separate category of (subjectively) reckless manslaughter. Some scenarios falling within that category would become second degree murder (intent to cause injury or fear of injury or risk of injury coupled with awareness that the conduct may cause death); the remainder would fall within gross negligence manslaughter. If this proposal were enacted, 'recklessness' could disappear from fatal offences. Secondly, the gross negligence must be as to death; gross negligence as to serious injury would not suffice. This would restate the common law as it has developed after *Adomako* above.

Conclusion

Lord Mustill in *Attorney-General's Reference (No. 3 of 1994)* [1998] AC 245 stated that 'the offence of manslaughter unites a group of crimes which have nothing in common except their name'. One might add that they also share the same *actus reus* and maximum sentence, but there is much sense in what Lord Mustill said, and that good sense is reflected in this book: diminished responsibility is akin to insanity and both are discussed in Chapter 9, while provocation (see earlier in this chapter) is a defence only to murder, discussed in Chapter 11. In such, bar the name, *actus reus* and sentence, voluntary and involuntary manslaughter are really separate offences, and the fact that they have the same name is apt to mislead.

Summary

In this chapter voluntary and involuntary manslaughter are considered. 'Voluntary' in this context means that the accused had malice aforethought, the *mens rea* of murder, but has a defence. Provocation is the one of the two principal forms of voluntary manslaughter (the other being diminished responsibility, which is considered in Chapter 9). Provocation occurs when the accused kills but (i) does so in hot blood and (ii) does not fall below the standard of a reasonable person. The main developments in the law revolve around the standard of the reasonable person, and current law draws a line between the gravity of the provocation and the level of self-control expected of a person in the modern world. In this context the debate in *Smith* (2000) HL and *Holley* (2005) PC is expounded. The defence, which applies to murder only, has come in for trenchant criticism over recent years, particularly on the basis that it is gender-biased: men may kill on a sudden impulse in response to provoking acts or words but women tend to have a 'slow burn' reaction; that is, they tend to kill when their victim is asleep or in a drunken stupor. Besides provocation and diminished responsibility there is a third form of voluntary manslaughter, killing in pursuance of a suicide pact. The standard example is when the accused and his victim, lovers, decide that they cannot live in an unforgiving world. The victim agrees to be killed by the accused; the accused kills the victim; but the accused then decides not to kill himself or herself.

Involuntary manslaughter is where the accused kills but does not have the *mens rea* of murder but does fall within two (or almost certainly three) definitions. One form of involuntary manslaughter is manslaughter by gross negligence; the second form is constructive manslaughter, which also goes by the name of unlawful act manslaughter, a name preferred by the author because it reminds the reader that there must be both an act (an omission will not suffice) and an act which is unlawful, i.e. criminal in its own right (though not all the cases are to that effect). The third form, which does seem to exist, is that of (subjectively) reckless manslaughter, a type of killing which only just falls short of murder.

The chapter concludes with a discussion of reform proposals.

- Provocation: Section 3 of the Homicide Act 1957 provides: 'Where on a charge on murder there is evidence on which the jury can find that the person charged was provoked (whether by things done or by things said or by both together) to lose his self-control, the question whether the provocation was enough to make a reasonable man do as he did shall be left to be determined by the jury; and in determining that question, the jury shall take into account everything both done and said according to the effect which, in their opinion, it would have had on a reasonable man.'

  Certain matters are clear on a reading of s 3: for example, it is a defence only to murder; perhaps more importantly, there are some matters which are unclear. What is provocation? Who bears the burden of proof? What is the outcome of a successful plea of provocation? Provocation consists of two stages: the first, subjective, test is whether the accused lost his or her self-control; the second, objective, one is whether a reasonable person might have lost his or her self-control. The burden of proof is on the prosecution to prove beyond reasonable doubt that the accused did not have the defence. The outcome of a successful plea is not that the accused is acquitted of murder but that he or she is convicted of manslaughter.

  Debate in this millennium has centred on the second test, the objective one, but it should not be forgotten that the first stage is often seen as being gender-based: women, it is said, are not strong enough to overpower men and therefore kill while men are drunk or asleep, by which time the female defendants are in control of their mind and are therefore not killing in the heat of the moment. Similarly, if provocation were restricted to the last act allegedly done by the victim, abused persons such as 'battered wives' may well not be able to rely on this defence because the last act of provocation was small and a jury might think it insufficient to excuse a killing; however, for some time the courts have permitted cumulative or last-straw provocation.

- Gross negligence manslaughter: This form of involuntary manslaughter occurs when the accused kills and does so in breach of a duty of care he or she owes to the victim, and that breach falls far short of the standard to be expected, and there is a risk of death. Where the accused is an expert such as a doctor performing his or her job, the standard is that of a reasonably competent person in that work.

- Unlawful act manslaughter (also known as constructive manslaughter): This is where the accused kills as a result of a crime (for which he or she performed the *actus reus* and usually at least had the *mens rea*), what he or she did was an act (not an omission) and the act was dangerous in the sense that all sober and reasonable people would say that what the accused did was likely to cause some harm.

  While the same act may give rise to both of these forms of involuntary manslaughter, they have different rules attached to them. For example, gross negligence manslaughter may be committed by an omission but unlawful act manslaughter may not; and in gross negligence manslaughter there must have been a risk of death but in unlawful act manslaughter it is sufficient that there was a risk of some injury, not even serious injury, never mind death.

- (Subjectively) reckless manslaughter: While no case definitively so rules, it is thought that there is an offence of (subjectively) reckless manslaughter when the accused foresees death or GBH as a possible consequence but nonetheless goes on and kills.

References

Reports

Criminal Law Revision Committee 14th Report, *Offences against the Person*, Cmnd 7844 (1980)

Home Office Consultation Paper, *Reforming the Law of Involuntary Manslaughter* (2000)

Judicial Studies Board Specimen Direction on Provocation (2003)

Law Commission Consultation Paper No. 135, *Involuntary Manslaughter* (1994)

Law Commission Consultation Paper No. 173, *Partial Defences to Murder* (2003)

Law Commission Consultation Paper No. 177, *A new Homicide Act for England & Wales?* (2005)

Law Commission Report No. 177, *A Criminal Code for England & Wales* (1989)

Law Commission Report No. 218, *Legislating the Criminal Code: Offences against the Person and General Principles* (1993)

Law Commission Report No. 227, *Legislating the Criminal Code: Involuntary Manslaughter* (1996)

Law Commission Report No. 290, *Partial Defences to Murder* (2004)

Law Commission Report No. 306, *Murder, Manslaughter and Infanticide* (2006)

Books

Gillespie, C. K. *Justifiable Homicide* (Ohio State University Press, 1989)

Horder, J. *Provocation and Responsibility* (Clarendon, 1991)

Yeo, S. *Fault in Homicide* (Federation Press, 1997)

Journals

Ashworth, A. 'The Doctrine of Provocation' [1976] CLJ 292

Ashworth, A. Casenote on *Weller* [2003] Crim LR 725

Dobson, P. Casenote on *Weller* 42 (2004) Student LR 20

Edwards, P. 'The erosion of the objective test in provocation' (2001) 23 JSWL 227

Mitchell, B. [1990] NLJ 935

Further reading

Ashworth, A. 'Sentencing for murder by provocation' [2004] Crim LR 501

Ashworth, A. and Mitchell, B. *Rethinking English Homicide Law* (Oxford University Press, 2000)

Bandalli, S. 'Provocation: A cautionary note' (1995) 22 JLS 398

Brown, H. 'Provocation as a defence to murder: to abolish or to reform?' (1999) 12 *Australian Feminist Law Journal* 137

Busuttil, A. and McCall Smith, A. 'Flight, stress and homicide' (1990) 54 JCL 257

Buxton, M. 'Sentencing in domestic homicide upon provocation' (2003) 11 *Feminist Legal Studies* 279

Buxton, R. J. 'By any unlawful act' (1966) 81 LQR 174

Carline, A. 'Women who kill their abusive partners: from sameness to gender construction' (2005) 26 Liverpool LR 13

Chalmers, J. 'Merging provocation and diminished responsibility: some reasons for scepticism' [2004] Crim LR 198

Davies, M. C. 'Leaving provocation to the jury: a homicidal muddle?' (1998) 62 JCL 374

Dressler, J. 'Why keep the provocation defense? Some reflections on a difficult subject' (2002) 86 Minn LR 959

Edwards, S. 'Battered women who kill' [1990] NLJ 1380

Edwards, S. 'Abolishing provocation and reframing self-defence' [2004] Crim LR 181

Edwards, S. 'Descent into murder: provocation's stricture – the prognosis for women who kill men who abuse them' (2007) 71 JCL 342

Freckleton, I. 'When plight makes right: the forensic abuse syndrome' (1994) 18 Crim LJ 29

Gardner, J. and Macklem, T. 'Compassion without respect: nine fallacies in *R v Smith*' [2001] Crim LR 623

Gardner, J. and Macklem, T. 'No provocation without responsibility: a reply to Mackay and Mitchell' [2004] Crim LR 213

Gardner, S. 'Manslaughter by gross negligence' (1995) 111 LQR 22

Golder, B. 'The homosexual advance defence and the law / body nexus' (2004) 11 E Law: Murdoch University Electronic Journal of Law, Pt I

Greene, J. 'A provocation defence for battered women who kill?' (1989–90) 12 Adel LR 145

Herring, J. and Palser, E. 'The duty of care in gross negligence manslaughter' [2007] Crim LR 24

Holton, R. and Shute, S. 'Self-control in the modern provocation defence' (2007) 27 JLS 49

Horder, J. 'Between provocation and diminished responsibility' (1999) 2 *King's College Law Journal* 143

Horder, J. 'Reshaping the subjective element in the provocation defence' (2005) 25 *Oxford Journal of Legal Studies 123*

Howe, A. 'More folk provoke their own demise' (1997) 19 Syd LR 376

Howe, A. 'Reforming Provocation' (1999) 12 *Australian Feminist Law Journal* 127

Howe, A. 'Provoking polemic – provoked killings and the ethical paradoxes of the postmodern feminist condition' (2004) *Feminist Legal Studies* 10: 39

Keating, H. 'The Law Commission's Report on Involuntary Manslaughter: the restoration of a serious crime' [1996] Crim LR 535

Law Reform Commission (Ireland) *Homicide: The Plea of Provocation*, Consultation Paper no. 27 (2003)

Law Commission (of New Zealand) *Some Criminal Defences with Particular Reference to Battered Defendants*, Report No. 73 (2004)

Leader-Elliott, I. 'Sex, race and provocation' (1993) 15 Syd LR 403

Mackay, R. and Mitchell, B. J. 'Provoking diminished responsibility: Two pleas merging into one' [2003] Crim LR 745

Mackay, R. and Mitchell B. J. 'Replacing provocation: More on a combined plea' [2004] Crim LR 219

Mackay, R. and Mitchell, B. J. 'But is this provocation? Some thoughts on the Law Commission's Report on Partial Defences to Murder' [2005] Crim LR 44

Macklem, T. and Gardner, J. 'Provocation and pluralism' (2001) 64 MLR 815

McSherry, B. 'It's a man's world: Claims of provocation and automatism in "intimate" homicide' [2005] MULR 28

Mitchell, B. 'Minding the gap in unlawful and dangerous act manslaughter: a moral defence of one-punch killers' (2008) 72 JCL 537

Mitchell, B. J., Mackay, R. D. and Brookbanks, W. J. 'Pleading for provoked killers: in defence of *Morgan Smith*' (2008) 124 LQR 675

Morgan, J. 'Provocation law and facts: Dead women tell no tales, tales are told about them' (2007) 21 MULR 237

Mousourakis, C. *Criminal Responsibility and Partial Excuses* (Ashgate, 1998)

Mytton, L. and Webley, L. 'Families and violence: making difference(s) visible, (2000) 7 *International Journal of the Legal Profession*' 273

Nicolson, D. 'Telling tales: Gender discrimination, gender construction and battered women who kill' (1995) 2 *Feminist Legal Studies* 185

Norrie, A. 'The structure of provocation' [2001] CLP 307

Nourse, V. 'Passion's progress' (1997) 106 Yale LJ 1331

Ormerod, D. C. Case comment on *Willoughby* [2005] Crim LR 389

Pasquale, S. de 'Provocation and the homosexual advance defence' [2002] MULR 6

Peiris, G. L. 'Involuntary manslaughter in the Commonwealth' (1985) 5 LS 21

Power, H. 'Provocation and culture' [2006] Crim LR 871

Quick, O. 'Prosecuting "gross" medical negligence: manslaughter, discretion and the Crown Prosecution Service' (2006) JLS 421

Reilly, A. 'The heart of the matter' (1997–98) 29 Ottawa LR 117

Rix, K. 'Battered woman syndrome and defence of provocation: Two women with something more in common' (2001) 12 *Journal of Forensic Psychiatry* 131

Spencer, J. R. 'Manslaughter by gross negligence' [1983] CLJ 187

Sullivan, G. R. 'Anger and excuse' (1993) 13 OJLS 421

Wasik, M. 'Cumulative provocation and domestic killings' [1982] Crim LR 29

Williams, G. 'Provocation and killing with compassion' (2001) 65 JCL 149

Williams, R. 'Policy and principle in drugs manslaughter cases' (2005) CLJ 66

Wilson, W. 'The structure of criminal homicide' [2006] Crim LR 471

Yeo, S. 'Resolving gender bias in criminal defences' (1993) 19 Monash ULR 104

Yeo, S. 'Sex, ethnicity, power of self-control and provocation revisited' (1996) 18 Syd LR 304

Yeo, S. 'The role of gender in the law of provocation' (1997) 26 A-ALR 431

Yeo, S. *Unrestrained Killings and the Law* (Oxford University Press, Delhi, 1998)

Horder, J. *Provocation and Responsibility* (Clarendon, 1991) is a monograph. The author contends that the defence should be abolished because it cannot be reconstituted in a gender-free way. For a contrary view, see C. Hall (1993) 2 Caribbean LR 23. There are a number of feminist writings on the topic. They include S. Lees in J. Radford and D. E. H. Russell (eds.), *Femicide: The Politics of Woman Killing* (OUP, 1992) and S. S. M. Edwards, *Sex and Gender in the Legal Process* (Blackstone Press, 1996), ch. 6. For a book which includes gendered killings, see F. Brookman, *Understanding Homicide* (Sage, 2005).

The latest Australian law reform proposals are contained in Victoria Law Reform Commission, *Defences to Homicide: Final Report*, 2004. For the Irish approach see Law Reform Commission, *Homicide: Murder and Involuntary Manslaughter*, Report no. 87, 2008.

For a recent discussion of 'homosexual advance defence' see A. Howe in (C. Stychin and D. Hermann, eds.), *Sexuality in the Legal Arena* (Athlone Press, 2000). For a US view see R. B. Mison 'Homophobia in manslaughter: the homosexual advance as insufficient provocation' (1992) 80 *California Law Review* 133. For a contrary view see J. Dressler, 'When "heterosexual" men kill "homosexual" men: reflections on provocation law, sexual advances, and the "reasonable man" standard' (1995) 85 JCL & Crim 726.

There is an overwhelming number of American law review articles on battered woman syndrome. One way into the literature is A. M. Coughlin 'Excusing women' (1994) 82 Calif LR 1. Her views, that the syndrome categorises women as lacking the self-control which men possess and therefore that it demeans women, have been criticised on the grounds that the syndrome is founded not on a distinction of gender but on society's response to the predicament in which women find themselves.

An exposition of the work of Lenore Walker appears in N. Z. Hilton (ed.), *Legal Responses to Wife Assault* (Sage, 1993) ch. 9. Her books include *The Battered Woman* (Harper & Row, 1979); *The Battered Woman Syndrome* (Springer, 2nd edn, 2000); and *Terrifying Love* (Harper & Row, 1989). Interestingly, she was a defence witness in the O. J. Simpson trial. For a criticism of battered persons' syndrome, see A. M. Dershowitz, *The Abuse Excuse and Other Cop-outs, Sob Stories and Evasions of Responsibility* (Little, Brown & Co, 1994). For a less polemic critique, see R. A. Schuller and N. Vidmar 'Battered woman syndrome, evidence in the courtroom' (1992) 16 *Law and Human Behavior* 273. For criticism of battered woman syndrome in the context of self-defence see J. Dressler 'Battered women, sleeping abusers, and criminal responsibility' (1997) 2 *Chicago Policy Review* 1.

Visit **www.mylawchamber.co.uk/jefferson** to access exam-style questions with answer guidance, multiple choice quizzes, live weblinks, an online glossary, and regular updates to the law.

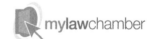

Use **Case Navigator** to read in full some of the key cases referenced in this chapter:

A-G for Jersey v *Holley* [2005] 2 AC 580

DPP v *Majewski* [1997] AC 433

R v *Adomako* [1995] AC 171

R v *G* [2003] UKHL 50; [2004] 1 AC 1034

R v *Pagett* (1983) 76 Cr. App. R 279

Non-fatal offences

Introduction

> The history of our law upon personal injuries is certainly not creditable to the legislature, and the result at which we have at present arrived is extremely clumsy.
>
> Sir James Fitzjames Stephen, *A History of the Criminal Law of England*, 1883, vol 3, 118.

The same may be said at the present day.

This chapter considers crimes against the person which do not result in death. Many but not all appear in the Offences Against the Person Act 1861 (hereinafter OAPA). Those offences which are considered are those most likely to be reviewed on a criminal law course. Assault on a constable in the execution of his duty, it is argued, properly belongs in constitutional law. This chapter also deals with the issue of consent. Two points to bear in mind throughout the discussion are that the same facts can give rise to more than one offence and that the crimes are defined in terms both of the fault element of the accused and the harmful consequences, but the relationship is not perfect. One is guilty of assault occasioning actual bodily harm even though one does not intend to do so and one is not reckless as to the result: *Savage* [1992] 1 AC 699.

Assault

'Assault' is used in two different senses: first as a generic term for the separate offences of assault and battery (this usage occurs in s 47 of the OAPA: see below); and secondly as a term denoting the crime of assault. The second use is sometimes called 'psychic assault' or 'technical assault'. Since there can be an assault without a battery, this section of this book uses the second meaning.

Both assault and battery have been held, contrary to earlier views, to be statutory offences: *DPP v Little* [1992] 1 QB 645 (DC), though this case was criticised for so holding in *Cross v DPP*, unreported, 20 June 1995 (CA). The Court of Appeal thought in *Haystead v Chief Constable of Derbyshire* [2000] 3 All ER 890 that assault and battery remained common law offences, but *DPP v Little* was not referred to. If *DPP v Little* is correct, this is the position. The charge should be one of assault (or battery) contrary to s 39 of the Criminal Justice Act 1988. Section 39 reads: 'Common assault and battery shall be summary offences and a person guilty of either of them shall be liable to a fine not exceeding level 5 on the standard scale, to imprisonment for a term not exceeding six months, or to both.' Currently, level 5 is up to £5,000. The allegation in the information should not be 'assault and battery', which is bad for duplicity (the legal phrase for saying that two separate offences cannot be contained in one charge), but 'assault and beat' or preferably 'assault by beating', both forms constituting only one offence. The outcome in *Little* is surprising. It had been thought that only the penalty was prescribed by statute, just as the penalty for murder is laid down by Parliament. The court said that assault and battery had been statutory offences since the enactment of s 47 of the OAPA, but that section simply stated the punishment. When Parliament abolished the common law penalty for murder (hanging) and substituted a different one (life imprisonment), it did not make it a statutory offence. *DPP v Little* does confirm that assault and battery are two separate offences. It was sometimes thought that assault had no separate existence, it was simply an attempted battery. The ruling by the Court of Appeal in *Notman* [1994] Crim LR 518 that assault is one offence committable either through (psychic) assault or (physical) battery is incorrect. The phrase 'common assault' is sometimes used. It means both (psychic) assault *and* battery, though sometimes it means only (psychic) assault.

James J defined assault in ***Fagan v MPC*** [1969] 1 QB 439 as 'any act which intentionally or possibly recklessly causes another person to apprehend immediate and unlawful violence'. The mental element now definitely includes recklessness. *Savage* (HL) confirmed this proposition. Robert Goff J used this definition of the *actus reus* in ***Collins v Wilcock*** [1984] 1 WLR 1172 (DC): 'an act which causes another person to apprehend the infliction of immediate, unlawful force on his person'. Whichever definition is used, the gist of the offence is the creation of fear in another's mind. If there is fear, there can be an assault. Examples include pointing a gun which may be loaded (***St George*** (1840) 173 ER 921). As long as there is fear, it does not matter that the gun was in fact unloaded, or as in ***Logdon*** [1976] Crim LR 121, the weapon was an imitation firearm. The accused is therefore guilty even though he could not carry out the threat in the way that the victim feared. *Logdon* demonstrates also that the accused is guilty even though he did not intend to execute the threat. Shaking a fist at the victim (***Stephens v Myers*** (1830) 172 ER 735) and threatening physical harm (***Mackie*** [1973] Crim LR 54) were assaults. If there is no apprehension of immediate harm, there is no assault. Examples would be: where the act is not seen, as when the victim is asleep; where the victim believes that the gun was unloaded (***Lamb*** [1967] 2 QB 981); where the victim knows by the accused's words that the threat will not take place (***Tuberville v Savage*** (1669) 86 ER 684, a civil case); or where the accused could not put his threat into effect for some time: the usual illustrations are shaking a fist while on a non-stop train at a person standing on the platform and doing the same to a person standing on the opposite bank of a fast-flowing and wide river where there is no bridge. Merely looking for a person is not an assault. The victim need fear only a battery, an offence which is committed by an accused who touches the victim and the victim does not consent. The victim need not fear serious injury.

The threat must be one which can be carried out immediately, though 'immediately' is read broadly. See also ***Ireland; Burstow*** in which Lord Steyn said that the immediacy requirement was satisfied by the accused's saying that 'I will be at your door in a minute or two'. Frightening a woman by looking into her bedsit at 11 at night causing her to fear violence was held to be immediate (it was open to the Justices to convict on these facts), despite the fact that the victim was behind a locked door and that the victim could have escaped in the time it would have taken for the accused to get to her: ***Smith v Chief***

Superintendent, Woking Police Station (1983) 76 Cr App R 234 (DC). Kerr LJ said that his remarks were limited to a case where the accused was 'immediately adjacent, albeit on the other side of a window'. It might also be doubted whether the accused intended to apply any force, whether immediately or otherwise. Surprisingly, Kerr LJ said that it would not be assault if the accused threatened someone in a locked car. Surely it should be an assault in both fact situations or neither. Possibly the case is explained that there is no crime specifically directed against voyeurs, and the offence of assault had to be stretched to cover the accused's conduct. In ***Lewis*** [1970] Crim LR 647, a case of assault occasioning actual bodily harm, the accused was guilty even though the victim, his wife, was on the other side of a locked door. The ***Smith*** case also demonstrates that the prosecution need not show exactly what the victim was afraid of. The requirement of immediate fear means that a threat to carry out violence a long time in the future does not amount to an assault, even though fear is present. There is, however, an offence of threatening to kill (OAPA, s 16). It must be said that the law is not clear as to how immediate the threat must be. The established rule was that the victim had to be put in fear of an immediate attack. Lord Steyn in ***Ireland; Burstow*** extended the requirement to causing the victim to apprehend that he possibly could be attacked in the immediate future. He spoke of a threat that violence would occur 'within a minute or two' but did not specify the width accorded to the requirement of a threat of imminent harm. The Court of Appeal in ***Constanza*** [1997] 2 Cr App R 492, which involved some 800 letters and numerous silent phone calls, spoke of 'fear of violence at some time not excluding the immediate future'. On the facts it is difficult to see that the victim was put in fear of *immediate violence* when she received many silent telephone calls and many letters from the accused. Rather she was put in *immediate fear* of violence, but that is not what the definition demands. It was only the last two letters which made the victim afraid. She was afraid when she received them but she did not fear that she would be immediately attacked. The accused might have been in a country far, far away. This scenario now falls within the Protection from Harassment Act 1997.

While no case so holds as *ratio*, a threat to set one's dog on the victim suffices. This was assumed in ***Dume*** (1986) *The Times* 16 October (CA). It follows that asking one's boyfriend to beat up one's enemy in the latter's presence may constitute an assault.

The threat must be an unlawful one. Therefore, a threat in self-defence, preventing crime, furthering arrest or lawful discipline is not an assault. Consent is dealt with below. It is often said that an assault and a battery can be committed only by an act and that an omission is not sufficient. However, in ***Fagan v MPC*** the court held the accused to be guilty when he inadvertently parked his car on a police officer's foot, realised what he had done, and refused to drive off. His omission was converted into an act by the means stated in Chapter 2. The continuing act of his sitting in the car which rested on the foot, coupled with his *mens rea*, rendered him liable. There was a series of events which were all part of one transaction. Nowadays ***Fagan v MPC*** could also be justified on the principle that the accused created a dangerous situation which he deliberately did not rectify. Since grievous bodily harm can be committed by an omission, it would be strange if assault and battery could not be. It is thought that a deliberate refusal to put a victim's mind at rest when the accused has unwittingly frightened him is an assault.

Ireland; Burstow [1998] AC 147

These two cases involving stalkers were heard together. In *Ireland* the accused made many telephone calls to three women. He remained silent when they answered the phone. They suffered psychological harm. He was charged with assault occasioning actual bodily harm. In *Burstow* the accused harassed a woman. As part of his campaign he too made silent phone calls. She suffered severe depression. He was charged with maliciously inflicting grievous bodily harm. Both were convicted and their appeals were dismissed. On further appeal, the House of Lords dismissed both appeals.

One issue raised in *Ireland* was whether verbally abusive or silent phone calls could constitute assault. *Constanza*, above, which was cited but not referred to by the House of Lords, held that written words could amount to an assault. As long as the victim apprehended fear, it did not matter how he came to apprehend fear. Words, letters and faxes were instanced. Famously in *Meade and Belt* (1823) 168 ER 1006 Holroyd J had said: 'no words or singing are equivalent to an assault'. Lord Steyn ruled to the contrary. 'The proposition that a gesture may amount to an assault, but that words can never suffice, is unrealistic and indefensible. There is no reason why something said should be incapable of causing an apprehension of immediate personal violence e.g. a man accosting a woman in a dark alley saying "Come with me or I will stab you." I would, therefore, reject the proposition that an assault can never be committed by words.' Indeed, if words could not constitute an assault, there would be no assault if the accused made threats to a blind person. That disposed of the question of whether an assault could be committed by words. In relation to silence, Lord Steyn stated that silence could constitute an assault, but whether it did so was a question of fact. 'As a matter of law the caller may be guilty of an assault: whether he is or not will depend on the circumstance and in particular on the impact of the caller's potentially menacing call or calls on the victim.' Accordingly, silence *may* constitute an assault but does not necessarily do so. This statement also resolved the issue whether the victim feared immediate personal violence: it was sufficient that she feared the possibility of immediate personal violence. There was no requirement that the victim feared an instantaneous attack. The Lords stressed that they were not ruling on the width of the concept of immediacy. What this case and *Constanza* seem to have done is to make the accused guilty if the victim fears that he may be attacked soon. This is a departure from earlier law which required a threat causing 'immediate' fear. Like *Constanza* the facts of *Ireland; Burstow* now fall within the Protection from Harassment Act 1998.

As stated above, words can negative (that is, render non-criminal) what would otherwise be an assault. In *Tuberville* v *Savage*, the accused laid his hand on his sword and said: 'If it were not assize time, I would not take such language.' The accused's words showed that he did not intend violence and the victim did not apprehend immediate personal violence. The same principle was applied in *Blake* v *Barnard* (1840) 173 ER 485. The accused said that he would blow the victim's brains out if he was not quiet. It may be that *Blake* v *Barnard* is incorrect. The threat was not as it was in *Tuberville* an extraneous condition (assize time), but was a conditional restraint on the victim's freedom of behaviour: that is an assault. One suggestion is that *Blake* v *Barnard* is badly reported and should not be followed in respect of there being no assault when there is a condition. Certainly in *Light* (1857) [1843–60] All ER Rep 934, the accused was seemingly guilty of an assault when he said: 'Were it not for the bloody policeman outside, I would split your head open.' *Light* is inconsistent with *Tuberville* v *Savage*. An alternative view is to say that the effect of the words is rendered nugatory by the overwhelming threat of violence of the situation. In *Light* the accused was holding a shovel over his wife's head at the time. The problem with the attempted reconciliation is that the accused in *Tuberville* v *Savage* had his hand on the sword.

The accused must cause the victim to apprehend immediate and unlawful personal violence. The principles of causation were discussed in Chapter 2.

The *mens rea* in assault is intention or recklessness, as stated by Lord Simon (dissenting) in **DPP v Morgan** [1976] AC 182, approved by Lord Elwyn-Jones CJ in **DPP v Majewski** [1977] AC 443. The House of Lords in **Savage**, above, confirmed that recklessness is of the **Cunningham** variety.

For a review of these concepts, see Chapter 2 on causation and Chapter 3 on recklessness.

In **Williams** (1983) [1987] 3 All ER 411, Lord Lane CJ held that 'the mental element necessary to constitute guilt is the intent to apply unlawful force to the victim. We do not believe that the mental element can be substantiated by simply showing an intent to apply force and no more.' It is sometimes said that assault is committed only when the accused has a hostile intention. There is, however, no need for any anger, spite or incivility. What hostility means in this context is that the accused must act without lawful excuse.

Threat to kill

Section 16 of the OAPA as amended creates the offence of threatening to kill without lawful excuse. An illustration is provided by a sentencing case. A threat to kill a foetus does not fall within s 16 because it is not a person in being for the purpose of murder. A threat to kill the foetus when it had been born, it is suggested, does fall within s 16. See **Tait** [1990] QB 290 (CA) where it was said, wrongly it is thought, that the threat to kill the foetus would not constitute this offence. It covers a threat to kill in the future. The threat may be implied as it was in **Solanke** [1970] 1 WLR 1 (CA): 'I do not wish to take her life but . . . I hope my children will be looked after.' The history between the parties may also be taken into account. **Williams** (1986) 84 Cr App R 299 (CA): the accused had repeatedly harassed and been violent to his ex-girlfriend.

Since assault requires an apprehension of immediate violence, a threat to injure in the future is not a criminal offence. Perhaps in the nineteenth century a threat to injure was not something which would be regarded as sufficiently serious to merit criminalisation. A modern view is that the victim of such a threat can seek official protection before the menace is executed. This lacuna in the law will be filled if the draft Criminal Code is enacted (see below). It is certainly anomalous that a threat to destroy or damage property is a crime but a threat to injure is not, and the proposed reform would cover only a threat to cause serious injury: a threat to impose less serious injury at some time in the future would remain non-criminal. At least the change would catch an accused who threatened to kneecap his victim if the latter did not do some act in the future.

The *mens rea* is the intention to cause the victim to apprehend that the threat will be carried out. A lawful excuse would occur when a person threatens to kill the man raping him or her.

The maximum penalty is 10 years' imprisonment, twice the length of assault occasioning actual bodily harm and maliciously inflicting grievous bodily harm or wounding.

Battery

The old definition of **battery** was that used in **Cole v Turner** (1705) 87 ER 907, 'the least touching of someone in anger'. Three more recent definitions are:

(a) 'The actual intended use of unlawful force to another person without his consent' (since then recklessness has been added to the *mens rea*), *per* Jones LJ in **Fagan v MPC**, above. The court in **Attorney-General's Reference (No. 6 of 1980)** [1981] 1 QB 715 added 'or any other lawful excuse' to that definition. 'Excuse' covers exceptions such as properly conducted games, lawful chastisement, reasonable surgery and the like. (It is uncertain what properly conducted games are: what about a wall of death?)

(b) 'The actual infliction of unlawful force on another person': Robert Goff J in **Collins v Wilcock**, above. Touching a woman on her shoulder was a battery.

(c) Apparently the most authoritative: 'Any intentional touching without the consent of that person and without lawful excuse. It need not necessarily be hostile or rude or aggressive, as some of the cases seem to indicate', *per* Lord Lane CJ in **Faulkner v Talbot** [1981] 1 WLR 1528 at 1536, which was approved by Lord Ackner in **Court** [1989] AC 28 at 41–42. Again, the mental element of recklessness should be added. (In fact, as Lord Goff, dissenting, said in **Court, Faulkner v Talbot** was a case on indecent assault, in which in most cases the sole mental element was intention: did the accused intend to assault in indecent circumstances? Indecent assault has since been abolished but the 'assault' part continues to apply.)

Statute has not defined battery, and the cases do not give a single definition.

The requirement of force means that a threat is not a battery. For example, causing psychiatric harm by a threat is not a battery because there is no touching. Using force to pull away from the victim is not a battery because it is not used *on* the victim.

Whether the accused did cause unlawful force is governed by the law of causation discussed in Chapter 2.

There is some debate whether hostility is a requirement. For example, in **Brown** [1994] AC 212 Lords Jauncey and Lowry spoke of hostility being a necessary ingredient. **Faulkner v Talbot, Collins v Wilcock** (a civil case) and Lord Goff in **Re F** [1990] 2 AC 1 (HL) do not require hostility. Perhaps the reference to hostility is another way of saying that touching is only a battery if it is unlawful. The *dicta* in **Brown** can be interpreted in this way. In that case the victims, masochists, had willingly consented to being sexually tortured by the defendants, sadists. It is difficult to demonstrate hostility on the facts. If the interpretation is correct, where there is consent to the causing of harm but the consent is not for an approved purpose, here sadomasochism, there is hostility, i.e. hostility is not a separate requirement. In **Collins v Wilcock** the touching was unlawful because a police constable has no power to restrain a person temporarily. Her powers in this regard do not exceed those of an ordinary citizen. The tort of trespass to the person does seem to require hostile contact, but the difference of hostility from unlawfulness is not clear. There is no need for hostility in the offence of indecent assault. In this context 'assault' includes battery. Accordingly, there should be no need for hostility in the crime of battery.

There is no need for an assault. One may batter an unconscious, sleeping or unsuspecting victim. Examples include: touching, throwing a stone which hits someone, tripping up, kicking, spitting on the victim, and throwing beer over the victim (**Savage** (1990) 91 Cr App R 317 (CA), which decision the House of Lords approved). Force may also be applied by setting a dog on the victim. In other words, the accused need not himself touch the victim. There must, however, be some form of contact. As Lord Steyn said in **Ireland; Burstow**, a silent phone call cannot amount to a battery because no force is applied.

Though the law is not entirely clear, it seems that the violence need not be directly inflicted. An old illustration deriving from civil law is digging a pit into which the victim falls. Another one is putting a bucket of water on top of a door which the victim will push open. The escape cases provide another example: the accused frightens the victim so much that she jumps out the window and is injured by coming into contact with the ground. In *Martin* (1881) 8 QBD 54 the accused called 'fire' in a theatre, causing the victims to be crushed against an iron bar into which they dashed. There are problems with this case discussed later, but it is thought, though some commentators disagree, that the accused would still be guilty nowadays. The Court of Appeal in *Spratt* did not hold *DPP v K* [1990] 1 WLR 1067 to be incorrect on the point that the injury was indirectly caused (for the facts see later). The injury, actual bodily harm occasioned by a battery, in *DPP v K* was indirectly caused, but the accused was guilty. The contrary view, that a battery must be directly inflicted, has the support of some commentators. They point out that while injury may be directly or indirectly caused or inflicted within ss 20 and 18 of the OAPA, there is little support in the cases for indirect causing being a battery. It would, however, be strange that a less serious offence could not be committed indirectly when more serious ones could be. If the accused tied a rope between two trees intending to decapitate the next cyclist who rode along a path, it would be absurd if he was guilty of an offence if the victim was killed or injured but not if she merely ran into the rope. The latest authority, *Haystead v Chief Constable of Derbyshire* [2000] 3 All ER 890, does not resolve the issue. The accused punched the complainant who dropped the child she was holding. It was held that he was guilty of battery on the child. The Divisional Court said that, even if a battery could be committed only by the direct application of force, the accused had had direct physical contact with the complainant which caused her to drop the child, which was the direct and immediate result of his punching her. *Obiter* it was suggested that force could be indirectly inflicted. The Divisional Court said: 'there is no difference in logic or good sense between the facts of this case and one where the defendant might have used a weapon to fell the child to the floor.' The force need not be applied on the victim's body: it can be on the clothes he is wearing: *Day* (1845) 173 ER 1042 and *Thomas* (1985) 81 Cr App R 331 (CA) *obiter*. It was suggested in *Thomas* that cutting the victim's clothes would be a battery even though he did not feel the snip. In *Fagan v MPC* (see above and Chapter 2), it was held to be a battery when the accused inadvertently applied force and wrongfully decided not to stop using it. If there is no violence, there is no battery. In *Walkden* (1845) 1 Cox CC 282, the accused put 'Spanish fly', an aphrodisiac, into the beer at a wedding reception. Since no force was applied, there was no battery. (The offence would be one of administering a noxious thing with intent to injure or annoy contrary to s 24 of the OAPA.) Similarly, putting out poison for a person to take is not a battery, again because no force is applied.

There was doubt whether an omission sufficed, even when there was a duty to act. In *Fagan v MPC*, above, the court said that a defendant was guilty when the whole conduct was considered, but he would not have been guilty if he had merely omitted to act. For example, if I fail to remove my body from the path of a blind person, I do not occasion a battery when she bumps into me. The facts of *DPP v K*, however, show that a battery can be committed by an omission, a failure to remove sulphuric acid from a hand dryer. The situation constituted a knowing failure to correct a dangerous situation which the accused has created, the area of law governed by *Miller* [1983] 2 AC 161 (HL). The Court of Appeal in *Spratt* did not criticise this part of *DPP v K* and both *Miller* and *DPP v K* were applied in *DPP v Santana-Bermudez* [2004] Crim LR 471 (see Chapter 2). The law now is that a battery can, subject to the ordinary rules stated in Chapter 2, be

See p 78 in Chapter 2 for a discussion of the *Miller* principle as applied in *DPP v Santana-Bermudez*.

committed by omission but it still remains the law that a 'mere' omission does not suffice. It would certainly be strange that an accused could be convicted of murder if the victim died but not of battery if she lived.

Consent is a defence to battery. It may be implied from the circumstances. For example, in a crowd one impliedly consents to some jostling. Whether the touching went beyond what is acceptable is a question of fact. One can tap a person to gain attention without being charged with battery: **Rawlings v Till** (1837) 150 ER 1042. A police officer who taps a suspect on the shoulder does not commit battery: **Donnelly v Jackman** [1970] 1 WLR 562. However, it was said in **Rawlings v Till** that physical restraint was a battery. Accordingly, if the accused takes hold of the victim's arm to restrain him there is a battery: **Collins v Wilcock**, above. It is not entirely clear whether touching is a battery, where the victim has indicated that he does not wish to be touched. There are other exceptions besides consent: lawful chastisement of a child, force used to effect an arrest, reasonable force in self-defence or to prevent crime.

The *mens rea* is intention to apply unlawful force or recklessness as to unlawful force: **Venna** [1976] QB 421. The House of Lords in **Savage** adopted the **Cunningham** approach to the definition of recklessness.

One question involving *mens rea* is this. The accused intends to commit a battery on the victim but does not get as far as touching her; instead she is made afraid and the accused commits the *actus reus* of assault. Can the *mens rea* of battery be added to create an offence? It is thought not because assault and battery are two separate crimes (**DPP v Little**, above) and one cannot aggregate one crime's *actus reus* with another's *mens rea* to create one offence.

Reform of assault and battery

By cl 75 of the draft Criminal Code, *A Criminal Code for England and Wales*, Law Com. No. 177, 1989,

> A person is guilty of assault if he intentionally or recklessly –
> (a) applies force to or causes an impact on the body of another; or
> (b) causes another to believe that any such force or impact is imminent,
> without the consent of the other or, where the act is likely or intended to cause personal harm, with or without consent.

The Criminal Law Revision Committee had recommended in its Fourteenth Report, *Offences Against the Person*, Cmnd 7844, 1980, that (psychic) assault should not be statutorily defined. The substance of a crime should be defined by Parliament as a point of principle. The width of 'applies force' is not clear. Does it cover stroking gently? If it does not, why should a victim be subjected to such behaviour if he does not consent? For the latest recommendations see the last section of this chapter.

Consent

The law does not prohibit all force on the person, but only the unlawful use of force. For example, parents may punish their children moderately. Surgeons may perform operations on their patients. The law is based on reasonableness, yet it may well not reflect public opinion. Swift J in **Donovan** [1934] 2 KB 498 (CCA) said that with some exceptions: 'It is an unlawful act to beat another person with such a degree of force that the infliction of bodily harm is a probable consequence and when such an act is proved, consent is immaterial.' The victim suffered bruising, which constitutes actual bodily harm. The basic rule was stated by Lord Lane CJ in *Attorney-General's Reference (No. 6 of 1980)* [1981] QB 715 (CA), where the victim suffered actual bodily harm in the form of a bloody nose: the accused is guilty of a crime even though the victim has consented 'if actual bodily harm is intended and/or caused'. This principle was approved by the House of Lords in the landmark case of *Brown* [1994] AC 212. It should be noted that Lord Lane CJ's proposition covered a situation where the accused does *not* intend and is *not* reckless as to occasioning actual bodily harm. It is sufficient that such harm occurs. The use of 'and/or' is a strange one. If correct, it means that an accused will not be able to rely on the victim's consent if he intends actual bodily harm but such injury does not occur. In principle, consent is a defence to assault and battery, as indeed the House of Lords held in *Brown* and, therefore, if no actual bodily harm is occasioned, the accused should not be guilty of assault occasioning actual bodily harm. Intending an offence is not committing an offence. A second criticism of 'and/or' looks at the words from the accused's *mens rea*. If actual bodily harm is occasioned, the phrase means that he is guilty even though he does not foresee an assault or a battery; in other words, he does not have the *mens rea* of the crime. This cannot be right!

To this rule there are exceptions. Those exceptions are difficult to state. Boxing is permissible, even though the aim is to knock someone out, while spanking, at issue in *Donovan*, is unlawful. Contrary to what has been suggested, the presence of a referee hardly explains the distinction. The result in *Donovan* will be preserved by cl 75 of the draft Criminal Code, quoted above. The relevance of consent is best dealt with by answering three questions: (a) What is the meaning of full or true consent? (b) Are there limitations on the classes of person who may give consent? (c) Are there any forms of behaviour to which the law provides that consent cannot be given? If the alleged consent falls foul of any of these principles, a crime is committed. Therefore, e.g., medical treatment is illegal if a mentally capable adult refuses it.

What is the meaning of true or full consent?

Consent may be express, but is usually implied. As we have seen in battery, consent may arise through custom. Consent to being tapped on the shoulder in the street, consent to jostling in a rugby match (rugby is the most dangerous sport played in the UK: a participant is four times more likely to be injured in rugby than in Association football) or on the football terraces, are implied. William Hardy was tried at the Old Bailey in 1994 for the manslaughter of an opponent in a rugby union match. The victim did not consent to the accused's alleged punching him in an off-the-ball incident. Canadian courts have been building up a jurisprudence based on a division between unintentional, instinctive or incidental to the game and other assaults. The former are permitted. There is also something of a line between professionals and amateurs. The former are taken to consent to more than the latter. In *Collins v Wilcock*, above, the court preferred to base such instances, as those occurring in sport, on 'a general exception embracing all physical contact which is generally acceptable in the ordinary conduct of daily life', not on implied consent. The same judge when he became Lord Goff said in *Re F*, above, that the implied consent approach led to difficulties when the 'victim' was young or mentally disordered. In all cases consent goes up to a certain point only. For example, if one consents to sexual intercourse, one does not consent to being strangled: *Sharmpal Singh* [1962]

AC 188 (PC). Submission is not consent, nor is consent obtained when the victim is drugged or drunk.

The old law was that only where there was deception as to the nature of the act or as to the identity of the accused was there consent. Accordingly, in **Clarence** (1888) 22 QBD 23, a woman's agreement to sexual intercourse with her husband meant that, surprising as it is to modern ears, he was not guilty of inflicting grievous bodily harm when he infected her with VD. She had consented to intercourse with him and would not have done so had she known of the disease, yet her consent was not vitiated by his omission to tell her of his bodily condition. (It may be inquired whether, if the wife knew of the VD, the law permitted the husband to infect her with it on the ground that she consented to his occasioning actual bodily harm to her. It is thought that the husband would be guilty under s 47 and consent would not be a defence, the argument being that there is no social benefit in the spread of VD.) The House of Lords discussed **Clarence** in **Ireland; Burstow**, above. Lord Steyn said that since that case was not about psychiatric injury, it was not useful in respect of s 20 of the OAPA. Since the facts the House of Lords was dealing with concerned psychiatric harm, anything said about inflicting physical harm was *obiter*. However, the House of Lords did hold that s 20 can be committed when no physical violence is applied directly or indirectly to the body of the victim. That is what occurred in **Clarence**. Accordingly, the Law Lords should not just have distinguished **Clarence**, but overruled it. Neither a wife nor anyone else can consent to the reckless infliction of serious harm. This was the strong view of the Court of Appeal in **Dica** [2004] QB 1257. The court held that where the victim is unaware of the fact that the accused is infected with a disease, here HIV/AIDS, and the latter had unprotected sexual intercourse with the former, the victim did not impliedly consent to the risk of being infected. If the victim was aware of the accused's condition, then the consent to sexual intercourse would be consent to the risk of infection and therefore a defence to s 20. **Dica** was explained in **Konzani** [2005] 2 Cr App R 198 (CA). Consent will only be effective if the victim gives informed consent. It is not informed consent if the victim does not know that the accused has the disease. Even where the victim knows that the accused is HIV positive, and thereby consents to the risk of being infected, the latter is guilty of GBH with intent to commit GBH contrary to s 18 of the OAPA. There was a second appeal in **Dica** [2005] All ER (D) 405 (July) after a retrial. The Court of Appeal dismissed the appeal and refused leave to appeal but did certify a point of law of general public importance: 'in what circumstances, if any, might a defendant who knows or believes that he is infected with a serious sexually transmitted infection and recklessly transmits it to another through consensual sexual activity be convicted of inflicting grievous bodily harm, contrary to s 20 of the Offences against the Person Act 1861?'

Another authority is **Richardson** [1998] 2 Cr App R 200 (CA). Patients did not know that the accused, a dentist, had been suspended from her duties. The patients knew her identity and were mistaken only as to her attributes, whether she was disqualified or not. Accordingly, their consent to dental treatment was valid. Fraud as to identity did not include a mistake as to attributes or qualifications. If the accused was not afforded the defence, she would have been guilty of assault occasioning actual bodily harm. The court, however, said that the dental treatment was reasonable. If so, where was the harm? Reasonable treatment, medical or dental, is not harm. **Richardson** is a doubtful decision. Surely, however, consent to treatment by a dentist does not cover consent to treatment by a disqualified dentist. Similar to **Richardson** is **Bolduc and Bird** (1967) 63 DLR (2nd) 82, a decision of the Supreme Court of Canada. A doctor brought a friend to a vaginal examination. It was held that there was no indecent assault. The patient was mistaken as to the identity of the friend, who was introduced as a trainee doctor, but not as to the nature of the examination. The accused was not guilty. The case of **Harms** [1944] 2 DLR 61 was distinguished. In that case the accused falsely represented sexual intercourse as a medical examination. He was guilty. There are English authorities similar to **Harms**. The dissent in **Bolduc and Bird** repays study: if consent is to a doctor and student, it is not to a doctor and friend. The case was distinguished by the majority of the Court of Appeal in **Maurantonio** (1968) 65 DLR (2nd) 674 on the grounds that one must take into account the circumstances which give meaning to the physical acts (such as the fact that the accused was not a doctor when he examined the victim). For more on consent in the context of rape, see Chapter 14.

Are there limitations on the classes of persons who can give consent?

Persons who do not understand the nature of the act cannot give consent. An example is the case of **Burrell v Harmer** [1967] Crim LR 169: boys of 12 and 13 could not consent to being tattooed. The Tattooing of Minors Act 1969 prohibits the tattooing of persons under 18. Mentally abnormal people cannot consent. Boys and girls cannot consent to indecent assault, no matter how willing they are: **McCormack** [1969] 2 QB 442. One effect of this area of law is that an accused is guilty even though he believed that the victim had consented to the activity. Another is that, although a boy cannot consent to his genitals being touched, he can consent to being touched on the arms and legs in order to pose for pornographic photographs. A person under 16 cannot consent to surgery, but the parent can on his behalf.

Are there any forms of behaviour to which the law provides that consent is no defence?

The law does not allow even an adult to do with his body as he wishes. It was said in **McShane** (1977) 66 Cr App R 97 (CA) that no consent can render a dangerous act innocent, but that statement is too broad. A person can consent to dangerous activities such as sport and surgery. There are some offences to which no matter how full the consent is, there is no defence.

(a) Murder and serious non-fatal offences (except for games, chastisement, etc): a person cannot consent to being killed, nor can one consent to grievous bodily harm, such as when one person was crucified – though not unto death – by the defendants driving six-inch nails through his palms. The House of Lords in **Brown** [1994] AC 212 held that consent was no defence to sado-masochists charged under ss 20 and 47 of the OAPA. The activities of the defendants, who were male homosexuals, included nailing a penis to a board and taping lighted matches to nipples. Any instruments were sterilised and wounds were dressed. The acts were videotaped and the videos were circulated. There were no permanent injuries, medical treatment was not needed, no one had complained of harm and the acts had been committed in private. There is some dispute as to whether the participants were truly consenting. The 'victims' were at times drugged, and the voyeurs watching the performances egged on the parties. It is not clear whether the 'victims' could freely refuse to engage in the activities. Their Lordships relied both on precedent and policy. The majority held that consent was not a defence to deeds which caused harm except in recognised circumstances such as boxing. Public health was at stake. Lord Jauncey thought that it was not in the public interest that a defence should be allowed to ss 20 and 47. Young men were likely to be corrupted. He said: 'It would appear to be good luck rather than good judgment which has prevented serious injury from occurring. Wounds can easily become septic if not properly treated, the free flow of blood from a person who is HIV positive or who has AIDS can infect another and an inflicter who is carried away by sexual excitement or by drink and drugs could very easily inflict pain and injury beyond the level to which the receiver had consented . . . when considering the public interest potential for harm is just as relevant as actual harm.' Lord Lowry refused to permit sado-masochism as a defence. Violence could get out of hand. Lord Templeman said that no defence should be afforded to persons who indulged in sado-masochism, which bred and glorified cruelty. Degradation was not a good reason to excuse such behaviour. Society (which partly comprises male homosexuals) was entitled to protection against such conduct. Violence in sex was violence. The sexual preferences of the participants did not affect that equation. The minority stressed that sexual behaviour was a sphere of private life in which the state should not intervene without good cause. Consent was presumed to be valid unless there was a good reason to the contrary. Paternalism was to be rejected in favour of liberty. People should be able to determine the satisfaction of their sexual needs. Before the criminal law intervened harm had to exist. There was no danger to life or limb. Public health was not affected. Young men were not corrupted. Any reform was for Parliament.

The starting-points of the majority and minority are so different that compromise is impossible. The men do not seem to have tried to recruit outsiders, but what they did was violent and it is possible that not all masochists consented with full knowledge of everything which was done to them. Vulnerable persons require protection whether or not they think they do. The alternative view is to say that private sexual behaviour among consenting adults is lawful, provided that it does not cause serious injury. *Brown* penalises people for expressing their sexuality in a certain way, sado-masochism, and unless the injuries are trifling, all such conduct is illegal. The outcome of *Brown* is that sado-masochists who intend to cause more than actual bodily harm must not give way to their urges; differently put, they must be celibate. Boxing can likewise be seen as a game of skill or as conduct, the aim of which is to cause serious harm. Yet boxing, a 'manly diversion', is lawful. The European Court of Human Rights ruled that on the facts of *Brown* the state was pursuing a lawful aim, the protection of health and morals, and that the law was necessary in a democratic society within Article 8 of the European Convention on Human Rights: *Laskey* (1997) 24 EHRR 39 (the name is that of one of the accused in *Brown*). The Court stated that 'The State is unquestionably entitled to . . . seek to regulate, through the operation of the criminal law, activities which involve the infliction of physical harm. This is so whether the activities in question occur in the course of sexual conduct or otherwise.'

A final comment on *Brown* is this. Under present law if the House of Lords had accepted that consent was a defence to non-serious injury, there is a problem with s 20. That section covers both grievous bodily harm and wounding. Wounding may or may not be serious injury, depending on the facts. If a person could consent to woundings which were not serious, then the line between offences to which consent is a defence and the others would be drawn in the middle of s 20! This result demonstrates the need for revision of s 20 to take out non-serious woundings, for as it stands it covers both serious and non-serious injuries.

In *Wilson* [1997] QB 47, which was approved in *Dica*, above, the Court of Appeal held that a person could consent to the burning of her husband's initials onto her buttocks. The reasoning was that the rule that there could be no consent to serious offences was subject to exceptions; one of those exceptions and one which had been recognised in *Brown* was tattooing; what the accused had done was no more dangerous than tattooing, therefore he was not guilty. The court considered what he had done equivalent to nose and tongue piercing, and was totally dissimilar to the activities in *Brown*. There was no reason of public policy to forbid this type of behaviour. The court considered that public policy did not demand that the accused's conduct should be criminalised. *Donovan*, above, was also distinguished. It is hard to distinguish the two cases; indeed, branding would appear to be worse than caning, yet the branding was lawful, the caning unlawful. If the distinction resides in the purpose of the activity, adornment of the body and sexual gratification, then contrary to the normal pronouncement of the courts, motive is an element in criminal law in this respect. The accused did not have an aggressive intent – but neither did the defendants in *Brown* – and it was his wife who instigated the branding. The court could just as easily have held that the consent was invalid because there was no good reason for what the husband did. Instead it seems that the court preferred to adopt what the minority had said in *Brown*. The court also based its decision on the privacy between married partners ('[c]onsensual activity between husband and wife, in the privacy of the matrimonial home, is not . . . normally a proper matter for criminal investigation, let alone criminal prosecution' (*per* Russell LJ)), but it is strange in modern times that the law is limited to such relationships. In the case next discussed, *Emmett*, the court rejected this analysis. Moreover, it is strange too that the victim required medical treatment in *Wilson* but the accused was acquitted, whereas the victims in *Brown* did not require treatment but the defendants were convicted. The defendants in *Brown* intended to inflict pain, whereas the accused in *Wilson* did not but the court did not use this reason to distinguish the cases.

The latest case on consent to sexual practices is *Emmett*, unreported, 18 June 1999, which was approved in *Dica* on the basis that what happened transgressed the boundary laid down in *Wilson*. The male accused semi-asphyxiated and poured lighter fuel onto the breast of his female partner, whom he later married. The Court of Appeal held that the accused did not have the defence of consent to a charge of assault occasioning actual bodily harm. *Brown* was applied, although it should be added that in *Brown* the violence was intended whereas it was not in *Emmett*. There was no difference between homosexual and heterosexual sado-masochism. *Wilson* was distinguished on the grounds that the injury, actual or potential, was less serious in that case. Where the line was to be drawn was not always easy to see but there was no doubt in *Emmett* that what the accused did went beyond the boundary of reasonable behaviour. Partial asphyxiation can lead to brain damage and even death; the burn was serious and painful and it became infected. *Brown* was applied as to the effect of the European Convention on Human Rights. Article 8 does not apply where the accused has gone beyond the permitted limit of consent. The court in *Emmett* said that *Wilson* and *Brown* were to be distinguished on the ground that in *Wilson* the facts were analogous to the recognised exception of tattooing whereas *Brown* did not fall within any exception and neither did *Emmett* itself.

The latest case on consent in sport is *Barnes* [2005] 1 WLR 910. Lord Woolf CJ said that a prosecution should be brought only when the accused's conduct was intentional or was so reckless that it went beyond what the victim could reasonably have consented to. Only in those circumstances could injuries be accounted as so grave as to constitute crimes. If the accused's behaviour was within the explicit or implicit rules of the game being played, that was a strong indication that the injury was not to be characterised as criminal. Whether the injury exceeded the threshold for being a crime depended on all the factors including whether the injury occurred during play or 'off the ball', the extent of the risk of injury, the type of sport, the level at which it was being played and (perhaps surprisingly) the accused's state of mind. Therefore, a foul can be consented to because it can be expected to occur in a football match; however, a bad foul may be conduct which one could not reasonably expect to occur on a soccer pitch. The court applied *Brown* when it held that sports were on public policy grounds an exception to the rule that no one could consent to the actual or more serious bodily harm.

A prize-fight is at least a battery: *Coney* (1882) 8 QBD 534. It is not an activity to which one can consent (even though at times more serious injuries are caused by boxing under the Queensberry Rules). One view of *Coney* is that it decided that prize-fighting was illegal and no one can consent to illegal acts. An alternative view is that *Coney* held that consent is no defence to acts which are intended or likely to cause injury, unless there was a good reason for them. The latter approach has been adopted in recent cases including *Brown*. In *Leach* (1969) *The Times*, 13 January, a man had himself crucified (though not to death). He could not consent to the wounds. In *Donovan* a girl could not consent to the infliction of six or seven weals on her bottom. It may be that the case is out of line with modern mores. Certainly the judges adopted a paternalistic attitude towards the victim, a 17-year-old girl. It might be thought that she understood what she was doing, and there was no permanent harm (cf. boxing where there may be). If *Donovan* is correct a bite during love-making would appear to be actual bodily harm. In *Boyea* [1992] Crim LR 574 the Court of Appeal stated, however, that the change in social attitudes since *Donovan* should be taken into account in determining whether or not injury during sexual activity was so trifling or transient that the victim could consent to it. The accused's twisting his hand in his victim's vagina went beyond behaviour to which she could consent. One modern view of *Donovan* is that the law was correctly stated but wrongly applied. Consent is a defence to battery, but not to assault occasioning actual bodily harm, yet the accused was convicted of common assault as well as indecent assault. In *Jones* (1986) 83 Cr App R 375, the Court of Appeal held that victims, even ones trying to run away, could consent to horseplay including throwing them nine or ten feet into the air, which resulted in a ruptured spleen and a broken arm, though the position would be different if the accused intended to cause harm. It may be wondered whether the risk of harm outweighed the public policy behind horseplay – boys will be boys. The harm was more serious than in *Donovan*, yet the accused was not guilty. Moreover, did the boys in *Jones* truly consent to such rough play? *Jones* looks like a case on bullying. Whether *Jones* is correct on its facts or not, this exception is well established and would cover, e.g., paintballing.

A summary of the law on consent to sexual practices can be stated thus:

(i)   one cannot consent to the intentional infliction of serious harm: *Brown*;

(ii) one can consent to being branded on the buttocks: *Wilson*;

(iii) however, *Emmett* shows that *Wilson* is restricted to activities in the nature of tattooing;

(iv) **Dica** holds that one can consent to the reckless infecting of oneself provided one knows of the risk but one cannot consent if one does not know the nature of the risk.

These propositions are subject to caveats.

(b) It used to be thought that sterilisation (perhaps only of a man) without just cause was unlawful as being contrary to the public interest. Denning LJ said so in the civil case of **Bravery v Bravery** [1954] 3 All ER 59. This possible restraint seems to have disappeared. Certainly one can consent to wounds in the course of surgery, at least it is thought to be so if there is a sound benefit, e.g. sex change. It is thought that both non-therapeutic (such as cosmetic surgery and sex changes) and therapeutic operations provide such a social benefit because of the psychological benefit. In this sense there is, it might be said, no harm and therefore no grievous or actual bodily harm. Presumably maiming oneself to avoid conscription in wartime remains a crime, as does an operation to change facial features to evade arrest. Ritual mutilation is a difficult issue. It is suggested that it is unlawful in England despite its legality in the 'victim's' country of origin: cf. the Prohibition of Female Circumcision Act 1985 and the Female Genital Mutilation Act 2003. Section 1(5) of the latter statute provides that custom or ritual does not give rise to a defence. It is suggested that flagellation for religious purposes may be consented to, whereas flagellation for sexual purposes may not. It is strange that the law may depend on the nature of the defendant's motive.

(c) Incest.

(d) Administration of drugs except for medical purposes: **Cato** [1976] 1 WLR 110.

The law on the issue of consent continues to change because it is based on public policy. In **Boyea**, above, the Court of Appeal said that more vigour was permissible nowadays than in the time of **Donovan** and in **Wilson** it was stated that: 'the law should develop upon a case by case basis rather than upon general propositions to which, in the changing times in which we live, exceptions may arise from time to time not expressly covered by authority'. If so, it is difficult to predict outcomes and uncertainty in law is not conducive to people knowing in advance whether what they are doing is illegal or not. For example, is **Wilson** itself a decision on body adornment (like tattooing) or is it an exception to **Brown** in the area of consensual sex? Is branding an exception like boxing or is **Wilson** part of a movement outflanking **Brown** by restricting it to its own facts? Would the law be different if the 'victim' was a homosexual? The court stated that public interest did not require what the husband did to be criminalised.

The Court of Appeal in **Attorney-General's Reference (No. 6 of 1980)**, above, said: 'It is not in the public interest that people should try to cause or should cause each other actual bodily harm for no good reason. Minor struggles are another matter. So . . . it is immaterial whether the act occurs in private or in public.' The question is not just whether the victim consented but also whether there was nothing contrary to the public interest in what the accused did. The phrase 'no good reason' is vague and unhelpful to citizens and advisers. Reasonable people may differ as to whether one type of behaviour, such as smacking a child or tattooing, is good or not. In **Brown** the majority apparently started from the proposition that all harm was criminal unless there was a good reason, whereas the minority proceeded from the basis that harm to which the victim consented was lawful unless there was a good reason for punishing the accused. It would be interesting to see how the same Lords of Appeal would approach boxing. If rough horseplay is permitted where true consent does not exist, why is not wounding where there is true consent? The court listed activities where consent was a defence, especially properly conducted sports, lawful chastisement (though how punishment can truly be said to be consented to is not explained), dangerous exhibitions (though why does public policy allow them? Is titillation a good reason?) and surgery. The court in *Jones* added horseplay. After *DPP v Smith* [2006] 1 WLR 1571 (Administrative Court), hairdressing must be added to the list. In *Aitken* [1992] 1 WLR 1006 the Court of Appeal extended horseplay between boys to setting light to white spirit poured over a colleague by RAF officers, causing severe burns – what a jolly jape! The acts were dangerous and the victim did not consent to the burns. Nevertheless, the court held that the victim did consent to this very rough horseplay. If such horseplay is acceptable, why is not sadomasochism? Moreover, these horseplay cases look like ones on bullying. *Aitken* was followed by the Court of Appeal in *Richardson* [1999] 1 Cr App R 392. The defendants and their victim were students who had been drinking. The former dropped the latter over a balcony. He suffered serious injuries. The court held that the defendants' drunken belief that the victim was consenting to the risk of harm provided them with a defence, a decision at odds with the usual rules on drunken mistakes.

A recent major authority is *Dica* [2004] QB 1257 (CA). It was held that women who knew that the accused was suffering from HIV/AIDS could validly consent to the risk of infection and therefore to the risk of GBH or death. (Similarly, they could consent to the risk of getting pregnant.) However, if the accused had concealed his infectious condition, the women had not consented. It would have been different if the accused had deliberately spread infection: he would have been guilty under s 18 of the Offences Against the Person Act 1861. The same applies to violence above actual bodily harm. The court in *Attorney-General's Reference (No. 6 of 1980)*, above, did not lay down a closed list: the public interest was the governing consideration. The House of Lords in *Brown* also thought that these exceptions depended on public policy and policy was a matter for Parliament, not for the courts. The open nature of the lists permits judges to control the infliction of harm for what they see as improper purposes. Yet the victims in *Jones* did not consent to their injuries and it is hard to believe that bullying serves a socially useful function, whereas the men in *Brown* allegedly did consent fully to the injuries, and the boys in *Jones* were taken to have consented to grievous bodily harm, whereas the men had no defence to the legal charge of actual bodily harm. It may be added that the victim in *Aitken* would not have been permitted by the law to consent to having others pour white spirit over his body and set it alight. Moreover, dangerous exhibitions such as bungee-jumping are permitted but not dangerous sexual practices: boxing is permitted, but not fights with fists. The law is in a mess. Why can one consent to rough horseplay but not masochism?

The position where the accused thinks the victim is consenting but in fact there is no consent was discussed in *Jones*, above, and the Court of Appeal held that the accused had a defence. It did not matter whether the accused's belief was formed unreasonably. As we have seen, the same surprisingly applies even though the accused was drunk: *Richardson*, above, an authority which, it is suggested, is wrong.

It is uncertain whether consent is no defence when the injury is *intentionally* caused or whether it is not also a defence when the harm is caused, but not intentionally. *Dicta* in *Brown* and *Attorney-General's Reference (No. 6 of 1980)* suggest the latter. *Dica* supports the former interpretation: consent is irrelevant where the actual bodily harm was both intended *and* caused.

The burden of proof of lack of consent lies on the prosecution: *Donovan, Attorney-General's Reference (No. 6 of 1980)*. A mistaken belief in consent is a defence, whether or not the belief was reasonably held: *Jones*, applying *Kimber* (on the then existing crime of indecent assault) and *Williams*, both above. See also under mistake.

If the accused lacked the *mens rea* for the offence, he is not guilty even though the victim has consented in fact to behaviour she could not in law consent to. In *Slingsby* [1995] Crim LR 570 (Crown Court) the accused was not guilty of constructive manslaughter because he gave no thought to any risk of injury when he penetrated the victim's anus and vagina with his hand and his ring cut her. He had no *mens rea* for the offence of wounding on which the charge was based. Therefore, he was not guilty of manslaughter. The issue of consent was irrelevant. This decision seems irreconcilable with the *dicta* noted two paragraphs above about harm caused unintentionally.

Reform of consent and other defences to assault and battery

In *Richardson* [1998] 2 Cr App R 200, referred to above, the Court of Appeal said: 'For the best part of a century the common law concept of consent in criminal law has been certain and clearly delineated. It is not for this Court to unwrite the law which has been settled for so long. This is an area in which it is to be hoped that the proposals of the Law Commission will be given an early opportunity for implementation.' Reform proposals from the Law Commission are contained in its Consultation Papers No. 134, *Consent and Offences Against the Person*, 1994 and No. 139, *Consent in the Criminal Law*, 1995. These Papers are the outcome of comments on the Consultation Paper which led to *Legislating the Criminal Code: Offences Against the Person and General Principles*, Law Com. No. 218, 1993 and of the House of Lords decision in *Brown*. The Law Commission had previously thought that defences to non-fatal offences could be left to common law development. These defences include surgery, dangerous exhibitions, properly conducted games and so on.

In Law Com. No. 218 the Law Commission put into cl 6(1) of the Criminal Law Bill its thinking that consent should be a defence to assault, when it consists of intentionally or recklessly applying force to or causing an impact on the body of another, but not to assault where the act is intended or likely to cause injury. This distinction encapsulates *Brown*. In the first of the Papers the Law Commission also considered that a line should be drawn between offences to which the 'victim', whether a willing participant or not, may consent and those to which he may not and that the line should be drawn between acts which are not intended or likely to cause injury ('actual bodily harm' in current terminology) and those which are. If the drawing of the line at this place is not supported, the Law Commission recommended drawing it between injury and serious injury, with the provisos: (a) the defence would not be available when the accused intended to cause serious injury; (b) it would be available if the victim had consented to serious injury but the accused had inflicted only non-serious harm; but (c) it would not be available if the accused knows that the victim is consenting to serious injury.

In the 1994 Paper, the Law Commission proposed that as at present 'consent' should be given its ordinary-language meaning but that, unlike current law, fraud as to any part of the deed (cf. the current law of rape) should be ineffective (with the effect that *Bolduc and Bird*, above, would be decided differently), as should consent obtained by force, threat of force, other threats (e.g. to demote the victim) and the exercise of authority (perhaps where a police constable tells his victim that he is entitled by reason of his office to punch the victim's face). Consent would not be available where the victim made a mistake and the accused knew of the error. The Law Commission suggested that young persons should be able to consent provided both that they did consent and they had 'sufficient understanding and intelligence to be capable of giving consent': for example, a child might be able to decide to have her ears pierced but not to be tattooed because she may understand the significance of the former but not of the latter. The different attitude of the Law Commission to some of these recommendations is noted below in the discussion of the 1995 Paper.

Besides consent the Law Commission looked also at matters which are often dealt with alongside consent. It proposed that if the rule is retained that consent is not a defence to acts intended or likely to cause injury, there should be exceptions only for ritual (male) circumcision, ear piercing (perhaps body piercing is meant, though there is no discussion of, e.g., nose and nipple piercing) and tattooing. Tribal scarring is not mentioned. Comment was invited about religious flagellation (though only the accused's motive in *Donovan* distinguishes his guilt from non-liability for religiously motivated beatings) and dangerous exhibitions, such as shooting a cigarette out of a victim's mouth and throwing knives around her body. After all, there is a risk of death in the William Tell scenario. The Law Commission noted that the current law on sport was unclear. With regard to properly organised sports and games except boxing and martial arts, the Law Commission considered that the intentional or reckless infliction of injury should be criminal. In cricket, bowling bouncers may therefore become illegal in circumstances where the batsman is ill-equipped to deal with them. The present law which permits rough horseplay should be abolished because it is not distinguishable from fighting. See *Aitken*, above. If, however, the law were amended to permit consent to injury, the sole exceptions should be sports and games.

The recommendations can be criticised from perspectives both of paternalism and personal autonomy, and there are instances where argument is conspicuously lacking: why is it obvious that ear piercing and tattooing are lawful? Both may lead to infection. The Law Commission left boxing to a special category. The purpose of boxing is to cause grievous bodily harm, and if the victim dies, the assailant would be guilty of murder. The Law Commission thought that boxing (and presumably kick-boxing, full-contact karate and the like), if it is to be non-criminal, should be placed in a special category based on public policy, but it did note that between 1945 and 1992 361 deaths had been caused worldwide by legal boxing. (The World Medical Association has called for a ban on boxing.) In the 1994 Paper there was no investigation into chastisement and medical treatment, both of which were said to 'raise complex issues of policy that go very far beyond the issues that we address. . . .' These omissions detracted from the force of the Paper. Perhaps the Law Commission shied away from these areas in order to have its proposals on the other matters accepted.

The 1995 Paper, unlike the 1994 one, included sections on lawful correction (though the Law Commission recognised that consent has very little to do with this issue and it made no recommendations), surgery, whether therapeutic or cosmetic (on the ground that it looks odd to omit this topic while including cosmetic body piercing), and boxing (recognising that it would similarly be strange to deal with martial arts while disregarding boxing). It did not consider consent in relation to other offences, such as theft and burglary, but the Law Commission proposed that the revisions should apply throughout criminal law. One theme of the 1995 Paper is that the Law Commission did not wish to be out of line with the wishes of Parliament whether expressed in statutes, in debates or in committee reports. For example, there should be no relaxation of the prohibition of euthanasia or female circumcision (on which now see the Female Genital Mutilation Act

2003), and boxing should not be outlawed. The Law Commission realised that this approach may result in 'what our critics may believe to be attitudes on related issues that are mutually inconsistent'. It sought ways of remedying these inconsistencies provided that they 'do not cut across prevailing Parliamentary culture, although we recognise that in the last resort we may simply have to live with them' (para 2.17). Boxing in particular could have been banned on several occasions but Parliament has chosen not to.

In brief, consent is to be lawful to any harm short of a seriously disabling injury. **Brown** would prospectively be overruled because the injuries were not seriously disabling. The purpose of the injury would be irrelevant. The 1994 Paper proposed to raise the level of the harm to which consent would provide a defence but did not clearly define that level. The 1995 Paper adopted the definition of Glanville Williams in 'Force, injury and serious injury' [1990] NLJ 1227, though his was a definition of 'serious injury' made in response to the failure of the draft Criminal Code to define that concept: a seriously disabling injury is one which:

(a) causes serious distress, and
(b) involves loss of a bodily member or organ, or permanent bodily injury or permanent functional impairment, or serious or permanent disfigurement, or severe or prolonged pain, or serious impairment of mental health, or prolonged unconsciousness. . . .

The Law Commission proposed that if a seriously disabling injury resulted, consent should be invalid on the ground that the victim had not truly consented to it because such harm is contrary to his interests. A major criticism of this proposal is that the level of harm to which the 'victim' can consent is high. A seriously disabling injury is not minor harm. No account is to be taken of whether the injury was remediable by surgery or not. Consent to lesser injuries would be allowed provided that it was valid and was consent to the type of injury caused. The Law Commission invited views on where the burden of proof should lie in relation to this defence.

The Law Commission sought to render ineffective any consent which was not given voluntarily. In respect of children, minors (i.e. persons who are under 18) must be able to understand what consent means. They should not be permitted to give consent if they were unable because of age or immaturity to make a decision on consent. The finder of fact would take into account the implications of the decision and the seriousness of the matter to which the minor allegedly gave consent. Children under 18 would not be allowed to consent to the infliction of pain on them for sexual or spiritual purposes. This would be in line with the law on anal intercourse. In respect of the mentally disabled, they would not be able to give consent if their disability rendered it impossible for them to make a decision on consent. Those who could not communicate consent, e.g. because they were unconscious or asleep, would also be incapable of consent. In criticism it may be said that consent even in other instances is not an unproblematic concept. In a relationship of power, such as a lecturer/student one, true consent may be lacking.

The Law Commission proposed to extend the law to cover a person who did not realise that the victim was not consenting when the lack of consent would have been obvious to a reasonable person and the accused was capable of appreciating that fact: 'it does not seem unreasonable to expect a person, before subjecting another to what will be a serious invasion of his or her bodily integrity if he or she does not consent to it, to make sure that he or she *does* consent to it' (para 7.25). The same rule would apply to sex crimes but not to property offences, which do not violate the victim's rights as much as non-fatal and sexual offences do. The distinction may be open to dispute, and the extension itself is not justified on a purely subjectivist approach. The proposed rule would also apply when a sexual offence was defined in terms of age. The defendant is to be guilty if it was obvious to a reasonable person that the victim was under the relevant age and the accused was capable of realising that fact if he had given any thought to it.

Consent should not be valid if there is deception as to the nature of the act or the identity of the other person. Possibly fraud should render consent invalid when the deception was as to freedom from sexually transmitted diseases and the Law Commission invited views on whether any other deception should nullify consent. A self-induced mistake as to the nature of the act or the identity (or perhaps freedom from a sexually transmitted disease and so on) would not provide a defence if the accused knew of the error. Non-disclosure of relevant facts would negate consent. Consent would exclude 'consent' given as a result of a threat to use force if the threat was to be carried out immediately or before the victim could free himself of the menace. There should be a crime of procuring consent by deception and the Law Commission invited views on whether there should be a crime of procuring consent by threats. It resiled from its proposition in its 1994 Paper that any fraud should negate consent because that law 'would be disproportionate', a phrase which it does not explain; instead the proposed offences would come into play. The accused would have a defence if he believed the victim to be consenting even though this was not the case, provided that the rule stated above did not apply.

Some issues of consent relate to the intentional causing of harm. Examples are surgery, tattooing, flagellation for religious reasons, male circumcision and ear piercing. Other aspects of the law are concerned with the risk of danger, not with the intentional causing of injury, e.g. dangerous exhibitions and some sports injuries. The risk must be one which is reasonable in the circumstances in which the accused acts.

The Law Commission invited views on whether the present age limit on tattooing, 18, should be retained and whether there should be any age limit for body piercing below the neck, branding and scarification when done for cultural or cosmetic reasons. Certainly hygiene controls should be tightened up. Male circumcision would continue to be lawful, and female circumcision unlawful.

In respect of boxing, the Law Commission was of the opinion that the question whether it should be legal was one for Parliament. It noted that Parliament had recently voted not to criminalise it. Clarkson, Keating and Cunningham, *Criminal Law: Text and Materials*, 6th edn (Thomson, 2007) pointedly comment (at p 17): '. . . by not allowing people to consent to seriously disabling injuries in the course of sadomasochism while not criminalising the same injuries in the course of, say, boxing, it is possible to assert that in reality the Law Commission has adopted a stance of paternalism hardened at the edges by legal moralism.' For other sports the Law Commission thought that 'a person should not be guilty of causing injury in the course of playing or practising a recognised sport *in accordance with the rules*' (emphasis added). This provision would, for example, cover fast bowlers in cricket and the playing of rugby football. Head-butting would obviously fall out with this stipulation. However, care will have to be taken in drafting the law because as stated, the mere fact that the accused was offside in football would make a non-criminal act into a criminal one. Dangerous exhibitions such as knife throwing would remain lawful but possibly there should be a lower age limit for victims.

The risk of harm to others is a factor which may render some activities unlawful even though there is consent. The Law Commission suggested that fighting should remain illegal. Horseplay, however, should not be unlawful unless a seriously disabling injury was caused. Presumably *Aitken*, above, would be overruled.

The Law Commission was of the view that consent to activities such as sport and surgery, which are normally seen as beneficial, should be accepted, provided that the rules are appropriately controlled, even though a seriously disabling injury occurs. Surgery is seen to occupy a special category. The 1994 Paper did not discuss the issue because it thought that surgery was not related to consent, but the 1995 Paper did because 'except in emergencies, the common law has never granted the medical profession the unqualified *legal right* to perform medical or surgical procedures irrespective of the patient's consent, even when the procedures are in the patient's best interests' (para 8.5). The Law Commission proposed to restate the medical exception thus: 'a person should not be guilty of an offence, notwithstanding that he or she causes injury to another, of whatever degree of seriousness, if such injury is caused during the course of proper medical treatment or care administered with the consent of that other person' (para 8.50). Medical treatment would cover *inter alia*: sterilisation, sex reassignment surgery, lawful abortions and cosmetic surgery. Treatment would be improper, e.g., when fingers are amputated to facilitate an insurance claim. Medical treatment would also cover properly approved medical research.

In the Home Office's Consultation Document, *Violence: Reforming the Offences against the Person Act 1861*, 1998, the government left the issue of consent to the common law. Once the Law Commission concluded its work on consent, there would be reform. There has been no government move since 1998.

Assault occasioning actual bodily harm

The OAPA 1861 consolidated several statutes dealing with non-fatal offences. The draftsman did not make the crimes formerly contained in those statutes consistent or create a hierarchy of offences. It is very much of a hotchpotch. Section 47 creates the offence of assault occasioning actual bodily harm (Fig. 13.1).

Actus reus

There is no definition of 'actual bodily harm' – surely all harm is actual! The term 'assault' covers both assault and battery, as was assumed in *DPP v Little*, above. An example from the cases is *Lewis* [1970] Crim LR 647. The accused threatened his wife, who was injured

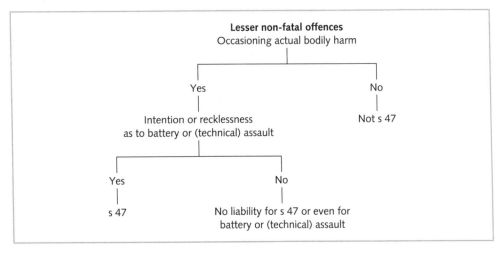

Figure 13.1 Lesser non-fatal offences

while escaping. 'Occasioning' means 'causing', a concept which is discussed in Chapter 2. A somewhat out-of-the-ordinary actual bodily harm was occasioned in *Savage*, above. The accused threw a glass of beer at the victim, the glass slipped from the accused's hand, hit the bar table and broke; a fragment of it flew off and cut the victim on the wrist. Throwing the beer was a battery and that battery had occasioned the actual bodily harm that the victim suffered.

According to *Saunders* [1985] Crim LR 230 (CA) grievous bodily harm means 'serious harm'. Actual bodily harm must mean something less than serious harm. In *Miller* [1954] 2 QB 282, Lynskey J said that the term 'includes any hurt or injury calculated [likely] to interfere with the health or comfort' of the victim. Hysterics fell within this definition. 'Hurt' alone is insufficient. A head-lock is painful but not actual bodily harm. 'Actual' seems to mean 'more than trivial' though *Taylor v Granville* [1978] Crim LR 482 said that it covered any harm, however slight. It covers bruises, grazes, black eyes and burns. In *Chan-Fook* [1994] 2 All ER 552 (CA) the accused suspected the victim of theft of his fiancée's ring. The victim felt humiliated and abused. The accused dragged him upstairs and locked him in a room. The victim, in fear of being assaulted, climbed out of a window and down a rope of knotted sheets. He fell, fracturing his wrist and dislocating his pelvis. Surprisingly the prosecution was based on the victim's fright, humiliation and distress, not on his physical injuries. The trial judge said, applying *Miller*, that a nervous and hysterical condition was actual bodily harm. The Court of Appeal allowed the appeal. 'Actual' meant not so trivial as to be wholly insignificant. 'Harm' was injury which goes beyond interference with the health or comfort of the victim while including injury to health such as infection with a disease. In other words, harm requires injury. 'Bodily' is not limited to harm to skin, flesh and bones, but includes injury to the nervous system and brain such as recognised and identifiable psychiatric harm, but not 'mere emotions or states of mind which are not themselves evidence of an identifiable clinical condition'. An hysterical condition, which according to *Miller* fell within the definition of actual bodily harm, no longer does. It did not cover fear, distress or panic. These are regarded as emotions, not harms. *Chan-Fook* was followed in *Dhaliwal* [2006] 2 Cr App R 348. Psychological injury which was not a recognised psychiatric condition was not 'bodily harm'. *Dhaliwal* is also known as *D*: see [2006] EWCA Crim 1139.

In *DPP v Smith* [2006] 1 WLR 1571 it was held that magistrates were entitled to find that cutting off a substantial amount of hair, a ponytail, could constitute actual bodily harm. The court rejected contentions that 'harm' could apply only to living material, that 'harm' requires pain, and that 'harm' applies only when the part injured will not regrow. The arguments against the ruling that cutting hair is actual bodily harm are these: (1) there is no 'hurt or injury' within *Miller*; (2) distress does not constitute actual bodily harm.

In *Morris* [1998] 1 Cr App R 386 it was held that sleeplessness, tearfulness, tension, and anxiety were not actual bodily harm. The court stated that fear of unlawful violence was the crime of assault, not of assault occasioning actual bodily harm; otherwise there was no difference between the two. It added that if psychiatric injury is relied on and is not admitted by the defence, expert evidence should be admitted. One of the issues raised in *Ireland; Burstow*, above, was whether 'bodily harm' in the OAPA included psychiatric illness. Lord Steyn said that, when drafting the OAPA, 'the Victorian legislator . . . would not have had in his mind psychiatric illness . . . But the subjective intention of the draftsman is immaterial. The only relevant inquiry is as to the sense of the words in the context in which they are used. Moreover, the Act of 1861 . . . must be interpreted in the light of the best current scientific application of the link between the body and the psychiatric injury.' He approved the ruling of the Court of Appeal in *Chan-Fook* that 'bodily' in the phrase 'bodily harm' does not restrict the definition to 'the skin, flesh and bones of the victim'. In the words of Hobhouse LJ: 'the body of the victim includes all parts of his body, including his organs, his nervous system and his brain. Bodily injury therefore may include injury to any of those parts of the body responsible for his mental and other faculties.' Accordingly, psychiatric illnesses were included, provided that they constituted 'some indentifiable clinical condition'. However, 'bodily harm' does not cover 'mere emotions such as fear or distress or panic'. The Court of Appeal in *Morris* held that psychiatric evidence of the nature of the victim's symptoms should be led when there was a non-physical assault which caused tension and sleeplessness. That type of evidence is needed to distinguish between the 'mere emotions' and psychiatric illness, such as 'a chronic anxiety state or depressive disorder'. Injuries can be aggregated to make the harm 'actual'. In *Smith* [1985] LSG Rep 198, four or five bruises caused by a belt were sufficient. In *Jones* [1981] Crim LR 119, minor abrasions and a bruise were held to be actual bodily harm, though the case was thought to be on the margins. Pain caused by a kick to the stomach with tenderness afterwards, but leaving no visible injury, was sufficient: *Reigate JJ, ex parte Counsell* (1983) 148 JP 193. In *Miller*, an injury to the state of a person's mind was enough (cf. *Dawson* (1985) 81 Cr App R 150 on manslaughter: shock is not harm unless physical injury is caused). *Chan-Fook* reminds us that there must be harm, even when the assault is on the victim's mind. Where there is a psychic assault, for the accused to be guilty that assault must cause the bodily harm: the apprehension of violence must cause the harm.

A recent authority is *T v DPP* [2003] Crim LR 622, which is also called *R (on the application of T) v DPP*. The accused kicked the victim momentarily unconscious. There were no contusions or other marks. The trial judge directed the jury according to the words of Swift J in *Donovan*, above: '. . ."bodily harm" has its ordinary meaning and includes any hurt or injury calculated [i.e. likely] to interfere with the health or comfort of the [victim]. Such hurt or injury need not be permanent, but must . . . be more than merely transient or trifling.' The jury convicted. The Divisional Court dismissed his appeal. Maurice Kay J, as he then was, said that Swift J's words were not to be treated as a statute but, in any case, while the injury here was 'transient' it was not 'trifling'. In other words, not to be actual bodily harm the injury had to be, as Swift J said, both transient *and* trifling. However, the main authority is *Chan-Fook*. The words in s 47 were ordinary ones. On the facts of the case loss of consciousness was 'harm'; the harm was 'bodily' because the victim's senses were impaired; and the harm was most definitely 'actual'. Therefore, the accused was rightly convicted.

Criticism of s 47 comes from academics. Glanville Williams wrote in 'Force, injury and serious injury' (1990) 140 NLJ 1227:

> What the Victorian draftsman intended by 'actual' is anyone's guess. He was evidently searching, unsuccessfully, for something between 'trivial' and 'serious'. The courts have not helped him by sensible pronouncements. They might have said that harm is not 'actual' unless it is something beyond the trivial, for which a charge of common assault is adequate; but they have not imposed even this degree of control. The question is held to be one for the unrestricted discretion of the jury or magistrates who are allowed to find that even a bruise is enough. In the scale of harms, a bruise is trivial. The offence under s 47 is relatively serious, carrying a possible sentence of five years. If only a bruise is caused, s 47 is an overcharge.

The penalty for s 18 is life imprisonment, substantially more than that for s 20, yet the harm may be the same: indeed, it could be less serious.

Mens rea

No mental element is expressly stated in s 47. In **Roberts** (1971) 56 Cr App R 95 (CA), an important case which was approved by the House of Lords in **Savage**, the court seems to have held that the *mens rea* is the same as for common law assault. After **Venna** [1976] QB 421, where the victim suffered a broken finger, that means that the accused is guilty if he intended to create or is reckless as to creating fear or as to touching and the outcome is actual bodily harm. On this approach the accused need not intend or be reckless as to actual bodily harm. On the facts of **Roberts** a person who assaults with the result that the victim tries to escape and suffers actual bodily harm is guilty of this offence, even though the accused did not foresee actual bodily harm. This issue is dealt with below.

The meaning of recklessness in s 47

In **DPP v K** [1990] 1 WLR 1067, the accused, a 15-year-old schoolboy, was using sulphuric acid in an experiment at school. Some splashed onto his hand. He washed it off in the lavatory. Unknown to the teacher he had taken with him a test tube of the acid to test its reaction with lavatory paper. While in the lavatory he heard footsteps, panicked and poured the acid into a dryer, intending to come back later to wash it out. Unfortunately another pupil came in, turned on the dryer and the acid splashed over his face, causing a scar. The Divisional Court directed the magistrates to convict. It held that s 47 could be committed indirectly: 'A defendant who pours a dangerous substance into a machine just as truly assaults the next user of the machine as if he himself switched the machine on.' Controversially the court held that **Caldwell** [1982] AC 341 (HL) applied to the mental element in s 47. **Cunningham** [1957] 2 QB 396 was not cited. Counsel agreed that **Caldwell** governed. The defence argument was solely that **Caldwell** could be distinguished on the grounds that in **DPP v K** there was a gap between the accused's act and the injury, an argument which the court rejected. The main criticism of **DPP v K** was in the words of Bennett and Hogan, 'Criminal law, criminal procedure and sentencing' All ER Rev 1990, 69, that it brought the 'thoughtlessly stupid' into the criminal law.

The Court of Appeal in **Spratt** overruled **DPP v K** on this point.

Spratt [1990] 1 WLR 1073

The accused fired shots from an air pistol from his flat. Two pellets hit a seven-year-old girl playing outside. He had not realised that there were people in the area, i.e. he gave no thought to the risk. The Court of Appeal quashed his conviction.

McCowan LJ held that:

> The history of the interpretation of the 1861 Act shows that, whether or not the word 'maliciously' appears in the section in question, the Courts have consistently held that the *mens rea* of every type of offence against the person covers both actual intent and recklessness, in the sense of taking the risk of harm ensuing with foresight that it might happen.

Venna was approved in **DPP v Majewski** [1977] AC 443 and seemingly by Lord Diplock himself in **Caldwell**. **Savage** (HL) confirms that **Cunningham** applies. **Caldwell** does not apply because 'maliciously' is a term of art with 'a special restricted meaning'. Any doubt as to the position was resolved by **G** [2004] 1 AC 1034 (HL) which held that **Caldwell** was wrong.

Does the accused have to intend to cause or be reckless as to causing actual bodily harm or is intention to recklessness as to battery sufficient?

In *Spratt*, though interpretations vary, the Court of Appeal seems to have required intentionally or recklessly occasioning actual bodily harm. In *Savage* (1990) 91 Cr App R 317, the same court (but a different division) on the same day said that intentionally or recklessly causing a battery was sufficient, as long as actual bodily harm occurred. In *Savage* the accused threw beer on the victim in a pub. She let go of the glass (whether deliberately or not is unknown) and the victim was cut by broken glass. She was held guilty under s 47. The battery was the consequence of her deliberate throwing of the beer as a result of which the victim was injured. There was no need to show that she foresaw the possibility of some harm. The stress was on causation, not recklessness: did the accused commit the assault which caused the actual bodily harm? The result is in line with *Roberts*, and is consistent with the decision if not the reasoning in *Spratt*, where the court seems to have been discussing the nature of recklessness, not whether there had to be *mens rea* as to the occasioning of actual bodily harm. Since *Roberts* was not mentioned in *Spratt* or in the next case, *DPP v Parmenter* [1992] 1 AC 699, those cases are *per incuriam*. The House of Lords in *Savage* approved *Roberts*.

In *Parmenter*, the Court of Appeal chose *Spratt* in preference to *Savage*. The court thought that the law was 'impenetrable' and called for the House of Lords to review it. The House of Lords in *Savage* approved the *Savage* (CA) approach. Lord Ackner said in *Savage*:

> The Court of Appeal in *Parmenter* was wrong in preferring the decision in *Spratt*. The decision in *Roberts* was correct. The verdict of assault occasioning actual bodily harm may be returned upon proof of an assault together with proof of the fact that actual bodily harm was occasioned by the assault. The prosecution are not obliged to prove that the defendant intended to cause some actual bodily harm or was reckless as to whether such harm would be caused.

'Occasioning' is an objective issue not dependent on the accused's state of mind. The law was made complex partly by *Mowatt* [1968] 1 QB 421. A person is guilty under s 20 of the OAPA (see later) when he does not foresee grievous bodily harm but does foresee some harm. According to *Savage*; *DPP v Parmenter* [1992] 1 AC 699 (HL) this definition applies to both ss 20 and 47. Mustill LJ said in *DPP v Parmenter* that, although the two offences are seen as different by defendants and lawyers, the *mens rea* is the same:

> If the *Cunningham* subjective test combined with the low level of intent prescribed by *Mowatt* is applied to s 47 in the same way as s 20, the moral overtones of the two offences become indistinguishable, and the differences between the two depend upon variations between the levels of physical injury which may often be the result of chance.

Both sections have the same maximum punishment, five years' imprisonment, yet s 20, which deals with maliciously inflicting grievous bodily harm, is seen as the more serious offence, yet that gravity may now depend on chance. Mustill LJ continued:

> The authorities can no longer live together and . . . the reason lies in a collision between two ideas, logically and morally sustainable in themselves, but mutually inconsistent, about whether the unforeseen consequences of a wrongful act should be punished according to the intent [*Cunningham*] or the consequences [*Mowatt*].

In other words, the accused is guilty not for what he intended to do or was reckless as to doing but for the result of his actions. This is a form of constructive liability in the same sense that liability for unlawful act manslaughter is constructive. Such liability is frowned upon by those people, sometimes called subjectivists, who hold that people should be punished according to their states of mind. The doctrine of constructive murder, by which an accused who killed in the course of a violent felony was guilty of murder, was abolished in 1957 and the Law Commission would like to abolish all forms of constructive criminality. In *Savage* it mattered whether the mental element was the intent to batter or assault rather than intent to cause actual bodily harm. The victim apprehended a battery and the accused foresaw such apprehension. She had the mental element of battery but did not foresee actual bodily harm. Such harm occurred through the accused's careless or accidental dropping of the glass. Nevertheless, she was guilty. She would also have been guilty if the harm had been done through the purely fortuitous circumstance that the glass had a defect in it which made it break easily. No wonder the House of Lords thought that the law was irrational.

Included offences

If the accused is charged with s 47, he cannot be convicted of common assault: *Mearns* (1990) 91 Cr App R 312 (CA) and *Savage* (HL). Assault and battery are summary offences (Criminal Justice Act 1988, s 39). A separate count for common assault must be added, and often is. The position was different before the statute. In all but exceptional cases, wounding will involve a battery. Therefore, on a charge of wounding (OAPA, s 20), one can convict of s 47 (*Savage* (CA) among other cases). Similarly, on a charge of inflicting grievous bodily harm, one can convict of s 47. The law is unsatisfactory.

Wounding and grievous bodily harm

Section 18 of the OAPA as amended reads:

> [w]hosoever shall unlawfully and maliciously by any means whatsoever wound or cause any grievous bodily harm to any person . . . with intent . . . to do some grievous bodily harm to any person or with intent to resist or prevent the lawful apprehension or detainer of any person shall be guilty . . .

Section 20 reads in part:

> [w]hosover shall unlawfully and maliciously wound or inflict any grievous bodily harm upon any person, either with or without any weapon or instrument shall be guilty . . .

Section 18 is the most serious non-fatal offence against the person, and differs from s 20 in the need for the ulterior intent ('with intent to') and in the different verbs for committing the grievous bodily harm (hereinafter GBH): 'cause' in s 18, 'inflict' in s 20 (Fig. 13.2). It should be noted that in s 18 the ulterior intent does not relate to wounding: the offence is not satisfied by wounding (or causing GBH) with intent to wound. Such facts fall within s 20 (if the GBH was inflicted). The phrase 'either with or without any weapon' makes s 20 pleonastic. Section 18 speaks of 'lawful' apprehension or detention. If the arrest is wrongful, the accused is not guilty. If the arrest is lawful but the accused believes it to be unlawful, he is guilty because he has made a mistake of law: *Bentley* (1850) 4 Cox CC 406. It might, however, be argued to the contrary that the

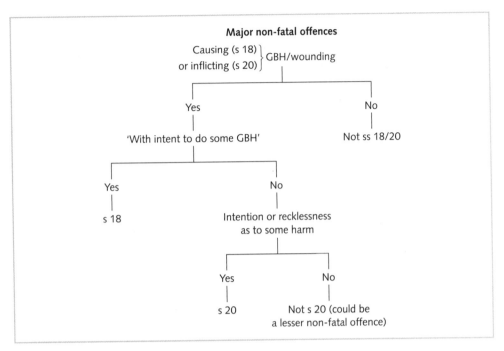

Figure 13.2 Major non-fatal offences

mistake is really one as to civil law, which does afford a defence, or that if the mistake is a factual one (e.g. was he a constable?) he should also not be convicted. (See Chapter 8 for discussion of mistake.) One result of the wording of s 18 should be noted. It is an offence to cause GBH with intent to prevent lawful apprehension. If the accused hits a constable while resisting arrest and the constable bangs his head on a kerbstone causing serious injury, he is guilty of GBH with intent. He need not intend GBH, yet he may be sentenced to any period of imprisonment, including for life.

The term 'unlawfully' in both sections exonerates a person who acts in self-defence or where there is consent or lawful chastisement. If the accused acts in defence of property, he is entitled to use reasonable force, force which would otherwise amount to GBH. It is hard to see how 'unlawfully' can operate with regard to some forms of s 18. One difference should be noted. Section 20 refers to 'upon any other person'; s 18 says 'to any person'. Section 18 could be interpreted as holding it to be illegal to wound or cause GBH to the accused himself, provided the ulterior intent is satisfied. Maiming oneself to avoid conscription in wartime, the example used above in relation to consent, would therefore be an offence contrary to s 18, but not to s 20.

Actus reus

A wound is a breach in the whole skin, a phrase which includes the internal lining of the mouth and the vagina and penis. It was so held in, among other cases, *JCC (A Minor)* v *Eisenhower* [1984] QB 331 (DC), where a ruptured blood vessel was held not to be a wound. A bruise is not a wound. It was thought that a wound requires a battery: *Taylor* (1869) LR 1 CCR 194 among other cases, except perhaps in 'extraordinary' circumstances: *Savage* (CA), above, which the House of Lords approved. Their Lordships did not give illustrations of these extraordinary circumstances. Perhaps an illustration of extraordinary facts would be a knife which is sent into the victim as a result of her touching a trip-wire. Since, as we shall shortly see, 'inflict' does not require an assault or battery, it might be expected that the same rule should apply to 'wound.' It is suggested that should the issue arise in the Lords, they would overrule this line of cases. The force is not directly applied by the person who set the trap but force is applied to the victim with the result that she is wounded. It is suggested that the rule that wounding requires a battery would not survive scrutiny nowadays in the House of Lords. There is no longer a condition that GBH must be caused by a battery, and the law should be the same for both.

It has been argued by William Wilson, *Criminal Law*, 3rd edn (Longman, 2008), 276, that 'wound' necessitates the accused to inflict a wound on the victim directly as with a knife; if so, causing the victim to run into a broken window on which he cut himself would not be a 'wound'. There is no judicial authority on this point.

In the context of murder the House of Lords held in **DPP v Smith** [1961] AC 290 that GBH meant 'really serious bodily harm'. This statement was applied to these offences in **Metharam** [1961] 3 All ER 200. However, the Court of Appeal in **Saunders**, above, held that 'really' did not add anything to 'serious'. That is, there were not three types of harm, 'really serious', 'serious' and 'non-serious', but just two, 'serious' and 'non-serious'. 'Really' meant 'actually', not 'very'. On the facts of **Saunders**, a broken nose was grievous harm.

Whether harm is grievous is judged by an objective test according to standards of usage and experience, not subjectively dependent on whether the jury would call it grievous if done to them: **Brown** [1998] Crim LR 485 (CA). Similarly, as **Brown** states, it is irrelevant what the victim thought about the injuries. In that case the accumulation of gross facial swelling, missing teeth, fracture of the nose, widespread lacerations and bruising was serious harm. However, what is grievous to one victim may not be grievous to another: **Bollom** [2004] 2 Cr App R 50 (CA). The court said that there was no requirement that the injuries be permanent, dangerous or life-threatening, but that injuries should be seen in the context of the victim. Injuries to a child or an elderly person may be more serious than the same injuries to 'a six-foot adult in the fullness of health'. On the facts, bruises which are harm to soft tissue, were capable of being grievous within the definition. They were superficial and would heal spontaneously, but whether the harm had lasting consequences or needed treatment was irrelevant to whether the harm was grievous. Extensive bruising and abrasions on a 17-month-old child were therefore capable of being grievous.

The jury should not ask whether each individual harm is very serious; instead the injuries should be added together to see whether as a whole they constitute GBH: **Grundy** [1989] Crim LR 502 (CA) and **Birmingham** [2002] EWCA Crim 2608. The same law applies to *actual* bodily harm. 'Bodily' and 'harm' presumably bear the same meaning as in the crime of assault occasioning actual bodily harm (see discussion). One effect is that 'bodily harm' covers psychiatric harm. In **Bullerton**, unreported, 1992 (CA), mentioned by R. Burns in 'GBH of the earhole' [1992] NLJ 1725, the accused, in order to stop obscene phone calls from the victim, attached a 'screech-box' to his phone. When the victim phoned, he was partly deafened and suffered tinnitus. The court seems not to have doubted that the results were grievous harm. In **Gelder** (1994) *The Times*, 25 May a man was convicted when the victim suffered sickness and diarrhoea as a result of his obscene phone calls. The Court of Appeal allowed the appeal (1994) *The Times*, 16 December, but only on the ground that the judge had wrongly instructed the jury on the mental element. The court did not rule whether GBH could be inflicted by phone.

It is a question of fact whether harm is serious. GBH covers situations where the skin is not broken as in **Wood** (1830) 172 ER 749, where a collar bone was broken. Conversely a wound is not necessarily GBH. An example is a pinprick. Sometimes the same facts are both GBH and wounding, such as when the accused chops off the victim's arm. It should be noted that a wound need not be a serious wound, yet the harm must be serious. It is difficult to accept that the law should treat a pinprick in the same way as a ruptured spleen.

The House of Lords in **Wilson** [1984] AC 242 overturned earlier authorities which held that 'inflict' in s 20 required an assault. 'Assault' is here used in the sense of battery. The House of Lords in **Savage** also thought that there can be infliction of GBH without a battery, as where the accused tampers with car brakes with the result that someone is seriously injured. An example, suggested in **Savage** by Lord Ackner, is inflicting GBH by creating panic. (Usually, however, there is a battery.) Most inflicting will involve an assault. For many years there has been debate as to the width of 'inflict' in s 20. These issues were raised in **Ireland; Burstow**, above. The first issue was whether or not s 20 required an assault (in the sense of a battery). The authorities were divided. Lord Steyn stated that s 20 does not require an assault on the basis that, if it did, words would have to be read into s 20 ('inflict *by assault* any grievous bodily harm'), whereas s 20 'works perfectly satisfactorily without any such implication'.

There is a problem arising from **Wilson**. Lord Roskill apparently believed that 'inflict' required the direct application of force to the victim or the doing of an act which directly resulted in force being applied to the victim's body. What is said is *dictum*. On this approach, to take an old example, if one dug a pit for the victim to fall into, one would be guilty under s 20 because, although one has not directly applied force to the victim, one has done an act which directly resulted in force being applied. One will have caused GBH within s 18, because 'cause' does not require the direct application of force. On the facts of **Martin**, above, the accused would be guilty of the more serious offence, s 18, and guilty of the less serious offence, s 20, for the same reason, but one is not guilty in the poisoning example because no force is used. The result is absurd. It would appear that the *dictum* is wrong. It could have been avoided by having the same verb in ss 18 and 20 or by the House of Lords in **Wilson** deciding that 'cause' and 'inflict' covered the same ground. The House of Lords took the point further: 'inflict' did not require direct application of force, but assault occasioning actual bodily harm and common assault did. Therefore, a person could be guilty of the most serious non-fatal assault but not of the lesser assaults! It is about time that the meaning of 'inflict' was settled. There are also problems with this definition of 'inflict' in s 20 with regard to s 23 of the OAPA, which creates the offence of administering a noxious thing '. . . so as thereby to inflict . . . any grievous bodily harm . . .' Administering poison requires neither a battery nor the application of force. Therefore 'inflict' in s 23 must be wider than 'inflict' in s 20. The OAPA is a mess but surely it is not such a mess. There seems to be little difference between the lack of a requirement of assault and the necessity for a direct application of force.

Another issue was whether s 20 required the direct or indirect application of force. The Lords held that no direct physical violence was necessary. Lord Steyn said:

> The problem is one of construction. The question is whether as a matter of current usage the contextual interpretation of 'inflict' can embrace the idea of one person inflicting psychiatric injury on another. One can without straining the language in any way answer that question in the affirmative. I am not saying that the words cause and inflict are exactly synonymous. They are not. What I am saying is that in the context of the Act of 1861 one can nowadays quite naturally speak of inflicting psychiatric injury.

In this way 'inflict' in s 20 and 'cause' in s 18 are of similar width, at least where psychiatric harm results. Lord Steyn thought it would be 'absurd' if 'cause' and 'inflict' were of different width. This interpretation was consistent with the hierarchy of non-fatal offences. As Lord Steyn said, 'the . . . approach should, so far as possible, be adopted which treats the ladder of offences as a coherent body of law'. One difference may be that 'cause' may be committed by omission, but 'inflict' cannot.

'Cause' in s 18 also does not require an assault: **Austin** (1973) 58 Cr App R 163. Perhaps 'cause' covers poisoning where the poison is left for the victim to take, whereas 'inflict' does not. 'Cause' thus does not require violence but 'inflict' does. A possible difference was suggested by Lord Hope in **Ireland; Burstow**. He said that 'inflict' denotes 'that the consequence of the act is something which the victim is likely to find unpleasant or harmful. The relationship between cause and effect, when the word "cause" is used, is neutral. It may embrace pleasure as well as pain.' If this statement is correct, the defendants in **Brown**, the sado-masochists, should not have been found guilty of a s 20 offence, but could have been convicted of a s 18 offence! It is suggested that whatever Lord Hope did mean by his comment, he did not intend to say that **Brown** was wrong. The law therefore remains uncertain as to whether there is a difference between 'cause' in s 18 and 'conflict' in s 20. The reader is reminded that the 1861 Act is a consolidation statute, bringing together laws from different Acts passed at different times and that no attempt was made to make the definitions consistent across the statute.

Mens rea

In both ss 18 and 20 the mental element is stated to be 'maliciously'. Section 18 requires proof of a further state of mind: 'with intent to do some grievous bodily harm'. Coleridge CJ said in **Martin** that 'maliciously' did not mean spitefully. It normally means in a statute 'intentionally or recklessly'. Negligence is insufficient. Yet one can be guilty of a more serious offence, manslaughter by gross negligence, by acting in a seriously careless fashion. As we have seen (Chapter 3), **Cunningham** [1957] 2 QB 396 held that on a charge of administering a noxious thing under s 23 of the OAPA recklessness was defined as: did the accused himself foresee the consequence? Though there is a *dictum* to the contrary in **Seymour**, above, this definition still applies to ss 18 and 20: **W v Dolbey** (1983) 88 Cr App R 1 (CA) (a case where the accused would not have been guilty under a test of objective recklessness because he considered whether there were pellets in his air rifle and decided that there were none), **Lynch** (1985) LEXIS, 14 January (CA), **Morrison** (1989) 89 Cr App R 17, and **Rainbird** [1989] Crim LR 505 (CA). Though the Court of Appeal in **Dume** (1986) *The Times*, 16 October, refused to say whether **W v Dolbey** was correct, there is now the House of Lords decision in **Savage** to the effect that it is.

The following cases exemplify this area of law.

See pp 110–16 in Chapter 3 for a review of Cunningham recklessness.

Lynch (1985) LEXIS, 14 January (CA)

During the night the accused fired his air gun out of the window of his first-floor flat. He was hoping to hit bottles he had placed on the roof of the garage opposite. A person standing in the garage was hit. The defendant contended that he thought that he was a good enough shot to hit only the bottles. He had put them in a place where the risk would be minimal and he had not pumped the gun the maximum number of times. It was held that the accused was aware of the probable consequences of firing the gun as he did.

Morrison (1989) 89 Cr App R 17

The victim, a detective constable, tried to arrest the accused. She grabbed his clothes. The accused dived through a window. The victim was brought into contact with the glass and serious lacerations were caused. The accused was charged with one form of s 18, wounding with intent to resist arrest. The court corrected the trial judge by holding that *Cunningham* applied. It expressed regret that English law recognised two forms of recklessness at that time.

Rainbird [1989] Crim LR 505 (CA)

The accused, a school caretaker, fired an air gun at some boys who were trespassing. He hit one of them. The trial judge seems to have mixed up the objective and *Cunningham* versions of recklessness. The Court of Appeal quashed the conviction, declaring that the subjective definition was necessary.

Brady [2006] EWCA Crim 2413

The accused, while having consumed alcohol and Ecstasy tablets, sat on a 44 inch high railing on a balcony above a dance floor. On the assumed facts, he fell on to one of the dancers, rendering her a paraplegic. The court held, applying *G* [2004] 1 AC 1034 (HL), that the accused was reckless for the purposes of s 20 if a significant risk of harm was obvious to him.

Though Diplock LJ said in *Mowatt*, above, that the accused was guilty when he should have foreseen harm, the foresight must be that of the accused, not of a reasonable person: *Grimshaw* [1984] Crim LR 108, *Parmenter* (CA) and *Savage* (HL), both above. In *Parmenter* the accused confessed to causing injuries to his three-month-old son, but said that he did not realise that what he was doing would injure him. Mustill LJ held that the accused himself must foresee some harm. The Court of Appeal in *Rushworth* (1992) 95 Cr App R 252 confirmed that the correct direction is to ask whether the accused might have foreseen some physical harm, not whether he *would* have foreseen harm. In *Savage*, above, Lord Ackner had used both concepts – the accused is guilty if he foresaw some harm might result and if he foresaw that some harm would result. *Rushworth* clarifies the law. On the facts the accused knew that some physical harm might result from his act of pushing a vibrator into a woman's vagina. The law was not that the accused had to foresee that some harm must result from what he did. The court in *Pearson* [1994] Crim LR 534 (CA) purported to follow *Rushworth* but at one point used the word 'would', as did the trial court in *DPP v A* [2001] Crim LR 140 (DC). If that were correct, the definition would constitute intent on one of the views of Woollin [1999] AC 82, discussed in Chapter 3. Professor Smith's comment on *Mowatt* at [1990] Crim LR 711 (case comment on *Savage*) is: 'We need some system of stamping a judicial health warning across certain pages of the law reports which have an unending capacity to mislead.' Though the *actus reus* comprises GBH or wounding, the *mens rea* for both is intention or recklessness as to physical harm.

Diplock LJ's statement in *Mowatt* that the harm foreseen need not be GBH so long as he foresaw some physical harm, however minor, was approved in *Sullivan* [1981] Crim LR 46 (CA), followed in *Jones*, above, and approved again in *Savage*; *DPP v Parmenter*.

In the light of the requirement of *physical* harm, it is surprising that a hoax caller was charged with GBH on the father of Abbie Humphreys, the baby who was abducted from a hospital in Nottingham in 1994. It is sufficient that the accused intends or is reckless as to causing some harm and GBH in fact results. The result is sometimes known as 'half *mens rea*'. The accused is guilty even though he did not intend, nor was he reckless as to the full *actus reus*, GBH. Whether the law should be this is a moot point. Commentators often say that the *actus reus* and *mens rea* should correspond, and they do not in s 20.

An intention to frighten is not by itself sufficient *mens rea* for s 20: **Sullivan**, above. For this reason it may be difficult to convict stalkers of the s 20 offence. Section 47 is, however, a possible charge provided that a recognised psychiatric illness is occasioned. Another possibility is a charge of s 20 where the accused intends to scare but foresees some psychiatric harm.

In s 18 the prosecution must prove that the accused acted with intent to do some GBH or resist arrest or prevent apprehension or detainer. In **Belfon** [1976] 3 All ER 46, the Court of Appeal held that this mental element was not satisfied by recklessness. In **Bryson** [1985] Crim LR 669 (CA), it was decided that the fact that harm was probable did not mean that the accused intended that harm. Intention bears the same meaning as in murder: **Bryson** and **Purcell** (1986) 83 Cr App R 45 (CA): see Chapter 3. As with regard to murder the jury should not be directed as to the definition of intent except in exceptional situations. In **Belfon**, a *dictum* of Lord Diplock in **Hyam v DPP** [1975] AC 55 that intent covered both desiring a consequence and knowing that a result was likely to happen was disapproved. Section 18 in summary requires intention. Foresight is insufficient. The different forms of the ulterior intent do not sit happily together in s 18: causing GBH with intent to do GBH may be more serious than causing GBH with intent to resist arrest yet the crime and punishment are the same.

Because s 18 is expressed in terms of 'cause GBH with intent to do GBH', the Court of Appeal in **Mowatt** opined that the term 'maliciously' was superfluous. The thinking is that if one intends GBH, one must foresee GBH as a probable or possible outcome. If, however, the indictment is based on GBH with intent to resist arrest, 'maliciously' is not superfluous. If the accused seriously harms an arresting officer, without 'maliciously' he would be guilty if he did not foresee any harm at all. By retaining 'maliciously' in the definition, the accused is not guilty unless he foresaw some harm. It has to be admitted that the law is in a mess.

Included offences

A person found not guilty under s 20 may be convicted under s 47: **Wilson**, approved by the House of Lords in **Savage**. While it is not possible to convict of a s 20 wounding, a s 47 actual bodily harm or common assault on a charge of s 18 (**Austin**, above), one may convict of a s 20 inflicting GBH: **Mandair** [1995] 1 AC 208 (HL). 'Causing' in s 18 covers all forms of 'inflicting' in s 20. A jury's verdict of causing GBH contrary to s 20, which the Court of Appeal had on this and previous occasions thought was a crime unknown to law, was to be read as meaning that causing GBH was contrary to s 20 because it consisted of inflicting GBH. The House of Lords emphasised that it was 'highly desirable' to use the actual words of the statute in the count and that if necessary alternative counts could be included in the indictment. **Mandair** has apparently been superseded by the ruling in **Ireland; Burstow** that there is little, if any, difference between 'cause' and 'inflict'.

Possessing anything with intent to commit an offence under the OAPA

Section 64 of the OAPA penalises any person who has 'in his possession ... any ... thing, with intent thereof' to commit an offence under the Act. The Law Commission's draft Criminal Code, Law Com. No. 177, 1989, does not include this crime. All remaining portions of the 1861 Act would be included in the Criminal Code. Therefore, s 64 would no longer serve a useful purpose. It does nevertheless seem a useful offence to catch persons who have not reached the stage of an attempt. An alternative view is that s 64 is restricted to explosives because it falls within the part of the Act dealing with explosives. On a literal reading, however, it is not so restricted.

Reform of ss 18, 20 and 47

Criminal law should work in practice. Clarkson and Keating 'Codification: Offences against the person under the draft Criminal Code' (1986) 50 JCL 405, at 415, wrote:

> Each of the non-fatal offences against the person is, to varying degrees, confused and uncertain ... [I]n relation to each other, they are incoherent and fail to represent a hierarchy of seriousness.

Reading such parts of the OAPA is more likely to confuse the student than enlighten him or her. It is possible to substitute all the terms in the sections and thereby produce an authoritative modern version of the crimes which gets rid of all the difficult and case-encrusted phraseology. The definition of concepts such as 'wound', 'cause', 'inflict', 'actual bodily harm' and 'grievous bodily harm' have to be gathered from the cases. The OAPA was a consolidation statute with no attempt made to grade the offences or fit them together. That said, since the Act dates from 1861 and, as stated, that was simply a consolidation Act, it is easy to see why modern judges find difficulty fitting modern methods into the 1861 statute. The telephone, e-mail, fax were not invented then. Similarly, HIV infection was unknown.

A Police–Crown Prosecution Service Working Group has drafted guidelines to distinguish among non-fatal offences including battery and attempted murder in an endeavour to ensure consistency of charges across the country. The first version was published in [1994] NLJ 1168 as *Charging Standards: Offences Against the Person*. A second version, *Offences Against the Person Charging Standard agreed by the Police and the Crown Prosecution Service*, was issued in 1996. An interesting point is that the guidelines at times adopt a charge below that stated in the texts. They classify, e.g., a graze as a battery not as actual bodily harm and put an undisplaced broken nose on the borderline between the two. Examples of actual bodily harm include broken teeth, extensive bruising, minor cuts which require stitching and minor bone fractures. The guidelines give as examples of GBH those injuries which require extensive surgery or a transfusion, permanent disabilities and significant visible disfigurement, and broken limb, skull, cheekbone and jaw injuries requiring lengthy treatment. There is a handy list of alternative verdicts, a topic which often creates difficulties in the courts. The aims of the Working Group are the choice of charges to reflect the nature of the attack, the provision of sufficient sentencing power and the facilitation of simple presentation of the case. Good administration of criminal justice is promoted. The guidelines have been criticised for channelling non-fatal offences into the magistrates' court where the chances of conviction are higher than in the Crown Court. The contrary argument is that the guidelines help to prevent a serious charge from being brought in the expectation that, as a result of plea bargaining, the accused will plead guilty to a lesser offence. Moreover, since Parliament has provided a hierarchy of offences, it is not legitimate that some other body should seek to lay down rules.

In its Fourteenth Report, *Offences Against the Person*, Cmnd 7844, 1980, the Criminal Law Revision Committee proposed replacing s 18 by 'intentionally' causing serious injury, s 20 by recklessly causing serious injury, and s 47 by intentionally or recklessly causing serious injury. The Criminal Code team adopted these proposals in the draft Criminal Code of 1985 (*Codification of the Criminal Law: A Report to the Law Commission* Law Com. No. 147). The 1989 version substitutes 'personal harm' for 'injury' (cll 70–72). By cl 6 'personal harm means harm to body or mind and includes pain and unconsciousness'. It covers cuts and bruises. There is no definition of 'serious', which is left to the triers of fact. No doubt there will be inconsistent decisions. Wounding is not dealt with separately. The crime will depend on whether the wound was serious harm or not.

Of the other offences adverted to in this chapter, the crime of threatening to kill is extended to threats to cause serious personal harm (cl 65); administering a substance without consent (cl 73) and assault to resist arrest (cl 77) are redrafted. The crime of assault with intent to rob, found in s 8 of the Theft Act 1968, is taken out of property offences and placed with offences against the person (cl 78). Intention and recklessness bear the same meaning throughout the draft Criminal Code. (See Chapter 3.)

In a roundabout way the defence of consent is preserved by cll 14(4) and 45(c). The exception of consent is expressly mentioned in assault (cl 75). No list of when consent is a defence was provided in relation to cll 70, 71, 72 and 75 because 'it is impossible to provide a comprehensive and closed list', a rather lame sentiment.

As the Court of Appeal said in *Lynsey* [1995] 2 Cr App R 667, 'Most, if not all, practitioners and commentators agree that the law concerning non-fatal offences against the person is in urgent need of comprehensive reform to simplify it, rationalise it, and make it trap-free . . . [B]ad laws cost money and clog up courts with better things to do.' Reform is a long time coming, even though the proposed changes would save money. This value-for-money approach was developed by the Law Commission in its proposals discussed in the next section.

The 1993 recommendations on assaults

The Law Commission made proposals for reforming crimes of violence in its Report No. 218, *Legislating the Criminal Code – Offences against the Person and General Principles*, 1993, which is based on the Criminal Law Revision Committee's Fourteenth Report, *Offences Against the Person*, Cmnd 7844, 1980, and the draft Criminal Code, Law Com. No. 177, 1989. The intention is to enact the draft Criminal Code in tranches, the first one being this area which was selected as being the one most in need of reform. The revised portions will be brought together into a Code.

The Law Commission followed its predecessors in noting that the law was inconsistent in substance and form and 'inefficient as a vehicle for controlling violence', e.g. even after *Savage* 'many aspects of the law are still obscure, and its application erratic'. Money was wasted in an attempt to find out the law and correct errors. The Law Commission estimated the costs of the trial and appeal in *Scarlett* [1993] 4 All ER 629 at £42,170 and the financial cost of the accused's imprisonment at some £7,000.

The proposals are as follows:

(a) Intent is defined as covering both 'purpose' and knowledge that a result 'would occur in the ordinary course of events if he [the defendant] were to succeed in his purpose of causing some other result'. The latter part of the definition catches the bomb-in-the-aeroplane scenario. The accused will not intend something which he wishes to avoid; e.g., a defendant will not intend to hurt a child when he throws her out of a window to escape a fire.

(b) Recklessness is defined in the subjective sense, awareness of a risk that a result will occur or awareness of a risk that a circumstance exists or will exist.

(c) Sections 18, 20 and 47 of the OAPA are to be repealed as unjust, ineffective, illogical, and seriously defective in terms of the hierarchy of harms and penalties, and incomprehensible to juries. A few illustrations will suffice. A person is guilty of s 18, a crime with a maximum sentence of life imprisonment, if his sole intention is to resist arrest. An accused is guilty of s 20 if he is reckless as to the risk of minor harm: *Mowatt* and *Savage*. The distinction between 'inflicting' in s 18 and 'causing' in s 20 is problematic. And the maximum punishment is the same for both s 20 and s 47 despite the difference in harm caused.

(d) In para 12.34 the Law Commission states: 'The interests both of justice and social protection would be much better served by a law that was (i) clearly and briefly stated; (ii) based on the injury intended or contemplated by the accused, and not on what he happened to cause; and (iii) governed by clear distinctions, expressed in modern and comprehensible language, between serious and less serious cases.' The new structure is based on (1) the abolition of the distinction between wounding and actual or GBH; (2) a distinction between serious and other injuries; and (3) a division between intentionally and recklessly causing injury. The effect, therefore, is the creation of three offences:

   (i) intentionally causing serious injury – maximum sentence life;
   (ii) recklessly causing serious injury – five years;
   (iii) intentionally or recklessly causing injury – three years. This would be the replacement for assault occasioning actual bodily harm. It could be used, for example, against stalkers when it is difficult to prove which of a series of acts caused the victim to be made afraid.

The Law Commission assures readers that these crimes would be 'just, simple, workable and effective in at least the great majority of cases' and that juries should have no difficulty understanding the wording. The enactment of these proposals would deal with the problems noted in the previous paragraph.

   Only intentionally causing serious injury could be committed by an omission to act.

(e) The term 'injury' is preferred to 'personal harm' in the draft Criminal Code as being apt to describe both physical and mental interference. 'Injury' is a term in ordinary use and juries should find no difficulty with it. In criticism it might be said that 'harm' is more apt than 'injury' to cover mental interference. The proposed law has been criticised for subsuming too broad a range of injuries within its definition of 'injury', on the ground that there is a moral difference between causing a slight injury and causing one just short of a serious injury.

(f) The law should continue to cover non-serious injuries.

(g) 'Serious' is not to be defined but left to the jury as in current law.

(h) Pain and unconsciousness are expressly mentioned as 'injury'. Wounding as a separate head of liability is abolished. Depending on the character of the wound it will be either a serious injury or an injury. This reform would remove the criticism that wounding is treated in the same fashion as grievous harm even when it does not amount to such harm.

(i) The transmission of diseases, such as AIDS, can be caught by the phrase 'impairment of a person's physical condition' in the definition of injury found in cl 18 of the Criminal Law Bill attached to the Report.

(j) Assault is defined in cl 6 of the Bill.

    (1) A person is guilty of the offence of assault if –

        (a) he intentionally or recklessly applies force to or causes an impact on the body of another –

            (i) without the consent of the other, or

            (ii) where the act is intended or likely to cause injury, with or without the consent of the other; or

        (b) he intentionally or recklessly, without the consent of the other, causes the other to believe that any such force or impact is imminent.

    (2) No such offence is committed if the force or impact, not being intended or likely to cause injury, is in the circumstances such as is generally acceptable in the ordinary conduct of daily life and the defendant does not know or believe that it is in fact unacceptable to the other person.

The term 'assault' thus covers both (psychic) assault and battery. Despite the Criminal Law Revision Committee's recommendation that assault did not need to be defined by Parliament, the Law Commission considered that it should be put on a statutory footing. Clause 6 is a restatement of cl 75 of the draft Criminal Code, quoted above.

(k) Section 16 of the OAPA, threats to kill, is extended to threats to cause serious injury. One criticism is that the maximum penalty for this offence is 10 years' imprisonment, whereas the maximum for recklessly causing serious injury is only five.

The issue of consent to violent non-sexual crimes is dealt with separately by the Law Commission in its Consultation Papers noted above.

The 1998 Home Office proposals

The Home Office issued a Consultation Document, *Violence: Reforming the Offences against the Person Act 1861*, in 1998. Attached was a draft Offences against the Person Bill. The principal non-fatal offences provisions are the following:

1(1)   A person is guilty of an offence if he intentionally causes serious injury to another.
      . . .

2(1)   A person is guilty of an offence if he recklessly causes serious injury to another.
      . . .

3(1)   A person is guilty of an offence if he intentionally or recklessly causes injury to another. . . .

4(1)   A person is guilty of an offence if –

(a) he intentionally or recklessly applies force to or causes an impact on the body of another, or

(b) he intentionally or recklessly causes the other to believe that any such force or impact is imminent.

(2) No such offence is committed if the force or impact, not being intended or likely to cause injury, is in the circumstances such as is generally acceptable in the ordinary conduct of daily life and the defendant does not know or believe that it is in fact unacceptable to the other person. . . .

10(1) A person is guilty of an offence if he makes to another a threat to cause the death of, or serious injury to, that other or a third person, intending that other to believe that it will be carried out. . . .

15(1) In this Act 'injury' means –

(a) physical injury, or

(b) mental injury.

(2) Physical injury does not include anything caused by disease but (subject to that) it includes pain, unconsciousness and any other impairment of a person's physical condition.

(3) Mental injury does not include anything caused by disease but (subject to that) it includes any impairment of a person's mental health.

(4) In its application to section 1 this section applies without the exceptions relating to things caused by disease.

The effect of cl 15(4) is that intentional transmission of disease resulting in serious injury will be a crime, but the intentional or reckless transmission of disease causing injury will not. Clause 10(1) extends the present offence of threat to kill to threat to cause serious injury. In relation to omissions, it should be noted that the offence of intentionally causing serious injury will be commitable by omission, but there will be no liability for recklessly causing serious injury or for intentionally or recklessly causing injury. Intent and recklessness are defined as in the 1993 Recommendations. Clause 18 provides that the offences are subject to any defence, lawful authority, justification or excuse. What these defences are is left to the common law.

As can easily be seen, the Home Office proposals are those of the Law Commission outlined in the previous section of this book. The then Home Secretary, Jack Straw, in his Foreword to the Consultation Document, stated that the aim was to reform 'out-moded and unclear Victorian legislation', thereby demonstrating 'this Government's commitment to modernising and improving the law'. This commitment awaits enactment.

The proposals have also come under criticism. First, there is what is sometimes called moral vacuity at the heart of the proposals; that is, ordinary people do not just take into account the *actus reus* and *mens rea* of the accused when they are assessing the gravity of his conduct. They also inquire into matters such as the way in which the injury was caused. For example, the weapon may be important or the fact that the accused tortured the victim. Secondly, there is the strange distinction between cll 1 and 2 on the one hand and 3 and 4 on the other. If, as the Law Commission thought, there is a moral distinction between intent and recklessness, why are the two combined in the lesser non-fatal offences? Thirdly, 'serious injury' is undefined. How serious is 'serious'? Moreover, it may be said that there is a vast difference between, say, a broken cheekbone and the loss of an arm, but both constitute serious injury. In that light, perhaps there should be several grades of serious injury. Fourthly, cl 10(3) excludes anxiety and distress from the ambit of 'impairment of a person's mental health'. However, minor physical harms remain within the definition of physical injury. So, minor mental injuries are not to be criminal, but minor physical ones are. For the sake of consistency the two should be brought into line. A fifth issue is that the revised definition of battery does not by its words ('force or impact') cover the situation where the accused's conduct is an omission, such as leaving one's hand on a knee on which it has rested accidentally, and where the accused's behaviour is unacceptable, but there is no force or impact, as when he strokes the victim's hair without consent.

Nevertheless, as the Conclusion to the Consultation Document states, the enactment of the draft Bill would create a more consistent hierarchy of offences than that which exists at present, and 'making the law more accessible in this way will help to smooth the passage of thousands of cases each year, enabling the citizen to understand the criminal offences more easily. . . . It should also make the task of judges, magistrates and juries more straightforward in the day to day administration of justice.' Unfortunately, work at the Home Office on reform of non-fatal offences appears to have stopped.

Summary

Non-fatal, non-sexual offences constitute the subject of this Chapter. The sequence is from the least serious, assault, up the 'ladder' of seriousness, through battery to assault occasioning actual bodily harm contrary to s 47 of the Offences Against the Person Act 1861 (OAPA) to malicious wounding or inflicting grievous bodily harm (GBH) contrary to s 20 OAPA to malicious wounding or causing GBH with intent to do some GBH contrary to s 18 OAPA. The defence of consent, both to assault and battery and exceptionally to more serious offences (cf. boxing), is considered. There is discussion of the case of the sado-masochists, **Brown** (1994), and the cases in which this authority has been applied and distinguished. Emphasis is placed on problems which students face, e.g. the two definitions of assault, the constructive nature of liability in ss 20 and 47, the possible distinction between 'inflicting' and 'causing' GBH. As ever, the chapter concludes with a consideration of reform proposals.

- Assault: Assault is the least serious non-fatal offence but care must be taken when reading the cases. This is because the term is used in two different but overlapping senses: first, as a separate offence concerned with making the victim afraid (in this sense assault is sometimes known as 'psychic' or 'technical' assault; secondly, as a generic term covering assault in the first sense and the discrete offence of battery. Assault is used here to mean the separate offence. The *actus reus* is causing another to apprehend immediate and unlawful personal violence and the *mens rea* is intentionally or (subjectively) recklessly causing another to apprehend immediate and unlawful personal violence. In relation to the *mens rea* the word 'subjectively' is put in brackets because even when objective recklessness existed, the law was always that the accused himself or herself had to foresee the relevant consequence.

  For many years it was said that one could not commit the crime by words alone but that rule has now gone; indeed, silent phone calls have in the quite recent past been classified as assaults (and therefore some instances of stalking are caught by this offence). The timescale of 'immediate' has been widened too recently and it now includes 'making someone afraid at some time not excluding the immediate future'; in this way phone calls are covered because the victim may not know where the caller is. However, words may negate what would otherwise be an assault. Modernising the words of the most famous authority on this point, 'I would shoot you dead if armed police weren't next to you', is not an assault. The word 'unlawful' is a reminder that some threats of immediate personal violence are not unlawful, e.g. a threat to hit someone may be a lawful threat in preventing crime.

- Threats to kill: Section 16 of the Offences Against the Person Act 1861 creates a specific offence dealing with threats to kill without a lawful excuse. The *mens rea* is intentionally causing the victim to apprehend that the threat to kill will be carried out.

- Battery: A battery is the intended or (subjectively) reckless use of force on a person without consent or other lawful excuse. There is no need for the direct infliction of force and an omission suffices as the *actus reus* where there is a duty to act. Hostility, it would seem, is not a requirement. The exception of lawful excuses covers for example lawful chastisement of children. Consent, which is noted next, is a defence.

- Consent: The basic rule is that consent is no defence to crimes more serious than a battery (e.g. to assault occasioning actual bodily harm) but there are several exceptions, including:

Boxing
Cosmetic surgery
Flagellation for religious purposes
Horseplay
Scarification
Sports within the rules of the particular sport
Sterilisation
Surgery
Tattooing

- Assault occasioning actual bodily harm: This is an offence contrary to s 47 of the Offences Against the Person Act 1861.
'Assault' bears its wider meaning of 'technical' or 'psychic' assault and the separate crime of battery.
'Actual' means 'more than trivial'.
'Bodily' does not just cover flesh and bones but also the psyche. It does not, however, include emotions such as distress or panic.
'Harm' means 'injury'.
More difficult is the *mens rea*, which is intention or recklessness as to assault (in its narrow sense of being an independent crime) or battery. There is no need for intent or recklessness as to actual bodily harm. As we have seen, murder's *mens rea* is somewhat similar: an intent to cause GBH suffices; and as we shall see, in s 20 of the 1861 statute intention or recklessness as to actual bodily harm constitutes the *mens rea*.

- Malicious wounding or inflicting grievous bodily harm: Section 20 of the Offences Against the Person Act 1861 creates the crime of malicious wounding or inflicting GBH. 'Bodily' and 'harm' have been defined above. 'Grievous' means 'really serious'. A 'wound' is a breach in all the layers of the skin. The *mens rea* is a trap for the unwary: it is intent or recklessness as to actual bodily harm: intent or recklessness as to GBH is not needed. It should be noted that both for the wounding and for the inflicting GBH versions of this offence, the *mens rea* is the same.

- Malicious wounding or causing GBH with intent to do some GBH (etc.): This crime is laid down in s 18 of the 1861 Act. Its main versions may be expanded as 'wounding with intent to do some GBH' and 'causing GBH with intent to do some GBH'. Therefore, s 18 does not include 'wounding with intent to wound'. One difference from s 20 is that the verb used in s 18 is 'cause' (GBH) whereas in s 20 it is 'inflict' (GBH). For many years it was thought that there was a distinction: if one left something for the victim to take, one may have caused GBH but not inflicted it. Modern thinking, however, is that the two verbs cover the same activities.

References

Reports

Criminal Law Revision Committee 14th Report, *Offences against the Person* (1980)

Home Office Consultation Document, *Violence: Reforming the Offences against the Person Act 1861* (1998)

Law Commission Consultation Paper no. 134, *Consent and Offences against the Person* (1994)

Law Commission Consultation Paper no. 139, *Consent in the Criminal Law* (1995)

Law Commission Report no. 177, *A Criminal Code for England & Wales* (1989)

Law Commission Report no. 218, *Legislating the Criminal Code: Offences against the Person and General Principles* (1993)

Police–Crown Prosecution Service Working Group, *Charging Standards: Offences against the Person* [1994] NLJ 1168

Books

Clarkson, C. M. V., Keating, H. and Cunningham, S. R. *Criminal Law: Text and Materials* 6th edn (Thomson, 2007)

Wilson, W. *Criminal Law* 3rd edn (Longman, 2008)

Journals

Bennett, G. and Hogan, B. 'Criminal law, criminal procedure and sentencing' (1990) All ER Rev 69

Burns, R. 'GBH of the earhole' [1992] NLJ 1725

Clarkson, C. M. V. and Keating, H. 'Codification: offences against the person under the draft Criminal Code' (1986) 50 JCL 405

Williams, G. 'Force, injury and serious injury' [1990] NLJ 1227

Further reading

Allen, M. J. 'Consent and assault' (1994) 58 JCL 183

Clarkson, C. M. V. 'Law Commission Report on offences against the person and general principles: (1) Violence and the Law Commission' [1994] Crim LR 324

Gardner, J. 'Rationality and the rule of law in offences against the person' (1994) CLJ 502

Gunn, M. and Ormerod, D. 'The legality of boxing' (1995) 15 LS 181

Hare, I. '*R v Savage, DPP v Parmenter* – a compelling case for the Code' (1993) 56 MLR 74

Horder, J. 'Rethinking non-fatal offences against the person' (1994) 14 OJLS 335

Horder, J. 'Reconsidering psychic assault' [1998] Crim LR 392

Livings, B. 'Legitimate sport or criminal assault' (2006) 70 JCL 495

McCutcheon, J. P. 'Sports violence, consent and the criminal law' (1994) 45 NILQ 267

Ormerod, D. C. 'Criminalising HIV transmission' (2001) 30 *Common Law World Review* 135

Ormerod, D. C. and Gunn, M. J. 'The legality of boxing' [1996] Crim LR 694

Reed, D. 'Court of Appeal: Offences against the person: Reckless transmission of HIV' (2005) 69 JCL 389

Roberts, P. 'Consent to injury: how far can you go?' (1997) 113 LQR 27

Roberts, P. 'The philosophical foundations of consent in the criminal law' (1997) 17 OJLS 389

Ryan, S. 'Reckless transmission of HIV: Knowledge and culpability' [2006] Crim LR 981

Shute, S. 'The Law Commission's second consultation paper on consent' [1996] Crim LR 685

Spencer, J. 'Retrial for reckless infection' (2005) 154 NLJ 762

Smith, J. C. 'Case comment on *Mandair*' [1994] Crim LR 667

Smith, J. C. 'Offences against the person: the Home Office Consultation Paper' [1998] Crim LR 317

Weait, M. 'Knowledge, autonomy and consent: *R v Konzani* [2005] Crim LR 763

Weait, M. 'Harm, consent and the limits of privacy' (2005) 13 *Feminist Legal Studies* 97

Williams, G. 'Force, injury and serious injury' [1990] NLJ 1227

Wilson, W. 'Consenting to personal injury: how far can you go?' (1995) 1 *Contemporary Issues in Law* 45

For a book on the assaults and HIV see M. Weait, *Intimacy and Responsibility: The Criminalisation of HIV Transmission* (Routledge-Cavendish, 2008)

Visit **www.mylawchamber.co.uk/jefferson** to access exam-style questions with answer guidance, multiple choice quizzes, live weblinks, an online glossary, and regular updates to the law.

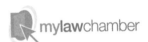

Use **Case Navigator** to read in full some of the key cases referenced in this chapter:

DPP v Majewski [1976] 2 All ER 142
DPP v Morgan [1975] 2 All ER 347
Fagan v Metropolitan Police Commissioner [1968] 3 All ER 442
R v Brown [1993] 2 All ER 75
R v Cunningham [1957] 2 All ER 412
R v G [2003] 4 All ER 765
R v Woollin [1998] 4 All ER 103

14

Rape and other sexual offences

Introduction to rape

Home Office statistics report that in 1995, 4,986 rapes of women were notified to the police and 150 of men. In 2004–5 there were 12,867 reported rapes of women and 1,135 of men. Meanwhile, the 2000 British Crime Survey estimated that there had been some 61,000 rapes in the previous year and that some three-quarters of women had been raped in their lifetime. The BCS deals not with crimes reported to the police but with figures derived from interviews. BCS figures are usually some four times greater than reported crimes. The Home Office sees the BCS figures as more accurate than totals reported to the police.

Although reports of **rape** increased steadily after World War II, a belief remained among victims that they would not be believed and would be treated unsympathetically; reporting levels of rape did not approach the actual figures (L. J. F. Smith, *Concerns About Rape*, Home Office Research Study No. 106, 1989). Changes initiated in the 1980s, such as police use of trained female officers, provision of victim examination suites, and liaison with victim support schemes, had gone some way towards reassuring victims that their complaints would be taken seriously and pursued, but reporting levels remained low.

L. J. F. Smith's detailed 1989 study revealed that in half of the cases there was actual or threatened violence, half of the victims were aged 16–24, and 60 per cent of offenders were aged 16–29. Only one-third of the perpetrators were total strangers, and 40 per cent were well known to the victims. There was some indication that rape by the husband was the most common form.

The research report *The Nature of Rape of Females in the Metropolitan Police District*, by Chandni Ruparel (Home Office Research Study 247, 2004), reports that 16 per cent of victims were under 16, and more than one-third were under 21. Some 6 per cent were rapes in which drugs were used, but in over 90 per cent of cases no weapon was involved. Of rapes by 'intimates', 64 per cent took place in the victim's home.

Although reporting rates have risen, there is great concern that the conviction rate for rape is low and falling. J. Harris and S. Grace, *A Question of Evidence? Investigating and Prosecuting Rape in the 1990s*, Home Office, 1999, found that fewer than 10 per cent of recorded rapes resulted in a successful prosecution. Home Office figures from 2003 reported the same proportion; in early 2005, they reported a conviction rate as low as

7 per cent; it is now below 6 per cent (L. Kelly, J. Lovett and L. Regan, *A Gap or a Chasm? Attrition in Reported Rape Cases*, Home Office Research Study 293, 2005).

The road to reform

In 1984 the Criminal Law Revision Committee proposed in its Report *Sexual Offences* that rape should remain a separate offence. The term 'rape' was established in popular language and marked a distinctive form of wrongdoing, partly because of the risk of pregnancy (though, of course, not all victims of rape can become pregnant). Other forms of penetration, e.g. with a bottle or via the anus, should continue not to be rape (although the latter became classified as rape in 1994 as a result of the Criminal Justice and Public Order Act of that year). The essence of the offence should continue to be the lack of consent, but what that phrase means should continue to be undefined, except that submission should expressly be a lack of consent. Misrepresentation as to the nature of the act should continue to be a factor which vitiates consent. Other forms of fraud should continue not to amount to lack of consent: the correct charge was obtaining intercourse by deception. The mental element was to be defined as knowing that the woman was not consenting or believing that she was not consenting. The proposed reform of what became s 1(3) of the 1956 Act, the partial abolition of the marital rape exemption (of course, the exemption has since been totally removed), and the abrogation of the immunity for boys are mentioned below. The draft Criminal Code, 1989, incorporates these proposals. The last two are already part of the law. The marital immunity is also to be withdrawn from the offences of procuring a woman to have intercourse by threats (cl 90: this would cover obtaining intercourse by threatening to dismiss from a job) or deception (cl 91) (these recommendations were enacted in 1994) and using an article to overpower for sexual purposes (cl 92). The Criminal Law Revision Committee made no recommendation but in the interests of consistency the Law Commission thought that the law should be the same as in rape. The Law Commission also proposed a clause (cl 88) stipulating that voluntary intoxication would continue not to be a defence to rape. The recommendations of the Criminal Law Revision Committee have been to some extent superseded by events, but its Report remains the last official investigation into the principles underlying this area of the law. Other reforms have been suggested: one which has considerable support is to put the legal burden of proof as to lack of consent onto the accused. Any mistake as to consent would then lie at his door.

The Law Commission in Consultation Paper No. 134, *Consent and Offences against the Person*, 1994, did not refer to sex crimes but it was persuaded by respondents to that Paper that it should do so, for it would be unsatisfactory to have two different laws on consent applying to a situation where a male beat up his partner in a sado-masochistic spree and then forced her to have sex with him. The Law Commission, in its Consultation Paper No. 139, *Consent in the Criminal Law*, 1995, wished to enact the Criminal Law Revision Committee's Fifteenth Report and the draft Criminal Code in order to state the law clearly. The general recommendations on consent are discussed in Chapter 13. The Law Commission invited views on whether a man should be criminally liable for having sexual intercourse with a person who did not consent when he had failed to realise that the victim was not consenting but the lack of consent would have been obvious to a reasonable person and the accused was capable of appreciating that it was. In other words, an objective interpretation was to be given to the *mens rea* as to lack of consent. This extension of the law was not to be made if the same rule did not apply to non-fatal offences. If the accused was to be liable, the Law Commission inquired whether the offence should be one of rape or whether a new crime of gross sexual invasion should be instituted. If the rule were adopted for rape (or for the new offence), it would also apply to indecent assault. In the words of the Law Commission, 'we think it arguable that in certain situations the potential harm to the other person may be so great as to justify the imposition of a positive duty to make minimal precautions to avoid it' (para 7.27). It is uncertain how much difference in practice the proposed amendment would make, but the symbolism would be important. The Law Commission also proposed that sexual intercourse gained by non-violent threats should not be rape (para 6.45). It is suggested that this proposal should be rejected. Rape is based on the lack of consent. This recommendation would destroy that basis where intercourse was obtained by a non-violent threat.

The Home Office announced in 1999 that a review of sexual offences would take place. The aims were to 'provide coherent and clear sex offences which protect individuals, especially children and the vulnerable, from abuse and exploitation' and to 'be fair and non-discriminatory in accordance with the European Convention on Human Rights and the Human Rights Act [1998]'. Parliament, in fits and starts, has over the past 20 years or so eliminated several discriminatory rules in relation to sex crimes. The obvious example is the equalisation in the age of consent for heterosexual and homosexual intercourse. The Sexual Offences Act 2003 carries through this policy (though not in respect of rape) in that soliciting prostitutes and kerb-crawling may be committed by both men and women. Prostitutes under the Act may also for the first time be male or female.

A Consultation Paper, *Setting the Boundaries: Reforming the Law on Sex Offences* was published by the Home Office in July 2000. It proposed in relation to rape that:

(a) rape should be retained as a separate offence with a maximum of life imprisonment;

(b) the crime should be extended to include penetration of the mouth; as in present law the slightest penetration would suffice; the law would for the avoidance of doubt cover female or male reconstructed genitalia;

(c) it would continue to include penetration only by a penis; other forms of sexual penetration of the anus or genitalia would be covered by a new crime of sexual assault by penetration, also with a maximum of life imprisonment; again the slightest penetration would suffice and surgically reconstructed genitalia would be included;

(d) there should not be a lesser form of rape ('date rape' or acquaintance rape) because there was no necessary difference in the trauma between rape by a stranger and rape by a friend or relation and in respect of date rape there was the additional detriment to the victim of betrayal of trust involving further psychological harm;

(e) consent would be redefined as 'free agreement' and a non-exhaustive list of examples where there was no such agreement would be provided;

(f) rape would continue to be committable recklessly as to the victim's consent and 'recklessly' would be defined as 'not caring less' (this is introducing objective recklessness: the accused will be guilty if he gives no thought to the victim's consent);

(g) the defence of honest belief should be excluded when the accused did not take all reasonable steps in the circumstances to ascertain free agreement, when he was in a state of self-induced intoxication and when he was reckless as to free agreement; some consultees were of the opinion that in all instances a mistaken belief as to consent should be accepted only if it was based on reasonable grounds.

It should be noted that although the Home Secretary had instructed the Sex Offences Review Committee to be non-discriminatory the offence of rape, even after these reforms, may only be committed by a man. This is not so in all jurisdictions. For example, in New South Wales the female can be the offender (and the offence includes penetration of orifices other than the vagina or anus and penetration by parts of the body or by implements). Though a woman cannot be guilty of rape, she may be guilty of assault by penetration (s 2 of the Sexual Offences Act 2003), if she, for example, penetrates the victim's anus; she may also be guilty of sexual assault (s 3) or causing another person to perform a sexual act without consent (s 4). The victim in ss 2–4 may be male and the perpetrator may be female.

The Home Secretary published *Protecting the Public*, Cm 5668, in 2002. It was proposed that where the victim was subjected to force or fear of force or to threats or fear of serious harm or serious detriment to himself, herself or another, or was abducted or unlawfully detained, or was unconscious, or was unable to communicate a decision because of physical disability, or agreement to sex was given by a third party, the burden of proving consent (on the balance of probabilities) should be on the accused. Reasonable belief would be needed for consent. Rape would cover penile penetration of the mouth.

The former requirement of the unlawful nature of the sexual intercourse

Until late 1994 (see the Criminal Justice and Public Order Act 1994, Part XI) the statutory definition of rape included the element that the intercourse was 'unlawful'. Until quite recently the sexual intercourse was unlawful if it took place outside marriage: *Chapman* [1959] 1 QB 100 (CA). However, in *R* [1992] 1 AC 599 the House of Lords ruled that the law no longer was that the husband was incapable in law of raping his wife. In the light of existing law it was surprising that the accused was prosecuted, for no crime seemed to exist. The principal speech was delivered by Lord Keith.

(a) The institutional writer Hale may have been correct to write in his *History of the Pleas of the Crown*, 1736, Vol. 1, 629, published by E. & R. Nutt and R. Gosling, that 'the husband cannot be guilty of a rape committed by himself upon his lawful wife, for by their mutual matrimonial consent and contract the wife hath given herself up in this kind unto her husband which she cannot retract'. However, the common law developed in accord with social, economic and cultural shifts. Marriage was now a partnership, and the wife was no longer a chattel. In the light of these changes, the idea that a woman had to have sexual intercourse with her husband, no matter how she felt or how her health was, was unacceptable. Accordingly, there was no justification for the marital exemption.

(b) The former state of the law had been undermined by the case law. In *Miller* [1954] 2 QB 282, it was held that the husband, while not guilty of rape, could be guilty of assault occasioning actual bodily harm. It was unrealistic, in Lord Keith's view, to separate the acts leading up to the sexual intercourse from the intercourse, and then find the husband guilty of the minor crime but not of the major one. Moreover, exceptions had been created which had cut into Hale's hard-and-fast rule. In *O'Brien* [1974] 3 All ER 663, the Court of Appeal held that the husband was guilty of rape when there was a decree nisi of divorce. In *Steele* (1976) 65 Cr App R 22 (CA), the husband was guilty when he had given an undertaking not to molest his wife. In

Roberts [1986] Crim LR 188 (CA), the husband was guilty where there was a formal separation order.

(c) The undermining of the marital exemption was, however, a common law development. In the statute there was the word 'unlawful'. To say that sexual intercourse outside marriage was unlawful was not the natural meaning of the word. The word was otiose, mere surplusage. The view that Parliament kept the word 'unlawful' in the 1976 Act to preserve the marital exemption with its exceptions was rejected. (This approach had been upheld by Rougier J in *J* [1991] 1 All ER 759 (Crown Court).) If asked in 1991, it might not have wished to preserve the exemption.

R may be criticised

(a) When it enacted the Sexual Offences (Amendment) Act 1976 Parliament rejected a clause which would have made rape within marriage illegal. *R* is therefore contrary to Parliament's intention. Law-making is for Parliament, not the judges, especially in controversial matters.

(b) Since Parliament did not change the law in 1976 the House of Lords have created an offence, something which they vowed they would not do (see Chapter 1).

(c) The offence of rape has been widened retrospectively. It has been applied to an accused who before this case would not have been guilty of rape. The European Court of Human Rights, however, ruled in *CR* v *UK* [1996] 1 FLR 434 (a case also called *SW* v *UK*) that the decision in *R* was not inconsistent with Article 7 of the European Convention on Human Rights, which prohibits retroactive criminal law. The European Convention's purpose was to impose dignity and freedom, both of which were promoted by the case of *R*.

(d) The Law Commission issued a Working Paper, *Rape Within Marriage*, Law Com. No. 116, 1989, where the options for reform were discussed. At the time of the decision in *R* the full Report was expected. The proposals of the Law Commission could have been enacted by Parliament, which through the Report would have seen the whole of the problem and not just the part at issue in *R*.

(e) Many cases have proceeded on the basis that 'unlawful' in the pre-1994 definition meant outside marriage. *Chapman*, a case on abducting girls contrary to s 19 of the Sexual Offences Act 1956 (since repealed), is one, as is *Jones* [1973] Crim LR 710 (CA) on abducting women contrary to s 17 of the same Act (also since repealed). The cases on the exceptions to the marital rape exemption assume that the rule exists. Some of those authorities are noted above. Others include *Clarke* [1949] 2 All ER 448, where the judge held that the marital exemption did not apply when the wife had obtained a non-cohabitation order in a separation order, and *Sharples* [1990] Crim LR 198 (Crown Court), where there was an undertaking not to have sexual intercourse. Another case showing that the courts recognised the marital exemption is *Cogan and Leak* [1976] QB 217 (CA), discussed in Chapter 5. The husband made his wife consent to sexual intercourse with a man who believed that the wife was consenting. That man was acquitted of rape on the grounds of honest mistake. The husband was convicted as principal to rape, with the other man being the innocent agent, i.e. he raped through the genitals of someone else. One difficulty in accepting that the husband was the principal party was the marital exemption rule. If the husband could in law rape his wife, criticism of *Cogan and Leak* would have been substantially less. As it was the court found a way round the marital exemption. Hale's proposition has been cut back by the exceptions to the marital exemption and in *Clarence* (1888) 22 QBD 23 the judges were *obiter* split on the crime, but it was accepted for 250 years.

(f) The word 'unlawful' must have meant something. It is not included in the crime of incest because a husband cannot commit that offence with his wife. Section 6 of the Sexual Offences Act 1956 (since repealed) dealt with unlawful sexual intercourse with a girl under 16. What if the accused is married by foreign law to a girl under 16? If 'unlawful' does not mean outside marriage, the husband is guilty of this offence if he has sexual intercourse in England with his wife. Surely that outcome is incorrect. A perhaps more contentious issue occurred in s 7 of the same Act (since repealed). It is a crime for a man to have unlawful sexual intercourse with a woman who is mentally defective. What if they are married? If 'unlawful' is surplusage, the husband is guilty.

Policy arguments against the marital exemption

(a) It is wholly unjust and contrary to common sense that a husband could go away for a lengthy period, come back, commit an act which would otherwise be rape on his wife, yet be found not guilty of rape.

(b) The Court of Appeal in *R* [1991] 2 All ER 257 thought it 'repugnant and illogical' that a husband could be punished for violence against the wife in the course of sexual intercourse to which she did not consent but could not be guilty of rape itself, especially when rape can be seen as a heinous form of violence. Whether the sexual intercourse without consent is by the husband, an acquaintance or a stranger, there may be a fear of sexually transmitted disease or pregnancy.

(c) The court also said that the law should not be based on fictions. It was a fiction that by marrying her husband the wife had consented to intercourse whenever he wanted it. That fiction was 'anachronistic and offensive'.

(d) It should not matter who the victim of the rape is: 'a rapist remains a rapist . . . irrespective of his relationship with the victim' (*per* Lord Lane CJ in *R* in the Court of Appeal). A husband can frighten and humiliate his wife just as much as a stranger can do to the same woman. Indeed it may be that marital rape is the most common form of rape.

(e) It is a fiction to say that at the wedding ceremony the wife surrenders her right to choose when and with whom to have sexual intercourse. Moreover, a woman who is cohabiting without marriage receives the protection of the law. Why should it make any difference that she is married?

(f) In the civil law the wife may refuse sexual intercourse when, e.g., her health would be endangered. It would be strange if criminal law were out of line.

(g) It could be argued that one effect of the marital immunity was that criminal law protected property more than persons. A husband can steal from his wife but could not rape her. Moreover, a husband can kidnap and falsely imprison his wife. It seems strange if he cannot rape her.

(h) The law is made consistent with Scottish law, which abolished the marital immunity in *S v HM Advocate* 1989 SLT 469. The court held, *inter alia*, that on marriage the wife does not irrevocably consent to sexual intercourse, that since she cannot in law consent to a major battery, she could not consent at one time to nonconsensual battery by intercourse at some time in the future, and that a charge of rape against the husband would not undermine domestic relations more than, e.g., a charge of indecent assault based on facts other than vaginal penetration. By late 1991 of the seven husbands tried for raping their wives in Scotland none had been convicted.

As J. A. Scutt commented 'Consent in rape: the problem of the marriage contract' (1977) 3 Monash ULR 255 at 288:

> Public policy surely requires protection of citizens, married or unmarried, from aggressive sexual acts; it also requires that potential defendants be treated alike . . . Again, public policy in upholding the marital relationship must be directed toward upholding those relationships wherein criminal acts are not committed by one spouse upon the other.

Indeed, the fact that the husband has foisted himself on his wife may demonstrate that the marriage has irretrievably broken down. The irretrievable breakdown of a marriage is the ground for divorce. There seems little point in using the very blunt instrument of marital immunity to patch up such a marriage. One problem which has not been addressed, however, is where does the victim go, whether married, cohabiting or otherwise, when she is a non-earner?

Reports of law reform institutions on the marital exemption

The Criminal Law Revision Committee's Fifteenth Report, *Sexual Offences*, Cmnd 9213, 1984, supported the marital immunity and the then-existing exceptions. The members concluded that liability should be extended to situations where the parties had ceased cohabiting. However, since there were problems of definition about cohabiting, the law should be left as it was. The minority view was that both sexes should be entitled to choose with whom they wished to have sexual intercourse. The majority view was that intercourse without consent but within marriage was not as serious as such intercourse out of marriage. The Law Commission's draft Criminal Code, Law Com. No. 177, 1989, would have re-enacted the marital exemption and the exceptions then current. The Law Commission members stated that they did not agree with the law as it then existed. The Law Commission dropped the term 'unlawful' from the definition of rape in order to reflect the law as it existed in 1989.

The Law Commission in its Working Paper, *Rape Within Marriage* above, disagreed with the opinion of the Criminal Law Revision Committee that non-consensual intercourse within marriage was not as heinous as such intercourse not within marriage. The Law Commission proposed to abolish the marital immunity. It thought that rape within marriage would not be more difficult to prove than rape between non-marrieds. Views were canvassed whether the immunity should totally disappear or the exceptions increased to include all situations where the spouses were living apart, and whether there should be a new crime where a husband had sexual intercourse with his wife without her consent. The Law Commission's view was that there should be no such offence because, if there was, there would be degrees of rape, yet rape was always a serious offence. The Law Commission also recommended the abolition of the marital immunity in s 2 of the Sexual Offences Act 1956 (procuring a woman to have unlawful sexual intercourse) and in s 3 (procuring a woman by false pretences). These amendments were made in 1994 (see the Criminal Justice and Public Order Act 1994, s 142 and Sch 11). The government of the time promised to look at the final Report urgently, though after *R* the Home Office stated that legislation was not imminent.

Boys and women as rapists and accessories

With effect from 20 September 1993 the Sexual Offences Act 1993 abolished the irrebuttable presumption that a boy under 14 was incapable of committing an offence involving sexual intercourse, whether anal or vaginal. A boy over 10 but under 14 can rely on the defence of infancy if he lacks mischievous discretion. A boy can be convicted of being a secondary party to rape: *Eldershaw* (1828) 172 ER 472.

A woman may be a secondary party to rape: *Ram and Ram* (1893) 17 Cox CC 609. She cannot commit rape.

The basic definition of rape

Section 1 of the Sexual Offences Act 2003 defines rape in this way:

  (1) A person (A) commits an offence if –
      (a) he intentionally penetrates the vagina, anus or mouth of another person (B) with his penis,
      (b) B does not consent to the penetration, and
      (c) A does not reasonably believe that B consents.
  (2) Whether a belief is reasonable is to be determined having regard to all the circumstances, including any steps A has taken to ascertain whether B consents.

This definition replaces that found in the Sexual Offences Act 1956, s 1, as amended, and s 1(1)(c) and (2) replace s 1(2) of the Sexual Offences (Amendment) Act 1976. The principal changes are that rape can now by committed by the penetration of the mouth by the penis (sometimes called 'oral rape') and that the *mens rea* is extended to include situations where the accused had an unreasonable belief in the victim's consent (overruling *DPP v Morgan* [1976] AC 182 for the purposes of rape). Section 2 of the 2003 Act creates the offence of assault by penetration and s 3 creates the offence of sexual assault, the replacement for indecent assault, and the mental element in both offences includes an unreasonable belief in the victim's consent. Section 4 creates the offence of causing a person to engage in sexual activity without consent. Sections 2–4 are discussed below.

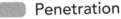 Introduction

The Act is based on, but not the same as, the Law Commission's Consultation Paper No. 139 on *Consent in the Criminal Law*, 1995, the Home Office Consultation Paper, *Setting the Boundaries*, 2000, and the White Paper, *Protecting the Public*, 2002. The government was concerned with finding the correct label for each offence it created so that an appropriate amount of stigma attached. The 2003 Act is the culmination of several changes in the law: in *R v R* [1992] 1 AC 599 (HL) it was held that husbands could rape their wives, even when they were cohabiting; since the Sexual Offences Act 1993 boys aged 10–14 can be guilty of rape; and by the Criminal Justice and Public Order Act 1994 rape was extended to include 'anal rape' of men and women as we have seen.

Penetration

The Act is restricted to penetration by the penis. Therefore, it can still only be committed by men. 'Penis' includes a surgically constructed penis and 'vagina' includes a surgically constructed vagina (s 79(3)). By s 79(9) 'vagina includes vulva', thereby confirming that the slightest penetration suffices. Rape is complete on penetration; however, if the victim consents to penetration but withdraws consent after penetration, the accused must in turn withdraw his penis, as s 79(2) makes clear ('penetration is a continuing act from entry to withdrawal'). It is uncertain how much time a man has to withdraw: the government's view was that he would have a reasonable time and whether or not the time he took was reasonable would be left to the juries' good sense. However, that is not what the statute says: there is on the face no defence of withdrawal within a reasonable time. Under the old law it did not have to be proved that the hymen was broken or that semen was ejaculated. The 2003 Act does not mention these rules but since the offence is complete on penetration, both rules apply under the new law.

Consent

Section 74 states in part: 'a person consents if he agrees by choice, and has freedom and capacity to make that choice.' The words 'choice', 'freedom' and 'capacity' are open-textured and reasonable juries may disagree as to their application to the facts. There is no need to prove active resistance. Similarly there is no requirement that the victim communicates his non-consent to the accused. By s 76 it is *conclusively* presumed that the victim did not consent and that the accused did not reasonably believe that he or she consented if '(a) the defendant intentionally deceived the complainant as to the nature or purpose of the relevant act; or (b) the defendant intentionally induced the complainant to consent to the relevant act by impersonating a person known personally to the complainant.' If there is no deception or inducement, s 76 does not apply. For example, the alleged victim may be mistaken as to 'the nature or purpose of the relevant act', but if the mistake was not brought about by the defendant's deception, the scenario does not fall within s 76. Compare a scenario where the accused persuades the victim to agree to intercourse as an expression of their undying love; however, the accused does not love the victim; if intercourse does take place, these facts fall within s 76 and constitute rape. Whether Parliament so intended may be doubtful. A case illustrative of s 76 is *Jheeta* [2007] EWCA Crim 1699. The accused lied to the victim, telling her that she must have sexual intercourse with him or she would be fined by the police. She was not deceived as to the nature or purpose of the activities. Note that to fall within s 76 the accused's deception or inducement must have been intentional. By s 75 there is a *rebuttable* presumption that the victim did not consent and that the accused did not reasonably believe in the victim's consent if the accused was using or threatening to use violence whether against the victim or some other person; if the complainant was being unlawfully detained; if he or she was 'asleep or otherwise unconscious'; if he or she was because of 'physical disability' unable to communicate consent; or if he or she had been administered a stupefying or overpowering substance. It is for the accused to rebut the presumption of lack of consent by leading sufficient evidence. It is not always clear why some matters are one of conclusive presumption (s 76) and some only of the evidential presumption. For example, surely if the accused gave the victim a stupefying drug in order to have intercourse with him or her, these facts should amount to a conclusive presumption that the victim did not consent. At present, furthermore, it is uncertain whether alcohol is a 'substance . . . which . . . was capable of causing or enabling the complainant to be stupefied or overpowered . . .' Similarly is the use of violence really not as bad as impersonating the victim's boyfriend? Section 75 provides for only a rebuttable presumption in the former case but s 76 states that the latter event falls within the irrebbutable presumption.

Accordingly there are three situations involving consent: the conclusive presumption in s 76; the rebuttable presumption in s 75; and the general rule, the default position, in s 74. There is no minimum age at which children can agree by choice to penetration but, as s 74 states, they must have 'capacity' to give agreement. If a child aged under 16 does freely agree, the crime is not one of rape itself but, for example, of rape of a child under 14 (s 5 of the 2003 Act; see also ss 6–15 of that statute, all of which deal with sexual offences against children). A mentally ill or mentally disabled person can consent if he or she does so within s 74. The problem again is one of 'capacity', and presumably he or she must be *Gillick*-competent (see *Gillick v West Norfolk and Wisbech AHA* [1986] AC 112 (HL)).

Further criticism of the distinction drawn in ss 75 and 76 may be made. For example, why is there a conclusive presumption against consent where the victim is deceived or there is impersonation, but only an evidential presumption where the victim has been drugged or is asleep?

Section 74 also applies in this situation: the victim is not so drunk that he or she is 'asleep or otherwise unconscious' (s 75(2)(d)) and is not voluntarily intoxicated (s 75(2)(f)) but is, say, loudly demanding sexual intercourse, i.e. he or she would not have been so acting, had he or she been sober; in other words, his or her inhibitions have been loosened by alcohol. In that event the jury must decide whether there is an agreement by choice to penetration and whether the victim had the freedom and capacity to make that choice. For example, in *Bree* [2007] 2 All ER 676 (CA), it was held that where the alleged victim was drunk but still capable of choosing whether to have intercourse or not, there was no rape. It may be difficult for a jury to decide these issues and it would not be surprising if juries came to different decisions. Such an outcome, however, is antithetical to justice for in one instance the accused is guilty of an offence with a maximum sentence of life imprisonment and in the other is not guilty of that offence. Section 74, however, does not prevent consent to sexual intercourse occurring when the accused does not reveal his HIV status: *B* [2006] EWCA Crim 1945.

Section 75 is largely self-explanatory but note that the paragraph dealing with violence does not apply if the accused makes a threat to destroy or damage property. Similarly, the provision does not apply if the threat is to inflict violence in the non-immediate future.

Section 76 is based on the common law, but the first point to make is that even if the facts do not fall within s 76, there can still be a lack of agreement within s 74. For example, to fall within s 76(2)(a) the accused must intentionally deceive the victim as to the nature or purpose of the penetration. If the victim is mistaken as to the nature or purpose but not because of the accused's deception, s 76(2)(c) does not apply but s 74 does. The application of s 76 may be illustrated by the facts of the following cases, all dating from before the 2003 statute.

Williams [1923] 1 KB 340: the accused persuaded the victim into agreeing to sexual intercourse by saying that the penetration would improve her breathing. Under both the old and the new law the accused is guilty of rape. He has intentionally, as s 76 requires, deceived her as to the 'nature' of the act. If the victim knew what sexual intercourse was but she was told by the accused that engaging in such conduct would improve her singing, there is deception as to the 'purpose' within s 76, though not as to the 'nature'.

Linekar [1995] 2 Cr App R 49: the victim, a prostitute, consented to sex with the accused for £25. The Court of Appeal held that the facts did not constitute rape: the accused's deception that he would pay her, but in fact he did not, did not invalidate her consent. She was deceived and thereby consented to the intercourse but she was not deceived as to the fact that what the parties did was sexual intercourse. There was no deception under the old law as to the nature of the act or the identity of the accused; similarly under the new law there is no deception as to the 'purpose' or as to the 'nature' of the act. This is what the Court of Appeal thought in *Jheeta*, above. However, there is a contrary argument. If it may be said that the nature of the act is 'paid-for sex', there is a conclusive presumption of lack of consent and the accused is guilty of rape. Presumably sex with a condom is different from sex without a condom too. Is sexual intercourse with an HIV positive person different from that with one who is not?

The facts of *Linekar* at the time would have fallen within s 3 of the Sexual Offences Act 1956. Section 4 of the 2003 Act, discussed below, is the replacement provision but it is so worded that the same definition of consent applies to it as to rape. Therefore, the difficulty with the current definition of rape also affects s 4.

Tabassum [2000] 2 Cr App R 328: this was a case on indecent assault. The Sexual Offences Act 2003 replaced this crime with the offence of sexual assault (s 3). In respect of the old and the new crime the law as to consent is the same as in the old and the new (respectively) offence of rape. The accused touched women's breasts, allegedly to show them how to conduct self-examinations. He had no medical training but he lied that he was a breast cancer specialist undertaking a breast cancer survey. The Court of Appeal held that the women consented to the nature of the act but not as to the quality; therefore, the accused was guilty. *Tabassum* was much criticised for drawing a distinction between nature and quality. Under the new law, however, the conviction is more securely grounded. The victims did not consent to the 'purpose' of the touching. Their consent was negated by the accused's deception as to the purpose of the act.

Section 76 also deals with the conclusive presumption of the lack of consent where there is a mistake as to identity. The person impersonated must be one 'known personally to the complainant'. Therefore, s 76 does not apply when the accused deceives the victim into believing that he is a rock star. Similarly, s 76 does not apply when the accused deceives the victim as to his wealth in order to achieve penetration. As with s 75, if s 76 does not apply, the general rule in s 74 applies. To use a pre-Act case as an example: in *Elbekkay* [1995] Crim LR 163 the victim thought that the accused was her boyfriend; he (the accused) did not impersonate him. Under the new law s 76 does not apply because there was no impersonation; however, s 74 does apply and a jury may well hold that the victim consented to sex with her boyfriend, not with the accused, and that therefore there was no agreement by choice within s 74.

Mens rea

The mental element consists of intentional penetration and the accused's lack of a reasonable belief that the victim is consenting. In relation to the first aspect, the phrase 'intentionally penetrates the vagina, anus or month' in s 1(1)(a) seems to require intention as to the penetration of an orifice which the accused intends to penetrate. If so, negligently penetrating the anus when one intended to penetrate the vagina does not give rise to rape. In relation to the second aspect the accused will have the mental element if he knows that the victim is not consenting, if he gives no thought as to whether or not he or she is consenting, and if he has no reasonable grounds for believing that he or she is consenting. *Morgan*, above, is overruled: the men did not believe on reasonable grounds that the woman was consenting. Sections 75 and 76, quoted above, apply to the lack of reasonable belief in consent. For example, there is a rebuttable presumption (s 75) that the accused does not have a reasonable belief in consent when the victim is asleep; and there is a conclusive presumption (s 76) when the accused deceives the victim as to the nature or purpose of the penetration or impersonates a person personally known to the complainant. Section 1(2), quoted above, instructs the jury to take into account all the circumstances, which include, presumably, nods and winks indicating a willingness to engage in sexual congress. 'Circumstances' is undefined. It is uncertain, for example, whether the accused can rely on previous occasions when the victim did consent. What about a culture where women are subservient to men's sexual demands? Are they to be treated as consenting and are the men to be deemed to have reasonable belief in the women's consent?

Sexual offences other than rape

The Sexual Offences Act 2003 establishes three offences which are in some respects drafted similarly to rape: assault by penetration, sexual assault and causing a person to engage in sexual activity without consent. These offences are considered next. There may be overlaps among them, and the alert reader should be able to construct scenarios where two, three or even four of the offences found in ss 1–4 of the 2003 Act occur. The 2003 Act also defines many other **sexual offences** including crimes against children and those suffering from learning difficulties, zoophilia, necrophilia, voyeurism and others, but these are not dealt with here.

Assault by penetration

Section 2(1) of the 2003 Act reads:

> A person (A) commits an offence if –
> (a) he intentionally penetrates the vagina or anus of another person (B) with a part of his body or anything else,
> (b) the penetration is sexual,
> (c) B does not consent to the penetration, and
> (d) A does not reasonably believe that B consents.

The maximum sentence on indictment is imprisonment for life: s 2(4). This offence is a partial replacement for the crime of indecent assault. The Home Office in *Setting the Boundaries*, 2000, concluded that ten years, the maximum sentence for indecent assault, was not long enough for the most serious sexual assaults. In terms of the maximum this crime is equivalent to rape.

The reasonableness of the belief as in rape 'is to be determined having regard to all the circumstances, including any steps A has taken to ascertain whether B consents': s 2(2). Also as in rape, the provisions in ss 75 (the rebuttable presumption of lack of consent) and 76 (irrebuttable presumption of lack of consent) apply. One effect is that if a doctor performs, say, a vaginal examination not for the purpose of medical treatment but for the purpose of sexual gratification, deception as to purpose falls within s 76. Indeed, the same activity such as penetration of the anus without consent falls within both the crime of rape and this offence. However, there are also differences: rape includes penetration of the mouth whereas this offence does not; this offence must be committed via a penetration which is sexual in nature, whereas rape need not be (though penetration by the penis is presumably sexual); rape turns on penetration by a penis whereas this offence does not (e.g. penetration by a carrot, bottle or brush handle suffices). This last point demonstrates that unlike rape this offence is not restricted to male defendants, and it should be noted that the maximum sentences for both offences is life imprisonment. **Whitta** [2006] EWCA Crim 2626 hold that liability is strict as to the identity of the victim. If the accused intends to penetrate one person digitally but makes a mistake as to the identity of the complainant, the fact that the intended victim would have consented to the penetration is irrelevant.

However, unlike rape the offence of assault by penetration is committed only when the assault was 'sexual'. By s 78:

> ... penetration, touching or any other activity is sexual if a reasonable person would consider that –
> (a) whatever its circumstances or any person's purpose in relation to it, it is because of its nature sexual, or
> (b) because of its nature it may be sexual and because of its circumstances or the purpose of any person in relation to it (or both) it is sexual.

The effect of s 78 is to exclude medical examinations from being 'sexual'. Where the penetration is not sexual in nature within either (a) or (b), the accused's purpose or the surrounding circumstances cannot make it 'sexual' within s 78. Therefore, the fact that the accused has a shoe fetish does not make the act of removing a shoe from a girl's foot into a sexual assault despite the sexual satisfaction the accused obtained from doing so. Similarly, touching the hem of a girl's skirt is not sexual despite the accused deriving sexual gratification in doing so. See, however, **H** [2005] Crim LR 735 on the post-2003 law. The court said that such fetishes may be 'sexual' within s 78. The position remains unclear.

Sexual assault

Section 3(1) of the 2003 Act creates the offence of sexual assault. By s 3(1):

> A person (A) commits an offence if –
> (a) he intentionally touches another person (B),
> (b) the touching is sexual,
> (c) B does not consent to the touching, and
> (d) A does not reasonably believe that B consents.

As in rape and assault by penetration the reasonableness of A's belief is determined by considering all the circumstances including any steps A took to ascertain whether B did consent; and as in rape and assault by penetration ss 75 and 76 apply. The definition of 'sexual' found in s 78, discussed above in relation to assault by penetration, applies. Section 3(1) applies to 'touching', which is defined in s 79(8) as including 'touching (a) with any part of the body, (b) with anything else, (c) through anything, and in particular includes touching amounting to penetration.' 'Assault' in s 3(1) really means 'battery'.

For an explanation of assault, see pp 525–29 in Chapter 13. 'Assault' in its technical or psychic sense (see Chapter 13) does not fall within s 3. Therefore, the same acts which constitute rape and assault by penetration can also constitute sexual assault. The maximum sentence, however, for this offence, on indictment, is ten years' imprisonment, whereas that for rape and assault by penetration is life imprisonment. The overlap is particularly acute in terms of sentence when it is known that the maximum sentence on summary conviction is six months' imprisonment or a fine not exceeding the statutory maximum, currently £5,000.

Reported cases on this offence as yet are rare and the main authority is *H*, above, where the Court of Appeal dismissed the accused's appeal. It held that since s 79(8) did not define 'touching' but merely stated that certain activities constituted 'touching', a person who touched the victim's clothes, here tracksuit bottoms near the righthand pocket, fell within the boundaries of the offence. The Court also rejected an argument that the touching was not sexual. Since the touching was not unequivocally sexual, s 78(b) applied. The jury had to consider whether the touching might be sexual; and, if so, whether the jury considered the touching to be sexual, taking into account the accused's (or any other person's) purpose and the circumstances.

Causing a person to engage in sexual activity without consent

Section 4(1) of the Sexual Offences Act 2003 creates the offence of causing a person to engage in sexual activity without consent. By it:

> A person (A) commits an offence if –
> (a) he intentionally causes another person (B) to engage in an activity,
> (b) the activity is sexual,
> (c) B does not consent to engaging in the activity, and
> (d) A does not reasonably believe that B consents.

Unlike s 3(1), there is no need for a touching. As may be expected, whether the belief is reasonable depends on all the circumstances including any steps taken by A to determine whether B consents; ss 75 and 76 apply; and the definition of 'sexual' noted above applies. The sexual activity may be one not between A and B but between B and someone else or something else. An example is forcing B to masturbate. The section is also satisfied where a woman forces a man to have sexual intercourse with her. It should be noted that s 4(1) may on the facts cover behaviour also caught by s 1(1), rape, s 2(1), assault by penetration, and s 3(1), sexual assault. For this reason there are complicated provisions as to sentence. By s 4(4):

> A person guilty of an offence under this section, if the activity caused involved –
> (a) penetration of B's anus or vagina,
> (b) penetration of B's mouth with a person's penis,
> (c) penetration of a person's anus or vagina with a part of B's body or by B with anything else, or
> (d) penetration of a person's mouth with B's penis,
> is liable, on conviction on indictment, to imprisonment for life.

Otherwise the maximum term is ten years on indictment and six months or a fine not exceeding the statutory maximum, currently £5,000, or both. One perhaps surprising effect of s 4(4) is that if the accused forces the victim to submit to penetration of the anus or vagina by a dog, the maximum sentence is life, but if the penetration is of the mouth, the maximum is ten years.

Summary

This chapter deals with some of the more important sex crimes, all of which were revised in the Sexual Offences Act 2003. The main focus is on rape but other linked offences such as sexual assault are considered. With regard to these crimes there is not just the problem of the *actus reus* (e.g. does sexual penetration cover penetration of an artificial vagina?) but also of the *mens rea*, which was changed in 2003, to include the state of mind of a man who decided on unreasonable grounds that the victim was consenting. Section 1(1) of the 2003 Act defines rape thus:

A person (A) commits an offence if –
(a) he intentionally penetrates the vagina, anus or mouth of another person (B) with his penis,
(b) B does not consent to the penetration, and
(c) A does not reasonably believe that B consents.

Sub-section (2) adds: 'Whether a belief is reasonable is to be determined having regard to all the circumstances, including any steps A has taken to ascertain whether B consents.'

Despite the difficulties of interpretation of the *actus reus* words, there is an even greater problem, that of consent. The current law revolves around three situations: in some situations lack of consent is irrebuttably presumed (s 76 of the Act); in other circumstances there is a rebuttable presumption of lack of consent (s 75 of the Act); and thirdly, there exist situations in which there is a lack of consent where neither s 76 nor s 75 applies. In this third scenario s 74 defines consent thus: 'a person consents if he agrees by choice, and has freedom and capacity to make that choice.'

Underlying this chapter is the extension of the law of rape over the last twenty or so years: married men may now be convicted: see the House of Lords decision in *R v R* at the start of the 1990s; boys used to be irrebuttably presumed not to be capable of sexual intercourse but that exception was abolished in the 1990s; rape, which previously had to be on a female victim, was extended to male victims in the mid-1990s and in turn buggery of a female without consent became rape; and the 2003 Act extends the coverage of rape from penetration of the vagina and anus to penetration of the mouth.

References

Reports

Criminal Law Revision Committee 15th Report, *Sexual Offences*, Cmnd 9213 (1984)

Home Office Consultation Paper, *Setting the Boundaries: Reforming the Law on Sex Offences* (2000)

Home Office White Paper, *Protecting the Public*, Cm 5668 (2002)

Law Commission Consultation Paper no. 134, *Consent and Offences against the Person* (1994)

Law Commission Consultation Paper no. 139, *Consent in the Criminal Law* (1995)

Law Commission Report no. 177, *A Criminal Code for England & Wales* (1989)

Law Commission Working Paper no. 116, *Rape within Marriage* (1989)

Books

Hale, M. *Pleas of the Crown* (E. & R. Nutt and R. Gooding, 1736)

Kelly, L., Lovett, J. and Regan, L. *A Gap or Chasm? Attrition in Reported Rape*, Home Office Research Study no. 293 (2005)

Ruparel, C. *The Nature of Rape of Females in the Metropolitan Police District*, Home Office Research Study no. 247 (2004)

Smith, L. J. F. *Concerns about Rape*, Home Office Research Study no. 106 (1989)

Journals

Scutt, J. A. 'Consent in rape: the problem of the marriage contract' (1977) 3 Monash ULR 255

Further reading

Amnesty International ICM opinion poll, *Stop violence against women* (2005)

Card, R. *Sexual Offences: The New Law* (Jordans, 2004)

Cowan, S. 'The trouble with drink: intoxication, (in)capacity and the evaporation of consent to sex' (2008) 41 Akron LR 899

Dingwall, G. 'Addressing the boundaries of consent in rape' (2002) 13 *King's College Law Journal* 71

Elliott, C. and de Than, C. 'The case for a rational reconstruction of consent in criminal law' (2007) 70 MLR 225

Finch, E. and Munro, V. G. 'Breaking boundaries? Sexual consent in the jury room' (2006) 26 LS 303

Gardner, J. and Shute, S. 'The wrongness of rape', in J. Horder (ed.), *Oxford Essays in Jurisprudence* 4th edn (Oxford University Press, 2000)

Gardner, S. 'Appreciating Olugboja' (1996) 16 LS 275

Gross, H. 'Rape, moralism and human rights' [2007] Crim LR 220

Her Majesty's Crown Prosecution Service and Her Majesty's Inspectorate of Constabulary *Without Consent – a Report on the Joint Review of the Investigation and Prosecution of Rape Offences* (2007)

Horder, J. (2001) 'How culpability can, and cannot, be denied in under-age sex crimes' Crim LR 15

Lacey, N. 'Beset by boundaries: The Home Office Review of sex offences' [2001] Crim LR 3

McGregor, J. *Is it Rape?* (Ashgate, 2005)

Munro, V. E. 'Concerning consent: standards of permissibility in sexual relations' (2005) 25 OJLS 335

Power, M. 'Towards a redefinition of the *mens rea* in rape' (2003) 23 OJLS 379

Rumney, P. 'The review of sex offences and rape law reform: another false dawn?' (2001) 64 MLR 890

Rumney, P. and Morgan-Taylor, M. 'Recognising the male victim: gender neutrality and the law of rape' (1997) 26 A-A LR 330

Schulhofer, S. 'Taking sexual autonomy seriously: rape law and beyond' (1992) 11 *Law and Philosophy* 35

Tadros, V. 'Rape without consent' (2006) 26 OJLS 449

Temkin, J. *Rape and the Legal Process* 2nd edn (Oxford University Press, 2002)

Temkin, J. and Ashworth, A. 'The Sexual Offences Act 2003: (1) Rape, sexual assaults and the problems of consent' [2004] Crim LR 328

Temkin, J. and Krahé, B. *Sexual Assault and the Justice Gap: A Question of Attitude* (Hart, 2008)

Wells, C. 'Law reform, rape and ideology' (1985) 12 JLS 63

For a symposium on consent, see (1996) 2 *Legal Theory* 89–164.

For the proposals for reform which led to the 2003 Act, see the Sex Offences Review Committee, *Setting the Boundaries*, 2 vols, Home Office, 2000. Volume 2 includes the Law Commission's Policy Paper, *Consent in Sex Offences*.

For current proposals for reform see Office for Criminal Justice Reform *Convicting Rapists and Protecting Victims – Justice for Victims of Rape*, 2006 and HM Crown Prosecution Service Inspectorate and HM Inspectorate of Constabulary, *Without Consent*, 2007.

For the view of the Scottish Law Commission see Discussion Paper 131, *Rape and Other Sexual Offences*, 2006.

Visit **www.mylawchamber.co.uk/jefferson** to access exam-style questions with answer guidance, multiple choice quizzes, live weblinks, an online glossary, and regular updates to the law.

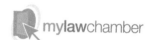

Use **Case Navigator** to read in full some of the key cases referenced in this chapter:

DPP v Morgan [1975] 2 All ER 347

15

Theft and robbery

Introduction to the Theft Act 1968

The Theft Act 1968 was based on the Eighth Report of the Criminal Law Revision Committee, *Theft and Related Offences*, Cmnd 2977, 1966. The Committee decided that the law required thorough overhauling because it was complex and failed to tackle several instances of dishonest dealing with property. The 1968 Act was to be a short, simple measure, a fresh start, free from technicalities and the first step towards codification of the criminal law. Old terminology such as larceny, larceny by a trick, false pretences and embezzlement were replaced by modern terms. The Committee replaced 'fraudulently converts' in the old law of larceny with 'dishonestly appropriates' in the new law of **theft** (para 35). No change in the meaning was intended. It is partly for this reason that *Gomez* [1993] AC 442 has been trenchantly criticised: it adopted a much wider meaning of appropriation than did the pre-1968 law. It may be argued that in simplifying Parliament left too much of the law to be worked out by the judges. Some words which had a fixed meaning under the old law were retained, e.g. 'receive' in handling, and 'menaces' in blackmail. Some parts of the new law are best explained by reference to the defects of the old, e.g. s 5(4) is difficult to understand without reference to *Moynes v Coopper* [1956] 1 QB 439. The court called for reform of the law to convict the accused and Parliament obliged.

Unfortunately the 1968 Act has not turned out in the way that its progenitors hoped. Interpretation of the Act has led to difficulties even in simple situations. For example, does one appropriate property for the purposes of theft when one touches it, takes it, or puts it in one's bag? Part of the Act, since repealed, was called by the Court of Appeal in *Royle* [1971] 1 WLR 1764 a 'judicial nightmare'. In *Hallam* [1995] Crim LR 323 the Court of Appeal said that the 1968 Act was in urgent need of simplification and modernisation because juries should not have to 'grapple with concepts couched in the arcane Franglais of "chose in action"' and public money should not be spent on 'hours of semantic argument divorced from the real merits of the case'. (Interestingly, the term 'chose in action' does not appear in the statute.) Offences overlap, and there are problems with key concepts such as dishonesty. Where the statute looks as if it does not cover certain forms of conduct the courts have sometimes read the statute widely to convict the 'manifestly guilty'. The phenomenon is especially common in theft when a charge would have been more appropriately brought under s 15, obtaining property by deception (since repealed).

Time is ripe for a thorough review of the Act. There are also difficulties in seeing how the Theft Act offences relate to civil law concepts, such as restitution and equity on which they are based. Despite criticism it is confidently asserted that criminal law judges cannot jettison civil law notions. Only by knowing when property belongs to another can one say that a person is or is not guilty of theft, and these concepts are civil law ones, not ones created *ad hoc*. As Lord Hobhouse put it in *Hinks* [2001] 2 AC 241: 'Section 5 and, particularly, s 5(4), demonstrates that the 1968 Act has been drafted so as to take account of and require reference to the civil law of property, contract and restitution.' Lord Diplock in *Treacy v DPP* [1971] AC 537 said that the Act was 'expressed in simple language as used and understood by ordinary literate men and women'. Interpretation of the statute has, however, been technical. Since some terms such as 'trust' are technical, a technical interpretation cannot always be avoided. For example, even a literate person may not know the meaning of 'equitable interest' in s 5(1). It is a question of law whether a certain legal relationship existed between the parties such as a trust: *Clowes (No. 2)* [1994] 2 All ER 316 (CA).

Moreover, changes in what constitutes property in civil law will have unforeseen consequences in criminal law. One debatable issue is that of property purchased with bribes, discussed below: see the consideration of *Attorney-General of Hong Kong v Reid* [1994] 1 AC 324 (PC) below. A simpler illustration is the consequential effect which would occur if trade secrets were held to be property in civil law. They would presumably also be property for the purpose of criminal law including the Theft Act 1968. The case of *Hinks*, discussed below, demonstrates, however, that even the House of Lords is willing to permit civil and criminal law to diverge.

The 2000 British Crime Survey estimated that in 1999 there were a little over 14.7 million crimes, of which some 1,284,000 were burglaries or attempted burglaries. There were about 1.7 million thefts. The authors, C. Kershaw *et al.* (Home Office Statistical Bulletin, 2000), estimated that only 23 per cent of offences are reported to the police. Some 95 per cent of all offences in England and Wales are property-related. S. Nicholas, D. Povey, A. Walker and C. Kershaw *Crime in England and Wales 2004–2005* (Home Office, 2005) said at p. 58 that there were 3,324,000 thefts.

Theft

Basic definition

Section 1(1) of the 1968 Theft Act contains a basic definition of theft: 'the appropriation of property belonging to another with the intention of permanently depriving [him] of it'. The *mens rea* is 'dishonesty' and 'the intention permanently to deprive'. The *actus reus* is 'appropriates', 'property' and 'belonging to another' (Fig. 15.1). Sections 2–6 offer partial or sometimes complete explanations of these concepts. The penalty is seven years' maximum imprisonment: Criminal Justice Act 1991, s 26(1), amending the Theft Act 1968, s 7. The alteration is the result of a recommendation in the White Paper, *Crime, Justice and Protecting the Public*, Cm 965, 1990, para 3.14. Previously the maximum had been 10 years.

Lack of consent to the appropriation by the owner need not be proved: *Lawrence v MPC* [1972] AC 626. Lack of consent is therefore not a constituent element in theft. It is, however, relevant to the other elements. If the owner agrees to the appropriation, the accused may not be dishonest. Moreover, once the elements of theft are satisfied, it does

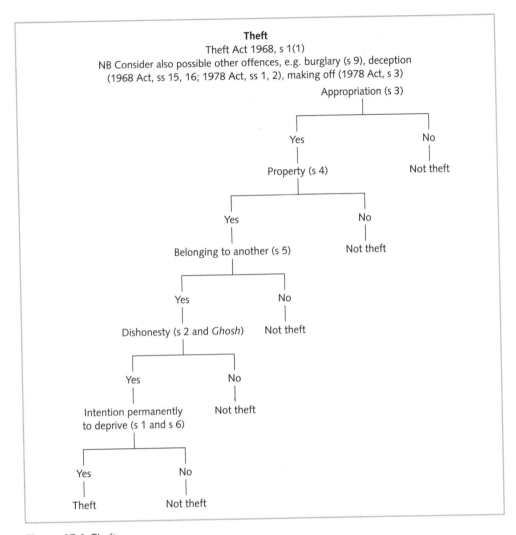

Figure 15.1 Theft

not matter that the victim has no civil law remedy. Because an appropriation of property belonging to another may be done by an honest person as well as a dishonest one, it is the *mens rea* of theft which is of great importance. The *actus reus* is 'neutral', contrary, it is suggested, to what Parliament intended. Performing the *actus reus* does not distinguish the thief from an innocent person. Dishonesty is now the crux of theft. For this reason it is considered before the *actus reus*, an arrangement which would normally be strange but one which is appropriate in the light of its importance.

It should be noted that theft forms part of the definition of the crimes of robbery, burglary and handling.

Dishonesty

Dishonesty replaced the concept of fraud in the previous law. Fraud was a legal concept, but dishonesty is largely a matter for the jury. It seems that the framers of the Theft Act

1968 wanted to update the terminology, but not to change the concept. Many of the offences under the Theft Act 1968 and all of those in the Theft Act 1978 require dishonesty. Even when dishonesty is not expressly mentioned, it may be an ingredient. For example, robbery requires a theft, which in turn requires dishonesty. One form of burglary consists of entering a building as a trespasser with intent to steal; again theft with its element of dishonesty is needed. A similar point can be made about going equipped, a crime contrary to s 25 of the 1968 Act. Perhaps half of all cases tried at the Crown Court involve dishonesty: the importance of this concept cannot be exaggerated.

The Act states in s 1(2): 'It is immaterial whether the appropriation is made with a view to gain or is made for the thief's own benefit.' A person can therefore steal property by destroying it and it is irrelevant that the item is of no use to the thief. In one case, **Welsh** [1974] RTR 478, the accused poured a sample of his own urine down a sink; the sample would have been tested. He was guilty of theft despite the fact he had poured it away. The Criminal Law Revision Committee's Eighth Report, *Theft and Related Offences*, Cmnd 2977, 1966, gave another example. The accused can be guilty of theft even though the property appropriated is useless to him. Section 1(2) also has the effect that, while in the general run of events the victim will have been made poorer by the accused's theft, there is no requirement for the victim to become poorer as a result of the theft: **Wheatley** v **Commissioner of Police of the British Virgin Islands** [2006] 1 WLR 1683 (PC), dealing with legislation identical to the Theft Act 1968. The appellant argued that the government had lost nothing when he made a contract with companies to re-erect a wall which had fallen down. The Privy Council advised that there could be dishonesty when a contract had been agreed on at an appropriate price.

(a) Section 2(1)

Dishonesty is partly defined in the statute. The Criminal Law Revision Committee did not totally define dishonesty because 'dishonesty is something which laymen can easily recognise when they see it' (at 20). By s 2(1) the accused is not dishonest if he:

s 2(1)(a) believes he has a legal right to deprive the victim of the property;

s 2(1)(b) believes that the victim would have consented to the appropriation of the property, if he had known of the circumstances;

s 2(1)(c) finds or otherwise appropriates property, when he believes that the owner, possessor or controller cannot reasonably be found.

Section 2(1)(a) gives the accused a defence if he makes a mistake of civil law. (If the accused does in fact have the right in law to deprive the owner of the property, there is no need to consider the effect of s 2(1)(a) because there is no *actus reus* of theft.) There is no need for the mistake to be a reasonable one. A mistake of criminal law does not bring s 2(1)(a) into play. Examples of (a) are a belief that the accused was allowed to borrow the item (**Kell** [1985] Crim LR 239 (CA)) and where the accused took pottery in lieu of wages (**Wootton** [1990] Crim LR 201 (CA)). A belief that the owner has consented to the appropriation falls within (a) above. A claim of a moral right to the asset does not fall within s 2(1)(a), but may be not dishonest within the principles to be discussed shortly. In **Forrester** [1992] Crim LR 793 (CA) the accused burst into a house in which he formerly had a tenancy. The landlord had retained his £200 deposit. The accused thought that the deposit was withheld unfairly because the landlord had no justification for asking him to leave. He took various items, intending to keep ones to the amount of over £200 in order to force the landlord to hand back the deposit. He would sell the items if the deposit was not returned, paying over the excess. Since he did not believe that he had a legal right, s 2(1)(a) did not apply. An example of (b) is *Flynn* [1970] Crim LR 118, where a cinema manager took £6 as an advance on his salary. Section 2(1)(b) provided that the accused is not guilty only when he believes the owner would have consented to the appropriation in the particular circumstances of the appropriation. A belief that a neighbour would have consented to your using her lawnmower to cut your lawn does not allow you to use it to mow the whole estate's verges. A person can be convicted of stealing from a company of which he is the controller. The company is separate from the controller and would not have consented to being divested of its property: *Attorney-General's Reference (No. 2 of 1982)* [1984] QB 624 (CA). As for (c), there will be an appropriation for the purposes of theft if the accused cannot at first discover the owner but later finds out the identity. In those circumstances whether the accused is dishonest falls outwith s 2(1) but within the principles discussed below.

An example of s 2(1)(c) is where clothing is left in a locker at a swimming pool. The local authority cannot readily trace the owner normally. It is not dishonest when it sells the clothes to defray expenses. It should also be noted that for the purposes of theft property may belong to more than one party. A lost golf ball may be owned by the golfer but possessed or controlled by the landowner. The golfer's name may not easily be discovered, but it may be easy to determine the landowner's identity. Section 2(1)(c) extends beyond people who find things to anyone who assumed one or more of the rights of the owner. If a cobbler repairs shoes and the owner does not reclaim them he is not dishonest if he sells them to recoup his expenses provided that he believes that 'the person to whom the property belongs cannot be discovered by taking reasonable steps'. The word 'cannot' has not been considered by the courts. It is suggested that it means 'cannot in the ordinary run of things'. It is often possible to find the owner by taking some steps, though what is reasonable is a matter for the jury. In any event if the accused does not fall within (c), he may fall within the general test, below.

Throughout s 2(1) an honest belief suffices. The accused does not, for instance, need to have reasonable grounds for his belief that the owner would have consented, had he known of the circumstances. An illustration is *Holden* [1991] Crim LR 478 (CA). The accused claimed that he had been granted permission by a supervisor to take scrap tyres from a certain firm. He had previously worked for the firm and was due to go back to it. He believed on those grounds that he had a legal right to the tyres.

This partial definition of dishonesty applies to theft and other Theft Act offences where theft is an ingredient. It does not, e.g., apply to the offence of abstracting electricity. The different definitions open up the possibility of divergent interpretations. Furthermore, in the Theft Act 1968 as enacted seven offences expressly mentioned dishonesty, but six do not. In blackmail the equivalent of dishonesty is an unwarranted demand. The Act has a further provision on dishonesty in theft. By s 2(2), 'A person's appropriation of property may be dishonest notwithstanding that he is willing to pay for the property.' Therefore, an individual can be guilty of theft even though he had £1,000 in his purse and said on arrest that he would pay for the items shoplifted. The Act states 'may be' because there may be circumstances in which an accused is otherwise honest, e.g. because the facts fall within s 2(1).

(b) Ghosh

Even if the accused does not fall within s 2(1), he may still be not dishonest for the purposes of the Act. The first major case in this area was *Feely* [1973] QB 530. The accused took money from his employers, intending to repay. The Court of Appeal ruled that outside s 2(1) the question of dishonesty was for the jury applying 'the current standards of ordinary decent people'. The jury does not consider whether the accused thought that what he had done was dishonest or not. For example, even if a person of high moral standards thought that what he was doing was dishonest, that state of mind is irrelevant. One looks to see whether ordinary decent people would consider it dishonest. The court said that dishonesty can be equated with immorality. The case itself was concerned with the substitution of money but was applied generally to other instances of dishonest conduct. With regard to the taking of money, the accused has the intention permanently to deprive the victim of the coins and notes actually taken, even though he means to replace them with an equivalent amount. The law was simple to state and was in accordance with **Brutus v Cozens** [1973] AC 854, where the House of Lords held that ordinary English words such as 'insulting' should be left for the jury. It is also in accord with the Eighth Report of the CLRC, *Theft and Related Offences*, Cmnd 2977, 1966, which was the basis of the Theft Act 1968. As stated at the start of this chapter, the Committee wished to substitute 'dishonestly' for 'fraudulently' because the former concept would be understood more easily by juries than the latter.

 Feely was applied to since repealed offences of obtaining by deception in **Greenstein** [1975] 1 WLR 1353 (CA). The same test applies now throughout the Theft Acts and in conspiracy to defraud and fraudulent trading. It is that stated in **Ghosh** [1982] QB 1053 (CA). The accused is dishonest if his conduct is dishonest according to the current standards of ordinary decent people and if the accused knows that his conduct is regarded as dishonest according to those standards. In **Ghosh**, the accused, a surgeon acting as a locum in a hospital, claimed fees for performing operations. Those fees were not owing to him. He was charged with dishonestly obtaining money by deception, contrary to s 15(1) of the 1968 Theft Act. He was found guilty and the Court of Appeal in a reserved judgment dismissed his appeal.

The twofold test was:

(a) The jury are to apply the 'ordinary standards of reasonable and honest people': if the accused is not dishonest by those standards he is not guilty.

(b) If he is dishonest by the first test: 'The jury must consider whether the defendant himself must have realised that what he was doing was by those standards dishonest.' The accused is dishonest if he acts in a way which he knows ordinary people would regard as dishonest. A juror should not ask whether what the accused did was dishonest by that juror's standards but by the standards of reasonable and honest people. A person who is fervently anti-vivisection should not use his own standards to judge an accused who broke into a laboratory to release rabbits. The court gave illustrations of ardent anti-vivisectionists who raided laboratories, and Robin Hood. The court thought that these people were dishonest, though reasonable jurors may disagree. On the **Ghosh** approach an accused who steals from the rich to give to the poor must be acquitted if he believes that reasonable people would regard what he did as not dishonest. Before **Ghosh** and its precursors the judge could rule that the evidence adduced was insufficient to negate dishonesty and Robin Hood would have been dishonest. The test should be put to the jury in the order stated: **Green** [1992] Crim LR 292 (CA). If the accused knows that what he is doing is illegal, he may still be acting honestly. Assume that there is an express or implied term in his contract of employment as a shop assistant that he will not take money from the till for his own purposes. He does so. He is liable for breach of contract and for the tort of conversion. Nevertheless, a jury might find that he was not acting dishonestly because ordinary decent people might so regard his behaviour. Some defendants may believe that using the contents of the stationery cupboard at work for their own purposes is not dishonest and may argue that they believe that ordinary decent people think the way they do. The fact that a witness believed the accused to be acting dishonestly is not conclusive: *Green*. While 'dishonesty' is an ordinary word, it is inappropriate to consider whether the accused himself thought that he was acting dishonestly. The jury does not, e.g., ask whether the defendant knew that he was acting recklessly when he is charged with a crime of recklessness. The standard should be an objective one.

The *Ghosh* definition applies to fraud offences: *Lockwood* [1986] Crim LR 244 (CA). The court said that the *Ghosh* test of 'reasonable and honest people' applied to businesspersons. There was no test of: how would a businessperson have reacted? The difference between *Feely* and *Ghosh* should be noted. In *Feely* the test of dishonesty was objective. In *Ghosh* the state of the mind of the accused is relevant. The court did not say why the test changed from 'ordinary decent people' to 'reasonable and honest people': are honest people different from ordinary ones? The test for dishonesty of 'reasonable and honest people' is circular. The test lays down a criterion of what might be called 'objective morality'. The jury looks both at the objective nature of the act and at the accused's own state of mind.

The same facts may fall within both s 2(1) and *Ghosh*. If the accused believes that the property he has appropriated is his own or if he believes that he is legally entitled to do as he did ('claim of right'), he is not dishonest under both. A *Ghosh* direction is sufficient: no reference need be made to s 2(1). If, however, he realised that what he was doing was dishonest by the standards of reasonable people, he is it seems honest within s 2(1) but dishonest under *Ghosh*. Such a scenario is unlikely to arise in practice.

A recent example of the application of *Ghosh* is *Atkinson* [2003] EWCA Crim 3031, [2004] Crim LR 226. The accused was charged with false accounting, an offence to which *Ghosh* applies. It was argued that she had submitted false claims relating to prescription forms. The first instance judge directed the jury that the accused would not be guilty if she was careless or acting under stress but would be if she 'knew that what she was doing would result in her submitting prescription forms containing false information'. The jury convicted and the Court of Appeal upheld the direction.

(c) Application and criticism of *Ghosh*

The *Ghosh* test may be quite difficult to explain to a jury. The jury embodies in one sense community values. The further away from those values the accused's beliefs are, the more likely he is to be acquitted. An accused who believes it is socially acceptable to eat a supermarket's food in the store and leave without paying for it is more likely to be acquitted than one who does not. Similarly, a person who believes it socially acceptable to keep overpayments from bookmakers or to take his employers' stationery home is entitled to be judged on his beliefs. It appears to be contrary to what the Criminal Law Revision Committee and Parliament intended when they established 'dishonesty' in the 1968 Act. There is a linked issue. If the law of theft exists to protect property, it is strange that it does not do so when the jury decides that the accused was not dishonest. Judges have the duty of interpreting the law and juries apply the law so interpreted to the facts but the *Ghosh* test places them in control of the former function as well as the latter. Furthermore, juries can reach inconsistent verdicts. What is dishonest in York may not be dishonest in London, and since dishonesty is judged by current standards, what was not dishonest in 1995 may be dishonest in 2010. Moreover, the *Ghosh* approach downgrades respect for property. There seems to be little evidence to support the view that 12 persons chosen at random can decide what is dishonest better than could Parliament or the judges. The decision creates a distinction between dishonesty in s 2(1) and dishonesty outside of it. Section 2(1) looks at the genuineness of the belief, not at the reasonableness of it. Under *Ghosh* the test is partly objective. In *Small* (1988) 86 Cr App R 170, the Court of Appeal held that unreasonable belief could be an honest belief, but reasonableness of the belief was 'a strong factor' in determining the honesty of the belief. With regard to blackmail the Criminal Law Revision Committee did not want a test that the accused's belief had to be reasonable because such could be out of line with the rest of the 1968 Act, yet *Feely* and *Ghosh* do just that in relation to dishonesty falling outside of s 2(1). Furthermore, some ordinary-language terms in the Act are matters of law, such as 'makes any . . . demand' in blackmail (*Treacy v DPP*, above). It may well be that when Parliament enacted the three exemptions from dishonesty, it intended there to be no others, but *Ghosh* creates an exception of undefined width. Countries which have adopted the English Theft Act as their model have not applied *Ghosh*. For example, in *Williams* [1985] NZLR 294 the Court of Appeal held that the test in New Zealand was subjective. An accused's belief in the morality of his conduct is a defence. The House of Lords has not had the opportunity of considering *Ghosh*.

The courts have held that if there is no evidence that the accused believed that he was not dishonest by the standards of ordinary people, the judge need not give a direction in *Ghosh* terms: *Roberts* (1987) 84 Cr App R 117 on handling; *Price* (1989) 90 Cr App R 409 on deception; *Miles* [1992] Crim LR 657 and *Buzalek* [1991] Crim LR 131 (CA) on fraudulent trading; *Wheelhouse* [1994] Crim LR 756 (CA) on burglary; and *Squire* [1990] Crim LR 341 on conspiracy to defraud. The same is also true of theft. A recent authority *Wood* [2002] EWCA Crim 832 the court stated that: 'the *Ghosh* direction . . . is best left only for that kind of case where there is a dispute about whether ordinary people would have different views from a defendant as to whether what he was doing was honest or not'. In other words, the whole *Ghosh* instruction is only needed where the accused asserts that what he did was not dishonest, no matter what others thought. After all shoplifting is dishonest according to current standards of ordinary decent people. It need not be decided in every case. Indeed in *Price* Lord Lane CJ said that in a majority of cases a *Ghosh* direction was inappropriate. In *O'Connell* (1992) 94 Cr App R 39, the accused had obtained several mortgage advances on houses. He said that he intended to repay the sums by renting out the dwellings or by selling them. He gave evidence that he did not regard the giving of a false name on an application form as being dishonest. The Court of Appeal held that the trial judge was incorrect to hold that such evidence should be excluded. By stating that he intended to fulfil his contractual obligations by repaying the loan, there arose the question whether he was dishonest in giving a false name. While the fulfilling of the obligations or the intention to repay is *per se* not dishonest it is evidence that the accused was not dishonest under *Ghosh*. *O'Connell* was applied in *Clarke*, unreported, 2 April 1996. The accused falsely represented that he had been a member of the Fraud Squad and a court bailiff, in order to secure work as a private investigator. The trial judge excluded evidence that the accused believed that he could do the work. The Court of Appeal held that such evidence was relevant to dishonesty. If the accused admits that his conduct was dishonest according to current standards of decent people, there is no need for a direction on this first part of the *Ghosh* test: *Thompson*, unreported, 1988 (CA).

Where the case is apt for a *Ghosh* direction, the whole test must be given, not just the first part: *Ravenshad* [1990] Crim LR 398 (CA) and *Brennan* [1990] Crim LR 118 (CA) (on handling). The fact that the accused was suspicious that barrels of lager were stolen was not sufficient. The exact words should preferably be given: *Ravenshad*, *Vosper* (1990) *The Times*, 16 February and *Hyam* [1997] Crim LR 419 (CA). To do so will as a minimum reduce appeals. The court in *Gohill v DPP* [2006] EWCA Crim 2894 held that no reasonable person would say that the manager of a tool hire shop was not dishonest when he allowed customers to borrow items for short periods of time without payment and he would alter the records to show that the items had been faulty or wrongly chosen. The case was remitted to determine whether he himself thought that what he did was dishonest by the ordinary standards of reasonable and honest people.

It should be noted that (a) where the accused's behaviour falls within s 2(1), *Ghosh* is irrelevant (*Wootton*, above); (b) the accused may act dishonestly even though he did something which the civil law allows him to do, such as retain the overpayment of a bet (*Gilks* [1972] 1 WLR 1341); and (c) as a result of *Lawrence v MPC*, above, and later cases a person may be dishonest despite the fact that the owner has consented to the appropriation.

In *Forrester*, above, the Court of Appeal left open the point whether an accused was not dishonest when he knew that what he was doing was unlawful. The general view of commentators is that under s 2(1)(a) and *Ghosh* it is the accused's belief that matters, not whether it is illegal in fact.

There was some discussion of dishonesty in *Hinks* [2001] 2 AC 241, which is noted below under 'Appropriation'. Lord Hutton dissented on the correct direction on dishonesty. The case involved an accused who induced a man with learning difficulties to transfer some £60,000 to her. She contended that he had given her the money of his own free will. Lord Hutton said that if her contention was correct, she was not dishonest. In cases with such facts he stated that the judge should instruct the jurors that they could not convict unless the donor lacked the mental capacity to make the gift and the donee knew of that incapacity. The direction is more specific than *Ghosh* and is tailored to the facts. It is suggested that Lord Hutton's speech is the way forward out of one of the uncertainties into which *Ghosh* put the law. It may take some time for precedents to build up, but in time the law will become more certain than it is at present, avoiding the charge that English law is inconsistent with the European Convention on Human Rights. See below for more on the Convention. However, it must be emphasised that Lord Hutton was dissenting and that the majority view in *Hinks* was that the issue of dishonesty when the issue does not fall within s 2(1) is resolved by *Ghosh*. The appellant's attempt to rely on Lord Hutton's remarks in *Wheatley v Commissioner of Police of the British Virgin Islands*, above, was firmly rejected by the Privy Council. On the facts *Ghosh* was applied, and the appellant was dishonest despite the fact that he, a government employee, had entered into a contract for a fair price for the re-erecting of a wall.

One academic point in *Ghosh* deserves consideration. Two problematical areas in modern-day criminal law are dishonesty and intention. With regard to the latter the House of Lords has stated that intention is an ordinary English word which in most eventualities the judge should leave undefined. The jury, however, does not ask whether the accused believed he was acting with the relevant state of mind, but under the Theft Acts as well as offences of fraud the jury must acquit if the accused believed that what he did was not dishonest by the standards of ordinary decent people. If the accused falls below that standard, it seems strange to inquire whether he knew that he fell below it. Both intention and dishonesty are questions for the jury, but are treated in different ways.

What the Court of Appeal wanted to do in **Ghosh** was to punish only those people to whom 'moral obloquy' was attached. To illustrate this proposition the court took the example of a person who comes to England and Wales from a country where public transport is free. In England and Wales public transport is not free but the foreigner believes it is. The court said that he was dishonest by the standards of ordinary decent people: 'His conduct, judged objectively by what he has done, is dishonest.' To exonerate him the court invented the second stage: did he believe that reasonable people would regard his behaviour as not dishonest? Surely, however, the court dealt with the first stage wrongly. The accused was not dishonest, judged objectively as well as subjectively. The question might be phrased as: do you believe it dishonest for a person not to pay a fare which he believes he does not owe? Unlike the Robin Hood example, the answer should be straightforward. If the foreigner is not dishonest at this first stage there is no need to ask the second question. Moreover, the hypothetical situation presented by the court is really one of mistake of fact. The foreigner thought that fares were not paid, whereas in truth they were. On the facts as he believed them to be he was not dishonest. The facts are not ones involving different beliefs about what is honest and what is not.

A more practical point is this. While it is often simple to say whether or not an accused is dishonest under the **Ghosh** test (e.g. it would not be difficult to hold that when he puts a frozen chicken into a large pocket on the inside of his coat he is dishonest), there are occasions where not all ordinary people would say that the accused was acting dishonestly. If he proposes to buy shares in an offer, has not enough money, but expects that the number of shares he will be allocated will be fewer than he asked for because of over-subscriptions, it is not self-evident to all that he is dishonest. Similarly, some people may think it dishonest to conceal the fact that a book is a valuable one whereas others may consider it honest. Certainly some people think it not dishonest to keep overpayments from shops and bookmakers, but others disagree.

(d) *Ghosh* and human rights

The law in **Ghosh** may come under attack as a result of the European Convention on Human Rights. Article 7, the rule against retroactivity, may come into play, because an accused may not be able to foresee when his behaviour will break the law: according to the European Court of Human Rights an offence cannot be defined by reference to moral obloquy, only by reference to the effect of the accused's behaviour. A Crown Court thought it was not incompatible in **Pattni** [2001] Crim LR 570 but that decision lacks authority and is concerned not with the Theft Acts offences but with another crime, cheating the Revenue. Possibly, the law in **Ghosh** may infringe Article 5(1), the right to liberty, because an accused may not foresee the possibility that what he did is dishonest for the purposes of English law. The European Court said *obiter* in **Hashman v UK** [2000] Crim LR 185 that the concept of dishonesty in the Theft Acts did not breach Article 5 but its mind was not on this issue.

(e) Reform of dishonesty

For the Law Commission's proposal to abolish dishonesty as a separate element in deception offences, see Chapter 16, below, which discusses Consultation Paper No. 155, *Legislating the Criminal Code: Fraud and Deception*, 1999. The Law Commission also agreed with the point made at the end of the previous paragraph, that the law in **Ghosh** is incompatible with Article 7 of the ECHR. However, in its Report No. 276, *Fraud*, 2002, the Law Commission resiled from its 1999 position. In para 5.18 it said: 'The fact that

Ghosh dishonesty leaves open a possibility of variance between cases with essentially similar facts is . . . a theoretical risk. Many years after its adoption, the *Ghosh* test remains, in practice, unproblematic. We also recognise the fact that the concept of dishonesty is now required in a very large number of criminal cases, so to reject it at this stage would have a far-reaching effect on the criminal justice system.'

Intention permanently to deprive

(a) Theft and borrowing

The second element of the *mens rea* in theft is the intention permanently to deprive. An intention to return sooner or later is not such an intent: *Warner* (1970) 55 Cr App R 93. As the Court of Appeal said, s 6 gives illustrations of 'intention permanently to deprive'; it does not water down the basic definition of theft found in s 1(1). To be precise, 'intention' and 'intention permanently to deprive' are not defined in the Act. Presumably 'intention' bears the same meaning as it does after *Woollin* [1999] AC 82. Section 6 merely gives three extensions to the concept of intent permanently to deprive: it does not define it. The word 'permanently' prevents most unauthorised borrowings being theft. Dishonest borrowings, even for a long time, are not theft. The Criminal Law Revision Committee justified non-liability in para 56 of *Theft and Related Offences*, Cmnd 2977, 1966. The moral considerations of dishonest borrowings were different from those of theft. Usually a borrowing is not as serious as a permanent taking. Such borrowings were not very common. Criminalising them would cover trivial matters, such as neighbours quarrelling over a lawnmower. To create a law would waste police time on minor matters. It would be especially hard on students. Additionally, it can nowadays be said (i.e. after the case of *Gomez*, above) that making dishonest borrowing into theft would place even more weight on the somewhat fragile concept of dishonesty than exists at present. Two instances of dishonest borrowing, removal of articles from buildings (s 11) and cars (s 12), are offences. The contrary arguments are these:

(a) If the crux of theft is the dishonest appropriation of another's property, the intention permanently to deprive seems otiose.

(b) The social importance of the accused's conduct does not depend on such an intention. After all there are many trivial thefts.

(c) If the victim wants the property during the time when the accused has dishonestly borrowed it, he cannot use it, whether or not the accused intends permanently to deprive. If a student wants this textbook for an exam in January, it is not to the point that he will get it back in February.

(d) Such an intent is not needed in most other Theft Acts offences such as obtaining a pecuniary advantage by deception (s 16).

(e) As we have seen, an intention to repay or substitute may be dishonest because the defendant cannot replace the very thing taken, yet if he intends to return the property itself, he is not guilty of theft because he does not have the intention permanently to deprive.

(f) Some items such as puffball skirts or gypsy tops are fashionable at one time but not trendy after; appropriating a child's toy and handing it back after its popularity has plummeted exemplifies the situation.

(g) It is not thought that the courts would be overwhelmed with cases.

The main argument to the contrary is that in respect of many items their value lies in the ability to use them at a particular time. Returning a lawnmower in February is no use when one wished to cut the grass over the previous summer.

Where there is no intent *permanently* to deprive, a conspiracy to defraud charge may lie. There may be one situation where an intention temporarily to deprive is caught by s 6(1). This possibility occurs where the victim has only an interest limited in time in the item and the accused intends to borrow it for longer than that person. For example, if the victim hires a skip from its owner for a week and the accused takes it away for longer than a week intending to return it, he has intended to deprive the victim of his whole interest. Towards him there is an intent permanently to deprive, and there is theft from him (though not from the owner).

(b) Section 6(1)

The concept is explained in s 6(1):

> A person appropriating property belonging to another without meaning the other permanently to lose the thing itself is nevertheless to be regarded as having the intention of permanently depriving the other of it if his intention is to treat the thing as his own to dispose of regardless of the other's rights; and a borrowing or lending of it may amount to so treating it if, but only if, the borrowing or lending is for a period and in circumstances making it equivalent to an outright taking or disposal.

The Court of Appeal in **Lloyd** [1985] QB 829 said that s 6 'sprouts obscurities at every phrase'. The basic thrust of it is that it should be looked at only exceptionally: **Lloyd**. Section 6(1) does not define intention permanently to deprive; instead it is a statutory extension of that concept. Most cases fall simply within s 1(1)'s basic definition of theft, which includes the phrase 'intention of permanently depriving', and there is no need to consider s 6. If I burn your £10 note, I do intend permanently to deprive you of it: one need not look to s 6(1) for guidance. Only in cases when the accused intends to return the property or it is not clear whether or not there is an intention permanently to deprive, where the accused acts 'without meaning the other permanently to lose the thing', need one look at s 6. If the accused intends the victim to get the property back, s 6(1) is relevant.

Lord Lane CJ thought that s 6(1) applied in only two circumstances, as can be seen from the wording of s 6(1): where the accused takes property and then offers it back to the owner (the so-called 'ransom' principle) and where the accused borrows or lends out the victim's property in circumstances 'equivalent to an outright taking or disposal'. It is also relevant where the accused deals with property in such a way that he knows that he is risking its loss: **Fernandes** [1996] 1 Cr App R 175 (CA), where the accused, a solicitor, invested money belonging to his clients in a firm of moneylenders, knowing the investment not to be a safe one. Otherwise only s 1(1) needs to be referred to. Therefore, s 6 is a deeming provision. According to **Warner**, s 6 clarifies and gives explanations of the requisite state of mind. In **Warner** the accused took a box of tools, intending to return them shortly. He was not guilty of theft because he had an intention to return, even though the handing back might be an indefinite period later. The Court of Appeal in **Fernandes** more recently said that the thrust of s 6 is the issue of whether the accused did intend 'to treat the thing as his own to dispose of regardless of the other's rights'. The rest of s 6(1) and (2) consists of illustrations of that issue. Auld LJ thought that Lord Lane CJ was wrong to restrict s 6(1) to the two situations he mentioned. Accordingly s 6(1) offers only a partial definition of 'intention of permanently depriving'.

(c) The interpretation of s 6(1)

Section 6 has been interpreted in the following ways. It speaks of intention permanently to deprive. There is no need for actual permanent deprivation; that is, s 6 belongs to *mens rea*, not *actus reus*. A person can be guilty of theft even though the owner gets the property back at some time. In the latter part of s 6(1) 'borrowing' is not restricted to a lender loaning something to a borrower. It covers a taking to which the victim has not agreed. In the first part selling the item back to the owner is treating it as one's own to dispose of regardless of the owner's rights.

The phrase 'equivalent to an outright taking' is obscure. It would seem to cover the situation where the accused takes the victim's umbrella dishonestly and the victim buys back the umbrella, not realising that it is his own. In ordinary language the accused does not intend to deprive the victim permanently of his umbrella, but s 6 deems there to be an intention permanently to deprive. The accused has appropriated one of the rights of the owner, the right to sell the article. This principle seems to have been applied in *Johnstone* [1982] Crim LR 454 (Crown Court). Two defendants were lorry drivers for a soft drinks company. They collected more bottles than they had accounted for. There was a deposit on each bottle. The bottles were dishonestly delivered to a shopkeeper, the third defendant, who was to get the deposits on the bottles from the company and share the money with the first two defendants. The bottles would therefore go back to the company, which would only pay one deposit on each bottle but the deposit would end up in the hands, not of the purchasers of the soft drinks, but of the defendants. The Recorder held that since the bottles would be returned to the company, the defendants did not intend to treat the bottles as their own to dispose of regardless of the company's rights. Therefore, there was no theft. If the accused takes the umbrella and leaves it on a bus, the victim is unlikely to get it back. The accused may have the requisite intent; if not s 6 can supply it. Another example may be a stolen cheque. In the ordinary course of banking the victim gets the cheque back but after encashment. It is no longer a valid cheque. The accused intends permanently to deprive the victim of a thing in action, the right to be paid the sum stated. The accused is deemed to have the intention permanently to deprive (see *Mulligan*, below).

The words 'to dispose of' are important. In *Cahill* [1993] Crim LR 141 one accused early one morning picked a newspaper out of a bundle outside a newsagent's. The second defendant had then picked it up. When a police car came level with them, the second accused dropped it. The first defendant said that the second was taking it to the police station because it was lost. (They had been drinking.) The court held that 'to dispose of' meant 'to get rid of', not 'to use'. The phrase must not be omitted when dealing with s 6(1). This issue is also noted in the next section of this book. If the accused intends to keep the thing until all the goodness or virtue has gone out of it that is equivalent to an outright taking. In *Lloyd* the accused had cinema films copied to be sold as videos and returned them. It was held that the virtue had not gone out of films as films. The public would still pay to see them at the cinema. The accused intended to cause loss to the cinema owners but that is not an intention permanently to deprive. To intend to use the property does not consitute an intent to deprive permanently. The position is different where the accused takes the victim's season ticket, uses it up and then hands it back. In those circumstances the accused has the intention permanently to deprive because of s 6(1). In *Bagshaw* [1988] Crim LR 321, the accused intended to return gas cylinders when he had finished with them. The court hinted that the accused was guilty of theft of the cylinders even though not all of the goodness had gone out of the property. They could on return have been refilled. (He should have been charged with theft of the gas.) There is debate whether in these circumstances s 6(1) is fulfilled. 'Equivalent to an outright taking' may cover a situation where the season ticket almost used up, but not where only one of the journeys is made or operas attended. The difficult, totally unresolved issue involves the situations in between. Lord Widgery CJ in *Lloyd* took a stronger view: '*all* its goodness or virtue' must go for s 6(1) to apply (emphasis added). The Court of Appeal, as stated above, held in *Fernandes* that s 6(1) was not restricted to two of the situations noted in this paragraph, attempting to sell the item back to the owner and giving it back when its value had been extinguished. The Court of Appeal had earlier spoken to similar effect in *Bagshaw*.

An example of intending to treat the thing as one's own to dispose of regardless of the other's rights is *Chan Man-sin* v *Attorney-General of Hong Kong* [1988] 1 All ER 1 (PC). The accused, an accountant, forged 10 cheques on two companies' bank accounts. He was charged with theft of the debt owed by the bank to its customers, the companies. The Privy Council rejected the argument that there was no theft because the companies had not been deprived of anything. He knew that the fraud would be uncovered. The companies stood to lose nothing. Their bank balances would not be affected. The Judicial Committee held that the accused purported to deal with the companies' property (the companies' accounts, things in action) regardless of their rights. Accordingly, the Hong Kong version of s 6(1) was satisfied. As a criticism it may be said that the Judicial Committee gave no weight to the words 'to dispose of' in s 6(1). See the next section in this book.

(d) Some examples of s 6(1) and its relationship with s 1(1)

Velumyl [1989] Crim LR 299 (CA)

The accused took £1,050 from a safe at work to lend to a friend. He expected to get the money back after the weekend. It was held that since the accused did not intend to return the particular banknotes, he had the intention permanently to deprive. His intention to repay the equivalent amount was relevant to dishonesty, not to the intention permanently to deprive. The same result will apply to petrol. You borrow my car, intending to replace the petrol you have used. You have the intention permanently to deprive me of the petrol. There is also nothing to stop this argument applying to things in action (see below for the definition of things in action). For example, if the accused obtains a mortgage loan by deception but intends to repay, since he cannot return the same thing in action, there is an intent permanently to deprive. Lord Goff in *Preddy* [1996] AC 815 declined to rule on this point.

Coffey [1987] Crim LR 498 (CA)

The accused obtained possession of machinery by a worthless cheque. He was charged with obtaining property by deception contrary to s 15 of the Theft Act 1968, which also requires an intention permanently to deprive. He claimed he intended to keep the machinery until a dispute with its owner had been settled. The court said that these facts gave rise to one of those rare cases where a direction on s 6(1) was needed. Did the accused intend that the period of his keeping the machinery would be so long as to amount to an outright taking? Was the accused treating the goods as his own to dispose of regardless of the owner's rights because the owner could get the machinery back only by giving in to the demands? The conviction was quashed because no such direction was given.

Scott [1987] Crim LR 235

The accused took a pair of curtains from a store. He returned them the next day, asking for a refund. It was held that he was treating the property as his own to dispose of regardless of the shop's rights contrary to s 6(1).

Mulligan [1990] STC 220 (CA)

Stolen Inland Revenue certificates about payment of tax were found in the accused's sock. It was alleged that the accused had stolen some of the vouchers in the book and sold them. The accused contended that the vouchers were worthless because their essential character had been destroyed. It was held that he had an intention permanently to deprive because he intended to sell them irrespective of the Revenue's rights, despite the fact that the vouchers would come back to the Revenue.

DPP v Lavender [1994] Crim LR 297 (DC)

The accused's conduct fell within s 6(1) when he removed doors from a council house which was being repaired and used them to replace doors on another council house where his girl-friend was the tenant. The court said that he intended to treat the doors as his own regardless of the owner's rights. A disposal covered dealing with property as in *Chan Man-sin v R*, above. The accused had done so. If this is correct, any moving of property is a disposal of it. One moot point is the meaning of 'to dispose of'. If the phrase means 'to get rid of', such as by burning or selling the doors he did not do so. See *Cahill*, above, which is inconsistent with *Lavender*. In *Cahill* the Court of Appeal accepted that 'to dispose of' meant 'to get rid of'. The accused did not get rid of the doors in *Lavender*. The point is aptly put by A. T. H. Smith, *Property Offences* (Sweet & Maxwell, 1994) para 6–33: 'one would not ordinarily say that a pianist disposes of his piano by playing it'. Yet such is the meaning attributed to the phrase in *DPP v Lavender*. Smith continued: '"dispose" as used in section 6 was fairly evidently used as the verb corresponding to "disposal", not disposition; indeed, sub-section (1) expressly links it with disposal ("equivalent to an outright disposal")'. On the view taken in *Lavender*, s 6(1) is otiose. By s 3(1) an intent to treat property as one's own is an appropriation.

Marshall [1998] 2 Cr App R 282

The defendants obtained London Underground tickets or Travelcards which had not expired. They argued that there was no intention permanently to deprive because London Underground would in due course get the items back. The tickets and cards remained the property of London Transport. The acquisition and resale of that property was an 'intention to treat the thing as his own to dispose of regardless of the other's rights', the rights being London Transport's exclusive right to sell tickets and Travelcards. It was irrelevant that the tickets and cards would come back to London Transport. Whether a jury would have found the defendants dishonest is debatable. The Court of Appeal did not discuss the logically prior question: to whom did this property belong at the time of the alleged appropriation? Whether the tickets and Travelcards belonged to London Underground is a matter of civil law. Who the owner is depends on the conditions of issue and whether these conditions were brought reasonably to the attention of the defendants. For further discussion see the 'ticket cases' in contract textbooks or Sir John Smith's article [1998] Crim LR 723.

(e) 'Intention', 'meaning' and 'the thing'

While no case has been discussed, 'intention' in the concept 'intention permanently to deprive' presumably bears that meaning which was discussed in Chapter 3.

Section 6(1) also includes the term 'meaning'. That term is another way of saying 'intending'.

The phrase 'the thing' means 'the property' mentioned in the opening words of s 6(1) and defined in s 4. If something is not property, the accused cannot have an intention permanently to deprive the owner of that property. In *Oxford v Moss* (1978) 68 Cr App R 183 (DC), an engineering student at a university read the contents of an examination paper. All the goodness and virtue went out of the paper by his action. The court held, however, that confidential information, i.e. the questions on the paper, was not property for the purpose of the Theft Act. Accordingly, the accused's behaviour did not amount to an intention permanently to deprive the owner of the information. If the accused had taken the paper itself, he would have been found guilty of theft of that piece of paper if he did not intend to return it, but that charge does not reflect the nub of what the accused did, namely cheat.

(f) Section 6(2)

Section 6(2) states:

> . . . where a person, having possession or control (lawfully or not) of property belonging to another, parts with the property under a condition as to its return which he may not be able to perform this (if done for purposes of his own and without the other's authority) amounts to treating the property as his own to dispose of regardless of the other's rights.

This subsection covers pawning property, intending to redeem it, without being able to guarantee that it will be returned, and gambling with the item. An alternative view is that the accused is guilty only if he foresaw that he might not be able to redeem the article, a proposition supported in *Fernandes*, above. This point awaits discussion. In either event the accused is guilty even though he does not *intend* permanently to deprive. It is in truth simply an example of the first part of s 6(1).

(g) The problem of conditional intention

Does the accused have the intention permanently to deprive when he has not made up his mind to keep the thing permanently? In *Easom* [1971] 2 QB 315, there was a spate of handbag-snatching in cinemas. A policewoman sat in a cinema with her bag attached to her wrist by cotton. A man sat next to her, took the bag and walked away. He opened the bag and found no money or other valuables. He discarded the bag and its contents. Edmund-Davies LJ said that conditional appropriation was not theft. The accused did not have the intention permanently to deprive at the relevant time. The charge nowadays would be one of attempted theft where the accused intended to steal anything of value or anything in a container such as a pocket, holdall or room. In criticism of *Easom* it might be said that the accused did intend permanently to deprive the owner at the time when he appropriated. This point was emphasised by the Full Court of the Supreme Court of Victoria in *Sharp v McCormick* [1986] VR 869, when it distinguished *Easom*. The accused was found with an item of apparatus for a car engine. The part belonged to his employers and he admitted dishonesty. His defence was that he intended to return it, should it have been the wrong size. Murray J said: 'If the facts in the present case establish that the defendant intended to keep the coil unless he *later* decided to return it then his intention *at the time of the appropriation* is sufficient to establish theft . . .'. The same might be said of the contents of the bag in **Easom**. It should be noted that certainly after **Gomez**, above, touching a handbag is an appropriation even though the accused has a conditional intent.

(h) Reform

The Law Commission, in its Consultation Paper No. 155, *Legislating the Criminal Code: Fraud and Deception*, 1999, provisionally proposed in the context of deception offences that temporary deprivations should be criminal unless, in its words, 'there is a significant countervailing argument'. The Commission's Report, *Fraud*, Law Com. No. 276, 2002, also proposed that obtaining property by deception (now repealed) should no longer require an intent permanently to deceive but no recommendation was made as to theft.

Appropriation

Under the old law of larceny the thing had to be carried away (asportation). Accordingly land could not be stolen. Now it can be, subject to the rules in s 4 (see below). The new word was 'appropriation', which it was hoped would be easily understood by the triers of fact. That hope has been dashed. Under present law an article can be stolen without being taken away. For example, if the accused puts his hand into the victim's pocket and grabs hold of a watch, there is an appropriation because of the definition found in s 3(1) of the Theft Act 1968: 'any assumption by a person of the rights of an owner amounts to an appropriation . . .'. The House of Lords in **Morris** [1984] AC 320 said that s 3 contained only a partial definition, as indeed did the Criminal Law Revision Committee in para 34 of the Eighth Report, *Theft and Related Offences*, Cmnd 2977, 1966. Therefore, a person may appropriate despite his actions not falling within s 3(1). Note also s 4(2)(d) noted below which states that severance of something forming part of land is an appropriation. One must, however, know that one is appropriating. An accused does not appropriate if his young son slips sweets into his shopping trolley at a supermarket.

(a) *Lawrence*

In **Lawrence** the House of Lords held that the accused can steal even though the victim consents to the taking. One can assume the rights of the owner even though the owner permitted one to do so. The House of Lords decision in **Lawrence**, that there may be theft despite the owner's consent, is applied generally to all forms of consent. In **Lawrence** the appropriation took place because an Italian student handed over extra money to a taxi-driver who had deceived him as to the taxi fare, but **Lawrence** is not restricted to instances where the accused appropriated by deception. Within the Theft Act there is an appropriation even though the owner consented to it. In **Rader** [1992] Crim LR 663 the Court of Appeal said that **Lawrence** applied even when the accused had taken the victim's money with his full consent. The victim gave him almost £10,000 on the latter's promise that he would return it on the due date with some sort of profit. The accused said that he was investing the money via an acquaintance in Miami, but that person had not repaid the money. His appeal was dismissed. The victim had consented to the taking but the facts constituted an appropriation.

(b) Morris

In **Morris** the accused took goods from the shelves of a self-service supermarket. He substituted lower price labels for those on the goods. He paid the lower price at the check-out but was then arrested and charged with theft. It should be noted that the accused would have had no defence to a charge of obtaining property by deception by switching the price labels. The question for the House of Lords was whether the swapping of the labels amounted to an appropriation. The principal speech was delivered by Lord Roskill. He said that the accused is guilty if he assumes *any* of the rights of the owner. He need not assume all of the rights. (Section 3(1) actually says 'any assumption . . . of the rights . . .', not 'any assumption of any right among the rights', is an appropriation. The construction of the phrase by the House of Lords is not the obvious interpretation. Only by knowing that this part of **Morris** represents the law can full weight be given to s 3(1).) The courts do not normally discuss which particular right has been assumed. The destruction of property or the accused's putting his hand over money in the victim's pocket will be an usurpation of one of the rights of the owner. This *dictum* was approved by the House of Lords in **Gomez** [1992] AC 442.

Academic criticism has been strong. Sir John Smith commented in 'Reforming the Theft Acts' (1996) 28 *Bracton Law Journal* 27 at 37, that in relation to this interpretation of s 3(1) 'Lord Keith thought this was obviously right. I think that, as a matter of statutory construction, it is obviously wrong . . .' Leigh in 'Some remarks on appropriation in the law of theft after *Morris*' (1985) 48 MLR 167 used the example of the accused's kicking a camel. He wrote that this act cannot be an appropriation. The law after **Morris** and **Gomez** is different. The camel-kicker is assuming one of the rights of the owner and therefore appropriates. There is no need for the accused to ride the camel into the sunset before an appropriation takes place.

This part of **Morris** was in turn approved in **Chan Man-sin v Attorney-General of Hong Kong**, above. A person who drew on someone's bank account was assuming the rights of the owner, and to be guilty the accused did not have to assume all rights of the owner. Presenting a cheque which was forged or otherwise not authorised constituted an appropriation, even though in law the transaction was a nullity and had no effect on the account holder's bank account because the bank would reimburse the loss. The English case of **Wille** (1988) 86 Cr App R 296 (CA) is to the same effect. A bank account was opened by a company. Each cheque had to be signed and countersigned. However, from the start the bank honoured cheques signed by one party only, the accused. It was held that by drawing on the company's bank account, the defendant had assumed the rights of an owner.

Morris also illustrates the proposition that the act by which the accused appropriates need not be the act by which he intends permanently to deprive. If an accused switches price labels on two items intending to pay a lower price for the higher priced item, he appropriates at that stage, even though he does not intend permanently to deprive until he reaches the cash till.

(c) Gomez

The principal authority on the definition of appropriation is **Gomez**.

Gomez [1992] AC 442

The accused, assistant manager of an electrical goods shop, agreed to supply items costing over £16,000 to a person in exchange for two stolen building society cheques. The accused and that person were acting together in a dishonest enterprise. The shop manager agreed to the transaction provided that the bank agreed that the cheques were acceptable. The accused later told the manager that the cheques were as good as cash, i.e. there was a fraudulent misrepresentation. The manager would not have agreed, had he known of the truth. The cheques were later dishonoured. The Court of Appeal held that there was no theft because the accused had not appropriated the property. The contract for the sale of goods was voidable not void, and had not been avoided when the goods were delivered. The manager had expressly authorised the goods to be removed. Accordingly, there was no misappropriation, and the conviction was quashed.

The House of Lords by a four to one majority reversed. The majority held that Lord Roskill had been incorrect to say *obiter* in **Morris**, above, that there was an appropriation only when the accused adversely interfered with or usurped one of the owner's rights. While adverse interference with or usurpation of the rights constituted one mode by which an appropriation may take place, the concept did not fully comprehend the situations in which an accused appropriated. Therefore, although the decision in **Morris** was correct, the reasoning was wrong: the law was wider than that stated in **Morris**. Applying **Lawrence**, above, the fact that the owner consented to the taking was irrelevant to the question whether or not there was an appropriation. Therefore, it did not matter that consent was induced by deception. Consent is not vitiated by fraud. Similarly, and contrary to Lord Roskill's *dictum*, the fact that the victim had expressly or impliedly authorised the accused to take an item was immaterial. Authorities which applied **Morris** were incorrect and those cases after **Morris** which sought to reconcile **Lawrence** and **Morris** were rejected. Therefore, an alleged fraudster did appropriate even though the victim consented to or authorised the transaction, and the House of Lords had been correct in **Lawrence** to hold that a conviction for theft was not dependent on the accused's appropriating without the consent of the owner. The Theft Act expressly noted where consent was relevant (e.g. in s 2(1)(b)). In the words of Lord Browne-Wilkinson 'appropriation' is 'an objective description of the act done irrespective of the mental state of either the owner or the accused'.

The dissenting judge, Lord Lowry, delivered a strong speech trenchantly criticising the decision of the majority. His criticisms were not answered by the majority. He said that as a matter of ordinary language appropriation meant 'take possession of, take to oneself, especially without authority'. It was a unilateral, not a consensual act. The majority had adopted the view that appropriation was a neutral term: a neutral act such as taking a can of beans from a supermarket shelf was converted into theft through the accused's state of mind. For them the lack of consent or authorisation by the owner was relevant only to *mens rea*, to dishonesty. For Lord Lowry it was by dictionary definition a constituent of appropriation. If he was wrong in his view that appropriation was not a neutral word, he said that if a meaning of a word in a statute was unclear, the report on which the statute was based would be looked at. In this instance the Theft Act 1968 was largely the work of the Criminal Law Revision Committee (Eighth Report, *Theft and Related Offences*, see above). The Report was to the effect that 'appropriation' was to bear its ordinary-language meaning. If the accused deceived the victim into handing over property, the proper charge was obtaining by deception, not theft. It was not theft because the definition of appropriation did not cover a situation where the victim consented to the taking. In other words property passed when the owner consented to the transfer and there was therefore no property to appropriate after the moment of transfer. Lord Lowry also said that **Lawrence** had been correct in holding that lack of consent was an extra element which the prosecution had to prove in theft but, while it was not an additional part of the *actus reus*, it was part and parcel of the definition of appropriation. Lord Lowry in summary may be said to have been protecting the honest shopper. Not until he did something wrongful with the goods did he appropriate. The majority said that both the honest shopper and the shoplifter appropriate. Innocence or guilt depends on their state of mind.

In Lord Lowry's view if the accused by deception induces the victim to transfer his entire right of ownership to him, he is not guilty of theft. If, however, the accused induces the owner to transfer (only) possession, he is. This distinction was the one drawn by the Criminal Law Revision Committee and endorsed by Parliament. The offence of obtaining property by deception was designed to cover situations where the accused had fraudulently obtained ownership. In most instances where there is deception the accused as buyer becomes the owner of the goods. For example, if there is a misrepresentation that the accused will pay for the item but in fact he will not, property nevertheless passes to him. It is only if there is a fundamental mistake of fact that property does not pass. The contractual effect of a non-fundamental mistake induced by deception is to render the contract not void but voidable. *Gomez* makes the accused into a thief even though he is the owner in civil law.

To summarise the criticism of *Gomez*, the accused should not have been convicted of theft because the words in the statute should have been construed in a case of ambiguity in favour of the accused; Parliament has enacted the Report of the Criminal Law Revision Committee, which was contrary to *Gomez*; and the House of Lords in *Morris* has decided differently from *Gomez*.

The implications of *Gomez* are profound.

(i)   Since appropriation is a neutral term, the guilt of the accused depends on his state of mind. The emphasis is on his dishonesty or lack of it. In theft the *mens rea* is of more importance than the *actus reus* and for that reason *mens rea* has been considered first in these pages. Unfortunately current law does not enable one to say that a certain form of conduct is dishonest in advance of trial. It may be that the law after *Gomez* is inconsistent with the European Convention on Human Rights. The concept of appropriation is very wide and that of dishonesty is uncertain at the margins. A person may not be able in advance to judge whether or not his conduct constitutes theft.

(ii)   While the facts of *Gomez* involved deception, the case is not limited to such facts. Appropriation occurs whether or not the accused has deceived the victim into transferring his property. An accused appropriates if he buys or hires property.

(iii) Since neutral facts may constitute an appropriation and since appropriation need involve the assumption of only one of the rights of the owner, appropriation after *Gomez* occurs at an earlier stage than it did under *Morris*. If the accused touches the can of beans mentioned above he appropriates. Under *Morris* he would not have appropriated until he did something inconsistent with the rights of the owner such as hiding the tin among other items in his own bag – simply taking the beans off the shelf would not have been an appropriation because the removal would have been impliedly authorised by the shopkeeper. This example illustrates how *Gomez* and *Morris* differ and how only the mental element in theft distinguishes the innocent from the guilty, the point made in (a) above. The example also demonstrates how far the law has been extended since 1968. Under the previous law, that of larceny, there had to be a taking away ('asportation') which was performed without the consent of the owner. Neither element is required in theft. The accused appropriates before he takes away and does so even though the owner consents. Facts which pre-1969 would have perhaps been attempted larceny are now definitely the full offence of theft. *Gomez* ensures that acts amount to appropriation when under the law prevailing previously they would at most be attempted theft and quite possibly not even that. If a British Rail luggage attendant puts a suitcase in a rack intending to steal it later, he nowadays appropriates it. Previously he was guilty of attempted theft and only then if the jury decided he had done a more than merely preparatory act. This outcome is sanctioned by reading 'the rights' as 'any of the rights', which is not what s 3(1) states. Theft is concerned with stealing property, not with stealing one of the rights in that property.

(iv) It may be that the police and store detectives will not arrest until the accused walks past the till or out of the shop without paying or puts the item into his pocket, but these actions are part of the proof of appropriation, not appropriation itself. They constitute evidence, not substantive law.

(v) *Gomez* led to an almost total overlap between theft and the former offence of obtaining property by deception where the accused has obtained the item by fraud. In these offences there are four common elements: property, belonging to another, dishonesty, and intention permanently to deprive. One element is similar: appropriation can cover the same facts as obtaining. One difference is that obtaining requires a deception whereas theft does not, but there is nothing to stop the bringing of a charge of theft where there is a deception. If there is any problem with proving deception, a theft charge will lie. An exception to this statement is that, in general, land cannot be stolen (see below) but it can be obtained by deception, the usual example being the accused's moving the boundary fence. The land gained is not stolen but the accused has gained it by deception. Though the same facts can give rise to both crimes it should be noted that the current maximum for theft is seven years' imprisonment, whereas that for obtaining property by deception before its repeal was 10 years. Lord Lowry has a strong point when he states that obtaining property by deception fulfils little or no function when almost all instances of the offence fall within theft. The practical effect of this point is that theft is now an 'included offence' so that if the prosecution cannot prove a deception, the accused may still be convicted of theft. In terms of statutory construction, it cannot be right that one major offence was intended by Parliament to swallow another. It is also argued that theft and deception are different concepts. Deception is concerned with the accused's doing something which affects the victim's mind: the latter is deceived. In theft the accused, to use a paradigm example, takes something from the victim. Since the rationales are different, the coverage of the crimes should be different too.

Contracts are voidable for fraud. In cases like *Lawrence*, *Gomez* and *Hinks* the contracts have not been avoided. Therefore, the property belongs to the defendant, who cannot by definition be guilty of theft of their own property. That is why the crime of obtaining property by deception was put into the Theft Act 1968. *Lawrence*, *Gomez* and *Hinks* destroyed the aim behind having two different offences.

(vi) Because consent is irrelevant, it no longer matters whether the effect of fraud on consent to the passing of property is to render a contract void or voidable.

(vii) One aspect of *Morris*, minor in comparison with the others, is that Lord Roskill said that a person who switched price labels in a shop out of mischief did not appropriate. This *dictum* was criticised because, applying Lord Roskill's *dictum*, he did interfere with or usurp the rights of the owner. Changing price tags was a right of the owner. Commentators said that the reason why the mischievous label-switcher was not guilty of the theft was not because he did not appropriate but because he was not dishonest. This reasoning was accepted in *Gomez*. A final comment is that the accused in *Morris* was after all convicted. By swapping the price labels and removing the items from the shelves he did appropriate. *A fortiori* he appropriates if one applies *Gomez*.

In *Gomez* the charge was theft but should have been obtaining property by deception. In order to convict the accused the concept of appropriation had to be stretched. Sir John Smith's comment that appropriation is now much wider than Parliament intended is a weighty one and his comment is yet weightier when it is noted that he was a member of the Criminal Law Revision Committee, the Report of which underlies the 1968 Act. The Committee's view is summarised in para 38a. 'Obtaining by false pretences is ordinarily thought of as different from theft, because in the former the owner in fact consents to part with his ownership; a bogus beggar is regarded as a rogue but not as a thief . . . To create a new offence of theft to include conduct which ordinary people would find difficult to regard as theft would be a mistake.' *Gomez* draws no distinction between a rogue and a thief, the accused who obtains fraudulently and the accused who appropriates by stealth. The crimes which an accused commits should be fairly labelled so that he can be appropriately punished. A taking by stealth is different from a taking with consent, even when consent is vitiated by fraud. The majority in *Gomez* refused to refer to the Report because there was clear House of Lords authority for the proposition that consent was irrelevant. The contrary argument is that *Lawrence* was not pellucid, that there was another House of Lords authority which seemed to decide differently, there was a string of Court of Appeal cases which sought to reconcile *Lawrence* and *Gomez*, and that anyway the House of Lords did not in *Lawrence* consider the Report. Only the dissentient, Lord Lowry, looked at the Report and by doing so he persuasively demonstrated that the majority ruling was inconsistent with the will of Parliament. Despite this criticism *Gomez* is wonderfully clear in its ruling. Its effect on appropriation from companies is discussed later. It will be seen that *Gomez* has also clarified the law in that area.

The argument from principle was pithily put by P. R. Glazebrook in 'Revising the Theft Acts' [1993] CLJ 191. 'Holding swindlers to be thieves does no injustice, will save much inconvenience in cases where it transpires only late in the day that a crook has resorted to deception, and avoids the extreme absurdity of denying the name of thief to those who misappropriate property received as a result of a mistake that they have induced while awarding it to those who had done nothing to bring about the mistaken transfer.' (The last phrase is a reference to s 5(4): see below.)

(viii) In *Gomez* there was a contract to sell the goods. Since the contract was voidable, the shopkeeper could have elected to treat the contract as subsisting and sue for the price. The buyer would then have the sole proprietary interest in the goods. In this scenario the purchaser's title to the goods would not have been disputable by anyone. Nevertheless this is presumably theft because all the elements are present at the moment of the purchase.

(ix) One consequence of *Gomez* is that the trial judge is saved from instructing the jury on civil law concepts such as the difference between void and voidable contracts. This point was made by Lord Steyn in *Hinks* [2001] 2 AC 241 (HL).

(d) *Gallasso*

On the day on which the speeches were delivered in *Gomez* the Court of Appeal heard argument in *Gallasso* (1994) 98 Cr App R 284. The accused, a nurse, became the house leader for a group of mentally handicapped adults. She opened trust accounts for each patient. She was the sole signatory and spent the money on various living expenses of the patients. Having opened three trust accounts for one patient, she *inter alia* withdrew sums over time from the third account. She was charged with theft of £1,800.32, the amount of a cheque she had deposited on opening the account. The jury convicted but the court allowed her appeal. Lloyd LJ giving the judgment said that if she had placed the cheque into her own account, she would have appropriated, but held that by paying a cheque for the patient into his account, she was not appropriating, no matter how dishonest she was. The court accepted the defence's contention that 'by paying in the cheques, the applicant was not assuming the rights of the owner. On the contrary, she was affirming those rights, by placing the cheque in trust accounts of which he was the named beneficiary.' The court either did not like *Gomez* or did not understand its implications.

Gallasso may be criticised for not applying *Gomez*.

(a) Lloyd LJ said that he was giving appropriation its ordinary meaning. Only the dissentient in *Gomez* gave that concept its dictionary meaning. The majority adopted what has come to be known as a 'neutral' definition.

(b) Lloyd LJ said that Lord Keith did not mean to say in *Gomez* that every touching was an appropriation. Lloyd LJ instanced a shopper who knocked an item from a shelf and then replaced it and a passer-by who picked up a lady's purse. He considered that such examples were not ones of appropriation. In the latter case he said that the passer-by would, however, appropriate if he ran away with the purse. Clarkson and Keating, *Criminal Law: Text and Materials*, 5th edn (Thomson, 2003) 762 comment: 'It is patently ridiculous to assert that picking up a dropped purse to hand it back to the owner is assuming the rights of the owner.' In criticism it may be said that appropriation does occur at the moment of the touching. It is suggested that Lord Keith meant to say exactly that. A person does assume the rights of the owner when he puts his hand on a tin of beans on the supermarket shelves. It is for this reason that dishonesty has to bear the weight which it does after *Gomez*. Dishonesty, not lack of appropriation, distinguished the passer-by who hands back the purse from the one who decamps with it. The external elements, the *actus reus*, are exactly the same whether the accused was an innocent shopper or a shoplifter. On the facts of *Gallasso* she appropriated the cheque by removing it from the envelope which it came in. Her *mens rea* makes her guilty of theft. Even though her action was impliedly authorised by the patient, even though it was only a preliminary stage in her withdrawing money from the account for her own purposes, she did appropriate for within s 3(1) she assumed (one of) the rights of the owner. Applying *Gomez* to *Gallasso* the accused appropriated by paying in the cheque.

(c) Lloyd LJ said that the accused was affirming the rights of the owner by paying the cheque into his account. However, if one applies *Gomez*, one appropriates goods by putting them into a basket provided by the shop. One is on these facts affirming the rights of the shop to the goods but one does assume one of the rights of the owner.

(d) There is a suggestion in the judgment ('the paying in was not a taking at all') that one can appropriate only if one takes the item, though Lloyd LJ did say that he was not incorporating the requirement of asportation (see above) into theft. However that may be, there exist some illustrations of appropriation which do not require a taking. If I sell your furniture, I appropriate even though I do not take or touch the property. Lord Keith in *Gomez* said that a person appropriates by switching price labels even when the item to be taken is not moved.

(e) The accused had possession of the victim's property at the time when she paid in the cheque. She did not need to 'take' it for she already had it. To use pre-Theft Act terminology, she converted the cheque. Since appropriation is the modern term for conversion, she appropriates the cheque by paying it in.

(f) The result which Lloyd LJ desired would have been obtained under *Morris*. The accused would not have adversely interfered with or usurped the rights of the owner before she withdrew cash for her own purposes. Her conduct until then would have been impliedly authorised by the patient. Only when she deviated from the authorisation did she appropriate under *Morris*. *Morris* has, however, gone and the reasoning in it is no longer applicable. Applying *Gomez* she appropriates.

In summary, *Gallasso* is wrong (and should not be followed) because an appropriation is simply a dealing with another's property. There need not be a nonconsensual dealing. For this reason it is suggested that Lloyd LJ was wrong to say that a hall-porter did not appropriate when he placed a suitcase under his desk, preliminarily to stealing it, in breach of hotel regulations which provided for the porter to lock it away. The accused in *Gallasso* did not just break the rules of the health authority which employed her, she also appropriated for the purposes of the law of theft. And if one were to consider *Gallasso* wrong, as from the viewpoint of precedent it is, the outcome exemplifies a point made above. The accused is guilty of theft at the point of paying in the cheque. She has not yet taken anything out of the account. Applying a combination of the law of attempt and *Morris* it is doubtful whether she would be guilty of attempted theft. After *Gomez*, however, she is guilty not merely of attempted theft but of the full offence of theft when she places the patient's cheque into his account.

(e) *Briggs*

The Court of Appeal in *Briggs* [2004] 1 Cr App R 34 held that appropriation required the accused to perform a physical act; deceiving the victim into transferring property was not an appropriation. As in *Gallasso* the court was seeking to restrict *Gomez*. Certainly it may be argued that in *Gomez* there was a physical appropriation. Possession of the goods was taken. (Similarly in *Hinks* the accused received the money: see below for a discussion of *Hinks*.) However, *Gomez* is not restricted to physical takings. Indeed, if it were, how would one be able to appropriate those intangibles which are property for the purposes of theft? The contention that theft was restricted to physical takings might have been arguable when the Theft Act 1968 came into force, but not in the twenty-first century, one might have thought. Amazingly the court did not refer to *Gomez* or *Hinks*; and Silber J said: 'it is not easy to see why an act of deceiving an owner to do something would fall within the meaning of "appropriation"', yet that is what *Gomez* holds.

(f) *Mazo* and *Kendrick*

The Court of Appeal also found difficulty in applying *Gomez* in *Mazo* [1997] 2 Cr App R 518. A lady's maid was given various items including £37,000 in cheques by her mistress, who was mentally incapable. The court allowed her appeal. The cheques were property, they belonged to another, the maid intended permanently to deprive, and the jury found that she was dishonest. Did she appropriate? By receiving the gifts she assumed all of the rights of the owner: she became the owner. Therefore, she ought to have been found guilty of theft. The actual outcome of the case raised the possibility that *Gomez* does not apply when in civil law the accused has a good title. The absurdity in the situation is that an accused can be found guilty of theft after *Gomez* despite the fact that he retains ownership even after a conviction for theft. Sir John Smith commented thus in his case comment on *Mazo* [1996] Crim LR 437: 'However all-embracing *Gomez* may seem, a line must be drawn where conviction of theft would cause a conflict with the civil law. . . . If the effect of the transaction is that [the accused] gets an absolute, indefeasible right to the property in question, it would be unacceptable for a criminal court to hold that the transaction amounted to a theft of the property by him. If [he] has a right to retain the property, or even to recover it from the alleged victim, it can hardly be held to be theft for him to take and keep it. Otherwise the civil law would be assisting [him] to recover or to retain the fruits of his crime.' There were two possible *ratios* to *Mazo*. First, a valid gift cannot constitute an appropriation. The cases in the next paragraph held that this proposition was wrong. Secondly, consent is relevant where the appropriation is not induced by fraud (deception). There is nothing in *Gomez* that supports this restriction, and the cases mentioned in the next paragraph do not support it.

Mazo was distinguished in *Kendrick* [1997] 2 Cr App R 524 (CA). The court stated that it was not being called upon to decide whether *Mazo* was correct in holding that a gift *inter vivos* could not constitute an appropriation (but it did call this ruling an 'apparent gloss' on *Gomez*, demonstrating that it thought *Mazo* to be incorrect). It held that the consent of the owner did not negate an appropriation. *Mazo* was distinguished as a case involving a person with reduced mental capacity, whereas *Kendrick* involved a person incapable of managing her own affairs.

(g) *Hinks*

The Court of Appeal in *Hinks* [2000] 1 Cr App R 1 ruled that a gift could be an appropriation. The concession by counsel in *Mazo* that it could not be an appropriation was wrong. Therefore, the act by which the accused gets ownership is an appropriation. The Criminal Law Revision Committee did not so intend. Contrary to the view of Sir John Smith, civil unlawfulness was not an element of theft. Whether the gift was validly made was irrelevant. Pitt LJ said: 'In relation to theft, one of the ingredients for a jury to consider is not whether there has been a gift, valid or otherwise, but whether there has been an appropriation.' As he earlier noted, the consent of the owner, the donor, is immaterial when determining appropriation. The court specifically rejected the analysis of Sir John Smith [1997] Crim LR 359 in his commentary on *Gomez* that the speech of Lord Browne-Wilkinson in *Gomez* has seen off all challenges to its authority. There is, however, a difference between *Hinks* and *Gomez*. In the former case the accused would not have been guilty of any offence, had the accused not been guilty of theft.

By a majority of three to two the House of Lords upheld the Court of Appeal decision in *Hinks* [2001] 2 AC 241 (HL). It applied *Lawrence* and *Gomez* to the following facts. The victim was a man of limited intelligence. He 'gave' his principal carer some £60,000 over a period in 1996. Her argument was that she received the money as gifts. Lord Steyn delivered the leading speech. He said that a person appropriates property belonging to another even though the victim transfers an indefeasible title to it and does not retain any interest in it. Therefore, the donee of a gift appropriates it by receiving it, and this is so despite the fact that in civil law the donor cannot get it back. The majority in *Gomez* had already held that an appropriation occurred even though the entire proprietary interest passed to the accused. Lord Steyn noted that *Gomez* was not restricted to situations in which an alleged fraud took place. He approved the statement of Rose LJ in the Court of Appeal that: 'Belief or lack of belief that the owner consented to the appropriation is relevant to dishonesty. But appropriation may occur even though the owner has consented to the property being taken.' He also rejected counsel's argument that an appropriation had to be an unlawful one. To accept it would be to interpolate a concept into the definition of theft, which had been 'carefully drafted'. In other words Parliament did not intend that the appropriation had to be an unlawful one. He furthermore rejected the contention that it was absurd that civil law and criminal law should reach different conclusions for they served different purposes. Counsel provided illustrations where the application of *Gomez* might be said to lead to unsettling outcomes: the accused was guilty of theft when he should not have been. An example is where the buyer of a painting believes it to be by a major artist when it is not and the seller knows of the mistake. Providing dishonesty can be proved, there is theft, even though in civil law there is an enforceable contract and if the buyer does not pay, the seller can sue for the price. Lord Steyn thought that the difficulties could be obviated by using the concept of dishonesty. On the facts the accused was dishonest. No one was likely to prosecute in marginal cases; and 'at the extremity of the application of legal rules there are sometimes results which may seem strange'. In his view, if a narrower conception of appropriation were adopted, 'the outcome is likely to place beyond the reach of the criminal law dishonest persons who should be found guilty of theft'. He was happy to reach the conclusion that appropriation bore a wide meaning for there was as a result no need to explain to juries civil law concepts such as indefeasibility and civil law unlawfuless. Finally he stated that *Gomez* does not lead to injustice in practice. 'The mental requirements of theft are an adequate protection against injustice.'

The minority forcefully dissented on the basis that where there was a valid gift, there was no dishonesty and therefore no theft, as *Mazo* had held. However, in *Kendrick* there was dishonesty because the accused knew that the donor was mentally incapable. Lord Hutton said that the judge should have directed the jury on whether the victim in *Hinks* was mentally capable. If he was, 'the defendant could not be found to be dishonest no matter how much they thought her conduct morally reprehensible'. If the victim was mentally incapable of making a valid gift, the *Ghosh* test applied. Similarly, if there was alleged to be undue influence or coercion, there would have to be a specific direction; if the gift was invalid for either reason, again *Ghosh* had to be applied. Lord Hobhouse said that 'the reasoning of the Court of Appeal . . . depends upon the disturbing acceptance that a criminal conviction and the imposition of custodial sanctions may be based upon conduct which involves no inherent illegality and may only be capable of being criticised on grounds of lack of morality.' One purpose of criminal law, however, was to define the boundary between criminality and immorality. Once the item had been given, there is no property belonging to another; 'the donee is not "assuming the rights of an owner": she already has them' and therefore there is no appropriation; even if the acceptance of the gift constitutes an appropriation, the accused is not dishonest because of s 2(1)(a); the accused does not intend to act regardless of the donor's rights within s 6(1) because he has relinquished those rights. 'The person who accepts a valid gift is simply conforming to the wishes of the owner.' There is no appropriation. On this approach, taking an article to the check-out in order to buy it is not an appropriation; it is merely complying with the implied request of the supermarket. In Lord Hobhouse's view *Mazo* was correct and *Kendrick* was wrong. He was strongly of the opinion that 'dishonestly appropriates' was one concept. There were not two, dishonesty and appropriation. A person does not 'dishonestly appropriate' if acts are done in relation to the property which are performed in accordance with the actual wishes or actual authority of the owner. Either there is no assumption of rights or there is no dishonesty. (Assuredly the accused may also be able to rely on s 2(1)(a): if he believes that he is legally entitled to the gift, he is not dishonest.) The position is different when there is fraud, misrepresentation, undue influence, cases falling within s 5(4) (where the victim has made a mistake and the accused is under a duty to restore) and cases falling within s 5(1) (where the victim retains an equitable interest).

Other problems with **Hinks** should be noted.

- First, the accused may not have been dishonest and accordingly could not have been guilty of theft.
- Secondly, if the gift was valid in civil law, then the owner could not recover it; if the owner used self-help to get it back, he could be sued by the alleged thief. It is unsatisfactory that the person who in civil law owns the property is in criminal law guilty of theft. Since civil law does not allow the owner to bring an action in respect of the gift, why should criminal law say that acceptance of a gift is an appropriation?
- Thirdly, in the law of handling, goods are no longer stolen when the owner loses the right to restitution. Therefore, there are no stolen goods and the crime of handling cannot take place. If on the facts of **Hinks** the owner never had such a right, how can it be said that the property is 'stolen'?
- Fourthly, Lord Steyn said that if criminal law and civil law were inconsistent, it may be that civil law was incorrect. However, the criminal law of theft exists to protect the civil law of property. If it is not, what exactly is the criminal law protecting? Coverage must be the same.
- Fifthly, if the victim took the property back dishonestly intending to keep it, he would be guilty of theft from the accused!
- Sixthly, the accused did not assume the rights of the owner: she *was* the owner.
- Finally, the Criminal Law Revision Committee, the Eighth Report, *Theft and Related Offences*, Cmnd 2977, 1966, which forms the basis of the Theft Act 1968, did not intend the law to be as stated by the majority in **Hinks**.

Academic criticism of **Hinks** reached its acme in E. Phillips, C. Walsh and P. Dobson, *Law Relating to Theft* (Cavendish, 2001, 43), who called the outcome of the case a 'horror'. They suggest (at 50) that **Hinks** breaches Article 6 of the European Convention on Human Rights, what may in American terms be called the 'void for vagueness' provision, because whether an accused is guilty of theft or not depends on his dishonesty or lack of it.

(h) Atakpu

One might have thought that **Gomez** would have widened the law in all respects. In one matter, however, it has narrowed it. The facts of **Atakpu** [1994] QB 69 (CA) exemplify this proposition. The defendants planned to hire expensive cars abroad, bring them to England, modify them and then sell them. English courts have no jurisdiction to try accused persons for thefts committed abroad. Where did the appropriation take place? The court held that appropriation occurred when the cars were hired. Therefore, there was no appropriation in England and the English courts lacked jurisdiction. Ward J said that it was incorrect to say that there could be one theft abroad and another in England (unless the defendants had lost possession abroad and then resumed it in England). The court was willing to consider the argument that theft was a continuing act (see below) but on the facts the theft was complete and did not continue for days after the appropriation. Since the issue did not arise on the facts, the court was unwilling to give a decided view on this point but did note that applying *Gomez* strictly, there was little scope for the doctrine of continuing appropriation. It is suggested that *Gomez* did not affect the law whether appropriation could be a continuing act. See the discussion of this point in robbery later in this chapter. The statements in *Atakpu* are *obiter*. Ward J said that the defendants were rogues but their conviction had to be quashed. It should be noted that under *Morris* the English courts would have had jurisdiction. A modification to a car would be an adverse interference with the owner's rights, and the modification would have taken place in England. Under *Gomez*, however, there was only one appropriation (there was no appropriation each time the accused touched the car), and that occurred abroad. Unlike the judges in its sister division in *Gallasso*, the Court of Appeal in *Atakpu* loyally followed, as it was obliged to, the decision in *Gomez*, despite doubts as to its effects. Incidentally, a charge of conspiring to steal money from buyers in England would have succeeded.

On the jurisdiction point, the English courts if *Atakpu*'s *ratio* is correct could still not try the offence of theft after the coming into force of the Criminal Justice Act 1993, s 2: no 'relevant event' occurred in England. No element to be proved before theft is committed occurred in England. However, the appellants were also charged with conspiracy to steal. By virtue of s 1A of the Criminal Law Act 1977, as inserted by s 5(1) of the 1993 Act, the courts have jurisdiction provided that what the men did was an offence under the law of the foreign law district. For criticism of *Atakpu*, see G.R. Sullivan and C. Warbrick 'Territoriality, theft and *Atakpu*' [1994] Crim LR 650 and 'Current developments: private international law' (1994) 43 ICLQ 464–465. They argue that the cars were not stolen abroad because stolen means 'stolen according to English domestic law'. Therefore the cars were stolen only when they were imported. In terms of the later part of s 3(1) the defendants came by the property (abroad) and kept or dealt with it (in England). The court therefore did have jurisdiction.

(i) Other examples of appropriation

As these examples illustrate, appropriation occurs when the accused deals in any way with the property. Damaging property belonging to another will amount to criminal damage but it is also an appropriation. As always, the reader should take care to consider that more than one crime can arise on the same facts.

(1) Taking the goods: *Stapylton v O'Callaghan* [1973] 2 All ER 782 (DC).

(2) Putting goods into the accused's shopping bag: *McPherson* [1973] Crim LR 191 (CA). After *Gomez* simply taking hold of the goods is an appropriation, even if the owner agrees to that. One cannot appropriate without assuming possession or control. As *Gomez* demonstrates it is irrelevant whether or not the accused deceived the victim. There is even an appropriation when the accused buys an item.

(3) Grabbing a handbag is an appropriation, even though the accused dropped the bag immediately and did not get away with it: *Corcoran v Anderton* (1980) 71 Cr App R 104 (DC).

(4) Taking money from a customer and not ringing up the price on the till: *Monaghan* [1979] Crim LR 673 (CA). (She is also guilty of false accounting, contrary to s 17 of

the Theft Act 1968.) It should be noted that the shop assistant was guilty of theft, and not just of attempted theft. She may never have decided to remove the money, and she did exactly what the shop had instructed her to do: put the money in the till. Her dishonesty was used to prove her appropriation. Under the old law of larceny she may not even have been guilty of attempted larceny. Indeed, it could be argued that there was only a preparatory step towards the full offence, and not a more than merely preparatory step, in which event she would not even have been guilty of the attempt. The law has been extended so that she is now guilty of theft. If it could not be proved that she intended to exercise control over those banknotes and coins the customer had given her but intended to take an equivalent amount, it is suggested that the offence is not theft but the attempt because she did not appropriate identifiable money. Again, a charge of false accounting appears to meet the facts better than theft does.

(5)   Deceiving the victim into handing over an extra £6 for a taxi-ride: *Lawrence v MPC* [1972] AC 626, above.

(6)   Deceiving a shop assistant into charging less: *Bhachu* (1977) 65 Cr App R 261 (CA). The assistant will also be guilty of theft if she was in league with the customer, e.g. *Pilgram v Rice-Smith* [1977] 1 WLR 671 (DC). A supermarket assistant, in cahoots with a customer, wrapped goods and deliberately understated the price. It was held that there was an appropriation by the assistant because she had no authority to deal with the goods in this way. She had assumed one of the rights of the owner, the right to put the price on items for sale. Within s 3(1) she had come by property, bacon and corned beef, innocently but she had assumed 'a right to it by keeping or dealing with [the property] as an owner.'

(7)   Getting a shopkeeper to cash a cheque sent to the accused by mistake: *Davis* (1989) 88 Cr App R 347 (CA).

(8)   Transferring export licences from one firm to another: *Attorney-General of Hong Kong v Chan Nai-Keung* [1987] 1 WLR 1339 (PC).

(9)   Presenting another's cheque, forging a cheque, or getting funds transferred from another's bank account into one's own: *Kohn* (1979) 69 Cr App R 395, discussed below, and *Wille*, above, even though the bank had no mandate to honour the cheque, and *Chan Man-sin v Attorney-General of Hong Kong* [1988] 1 All ER 1, where the cheques were not binding on the company because they were forged. Yet compare the civil law. In *Tai Hing Cotton Mill Ltd v Liu Chong Hing Bank Ltd* [1986] AC 80 (PC) an account was debited because of a forged cheque. The debit was void because the bank had authority to pay only against valid cheques. Honouring a forged cheque is a nullity. The bank had to pay for the account-holder's loss. Therefore, the account-holder lost nothing. The Privy Council in *Chan Man-sin*, where a company's accountant wrote unauthorised cheques to withdraw money from the bank accounts of two companies, advised that the owner of a credit at the bank or of a right to draw on an account 'has, clearly, the right as owner to draw by means of a properly completed negotiable instrument or order to pay and it is . . . beyond argument that one who draws, presents and negotiates a cheque on a particular bank account is assuming the rights of the owner . . . It is . . . entirely immaterial that the end result of the transaction may be a legal nullity, for it is not possible to read into [the Hong Kong version of s 3(1)] any requirement that the assumption of rights there envisaged should have a legally efficacious result.' In other words, the accused appropriates even though the owner's rights

against the bank are not reduced. He is doing something which only the owner is permitted to do. Since only the account-holder has the right to draw a cheque, the accused appropriates by doing so: *ex parte Osman* [1990] 1 WLR 277 (DC) and *Ngan* [1998] 1 Cr App R 331 (CA). To the contrary is *Hilton* [1997] 2 Cr App R 445 (CA) where it was held that there had to be a transfer of funds for the accused to be guilty. The Court said that the transfer had to be complete before there could be an appropriation. In the words of Evans LJ: '. . . where property consists of a credit balance . . . then the defendant appropriates it by assuming the rights of the owner of the balance and so causing the transfer to be made out of the account. His instructions to the bank to make the transfer, whether given by cheque or otherwise, are the key which sets the relevant inter-bank (or inter-account) machinery in motion. The fact that the transfer is made is enough to complete the offence . . .'. This is inconsistent with the earlier authority of *ex parte Osman* and the later one of *Ngan*. It is suggested that *Hilton* is wrong on this point. The rest of *Hilton*, in particular the court's ruling that the chair of a charity appropriated when he sent faxes to a bank asking it to transfer money from the charity account to another one and when he presented a cheque on the charity's account to move money into the other account is correct. The Court of Appeal held that he had appropriated a thing in action, the right of the charity to sue the bank. It does not matter that the owner's property is not affected by the accused's assumption of one of his rights. Simply signing a cheque is not theft, but attempted theft: *Ngan*.

This situation, where the accused has his account credited and the victim's debited, should be contrasted with the situation where he uses a bank card to debit his account, knowing that he does not have enough money to meet the price. In this situation the bank is obliged to honour the cheque if the accused goes through the correct procedure. Since there is no money in the account, there is no property, no debt (a thing in action) to steal (see *Kohn*, discussed below). Moreover, there is no appropriation. The bank was legally obliged to meet the cheque; therefore, no right of an owner had been assumed: *Navvabi* [1986] 1 WLR 1311 (CA), which illustrates a very important principle. See (10) below.

(10) Sending a telex to a bank asking it to transfer funds: *ex parte Osman*. There was not merely an attempt to appropriate, but an appropriation. The accused had assumed the rights of a customer to have the cheque met. A contrasting case is *Navvabi* [1986] 1 WLR 1311 (CA), where *Kohn* was applied. The accused drew by cheque card on a bank balance which he knew had insufficient funds to meet the sum. It was held that there was no appropriation because there was no identifiable property, merely a contractual right against the bank. There was no thing in action. Therefore, the accused had not assumed any of the rights of the owner, the bank. There was no appropriation. This is an important principle. The correct charge is one of fraud contrary to the Fraud Act 2006.

(11) Assuming rights over property which one has previously taken but then abandoned: *Starling* [1969] Crim LR 556 (CA), a case on larceny but the law is unchanged.

(12) Destroying property is appropriation.

Even if the accused is not in possession there may be an appropriation, as indeed was the case in *ex parte Osman*. It did not matter whether the bank complied with the demand; it sufficed that the accused pretended to be exercising one of the rights of the owner. That right was one to have cheques or instructions as to his account met.

Section 3(1) does not mention possession and therefore it is not restricted to situations where the accused becomes possessed of property. An illustration is **Pitham and Hehl** (1976) 65 Cr App R 45 (CA). An acquaintance of the victim offered to sell furniture to third parties. The furniture belonged to a man in prison, and the acquaintance was not in possession. It was held (the court seemingly assuming that the acquaintance held himself out as owner, though the actual facts tell a different story, which is one of joint theft by the acquaintance and the third parties) that by the offer to sell, the acquaintance was assuming one of the rights of the owner, the right to sell. If the intended buyer has refused to purchase, the owner of the furniture would not have lost any property but, according to the ratio, the accused would still have been guilty. The victim is still the owner and the purported sale interferes with his proprietary rights. In **Pitham** the acquaintance was at the scene of the sale but presumably he would still have been guilty, had he been 100 miles away and the owner was in possession of the goods. (If another person dishonestly agreed to buy, he will be guilty of handling stolen goods.) There is debate whether there is an appropriation in such circumstances. Glanville Williams, *Textbook of Criminal Law*, 2nd edn (Stevens, 1983) 764, criticised **Pitham**: if a butler invites the maid to join him in stealing the Duke's silver when he has found the key to the safe, surely he has not at that time appropriated the silver. It is very strange that one of the attributes of property is that a non-owner has the right to sell it!

The civil case of **Dobson v General Accident Fire and Life Assurance Corp plc** [1990] QB 274 (CA) illustrates the proposition that the defendant assumes one of the rights of the owner by acquiring ownership. The owner of a watch and a ring sold them to a rogue over the telephone. The next day the rogue paid for the articles by a bad cheque. Therefore, at the time of acquiring ownership he did not have possession. Nevertheless, he had assumed one of the rights of the owner, ownership. Alternatively, if by civil law ownership did not pass at that moment but only on payment the rogue appropriated then.

(j) 'Come by the property'

Section 3(1) deems there to be an appropriation where the accused 'has come by the property (innocently or not) without stealing it'. (If the accused does come by the property by stealing it, these later words in s 3(1) do not apply and any later assumption will not be an appropriation. This phrase prevents a thief from becoming a thief again each time he deals with an item.) There is an appropriation where in those circumstances he later assumes 'a right to it by keeping or dealing with it as owner'. The use of the phrase 'later assumption' demonstrates that when the accused 'comes by' property, he appropriates it, i.e. there are two appropriations. If the accused hired a car and then sold it, the later words of s 3(1) apply. Another example is when a drunken student takes a flashing yellow light from a road excavation, puts it into his bedroom, wakes up to discover it there, and decides to keep it. He has come by the property without stealing it and has later assumed a right to it by keeping it. In **Rader** [1992] Crim LR 663, discussed above, the accused was given money, i.e. he 'came by' it. Then he used it for his own purposes. It is likely that most of the situations where s 3(1) applies are ones where the accused has been overpaid. An example where the latter part of s 3(1) did not apply is **Broom v Crowther** (1984) 148 JP 592 (DC). The accused bought a theodolite, suspecting that it was stolen. He then found out that it was indeed stolen. He left it in his bedroom while he decided what to do with it. It was held that there was no appropriation while he was making up his mind. There would be an appropriation once he had decided to keep it. Therefore, one can appropriate by making up one's mind – a far cry from asportation.

Broom v *Crowther* shows that one can appropriate by an omission, though as Leggatt LJ said in *Ngan*, above, it may be difficult to prove that the accused did intend to keep property as owner when he simply refrained from doing anything. If the accused kept the item he has appropriated it even though he has not done anything physically with it. Within s 3(1) he has assumed a right to it 'by keeping . . . it as owner'. The case also demonstrates the purpose of s 3(1). An innocent first appropriation would have become an unlawful second appropriation if the accused has exercised any of the owner's rights. (The facts of *Broom* v *Crowther* actually fall within s 3(2), which is discussed next, because the accused was a bona fide purchaser.) The cases are not helpful as to the last words in s 3(1): 'dealing with it as owner.' It is suggested that this phrase includes a situation where the accused sells the item, swaps it, spends it, eats it and the like.

(k) The bona fide purchaser for value without notice

One person who would otherwise appropriate is exempted by s 3(2).

> Where property or a right or interest in property is or purports to be transferred for value to a person acting in good faith, no later assumption by him of rights which he believed himself to be acquiring shall, by reason of any defect in the transferor's title, amount to theft of the property.

An example of the application of s 3(2) is *Adams* [1993] Crim LR 72 (CA). The accused, a motorcycle enthusiast, bought for £350 parts which had been stolen. He was told they came from a motorcycle written off in a crash. He did not begin to suspect that the parts had been stolen until two or three days after acquisition. There was no *actus reus* at the moment of acquiring the parts. Another illustration is *Wheeler* (1991) 92 Cr App R 279. The stallholder received the medal in the course of sale. His later sale of it was protected by s 3(2). Protection is given only to Equity's Darling. A person who is given property cannot rely on s 3(2) if he later discovers that the property was stolen. Similarly a person who is not dishonest when he acquires goods is guilty of theft if he later discovers the identity of the owner and then he keeps or alienates the property. Protection is not given by s 3(2) to honest finders who turn dishonest. If the accused was a bona fide purchaser for value without notice, finds out about the defect in title and then sells the item, he will be guilty of obtaining the price by deception and of theft under *Gomez* because he is not entitled to sell the goods.

(l) Appropriation as a continuing act

Appropriation may be a continuing act. In *Hale* (1978) 68 Cr App R 415 (CA), the accused, wearing stocking masks, went into the victim's house, took her jewellery box, and tied her up. The court held that the theft was not over by the time the lady was tied up. They were therefore guilty of robbery when they used force seconds after seizing the property. Because the courts have held that appropriation does not occur instantaneously they have been able to expand and contract the term to catch those who are 'manifestly guilty'. *Hale* was a case on robbery. The accused is not guilty of that offence if force or threat of force is not used at the time of the theft. Therefore, to catch the accused the appropriation must be read as a continuing act to include situations where the taking is not by force but there is a struggle afterwards. However, the accused is not guilty of the offence of handling if the *actus reus* is committed otherwise than 'in the course of the stealing'. That phrase is read narrowly to convict the accused of handling rather than theft, handling being a more serious offence than theft. Such a construction explains *Pitham*. The accused appropriated property by offering the furniture for sale. At that moment it became stolen property. When his confederates took delivery of it, they received it for the purposes of the crime of handling because their handling was not in the course of stealing. The theft was already, as it were, completed. (See Chapter 17 for explanation of handling.) What is certain is that the theft is over at some point: *Atakpu*, above. Importing or selling the cars did not constitute an appropriation because they had been appropriated when the defendant hired them abroad.

(m) Theft by partners, co-owners, directors and sole controllers of companies

Where the director or directors is or are not in sole control of the company, there is no difficulty in holding that he or they can appropriate from the company and the property belong to another. For example, in *R (on the Application of R)* v *Snaresbrook Crown Court* (2001), *The Times*, 12 July, the Administrative Court rejected an application for a judicial review of the decision of a Crown Court judge that a director could dishonestly appropriate corporate property with the intention of permanently depriving the company of it even though he was the directing mind and will of the company and therefore the company had consented to the appropriation. He assumed the rights of the owner when the company's money was transferred from its bank account into another account; the company's consent was, applying *Gomez*, irrelevant. Similarly a partner can appropriate partnership property (*Bonner* [1970] 1 WLR 838 (CA), rejecting an argument that since one partner is not liable in tort for conversion, he cannot be guilty of theft), and a co-owner such as a member of a club can appropriate property from the other co-owners as occurs when he sells the item. In these instances the company, the other partners and co-owners have a proprietary right to the property within s 5(1). *Gomez*, above, confirms *obiter* the view taken in *Philippou* (1989) 89 Cr App R 290 (CA) that despite persons being the sole directors and sole shareholders of a company they could appropriate from it by misusing corporate assets. It does not matter that they, through their being sole controllers of the company, did give the company's assent to the misappropriation. Accordingly when the accused used their company's money to buy a Spanish building, they did appropriate. If the approach of the dissentient were adopted, sole controllers would not be guilty because the persons entitled to consent to the transfer of the asset did consent. Sole controllers may, however, not be guilty of theft because they may not be dishonest. (The *ratio* of *Philippou* is incorrect because *Morris* was applied, but the principle in it that sole controllers can appropriate is correct.) Since owners can be found guilty of stealing their own property (see the discussion of 'Belonging to another' below), policy dictates that partners, other co-owners and sole controllers, should also be liable.

Property

The second element of the *actus reus* of theft is property. Section 4(1) gives a broad definition of property: 'money and all other property, real or personal, including things in action and other intangible property'. Whether something is property is determined by the civil law: criminal law has no separate definition. 'Money' includes foreign money but it excludes out-of-date currency. A thing in action is property without physical existence (and therefore cannot be seen or touched) which can, however, be enforced by legal action, such as the right to sue to recover a debt. Cheques, direct debits and credit cards give rise to things in action. Copyright is a thing in action and therefore if the accused purports to sell copyright in this book, appropriation occurs. (However, infringement is not theft because there is no intent permanently to deprive.) A right by contract to overdraw a bank account is also a thing in action. Rights of way are property which can be stolen by dishonestly conveying the property to another. In *Marshall* [1998] 2 Cr App R 282 (discussed above) the Court of Appeal thought that London Underground, which they held had an exclusive right to sell tickets, had a right of action over its tickets to prevent their being used by persons who did not buy them. If so, people who pass on unexpired bus tickets or parking tickets will, depending on their *mens rea*, be guilty of theft. Intangible property, which by definition cannot be touched, can be appropriated by the accused's assuming any of the owner's rights. (See also (c) below.)

Some forms of intellectual property such as patents (and applications for patents) are also covered. A patent is in civil law not a thing in action but personal property. An invention over which there is no patent is intangible property and therefore can be stolen. Therefore, *in this respect*, confidential information is property. However, *Oxford* v *Moss* (1978) 68 Cr App R 183, above, held that confidential information such as exam questions is not property for the purposes of the Theft Act. Information such as trade secrets does contain at least some constituents of property. For example, they can be bequeathed and sold. Nevertheless, because a trade secret is not property for the purposes of civil law, it cannot be stolen. Other offences, in particular conspiracy to defraud, may be committed. (The Law Commission proposes a specific separate offence to deal with the use or disclosure of trade secrets: see Consultation Paper No. 150, *Misuse of Trade Secrets*, 1997.)

Services are not property. Therefore, a ride in a taxi cannot be stolen. The Criminal Law Revision Committee's Eighth Report, *Theft and Related Offences*, Cmnd 2977, 1966, 39, said that electricity could not be stolen because it was not a substance and the Divisional Court held so in *Low* v *Blease* [1975] Crim LR 513 where the accused was not guilty of theft when he used a telephone; instead a separate offence, s 13, abstracting electricity, was created. One effect of the law should be noted. A person who having entered part of a building as a trespasser and then steals is a burglar, but one who turns on an electric fire is not, despite electricity's being a valuable commodity. A battery can be stolen but not the electricity it contains despite the battery's uselessness without electricity. Water flowing freely whether underground or overground cannot be stolen.

At common law a human corpse and body parts could not be stolen because there was no 'property' in them, but anatomical specimens can be stolen: *Kelly* [1999] QB 621 (CA). The distinction is that such specimens 'have acquired different attributes by virtue of skill, such as dissection or preservation techniques, for exhibition or teaching purposes'. These uncertainties should be cleared up. Certainly a sample of blood (*Rothery* [1976] RTR 550 (CA)) and of urine (*Welsh* [1974] RTR 478 (CA)) can be stolen. In fact, in *Rothery* the accused was found guilty of theft of the container which held the blood, but if urine can be stolen, so can blood. Presumably also sperm in a sperm bank, human eggs and human organs for transplant can be stolen. Whether a body kept in a store for medical students' use is property is debatable. Burke and Hare and other 'resurrection men' would not be guilty of theft if the events took place on English soil at the present time. It is suggested that the common law rule that a human body cannot be stolen will over time become so encrusted with exceptions that Parliament will abolish it. Whatever the position with corpses live human beings cannot be stolen.

Some examples

As the trade secrets example above demonstrates, if there is no property in civil law there is no property for the purposes of the law of theft. Some examples as to what constitutes property follow:

(a) Property covers export quotas: *Attorney-General of Hong Kong* v *Chan Nai-Keung*, above. They are intangible property, not a thing in action.

(b) If a first person owes the victim a sum of money, the accused forges an assignment from the victim to him, and the first person pays the accused, the accused has stolen property (and obtained it by deception).

(c) A patent is not a thing in action (Patents Act 1977, s 30(1)) but it is intangible property. The same is true of an unpatented invention (s 7(2)(b) of that Act).

(d) A difficult topic is cheques. If a company secretary uses company cheques to settle his own debts, he has stolen the company's credit balance as well as the cheque itself. While there has been development, the principal authority remains *Kohn*.

Kohn (1979) 69 Cr App R 395

The accused, an accountant, drew cheques on his employer's account. He was guilty of theft. The causing of the bank account to be reduced was appropriation, and the account was property.

The court held that debiting an account which is not overdrawn or one where the overdrawing is within the agreed limit (a credit facility) is theft because the bank has an obligation to meet the drawing. That obligation is enforceable by action. Therefore, it is a debt, a thing in action, which is property. Causing a bank to transfer money out of one account into another, e.g. by drawing a cheque on the first account, was theft of a credit balance, as where the chair of a charity caused its account to be debited and his to be credited. (In *Chan Man-sin* v *Attorney-General of Hong Kong*, above, the thing in action was said to be the benefit of the contract with the bank.) However, drawing on an overdrawn account or an account overdrawn beyond the agreed credit limit does not amount to the appropriation of property because the bank has no obligation to meet the drawing. The accused has not appropriated a thing in action, because the bank did not owe the money to anyone. The charge should be attempted theft or obtaining a pecuniary advantage by deception.

The problem is, however, this. If the accused gets a transfer of funds from the victim, it is a thing in action but it never existed before it was drawn up. Therefore, it never belonged to anyone but the accused. It was not property belonging to another. In *Preddy* [1996] AC 815 it was held that cheques cannot be stolen where the accused induces the victim to write a cheque in his favour, though it remains to be seen whether the courts would accept the late Sir John Smith's suggestion that a cheque is a valuable security, which can be stolen: 'Obtaining cheques by deception' [1997] Crim LR 396. Cases have, however, distinguished *Preddy* as being an authority on the now repealed law of obtaining. In *Williams* [2001] 1 Cr App R 362, the accused dishonestly overcharged for building work. The victims sent cheques to him. He paid them into his bank account. The Court of Appeal held that he was guilty of theft of the thing in action, the right to sue on the cheque, belonging to the person who had signed the cheque. The court said that appropriation occurred when the accused by presenting the cheque reduced the victim's account. The accused has extinguished the victim's rights. The court stressed that *Preddy* had not affected *Kohn*. If the victim's account is in credit, the accused's reducing of the credit constitutes an appropriation. It should be noted that the victims' bank accounts were in credit. If they had been in the red, there would have been no thing in action to steal, as *Kohn* demonstrates. It is different if the accused gets a cheque drawn by another for the victim's benefit. In this example the thing in action did exist before the appropriation. It did belong to another and so could be stolen. The obvious charge in these situations is that of obtaining a money transfer by deception.

One possible way round these difficulties is to say that a cheque is not just a piece of paper (which is property), but is also a valuable security, which can be stolen too.

Cheques, telexes and appropriation

Kohn was approved in **Thompson** [1984] 1 WLR 962, **Doole** [1985] Crim LR 450, **Chan Man-sin**, above, and **ex parte Osman**, above. An alternative view is found in **Wille**, above. The accused, a company director, drew cheques on the company's account and used the money for his own purposes. The cheques had not been countersigned, and it was arguable that the bank had no authority to honour them. The Court of Appeal, however, held that the lack of authority was irrelevant, and the accused had appropriated the credit balance, which was a thing in action, by drawing the cheques. This case was approved in **Chan Man-sin**. One problem with cheques is: when does the appropriation take place? Does it occur on withdrawal or when the entry is made in the bank's books, i.e. when the account is debited? What happens when the account is in the black at the time of presentation but in the red when the bank honours the withdrawal? If the latter applies, there is no thing in action and so no property to steal. **Kohn, Tomsett** [1985] Crim LR 369 (CA) and **Doole** support that view. For example, in **Tomsett**, the accused, a telex operator employed by a bank in England, diverted money sent by his bank to New York. The court held that the money was appropriated only when the telex took effect. Since the telex did not take effect in England, the English courts had no jurisdiction at the time. Jurisdiction is now available under the Criminal Justice Act 1993. **Navvabi** [1986] 1 WLR 1311 (CA) said that **Kohn** was *obiter* on this point. The Privy Council refused to decide this point in **Chan Man-sin**, where the accused assumed the rights of the owner by drawing on the account. **Ex parte Osman** held that the sending of a telex amounted to an appropriation. (See also **Ngan**, above.) Therefore, theft was complete at that moment, contrary to **Tomsett**. The Divisional Court in **ex parte Osman** refused to follow **Tomsett**, where it was held that the bank had to comply with the instruction to debit one account and credit another. (It was thought in **Tomsett** that there can be an appropriation only when the accused's act affected the property but the concept bears a wider meaning than that.) **Tomsett** was said not to be binding because the prosecution did not wish to argue the view accepted in **ex parte Osman**, even though the court had invited counsel to do so. See also the section on **Atakpu**, above. In point of interpretation the line taken in **ex parte Osman** looks correct. Under **Morris** and **Gomez** any assumption of any of the rights of the owner suffices, and there is no need to prove that the accused deprived the owner of anything. Accordingly a preparatory act can be an appropriation (cf. the law of attempt)!

If an accused steals a cheque, he might appear to be guilty of theft of a piece of paper. The difficulty here is that the accused may not have an intent permanently to deprive. It is certainly arguable that when the cheque is returned, its virtue or value remains. It is still a piece of paper, both before and after the bank stamped it as having been accepted. Lord Goff accepted this argument in **Preddy**. Surprisingly the Court of Appeal in **Graham** [1997] 1 Cr App R 302 treated this *dictum* as *ratio* and in **Clark** [2001] Crim LR 572 the same court somewhat reluctantly held that it was bound by **Graham**, which held that there was no offence of obtaining a cheque by deception. See the next chapter for a discussion of cheques as 'property belonging to another'.

Prosecutors should be aware of the offence of procuring the execution of a valuable security. Cheques are valuable securities, whether they constitute consideration in contract law or not. Since they are, they are property. If the accused acquires a cheque and uses it to obtain money from the victim's account, he has appropriated the cheque. This argument has not yet been adopted by the courts in relation either to theft or to obtaining by deception, though in **Graham** the judges thought that it was highly persuasive.

Land, flora and fauna

By s 4(2) of the Theft Act 1968:

A person cannot steal land, or things forming part of land and severed from it by him or by his direction, except . . .

(a) when he is a trustee or personal representative, or is authorised by power of attorney, or as a liquidator of a company, or otherwise, to sell or dispose of land belonging to another, and he appropriates the land or anything forming part of it by dealing with it in breach of the confidence reposed in him; or

(b) when he is not in possession of the land and appropriates anything forming part of the land by severing it or causing it to be severed, or after it has been severed; or

(c) when, being in possession of the land under a tenancy, he appropriates the whole or part of any fixture or structure let to be used with the land . . .

The basic rule is therefore that land cannot be stolen, but there are exceptions. An example of (a) is where a trustee sells a plot of land for his own purposes. The Act is not limited to express trustees. Constructive trustees are presumably covered. An example of (b) is where one farmer grazes cattle on the victim's land without the latter's consent. The farmer has caused to be severed something which forms part of the land. Lead on a church roof is property for this purpose. Soil is land. Manure spread on land is land; manure in a dung heap is personal property. A person who trespasses on land to pick fruit falls under (b) but may have a defence under s 4(3); if, however, the accused gains possession of the land and then picks fruit, there is no theft since he is in possession of the land and (b) demands that he is not in possession.

There may be difficulties knowing what forms part of the land and what does not. Before the 1968 Act a hut that was bolted onto a concrete base was held not to be part of the land, whereas the concrete base, *obiter*, was. A fixed caravan may be part of the land but a mobile one is not. Grazing cattle on land will cause the grass, part of the land, to be severed. Under (b) the extension of a boundary fence does not steal the land enclosed because there is no severance.

Under (c) an accused will be guilty of theft (provided all the other ingredients of theft are satisfied) if he, the tenant, hacks out an Adam fireplace for whatever purpose. There is no need for severance. If, however, the person in possession of the house is not a tenant but a licensee or squatter, s 4(2)(c) does not apply and he will not be guilty of theft of the fireplace! And by being in possession s 4(2)(b) does not apply. The law is in need of reform to bring about consistency between tenants and licensees and squatters (provided squatters are held to be in possession of the land). Section 4(2)(c) applies only to the person in possession under a tenancy. Therefore, the tenant's partner does not fall under this paragraph if he appropriates a fixture. Section 4(2)(b) is, however, applicable but only when the fixture has been severed from the land. Accordingly under (c) the tenant is guilty at the time of appropriation, the partner is guilty under (b) only on severance. A tenant who picks fruit does not commit theft because fruit is not a 'fixture or structure'. A 'structure' includes a shed and a garage; a 'fixture' includes bathroom ware and central heating radiators.

Under a later part of s 4(2) land does not include incorporeal hereditaments such as easements and profits, which can therefore be stolen because these are property falling within s 4(1).

> A person who picks mushrooms growing wild on any land, or who picks flowers, fruit or foliage from a plant growing wild on any land, does not (although not in possession of the land), steal what he picks, unless he does it for reward or for sale or other commercial purpose.
>
> For purposes of this subsection 'mushroom' includes any fungus, and 'plant' includes any shrub or tree (s 4(3)).

Under s 4(3) the accused is guilty only if he has a commercial purpose. If the accused picks mistletoe to sell in the streets at Christmas, he is guilty, provided the other elements of theft are satisfied. The commercial purpose assuredly must exist at the time of the picking. If the accused picks wild strawberries and later decides to sell them to the Ritz, he is not appropriating property within s 4(3). Possibly a one-off sale cannot be described as being 'for a commercial purpose'. With regard to plants s 4(3) will be satisfied if they are picked for a commercial purpose. If, however, a whole plant is dug out, s 4(2) comes into play because the plant forms part of the land and is stolen by severing it (s 4(2)(b)). Moreover, one does not 'pick . . . from a plant' if one picks the whole plant or if one lops and tops a tree.

> Wild creatures, tamed or untamed, shall be regarded as property; but a person cannot steal a wild creature not tamed nor ordinarily kept in captivity, or the carcase of any such creature, unless either it has been reduced into possession by or on behalf of another person and possession of it has not since been lost or abandoned, or another person is in course of reducing it into possession (s 4(4)).

In s 4(4) there is no need for a commercial purpose. An example is the taking of animals kept in captivity in a wild life safari park. The animal is one normally kept in captivity and remains so even though it has escaped from the park. The accused who appropriates a grouse hidden by a poacher to be collected later will be guilty of theft (provided the other elements exist), even though he does not intend to sell it in a pub. The accused steals the grouse from both the poacher and the landowner. Under the law of larceny before the Theft Act 1968 it was held that a person was not in possession of mussels growing naturally when he raked them over. Therefore, when a second person took the mussels he did not steal them. Such is also the law after 1968.

Belonging to another

By s 5(1) of the Theft Act 1968:

> [p]roperty shall be regarded as belonging to any person having possession or control of it, or having in it any proprietary right or interest (not being an equitable interest arising only from an agreement to transfer or grant an interest).

A thief may therefore steal from several people: the owner, the possessor and the person in physical control. For this reason the owner may be guilty of theft from the possessor or controller. 'Belonging to' refers not just to ownership as it normally does, but extends beyond to possession and control. Property which is about to be destroyed nevertheless belongs to another. An example is misappropriating property which is on the point of being burnt in a municipal incinerator. The seller retains the legal interest. If he then sells the property to a second buyer, he does not steal from the first purchaser. An example of the application of the term 'control' in s 5(1) is **Woodman**.

Woodman [1974] QB 754 (CA)

A company sold off all the scrap metal on the site of its disused factory but retained control of the site. It did not know that the purchaser of the scrap had left some behind. The accused removed some of the metal. It was held that he was properly indicted with stealing from the company because a person or company in control of the site is deemed *prima facie* to have control over things on the land. The company retained control because it intended to exclude others by surrounding the site with barbed wire and erecting warning notices. (The presumption that the owner had control over items on the land would, however, be rebutted where a third party had hidden drugs or explosives on the land.) **Woodman** demonstrates that the owner need not know he owns the property and that the owner need not even know that he possesses it.

The same argument will apply to lost golf balls. The balls belong to the club. It seems that rubbish left in a skip belongs to the skip-owner and rubbish in dustbins belongs to the local authority. Property buried in the soil belongs to the occupier. Items abandoned and not owned by anyone no longer belong to another and so cannot be stolen. An illustration would be a newspaper left in the street. Section 5(1) does, not, however, cover the following facts. The accused purchases goods from the victim without dishonesty. He now has ownership and possession. At that point he decides to keep the goods but not to pay for them. The items are now his, not property belonging to another. Therefore, he is not guilty of theft despite his dishonesty, his intent permanently to deprive and his appropriation.

Gomez, above, exemplifies another situation covered by s 5(1). If an accused gets hold of property by misrepresentation, in contract law the transaction is voidable for fraud. In criminal law terms the property still 'belongs to another' and can therefore be stolen despite the accused's having a (voidable) title.

The phrase in brackets in s 5(1) excludes from 'belonging to another' the following situation. The accused agrees to transfer shares to the victim but before doing so he transfers them to a third party. The victim has only an equitable interest, and the accused is not guilty of theft of the shares. The accused may, however, be guilty of theft of the money or of obtaining the money by deception. The principal equitable interest referred to arises under an agreement to buy and sell land. The seller retains the legal interests, the buyer acquires an equitable interest. If the vendor then sells to a third party, he is not guilty of theft.

There is a *dictum* in **Edwards v Ddin** [1976] 1 WLR 942 (DC) that s 5 offers only a partial definition of 'belonging to another', but the statement is probably incorrect. Section 5(1) has been interpreted in the following ways:

(a) It does not cover cases where under the civil law the entire proprietary interest in the goods has passed. If there is a contract and the seller has delivered to the buyer, the latter obtains ownership even though he has not paid for the item. The principal case is **Edwards v Ddin**. A driver had his tank filled with petrol. He then (the facts are not clear – perhaps he all the time intended to drive out without paying) decided not to pay and drove away. By virtue of the Sale of Goods Act 1979, s 18, at the moment of driving off the petrol no longer belonged to the garage. Therefore, it was not property 'belonging to another', and so could not be subject to theft. (If, however, the accused intended all along to drive off without paying, he has obtained the petrol by deception: **McHugh** (1977) 64 Cr App R 92 (CA). There is no doubt nowadays that there is an appropriation despite the garage owner's desire that a motorist put the petrol into the tank.) At a self-service petrol station it is suggested that the same principle applies. The property passes and therefore the accused is not guilty of theft. **McHugh** is *contra*, but seems incorrect. The same principle applies to the accused who eats a meal in a restaurant and then decides to leave without paying: **Corcoran v Whent** [1977] Crim LR 52 (DC). As well as there being no theft, the accused has not obtained property, the petrol or the food, *by* deception because he obtained the property before the deception. Parliament has filled this gap by creating the offence of making off without payment in s 3 of the Theft Act 1978. It should be remembered that the position is different in a shop, whether self-service or otherwise, where ownership does not pass to the alleged thief, the buyer, until the goods have been paid for even if the buyer obtains possession before payment. In this case the seller retains ownership, the 'proprietary right' within s 5(1), and so the goods belong to another and can be stolen.

An easier case is **Walker** [1984] Crim LR 112 (CA). The victim bought a video from the accused. It was defective and he took it for repair to the accused, who sold it. The accused's conviction was quashed because the judge had not explained to the jury that the sale amounted to theft only if the victim had a 'proprietary right or interest' in the video. The victim had served on the accused a summons for return of the purchase price. Doing so rescinded the contract of sale, and the accused regained full ownership of the video recorder. A charge of attempted theft would have succeeded.

(b) The interests under s 5(1) include liens and bailments at will: **Turner (No. 2)** [1971] 1 WLR 901 (CA). In **Turner (No. 2)** the accused left his car at the victim's garage for repair. After it had been repaired, he drove away without paying. In civil law the victim had a 'lien' over the car, which meant that he was entitled to keep the car until the repairs had been paid for. (The same rule applies to cobblers and ship repairers.) The trial judge instructed the jury to ignore the concept of a lien. On that approach the repairer was a bailee at will. The Court of Appeal, upholding the judge's direction and expressly stating that its decision was not based on the existence of a lien, held that the owner had stolen his own car because the victim had been deprived of 'possession or control of it' within the terms of the statute. The jury had only to see whether the accused had in fact deprived the other of possession. Therefore, even though in civil law the bailee at will's right was inferior to that of the owner, the latter could steal from the former. Therefore, the owner, the person with the right to immediate possession, is guilty of theft when he exercises that right! A bailee at will cannot prevent a bailor from getting the item back, yet doing so is theft. Accordingly, in civil law the bailor may recapture the property but his doing so is appropriating property belonging to another. This means that if a person lends the next-door neighbour his lawn mower, then depending on his state of mind he may be guilty of theft when he takes it back without telling the owner what he has done. Moreover, the bailor may well not be dishonest, and it cannot be said that he intends permanently to deprive the bailee of his property in the item because a bailee does not have any interest in it. The case has been heavily criticised on these grounds. Had there been a lien, the position would have been different, because the car repairer would have had a right to the property. It was unfortunate that the Court of Appeal had to work on the basis that the garage had only a bailment at will because of the trial judge's instruction. It is suggested that rather than use civil law terms such as liens and bailments at will judges should refer to the words used in s 5(1): did the victim have 'possession or control' of the property? On the facts of *Turner (No. 2)* there was no doubt on that score.

It is thought that there is no theft where the owner recovers an impounded car because the police have no legal right to retain it: *Meredith* [1973] Crim LR 253, *per* Judge Da Cunha. (The accused was also not dishonest.) The police's power lawfully to remove obstructions did not include a power to keep the car from the owner. However, the judge should surely have said that for the purposes of theft, as indeed s 5(1) states, property can be stolen from people who have possession or control over it such as the police had on these facts.

There is no theft where the accused induces a testatrix to revoke her will and make another, for there is no proprietary interest in the executors: *Tillings* [1985] Crim LR 393. The intended beneficiaries did not at the time of the revocation have property in the items which they would have received under the former will. In *Hancock* [1990] 2 QB 242 it had not been decided whether coins were treasure trove or not under law which was abolished in 1996. The answer to that question would mean that they belonged either to the Crown or not. The accused, the finder, was not guilty of theft because at the moment of appropriation the coins were not property belonging to another. The Crown's right had not been proved. It is therefore not such property where there is only in the alleged owners a claim to a proprietary interest. There is also authority for the proposition that for the purposes of s 5(1) a copyright owner does not have a proprietary interest in the item copied: *Storrow* [1983] Crim LR 332 (Crown Court).

(c) In *Shadrokh-Cigari* [1988] Crim LR 465 (CA), a bank made a mistake of fact and the accused received money. The bank retained an equitable right to the money. Therefore, it belonged to them within s 5(1). Presumably the reason why the bank has an equitable proprietary interest is that the law imposes a constructive trust. There is, however, the contrary authority of *Attorney-General's Reference (No. 1 of 1985)* [1986] QB 491 (CA), where the manager of a tied pub sold beer as that of the brewery when he had purchased it elsewhere. The court held that, even if there was a constructive trust of the secret profit, such did not create an equitable interest in the brewery. It thought that in any case there was no constructive trust because the making of a secret profit by a fiduciary, as the manager was, did not give rise to any trust. Furthermore, trusts cannot exist without there existing property to which the trust attaches, and no separate property was to be found in the profit. The case has been criticised for deciding that there is no constructive trust where the accused uses the victim's facilities to make a secret profit and for holding that a constructive trust is not a proprietary right or interest within s 5(1). Civil law developments since 1985 tend towards showing that there is a constructive trust when property is obtained by fraud. The profit made from selling cheaper alcoholic drinks at the normal suppliers' price was surely property which could be the subject of a trust. Whether *Shadrokh-Cigari* is correct on the equitable interest point, the decision does point up the fact that there is no need to refer to s 5(4), on which see below, where the owner retains ownership but has transferred possession to the alleged thief. The property still belongs to another within s 5(1) and accordingly can be stolen by him. If the owner makes a mistake as to the identity of the accused and that error is fundamental at civil law, ownership of the property is not transferred and the owner retains the proprietary right. See also below.

The **Reference** case was distinguished by the Divisional Court in **Re Holmes** [2005] 1 WLR 1857 as being a case on secret profits, whereas **Re Holmes** concerned the fraudulent acquisition of property.

(d) A thief has 'possession or control' within s 5(1). 'Possession or control' need not be lawful possession or control: **Turner (No. 2)**, above, and **Kelly** [1999] QB 621. Therefore, a second thief can steal from the first: **Meech** [1974] QB 549 (CA). (Another aspect of **Meech** was impliedly overruled in **Gomez**, above, but the point stands.) It does not matter that the owner has a better right to possession than either of the thieves.

(e) In **Clowes (No. 2)** [1994] 2 All ER 316, one of the accused mixed his own money with that of investors. The Court of Appeal said that there was a trust between him and them. They were in civil law entitled to a first charge on the mixed fund. When he removed £14,000 from the fund, he appropriated a sum in which they had an equitable interest. Accordingly, he had appropriated an interest in property. The definition in s 5(1) was satisfied. The court rejected the contention that there was a presumption that he had withdrawn his own money first from the mixed fund.

(f) If the accused takes property which previously was owned by a dead person, that property belongs to those entitled under the will or on intestacy (or if none, the Crown).

Trusts

Section 5(2)–(4) deal with cases where property belongs to the accused before he dishonestly appropriates it. By s 5(2):

> [w]here property is subject to a trust, the persons to whom it belongs shall be regarded as including any person having a right to enforce the trust, and an intention to defeat the trust shall be regarded accordingly as an intention to deprive of the property any person having that right.

Normally theft by a trustee from a trust will fall within s 5(1). The trustee has a legal interest in the property; the beneficiaries have an equitable interest. Section 5(2) deems the property to belong to the beneficiaries. (Similarly appropriation by an executor will be theft because the legatees have an equitable proprietary interest within s 5(1).) Where the trust does not have identified beneficiaries, such as a charitable trust, s 5(2) applies. The Attorney-General is the person who enforces charitable trusts, and by s 5(2) a theft by a trustee of such a trust is a theft from him. Section 5(2) covers constructive trusts. If Lord Browne-Wilkinson was correct to say in **Westdeutsche Landesbank Girozentrale v Islington Borough Council** [1996] AC 669 (HL), a civil case, that if property is obtained by deception, there is a constructive trust imposed on the recipient, the victim has an equitable interest, and s 5(2) applies.

Where a trustee is charged, not with theft from the intended beneficiaries, but with theft from the public who gave them the money, the public have parted with the whole proprietary interest; therefore, it no longer belongs to them but to the trustees. They are the legal owners. Therefore, the trustees do not steal from the public when they appropriate the money for themselves: **Dyke** [2002] 1 Cr App R 404 (CA). What the court missed, however, was s 5(2). The Attorney-General is the person charged with enforcing charitable trusts. Therefore, he is the owner for the purposes of s 5(2) and the money, again by s 5(2), was stolen from him.

Receipt of property and duty to retain and deal

By s 5(3):

[w]here a person receives property from or on account of another, and is under an obligation to the other to retain and deal with that property or its proceeds in a particular way, the property or proceeds shall be regarded (as against him) as belonging to the other.

The first point to make about s 5(3) is that it is really a fall-back provision. If the victim has a legal or equitable interest in the property or its proceeds, s 5(1) applies too. If a person obtains property under a trust, it belongs to the beneficiary and s 5(1) applies. The same is true of a bailment. The bailor retains property in the item and again s 5(1) governs. Whether the victim has a legal or equitable interest may turn on whether a constructive trust occurs. There is also an overlap between s 5(1) and (3) when a fiduciary has a legal interest in the property. In other words, the same facts can fall within both s 5(1) and s 5(3). If it is uncertain whether the victim had a proprietary interest, s 5(3) comes into play. *A fortiori* it applies where there is no legal or equitable interest. Section 5(3) requires the jury under the judge's instruction to consider questions of civil law. There has to be an obligation to retain and deal as laid down by civil law: *Breaks* [1998] Crim LR 349 (CA). The trial judge was wrong to rule that s 5(3) avoided civil law. There is no criminal rule which determines whether or not the accused 'is under an obligation . . . to . . . deal, with that property . . . in a particular way.'

Section 5(3) has been interpreted in the following ways.

(a) The accused himself must know of the obligation. It is insufficient that his agent knew: *Wills* (1991) 92 Cr App R 297 (CA).

(b) The principal problem is understanding the need for particular arrangements. The basic rule is that s 5(3) applies only where the victim has imposed particular arrangements on the accused. The main authority is *Hall*.

Hall [1973] QB 126 (CA)

The accused, a travel agent, received money from clients. He did not arrange trips and could not repay the money. It was held that he was not guilty of theft because there was no such special arrangement as would give rise to the obligation in s 5(3).

Hall is surprising. One might expect one's money to be used to buy holidays, but that is not what happens. The money can be mixed with other money, e.g. to pay the electricity bill. The money is not kept separate. It is not those coins and notes which are to be handed over. Accordingly, the mere fact that there is a contractual obligation does not mean that the accused is under a duty to retain and deal with the property. (If the accused is dishonest from the start, he will appropriate on receiving the money and therefore be guilty of theft at that moment; in these circumstances there is no need to rely on s 5(3).) The position has been held to apply to an insurance agent, who was under no duty to hand those notes and coins to the company (*Robinson* [1977] Crim LR 173 (CA)), to a person who received premia to buy insurance (*Breaks* [1998] Crim LR 349 (CA)) and to a person in receipt of housing benefit, who was under no legal obligation to use the money to pay off rent arrears (*DPP v Huskinson* [1988] Crim LR 620), even though that was the purpose for which the accused received the benefit. In *Dyke*, above, the Court of Appeal held that where a person collects money on behalf of a charity, property passes from the donors to the charity. Therefore, if a trustee misappropriates that money, s 5(3) applies because he is under an obligation to deal with the money in a particular way, to hand it over to the charity. The court allowed the appeal because the accused had been charged with theft from the donors, and not with theft from the beneficiaries of the trust. However, circumstances alter cases. In *Re Kumar* [2000] Crim LR 504 the accused was also a travel agent, but he was subject to a trust that he would, after deducting commission, transfer money from the agency's account to another body. The Divisional Court held that he was under an obligation to retain and deal with the money in a particular way.

In *Attorney-General's Reference (No. 1 of 1985)*, above, the accused sold other beer than that of the brewery to which he was tied and made a profit for himself. It looks like s 5(3) should apply: the profit should be paid over to the brewery, because there was a constructive trust which created an equitable interest. He was accountable for the profit. It was held that he was not a trustee of the money for the brewers and therefore he was under no obligation to deal with it in a certain way. Section 5(3) was inapplicable. The same reasoning presumably applies to bribes. The law may, however, be on the point of turning. In *Attorney-General of Hong Kong v Reid* [1994] 1 AC 324, a civil case, the Privy Council was faced with a defendant, a New Zealander, who was the acting DPP for Hong Kong. It was conceded that he was a fiduciary. He had been taking bribes to obstruct prosecutions. The Crown sought to exercise proprietary rights over property which the defendant had bought in New Zealand with the proceeds. English civil law provides that breaches of fiduciary duty which involve misapplication of existing trust property result in the property acquired being held on trust, whereas other breaches result in the property not being held on trust: the remedy is an account, a personal remedy not a proprietary one, and the relationship is treated as one of debtor and creditor: *Lister v Stubbs* (1890) 45 Ch D 1 (CA). For example in *Lister* the actual banknotes of the bribe belonged to the bribee; he had to account for the amount of the bribe. In a criminal case a bribe to a turnstile-operator at Wembley was held not to give rise to a charge of theft of the bribe. He was not a fiduciary. There is no property which can be stolen. (The defendant may be liable for breach of contract.) The Privy Council held that *Lister v Stubbs* was incorrect. Reid was such a senior employee that he was a fiduciary and as such was a constructive trustee, holding the property for the Crown, the beneficiary. The effect on criminal law is this. If *Lister* is correct, a person who has been bribed is not guilty of theft, no matter how dishonest he is. If it is wrong, an employee, say, who is bribed is guilty of theft of that sum from his employers provided that in civil law he is a fiduciary. There is property which can be stolen. *Attorney-General's Reference (No. 1 of 1985)*, above, which relied on *Lister v Stubbs*, will be overruled. There will now be a resulting trust where the salaried manager of a tied house sells his own beer. One difficulty with this argument may be that, as *Attorney-General's Reference (No. 1 of 1985)* held, a constructive trust does not create a 'proprietary right or interest' within s 5(1). The profit is not a separate item of property. The contrary contention is that there is a notional (equitable) interest in the employers. A constructive trust creates an equitable proprietary interest. Section 5(1) applies to 'any proprietary . . . interest'. Therefore, a constructive trust falls within s 5(1). A second difficulty is that Lord Wilberforce in *Tarling v Government of the Republic of Singapore* (1978) 70 Cr App R 77 (HL) said: 'The making of a secret profit is no criminal offence.' We await developments. It should be noted that even if the accused is not guilty of theft, he may be convicted of an offence of corruption. If *Reid* is followed, the decision would be an example of how changes to civil law affect criminal law. From the viewpoint of precedent, in cases on provocation the Court of Appeal held that it is bound by its own decisions and not by the advice of the Privy Council. It is uncertain whether it would similarly rule in respect of this area of the law.

The position is different where there are particular arrangements. The law is illustrated by the pre-Theft Act case of *Hassall* (1861) 169 ER 1302 where the treasurer of a Christmas club did not spend the money on Christmas treats. In *Wain* [1995] 2 Cr App R 660 (CA) the accused organised events which raised nearly £3,000 for charity. He put the money into his own bank account and withdrew money from that account. The court held that the accused was under a duty to retain the money in his bank account, the proceeds of the specific notes and coins raised for charity, because s 5(3) applied. (Indeed, there might have been a duty to retain the specific notes and coins for the benefit of the charity.) The case of *Lewis v Lethbridge* [1987] Crim LR 59 where the Divisional Court had held that sponsorship money did not belong to the charity by virtue of s 5(3) was overruled. The court held that there is an obligation because the donors impose a trust on the recipient to give the money to the charity. It does not matter that there is no rule imposed by the charity that recipients hand over the specific notes and coins. In *Klineberg* [1999] 1 Cr App R 427 (CA) there was an obligation imposing particular arrangements when purchasers of timeshares paid money into a trust which was charged with the duty of safeguarding moneys. *Klineberg* was applied in *Floyd v DPP* [2000] Crim 411 (DC). An agent for a firm supplying hampers was under a duty to send the money she had collected from her colleagues to the firm. The court held that the prosecution did not have to prove that the firm had a legal or equitable interest in the money collected by the accused. However, what the court did not inquire into was the source of the obligation to deal with the money in a particular way. There was no contract between the parties that she should transmit the money to the company. If contract was not the source of the duty, it is difficult to see how the duty arose.

In *Davidge v Bunnett* [1984] Crim LR 297 (DC), which was approved in *Wain*, the accused was given money by her flatmates to pay the gas bill. She spent it on other things. She was held to be guilty of theft. She was under a duty to use the money to pay the gas bills (cf. *Hall*, where the accused was not under a duty to use that money for that holiday). On the facts of *Rader* given above the accused was under a duty to invest the money in a way that would yield a profit for the victim. The court distinguished *Hall*. The Court of Appeal in *McHugh* (1993) 97 Cr App R 335 spoke of s 5(3) applying where there was a legal arrangement whereby the victim's money was to be kept separate from the accused's. It should be noted that s 5(3) does, however, apply where the accused has put the money he received into his own bank account, as *Wain* demonstrates. In *Brewster* (1979) 69 Cr App R 375 (CA), an insurance agent was guilty of theft of the premiums because the money had to be handed over to the companies he worked for under the terms of his contract. Therefore, he was under an obligation to deal with the money in a particular way, that obligation being constituted by the contract. The fact that the firms allowed him to use the money for his own purposes and replace it was merely an indulgence. *Robinson*, above, also concerned an insurance agent, but there was no such obligation. In *Crown Prosecution Service, ex parte Judd*, unreported, 1 November 1999, the Divisional Court held that money received in weekly instalments from five colleagues at work belonged to the mail order company for which the accused had collected. There was no need for an express contract to that effect. In *Wakeman v Farrar* [1974] Crim LR 136 (DC), the accused received a warning that he must return a lost cheque after he had received an over-the-counter payment from the Department of Health and Social Security. The cheque was thereby subject to a legal obligation within s 5(3). In *Hallam* [1995] Crim LR 323 the Court of Appeal held that two defendants, financial advisers, who did not invest money on behalf of investors, fell within s 5(3) because the victims retained an equitable interest in the cheques they drew and the proceeds of the cheques.

(c) On analogy with *Gilks* [1972] 1 WLR 1341 on s 5(4) the obligation in s 5(3) must be a legally enforceable one, and this proposition was apparently accepted in *Meech* [1974] QB 549 (CA) and *Mainwaring* (1981) 74 Cr App R 99 (CA). That the obligation had to be legally enforceable was accepted in *Williams* [1995] Crim LR 77 (CA). An example of a non-legally enforceable obligation is a gambling debt. (However, a bet on the Tote is legally enforceable because the Tote can neither win nor lose, and there is accordingly no wager.) *Cullen*, unreported, 1974, seems to be contrary to cases such as *Mainwaring*. A mistress was given money to buy food. The court thought that there was a legal obligation, which she breached by spending the money on herself. As a matter of contract law, however, the outcome would have been different. There would have been no contract but a non-binding domestic arrangement. She therefore would not have been liable for breach of contract. The result looks odd: she is guilty in criminal law but not liable in civil law. Whether there is a legal obligation is a question for the judge: *Mainwaring* and *Dubar* [1994] 1 WLR 1484 *obiter* (Courts-Martial Appeal Court), among other cases. Cases which state that the question whether there is an obligation is one for the jury are incorrect, as are ones which state that there is no need for the jury to consider matters of civil law. The jury's task is to see whether the duty arose on the facts.

(d) *Meech* held that the accused was under an obligation to retain and deal with a cheque if he believed that he was under such a duty, though in fact he was not. In the light of the need for a legal obligation *Meech* looks incorrect on this point. In *Meech* the victim obtained a cheque by fraud. The accused cashed it for him. The accused and a couple of friends staged a false robbery of the accused in order not to have to pay over the money. The Court of Appeal held that the accused was under an obligation despite the victim's inability to enforce the obligation because he had obtained the cheque fraudulently. Section 5(3) says 'is under an obligation', not 'believes himself to be under an obligation'. A charge of attempted theft should have been brought.

(e) Where there is a trust, s 5(3) will apply (as well as s 5(2)). In *Arnold* [1997] 4 All ER 1 the Court of Appeal held that s 5(3) applied to relationships falling short of trusteeship. It covered the relationship of a franchisor and franchisee where the former had received from the latter bills of exchange and he had then discounted them. The bills of exchange were property which belonged to another within s 5(3). It did not matter that they had only temporarily been in the hands of the franchisees or that the relationship between the parties was a contractual one. The court held that s 5(3) applied, even though the accused retained the property throughout the dealings. For comment, see Sir John Smith in his case comment on *Malone* [1998] Crim LR 834.

(f) Section 5(3) applies when there is an obligation in respect of 'that property or its proceeds'. In *Klineberg*, above, the court held that when the purchasers of timeshare apartments paid by cash or by cheques, the defendants were under an obligation to retain the funds; in the case of bank transfers from the purchasers to the defendants, the latter had come by the property and were also under the same obligation. The new credit was 'proceeds' of property. However, this analysis fails to take account of *Preddy* [1996] AC 815. Bank transfers create a new thing in action. There is no transfer.

Receiving by mistake and obligation to restore

By s 5(4):

> [w]here a person gets property by another's mistake and is under an obligation to make restoration (in whole or in part) of the property or its proceeds or the value thereof, then to the extent of that obligation the property or proceeds shall be regarded (as against him) as belonging to the person entitled to restoration, and an intention not to make restoration shall be regarded accordingly as an intention to deprive that person of the property or proceeds.

Section s 5(4) applies where the victim has made a mistake. The mistake need not have been induced by the accused. Section 5(4) comes into play only if the accused is under a legal duty to restore. If there is no such obligation, but, say, a duty to pay the price of an article, s 5(4) does not apply. One way of approaching s 5(4) is to hold that ownership of goods is not transferred to the alleged thief in situations where under civil law it would not have passed. Therefore, s 5(4) does not apply where under civil law ownership would not have been transferred. Ownership would not have been transferred where the mistake is so fundamental that the transaction is void such as when there is a mistake caused by fraud as to the relevant identity of the recipient. In this event, s 5(1) applies. In *Williams* [1980] Crim LR 589 (CA) it was held that there was a fundamental mistake in the mind of a cashier at a bureau de change when the accused proffered obsolete foreign currency, knowing it to be obsolete, and the cashier took it, not knowing it was obsolete. When the cashier handed over money in exchange, no property passed to the accused. That money remained property belonging to another within s 5(1). If s 5(4) does not apply to such mistakes, what is left? Therefore, s 5(4) applies to voidable contracts; that is, where the mistake is not so fundamental that the contract is void. Ownership passes to the alleged thief under a voidable contract and remains with him until the contract is avoided by the innocent party. Section 5(4) deems ownership to remain with the victim. Section 5(4) is not needed for void contracts because ownership remains with the victim.

This reading derives support from the legislative history of the provision. The aim was to reverse the decision in *Moynes v Coopper*, above. The employee received a pay packet which contained an overpayment. The amount should have been reduced because he had received an advance on his wages. He later discovered the overpayment and spent the money. He was not guilty of the offence, which is now theft, but would now be so because of s 5(4) where the innocent party's belief is classified as a non-fundamental one. Under civil law the accused is under a duty to make restitution ('an obligation to make restitution'). Section 5(4) is applicable and the accused is guilty of theft of the excess. This effect of s 5(4) can be seen from *Attorney-General's Reference (No. 1 of 1983)* [1985] QB 182. The accused was overpaid, the money going into her current account. The Court of Appeal held that she had acquired something, a right of action against the bank, by mistake and she was under a duty to make restoration of the value of the property she had received. The case demonstrates that s 5(4) applies to intangible property (the debt) as well as tangible property. The court considered, however, that the criminal law should not normally be used in such situations. Possibly she did not appropriate. The Court of

Appeal did not discuss this issue. If she kept her account above the sum wrongly paid to her, by civil law she would be deemed to have spent her own money when withdrawing from the account. Her omission to inform the authorities that she had been overpaid was not an act and on general principles a failure to act does not normally constitute the *actus reus* of an offence.

Another approach to s 5(4) is to argue thus: s 5(4) applies only if the contract is void. If the contract is voidable, there is no 'obligation to make restoration' because the obligation does not arise until the innocent party elects to avoid the contract. There is only a potential, not an actual, obligation. The accused *is* not under an obligation. The contrary contention is that there is a legal obligation even though it depends on the innocent party's making the election.

Certainly s 5(4) applies where property does pass. There is deemed to be property still owned by the victim, and the accused is under a duty to restore.

In *Chase Manhattan Bank NA* v *Israel-British Bank NA* [1981] Ch 105, a civil case, it was held that the innocent party to an overpayment retains an equitable right where the overpayment was brought about by a mistake of fact. Therefore, s 5(1) applies and there is no need to rely on s 5(4). The case has been criticised in the House of Lords but not overruled. The Court of Appeal in its criminal guise adopted this understanding of the law in *Shadrokh-Cigari*, above, but also held that s 5(4) was another way to the same result since there was also an obligation to make restoration. In *Shadrokh-Cigari* a bank erroneously transferred money to an account of a child, whose guardian the accused was. He knew that the bank had made a mistake. He persuaded the child to sign mandates authorising the bank to issue drafts in his favour. Either the bank retained an equitable interest in the drafts within s 5(1) or the accused was under a duty to restore within s 5(4). It must be said that as a matter of civil law the existence of an equitable proprietary interest is unclear. If, however, *Shadrokh-Cigari* is correct, there is no problem with instances of overpayment such as *Stalham* [1993] Crim LR 310. The debt owed by the bank to the accused belongs in equity to the employers. The accused appropriated her employers' equitable interest. If *Chase Manhattan* is wrong, as seems to be the view after *Westdeutsche Landesbank Girozentrale* v *Islington Borough Council* [1996] AC 669, at least where the recipient does not know of the error, there is still a route to conviction via s 5(4). The reasoning behind *Shadrokh-Cigari* was applied in *Webster* [2006] EWCA Crim 2894. A soldier erroneously received a second medal for service in Iraq. He gave it to the accused, who sold it on an internet auction site. The court held that because of the fundamental error in sending the second medal, the Crown retained an equitable interest, therefore s 5(1) applied with the result that there was no need to rely on s 5(4). If *Shadrokh-Cigari* is correct, then the purpose behind s 5(4), the deeming of overpaid money to belong to the giver, has been destroyed, for s 5(4) is not needed when the facts fall within s 5(1). The Court of Appeal in *Ngan* [1998] 1 Cr App R 331 relied on s 5(4) where the accused's account had been credited with the victim's cheques because the bank made a mistake. It did not discuss whether or not a constructive trust existed.

Under s 5(4) the obligation must be a legally enforceable one: *Gilks*, above. A gambling debt is not legally enforceable. Therefore, if a bookmaker pays out money in the mistaken belief that a certain horse has won, s 5(4) is inappropriate. Ownership of the money, it was then thought, did not pass. Therefore, the money remained property belonging to another. (Civil law appears to be, however, that property does pass to the winner of a bet.) Under *Gomez* the accused nowadays appropriated when he took the money from the bookmaker's even though the clerk gave it to him. If it was not until later that the accused discovered that he had been overpaid, it is suggested that the money no longer belongs to another because ownership of it passes on payment. On the understanding that **Shadrokh-Cigari** is correct, the bookmaker in **Gilks** retained an equitable interest in the money which the assistant manager mistakenly overpaid, and s 5(1) applied.

'Proceeds' in s 5(4) covers money received from a third party who had cashed a cheque for the accused.

Davis (1989) 88 Cr App R 347 (CA)

The accused received cheques for housing benefit from his local authority. He was not entitled to that benefit. He cashed the cheques. The court held that he had obtained the paper on which the cheques were written by mistake. He was under a legal duty to make restoration. He did not do so but converted the cheques into money, which constituted the proceeds of the property. By s 5(4) the money belonged to another.

The accused had also for a time received two housing benefit cheques for the same period. It was uncertain to which of the cheques he was or was not entitled. The court held that the accused was under an obligation to restore such of the proceeds as belonged to another.

Section 5(4) covers property, proceeds and 'the value thereof' whereas s 5(3) refers only to 'property or its proceeds'. In **Dubar**, above, the accused received money from a fellow member of the armed forces. The obligation was to find a second-hand car for him. If the accused did not become dishonest until all the money had been spent and no proceeds of that money survived, s 5(3) could not apply.

Robbery

Introduction

This offence may be seen as a crime against both property and the person. By s 8(1) of the Theft Act 1968:

> [a] person is guilty of **robbery** if he steals, and immediately before or at the time of doing so, and in order to do so, he uses any force on any person or puts or seeks to put any person in fear of being then and there subjected to force.

For an explanation of assault, see pp 525–29 in Chapter 13.

The maximum sentence is life imprisonment (s 8(2)). Robbery covers both serious crimes and facts which are not as serious as some thefts. There is also a separate crime of assault with intent to rob. 'Assault' covers both psychic (for definition see Chapter 13) assault and battery. There is no requirement that the victim is in fact put in fear of force: **R v DPP** [2007] EWHC 739 (Admin).

Robbery is essentially an aggravated form of theft. All the elements of theft must be proved before a conviction may be secured for this offence. An accused is therefore not guilty of robbery if he believes that he has a legal right to deprive the victim of the property. In **Robinson** [1977] Crim LR 173 (CA), the accused demanded that the victim repay a debt owed by the victim's wife to him. He had a knife to reinforce his demand. The court held that the facts did not constitute robbery because the accused was not dishonest, because he thought he had a legal right to the money (see the discussion of s 2(1)(a) above). In **Forrester** [1992] Crim LR 793, the accused had no claim of right and applying

Ghosh he was dishonest. All the other elements of theft were present. He used force by knocking off balance his victim, who was also kept under restraint, and the force was used immediately before stealing and in order to do so. There is a *dictum* that 'steals' does not mean the same as it does in *Ghosh* but it would be strange if it did not. The *Ghosh* test of dishonesty and the *Gomez* test of appropriation apply.

The *Criminal Statistics, England and Wales 2000*, Home Office, 2001, stated that there were some 66,200 reported instances of robbery. V. Harrington and P. Mayhew, *Mobile Phone Thefts*, Home Office Research Study 235, 2001, stated that 28 per cent of robberies involved the appropriation of mobiles. The British Crime Survey estimated that some 362,000 robberies occurred in 2001–02, of which 43 per cent involved mobiles. There were 88,710 reported instances of robbery in 2004–05, but the British Crime Survey estimated 255,000 in the same period. Certainly the number of robberies has fallen more or less every year since 1995.

The *actus reus*

'Force' is an ordinary English word, apparently chosen because it is comprehensible to lay people. It is for the jury to determine its meaning: *Dawson* (1976) 64 Cr App R 170 (CA). Whether jostling is force is for the jury. The Court of Appeal approved this approach in *Clouden* [1987] Crim LR 56.

The force must be used *in order to* steal, as s 8(1) states. In *Donaghy* [1981] Crim LR 644 (Crown Court), the accused ordered a taxi-driver to take him from Newmarket to London and made threats to his life. Once in London he stole £22 from the driver. He was held not guilty of robbery because the threats were not made in order to take the money. If a person is engaged in a fight, knocks down the victim, and then decides to take her purse, he has not used force in order to steal. The force enables him to steal, but the definition of robbery is not satisfied because the force is not used *in order to* steal.

The force must be used 'on' the person. An example is putting a hand over the victim's mouth to stop her screaming: *Hale* (1978) 68 Cr App R 415 (CA). It should also be noted that this action amounted to 'force'. It has been suggested that 'on' means 'against' and therefore it is not robbery if the accused snatches the victim's bag unless the victim retains hold or recovers it and there is a fight. Perhaps this distinction is too little to bear the weight placed on it. The section states 'on any person' not 'against'. In *Corcoran v Anderton* (1980) 71 Cr App R 104 (DC), there was robbery where a handbag was tugged away from the victim, even though she did not lose control. This case exemplifies that an accused is guilty of robbery even though he has not succeeded in his purpose. In *Clouden* snatching a basket out of the victim's hands was robbery. It is certain that the Criminal Law Revision Committee, the Report of which formed the basis of the Theft Act (*Theft and Related Offences*, Cmnd 2977, 1966), would not have wanted such a result but would have preferred the outcome to be theft (see para 65). The Court of Appeal did not resort to the Report in *Clouden* despite the provision's being ambiguous. Simple pickpocketing or slipping one's hand into a bag and removing a purse is theft because no force is used on the victim. Nevertheless, since the meaning of 'force' is left to the jury, it is possible that some juries might conclude that force has been used on a person. A maximum sentence of life imprisonment for pulling a handbag from a victim's grasp would seem to be excessive.

The force must be used 'immediately before or at the time of' the theft. It is not robbery, wrote the Criminal Law Revision Committee in the same paragraph, where the accused uses force to escape. If, however, 'appropriation' in the definition of theft is a continuing act, the accused may be convicted of robbery if there is a force during a struggle to escape: *Hale*, approved in *Gregory* (1982) 77 Cr App R 41 (CA). Therefore, robbery is seen as a continuing act. It seems that whether the accused is guilty of robbery if he uses force when escaping is a question for the jury: *Hale* (unreported on this point). In *Lockley* [1995] 2 Cr App R 554 the Court of Appeal held that *Gomez* had not affected *Hale*. Appropriation was not over at the moment when the accused took cans of beer but was continuing when at a later stage he used violence against the off-licence shopkeeper who has challenged him. *Gomez* related to the issue whether there was an appropriation when the victim consented to the accused's assumption of his rights, not whether appropriation was a continuing act. The accused's conviction was upheld. Accordingly whether there is a robbery depends on whether the force or threat of force is used while the accused is still 'on the job'.

It is immaterial that the accused uses force on some person other than the one from whom he takes the item. If the accused uses force on a railway signalman to make him stop a train, it is robbery if the accused steals from the train.

Section 8(1) covers not only force but the threat of force. The threat must be one which puts the victim 'then and there' in fear of force. A threat of future force is not sufficient. In those circumstances a charge of blackmail is appropriate. The subsection also covers where the accused 'seeks to put' a person in fear of force. An example is threatening a deaf person. The victim need not actually be made afraid. An example of this type of robbery was briefly noted in *The Guardian*, 1 March 1994, where a Mr Muldownie was jailed by the Southwark Crown Court for brandishing a syringe which he said contained his blood contaminated with HIV.

Mens rea

Besides the mental element required for theft, it is probable that the force must be applied intentionally or at least recklessly and that the accused must be aware that the force is being used on a person. The force or threat of force must be done 'in order to' steal. This is a *mens rea* term. As stated above in the discussion of *Robinson*, if the *mens rea* of theft does not exist robbery is not committed, even though the accused in that case used a knife to get the money he was owed.

Reform

The Law Commission's draft Criminal Code, Law Com. No. 177, 1989, is a restatement of present law. 'The aim has been to achieve consistency with Code style and method in point of language, presentation and clarity of statement, without affecting substance' (at 270). One minor change is that the crime of assault with intent to rob, at present found in s 8, is transferred out of the part of the draft Criminal Code dealing with property offences to the part dealing with offences against the person (cl 78); however, in its Report No. 218, *Legislating the Criminal Code – Offences Against the Person and General Principles*, 1993, the Law Commission considered that the offence should not be part of the Criminal Law Bill in which revised non-fatal offences including assault are found. The Law Commission accepted that both the 1968 and 1978 Theft Acts and the case law on them are thought by some to be 'seriously defective', but the draft Criminal Code was a restatement, not a Code to reform the substance of the law. In 1995 the Law Commission commenced work on offences of dishonesty but progress has been slow.

Summary

Chapter 15 is the first of four dealing with offences against property. It lays out the definitions of theft and robbery. Theft is the dishonest appropriation of property belonging to another with the intention of permanently depriving the other of it. Robbery is basically theft plus violence or the threat of violence. The main debates in the law of theft are whether any dealing with property amounts to appropriation and which behaviour constitutes dishonesty. Appropriation is defined in part in the Theft Act 1968, s 3(1), but the courts, in particular the House of Lords, have expanded that definition, contrary to Parliament's intention, to cover being given property with the consent of the owner (***Gomez*** [1993] AC 442) and receiving property as a gift (***Hinks*** [2001] 2 AC 241). The result is that if you, an honest shopper, take a tin of beans from your local supermarket for your supper, you satisfy four of the five elements of theft: 'take' = appropriation; 'a tin of beans' = 'property'; 'from your local supermarket' = the property belongs to another; 'for your supper' = 'with the intention of permanently depriving the other of it' within the basic definition of theft found in s 1(1) of the 1968 statute. You are not guilty of theft because you are not dishonest. However, the definition of dishonesty as found in s 2(1) of the Act *and* in ***Ghosh*** [1982] QB 1053 is not always easy to apply and it is a question for the jury whether or not the accused was dishonest. These are not the only issues in theft. Students may be interested to know that the confidential information contained in an exam paper before it is sat is not property for the purposes of s 4(1) of the Act and therefore it cannot be stolen (but the paper on which the questions are written can be)! Another issue which students often get wrong is whether the facts fall within s 6(1) of the Act, intention permanently to deprive. Normally s 6(1) is not needed because the thief usually intends the victim not to get the item stolen back; however, s 6(1) comes into play when the accused intends that the victim should get the property back, as when she means at the time of the appropriation to return a football season ticket once the season is over.

- Theft – the basic definition: Section 1(1) of the Theft Act 1968 prohibits the (i) dishonest (ii) appropriation of (iii) property (iv) belonging to another (v) with the intention of permanently depriving the other of it. Sections 2–6 treat of those concepts in order. There is no need for the accused to act with a view to gain, and there is no need for the thief to receive any benefit from the theft: s 1(2).

- Dishonesty: Unlike in the rest of this book the *mens rea* is dealt with before the *actus reus*. This is because it is the *mens rea* which converts an otherwise innocuous *actus reus* into the crime of theft. If you take a can of beans from your local supermarket, you have committed the *actus reus* of theft, the appropriation ('take') of property ('a can of beans') belonging to another (the 'local supermarket'). Indeed, even one of the elements of the *mens rea*, intent permanently to deprive, does not distinguish the thief from the honest shopper, for presumably both intend to eat the beans. The distinction lies in the 'dishonesty' element. Section 2(1) gives a partial definition of when the accused is NOT dishonest:

  belief in a legal right to deprive the other
  belief that the victim would have consented, had he or she known of the true circumstances, and
  belief that the owner cannot be found by taking reasonable steps.

  Even outside s 2(1), however, an accused will be not dishonest if he or she was not dishonest by the standards of ordinary decent people, or if he or she was so dishonest, he or she did not know that what he or she was doing was dishonest by those standards.

- Intention permanently to deprive (IPD): An error often committed by students is to think that s 6(1) defines IPD – it does not! Section 6(1) is used only where the accused intends that the victim should get the item back; otherwise the basic definition in s 1(1) is all that is needed. For example, if I take your coat and use it as the basis for a fire, I do intend to deprive you of it permanently. Indeed, s 6(1) does NOT apply because I do not mean you to get the coat back. In sum, s 6(1) applies only when it says it applies: 'without meaning the other permanently to lose the thing itself'. It governs two situations, both of which are ones in which the accused does intend that the victim gets the item back: 'his intention is to treat the thing as his own to dispose of regardless of the other's rights' and 'a borrowing or lending of it [the property] may amount to so treating it if, but only if, the borrowing or lending is for a period and in circumstances making it equivalent to an outright taking or disposal.'

- Appropriation: Section 3(1) of the Theft Act 1968 states that appropriation consists of 'any assumption by a person of the rights of an owner . . .'. 'The rights' has been construed as meaning 'any of the rights'; and appropriation covers not just taking but receiving, including receiving something as a gift, a far-fetched judicial construction one may think. If one deceives another into giving one an item of property, one also appropriates. Indeed, the stage has been reached where it can be said that any dealing with property (even honestly) is an appropriation. There is no need for a misappropriation.

  One person who would otherwise appropriate is exempted by s 3(2), the bona fide purchaser for value without notice.

- Property: Section 4(1) provides that 'money and all other property, real or personal, including things in action and other intangible property' constitutes property. The section may be read as 'property = property' but a better equation is: 'property for the purposes of the criminal law of theft = property for the purposes of civil law'; therefore anything which is property at civil law is also property for the purposes of theft, and the corollary is that what is not property at civil law is also not property for theft (e.g. confidential information such as that found on an exam paper). A thing in action is something which does not physically exist but which may be enforced by legal action, e.g. a debt. Intangible property includes patents and export quotas: they can be appropriated by the accused's transferring them from the victim to a third party. At common law a human body cannot be stolen but the exceptions are growing and include body parts which have had work done on them, e.g. anatomical specimens. There is much law on cheques but the basic rules are these: drawing a cheque on an account in credit or on an account which is within the agreed overdraft limit creates a debt, which is property, as we have seen; however, drawing a cheque on an account which is beyond the overdraft limit does not create a debt because the bank is not obliged in law to meet the cheque and therefore in this case there is no debt which may be the subject of a theft charge.

  Section 4(2) states that land and things forming part of the land cannot be stolen except:
  (a) when he is a trustee or personal representative, or is authorised by power of attorney, or as a liquidator of a company, or otherwise, to sell or dispose of land belonging to another, and he appropriates the land or anything forming part of it by dealing with it in breach of the confidence reposed in him; or

(b) when he is not in possession of the land and appropriates anything forming part of it by severing it or causing it to be severed, or after it has been severed; or

(c) when, being in possession of the land under a tenancy, he appropriates the whole or part of any fixture or structure let to be used with the land . . .

Readers if students may be interested to know that (c) exempts them from theft if they appropriate as licensees but not as tenants. Land Law is useful in Criminal Law!

Section 4(3) exempts those who pick fungi, 'flowers, fruit or foliage from a plant growing wild on any land' unless they do so 'for reward or for sale or for any other commercial purpose'. Note that 'plant' includes 'any shrub or tree' and that the exemption is restricted to picking FROM a plant: therefore, digging up the whole plant does not give rise to the s 4(2) exception.

Section 4(4) exempts poachers from liability for theft but the provision is complex and best not summarised but written out: 'Wild creatures, tamed or untamed, shall be regarded as property; but a person cannot steal a wild creature not tamed not ordinarily kept in captivity, or the carcase of any such creature, unless either it has been reduced into possession by or on behalf of another person and possession of it has not since been lost or abandoned or another person is in the course of reducing it into possession.' If one follows the terms of s 4(4), one can see that while a poacher cannot steal, a poacher can steal from a poacher. Note that there are other offences dealing with poachers. Unlike s 4(3), s 4(4) is not limited to commercial purposes.

- Belonging to another: The main provision is s 5(1), which states that property belongs to 'any person having possession or control of it, or having any proprietary right or interest (not being an equitable interest arising only from an agreement to transfer or grant an interest).' There are several matters worth noting. First, the thief may steal from the owner ('any person . . . having a proprietary right . . .') or the possessor or the controller or any two or more of these potential victims. Indeed, a thief may, because of s 5(1), steal from another thief. Secondly, unless the equitable interest falls within the phrase in brackets, it falls within s 5(1). Therefore, a trustee, who has the legal interest, may steal from a beneficiary, who has the equitable interest.

Section 5(2) ensures that persons who appropriate assets subject to charitable trusts are deemed to be thieves, if all the other elements of the offence are satisfied.

Section 5(3) is another deeming provision. By it 'if a person receives property from or on account of another, and is under an obligation to retain and deal with that property or its proceeds in a particular way, the property or proceeds shall be regarded . . . as belonging to the other.' The principal trap for the unwary is the concept of 'an obligation to . . . deal with in a particular way'. Unless this condition is satisfied, s 5(3) does not apply. For example, if students share a flat and one, the victim, gives another, the accused, money to be paid towards the gas bill, as long as the other does pay the gas bill, he or she need not use that exact money for the bill. In that case, if the student uses the money given on wine, women (or men) and song, s 5(3) does not apply and the accused is not guilty of theft, no matter how dishonest he or she was. However, if the victim impresses on the accused that THIS money must be used to pay off the bill, then s 5(3) does apply for now the accused is under a duty to use that money in a particular way.

Section 5(4) is also a deeming provision. By it 'where a person gets property by another's mistake and is under an obligation to make restoration . . . of the property or its proceeds or the value thereof, then . . . the property or proceeds shall be regarded . . . as belonging to the person entitled to restoration . . .' This subsection is obviously about situations where the accused has received the victim's property through the latter's mistake but it should be noted that most, if not all, such scenarios fall also within s 5(1); the other major noteworthy point concerns the interpretation of s 5(4) and may be put in this way: the fact that the accused has received property by mistake does not automatically mean that he or she is under a duty to restore; whether there is such an obligation depends on the civil law of restitution.

● Robbery: The offence of robbery, contrary to s 8(1) of the Theft Act 1968, may be seen as one of 'theft plus': that is, all the elements of theft must be proved plus either force or the threat of force. The subsection reads: 'a person is guilty of robbery if he steals, and immediately before or at the time of doing so, and in order to do so, he uses any force on any person or puts or seeks to put any person in fear of being then and there subjected to force.' One of the points of interpretation that should be noted is that s 8(1) applies where the force or threat of force is on a person other than the victim of the theft.

Refences

Reports

Criminal Law Revision Committee 8th Report, *Theft and Related Offences*, Cmnd 2977 (1966)

Home Office *Criminal Statistics, England & Wales 2000* (2001)

Home Office White Paper, *Crime, Justice and Protecting the Public*, Cm 965 (1990)

Law Commission Consultation Paper No. 150, *Misuse of Trade Secrets* (1997)

Law Commission Consultation Paper No. 155, *Legislating the Criminal Code: Fraud and Deception* (1999)

Law Commission Report No. 177, *A Criminal Code for England & Wales* (1989)

Law Commission Report No. 218, *Legislating the Criminal Code: Offences against the Person and General Principles* (1993)

Law Commission Report No. 276, *Fraud* (2002)

Books

Clarkson, C. M. V. and Keating, H. *Criminal Law: Text and Materials* 5th edn (Thomson, 2003)

Harington, V. and Mayhew, P. *Mobile Phone Thefts*, Home Office Research Study No. 235 (2001)

Nicholas, S., Povey, D., Walker, A. and Kershaw, C. *Crime in England & Wales 2004–05* (Home Office, 2005)

Philips, E., Walsh, C. and Dobson, P. *Law Relating to Theft* (Cavendish, 2001)

Journals

Glazebrook, P. R. 'Revising the Theft Acts' [1993] CLJ 191

Smith, J. C. 'Reforming the Theft Acts' (1996) 28 *Bracton Law Journal* 27

Sullivan, G. R. and Warbrick, C. 'Current developments: private international law' (1994) 43 ICLQ 464

Sullivan, G. R. and Warbrick, C. 'Territoriality, theft and *Atakpu*' Crim LR 650 [1994]

Further reading

Campbell, K. 'The test for dishonesty in *R v Ghosh* [1984] CLJ 349

Elliott, D. W. 'Dishonesty in theft – a dispensable concept' [1982] Crim LR 395

Gardner, S. 'Property and theft' [1998] Crim LR 35

Griew, E. 'Dishonesty: the objections to *Feely* and *Ghosh*' [1985] Crim LR 341

Griew, E. 'Stealing and obtaining bank credits' [1986] Crim LR 356

Halpin, A. 'The test for dishonesty' [1996] Crim LR 283

Hammond, G. '*R v Stewart*: the final judgment?' (1989) 11 Sup Ct LR 21

Kershaw, C. *et al. The 2000 British Crime Survey* (Home Office Statistical Bulletin, 2000)

Melissaris, E. 'The concept of appropriation and the law of theft' (2007) 70 MLR 581

Shute, S. 'Appropriation and the law of theft' [2002] Crim LR 445

Simester, A. P. and Sullivan, G. R. 'On the nature and rationale of property offences' in (eds) Duff and Green *Defining Crimes: Essays on the Special Part of Criminal Law* (Oxford University Press, 2005)

Smith, J.C. 'The sad fate of the Theft Act 1968' in W. Swadling and G. Jones (eds) *The Search for Principle* (Oxford University Press, 1999)

Smith, J.C. [2001] Crim LR 573 (for case comment on *Clark*)

Stannard, J. 'Fools rush in – the meaning of s 6 of the Theft Act' (1979) 30 NILQ 225

Williams, G. 'Temporary appropriation should be theft' [1981] Crim LR 129

Williams, G. 'Innocuously dipping into trust funds' (1985) 5 LS 183

The principal modern work on this and the next two chapters is A. T. H. Smith, '*Property Offences*' (Sweet & Maxwell, 1994). For a simpler and more modern work see E. Phillips, C. Walsh and P. Dobson, *Law Relating to Theft* (Cavendish, 2001).

J. C. Smith, *The Law of Theft*, has been updated by D. Ornerod and D. Williams (Oxford University Press, 9th edn, 2007). It is now published as *Smith's Law of Theft*.

Visit **www.mylawchamber.co.uk/jefferson** to access exam-style questions with answer guidance, multiple choice quizzes, live weblinks, an online glossary, and regular updates to the law.

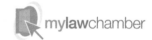

Use **Case Navigator** to read in full some of the key cases referenced in this chapter:

R v Ghosh [1982] 2 All ER 689
R v Woollin [1998] 4 All ER 103

16

Fraud, making off without payment

Introduction

The Theft Act 1968 created five offences of obtaining by deception, of which the most important were obtaining property by deception (s 15) and obtaining a pecuniary advantage by deception (s 16). Section 15A was inserted into the 1968 Act by the Theft (Amendment) Act 1996. It created the offence of obtaining a money transfer by deception. Part of s 16 was abolished by the Theft Act 1978, which created three offences: obtaining services by deception (s 1), evading liability by deception (s 2), and making off without payment (s 3). The s 3 crime does not require deception and is treated separately.

The Fraud Act 2006 carne into force. The Act replaced all the deception offences, namely ss 15, 15A and 16 of the Theft Act 1968 and ss 1 and 2 of the Theft Act 1978. Because the crime of making off is not an offence of deception, s 3 of the Theft Act 1978 (making off) is unaffected. The Act creates one offence of fraud (s 1) but that is committed in three ways: by false representation (s 2), by failing to disclose information (s 3), and by abuse of position (s 4).

The Fraud Act 2006

The new offence of fraud

This statute came into force on the 15 January 2007. The Act creates the general offence of fraud, which is punishable on indictment to a maximum of ten years' imprisonment or an unlimited fine or both; the maximum on summary conviction is 12 months' imprisonment or a fine not exceeding the current maximum (£5,000) or both. The offence may be committed in three ways, which are laid down in ss 2–4 of the Act. There is no need for the financial interests of the victim to be imperilled. The Home Office's Criminal Law Policy Unit in *Fraud Law Reform: Government Response to Consultations* (2006) at para. 12 stated that the offence did not breach Article 7 of the European Convention on Human Rights. The Act repeals and replaces all the offences of obtaining by deception found in the Theft Acts 1968–78.

Fraud by false representation (s 2)

Section 2(1) states:

> A person is in breach of this section if he –
> (a) dishonestly makes a false representation, and
> (b) intends, by making the representation –
>   (i) to make a gain for himself or another, or
>   (ii) to cause loss to another or to expose another to a risk of loss.

There is no need for the intended victim to be deceived. Unlike its predecessor, fraud is a conduct, not a result, crime. There is also no requirement, unlike the previous law, for anyone to be deceived. By s 2(3) a representation means 'any representation as to fact or as to law, including a representation as to the state of mind of – (a) the person making the representation, or (b) any other person.' There is no actual definition of 'representation'. The representation may be express or implied: s 2(4). An example is the famous second-hand car dealer's 'it's a good little runner'. This is not just a statement of opinion but an implied representation as to fact: 'it is my honest opinion that this car is a good little runner'. By s 2(2) a representation is false if '(a) it is untrue or misleading, and (b) the person making it knows that it is, or might be, untrue or misleading.' Section 2 goes on to cover deception of machines: '. . . a representation may be regarded as made if it (or anything implying it) is submitted in any form to any system or device designed to receive, convey or respond to communication (with or without human intervention).' This provision means that unlike earlier law a fraud may be committed where a machine is 'deceived'.

Gain and loss are defined in s 5, which also applies to ss 3 and 4 (see below). By s 5(2), which is very similar to s 34(2)(a) of the Theft Act 1968, discussed in the next chapter. ' "Gain" and "loss" – (a) extend only to gain and loss in money or other property; (b) include any such gain whether temporary or permanent; and "property" means any property whether real or personal (including things in action and other tangible property).' For an explanation of 'things in action' see Chapter 15. 'Gain' is further defined as 'a gain by keeping what one has, as well as a gain by getting what one does not have.' (s 5(3)). 'Gain' covers getting what the victim legally owes to the accused. Similarly, by s 5(4) 'loss' includes 'a loss by not getting what one might get, as well as a loss by parting with what one has.' Because there need be no actual gain or loss, fraud can be seen as an inchoate offence.

See p 615 in Chapter 15 for an explanation of 'things in action'.

Throughout the 2006 Act 'dishonestly' bears its **Ghosh** [1982] QB 1053 definition: see Chapter 15, but note that s 2(1) of the Theft Act 1968 does not apply to the offence of fraud. The other elements of the *mens rea* are intending to make a gain or lack a loss and knowledge that the representation is or may be false.

For more on the *Ghosh* definition of dishonesty, see pp 587–89 in Chapter 15.

This revision to the previous law gets rid of the difficulty of proving that the deception operated on the mind of the victim and thereby resolves the difficulties posed by **MPC v Charles** [1977] AC 177 and **Lambie** [1981] 2 All ER 776, discussed above, where the persons accepting the cheque card and credit card respectively were indifferent to the creditworthiness of the accused because the issuer of the cards would make up any loss. Making false applications, e.g. for mortgages, falls within s 2(1). There is no need for the victim to rely on the representation; the crime is complete once the false representation is made. Section 2(1) also deals with an increasingly common problem, that of 'phishing', i.e. the accused sends out requests over the internet for victims to reregister their accounts at a replica website with a view to emptying the victim's account. Section 2(1) even covers situations where the accused has obtained the entire proprietary interest before he makes a representation. For example, a driver put petrol into his tank. In civil law he owns it. He then falsely represents that his company will pay. Another charge possible on these facts is s 3 of the Theft Act 1978, making off.

In respect of the definition of 'property', which is similar to that laid down in s 4(1) of the Theft Act 1968, the government rejected an extension to 'confidential financial data', but where the accused intends to make a gain, e.g. through the exploitation of the information which he has accessed, the crime is committed.

In relation to the *mens rea* it should be noted that 'know that it . . . might be' in s 2(2) is the equivalent to subjective recklessness as discussed in Chapter 3 but there is no requirement that it was unreasonable for the accused to take the risk.

Fraud by failing to disclose information (s 3)

The second way in which the offence of fraud may be committed is when the accused (s 3(1)):

(a) dishonestly fails to disclose to another person information which he is under a legal duty to disclose,
(b) intends, by failing to disclose the information –
  (i) to make a gain for himself or another, or
  (ii) to cause loss to another or to expose another to a risk of loss.

The matters covered by s 3 may also fall within s 2. It should be noted that there must be a legal duty to disclose and therefore a moral duty to disclose is insufficient. Furthermore, there need be no deception. There is no definition of 'information'.

The *mens rea* besides dishonesty is the intent to make a gain or cause a loss or to expose to the risk of loss. 'Gain' and 'loss' bear the same definition as in s 2, noted above.

Fraud by abuse of position (s 4)

Section 4(1) provides the third manner in which fraud may be committed:

A person is in breach of this section if he –
(a) occupies a position in which he is expected to safeguard, or not to act against, the financial interests of another person,
(b) dishonestly abuses that position, and
(c) intends, by means of abuse of that position,
  (i) to make a gain for himself or another, or
  (ii) to cause loss to another or to expose another to a risk of loss.

It is expressly provided by s 4(2) that abuse of position includes an omission to act. There is, however, no definition of 'abuse'. There need be no deception. Among persons covered by s 4(1) are government officials and those taking care of the elderly. There is no restriction as there is in s 3(1) to persons who are under a legal duty to disclose information. There is no need for the abuse to be carried out secretly (contrary to the recommendation of the Law Commission). 'Abuse', 'position' and 'financial interests' are not defined.

The *mens rea* is the same as in s 3.

Supplementary provisions to the offence of fraud

Sections 6 and 7 create the offences of possessing articles for use in frauds and making or supplying articles for use in frauds respectively. Section 6 replaces in part s 25 of the Theft Act 1968 (going equipped), discussed in Chapter 17, which is now restricted to going equipped for theft or burglary. Unlike s 25, s 6 applies whether or not the accused is at his 'place of abode'. Therefore, a home computer falls within s 6. Section 6(1) reads:

> A person is guilty of an offence if he has in his possession or under his control any article for use in the course of or in connection with any fraud.

The maximum sentence is five years' imprisonment, whereas it is three years for going equipped.

Section 6(1) does not apply to any article which may be used for fraud but only to an article intended to be used for fraud. There is no need to prove that the article is to be used for any particular fraud, and the accused need not intend to use the item in a fraud committed by himself. It is arguable that the accused has control over information on the internet which he can download. An example of an article caught by s 6 is that of a blank plastic card which the accused intends to make into a false credit card. Section 6 has no express *mens rea*. However, 'possession' requires some mental element: one does not possess something one is unaware of; presumably also the accused must be aware of the nature of the article i.e. that it may be used 'in the course of or in connection with any fraud.'

Section 7(1) provides:

> A person is guilty of an offence if he makes, adapts, supplies or offers to supply any article –
> (a) knowing that it is designed or adapted for use in the course of or in connection with fraud, or
> (b) intending it to be used to commit, or assist in the commission of, fraud.

By s 8(1), 'article' in ss 6 and 7 includes 'any program or data held in electronic form.' It is uncertain whether these sections are restricted to fraud under the 2006 Act.

Obtaining services dishonestly

Section 11 of the 2006 Act creates the offence of obtaining services dishonestly. Unlike previous law there is no requirement of a deception. Section 11(1) reads:

> A person is guilty of an offence . . . if he obtains services for himself or another –
> (a) by a dishonest act, and
> (b) in breach of subsection (2).

There is no definition of both 'obtain' and 'services'. Dishonesty is defined according to *Ghosh* [1982] QB 1057, which is explained in the chapter on theft. It would seem that because of the reference to 'act' this offence cannot be committed by an omission.

Subsection (2) provides:

> A person obtains services in breach of this subsection if –
> (a) they were made available on the basis that payment has been, or is being or will be made for or in respect of them,
> (b) he obtains them without any payment having been made for or in respect of them or without payment having been made in full, and

(c) when he obtains them, he knows –

    (i) that they are being made available on the basis described in paragraph (a), or

    (ii) that they might be,

but intends that payment will not be made, or will not be made in full.

The maximum sentence for this offence if tried on indictment is five years' imprisonment or an unlimited fine or both (s 11(3)). Unlike its predecessor, s 11(1) does not require any deception.

One aim behind s 11(1) is that services made by automatic means are covered. Previous law was that machines could not be deceived. For example, giving false credit card details are covered. However, it is not restricted to machines. Therefore, both opening a bank account dishonestly through a bank official and downloading music dishonestly from the Web are covered. Similarly covered is using a device to watch pay-per-view TV free of charge. The obvious situation covered by this offence which was not covered by its predecessor, obtaining services by deception, is sneaking into a football ground to watch a match free of charge. The crime is restricted to the obtaining of services. If services are not obtained, a charge of attempting to obtain services may be available. There is no definition of 'services' except that they must be 'paid for' ones. Therefore, gratuitous services are not caught by s 11(1), though the general fraud offence may apply. It should be noted that s 11(1) applies only where there is no intent to pay either in full or partly. Therefore, parents who lie about the religion of their child in order to get him or her into a fee-paying faith school are not guilty of this offence if they intend to pay. This example is that of the Law Commission in its *Report on Fraud*.

The *mens rea* besides dishonesty is knowledge that the services are to be paid for, and either an intent not to pay at all or an intent not to pay in full. Dishonesty is defined in the usual way.

Conclusion: conspiracy to defraud

The government refused to take the opportunity to repeal the common law crime of conspiracy to defraud (see Chapter 10 of this book). A large minority of the consultees to the consultation exercise preferred to see the offence abolished because it was illogical that two people could be guilty of an offence when a single person doing the same act would not be; moreover, the crime is so broad that it covered potentially agreements to do things which ought not to be criminal, and the width of the offence is uncertain. The government, however, decided that (para. 40 of the government's *Fraud Law Reform*, noted above) '. . . at least until we have experience of how the new offences operate in practice, it would be rash to repeal conspiracy to defraud as it provides flexibility in dealing with a wide variety of frauds. . . . [I]t was not clear that the new offences could successfully replace it in every case, especially bearing in mind developing technology and possible new types of fraud.' The government, however, remains committed to the long-term repeal of the crime and will review it on publication of the Law Commission's Report on assisting and encouraging crime and after the Fraud Act 2006 has bedded down.

Making off without payment

Making off without payment is covered in Section 3 of the Theft Act 1978 which provides:

(1) Subject to subsection (3) below, a person who, knowing that payment on the spot for any goods supplied or service done is required or expected from him, dishonestly

makes off without having paid as required or expected and with intent to avoid payment of the amount due shall be guilty of an offence.

(2) For purposes of this section 'payment on the spot' includes payment at the time of collecting goods on which work has been done or in respect of which service has been provided.

(3) Subsection (1) above shall not apply where the supply of the goods or the doing of the service is contrary to law, or where the service done is such that payment is not legally enforceable.

Points of interpretation

'This is not an easy section to construe': *Allen* [1985] 1 WLR 50 (CA). The omission of a definition of 'service' in s 3 is inexplicable.

(a) The principal difference between this offence and the others in this chapter is that the accused is guilty of making off whether or not he deceived anyone. Where there is a deception, s 3 and the deception offences will both apply.

(b) Section 3 is restricted to legally enforceable payments (s 3(3)). The offence in s 3 will not be committed by an accused who walks away from a betting shop or brothel. The Criminal Law Revision Committee (Thirteenth Report, *Section 16 of the Theft Act 1968*, Cmnd 6733, 1977) considered that s 3 would not apply if the accused did not intend to pay from the start of the transaction. The last phrase in s 3(3) should be noted. Section 3(3) does not apply to goods. Therefore if the victim supplies goods to the accused, a s 3 charge is available even though the contract between the parties is not enforceable. The provision of non-necessary items to a minor falls within this exception.

(c) The 'payment' need not be by money. If a restaurant accepts luncheon vouchers, 'payment on the spot' in s 3(1) applies.

(d) Dishonesty need not be present at the start of the transaction. It is sufficient that there exists dishonesty at the time of making off. Section 3 covers the situation where the accused goes into a restaurant or petrol station intending to pay but leaves without doing so.

(e) The phrase 'with intent to avoid payment' is read as meaning 'with intent never to pay': *Allen* [1985] AC 1029 (HL). On the facts the accused was not guilty if he intended merely to delay paying a hotel bill of £1,286. He told the hotel that he was in financial difficulties and surrendered his passport to it. The effect of *Allen* would appear to undermine the thrust of the crime. The accused will after *Allen* be guilty if he simply vanishes with no intent to repay. It is thought that *Allen* undermines the rationale behind s 3. It may be hard to prove that the accused never intended to return to pay.

(f) It is uncertain whether s 3 covers the giving of worthless cheques. It is sometimes thought that it does. The accused has not paid as 'required or expected'. However, in *Hammond* [1982] Crim LR 611 (Crown Court), a judge ruled that if the victim accepts a cheque without a guarantee card, he knows that he is taking a risk. The accused is therefore not guilty of this offence if he drafts a worthless cheque. One argument is that payment by a worthless cheque does not satisfy the requirement in s 3(1) that the creditor is 'paid' because the victim takes it in conditional satisfaction of the debt. On the other hand, the creditor does expect a valuable cheque. Therefore, payment by a dud cheque is not payment as 'required or expected' within s 3(1). If the accused merely intends to defer paying, s 3 is inapplicable for the reason stated in (e).

(g) Section 3 does not cover the moonlighting tenant. The rent is payable 'then' but not 'there'.

(h) *Troughton v Metropolitan Police* [1987] Crim LR 138 (DC) illustrates a nice point. A very drunk accused did not give his name and address to the taxi-driver. The cab driver drove to a police station. The court held that the driver was in breach of contract through not completing the journey (in civil law terms there was an entire contract). Therefore, he could not legally demand the fare. The accused was never bound to pay on the spot for the service. He was not guilty. Accordingly, within s 3 it is not enough that the victim expects or requires the accused to pay. The payment must be legally due.

(i) Where is 'the spot'? In *Brooks* (1982) 76 Cr App R 66, the Court of Appeal determined that 'the spot' meant the place where payment was required. In a restaurant that place was the cash desk. There was no need for the accused to reach the restaurant door. In an underground system 'the spot' includes the gate at the exit. In *McDavitt* [1981] Crim LR 843, it was held at Crown Court level that the accused was guilty of the attempt if he had not yet reached 'the spot'. In *Aziz* [1993] Crim LR 708 (CA) the defence argued that in relation to a taxi ride 'the spot' was at the end of the ride. The driver had reached that spot but had driven off to a police station when the defendants refused to pay. The court held that when they ran off from the cab, they had departed from the spot. Payment was expected when the taxi reached the destination specified. The court held that the trial judge had properly directed the jury that the driver continued to require payment after reaching the destination and driving off to the police station. The place of the spot could differ according to circumstances and it is a question of fact whether the accused has departed from the spot.

(j) Section 3 stipulates that the accused must make off. It is moot whether that phrase covers a situation where the accused departs with the victim's consent. For instance, if the defendant tells a taxi-driver that he must get money from his flat and the driver agrees, does he make off? In *Hammond*, above, it was said that there was no making off when the creditor allowed the accused to leave. In *Brooks* the Court of Appeal decided that there was no need for the accused to make off stealthily, and that the words 'dishonestly makes off' usually required no explanation because they bore their 'ordinary natural meaning'. If so, *Hammond* would appear to be wrong. An accused does make off even when he has the creditor's consent to leave.

(k) A shoplifter in a shop where goods are served will be guilty of this offence and theft when the item is given to him. In a self-service shop, however, goods are, it is thought, not 'supplied' to him within s 3(1). He will in any event be guilty of theft. It had been suggested that 'supplied' means 'available for purchase' or is to be read as including 'supplied to himself'. If this interpretation is correct, the accused is guilty of this offence. If the accused receives ham from the meat stall in a supermarket he is guilty if he makes off before paying at the cash desk. Similarly, the accused is guilty where ownership passes on delivery such as when food is eaten or petrol put into the tank. However, the accused who sneaks out of a cinema which he has sneaked into is not guilty: no service has been 'done'.

(l) There is no definition of service. It is suggested that the ordinary language definition is the one to be used. The same point can be made about 'goods'. One might have expected an incorporation of the definition of 'goods' used for the purposes of the offence of handling.

(m) It is suggested that the accused who can be traced (e.g. he has put his real name and address on the back of a cheque) can still be guilty of making off. There is no restriction in the definition to persons who cannot easily be traced. The opposing argument is that the section applies only when the accused has done something which makes him harder to trace.

(n) The supplying or service need not take place before the payment is required. Payment is required on one-man buses before getting on the bus, but a s 3 offence can be committed if the accused stands by the driver, looking through his purse, and jumping off before paying.

If the accused obtains credit, even when the obtaining was dishonest and by deception, he is not guilty of this offence because 'payment on the spot . . . is [not] required or expected': **Vincent** [2001] 1 WLR 1172 (CA). The accused contended that two hotel proprietors had agreed that payment due could be postponed. The court held that 'payment on the spot' was not required even though the accused may have obtained the agreements by deception. The reason why payment was not required or expected was irrelevant. The court also said that 's 3(1) is . . . intended to create a simple and straightforward offence'. Therefore, any attempt to complicate matters should be eschewed. The correct charge nowadays is that of false representation contrary to the Fraud Act 2006 s 2. There is an overlap between s 3(1) of the 1978 Act and s 2(1) of the 2006 Act. Section 2(1) can be committed even when the accused has received ownership of the property *before* making the false representation. For example, to use a common illustration, if the accused puts petrol into his tank, under civil law he has obtained the entire proprietary interest in it; if he then says that his company will pay for it by asking for it to be put on the company's account but the petrol is to be used for private purposes, and this is not contractually permitted, then both making off and fraud are committed.

Summary

Making off (without payment) is the exceptional crime in this chapter: it is not one involving the element of fraud. The definition is found in s 3(1) of the Theft Act 1978: '. . . a person who, knowing that payment on the spot for any goods supplied or service done is required or expected from him, dishonestly makes off without having paid as required or expected and with intent to avoid payment of the amount due shall be guilty of an offence.' The crime is limited to legally enforceable services and supplies. Dishonesty is defined as in **Ghosh** (see Chapter 15).

References

Reports

Criminal Law Revision Committee 13th Report, *Section 16 of the Theft Act 1968*, Cmnd 6733 (1977)

Home Office Criminal Law Policy Unit, *Fraud Law Reform: Government's Response to Consultations* (2006)

Law Commission Consultation Paper No. 155, *Legislating the Criminal Code: Fraud and Deception* (1999)

Law Commission Report No. 177, *A Criminal Code for England & Wales* (1989)

Further reading

Attorney-General, *Guidance on the Use of the Common Law Offence of Conspiracy to Defraud*, (2007)

Home Office *Fraud Law Reform* (2004)

Home Office *Fraud Law Reform: Government Response to Consultations* (2006)

Kiernan, P. and Scanlan, G. 'Fraud and the Law Commission: The future of dishonesty' (2003) 24 Co. Law 4

Liberty, *Liberty's Response to the Home Office Consultation on Fraud Law Reform* (2004)

Ormerod, D. 'A bit of a con? The Law Commission's Consultation Paper on fraud' [1999] Crim LR 789

Ormerod, D. 'The Fraud Act 2006 – Criminalising lying' [2007] Crim LR 193

Peck, M. *The Fraud Bill [HL]*, Research Paper 06/31, House of Commons Library (2006)

Sullivan, G. R. 'Fraud: the latest Law Commission proposals' (2003) 67 JCL 139, which should be read together with the next entries:

Sullivan, G. R. 'Fraud and the efficacy of the criminal law: a proposal for a wide residual offence' [1985] Crim LR 616;

Sullivan, G. R. 'Reforming the substantive law of fraud' (1988) 52 JCL 288; and

Sullivan, G. R. 'Framing an acceptable general offence of fraud' (1989) 53 JCL 92

Visit **www.mylawchamber.co.uk/jefferson** to access exam-style questions with answer guidance, multiple choice quizzes, live weblinks, an online glossary, and regular updates to the law.

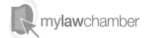

Use **Case Navigator** to read in full some of the key cases referenced in this chapter:

R v Ghosh [1982] 2 All ER 689

17

Blackmail, burglary, going equipped, handling

Blackmail

Introduction

The term blackmail seems to derive from an old English word 'mail', meaning tribute or rents paid in work, goods, crops or base metal ('black'). There is no racist connotation. If the threat is one of violence, blackmail may be classified both as a property offence and a crime against the person. By s 21(1) of the Theft Act 1968:

> [a] person is guilty of blackmail if, with a view to gain for himself or another or with intent to cause loss to another, he makes any unwarranted demand with menaces; and for this purpose a demand with menaces is unwarranted unless the person making it does so in the belief –
> (a) that he had reasonable grounds for making the demand; and
> (b) that the use of the menaces is a proper means of reinforcing the demand.

The framework is that a demand concerning an economic matter is blackmail, but there is an exception that it was warranted. This exception is the equivalent of lack of dishonesty in other parts of the Act.

Blackmail and theft may overlap. If the accused forces the victim to deliver property by threats, he has appropriated it within s 3(1) of the 1968 Act and he has also made an unwarranted demand with menaces. If, however, he does not just oblige the victim to hand over property but makes him act in such a way (e.g. makes him sell it) that in civil law the victim transfers to him the ownership of the item, the question whether he is guilty of theft depends on the present state of the civil law. If duress renders the contract voidable, the victim would transfer ownership and the property would belong to the accused. Therefore, he would not be guilty of theft. If the effect is to render it void, no property is transferred, and the accused is guilty. Because of the lack of clarity in the civil law, it is suggested that in this situation he should be charged with blackmail. In this offence the accused is guilty whether or not he has acquired the entire proprietary interests over the asset.

Getting property by threatening immediate force (e.g. 'your money or your life') may be both blackmail and robbery. The usual charge is robbery. If the threat is to beat up the victim later, the facts do not constitute robbery because the victim was not put in fear of being 'then and there subjected to force'. In blackmail the demand must be to make a gain

See pp 631–33 in Chapter 15 for an explanation of robbery.

or loss, whereas in robbery the threat is made to get property. Blackmail occurs as soon as the demand is made, whereas robbery requires an appropriation. Blackmail requires menaces, whereas robbery is dependent on the threat or use of force. Accordingly, using force without threat is robbery, only because there must be menaces in blackmail. Menaces other than threats of immediate force cannot be robbery, only blackmail.

The paradox of blackmail

If the accused asks his victim 'Will you give me money?' that is not a crime. If the accused said to his victim, 'I will tell your husband that you have been committing adultery', that too is no crime. If, however, the two are run together thus: 'Unless you give me money, I will tell your husband you are an adulteress', that is a crime. Two non-crimes added together create the offence of blackmail. This startling proposition is sometimes known as 'the paradox of blackmail'.

The *actus reus*

A major part of the *actus reus* is 'a demand with menaces'. Making the demand is sufficient. The prosecution need not prove that the victim complied or that the accused obtained anything by his threat.

Demand

> The nature of the act or omission demanded is immaterial and it is also immaterial whether the menaces relate to action to be taken by the person making the demand. (s 21(2))

The word is defined as in ordinary language: ***Treacy v DPP*** [1971] AC 537 (HL). A demand couched in polite terms is still a demand. It may be made by words or impliedly. Actions will suffice, at least if 'an ordinary reasonable man' would realise that a demand was being made: ***Collister*** (1955) 39 Cr App R 100, a case which would probably be followed today. A demand is made when and where a letter containing it is posted (***Treacy***, by a 3:2 majority), and probably continues to be made until it is read by the victim (***Treacy*** 5:0, but *obiter*). A demand by fax will be made when the fax is sent. It was once thought that blackmail could not be attempted because blackmail itself is in the nature of an offence of attempt, an attempt to obtain property. It seems absurd to charge attempting to attempt to obtain property. It is, however, suggested that such a charge does exist. In *The Theft Acts 1968–1978*, 7th edn (Sweet & Maxwell, 1995) 225, E. Griew wrote:

> [i]f a blackmailing demand is 'made' as soon as it is spoken or dispatched beyond recall, the possibility of a case of attempted blackmail is limited to fanciful situations such as where [the accused] is affected by a stammer or interrupted in the act of posting.

Blackmail is complete on the making of the demand. The offence is therefore committed when the accused makes the demand even though the victim is deaf.

Menaces

The term does not cover only threats of violence but anything detrimental or unpleasant according to Lord Wright in the civil case of ***Thorne v MTA*** [1937] AC 797. Despite that wide definition, 'menaces' is stronger than 'threats'. It bears the meaning it has in ordinary language: ***Lawrence and Pomroy*** (1971) 57 Cr App R 64. By that, the court meant that there was no need for the judge to define the term to the jury, at least in the general run of cases. The Appeal Court was not saying that the ordinary-language meaning of 'menaces' was a detriment for the term does seem restricted in ordinary language to threats of violence. In *Garwood* [1987] 1 All ER 1032, the accused, believing that the victim had burgled his house, aggressively demanded £10 'to make it quits'. The victim gave him the money. The Court of Appeal held that menaces did not exist unless (a) they would affect the mind of a reasonable person or (b) did affect the mind of the victim and the accused knew that his actions were likely to have such an effect. The accused, therefore, is guilty of blackmail against a timorous person, when a reasonable person would not have been frightened, only if he knew of the timidity. Trivial threats are not menaces: *Harry* [1974] Crim LR 32. A student who offered shopowners immunity from the activities of rag week in return for donations to charity was held by the trial judge not to have used menaces.

Gain or loss

Gain and loss are to be construed as extending only to gain or loss in money or other property, but as extending to any such gain or loss whether temporary or permanent; and
(i) 'gain' includes a gain by keeping what one has, as well as a gain by getting what one has not; and
(ii) 'loss' includes a loss by not getting what one might get, as well as a loss by parting with what one had. (Theft Act 1968, s 34(2)(a))

'Gain' and 'loss' bear wide meanings. By s 21(1), above, the gain or loss need not be for the accused or to the victim. The gain or loss need not be permanent. It is sufficient that, e.g., the accused is allowed to borrow something. However, this definition shows that blackmail protects economic interests. Accordingly, it is not blackmail where the accused extorts oral sex from the victim because that is not 'money or other property'. (A different result has been reached in some US states, the blackmail statutes of which are couched differently, e.g. Iowa: *State v Todd* (1900) 82 NW 322.) Similarly, it is not blackmail where the accused extorts a position of honour or release from lawful custody. English cases are few, but a threat to get back money owing to the accused falls within s 34(2)(a)(i) because it is a 'gain': *Parkes* [1973] Crim LR 358; and a threat by a person suffering from osteoarthritis to a doctor that he would shoot him unless he was given a pain-killing injection was held to be blackmail in *Bevans* (1988) 87 Cr App R 64 (CA). The drug which the doctor used under threat was property. The outcome is somewhat stretched. What the accused really obtained was a pain-killing injection. While a demand for sex is not blackmail, a demand for money in return for not disclosing that the accused has indulged in such behaviour would be because the gain would be money within s 34(2)(a). If the conduct falls within s 34(2) it does not matter that the accused's purpose was not economic gain. In *Bevans* the drug was demanded in order to relieve pain but the thing obtained, the gain, was something which he had not got. Most cases involve gains to the accused but the definition extends to loss to others. A threat to the victim that she must throw away her wedding ring falls within (ii) above.

Permitted demands with menaces

It is not blackmail where the accused believes he has reasonable grounds for making the demand *and* believes the use of menaces is a proper means of reinforcing the demand. The requirement of belief relates to the accused's own belief. He does not have to believe on reasonable grounds that he has reasonable grounds for making the demand and so on: *Lambert* [1972] Crim LR 422, where the accused threatened to tell the victim's employers of his affair with the accused's wife unless the victim paid him £250 for his rights to his wife. The jury acquitted him. In *Harvey* (1981) 72 Cr App R 139, the Court of Appeal ruled that 'proper' was wider than 'lawful' and held that whether a threat to kill, rape or maim (the accused not knowing that killing, raping and maiming are breaches of the criminal law) was a proper means of reinforcing the demand was a question for the jury, as was the question whether the accused believed that he had reasonable grounds. Bingham LJ said: 'It matters not what the reasonable man, or any man other than the defendant, would believe save in so far as that may throw light on what the defendant in fact believed.' However, the court held that the accused does not have this exception when he knows that what he proposes to do is a crime. Accordingly 'a fanatic or deranged idealist' has no defence when he knows or believes that what he is doing is a crime but is justified by the end to be achieved. The accused's own standards are not used to assess whether his means were 'proper'. Instead his standards are judged against those of society. The statute is not so worded, and *Harvey* may be incorrect on this point. It may be in respect of a petty offence that the accused believed that what he was doing was generally acceptable even though it was a crime. *Harvey* is inconsistent with *Lambert*'s thrust. If the accused is not guilty when he believes (whether on reasonable grounds or not) that he has reasonable grounds for making the demand, should he also not be guilty when he believes that the means of reinforcing the demand is proper? The Criminal Law Revision Committee, Eighth Report, *Theft and Related Offences*, Cmnd 2977, 1966, para 123, goes against *Lambert* in that it would have given a defence only when the accused's act was 'morally and socially acceptable'. The requirement of belief in social acceptability means in theory that if the accused has low standards of morality, he will not be convicted, but if he has high standards, he will be! The requirement of 'proper means' covers where the accused demands what he believes to be his: such would not be robbery but can be blackmail.

A case which might now be determined differently because of this exception is *Dymond* [1920] 2 KB 260. The victim of a sexual assault threatened to tell the town of the crime unless she was paid money. Before the Act she was guilty. After the Act she might have believed that she had reasonable grounds for making her demand and that her threat was a proper means of reinforcing the demand.

Mens rea

There are three elements:

(a) an intent to make a demand with menaces;

(b) a view to gain for himself or another, or intent to cause loss to another;

(c) either no belief that he has reasonable grounds for making the demand or no belief that the use of menaces is a proper form of reinforcing the demand.

'A view to' is a way of phrasing 'intent'.

Burglary

Introduction

This offence may be seen as one which is directed against 'criminal trespass' to the home and other buildings such as factories and shops. At a deeper level it safeguards the feelings of those whose houses have been entered and one aim of the offence may be to prevent violence between householders and burglars. By s 9 of the Theft Act 1968, as amended:

(1) A person is guilty of **burglary** if –
   (a) he enters any building or part of a building as a trespasser and with intent to commit any such offence as is mentioned in subsection (2) below; or
   (b) having entered any building or part of a building as a trespasser he steals or attempts to steal anything in the building or that part of it or inflicts or attempts to inflict on any person therein any grievous bodily harm.

(2) The offences referred to in subsection (1) above are offences of stealing anything in the building or part of a building in question, of inflicting on any person therein any grievous bodily harm therein, and of doing unlawful damage to the building or anything therein.

Until the coming into force of the Sexual Offences Act 2003, s 9(2) of the Theft Act, as amended by s 142 of the Criminal Justice and Public Order Act 1994 contained the words 'or raping any person' after 'grievous bodily harm'. The 2003 Act, s 63, replaced this form of burglary with a specific sex crime. The accused must be a trespasser on premises, he or she must intend to commit 'a relevant sexual offence on the premises'; and he or she must know, or be reckless as to whether, he or she is trespassing. A 'relevant sexual offence' includes rape.

The maximum penalty is 14 years' imprisonment in the case of burglary in a dwelling and 10 years elsewhere, such as a shop, after conviction on indictment. It is unclear whether the accused is guilty of the more serious offence only if he knows that what he entered was a dwelling. An interesting aspect of the sentence is that an accused is guilty under s 9(1)(a) even though he has not yet even attempted to steal in a house and is liable to 14 years' imprisonment, yet if he does actually steal, the maximum sentence for theft is seven years. The difference between 'dwelling' and other buildings was introduced in 1991. There has not been a problem so far in distinguishing the two. A flat is undoubtedly a dwelling, but what of a house in the process of construction? It is uncertain whether the accused is subject to the higher penalty only if he knew that what he entered was a dwelling or whether it is sufficient that the building he entered was in fact a dwelling, whether he knew it to be so or not. Since, if the accused trespasses in a building and intends to steal (but has not yet stolen), he is guilty of burglary, a maximum sentence of 14 years looks excessive in relation to the harm.

In s 9(1)(a) it is not necessary to show that the accused intended to take a specific object or even that that object was in the building: *Attorney-General's References (Nos 1 and 2 of 1979)* [1980] QB 180 (CA). Section 9(1)(a) is really an inchoate offence. However, it seems that the accused must know or believe that the item or the person is in the building. In other words, at the time of the entry the accused must intend to commit the further offence against the person or thing who or which is therein. What is more certain is that an accused is guilty of burglary if he enters with intent to commit the relevant offence on a person or thing whom or which he will remove to another place where he will commit the offence.

By sub-s (4) 'building' includes inhabited vehicles and vessels. The later part of sub-s (4) is to the effect that a vehicle or vessel remains inhabited even if no one is living there at the time of the burglary. An 'inhabited vehicle' includes a caravan. It is uncertain whether it covers a caravanette, a vehicle which can be used as an ordinary car or as a motorised caravan. It seems a little inept to consider the crime to be burglary when the caravanette is being used as a holiday home and theft when it is not. A Crown Court held in **B & S v Leathley** [1979] Crim LR 314 that a large freezer container resting on railway sleepers in a farmyard was a building. It does not include an articulated trailer used as a store despite its having electric power, steps up to it, and lockable shutters: **Norfolk Constabulary v Seekings** [1986] Crim LR 167. Both the container and the trailer were being used as an extra store for shops. It does seem strange that burglary could be committed in the first instance but not the second. The accused would have been convicted had someone been living in the trailer, which would then have been an inhabited vehicle. A tent will not be a building, nor, it is thought, will a phone kiosk or a mobile shop or mobile library. A camper van is debatable. There may also be problems with buildings in the course of construction. Is a house being erected only a building when its roof is on? 'Part of a building' can also give rise to problems. In **Walkington** [1979] 2 All ER 716 (CA), the accused was guilty under s 9(1)(a) when he went into a three-sided partition in the middle of a shop where the till was. The area inside the partition was 'part of a building'. There need be no physical separation between one part of a building and another. A sign is sufficient. There may be difficulties in determining whether the accused has entered a part of a building. If he enters a shop, hides in a corner, comes out when the members of staff have gone home, and steals some items, is he a burglar? In the evening when he comes out, is his previously lawful presence converted into a trespassory entrance? Is he guilty only when he crosses some notional line?

Paragraphs (a) and (b) create separate offences. It was thought that a person charged under one paragraph may not be convicted under the other: **Hollis** [1971] Crim LR 525 (CA). However, the same fact situation may give rise to either offence: **Taylor** [1979] Crim LR 649. Therefore, a person only charged under s 9(1)(b) may be convicted under s 9(1)(a) because the former includes the latter when the accused is charged with entering with intent to steal or inflict grievous bodily harm: see **Whiting** (1987) 85 Cr App R 78. This ruling applies even though on the facts it very probably is that the accused did not intend the further offence until he was in the building. A person charged only under s 9(1)(a) cannot be convicted under s 9(1)(b).

For a definition of grievous bodily harm, see pp 552–53 in Chapter 13.

In s 9(1)(a) the statute speaks of 'offence' of grievous bodily harm. It has been said that in s 9(1)(b), which does not mention the term 'offence', grievous bodily harm does not necessarily mean the offences found in ss 20 and 23 of the Offences Against the Person Act 1861: **Jenkins** [1983] 1 All ER 993, a Court of Appeal decision. (Section 18 requires the *causing* of grievous bodily harm. Presumably Parliament meant to include this offence but the paragraph is not well drafted.) It would certainly be strange if the accused could be guilty of this form of burglary if he accidentally or indeed lawfully inflicted the harm, for all other ulterior offences in burglary require intent. It was sufficient in **Jenkins** that the victim was so shocked by the accused's presence that the victim suffered a stroke. There was no need for an assault. The accused need not know that the victim was present. An alternative reading of **Jenkins** is to say that s 9(1)(b) does require an offence involving the infliction of grievous bodily harm but the prosecution need not specify the offence. The House of Lords reversed, but not on this point (**MPC v Wilson** [1984] AC 242). It is suggested that **Jenkins** should not be followed. If the accused inflicts grievous bodily harm on the victim without intending to do so and without being subjectively reckless, he is not guilty of a non-fatal offence. It would be strange if he were guilty of burglary on those facts. Moreover it seems to be a draftsman's error that the word 'offence' is omitted in s 9(1)(b), especially as it is found in s 9(1)(a). Finally, burglary is a serious offence but the ruling in **Jenkins** inappropriately makes it a strict one in respect of grievous bodily harm. The draft Criminal Code, 1989, cl 147, would clear up this difficulty by requiring an offence of grievous bodily harm.

A possible difficulty which requires resolution is whether the accused is guilty of burglary when he kills. Does 'inflicts' or 'inflicting' cover murder? A strict constructionalist would argue that the offence cannot be so read, but surely no court would so rule. A court might reason that the infliction of harm is a step on the way to killing and that the less (grievous bodily harm) includes the greater (murder).

Another difficulty is the omission of other offences. Fraud is not listed in s 9(2). Therefore, trespassory entry in order to obtain a watch by fraud is not burglary, though the likelihood is that the fraud may also be theft. This result is an unexpected outcome of **Gomez**. If there is no 'offence' there will, subject to the grievous bodily harm point, be no burglary. A simple illustration is where the accused enters a house as a trespasser with intent to resume possession of an item to which he has a lawful claim. There is no theft and thus no burglary.

The *actus reus*

For both types of burglary the accused must enter a building or part of one as a trespasser. Edmund-Davies LJ in an extempore judgment said that the accused has to make 'an effective and substantial entry': **Collins** [1973] QB 100, the case of the 'socks maniac'. Fortunately or unfortunately this case, well-known to generations of law students, has been deprived of some of its reasoning by the fact that entry into a building or part of one as a trespasser with intent to rape no longer is burglary. Nevertheless, its authoritativeness on the *actus reus* of trespass and the *mens rea* of the offence remains undiminished.

Collins [1973] QB 100

The accused, having taken drink, determined upon sexual intercourse. He placed a ladder against an upper window, climbed up, and saw a naked woman on the bed. He climbed down and removed all his clothing except for his socks, which he left on in order to make a quick getaway. He climbed up and at some point he was beckoned in. Intercourse took place. The woman, who had earlier thought that the male was her boyfriend, discovered that it was not. The question was whether any part of his anatomy had made an effective and substantial entry (into the building) at the moment she beckoned him in. Until the Sexual Offences Act 2003 entry as a trespasser to commit rape was one form of burglary.

On the facts the answer was not certain.

The Court of Appeal in **Brown** [1985] Crim LR 212 widened the **Collins** definition by holding that the entry had to be effective, but need not be substantial. The question whether the entry was effective was for the jury. There was no need for the whole of the accused's body to be in the building: the top half was in a shop-front display, the bottom half outside. In **Ryan** [1996] Crim LR 320 the accused had his head and right arm inside a house but he was trapped by the neck by the window. The Court of Appeal applied **Brown**. There was evidence on which a jury could find that the accused had entered. The accused had entered a building even though only part of the body was within the building and even though he could not do anything 'effective' in the position in which he was caught. 'Effective' therefore does not mean 'effective to commit the ulterior offence'. This ruling seems right in principle. After all a person can be guilty of burglary with intent to rape when there is no person present in the building.

It is thought that 'effective' relates to the entry, not to the possibility of theft, etc. The problem is this: if the accused's intention is unlawful damage and he is in the same position as in *Brown* with the top half of his body in the building, is his entry therein effective for the purposes of the unlawful damage form of burglary? On the wording of the statute it would seem that an effective entry into the building is sufficient without the accused's going so far as to be in a position to effect his ulterior intent. *Ryan* confirmed this supposition. It may be that *Brown* and *Ryan* are leading to a position where entry need not be effective just as it need not be substantial.

It is questionable whether the accused has entered if he inserts a key into a lock or puts his hand through a window. Under the pre-Theft Act law it was sufficient if any part of the accused's body was inside. *Collins* and *Brown* scotch that notion (a charge of attempted burglary is available), but uncertainty remains whether inserting an implement into the premises is sufficient. It was under the old law if done in pursuance of the ulterior intent, not if done simply to gain access. Perhaps the same rule stands. The *Daily Telegraph*, 4 March 1979, notes a case where transvestites who hooked dresses through letter boxes pleaded guilty to burglary in a magistrates' court, even though no part of their bodies was through the letter boxes. This case may be inconsistent with *Collins* and *Brown*. The wording of the Act supports the view that the accused is not guilty: '*He* enters' and 'having entered . . . *he*' (emphasis added). It must be the accused or at least some part of him who enters. It would be helpful if this point were resolved.

If an accused is pushed into a building, it is suggested that he does not enter as a trespasser because an involuntary entry is no trespass. Furthermore, one cannot 'enter' by an omission. Therefore, burglary is one of those offences which require an act.

Trespassing means entry without the consent of the owner, express or implied. The accused must enter as a trespasser. Stealing does not convert a lawful entry into trespass. On the facts of *Collins* the accused did not know that the woman had made a mistake and he was not entering as a trespasser. If the owner's daughter invites the accused into her bedroom for the purpose of sexual intercourse, he is not trespassing. The Court of Appeal held that it was not only the occupier who could license entry but also her child. It will, however, be trespass if she had no authority to issue that invitation. In *Jones and Smith* [1976] 1 WLR 672 (CA), the occupier's son had general permission to enter the house but he did not have permission to come in with a friend to steal two televisions, despite the father's saying that his son would never be a trespasser in his house. The limits of permission were exceeded. The same rule applies in shops provided that the accused had the ulterior intent before entering the shop, it is thought. Therefore, many shoplifters are burglars. If the accused made his mind up to steal only on seeing the goods displayed in the shop, he is not guilty under s 9(1)(a) because he has not entered the shop, or a forbidden part of the shop, as a trespasser. *Jones and Smith* may be inconsistent with *Collins*, where the accused should, applying the *ratio* of *Jones and Smith* (retrospectively), have been held to be a trespasser because he exceeded his permission to enter. (If so, it would not have mattered whether any part of his male anatomy had intruded into the daughter's bedroom before she invited him to engage in sexual congress. He had trespassed because he had exceeded the invitation to enter because he intended to rape (as the definition of burglary then provided) unless the victim consented.) The point was not seen in *Collins*, which would seem to be incorrect on this issue. The son's friend could have been convicted of burglary with the son's being found guilty of being a secondary party to that crime. A possible reconciliation is to argue that in *Collins* the accused's intent was to rape, if necessary, whereas in *Jones and Smith* there was no 'if necessary' about the intent to steal. This definition is narrower than that in the tort of trespass. *Jones and Smith* looks like a simple theft case and the defendants should be so charged. This approach is supported by *Walkington* (above). The Court of Appeal would not have needed to debate whether the place the accused had entered was part of a building if all shoplifters are trespassers from their first entry into the building (if they have intent at that stage). The accused will be trespassing if he enters fraudulently, e.g. by falsely claiming that he is a police officer investigating crime. A person who would otherwise enter lawfully is a trespasser if he enters for an unauthorised purpose such as theft. Despite this criticism of *Jones and Smith* it remains authoritative.

Where the offence is of the s 9(1)(b) type, the attempt or full crime must be proved. Abstracting electricity is not theft. Therefore, the accused who enters a building as a trespasser and turns on the electric fire is not guilty of this form of burglary.

Mens rea

The accused must deliberately enter knowing that he is a trespasser: *Collins*; *Jones and Smith*. Perhaps recklessness is sufficient: *Collins*. The court in *Jones and Smith* was clear that recklessness was sufficient. Presumably recklessness bears the meaning of *Cunningham* [1957] 2 QB 396. The conviction was quashed in *Collins* because the trial judge did not direct the jury as to the mental element in relation to trespass. Where the charge is under s 9(1)(a), there must also be the ulterior intent. No theft, GBH or criminal damage need occur. This further intent may be conditional. Under s 9(1)(b) the accused must have the *mens rea* of the completed crime, e.g. grievous bodily harm requires intention or recklessness in the *Cunningham* form as to the infliction of some harm, though see the discussion of *Jenkins*, above. The term 'with intent' in s 9(1)(a) would seem to require purpose, a narrower meaning than intent in murder (see Chapter 3). There is no explanation why s 9(1)(a) covers intent to commit criminal damage but s 9(1)(b) does not include the completed offences. Burglars often wreak havoc and one would have thought it prudent to include criminal damage in that paragraph.

Aggravated burglary (s 10)

This offence occurs when the accused has with him a firearm, imitation firearm, weapon of offence, or explosive. The time at which he must have it with him is the time when he stole etc., if the burglary is the s 9(1)(b) type: *O'Leary* (1986) 82 Cr App R 341 (CA), which was applied in *Kelly* (1993) 157 JP 845 (CA). In the latter case the accused had a screwdriver with him which he used to gain entry and used it as a weapon of offence to threaten a young couple at the time of the theft of a video recorder. He was guilty. For criticism see J. C. Smith in his case comment [1993] Crim LR 765. In *Francis* [1982] Crim LR 363, the accused had a stick with him when he demanded entry into a house, but not when he was stealing from a room. He did not intend to steal when he entered the house. The Court of Appeal held that the crime was not aggravated burglary. For the purposes of the s 9(1)(a) type, the relevant time is that of entry. If the act of theft etc. is over and the accused picks up a weapon in order to make good his getaway, it is suggested that the facts do not constitute burglary in its aggravated (or even simple) form. The burglary is complete once the underlying offence is complete. Nevertheless, it is possible that a court may hold that burglary is a continuing offence with the result that, contrary to what has been argued, the accused is guilty of this offence.

A weapon of offence is defined in s 10(1)(b) as 'any article made or adapted for use for causing injury to or incapacitating a person or intended by the person having it with him for such use'. A screwdriver falls within this definition, which is wider than that in s 1(4) of the Prevention of Crime Act 1953, in relation to offensive weapons, for it includes incapacitating articles such as handcuffs and rope (to tie up security guards) as suggested by the Criminal Law Revision Committee's Eighth Report, *Theft and Related Offences*, Cmnd 2977, 1966, 128. 'Firearm' includes an airgun: s 10(1)(a). An imitation firearm means 'anything which has the appearance of being a firearm' (s 10(1)(a)).

The prosecution does not have to show that the weapon of offence was intended to be used during the burglary. As Potts J said in *Kelly*, above, s 10 'is directed at the use of articles which aggravate the offence of simple burglary, so as to render the offender punishable with imprisonment for life'. In fact s 10 is not directed at the use of the article but at its presence. Section 10's aim is to prevent use by penalising a person who has a weapon on him. It is not directed at the spontaneous grabbing of a weapon. In *Stones* [1989] 1 WLR 156 (CA), Glidewell LJ said that: 'The mischief at which the section is clearly aimed is that if a burglar has a weapon which he intends to use to injure some person unconnected with the premises burgled, he may nevertheless be tempted to use it if challenged during the course of the burglary and put under sufficient pressure.' The court did not state why they thought this was the mischief, and the Criminal Law Revision Committee's Report considered aggravated burglary was aimed at instances where the accused intends to use or threaten the use of weapons in order to steal. The Committee also stated that this offence was aimed at deterring those whose activities frightened householders. Burglary with weapons can lead to violence and death. For these reasons the maximum sentence is life imprisonment. A conditional intent to use the firearm, etc., should the need arise, suffices for liability.

The accused is not guilty of s 10 if he uses a weapon to gain entry but does not take it in with him. In *Klass* [1998] 1 Cr App R 453 (CA) the accused smashed the window of a caravan with a pole; the occupier came outside and the accused beat him with the pole. These facts do not constitute aggravated burglary.

The accused must know that he has the prohibited article. If a knife is planted on him, he is not guilty. The outcome is the same if he has forgotten that he has a knife on him.

One last point on s 10: the prohibited articles form the mnemonic 'wife' – Weapon of offence, Imitation firearm, Firearm, Explosive!

Going equipped

Introduction

By s 25 of the Theft Act 1968 as amended by the Fraud Act 2006:

> [a] person shall be guilty of an offence if, when not at his place of abode, he has with him any article for use in the course of or in connection with any burglary or theft.

This offence is often known as 'going equipped'. This term appears in the side-note. The crime is one aimed at stopping the accused from committing offences even before he has attempted to steal. Since one can attempt to go equipped, the range of s 25 together with its inchoate offence is broad. The crime could be called a 'double inchoate' or 'double preparatory' one. Moreover, there is no need for the accused to be on his way to a burglary or theft. If he has his bag marked 'swag' in the back of his car, he is guilty of this offence, even if, say, he is driving the car to the Channel Tunnel for a holiday.

Section 25 used to cover going equipped to cheat, but that offence is now governed by the Fraud Act 2006, which is discussed in the previous chapter.

Actus reus

The accused must have with him an article. Since the article need not be made or adapted for burglary or stealing it bears a wide meaning. The Criminal Law Revision Committee's Eighth Report, *Theft and Related Offences*, 1966, Cmnd 2977, which formed the basis of the Theft Act 1968, said that a getaway car was an 'article for use . . . in connection with any burglary, theft or cheat'. (As originally drafted s 25 included articles to be used for cheating. Many of the cases below involved cheating but their principles are not affected by the deletion of 'cheating' from s 25.) Where the accused had Kenyan five shilling pieces which were the same shape, size and weight as 50p pieces (but worth less) for use in slot machines, he was guilty of this offence: *Goodwin* [1996] Crim LR 262 (CA). (He would also be guilty of theft of any winnings.) A pair of gloves which a burglar uses to prevent his fingerprints getting onto panes of glass falls within the definition. A shirt is an article, so *In the matter of McAngus* [1994] Crim LR 602 (DC) one with a false label specifying wrongly that it was made in America was an article made for cheating. A bottle of wine was sufficient in *Doukas* [1978] 1 All ER 1061 (CA), which was approved in *Cook* (1988) 83 Cr App R 339. In *Minor v CPS* (1988) 86 Cr App R 378, a piece of tubing with which to syphon petrol was held by the Divisional Court to be an 'article'. In *Rashid* [1977] 2 All ER 237 (CA) a sliced loaf and some tomatoes fell within 'any article', though the court held the accused not to be guilty on the facts because train passengers would not care whether sandwiches were provided by British Rail or the steward personally, a questionable decision in the light of *Doukas* and *Cooke* [1986] AC 909 (HL). The question whether a customer knowing of the facts would have taken part in the fraud is one for the jury. It should not be assumed that people did not care whose sandwiches they were buying in a BR buffet.

The phrase 'with him' may cover articles which the accused does not have on his person but does have under his control a short way off. The phrase 'has with him' seems to exclude articles picked up for immediate use. For example, if the accused was reconnoitring a home preparatory to burglary, he may not be guilty of this offence if he picks up some ladders which he has found in the garden. Nevertheless, the accused in *Minor v CPS* was guilty when he did not take the articles for syphoning petrol, a tube and two empty petrol cans, from his home but (apparently) found them near the car the petrol cap of which he was removing. It is suggested that the court did not give sufficient weight to the phrase 'has with him', which seems to require something more than picking up an article at or near the scene of the ulterior offence. He was not 'going equipped'. See also the previous section ('Aggravated burglary (s 10)') where the same phrase is discussed.

'Place of abode' means the accused's home and no doubt his garage.

The term 'theft' covers both theft and taking a conveyance (s 12). There is no need for any theft to occur. This definition is found in s 25(5).

The side-note says that the crime is 'going equipped' but there is no need for the accused to go anywhere with the article provided that he is not at his place of abode, as *McAngus*, above, demonstrates. The accused was in a bonded warehouse, selling shirts to two persons who happened to be undercover agents. *McAngus* also shows that the persons the accused intended to cheat need not in fact be deceived.

'In connection with' imports a requirement of proximity. In *Mansfield* [1975] Crim LR 101 (CA) it was held that having with one a driving licence in order to get a job in which one would have an opportunity to steal was too remote from the crime of theft. Thus one is not guilty under s 25(1). However, in *McAngus* showing shirts was proximate to cheating.

Mens rea

None is stated in the subsection, but it is assumed that the accused must intend to use the article in the course of or in connection with the burglary or theft, and he must know that he has the article with him. In *Hargreaves* [1985] Crim LR 243, the accused had a piece of wire adapted to clock up credits on gaming machines. The Court of Appeal held that he was not guilty when he had not decided whether to use it or not. The court did say that an intention to use the article, should a suitable opportunity arise, would be sufficient *mens rea*. A conditional intent is sufficient. If the accused intends to burgle only if he finds something worth stealing, this crime applies.

Perhaps the principal authority is *Ellames* [1974] 3 All ER 130 (CA). The accused had been involved in a robbery. He had with him masks, gloves, and guns. It was held that he was not guilty. Section 25 deals with preparation for crime, not what occurs after crimes. The court said, however, *obiter*, that he would be guilty of the offence if he was storing the articles for use by others (i.e. 'use' need not be his use) or if the accused intended to use the article for any burglary. It did not have to be proved that the accused intended to use the article for a particular burglary, theft or cheat. The court said, moreover, that 'in connection with' covered using an article to escape from the scene of a crime.

Handling

Section 22(1) of the Theft Act 1968 stipulates:

> [a] person handles stolen goods if (otherwise than in the course of the stealing) knowing or believing them to be stolen goods he dishonestly receives the goods, or dishonestly undertakes or assists in their retention, removal, disposal or realisation by or for the benefit of another person, or if he arranges to do so.

This crime is aimed at making theft harder to carry out successfully and less profitable: *Tokeley-Parry* [1999] Crim LR 578 (CA). Before 1968 only 'receiving' was a crime. Now there are 18 ways in which the offence of handling may be committed: see *Nicklin* [1977] 2 All ER 444 (CA) – there is only one crime but several ways of committing it. A *dictum* to the contrary in *Bloxham* [1983] 1 AC 109 (HL) seems to be wrong.

The main division is that between receiving and the rest of the subsection: *per* Lord Bridge in *Bloxham*. The second part is often charged as a single count embodying such words of the subsection as are appropriate to the facts: *Deakin* [1972] 3 All ER 803 (CA), *Bloxham*. If one is charged under one part, one cannot be convicted under the other: *Nicklin*. The effect is that if it is unclear as to which form the handling took, the indictment should have separate counts for each possible form.

All the elements of the offence must be contemporaneous. In *Brook* [1993] Crim LR 455 (CA) a husband was given a bag containing stolen cheque books and cards by his wife. She said she had found the bag in a public lavatory. The accused left the bag in the back of the car until he decided what to do. The court in quashing his conviction held that he was guilty only if at the time of the handling he believed the goods to be stolen. A later handling could not be added to an earlier receipt.

The rationale of handling is that if handlers did not exist, there would be fewer thieves. Thieves would be less able to realise even part of the value of what they had stolen. In the words of the Criminal Law Revision Committee's Eighth Report, *Theft and Related Offences*, 1966, para 127, the aim behind the crime of handling is 'to combat theft by making it more difficult and less profitable to dispose of stolen property'. In some senses handling can be seen as a secondary offence to theft.

Actus reus

Handling is a term of art. There is no need for the accused actually to touch the goods, and he may touch the goods without being a handler. There is also no requirement that the accused makes a profit out of the transaction.

Section 34(2)(b)

By s 34(2)(b) of the Theft Act 1968:

> [g]oods, except insofar as the context otherwise requires, includes money and every other description of property except land, and includes things severed from the land by stealing.

The definition of 'goods' is very much like that of 'property' in theft except for land which cannot be handled unless severance has taken place. Things in action are covered: ***Attorney-General's Reference (No. 4 of 1979)*** [1981] 1 All ER 1193: balance in a bank account. They fall within 'every other description of property'. On the facts money taken from a bank account is 'proceeds' for the purposes of handling if the account derives (at least in part) from stolen money or other goods and if the money taken out is (again at least in part) derived from the proceeds of the stolen money or other goods. Accordingly if a thief pays money he has stolen into a bank account he has opened for this purpose and assigns the debt to the accused, the latter is guilty of handling if he has the *mens rea*. As will be seen, 'handling' covers retention, removal, disposal and realisation and any of these can happen to intangibles.

Section 24

By s 24 (as amended) of the Theft Act 1968 goods are stolen for the purposes of handling if any one of four conditions is fulfilled:

(a) they have been stolen contrary to s 1;

(b) they have been obtained by fraud contrary to the Fraud Act 2006;

(c) they have been obtained by blackmail contrary to s 21;

(d) they consist of money which has been dishonestly withdrawn from a wrongful credit (for the crime of dishonestly retaining a wrongful credit, see below);

(e) they have been subject to an act done in a foreign country which both was a crime in that country and, had it occurred in England, would have been theft, obtaining by deception (including obtaining a money transfer by deception) or blackmail in this country.

Goods which are stolen contrary to s 1 include those obtained by robbery and burglary provided that the robbery or burglary include a theft.

Condition (e) is aimed at preventing persons acting in England for goods stolen abroad. 'Country' is used in its conflict of laws sense. Therefore, Scotland is a foreign country because it forms a law district separate from England and Wales. The fact that the item was stolen within the meaning of the foreign law must be proved, even though theft, blackmail and fraud are probably crimes in every law district (the width may vary), especially within western Europe: *Ofori (No. 2)* (1994) 99 Cr App R 223 (CA). It is interesting to note that in a civil case where the parties do not plead foreign law, English domestic law is applied. It is uncertain why only these four crimes were chosen. One might have expected that the law would apply to the proceeds of any crime. If there is no theft within the s 24 definition such as occurs when the accused is insane, there is no offence of handling. (A charge of attempted handling is, however, possible.) The person who would otherwise be the handler is the thief. If the goods are not 'stolen' within the wide definition in s 24, there is no crime of handling. Other jurisdictions have a wider definition. For example, in New Zealand the goods which are the subject of handling need only be 'obtained by any crime'.

The offence of handling extends to the proceeds of the stolen goods: s 24(2). If the accused, a fence, sells an item, the money he receives is the proceeds of the sale, and he is the handler of that money. Similarly, if the thief steals a pig and slaughters it, the accused who receives the pork can be guilty of handling it. The goods must actually have been stolen at the time of the offence. It is not enough that he believes them to have been stolen: *Haughton v Smith* [1975] AC 476 (HL). A person who mistakenly believes the goods to be stolen is therefore not guilty of handling – charge the attempt.

And see s 24(3):

> [n]o goods shall be regarded as having continued to be stolen after they have been returned to the person from whom they were stolen or to other lawful possession or custody or after that person and any other person claiming through him have otherwise ceased as regards these goods to have any right to restitution in respect of the theft.

So goods once stolen cease to be so on restoration. They also cease to be stolen when taken into police possession: *Attorney-General's Reference (No. 1 of 1974)* [1976] QB 744. Possibly this was not the intention of Parliament, for 'restored' seems inappropriate to describe the situation where goods have come into the police's possession. The goods must have been reduced into the custody of the police.

Attorney-General's Reference (No. 1 of 1974)

A constable reported that goods on the back seat of a car were stolen. He removed the rotor arm and kept watch on the car. The Court of Appeal held that whether the officer had taken possession was a question for the jury, and that the answer depended on whether he had made his mind up to take possession so that they would not be removed, or whether he had an open mind and merely wanted to stop the driver getting away without being questioned. Accordingly, whether the property is reduced into possession depends on the intention of the person in control of it. (If the alleged handler is not guilty because the item has been reduced into the possession of the police, he may well be guilty of attempted handling or theft.)

The case is to be distinguished from *Haughton v Smith* [1975] AC 476 on the ground that in that case the prosecution conceded, perhaps wrongly, that the goods had been reduced into the police's possession.

A similar case is *GLC Police Commissioner v Strecker* (1980) 71 Cr App R 113 (DC) – initialling goods to indicate that they had been stolen did not indicate possession. Goods will cease to be stolen, e.g., if the victim's property is sold to a bona fide purchaser for value without notice by the person who obtained it by deception.

Handling

Handling may be done in several distinct ways. It is easier to divide up s 22 than to look at it all at once. Handling means:

(a) receiving the goods (which was the form of this offence before the Theft Act 1968);

(b) undertaking the retention, removal, disposal or realisation of the goods by or for the benefit of another person;

(c) assisting in their retention etc.; or

(d) arranging to do any of these things.

The phrase 'by or for the benefit of another person' applies to each preceding word denoting handling: i.e. to retention, removal, disposal and revaluation (but not to receiving): *Sloggett* [1972] 1 QB 430. The other person must be someone who is not jointly charged with the handling. 'Receiving' means acquiring possession or control of the goods. The accused need not have physical possession of the goods. Finding stolen goods is not 'receiving' them: *Haider* (1985) LEXIS 22 March (CA). The accused must 'receive' them from another. One does not 'receive' when one is bargaining with a thief over the price. Receiving covers obtaining possession or control. One can control something without being in physical possession of it, as when one's employee has it. 'Retention' connotes a positive act such as concealment or misleading the police: *Kanwar* [1982] 2 All ER 528. It does not matter that the lies do not in fact deceive the police. It does not cover simply keeping goods after the accused has discovered that they have been stolen: *Broom v Crowther* (1984) 148 JP 592. It is thought, however, that receiving covers the situation where the accused has taken goods out of the thief's possession without consent. 'Disposal' covers dumping, giving away and destruction. It has been suggested that 'disposal' is limited to alienation of the asset but that is not the natural meaning. A buyer is not involved in the 'realisation' of stolen goods: *Bloxham*, above. The term does cover the sale or exchange of goods, according to *Bloxham*. 'Assisting' is based on a positive act of encouragement or helping. The fact that the accused's wife spent money on their flat does not mean that he assisted in the disposal of money stolen by the wife: *Coleman* [1986] Crim LR 56. He did not arrange or help in the disposal of the money. He would have been convicted, had he instructed his wife to use the money to buy certain items. 'Assisting' is thus a narrow term. In *Burroughes*, unreported, 29 November 2000, the Court of Appeal said that 'assisting' connoted concealing the goods, making them more difficult to identify, holding them pending disposal and doing some other act which was part of the chain of handling. It does not cover using stolen property, here a stolen heater, left in one's father's garage: *Sanders* (1982) 75 Cr App R 84. A mere refusal to answer police questions does not constitute 'assisting'. However, telling lies to the police is assisting in the retention of stolen goods: *Kanwar*, above.

Arranging to receive is really an inchoate offence. The accused is guilty of handling at an early stage. Before the Theft Act 1968 the accused would at most be found guilty of attempted receiving. Now he is guilty of the full offence of handling. Arranging to receive goods before they have been stolen does not amount to handling: *Park* (1988) 87 Cr App R 164 (CA), because 'guilty knowledge must exist at the time when the offence is committed'. The goods have to be stolen before the offence is committed. A charge of conspiracy to handle would succeed on these facts. Incitement and secondary participation (abetting) are other possible crimes. The court in *Park* also held that there must be specified goods which have been stolen before the crime of handling takes place. This holding means that a fence who has an arrangement with a thief to take whatever the latter brings along is not a handler. It is suggested that in the light of the policy of getting rid of fences *Park* is incorrect on this point.

May a person handle by an omission?

The words 'receiving', 'undertaking' and 'arranging' all seem to suggest a positive act, but 'assisting' covers omissions, provided that there is a legal duty to act: *Brown* [1970] 1 QB 105 (CA) – allowing another to place stolen goods on his property. The court ruled that '"retain" means "to keep possession of, not lose, continue to have"'. On the facts of *Brown* the accused was not guilty because he did not have a duty to reveal the fact that there were stolen goods on his premises. *Brown* was followed in *Pitchley* (1972) 57 Cr App R 30 (CA), where the accused was under a duty to withdraw money from his bank account and return it to the owner. He assisted in the retention of stolen money for the benefit of the thief, his son. The court held that 'retain' covers 'keep possession of'.

'Otherwise than in the course of stealing'

These words ensure that not every thief is also a handler but many will be. If the thief after having stolen assists another to sell the property, he will be a handler too. The phrase contemplates that the 'course of stealing' extends beyond the point and moment of theft. Only if the issue, whether the accused is really the thief or the handler, is live, need the phrase be proved by the prosecution: see *Cash* [1985] QB 801 (CA), approving *Griffiths* (1974) 60 Cr App R 14 (CA), and *Attorney-General of Hong Kong* v *Yip Kai-foon* [1988] AC 642 (PC). It is strange that Parliament's words are disregarded. In *Greaves* (1987) *The Times*, 11 July, it was held that it was a question for the jury whether a gap of 17 days between burglary and handling meant that the accused was not the burglar and so could be convicted of handling. Often a handler will also be a thief. If the accused sells stolen property, he appropriates it, and there is little difficulty in proving the *mens rea* of theft.

The phrase 'otherwise than in the course of stealing' does not solve every issue of the relationship between theft and handling. The problem is complex. In *Pitham and Hehl* (1976) 65 Cr App R 45, a person took the two defendants to his friend's house and sold them the furniture of his friend who was in prison. Were the defendants guilty of handling? They could only be so if the seller had stolen the goods. The Court of Appeal held that he had appropriated the goods for the purposes of theft when he showed them the goods and invited them to buy. Accordingly, he was a thief. Therefore, the defendants could be convicted as handlers. The Court of Appeal in *Gregory* (1983) 77 Cr App R 41 considered this case to be one of 'instantaneous appropriation', yet *Pitham and Hehl* does look like a case where the course of stealing was not complete at the time when the defendants got their hands on the furniture. This case has come under much criticism. Cases concerning robbery suggest that stealing continues beyond the moment of appropriation but *Gomez* [1993] AC 442 seems to lay down the rule that appropriation is instantaneous. Another way of thinking is to say that even though appropriation is instantaneous, theft is not and can be a continuing activity. Therefore, 'in the course of stealing' extends beyond the moment of appropriation.

For a definition of bona fide purchaser, see p 614 in Chapter 15.

One difference between theft and handling is that the bona fide purchaser of goods is not guilty of theft when he later discovers that they were stolen (s 3(2)). However, if he gets the goods, finds out that they are stolen, and sells them, he is guilty of handling. When the accused handles, he appropriates for the purposes of theft, and so will be guilty of theft, but the phrase in brackets ensures that it is not this theft which matters for this purpose but the original theft.

Though not resolving all problems, the Court of Appeal in **Shelton** (1986) 83 Cr App R 379 held in accordance with previous practice: (a) if there is doubt as to whether the appropriate charge is theft or handling, both can be charged; (b) the jury should be directed that a handler may also be a thief but he cannot be convicted of both in relation to the same property at the same time; and (c) if the jury cannot agree whether theft or handling has been proved, the jury should be discharged. The Privy Council in **Yip Kai-foon** went a little further. If there are alternative theft and handling counts, the jurors should not be instructed to convict of the offence which it seems more probable to them that the accused committed. They should look first at theft. If theft is not proved beyond reasonable doubt, they should consider handling. If handling is not proved, the accused is not guilty of either, even though the jury thought that he was definitely guilty of one of them. **Yip Kai-foon** was applied by the Court of Appeal in **Foreman** [1991] Crim LR 702 and by the Divisional Court in **Ryan v DPP** (1994) 158 JP 485. The court in the latter case held that the prosecution does not have to disprove theft before the triers of fact can consider handling. Professor Smith's comments on the case [1991] Crim LR 704 are noteworthy:

> The jury may well be sure that the defendant is guilty either of theft or of handling but quite unable to decide which. In **Yip Kai-foon** the Privy Council rejected the solution which has been adopted in some jurisdictions of directing the jury to convict of the offence which they consider to be more probable. Such a solution 'detracts, or may be thought to detract, from the obligation of the jury to be satisfied beyond reasonable doubt that the accused is guilty of the particular offence, before they enter such a verdict'. But if that solution is objectionable, the one adopted is more so.
>
> Suppose that the jury, having been directed in accordance with the present decision, consider first the robbery charge, as instructed. They conclude that the defendant was probably guilty of robbery. But they are not satisfied beyond reasonable doubt so they decide, quite properly, to acquit of robbery. When they turn to the handling charge they must presume that he is not guilty of robbery; and, if they are quite satisfied that he must have been guilty of the one offence or the other, they are bound to conclude that he was guilty of handling. That is, they must convict him of the offence which they think he probably did not commit. The result is entirely arbitrary. If the jury were to consider the handling count first they would reach the conclusion that he was guilty of the robbery. It is not clear why the theft or robbery count should be considered before that of handling except that the theft or robbery must have come first in time. The solution rejected in **Yip Kai-foon** of directing the jury to convict of the offence which they consider to be the more probable is, at least, rational and less potentially repugnant to the principle that the prosecution must prove its case.

(Of course since we do not know what happens in the jury room – and it is illegal to find out – the likelihood is that the jury will disregard the law and convict the accused of one offence or the other, hardly the best possible outcome.) Perhaps there should be a review of possible alternative verdicts under the Theft Acts. Professor A. T. H. Smith suggested the following in *Property Offences* (Sweet & Maxwell, 1994) para 30–77: 'there can be no objection to a conviction of theft either on the basis that the defendant was the original thief, or that he stole when he acquired the goods as a handler. Where the jury is in doubt, therefore, they should convict of theft.'

Shelton points out that handling is a more serious offence than theft, which has a maximum penalty of seven years' imprisonment, and has a maximum of 14 years' imprisonment. Handling is a serious offence because handling encourages thieves. It is, in the words of the Criminal Law Revision Committee's Eighth Report, *Theft and Related*

Offences, Cmnd 2977, 1966, para 127, 'to combat theft by making it more difficult and less profitable to dispose of stolen property'.

The High Court of Australia in **Gilson v R** (1991) 172 CLR 353 rejected the advice of the Privy Council in **Yip Kai-foon**. The majority held that, where the accused was charged with theft and handling alternatively, if the jury was satisfied that he was guilty of one or the other but not sure which, the verdict is that he is guilty of the less serious offence. The standard of seriousness is normally the maximum sentence.

Mens rea

It must be proved that the accused handled the goods 'knowing or believing them to be stolen goods' and that he acted dishonestly. Knowledge must be proved at the time of the handling: **Atwal v Massey** [1971] 3 All ER 881. Finding out that the goods were stolen after receipt is not handling, but if the accused then, e.g., sells them, he may have arranged for their disposal for the benefit of another and so handle. (It could also be theft, where there is no need for the disposal to be for the benefit of another.) The test of 'knowing or believing' is subjective: **Atwal**, **Stagg** [1978] Crim LR 227. Constructive knowledge, i.e. that the accused ought to have known that goods were stolen, is insufficient: **Bellenie** [1980] Crim LR 137. The accused must know or believe that the goods are stolen, not that they may be stolen. Whether the accused did believe that the goods were stolen is a matter for the jury.

One of the leading authorities is **Hall** (1985) 81 Cr App R 160. The Court of Appeal held:

> [a] man may be said to know that goods are stolen when he is told by someone with first hand knowledge . . . that such is the case . . . Belief . . . may be said to be the state of mind of a person who says to himself: 'I cannot say I know for certain that these goods are stolen, but there can be no other reasonable conclusion in the light of circumstances . . .' What is not enough . . . is mere suspicion.

This definition of 'believing' appears narrow. Certainly suspicion is most definitely not belief. It does not include thinking that something is probably true, a state of mind which may be part of 'believing' in ordinary language. Thinking that something is more likely than not stolen is not 'believing': **Reader** (1978) 66 Cr App R 33. The test for belief is subjective. It is not to the point that a reasonable person might have believed that the goods were stolen: **Brook**, above. There is no need for this direction to be given if the issue is solely one of belief, for 'believing' is an ordinary word and its scope is a matter for the jury. Only if the distinction is between belief and suspicion is it 'prudent' to give it: **Toor** (1987) 85 Cr App R 116 (CA) following **Harris** (1987) 84 Cr App R 75 (CA). The point seems to be that 'knowing or believing' are simple words which do not in the ordinary run of things require an explanation.

As stated in **Hall** suspicion is insufficient. **Grainge** [1974] 1 All ER 928 (CA) had so held previously. The Court of Appeal held in **Forsyth** [1997] 2 Cr App R 299 that judges should not instruct juries that 'mere suspicion' is insufficient *mens rea*, for doing so might lead them into thinking that 'great suspicion' is sufficient. Whatever the degree of suspicion, no amount of it constitutes 'believing'. 'Belief is the mental acceptance of a fact as true or existing.' 'Believing' is an ordinary English word which should be left to the jury. Nor is it enough if the accused acted with wilful blindness, even though in some areas of criminal law wilful blindness is treated as knowledge: **Griffiths** (1968) 49 Cr App R 279, above, **Pethick** [1980] Crim LR 242 and **Moys** (1984) 79 Cr App R 72. This ruling is contrary to the wishes of the Criminal Law Revision Committee's Eighth Report, *Theft and Related Offences*, Cmnd 2977, 1966, on which the 1968 Act is based. The members considered that an accused who bought items in a pub at a substantial undervalue ('ridiculously low price') did believe that they were stolen. In the words of the CLRC 'the man . . . may not *know* [their emphasis] that the goods are stolen, and he may take the precaution of asking no questions. Yet it may be clear on the evidence that he believes that the goods were stolen.' In *McDonald* (1980) 70 Cr App R 288 it was held that a jury could infer that a TV set was known or believed to have been stolen when the accused paid a third of its shop price in a betting shop to an unnamed individual. The Court of Appeal in *Griffiths* said that a jury could infer knowledge or belief from suspicion. The cynic might say that the upshot of this law is that since the question of belief is one for the jury, there is nothing to stop a jury from inferring belief from suspicion.

It is handling if the accused knows or believes the goods to be stolen. He need not know the identity of the thief or of the owner or the nature of the goods: *McCullum* (1973) 57 Cr App R 645, where the goods were in a locked suitcase.

The question of dishonesty is settled by reference to *Ghosh* [1982] QB 1053 (see under 'Theft'). The three forms of 'not dishonesty' found in s 2(1) do not apply but they would presumably always be not dishonest under *Ghosh*. *Roberts* (1987) 84 Cr App R 117 held that the second stage of the *Ghosh* test does not have to be given in handling cases if there is no evidence that the accused did believe that he was not dishonest by the standards of ordinary decent people. On the facts *Roberts* looks incorrectly decided. His argument was that he was a businessperson who was trying to return two paintings for what he called a 'commission', and that this behaviour was not dishonest. The court held that no jury would find that selling back stolen items was not dishonest but it is suggested that the appellant's argument ought to be left to the jury. It will be rare for a person who is handling stolen goods, knowing or believing them to be stolen, not to be dishonest but if he is keeping stolen goods in readiness to hand them over to the police, he is not dishonest.

For more on the *Ghosh* definition of dishonesty, see pp 587–89 in Chapter 15.

Dishonestly retaining a wrongful credit

The Theft (Amendment) Act 1996 inserted s 24A into the Theft Act 1968 and in turn s 24A has been amended by the Fraud Act 2006. By it a person is guilty of a crime if 'a wrongful credit has been made to an account kept by him or in respect of which he has any right or interest, he knows or believes that the credit is wrong, and he dishonestly fails to take such steps as are reasonable in the circumstances to secure that the credit is cancelled'. Section 24A(2A) as inserted by the Fraud Act 2006 reads:

A credit to an account is wrongful to the extent that it derives from –
(a) theft;
(b) blackmail;
(c) fraud (contrary to s 1 of the Fraud Act 2006); or
(d) stolen goods.

It does not matter that the account was overdrawn before or indeed after the credit arrived in it.

The principal fact situation covered by s 24A is where one accused has procured the crediting of another accused's account, but it also covers the situation where one accused has procured the victim to credit his account. In the latter scenario, if the accused does not take the steps mentioned, he is guilty of this offence. In both scenarios the accused is guilty even though he has done nothing in respect of his account. Presumably he will avoid liability if he tells the police about the credit. It is suggested, however, that simply spending the money on wine, women (or men) and song does not amount to steps securing that the credit is cancelled. It is a pity that this interpretation is not expressly stated in s 24A.

The maximum sentence is ten years' imprisonment.

Reform

If enacted, the draft Criminal Code, Law Com. Report No. 177, 1989, will contain the offences of burglary (cl 147), aggravated burglary (cl 148), blackmail (cl 154), handling (cl 172 as expanded in cl 174), and going equipped (cl 175). Blackmail and handling are unchanged. Burglary is very slightly redefined in its s 9(1)(b) form to correct the possible anomaly revealed in *Jenkins*, above, that the infliction of grievous bodily harm need not amount to an offence. Accordingly the accused is at present guilty if he negligently caused such injury. The paragraph is restated to ensure that an offence including the *mens rea* is required in order to convict of this form of burglary. By cl 18(a) 'knowingly' includes a situation where the accused 'avoids taking steps that might confirm his belief' that a circumstance exists. This reform would extend present law. Clause 172 is also redrafted to clarify the law and reads:

> [a] person is guilty of handling stolen goods if (otherwise than in the course of the stealing) knowing or believing them to be stolen goods, he dishonestly –
> (a) receives or arranges to receive the goods; or
> (b) undertakes or arranges to undertake their retention, removal, disposal or realisation for the benefit of another; or
> (c) assists or arranges to assist in their retention, removal, disposal or realisation by another.

The enactment of the Theft Act 1978 and the Theft (Amendment) Act 1996 as well as the numerous cases on the Theft Act 1968 demonstrate the need for a thorough reform of the law.

Summary

This chapter considers several offences against property, all of which are found in the Theft Act 1968: blackmail, burglary, going equipped, and handling.

- **Blackmail**: Blackmail contrary to s 21(1) of the Theft Act 1968 is based on a demand with menaces: 'a person is guilty of blackmail if, with a view to gain for himself or another or with intent to cause loss to another, he makes any unwarranted demand with menaces; and for this purpose a demand with menaces is unwarranted unless the person making it does so in the belief –
  (a) that he had reasonable grounds for making the demand; and
  (b) that the use of the menaces is a proper means of reinforcing the demand.'
- **Burglary**: Burglary contrary to s 9 of the Theft Act 1968 comprises of two offences: entering a building or part of one with intent to steal, commit grievous bodily harm or cause criminal damage; and having entered a building or part of one, the accused

steals, attempts to steal, commits criminal damage or attempts to cause criminal damage. The former crime of burglary which consisted of the accused's entering a building or part of one with intent to rape is now found in the Sexual Offences Act 2003 in a broadened form. A building must, it seems, have some sort of permanence.

- **Going equipped**: Going equipped is the crime of having with one 'any article for use in the course of or in connection with any burglary or theft' provided that the accused is not 'at his place of abode.' It is a crime contrary to s 25 of the Theft Act 1968 as amended by the Fraud Act 2006. It resembles inchoate crimes discussed in Chapter 10: the defendant is guilty even though she has not (as yet) burgled, stolen or committed an offence of cheating.

- **Handling**: The final crime in this chapter is that of handling contrary to s 22(1) of the Theft Act 1968, which states: 'A person handles stolen goods if (otherwise than in the course of the stealing) knowing or believing them to be stolen goods he dishonestly receives the goods, or dishonestly undertakes or assists in their retention, removal, disposal or realisation by or for the benefit of another person, or if he arranges to do so.' There are 18 ways of committing this offence, as a close reading of s 22(1) reveals. 'Handling' is a term of art: one can handle stolen goods without touching them. 'Goods' are defined in s 34(2)(b) as including 'money and every other description of property except land, and includes things severed from the land by stealing.' 'Stolen' is wider than theft and covers obtained by fraud and by blackmail. The phrase 'otherwise than in the course of stealing' exempts the thief during theft from the crime of handling.

References

Reports

Criminal Law Revision Committee 8th Report, *Crime and Related Offences*, Cmnd 2977 (1966)

Law Commission Report No. 177, *A Criminal Code for England & Wales* (1989)

Books

Griew, E. *The Theft Acts 1968–1978* (Sweet & Maxwell, 1997)

Smith, A. T. H. *Property Offences* (Sweet & Maxwell, 1994)

Journals

Smith, J. C. Casenote on *Kelly* Crim [1993] LR 765

Further reading

Lamond, G. 'Coercion, threats and the puzzle of blackmail' in D. P. Simester and A. T. H. Smith (eds) *Harm and Culpability* (Oxford University Press, 1996)

Reville, N. J. 'Mischief of aggravated burglary' [1989] NLJ 835

Spencer, J. R. 'Handling, theft and the mala fide purchaser' [1985] Crim LR 92 and 440

Williams, G. 'Handling, theft and the purchaser who takes a chance' [1985] Crim LR 432

There is a symposium on blackmail in (1993) 41 UPaLR.

Visit **www.mylawchamber.co.uk/jefferson** to access exam-style questions with answer guidance, multiple choice quizzes, live weblinks, an online glossary, and regular updates to the law.

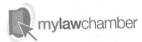

Use **Case Navigator** to read in full some of the key cases referenced in this chapter:

R v *Cunningham* [1957] 2 All ER 412
R v *Ghosh* [1982] 2 All ER 689

18

Criminal damage

Introduction

Criminal damage is based on the 1971 Act of the same name, by which Parliament simplified the law. It is normally seen as an offence against property dealing with vandalism and suchlike, but it is in part a crime which deals with the protection of people and can deal with the maintenance of public order, as occurs when rioters burn down American-owned coffee shops.

The 'simple' and 'aggravated' forms

It is an offence for a person without lawful excuse to destroy or damage property belonging to another with intent to destroy or damage the property or being reckless as to whether that property is destroyed or damaged: s 1(1). The maximum sentence is 10 years' imprisonment. This type of crime is sometimes known as the 'simple' form of criminal damage. The 'aggravated' form, with a maximum of life imprisonment, is the simple form of the offence without the restriction on who owns the property (the defendant may own it or he may damage the victim's property with the latter's consent, as in *Merrick* [1996] 1 Cr App R 130 (CA)) but with the addition of a further *mens rea*: the accused must also intend by the destruction or damage to endanger another's life or he must be reckless as to whether life is endangered thereby: s 1(2). There is no need to show that life was in fact endangered: *Parker* [1993] Crim LR 856 (CA). This aggravated form could be seen as an offence against the person, rather than an offence against property. Recklessness as to whether life is endangered is sufficient. Furthermore the defence of lawful excuse, s 5, does not apply to the aggravated form (including arson contrary to s 1(2)). Nevertheless, though s 5 does not apply to s 1(2), that subsection still provides for a defence of lawful excuse. The sort of happening which would be covered by s 1(2)'s 'lawful excuse' provision would be where the accused uses a weapon in self-defence against the victim, whose life he thereby intends to endanger. There would be a lawful excuse if the accused damaged the article. No doubt this behaviour would rarely be charged as criminal damage. (A man the author once met on holiday had been tried at the Old Bailey for murder when he killed a burglar with a spear he had grabbed off his wall. If the spear had been broken, he could nowadays be charged under s 1(2), but he would have this defence.) It should be noted that while there is no general defence of endangering life, s 1(2) creates an offence when the endangering is caused by criminal damage.

Arson

If the destruction or damage is caused by fire, the offence is arson: s 1(3). The fire need not be a major one: it suffices that the slightest damage is caused by the fire. The maximum penalty is life imprisonment. Section 1(3) reads: 'An offence committed under this section by destroying or damaging property by fire shall be charged as arson.' Section 1(3) applies to both s 1(1) and s 1(2). The charge is arson contrary to s 1(1) (or s 1(2)) and s 1(3) of the Criminal Damage Act 1971. The restrictions in s 1(1) and s 1(2) also apply where the cause of the damage is fire, e.g. if the property belongs to the accused, there is no charge possible under s 1(1) and s 1(3). It should be noted that the maximum sentence in s 1(3) applies even though the sole difference between the 'simple' offence and s 1(3) is that the damage was caused by fire. Presumably the accused must intend to cause, or be reckless as to causing, damage by fire. If, for instance, he intends a bomb to explode, but the damage is in fact occasioned by fire, he is not guilty under s 1(3). This point, however, is not settled. The Law Commission in its Report No. 29, *Offences of Damage to Property*, 1970, recommended the abolition of the separate offence of arson, but Parliament disagreed. The charge of arson was retained because of the public's desire to stigmatise the defendant who set light to property. Another reason was given by the Law Commission, the Report of which led to the 1971 statute. Fires were often started by the mentally ill. Finding them guilty of an offence for which the maximum sentence was life imprisonment could result in safeguarding the public. The contrary argument on this point is easily put: pyromaniacs by definition cannot stop themselves causing fires and prison is unlikely to cure them.

Despite the mandatory words in s 1(7) ('shall be charged as arson'), according to the Court of Appeal in **Drayton** [2005] EWCA Crim 2013 there is no need to charge criminal damage by fire as 'arson'. It is sufficient that the charge is one of criminal damage by fire.

Steer

In the aggravated form the prosecution must show that the destruction of or damage to property caused the danger to life; it is not sufficient to show that the danger to life resulted from the act which caused the damage or destruction.

Steer [1988] AC 111 (HL)

The accused went to the home of his former business partner, against whom he had a grudge, and fired several shots at the house, breaking the bedroom window. No injuries were caused. He was held not guilty of s 1(2). That subsection applies only if the property damaged caused life to be endangered. Danger came from the shots, not from the damage to property. The subsection applies only if it is 'by the . . . damage' that the danger is caused.

The result would have been different if flying glass had been proved to be dangerous to life. Lord Bridge said: 'It is not the match, the flaming firebrand or other inflammatory material which the arsonist uses to start the fire which causes danger to life; it is the ensuing conflagration which occurs as the property which has been set on fire is damaged or destroyed.' A similar case is **Asquith** [1995] 1 Cr App R 492 (CA), which is called **Webster** in [1995] 2 All ER 168. The defendants pushed a very heavy stone off a bridge on to a train. The stone caused bits of the roof to fall on the passengers but did not itself come through the roof. In the words of Lord Taylor CJ:

> The effect of the statute may be thought strange. If the defendant's intention is that the stone itself should crash through the roof of a train or motor vehicle and thereby directly injure a passenger or if he was reckless only as to that outcome, the section would not bite . . . If, however, the defendant intended or was reckless that the stone would smash the roof of the train or vehicle so that metal or wood struts from the roof would or obviously might descend upon a passenger, endangering life, he would surely be guilty. This may seem to many a dismal distinction.

On the facts if the defendants intended to endanger the lives of the passengers by the stone, they were not guilty of intending to endanger life but they were reckless as to endangering life by bringing down the roof.

Steer was distinguished in ***Dudley*** [1989] Crim LR 57 (CA). The accused threw a fire-bomb at the victim's house. The fire was quickly extinguished, with only trivial damage caused. The accused was found to be guilty of the aggravated offence. It did not matter that only minor damage was caused. The defendant did act with the intention to endanger life. That is, indeed, how this offence is defined: by reference to intent or recklessness, not by reference to the harm caused. *Steer* was a case where the actual and intended damage were the same, and the accused did not have the further or ulterior intent specified in s 1(2).

Actus reus

In both the simple and aggravated forms, part of the *actus reus* is destruction or damage of property of a tangible nature. In the 'simple' form the property must belong to another. 'Belonging to another' is defined in such a way that, although the accused may own and possess the property, it belongs to someone else for the purposes of this offence. Accordingly, the accused can be guilty of the 'simple' offence in some situations, even though he owns the property. When property belongs to another is defined in s 10(2):

(a) Where another has custody or control. An example is ***Pike v Morrison*** [1981] Crim LR 492. A person who ran his mother's home could be said to have custody of it (*obiter*). It is not certain whether 'custody' is preferred to 'possession' which appeared in the 1968 Theft Act. It is suggested that 'custody' means that the accused has physical control over the item, whereas 'control' means that he has the right to tell others what to do with it.

(b) Where a person has a proprietary right or interest over the property (but not where that right or interest arose from a contract for the sale of land).

(c) Where a person has a charge over the property. (A charge is a proprietary right or interest such as a mortgagor has: this exception falls within the second one.) Presumably restrictive covenants and equitable easements are included.

(d) By s 10(3), property subject to a trust belongs to any person having a right to enforce the trust.

(e) Subsections 5(3) and (4) of the Theft Act 1968 do not apply to criminal damage.

Points (b), (c) and (d) relate to civil law, to which the reader is referred.

If damage is to property which falls outside these circumstances, the accused will not be guilty of the 'simple' offence if he destroys or damages his own property. For example, he smashes a bottle of wine he has just bought: not guilty. Similarly, if he crashes his own car to claim off the insurance – not guilty of this offence: the charge would be obtaining property by deception. The accused is not guilty because the insurers have no proprietary interest in the car. He would, however, be guilty of the more serious offence under s 1(2), (3), if he set light to his own car intending to endanger the life of a joy-rider: the restriction to 'belonging to another' applies to s 1(1), not s 1(2). It should be realised that a person's dishonesty is irrelevant in criminal damage.

What, then, is **property**? There is a wide definition in s 10(1). The following should be noted:

(a) unlike the Theft Act 1968, there is no difference between land and other property with the result that agricultural land which the accused has incorporated into his garden has been criminally damaged;

(b) intangible property is excluded – the essence of criminal damage is damage to a physical thing, though the damage itself need not be tangible (but see below for computer programs);

(c) also excluded are wild mushrooms and wild flowers, fruit and foliage – one can squash wild mushrooms as much as one likes: there is no test of commercial purpose as exists in the Theft Act;

(d) the same rules apply to wild animals as occur in the Theft Act (badgers are not property within the 1971 Act when they are lured into traps: *Cresswell v DPP* [2006] EWHC 337 (Divisional Court);

(e) it would seem that water flowing naturally over or under land cannot be criminally damaged, but it can be if reduced into possession, for example, in a reservoir;

(f) confidential information such as trade secrets cannot be damaged. It is not property.

In relation to (c), the comment by N. Lacey *et al.*, *Reconstructing Criminal Law*, 3rd edn (LexisNexis, 2003) 406, is noteworthy: 'the image of criminal damage which the Act reproduces is the image of the destruction of tangible goods – the smashed bus shelter, the indelible inner city graffiti, the vandalised car. . . . The polluted air or river . . . [is] apparently excluded from the definition.'

A simple illustration is the printed circuit card in *Cox v Riley* (1986) 83 Cr App R 291 (DC). Other examples occur in the following paragraphs dealing with destruction and damage. Neither of those terms is defined in the Criminal Damage Act or in the Law Commission Report No. 29, *Offences of Damage to Property*, 1970, on which the statute is based.

Destroy

This term does not add anything to 'damage'. If one destroys property, one damages it. It may have been included to forestall the argument that 'damage' does not cover 'destroy'. The Divisional Court in *Barnet LBC v Eastern Electricity Board* [1973] 2 All ER 319, a case on town and country planning legislation, stated that: 'The act of destruction must be one having at least the elements of finality and totality about it.' Killing a pet is destruction of it.

Damage

Property is damaged if it is rendered imperfect or inoperative, or if the harm impairs its usefulness or value: *A (A Juvenile) v R* [1978] Crim LR 689 (Crown Court). Spitting on the back of a police sergeant's uniform was not criminal damage because the saliva could be wiped off. The raincoat was service issue, designed not to be affected by the British weather. (No doubt it would be different with a silk coat.) However, the Divisional Court in *Roe* v *Kingerlee* [1986] Crim LR 735 disagreed with the reasoning in *A* v *R*. The court held that magistrates were wrong to hold that graffiti made from mud smeared on the walls of a police cell could not amount to damage. In *Morphitis* v *Salmon* [1990] Crim LR 48, the Divisional Court held *obiter* that damage included 'not only permanent or temporary physical harm but also permanent or temporary impairment of value or usefulness'. Scratching a scaffolding bar was not criminal damage but merely an incident of normal use of scaffolding components. The accused could have been charged with damage through dismantling the barrier of which the bar formed a part. Some examples are:

Faik [2005] EWCA Crim 2381 – stuffing a blanket down the lavatory and flushing the cistern. The blanket was wet and had to be dried and cleaned; the police cell and two adjoining cells had to be cleaned. The accused was guilty of criminal damage.

Henderson, unreported, 29 November 1984 (CA) – rubbish dumped on a building site. The court applied the *Concise Oxford Dictionary* definition of damage as 'injury impairing value or usefulness'. The value and usefulness of the land were both impaired, even though the land beneath was not harmed by the rubbish.

Cox v *Riley* (above) – damaging a plastic circuit card thereby erasing a computer program (the program was intangible and not covered by the Act). D. Ormerod (ed.) Smith and Hogan, *Criminal Law*, 12th edn (OUP, 2008) 982, states: 'what is contemplated . . . is some physical harm, impairment or deterioration. This will usually be capable of being perceived by the senses'. Martin Wasik suggested in 'Criminal damage/criminal mischief' (1988) 17 A-ALR 37, 40, that the present law should be extended to data but the Computer Misuse Act 1990 ended that possible road to reform. (See comment after the next case.)

Whiteley (1991) 93 Cr App R 25: a computer hacker gained access to a system called JANET, the Joint Academic Network, which links institutions of higher education. He got to know his way around the files which were stored on large metal magnetic disks. He added and deleted files and changed the password of authorised users. He wiped the files containing his use of the system and even deleted the program designed to catch him. He was charged with, among other things, damaging the disks by altering their magnetic particles. He contended that the functions of the disks were not altered by him; they did not suffer physical damage; any destruction or damage was to information on the disk; such damage did not damage or impair the usefulness of the disk. Lord Lane CJ in a reserved judgment in the Court of Appeal held:

> [w]hat the Act requires . . . is that tangible property has been damaged, not necessarily that the damage itself should be tangible . . . [T]he magnetic particles upon the metal discs [*sic*] were a part of the discs and if the appellant was proved to have intentionally and without lawful excuse altered the particles in such a way as to cause impairment of the value or usefulness of the disc to the owner, there would be damage . . .

He continued by summarising the law.

> Any alteration to the physical nature of the property concerned may amount to damage. Whether it does so or not will depend upon the effect that the alteration has had upon the legitimate operator . . . If the hacker's actions do not go beyond, for example, mere tinkering with an otherwise empty disc, no damage would be established. Where, on the other hand, the interference with the disc amounts to an impairment of the value or usefulness of the disc to the owner, then the necessary damage is established.s

Note the emphasis on the effect of the alleged damage to the operator.

The difficulties which arose in *Cox v Riley* and *Whiteley* are in part dealt with by s 3(6) of the Computer Misuse Act 1990. (Note that the Act applies only to computers, and not, for example, to videos or DVDs.)

> For the purpose of the Criminal Damage Act 1971 a modification of the contents of a computer shall not be regarded as damaging any computer or computer storage medium unless its effect on that computer or computer storage medium impairs its physical condition.

This provision will become s 10(5) of the Criminal Damage Act 1971 with the substitution of 'this Act' for 'the Criminal Damage Act 1971' when the Police and Justice Act 2006, Sch 14, para 2, is brought into force (and s 3(6) will be repealed).

The effect on *Cox v Riley* was to make the accused now guilty under this Act and not the 1971 one, if the damage did not impair the physical condition of the circuit card. The offence under the 1990 Act can only be committed intentionally, whereas criminal damage may be committed recklessly. In the event of both charges being possible, there is a higher penalty for criminal damage on indictment than for conviction of computer misuse. It might have been more sensible to amend the Criminal Damage Act 1971 directly than to declare in a different statute that the accused is not guilty under that Act. When the 2006 Act comes into effect, *Cox v Riley* and *Whiteley* will be crimes under the revised s 3 of the 1990 Act, 'unauthorised acts with intent to impair or recklessness as impairing, operation of computer etc.' If the effect of the act of the accused is to change a program which leads to physical damage, that damage can be prosecuted against under the 1971 Act.

The court in *Whiteley* approved *Tacey* (1821) 168 ER 893 and *Fisher* (1865) LR 1 CCR 7 from before the 1971 Act. *Fisher* was also approved in *Cox v Riley*: tampering with part of a machine was malicious damage and would now be criminal damage. In *Lloyd v DPP* [1992] 1 All ER 982 (DC) the cutting of two padlocks which secured a wheel-clamp to his car, which he had parked in a private car park which had notices stating that clamps were in use and removable only on payment of a fine of £25, was criminal damage. Could it be argued that by attaching the clamp to the wheel the clampers had rendered the car unusable and thus criminally damaged it? It is thought not. The accused has been deprived of use of his car, and that is not criminal damage. If the accused threw away the key to a shop door, one would not say that the shop has been criminally damaged. There was no damage, it was stated, to the car in *Lloyd v DPP* despite the fact that it could not immediately be driven away. The case from this viewpoint resembles the next case. Had there been damage, the question would then be: did the clampers have a lawful excuse? See below. The same principles apply to the situation where the landowner arranges for a sticker to be placed on a trespassing driver's windscreen.

In fact this also happened in *Lloyd v DPP*. The sticker cannot be removed without considerable time and effort. The court held that this was not criminal damage. In *Drake v DPP* [1994] Crim LR 855 the Divisional Court justified this holding by saying that the use of stickers and wheel-clamps did not interfere with the integrity of the car. That is the distinction between what is and what is not criminal damage.

In *Tacey* removing an essential part from a machine was sufficient even though the part, an iron bar, could easily be put back in position. Also amounting to criminal damage would be so running a machine that impairment results (*Norris* (1840) 173 ER 819) and trampling on grass (*Gayford v Chouler* [1898] 1 QB 316). However, simply trespassing on land will not amount to criminal damage: *Eley v Lytle* (1885) 2 TLR 44. In the case of arson, it is presumably sufficient that, for example, wood is charred, but it will not be criminal damage if it is blackened, though after **Whiteley** (above) the result may be different depending on the owner's use for the wood. Perhaps the result in **Henderson** (above) would have been different if the land was not about to be used for building but was waste.

Five other matters should be noted:

(a) Damage need not be permanent, nor need it result in a loss which can be quantified in monetary terms. In **Hardman v Chief Constable of Avon** [1986] Crim LR 330, a Crown Court held it irrelevant that the pavement on which CND members had painted human silhouettes on Hiroshima Day could be restored to its original condition.

(b) **Hardman** also demonstrates that a good motive does not excuse.

(c) The question whether property is damaged or not is one for the triers of fact. Whitewashing over National Front slogans does not necessarily amount to damage: **Fancy** [1980] Crim LR 171 (DC). Another court could, however, rule that it was. The wall was already white and it is arguable that there was no intent to cause criminal damage, but the accused's *mens rea* does even then depend on the uncertain scope of 'damage'. It is uncertain also how far **Fancy** extends. If the accused improves something, can it be said that he has criminally damaged it?

(d) The method of destruction or damage does not matter. It could for instance be chemical, as in dissolving something in an acid bath, or it could be by fire, as in burning a house down.

(e) The same fact situation can give rise to both theft and criminal damage, as when the accused takes the victim's car and sets fire to it.

The defence of lawful excuse (s 5)

Apart from any other defence the accused may have, such as mistake, he may have a lawful excuse. For the purpose of the 'simple' offence, s 1(1), s 5 grants him a defence if:

(a) he believed that the person whom he believed entitled to consent to the destruction or damage of the property would have consented, had he known of the circumstances (s 5(2)(a)); *or*

(b) he acted 'in order to protect' the property of himself or another, or a right or interest in property and he believed that
   (i) the property, right, or interest was in immediate need of protection, and
   (ii) the means adopted were reasonable, having regard to all the circumstances (s 5(2)(b)).

An example of s 5(2)(a) is **Denton** [1982] 1 All ER 65 (CA). The accused set fire to a cotton mill on the request of his employer, who wished to claim the insurance money. His conviction was quashed. He believed the person entitled to consent did consent. (A possible charge here is conspiracy to defraud.) If the accused burns his own property in order to claim insurance money, he is not guilty under s 1(1) because he has not destroyed property belonging to another.

An example of how s 5(2)(b) is used is **Mitchell** [2004] Crim LR 139 (CA). The accused had his car wheel-clamped. He cut through the clamp. He could not rely on s 5(2)(b) because his car was in immediate need of protection.

In s 5(2) 'right' covers a right of way: ***Chamberlain v Lindon*** [1998] 2 All ER 538 (DC). The accused was held to be protecting it when he demolished a wall and that right was in immediate need of protection because it was being obstructed. Whether what he was doing was lawful in civil law was irrelevant: if the facts fell within s 5(2), he had a defence.

Points to note

(a) It is immaterial whether or not the belief was justified, as long as it was honestly held (s 5(3)). The test, therefore, is subjective.

(b) As stated, the defence in s 5 does not apply to s 1(2), the aggravated offence. There is, however, a defence of lawful excuse to s 1(2), but it is not defined by reference to s 5. An example is smashing a coal shovel over the head of a person who is attempting to burgle one's house. One intends to damage property with intent to endanger life but, provided the force used is reasonable, one has a s 5 defence.

(c) The burden of proof lies on the prosecution, which must disprove the lawful excuse.

(d) The difficult principle to understand in this topic is this: s 5 is construed to give a defence to persons intoxicated. In ***Jaggard v Dickinson*** [1981] QB 527 (well discussed by Glanville Williams 'Two nocturnal blunders' (1990) 140 NLJ 1564, who ably contrasts the instant case with ***Gannon*** (1987) 87 Cr App R 254), a magistrates' court held that the accused could not rely on the defence of lawful excuse because her belief that the person entitled to consent to the damage would have consented was brought about by alcohol. Since the crime was one of basic intent (see the section on intoxication), she had no defence. The Divisional Court reversed the magistrates' court's decision. It held that her defence was based on her state of belief, *not* upon her drunkenness. The intoxication merely explained her belief. The Act does not provide that the accused's belief must be a sober one. Therefore, drunkenness giving rise to a belief in the owner's consent establishes this defence.

> See Chapter 8 for an explanation of intoxication. There is a diagram illustrating this on p 308.

The contrasting position is where the accused puts forward evidence that he did not have the *mens rea* of recklessness because he was drunk. ***MPC v Caldwell*** [1982] AC 341 decided that intoxication not merely does not negative recklessness, it supplies it. Therefore, he has no defence to a charge of criminal damage if while drunk he sets light to a hotel. Accordingly, while drunkenness can explain why the accused believed as he did and so provide the basis for a lawful excuse, it leads to a conviction for recklessly causing criminal damage. The prosecution has shown recklessness, but he may have a lawful excuse.

(e) If the accused who is not drunk destroys property, believing it to be his own, the defence is not lawful excuse but is a failure to prove part of the offence: ***Smith*** [1974] QB 354. (See also Chapter 8 on mistake.)

(f) Section 5 is not exhaustive of lawful defences. Any other defence, such as self-defence, remains: s 5(5). Section 5(2) notes that there can be a lawful excuse as a defence in areas falling outside the terms of s 5(2). The Divisional Court in ***Stear v Scott*** (1984) LEXIS, 28 March, rejected the contention that breaking off a wheel clamp was such an excuse.

(g) It is not a lawful excuse for defendants to cut the wire at an airforce base in order to show their opposition to nuclear weapons, even if they subjectively believed that their actions fitted within s 5: ***Ashford*** [1988] Crim LR 682 (CA). They argued that the reduction of the risk of the use of nuclear weapons would protect property in England because the risk of retaliation would be reduced. The court held that the test of whether the accused was acting 'in order to protect property' was objective. *Ashford* was followed in *Kelleher*, 20 November 2003, unreported. The accused knocked the head off a statue of Baroness Thatcher in a protest against the influence multinational companies had over the policies of democratic governments and over the policies of the governments of the USA and UK, which he believed made the world a more dangerous place to live in and which would lead to the destruction of this planet. The accused was not acting 'in order to protect property'; whether he subjectively believed he was was irrelevant. This ruling is inconsistent with the wording of s 5, which looks at the accused's own (subjective) belief. In *Hill* (1989) 89 Cr App R 74, the Court of Appeal held that the act of cutting the wire with a hacksaw was too remote from the prevention of nuclear war. The property was not 'in immediate need of protection'. Therefore, it did not matter that the defendants believed they were acting 'in order to protect property belonging to another'. In *Chamberlain* v *Lindon* (above) the right of way was in immediate need of protection because the obstruction would otherwise continue until litigation had resolved the matter several years in the future. *Hill* also confirmed that the test was objective. The Divisional Court in *Chamberlain* v *Lindon* applied *Hill*.

This interpretation is contrary to the recommendation of the Law Commission (above), which proposed a subjective test. The phrase 'in order to' looks at the mind of the accused. It is interesting to note that the Court of Appeal has here made a subjective test into an objective one, whereas in self-defence it once made an objective test into a subjective one: *Scarlett* [1993] 4 All ER 629, though it later recanted and reinstated the objective test. A belief that God ordered the accused, a vicar, to write words from the Bible on a concrete pillar to protest against the use of force by the coalition against Iraq was not a lawful excuse: *Blake* v *DPP* (1992) 93 Cr App R 169 (DC). The law of England overrode the law of God. Belief in the consent of God to damage did not constitute a valid excuse. (Section 5(2)(a) requires a person to consent and it is moot whether God, if He exists, is a person.) The act, moreover, was not objectively capable of protecting property. It was too remote from protecting property in the Gulf States. The subjective belief that he was acting within s 5(2)(b) was irrelevant. A similar ruling was made in *Jones* v *Gloucestershire Crown Prosecution Service* [2005] QB 259. The defendants contended that they had a defence within s 5(2)(b) when they damaged property at RAF Fairford in order to demonstrate their belief that the war in Iraq was illegal. They argued that they had acted to preserve their homes and the homes of friends. The court held that none of the defendants could reasonably believe that cutting wire around the base could reasonably protect those houses. This is an objective test. The court held that the sole objective test was: 'could the act be said to be done in order to protect property?' All the other tests in s 5(2)(b) were subjective. In criticism it must be said that the paragraph is phrased in subjective terms. The courts have read in an objective limitation, a limitation impossible to square with the requirement that the accused acts 'in order to' protect property. There is, of course, nothing to prevent a Crown Court jury from not following a judge's direction and applying a subjective test.

The court in the *Jones* case summarised the law thus: the accused has a defence if

(i) he acted in order to prevent damage to property, whether his own or another's. This test requires an answer to the question: 'could the act done be said to be done in order to protect property? . . .';

(ii) at the time he acted, he believed that the property was in immediate need of protection; and

(iii) he believed that the means adopted or proposed to be adopted were or would be reasonable having regard to all the circumstances;

(iv) in determining the answers to (ii) and (iii), it is immaterial whether the belief was justified, provided that it was honestly held.

The first test alone is objective.

(h) The act must be done in order to protect property. In **Hunt** (1977) 66 Cr App R 105, the accused, husband of the deputy warden of a block of flats, set fire to bedding in order to show that the alarm system was inadequate. He did show that the alarms did not work. His appeal was dismissed. His intention was not to protect property, but to reveal defects in the alarm system. His subjective belief was irrelevant. The Act must not be too remote from the protection of property. **Hunt** was applied in **Blake v DPP**, above. A belief that property may at some time in the future be damaged does not constitute a belief that it is in immediate need of protection: **Johnson v DPP** [1994] Crim LR 673 (DC). It is irrelevant though the accused believed that a certain date in the future is immediate. The court also held that the purpose of the accused in breaking locks was to bring in his furniture, not to protect it, when he was squatting. The phrase 'in order to . . .' in s 5(2)(b) means 'purpose': his purpose must have been to protect property to give rise to this defence. This objective reading of 'in order to' is criticised in (g) above.

(i) As stated above, s 5(2) is restricted to the protection of property. Therefore, it does not apply to the protection of a person, even a child: **Baker** [1997] Crim LR 497 (CA).

(j) The Court of Appeal in **Jones** [2005] QB 259 rejected the argument that the accused must act to prevent *unlawful* damage. He is allowed to act to prevent lawful damage. This issue was not the subject of the appeal to the Lords [2006] UKHL 16.

The draft Criminal Code 1989, cl 185(1)(a), would extend the present s 5 to cover 'doing an act which . . . is immediately necessary and reasonable to protect himself or another from unlawful force or injury'. This recommendation would give consistency of treatment to the protection of persons and property: **Baker**. The Law Commission would revise s 5(2)(b) so that the force used is objectively reasonable as in the current law on self-defence: *Legislating the Criminal Code – Offences against the Person and General Principles*, Report No. 218, 1993. This recommendation would bring the law into line with that of the protection of people in the law of self-defence.

Mens rea

Recklessness is notorious for its different meanings in English law according to the subject matter (*per* Auld LJ in **Nugent v Michael Goss Aviation Ltd** (2000) The Times, 10 May (CA)).

For a review of *Caldwell*, see pp 110–16 in Chapter 3 and pp 313–15 in Chapter 8.

MPC v Caldwell, which has been mentioned above in relation to drunkenness and criminal damage, was for a decade thought to be the most important case in modern English criminal law. In relation to intoxication, the House of Lords held that where the charge was one of recklessly causing criminal damage the mental element of recklessness existed when the accused was drunk. In relation to recklessness, the accused had this mental element in criminal damage not just when he himself foresaw an unjustifiable obvious risk of damage occurring, but also when a reasonable person would have foreseen that risk.

The former state of mind is sometimes called 'subjective recklessness', the latter 'object-ive recklessness'. Subjective recklessness is often called '*Cunningham* recklessness' after the CCA case which is the classic authority. Objective recklessness is often called '*Caldwell* recklessness'. What the House of Lords said is stated in the next paragraph. It should be remembered that in criminal damage there is an alternative mental state, intention, which was dealt with above. Since in both the aggravated and the simple forms, recklessness is sufficient, the definition of intent is not as important in criminal damage as in murder, where the sole requisite *mens rea* is intention. Besides intention or recklessness as to the destruction or damage, in the simple offence the accused must know that the property belongs to another. In criminal damage, the mental element (omitting knowledge that the property belongs to another in the simple offence) can be stated thus:

(a) 'simple offence' (s 1(1)):
    (i)   intentionally causing criminal damage; and
    (ii) recklessly causing criminal damage;

(b) 'aggravated offence' (s 1(2)):
    (i)   intentionally causing criminal damage with intent to endanger life;
    (ii) intentionally causing criminal damage being reckless as to whether life is endangered;
    (iii) recklessly causing criminal damage with intent to endanger life; and
    (iv) recklessly causing criminal damage being reckless as to whether life is endangered.

Form (b)(iii) must be rare.

The facts of *Caldwell* were simple. The accused, who bore a grudge against the victim, set fire to the victim's hotel. The accused was drunk. Lord Diplock in a model direction gave what he himself described as an appropriate instruction, that recklessness through-out criminal damage was to be defined as follows. The accused was guilty if:

(1) he does an act which in fact creates an obvious risk that property will be destroyed or damaged and
(2) when he does the act he either has not given any thought to the possibility of there being any such risk or has recognised that there was some risk involved and has nonetheless gone on to do it.

Lord Diplock considered that the two states of mind in (2) were not practically distin-guishable, yet the difference has marked criminal law over many years. Indeed Lord Goff in *Reid* [1992] 1 WLR 793 went further and said that in many situations a driver who failed to think was more blameworthy than one who considered the existence of a risk but disregarded it. This direction came under severe criticism (see previous editions of this book) and was 'departed from', in other words overruled, by the House of Lords in *G* [2004] 1 AC 1034. For further details of recklessness in modern law see Chapter 3. Not surprisingly Rose LJ said in *Cooper* [2004] EWCA Crim 1382: 'It is now, in the light of *G*, incumbent on a trial judge to direct a jury, in a case of this kind [criminal damage], that the risk of danger to life was significant to the defendant.' The accused, who had learn-ing difficulties, lived in a hostel for those with mental health problems. He set light to the underside of a mattress in his room, using lighter fuel as accelerant. His conviction was quashed because the trial judge had directed the jury in *Caldwell* terms. Other con-victions had to be quashed because between the judge's direction and the appeal, *G* had overruled *Caldwell*. See *Castle* [2004] EWCA Crim 2758 in which the court held that in respect of aggravated criminal damage being reckless as to whether life was endangered that the accused was reckless as to a consequence when he was aware of a risk that it might occur and that an accused was reckless as to a circumstance when he was aware of a risk that it existed or would exist.

Transferred malice

See pp 123–26 in Chapter 3 for an explanation of the doctrine of transferred malice.

An issue of transferred malice (see Chapter 3) may arise in the crime of intentionally or recklessly causing criminal damage. The intention or recklessness need not be directed at a particular piece of property which was damaged as long as the accused intended to damage some property or was reckless as to the damage. For example, if the accused threw a stone at a car, intending to damage it, but missed and broke a shop window, he is guilty of criminal damage. He has the intent necessary in relation to the window as he intended to damage another's property. However, he will not necessarily be guilty under s 1(1) if he threw a stone at his own car intending to damage it but broke the window. His intention is not transferred: he has no 'malice' to transfer. Whether he is guilty of criminal damage depends now on whether he acted recklessly.

Creating a dangerous situation and not dealing with it

In *Miller* [1983] 2 AC 161, the accused, a squatter, lit a cigarette, lay down on a mattress, and fell asleep. The cigarette fell onto the mattress. He woke up and saw it smouldering. He went into another room and fell asleep again. The house caught fire. He was charged with arson. He contended that all he had done amounted to an omission, a failure to put the fire out, and that did not constitute the *actus reus* of criminal damage. (See Chapter 2 for more about omissions.) The House of Lords held that the accused was guilty. Lord Diplock criticised the use of the term '*actus reus*' because that phrase made one believe that in the criminal law the accused was guilty only if he had *acted*. He said that he was guilty if his *conduct* had caused the damage. In this instance it had. The defendant had failed to take measures to stop the danger he had created. Since he also had the required mental element in that he was aware that the fire presented an obvious risk of damaging the house, he was under a responsibility to put out the fire: since he did not do so, he was guilty.

As in *Caldwell*, Lord Diplock gave a model direction:

> The accused is guilty of the offence under s 1(1) of the 1971 Act if, when he does become aware that the events in question have happened as a result of his own act, he does not try to prevent or reduce the risk of damage by his own efforts or if necessary by sending for help from the fire brigade and the reason why he does not is either because he has not given any thought to the possibility of there being any such risk or, because having recognised that there was some risk involved, he has decided not to try to prevent or reduce it.

Accordingly, the accused must be aware of the circumstances, but he need not realise that he ought to do something. Applying *Miller* the accused would not be guilty if he watched a fire which someone else had started. The width of *Miller* is a little uncertain, but presumably it would cover the 'hit-and-run' driver who leaves his victim unconscious at the side of the road.

The effect of intoxication in a *Miller* situation was discussed in *Cullen* [1993] Crim LR 936 (CA). The accused had taken a large dose of sedatives and a large amount of alcohol.

He set fire to material in his room in a hostel. The court applied *Miller* and *Caldwell*. He had caused criminal damage. If he did not appreciate the risk because he was drunk, he was guilty because he was to be judged on how he would have reacted to the fire, had he been sober. If he had been sober, he would immediately have put the fire out. He was thus guilty.

Custody or control of anything with intent to destroy or damage

Section 3 of the Criminal Damage Act 1971 reads:

> A person who has anything in his custody or under his control intending without lawful excuse to use it or cause or permit another to use it –
> (a) to destroy or damage any property belonging to some other person; or
> (b) to destroy or damage his own or the user's property in a way which he knows is likely to endanger the life of some other person
> shall be guilty of an offence.

It is sufficient that the accused intends to use the thing at some future time. There is no need for an intent to make immediate use. 'Anything', which is not defined in the Act, would seem to be just that, anything. The Law Commission gave two examples: a hammer and a box of matches. In *Hill* (1989) 89 Cr App R 74, see above, a hacksaw blade fell within 'anything'. The lawful excuse defence in s 5 does not apply to s 3 if the offence falls within (b); it does if it falls within (a). Section 3 is a preliminary offence. It covers a situation where the crime of attempted criminal damage does not apply because of the narrowness of the definition of attempt. This offence enables the police to intervene at an early stage to prevent criminal damage. As will be seen in Chapter 10, the trial judge has power to withdraw the issue of attempt from the jury and may do so in circumstances where most juries would convict such as when the accused is near the entrance of the Post Office he intended to steal from. Section 3 would catch the accused at this stage if he intended to cause criminal damage as a preliminary to the theft or robbery. Surprisingly there is no equivalent offence in the area of non-fatal offences: the accused would not be liable until he had done a more than merely preparatory act. In the interests of crime prevention it is suggested that s 3 could be generalised to apply beyond criminal damage, thereby protecting the public more than the law of attempts does at present. The mental element is 'intending'. In this context only direct intent (see the previous chapter) is included because it must be the accused's purpose to destroy or damage. The accused is guilty of this offence if he intended to use the 'thing' should it prove necessary: *Buckingham* (1976) 63 Cr App R 159 (CA). This ruling is in line with the law on possessing explosives.

In this context one should note the offences in s 38 of the Public Order Act 1986. Section 38(1) provides:

> It is an offence for a person with the intention – (a) of causing public alarm or anxiety, or (b) of causing injury to members of the public consuming or using the goods, or (c) of causing economic loss to any person by reason of the goods being shunned by members of the public, or (d) of causing economic loss to any person by reason of steps to avoid any such alarm or anxiety, injury or loss, to contaminate or interfere with goods, or make it appear that goods have been contaminated or interfered with, or to place goods which have

been contaminated or interfered with, or which appear to have been contaminated or interfered with, in a place where goods of that description are consumed, used, sold or otherwise supplied.

It is not sufficient that the accused foresaw alarm. Intention is necessary.

Section 38(2) creates the offence of threatening to do any of the above. Section 38(3) penalises the possession of materials for contamination. Accordingly, the accused who has with him razor blades which he intends to put into baby food is guilty of this offence.

The government thought that the offences of criminal damage and administering a noxious thing (Offences Against the Person Act 1861, s 23) were insufficient to get at the mischief. The offences are triable either way, with a maximum of 10 years' imprisonment on indictment.

Threats to destroy or damage property

This offence is created by s 2 of the Criminal Damage Act 1971. The *mens rea* is the intent to make the threat; there is no need to intend to carry it out. It need not be shown that the victim was made afraid. Section 2(1) reads:

> A person who without lawful excuse makes to another a threat, intending that the other would fear it would be carried out –
> (a) to destroy or damage any property belonging to that other or a third person; or
> (b) to destroy or damage his own property in a way which he knows is likely to endanger the life of that other or a third person
> shall be guilty . . .

There is no restriction of the form of the threat. It may be made orally or in writing, expressly or impliedly. A threat is made when it is uttered. There is no need for the victim to receive or understand the threat. The threat need not be one of immediate harm.

If the threat is one to do an act which falls within s 1(1), the 'simple' offence, the s 5 definition of 'lawful excuse' applies (see above). If it is one to do a s 1(2) offence, that definition does not apply.

Cases are rare but a recent one is *Cakmak* [2002] Crim LR 581. Six defendants threatened to set fire to themselves if an attempt was made to storm the two pods of the 'London Eye' which they had taken over in a protest against human rights abuses in Turkey. The Court of Appeal quashed the convictions because the trial judge had not properly directed the jury that there had to be a threat to destroy or damage the property of another. On the facts there was a threat to another, the controller of the 'Eye', and the defendants intended to damage the attraction.

Summary

This final chapter has as its subject the offence of criminal damage. There are two types of criminal damage crime: 'simple' criminal damage, which is where the accused intentionally or recklessly destroys or damages property belonging to another, a crime contrary to s 1(1) of the Act; and 'aggravated' criminal damage where the accused intentionally or recklessly destroys or damages any property (including property belonging to the accused herself) with intent to endanger life or being reckless as to whether life will be endangered contrary to s 1(2) of the Act. Where either form of criminal damage is caused by fire, it should be charged as arson: s 1(3).

To the 'simple' form of the offence there is a defence of lawful excuse: see s 5(1).

The chapter concludes with a discussion of the crimes of custody or control of anything with intent to destroy or damage, an offence contrary to s 3 of the 1971 Act, and threats to destroy or damage property contrary to s 2(1) of the Act.

References

Reports

Law Commission Report no. 29, *Offences of Damage to Property* (1970)

Law Commission Report no. 177, *A Criminal Code for England & Wales* (1989)

Law Commission Report no. 218, *Legislating the Criminal Code: Offences against the Person and General Principles* (1993)

Books

Smith, J. C. and Hogan, B. *Criminal Law* (ed. D. Ormerod) 12th edn (Oxford University Press, 2008)

Journals

Wasik, M. 'Criminal damage/criminal mischief' (1988) 17 A-ALR 37

Further reading

Elliott, D. W. 'Endangering life by destroying or damaging property' [1988] Crim LR 403

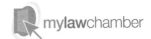

Glossary

actual bodily harm injury which is more serious than a touching but less serious than grievous bodily harm (q.v.). 'Bodily' is read widely to cover not just the flesh and bones but also psychiatric matters. The crime of assault occasioning actual bodily harm is contrary to s 47 of the Offences Against the Person Act 1861.

actus reus this Latin term means the act, omission or state of affairs required by the offence. It is distinguished from the *mens rea* or mental element of the crime. The *actus reus* differs from crime to crime. For example, in theft it comprises three elements: appropriation, property and belonging to another.

age the age of criminal responsibility is 10. The Crime and Disorder Act 1998, s 34, abolished the previous law of mischievous discretion which applied to those above 10 and below 14.

aiding and abetting helping or encouraging

arson this is the crime of criminal damage by fire. It is contrary to s 1(1) and s 1(3) of the Criminal Damage Act 1971 when the accused did not intend to endanger life or was reckless as to endangering life and contrary to s 1(2) and s 1(3) when he did.

assault in criminal law this word bears two meanings. The first, narrower definition is the intentional or reckless causing of the victim to apprehend immediate and unlawful violence. This type of assault is sometimes known as psychic or technical assault. The second, wider meaning covers both the first type of assault and the crime of battery (q.v.). It is in this second sense that 'assault' is used in the offence of assault occasioning actual bodily harm contrary to s 47 of the Offences Against the Person Act 1861. The offence of 'psychic' or 'technical' assault is, the Divisional Court has ruled, contrary to s 36 of the Criminal Justice Act 1988.

attempts most indictable offences (i.e. those triable in the Crown Court) are committable as attempted crimes when the accused intends to commit the offence and performs a 'more than merely preparatory' step on the way towards committing the offence. For example, I, having made my mind up to kill you, am stopped from shooting you dead just before I pull the trigger. I intend to kill you and I have performed a more than merely preparatory step on the way towards killing you. Similarly, if I shoot to kill but miss, I can be found guilty of attempted murder. It should be noted that the crime of attempted murder's *mens rea* is intent to kill even though murder itself may be committed by either an intent to kill or an intent to cause grievous bodily harm. All attempts are contrary to the Criminal Attempts Act 1981.

automatism this is a defence to all offences and occurs where the accused is not in control of his or her bodily actions: the defendant has acted involuntarily. There is debate as to whether the accused does not have the *actus reus* for the offence or does not have the *mens rea* or has a defence; or (and this is the view taken by the writer) whether there is something preliminary to *actus reus*, *mens rea* and any defence, namely that the prosecution has to prove that the defendant acted voluntarily: if the accused has not so acted, he or she is not guilty at that point, i.e. before there is any need to prove the *actus reus* and *mens rea*. Whichever theory is preferred, the outcome is the same: the accused is not guilty.

basic intent offences these are crimes to which intoxication is not a defence, e.g. manslaughter.

battery this crime occurs when the accused intentionally or recklessly touches another person without consent. The Divisional Court has held that battery is contrary to the Criminal Justice Act 1988, s 36.

beyond reasonable doubt this phrase represents the criminal law burden of proof. The prosecution must prove each element of the offence in such a manner that the jury (in the Crown Court) or the magistrates (Justices of the Peace) or District Judge Magistrates' Court, formerly a stipendiary, in the magistates' courts are sure that the accused committed the offence.

blackmail this is defined in s 21(1) of the Theft Act 1968 as taking place when 'with a view to gain for himself or another or with intent to cause loss to another, he [the accused] makes any unwarranted demand with menaces; and for this purpose a demand with menaces is unwarranted unless the person making it does so in the belief – (a) that he had reasonable grounds for making the demand; and (b) that the use of the menaces is a proper means of reinforcing the demand.'

burden of proof in criminal law it is normally the prosecution which has to establish that the offence took place. This principle extends even to most defences. For example, the prosecution has to prove that the accused is not afforded the defence of provocation. The exceptions to the rule about defences are insanity (because every person is according to the law of insanity presumed to be sane) and diminished responsibility (because Parliament has so ruled: see s 2(2) of the Homicide Act 1957). The third exception, found in s 101 of the Magistrates' Courts Act 1980, is where the crime is defined in terms of an offence followed by an exception. Where the burden of proof is on the defendant, the standard of proof is the civil law one of 'on the balance of probabilities'. The current controversy is whether these so-called 'reverse onus' of proof exceptions are justifiable under Article 6 of the European Convention on Human Rights.

burglary this is an offence contrary to s 9 of the Theft Act 1968. Better put, s 9 is divided into two ways of committing the crime and there are two crimes, dependent where the accused is in relation to the building or part of one she wishes to enter or has entered. The two ways of committing burglary are:

1. entering a building or part of a building as a trespasser with intent to commit one of three crimes: theft, grievous bodily harm and criminal damage;

2. having entered a building or part of one as a trespasser, stealing or attempting to steal or committing grievous bodily harm or attempting to do so.

If the building is a dwelling place, the maximum sentence is 14 years' imprisonment; if it is not a dwelling place, the maximum is 10 years.

The case which generations of law students loved for its facts, *Collins* (1973) CA, involved the crime of burglary as it then existed: it then covered entry as a trespasser with intent to rape. This crime was abolished and replaced by a wider crime with the Sexual Offences Act 2003.

causation in criminal law it is usual to state that whether the accused caused a certain consequence depends on two issues, causation in fact (also known as factual causation and 'but for' causation) and causation in law (sometimes called legal causation). The prosecution must prove both beyond reasonable doubt. See also eggshell skull rule.

children see age.

coercion see marital coercion.

conduct crimes offences where only the forbidden behaviour is to be proved such as the offence of dangerous driving.

consent the basic rule is that consent is a defence to assault and battery but not to more serious offences such as wounding with intent to cause grievous bodily harm. The leading authority is *Brown* (1993) HL. To this rule there are several exceptions including 'manly sports' such as boxing, horseplay, flagellation for religious purposes, and branding one's initials onto one's wife's buttocks (!).

conspiracy this offence is known as an 'inchoate' one, i.e. it occurs before the principal offence takes place. For example, there may be a conspiracy to murder at a time before the murder itself takes place. Conspiracy is based on an agreement to do an unlawful act. If the unlawful act is a crime, the offence is one contrary to the Criminal Law Act 1977, s 1(1), as amended. There are one or two common law conspiracy offences, the main one being conspiracy to defraud: one can be guilty of this offence even though the object is not in itself criminal.

constructive manslaughter a person is guilty of this form of manslaughter if she kills as a result of committing a crime which is seen objectively as being dangerous. The term 'dangerous' in this context means: one which 'all sober and reasonable people would inevitably recognise must subject the other person to, at least, the risk of some harm resulting therefrom, albeit not serious harm' (per Edmund Davies LJ, *Church* [1966] 1 QB 59 (CCA).

contributory negligence is not a defence in Criminal Law.

corporate liability at times a company may be responsible for the crimes of others. The controversial method of so doing is via the doctrine of identification, i.e. the company is criminally liable for the acts and omissions of high-ranking officers of the company. Those officers are identified as being the company; in other words, they are the company.

counselling advising on the commission of an offence.

criminal damage this offence occurs when the accused destroys or damages property. It comprises two different offences. The first is contrary to s 1(1) of the Criminal Damage Act 1971: the accused intentionally or recklessly destroys or damages property *belonging to another*. This crime is sometimes known as 'simple' criminal damage. Section 1(2) creates what may be called 'aggravated' criminal damage. This crime occurs when the accused intentionally or recklessly destroys or damages property *whether belonging to another or not*, intending to destroy or damage property or being reckless as to whether property is destroyed or damaged.

deception misrepresentation, fraud, telling lies. See also fraud.

diminished responsibility this defence found in s 2(1) of the Homicide Act 1957 has the effect of reducing murder to (voluntary) manslaughter. It comprises three elements: an abnormality of mind, a certain cause (which must be one of those stated in s 2(1)), and that abnormal mind must have led to a 'substantial impairment' of the accused's 'mental responsibility' for the killing. Note that this defence is a defence only to murder and that the burden of proof is on the accused; however, the standard of proof is the civil law one of 'on the balance of probabilities'.

drunkenness as a defence see intoxication.

duress this is a defence to all offences except murder, attempted murder and 'some forms of treason', as the authorities put it. The width of the defence has recently been tightened by *Hasan* [2005] 2 AC 467 HL. This defence is sometimes called duress *per minas* (by threats) to distinguish it from the next entry where the threat is not caused by a human being. It takes the form of 'do this or else' and has a human source, e.g. 'I will seriously harm your mother unless you take part in a bank robbery.'

duress of circumstances this is a defence with similar boundaries to that of duress but the foundation for the defence is an emergency (e.g. 'drive through red lights to escape armed robbers') rather than 'unless you break the law, I will kill your children,' which is the form duress takes.

eggshell skull rule this is one of the 'rules' of causation. It is also known as 'you must take your victim as you find him.' It means that if the victim is physically or psychologically 'weak', the accused is responsible in criminal law just as in tort law for the injuries or death caused by a blow to him or her, even though the victim would not otherwise have suffered death or injury. For instance, assume that I am attacking you. Unknown to me, your skull is weak and when I hit you there with a brick, you die, then even though you would have lived, had you not had a thin skull, I have caused your death and I have done so whether or not I (or anyone else including the victim) knew of the thinness of your skull.

excuse this is a type of defence where the accused is not justified in doing as she did but has a defence personal to her, e.g. 'at the time of the killing, I was insane.'

fitness to plead see unfitness to plead.

fraud there were several offences of fraud in criminal law. The main ones are obtaining property by deception (s 15 Theft Act 1968), obtaining a pecuniary advantage by deception (s 16 of the same), obtaining services by deception (s 1 of the Theft Act 1978) and evading liability by deception (s 2 of the same). These have been replaced by the Fraud Act 2006.

going equipped this crime, contrary to s 25 of the Theft Act 1968, as amended by the Fraud Act 2006, takes place when the accused has with him otherwise than at his 'place of abode' 'any article for use in the course of or in connection with any burglary or theft.'

grievous bodily harm (GBH) this is injury to the person, whether to the body or to the psyche, which is more serious than 'actual' bodily harm (but which does not result in death). Examples include the effects of chopping someone's arm off, gouging out the victim's eye, and shooting someone in a vital organ. The Offences Against the Person Act 1861 contains two GBH offences: in brief, maliciously causing GBH with intent to do some GBH (s 18) and maliciously inflicting GBH (s 20).

gross negligence this is carelessness which is so bad that it deserves being called criminal. See *Adomako* [1995] 1 AC 171 (HL).

handling this is a crime contrary to s 22(1) of the Theft Act 1968, which reads: 'A person handles stolen goods if (otherwise than in the course of the stealing) knowing or believing them to be stolen goods he dishonestly receives the goods, or dishonestly undertakes or assists in their retention, removal, disposal or realisation by or for the benefit of another person, or if he arranges to do so.' 'Goods' according to s 34(1) 'includes money and every other description of property except land, and includes things severed from the land by stealing.' The word 'stolen' in this definition is not restricted to goods which have been stolen contrary to s 1(1) of the 1968 Theft Act but extends e.g. to goods obtained by fraud and by blackmail. Whether the accused is dishonest is determined by the *Ghosh* [1982] QB 1053 (CA) test.

homicide this is the generic term for killing a human being. The main homicide offences are murder and manslaughter.

inchoate offences these crimes are ones in which the principal offence has not (yet) been committed. An example is the crime of attempt (q.v.). The other two inchoate offences are incitement and conspiracy. It should be noted that other offences take the form of inchoate offences. For example, burglary contrary to s 9(1) of the Theft Act 1968 includes entry as a trespasser with intent to steal. The accused is guilty of this offence even though she has not yet stolen any property.

incitement this is a common law offence whereby the accused seeks to persuade in whatever manner the main offender to commit a crime. During the current edition of this book it is likely that this crime will be replaced by the offence of encouraging or assisting crime.

infanticide this offence is where a woman causes the death of her child who is aged under 12 months 'but at the time of the act or omission the balance of her mind was disturbed by reason of her not having fully recovered from the effect of giving birth to the child or by reason of the effect of lactation consequent upon the birth of the child'. In those circumstances the crime is infanticide, a form of manslaughter, and not murder.

insanity an accused has the defence of insanity to any offence if she proves on the balance of probabilities that at the time of the offence she (i) was suffering from a disease of the mind (ii) which caused a defence of reason and (iii) either (a) did not know the nature and quality of the act or (b) did not know that what she was doing was wrong. This statement of the law derives from *M'Naghten* (1843) 8 ER 718. For insanity at the time of the trial see unfitness to plead.

intent(ion) in criminal law this term bears two different meanings depending on the crime charged. The narrow meaning is 'aim' or 'purpose'. This definition is sometimes known as direct intent. The other meaning both covers the first meaning and may cover the situation where the accused foresees a consequence as virtually certain, as occurs when the accused explodes a bomb on a plane at 30,000 feet, wishing to claim on the insurance. Here she would be very happy if the plane victims survived – it is not her aim to kill them – but she knows that it is virtually certain that they will be killed. The definition says 'may cover' because it is a question for the jury looking at all the facts in deciding whether the accused did intend to kill. The principal authority on intent in this second, wider meaning is **Woollin** [1999] 1 AC 82 HL, which is a case on murder. The term sometimes used for the scenario where the accused foresees a situation as virtually certain is 'oblique intent'.

intoxication whether it is caused by alcohol or drugs, intoxication is a defence to specific intent offences such as murder but not to basic intent offences such as manslaughter. The distinction between basic and specific intent offences is controversial. See this textbook for details.

involuntary manslaughter see manslaughter.

joint enterprise an agreement by two or more to carry out a common purpose.

justification in criminal legal theory this term denotes a defence where the accused's conduct was praiseworthy or at least permissible. An example is the defence of the use of reasonable force in self-defence.

making off without payment this offence, contrary to s 3 of the Theft Act 1978, occurs when the accused, 'knowing that payment on the spot for any goods supplied or service done is required or expected from him, dishonestly makes off without having paid as required or expected and with intent to avoid payment of the amount due.' An example is where the defendant drives into a petrol station, intending to pay, changes her mind about paying after the petrol is put into the tank and drives off. Where the spot is will vary with the facts but in a restaurant it may be the point where the accused is to pay, often nowadays the table where the meal was eaten. Dishonesty bears its **Ghosh** [1982] QB 1053 CA definition. The HL in **Allen** [1985] AC 1029 held that the accused must intend to deprive *permanently*.

malice aforethought this is the *mens rea* of murder. It comprises the intent to kill and the intent to commit grievous bodily harm. It should be noted that no 'aforethought', i.e. premeditation, is needed and no malice, i.e. spite, is needed.

manslaughter this is best seen as two different offences. The first type, voluntary manslaughter, occurs when the accused has malice aforethought and kills but has one of the defences found in ss 2–4 of the Homicide Act 1957: diminished responsibility, provocation and killing in pursuance of a suicide pact respectively. The second type, involuntary manslaughter, takes place when the accused kills either by an unlawful act ('constructive manslaughter') or when the accused kills through his or her gross negligence. There is also almost certainly a crime of (subjectively) reckless manslaughter.

marital coercion this is a defence available to wives only who commit an offence under the domination of their husband. The boundaries of the defence are similar to but seemingly wider than duress.

mens rea this Latin term, sometimes translated as 'guilty mind', is the mental element required by the crime. The mental element varies from crime to crime. For example, the accused is guilty of theft if she appropriates property belonging to another only when she does so dishonestly and with the intention permanently to deprive. The concepts of 'dishonesty' and 'with the intention permanently to deprive' form the *mens rea* of theft. When added to the *actus reus* of the offence, there is the crime of theft.

mistake the general rules are that a mistake as to law is no defence but a mistake as to an element of the crime is a defence; however, the mistake, to be a defence, must be one as to a relevant element. Take the following illustration. Parliament has created an offence of selling 'bad' meat; the accused sells a piece of lamb, not knowing that it is 'bad'; therefore, she has made a mistake as to whether the meat is of the correct quality; if, however, the offence is a strict liability one as to the badness or otherwise of the meat, then the accused is guilty because it is irrelevant whether she knew the meat to be 'bad' or not.

murder this, often thought to be the most serious crime, is committed when the accused causes the death of the victim with malice aforethought. The victim must be alive and not an enemy alien in time of battle. The former rule that the victim had to die within a year and a day of the attack was abolished in 1996. There are several defences to murder, both those which are defences only to murder such as provocation and diminished responsibility and those which apply to all defences including murder such as self-defence. The defences of duress (by threats) and duress of circumstances do not apply to murder.

necessity there is debate in English law as to whether necessity exists as a defence and, if so, what its boundaries are. One view is that there is no defence at all; another is that there is a defence but it is restricted in its application in that it does not apply to murder, attempted murder and 'some forms of treason' (i.e. the same crimes to which duress is not a defence); and a third view is that it is a defence to all offences. This debate in part turns on the definition of necessity. If necessity is seen as a justification, it is defined as having a choice between committing a less serious crime and a more serious one and choosing to commit the less serious one. For example, the accused is faced with the choice between shooting dead a bomber (murder unless there is a defence) or letting the terrorist explode the bomb on public transport. The difficulties underlying this defence are exacerbated by the inconsistent use of terminology by the courts: sometimes, for instance, necessity is seen as a synonym for duress of circumstances.

novus actus interveniens there may be an act supervening between what the accused has done and the injury or damage. Where that act breaks the chain of causation, it is known as '*novus actus interveniens*'.

obtaining by deception see fraud.

omissions sometimes an accused is criminally liable for not doing something. An example is murder: if one deliberately starves one's victim, one is guilty of murder.

prevention of crime by s 3(1) of the Criminal Law Act 1967 the use of force is justified if done in the prevention of crime. There is a large overlap with the common law defence of self-defence. In both defences the force must be necessary and proportionate.

procuring instigating an offence.

property for the purposes of the Theft Act 1968 property is defined in s 4(1) of the Act as 'money and all other property, real or personal, including things in action or other intangible property'. This definition applies to both the offence of theft itself and to the crime of fraud. For the purposes of criminal damage property is defined in s 10(1) of the Criminal Damage Act 1971 as 'property of a tangible nature, whether real or personal, including money and – (a) including wild creatures which have been tamed or are ordinarily kept in captivity, and any other wild creature or their carcasses if, but only if, they have been reduced into possession which has not been lost or abandoned or are in the course of being reduced into possession; but (b) not including mushrooms growing wild on any land or flowers, fruit or foliage of a plant growing wild on any land.'

provocation this specific defence, partly defined in s 3(1) of the Homicide Act 1957, is a defence only to murder. It applies where the accused has killed in the heat of the moment (read to include cumulative provocation) as a result of something said or done and a reasonable person might have done as she did. Though provocation is called a defence, the burden of proof lies on the prosecution to disprove it beyond reasonable doubt.

rape this crime, which can be committed only by men, consists according to s 1(1) of the Sexual Offences Act 2003 in the penile penetration of the vagina, anus or mouth of the victim (whether male or female) without consent. The mental element as to consent is that the accused did not have reasonable belief in the victim's consent.

recklessness the definition of recklessness in criminal law was settled by the House of Lords in *G* (2004). It means that the accused has foreseen that a consequence may occur but has nonetheless gone on with his or her conduct. The risk of that consequence's occurring must be an unjustifiable one.

result crimes these are offences which the accused is not guilty of unless the prosecution can prove that her act or omission caused the consequence stated in the definition of the offence. For example, the result in murder is the death of the victim. If there is no death, murder is not committed (though attempted murder is a possible crime).

robbery this offence is committed where the accused, while stealing, uses force on any person (whether the victim of the theft or not) or puts or seeks to put any person (similarly) in fear of force. See s 8 of the Theft Act 1968 for the full definition.

secondary participation not just is the perpetrator guilty of an offence (as the principal offender) but also those who help and encourage may be guilty as secondary parties. These accused are liable as aiders, abettors, counsellors, and procurers.

self-defence this is a defence to all offences. It covers the defence of oneself, of others and of property. The force used must be necessary and proportionate. It largely overlaps with prevention of crime. One difference is that in the defence of prevention of crime the force must, as may be evident, be used to prevent an offence; if the victim of the alleged defence would not be a criminal, e.g. because she is an infant (under the age of 10) or has the defence of insanity, then the user of force, the accused, cannot be acting to prevent crime but may have the defence of self-defence.

sexual offences these crimes are almost all contrary to the Sexual Offences Act 2003. The most serious one is rape.

specific intent offences these are crimes to which intoxication is a defence, e.g. murder and theft.

spouses husband and wives may be guilty of most offences but not conspiracy; however, if the agreement to commit an offence is made by the wife, husband and a third party, all may be criminally liable.

status offences these are crimes where the *actus reus* consists of no voluntary action on the part of the accused. The most famous case involving such an offence is *Larsonneur* (1933) 24 Cr App R 74 (CCA).

stealing this is the offence of theft.

strict liability many offences in English law are ones where the prosecution does not have to prove *mens rea* as to one or more elements of the *actus reus*. An example is a butcher who is charged with the crime of 'selling bad meat'. If she is guilty of the crime even when she does not know that the meat she is selling is 'bad', the part of the *actus reus* of 'bad' in the crime of selling bad meat has no *mens rea* attached to it: this element of the offence is 'strict' and the offence is one of strict liability. Note that all the other elements of the *actus reus* have *mens rea* attached to them: the butcher must know that what she is doing is 'selling' and must know that she is selling 'meat'; nevertheless, because one element is 'strict', the whole crime is known as an offence of strict liability.

theft this offence, contrary to s 1(1) of the Theft Act 1968, occurs when the accused dishonestly appropriates property belonging to another with the intention of permanently depriving the other of it. The maximum sentence is seven years' imprisonment (s 7 of the 1968 Act).

transferred malice this so-called doctrine applies where in simple terms the accused attacks one human being (or thing), misses him, and hits another (or another thing). For example, I shoot at you intending to kill you but I miss and kill your friend standing at your side. My intent ('malice') against you is transferred from you to your friend. The crime will be one of murder: I intended to kill and I did kill. Note that the doctrine does not apply between people and things (or vice versa). For instance, I intend to shoot you dead, but miss and my bullet breaks a window. My 'malice' against you, a human being, cannot be transferred against a thing, the window, to make me guilty of criminal damage. I may, however, be guilty of attempted murder and reckless criminal damage.

unfitness to plead this is a defence to all offences and applies when the accused is insane at the time of the trial. Note that insanity at the time of the offence constitutes the defence of insanity.

unlawful act manslaughter see constructive manslaughter.

vicarious liability rarely in criminal law may one person be responsible for the criminal acts and omissions of another person or of an organisation, but when he or she is, he or she is said to be vicariously liable. For readers who know the tort doctrine of vicarious liability, it must be emphasised that the criminal law doctrine is much narrower.

voluntary manslaughter see manslaughter.

wounding this is defined as a breach of both layers of the skin. There are two offences of wounding: one contrary to s 18 of the Offences against the Person Act 1861 (wounding with intent) and one contrary to s 20 (malicious wounding).

Index

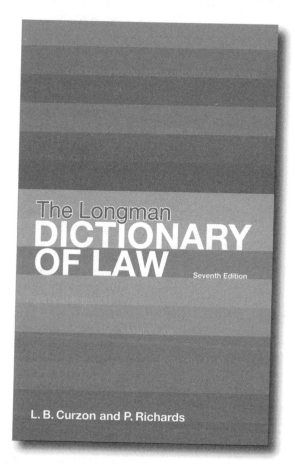